PROFILE DRUGS

Name of Drug	Classification	Page
acetaminophen (Tylenol, and others)	Nonopioid analgesic; NSAID	208
acyclovir (Zovirax)	Antiviral	435
alteplase (Activase)	Thrombolytic	245
aminocaproic acid (Amicar)	Hemostatic	247
amiodarone (Cardarone)	Potassium channel blocker	306
amphotericin B (Fungizone)	Systemic antifungal	425
aspirin (Acetylsalicylic acid, ASA, and others)	NSAID; salicylate	204
atenolol (Tenormin)	Beta-adrenergic blocker	321
atorvastatin (Lipitor)	HMG CoA reductase inhibitor (statin)	354
atropine	Anticholinergic	95
beclomethasone (Beclovent and others)	Anti-inflammatory agent; glucocorticoid	479
benzocaine (Solarcaine and others)	Local anesthetic	630
benztropine (Cogentin)	Anticholinergic	164
bethanechol (Urecholine)	Parasympathomimetic	93
calcitriol (Calcijex, Rocaltrol)	Vitamin	608
calcium gluconate (Kalcinate)	Electrolyte; calcium supplement	608
carvedilol (Coreg)	Beta-adrenergic blocker	289
cefotaxime (Claforan)	Cephalosporin	403
chlorothiazide (Diuril)	Diuretic; thiazide	530
chlorpromazine (Thorazine)	Antipsychotic; phenothiazine	154
cholestyramine (Questran)	Bile acid sequestrant	355
ciprofloxacin (Cipro)	Fluoroquinolone	409
clozapine (Clozaril)	Antipsychotic; atypical	158
colchicine	Uric acid inhibitor	616
conjugated estrogens (Premarin) and conjugated estrogens with medroxyprogesterone (Prempro)	Hormone replacement therapy	581
cyanocobalamin (Cyanabin and others)	Vitamin	513
cyclobenzaprine (Cycloflex, Flexeril)	Skeletal muscle relaxant; central-acting	600
cyclophosphamide (Cytoxan)	Antineoplastic; alkylating agent	451
cyclosporine (Neoral, Sandimmune)	Immunosuppressant	387
dantrolene sodium (Dantrium)	Skeletal muscle relaxant; direct-acting	604
diazepam (Valium)	Benzodiazepine	182
digoxin (Lanoxin)	Cardiac glycoside	285
diltiazem (Cardizem)	Calcium channel blocker	323
diphenhydramine (Benadryl and others)	H_1-receptor blocker (antihistamine); first-generation/sedating	377
diphenoxylate with atropine (Lomotil and others)	Antidiarrheal	502
donepezil	Acetylcholine inhibitor	167
dopamine (Dopastat, Inotropin)	Cardiotonic agent	338
doxazosin (Cardura)	Adrenergic blocker	270
doxorubicin (Adriamycin)	Antitumor antibiotic	456
enalapril (Vasotec)	Renin-angiotensin pathway modifier	268
epinephrine (Adrenalin)	Vasoconstrictor/sympathomimetic	342
epoetin alfa (Epogen Procrit)	Hematopoietic growth factor	461
erythromycin (E-mycin, Erythrocin)	Macrolide	406
ethinyl estradiol with norethindrone (Ortho-Novum 1/35)	Oral contraceptive	579
ethosuximide (Zarontin)	Anticonvulsant; succinimide	186
etidronate (Didronel)	Biphosphonate	612
ferrous sulfate (Ferralyn and others)	Mineral	516
fexofenadine (Allegra)	H_1-receptor blocker (antihistamine); second-generation/nonsedating	378
finasteride (Proscar)	Benign prostatic hypertrophy agent	590
fluoxetine (Prozac)	Antidepressant; selective serotonin-reuptake inhibitor	135
fluticasone (Flonase)	Intranasal glucocorticoid	380
furosemide (Lasix)	Loop diuretic	287
gemfibrozil (Lopid)	Fibric acid agent (fibrate)	357
gentamicin (Garamycin)	Aminoglycoside	407
glipizide (Glucotrol)	Oral hypoglycemic	555
haloperidol (Haldol)	Antipsychotic; nonphenothiazine	155
halothane (Fluothane)	Volatile anesthetic	225
heparin (Heplock)	Anticoagulant	242
Hepatitis B vaccine (Recombivax HB)	Vaccine	386
hydralazine (Apresoline)	Direct-acting vasodilator	271
hydrochlorothiazide (HydroDIURIL)	Diuretic	261
hydrocortisone (Aeroseb-HC and others)	Systemic glucocortisoid	564
hydroxychloroquine sulfate (Plaquenil Sulfate)	Anti-inflammatory; antimalarial	615

PROFILE DRUGS *(continued)*

imipramine (Tofranil)	Antidepressant; tricyclic antidepressant	131
interferon alfa 2 (Roferon-A, Intron A)	Biologic response modifier	461
isoniazid (INH)	Antitubercular agent	414
isosorbide mononitrate (Isordil)	Vasodilator	289
isotretinoin (Accutane)	Antiacne agent; retinoid	632
latanoprost (Xalatan)	Prostaglandin	645
levodopa (Larodopa)	Dopaminergic agent	163
levothyroxine (Synthroid)	Thyroid agent	560
lidocaine (Xylocaine)	Local anesthetic; amide	220
lindane (Kwell)	Antiparasitic; scabicide	628
lisinopril (Prinivil)	ACE inhibitor	286
lithium (Eskalith)	Bipolar disorder agent; mood stabilizer	139
lorazepam (Ativan)	Benzodiazepine	117
medroxyprogesterone (PremOro)	Dysfunctional uterine bleeding agent; progestin	583
methotrexate (Mexate)	Antimetabolite	455
methylphenidate (Ritalin)	CNS stimulant for ADHD	142
metoprolol (Lopressor)	Beta-adrenergic blocker	326
metronidazole (Flagyl)	Antiprotozoal	437
milrinone (Primacor)	Phosphodiesterase inhibitor	288
morphine (Astramorph PF and others)	Opioid agonist	199
naloxone (Narcan)	Opioid-antagonist	200
naproxyn (Naprosyn) and naproxen sodium (Aleve, Anaprox)	Nonsteroidal anti-inflammatory drug (NSAID)	370
nifedipine (Procardia)	Calcium channel blocker	265
nitroglycerin (Nitrostat)	Organic nitrate; vasodilator	319
nitrous oxide	General anesthetic; gas	224
norepinephrine (Levarterenol)	Vasoconstrictor/sympathomimetic	337
normal serum albumin (Albuminar and others)	Fluid replacement agent; colloid	339
nystatin (Mycostatin)	Superficial antifungal	425
omeprazole (Prilosec)	Proton pump inhibitor	496
oxymetazoline (Afrin and others)	Sympathomimetic; decongestant	382
oxytocin (Pitocin, Syntocinon)	Uterine stimulant and relaxant; oxytocic	585
penicillin G (Pentids)	Penicillin	403
phenelzine (Nardil)	Antidepressant; monamine oxidase inhibitor	137
phenylephrine (Neo-Synephrine)	Sympathomimetic	098
phenobarbital (Luminal)	Anticonvulsant; barbiturate	182
phenytoin (Dilantin)	Anticonvulsant; hydantoin	185
potassium chloride	Electrolyte	538
prazosin (Minipress)	Adrenergic blocker	101
prednisone (Meticorten and others)	Systemic glucocorticoid	373
prochlorperazine (Compazine)	Antiemetic	503
propranolol (Inderal)	Beta-adrenergic blocker	305
propylthiouracil (Propacil)	Antithyroid agent	562
psyllium mucilloid (Metamucil and others)	Laxative	500
quinidine (Quinidex)	Sodium channel blocker	304
raloxifene (Evista)	Hormone; estrogen blocker	612
ranitidine (Zantac)	H_2-receptor blocker	494
regular insulin (Humulin R, Novolin R, and others)	Insulin	550
reteplase (Retevase)	Thrombolytic	325
salmeterol (Serevent)	Bronchodilator; beta-adrenergic agent	476
sibutramine (Meridia)	Anorexiant	504
sildenafil (Viagra)	Erectile dysfunction agent	588
sodium bicarbonate	Acid-base agent	537
spironolactone (Aldactone)	Diuretic; potassium-sparing	532
succinylcholine (Anectine)	Neuromuscular blocking agent	228
sumatriptan (Imitrex)	Antimigraine agent; triptan	210
tamoxifen (Nolvadex)	Antineoplastic; hormone antagonist	459
testosterone base (Andro and others)	Male hypogonadism agent; androgen	587
tetracycline HCl (Achromycin and others)	Tetracycline	405
thiopental (Pentothal)	IV anesthetic	226
ticlopidine (Ticlid)	Anticoagulant; antiplatelet agent	244
timolol (Timoptic, Timoptic XE)	Beta-adrenergic blocker	647
trimethoprim-sulfamethoxazole (Bactrim, Septra)	Sulfonamide	410
valproic acid (Depakene)	Anticonvulsant	185
vancomycin (Vancocin)	Miscellaneous antibacterial	410
verapamil (Calan)	Calcium channel blocker	307
vincristine (Oncovin)	Antineoplastic; plant alkaloid/natural product	459
warfarin (Coumadin)	Anticoagulant	243
zidovudine (Retrovir, AZT)	Antiviral; nucleoside reverse transcriptase inhibitor	429
zolpidem (Ambien)	Nonbarbiturate CNS depressant	119

CORE CONCEPTS IN PHARMACOLOGY

SECOND EDITION

LELAND NORMAN HOLLAND, JR., PHD

Associate Academic Dean and Dean, College of Arts and Sciences
Southeastern University
Lakeland, Florida

MICHAEL PATRICK ADAMS, PHD, RT(R)

Dean of Health Occupations
Pasco-Hernando Community College
New Port Richey, Florida

Nursing Consultant:
Jeanine Brice, RN, MSN
Pasco-Hernando Community College
New Port Richey, FL

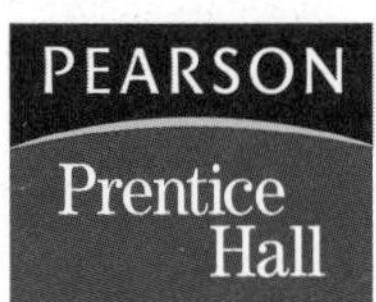

Upper Saddle River, New Jersey 07458

Library of Congress Cataloging-in-Publication Data
Holland, Leland Norman
Core concepts in pharmacology / Leland Norman Holland, Michael Patrick Adams.— 2nd ed.
p. ; cm.
Includes bibliographical references and index.
ISBN 0-13-171473-2
1. Pharmacology—Outlines, syllabi, etc. I. Adams, Michael II. Title.
[DNLM: 1. Pharmaceutical Preparations—Handbooks. 2. Drug Therapy—Handbooks. QV 39 H736c 2007]
RM301.14.H655 2007
615′ .1—dc22 2005035390

DEDICATION

I would like to acknowledge the willful encouragement of Farrell and Norma Jean Stalcup. I dedicate this book to my beloved wife, Karen, and my three wonderful children, Alexandria Noelle, my double-deuce daughter; Caleb Jaymes, my number one son; and Joshua Nathaniel, my number three "O"!

LNH

I dedicate this book to my wife, Kim, and my daughter Kimberly Michelle Valiance, who supported me through the endless hours of creativity and preparation that culminated in this work.

MPA

COVER ILLUSTRATION

Photomicrograph of codeine, an alkaloid obtained from opium or prepared from morphine by methylation. Used as a narcotic analgesic and as an antitussive. Copyright © Lars Bech/Phototake—All rights reserved.

Publisher: Julie Levin Alexander
Assistant to the Publisher: Regina Bruno
Editor-in-Chief: Maura Connor
Managing Editor Development: Marilyn Meserve
Developmental Editor: Elena Mauceri/Jennifer Maybin
Senior Media Development Editor: John J. Jordan
Associate Editor: Michael Giacobbe
Director of Production & Manufacturing: Bruce Johnson
Managing Production Editor: Patrick Walsh
Production Liaison: Nicholas Radhuber
Production Editor: Emily Bush, Carlisle Publishing Services
Manufacturing Manager: Ilene Sanford
Design Director: Cheryl Asherman
Senior Design Coordinator: Maria Guglielmo
Interior Designer: Wanda Espana
Cover Designer: Wanda Espana
Cover and Interior Illustration: Lars Bech/Phototake
Electronic Art Creation: Precision Graphics
Manager of New Media Production: Amy Peltier
New Media Production: CD Design and Programming: Red Frog; Dosage Calculator: Silverchair Science & Communications
New Media Project Manager: Tina Rudowski
Director of Marketing: Karen Allman
Senior Marketing Manager: Francisco Del Castillo
Marketing Coordinator: Michael Sirinides
Composition: Carlisle Publishing Services
Cover Printer: Phoenix Color
Printer/Binder: Banta

Pearson Education Ltd.
Pearson Education Australia PTY, Limited
Pearson Education Singapore, Pte. Ltd.
Pearson Education North Asia Ltd.
Pearson Education Canada, Ltd.
Pearson Educatión de Mexico, S.A. de C.V.
Pearson Education—Japan
Pearson Education Malaysia, Pte. Ltd
Pearson Education, Upper Saddle River, NJ

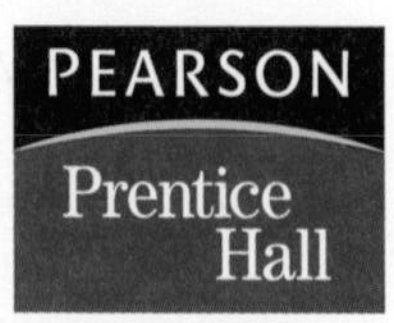

10 9 8 7 6 5 4 3 2
ISBN 0-13-171473-2

ABOUT THE AUTHORS

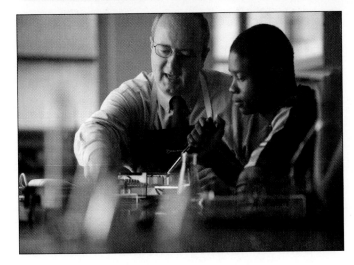

Leland Norman Holland, Jr., PhD (Norm), is the Associate Academic Dean and Dean of the College of Arts and Sciences at Southeastern University in Lakeland, Florida. He is actively involved in teaching and helping students prepare for service in various health professions including medicine, nursing, dentistry, and allied health. He has taught pharmacology over the course of 15 years at both the undergraduate and graduate level. He is very much dedicated to the success of students preparing for work–life readiness. He comes to the teaching profession after spending several years doing basic science research at the VA Hospital in Augusta, Georgia, and the Medical College of Georgia where he received his PhD in Pharmacology.

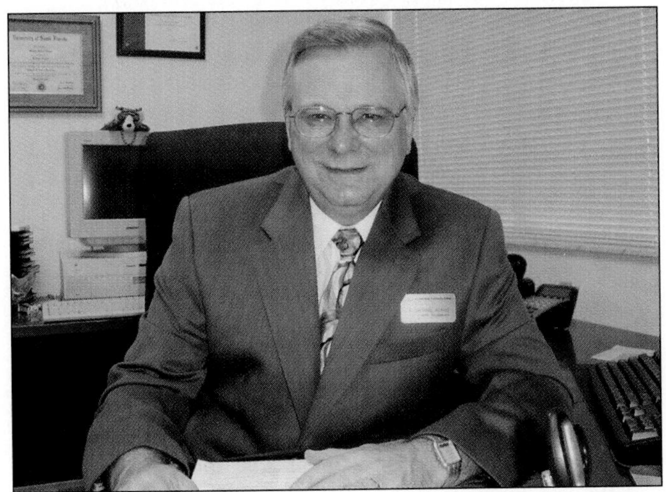

Michael Patrick Adams, PhD, RT(R), is the Dean of Health Occupations at Pasco-Hernando Community College. He is an accomplished educator, author, and national speaker. The National Institute for Staff and Organizational Development in Austin, Texas named Dr. Adams a Master Teacher. He has been registered by the American Registry of Radiologic Technologists for over 30 years. Dr. Adams obtained his Master's degree in Pharmacology from Michigan State University and his Doctorate in Education at the University of South Florida.

PREFACE

Pharmacology is one of the most challenging subjects for those embarking on careers in the health sciences. By its very nature, pharmacology is an interdisciplinary subject, borrowing concepts from a wide variety of the natural and applied sciences. Prediction of drug action, the ultimate goal in the study of pharmacology, requires a thorough knowledge of anatomy, physiology, chemistry, and pathology as well as the social sciences of psychology and sociology. It is the interdisciplinary nature of pharmacology that makes the subject difficult to learn, but fascinating to study.

This text presents pharmacology from an interdisciplinary perspective. The text draws upon core concepts of anatomy, physiology, and pathology to make drug therapy understandable. The text does not assume that the student comes to the course with a strong background in the natural or applied sciences. Although it is true that many students have prerequisite courses prior to attempting introductory pharmacology, such courses may have been taken many years prior to the current course. The prerequisite science knowledge necessary for understanding drug therapy is reviewed prior to presenting the core concepts in pharmacology.

APPROACH AND RATIONALE

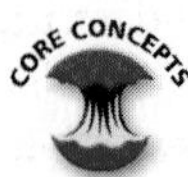

Core Concepts

The authors have created a concise means of communicating the most important pharmacologic information to the student. Through the use of numbered **Core Concepts,** the student is able to quickly identify key ideas. These core concepts are stated at the beginning of each chapter, so that the student can get an overview of what is to be learned. They are repeated at the end of the chapter, with a brief summary of the important concepts.

Disease and Body System Approach

Core Concepts in Pharmacology is organized according to body systems and diseases. This clearly places the drugs in context with how they are used therapeutically. The student is able to easily locate all relevant anatomy, physiology, pathology, and pharmacology in the same chapter in which the drugs are discussed.

Prototype Approach to Drug Therapy

The vast number of drugs taught in a pharmacology course is staggering. To facilitate learning, a prototype approach is used in which the one or two most representative drugs in each classification are introduced in detail. **Drug Profile** boxes are used to clearly indicate these important medications.

Pharmacology as a Visual Discipline

For nearly all students, learning is a highly visual process. *Core Concepts in Pharmacology* is the first pharmacology text to incorporate **Mechanism in Action,** which uses computer animations to clearly demonstrate drug action. A colorful grahic of the animation is included in many of the Drug Profile boxes, as well as a description of the drug action. The complete animation, including audio narrations that describe each step of the mechanism, are provided on the included student CD-ROM. The text also incorporates generous use of figures and diagrams to illustrate and summarize key concepts.

Focused Nursing Content

This text provides focused nursing content, which allows students to quickly find the essential content for safe, effective drug therapy. Forty-five **Nursing Process Focus** flowcharts provide a succinct, easy-to-read view of the most commonly prescribed drug classes. Need-to-know nursing actions are presented in a format that reflects the "flow" of the Nursing Process: nursing assessment, potential nursing diagnoses, planning, interventions, patient education and discharge planning, and evaluation. Rationales for interventions are included in parentheses. The Nursing Process Focus flowcharts identify clearly what nursing actions are most important. A Nursing Process Focus for every profile drug can be found on the Companion Website (www.prenhall.com/holland). The is provided at the bottom of each Drug Profile box to remind the student that this content can be found on the Companion Website.

Patient Education is an important nursing intervention. In addition to the patient education in the Nursing Process Focus flowcharts, **Patients Need to Know** boxes assist the nurse in imparting essential information to the patient and caregiver.

Integrated rationales for nursing actions provide the physiology of the drug action to answer the "why" of nursing interventions. This is key to developing critical thinking skills.

Lifespan Facts provide important **pediatric** and **geriatric** considerations for drug therapy. Vital **bioterrorism** and **poisoning** content is integrated into appropriate chapters to help students prepare for this new fact of life. In addition, **enteral** and **parenteral nutrition** content has been added to Chapter 27.

The Nurse as Teacher

It is not sufficient for a nurse to learn pharmacology. He or she must also have the ability to communicate this knowledge to patients and other members of the public. To help the student communicate about pharmacology, each chapter contains concise **Patients Need to Know** boxes that apply fundamental patient care principles to pharmacology.

Holistic Pharmacology

Core Concepts in Pharmacology approaches pharmacology from a holistic perspective. Throughout the text, the relationship of lifestyle habits such as proper body weight, exercise, and nutrition to pharmacology are discussed. Most chapters contain a **Natural Alternative** feature that presents a popular herbal or dietary supplement that may be considered along with conventional drugs. Note that we are not recommending any therapies or supplements in these features, only informing the practitioner of alternatives that patients may be using, and alerting them to any potential interactions. The **FastFacts** feature puts the disease in a social and economic perspective.

Medical Terminology

Pharmacology and other medical sciences use a unique language that can be overwhelming for beginning students. In each chapter of *Core Concepts in Pharmacology* key terms are defined at the beginning of each chapter, with the page number on which the first reference to the word can be found. **Key terms** are placed in blue boldface type throughout the text. **Word roots** are included in the margins to help the student identify prefixes and suffixes essential to medical word-building. Since pronunciation of medical terms is often difficult, a phonetic pronunciation is provided for difficult terms. In the drug tables, phonetic pronunciations are also provided for the generic name of each drug. An audio glossary can be found on the Student CD-ROM as well as the Companion Website.

Integrated Media

MediaLink boxes are included at the beginning of each chapter. This feature guides the student to resources, interactive exercises, and animations for that chapter on the Student CD-ROM and Companion Website. **MediaLinks** serve as a gateway to additional learning by inviting the student to perform specific web activities or to consult the accompanying CD-ROM.

Reinforcement and Review

Each chapter concludes with features to reinforce and enhance student learning. The **Chapter Review** section consists of a summary of the most important concepts in each chapter (**Core Concepts Summary**). The **Key Terms** list provides a summary of the important terms from the chapter. NCLEX–PN®-style **Review Questions** help the student review the chapter material and practice their test-taking skills. **Case Study** questions help the student to apply pharmacology to patient care. Answers for the Review Questions and Case Study questions can be found in Appendix B. Answer rationales for the NCLEX-PN® Review Questions are available in the Instructor's Resource Manual, as well. Finally, **Further Study** is a handy listing of cross-references within the chapter and the topics to which they apply.

COMPLETE TEACHING AND LEARNING PACKAGE

To enhance the teaching and learning process, an attractive media-focused supplements package for both students and faculty has been developed in close correlation with *Core Concepts in Pharmacology.* The full complement of supplemental teaching materials is available to all qualified instructors from your Prentice Hall Health Sales Representative.

Student CD-ROM. The Student CD-ROM is packaged with each copy of the textbook. It provides 30 animations showing how drug action occurs at the cellular and system levels. These animations build upon the *Mechanism in Action* feature in the textbook and help students visualize these difficult concepts. The CD-ROM also includes NCLEX–PN® Review Questions that emphasize application of care and patient education related to drug administration. Students can test their knowledge and gain immediate feedback through rationales for right and wrong answers. In addition, Concept Review questions provide students an additional opportunity for checking their knowledge. Students will also find the audio glossary and objectives useful for review. Finally, the CD-ROM allows access to the Companion Website described in the following text (Internet connection required).

Student Workbook. A Student Workbook for *Core Concepts in Pharmacology* has been developed to closely parallel the text. The Workbook contains a variety of question types and a large number of practice questions and learning activities. Other study aids may be found at the Companion Website.

Instructor's Resource Manual. This manual contains a wealth of material to help faculty plan and manage the pharmacology course. It includes Chapter Overviews, Lecture Suggestions and Outlines, Learning Objectives, a complete Test Bank, Teaching Tips, and more for each chapter. The IRM also guides faculty how to assign and use the text-specific Companion Website, www.prenhall.com/holland, and the CD-ROM that accompany the textbook.

Instructor's Resource CD-ROM. New to this package, the Instructor's Resources CD-ROM provides many resources in an electronic format. First, the CD-ROM includes the complete Test Bank in Test-Gen format. Second, it includes a comprehensive collection of images from the textbook in PowerPoint format, so faculty can easily import these photographs and illustrations into their own classroom lecture presentations. Finally, the CD-ROM provides instructors with access to the same animations that appear on the Student CD-ROM, so faculty can incorporate these visual accents into their lectures.

Companion Website and Syllabus Manager®. Students and faculty will both benefit from the free Companion Website at www.prenhall.com/holland. This website serves as a text-specific, interactive online workbook to *Core Concepts in Pharmacology.* The Companion Website includes modules for Objectives, Audio Glossary, Chapter Summary for lecture notes, NCLEX-PN® Review Questions, Case Studies, Care Plan activities, Message Board discussion questions, Web Links, Nursing Tools, and more. Instructors adopting this textbook for their courses have free access to an online Syllabus Manager with a whole host of features that facilitate the students' use of this Companion Website and allow faculty to post their syllabi online for their students. For more information or a demonstration of Syllabus Manager, please contact your Prentice Hall Health Sales Representative or go online to www.prenhall.com/demo.

ACKNOWLEDGMENTS

We are grateful to all the educators who reviewed the manuscript of this text. Their insights, suggestions, and eye for detail helped us prepare a more relevant and useful book, one that focuses on the essential components of learning in the field of pharmacology.

Carol Alexander, MSN, RN
Palm Beach Community College
Lake Worth, Florida

Cheryll Alt, RN, BSN
Montana State University
Great Falls College of Technology
Great Falls, Montana

Linda Arnold, RN, MSN
Ivy Tech State College, Bloomington
Bloomington, Indiana

Carol Dean Baker, RN, MSN
Georgia College & State University
Milledgeville, Georgia

Faye Baker, RN, MSN
Wallace Community College, Sparks Campus
Eufaula, Alabama

Heidi Hartenstein Benoit, RN, BSN, MS
Lafayette General Medical Center
Lafayette, Louisiana

Korbi Berryhill, RN, BA, CRRN
South Plains College
Lubbock, Texas

Cora Beute, RN, MSN, BC
Grand Rapids Community College
Grand Rapids, Michigan

Paula Bostwick, RN, MSN
Ivy Tech State College Northeast
Fort Wayne, Indiana

Yvonne Broussard
Lafayette General Medical Center
Lafayette, Louisiana

Victoria Brown, RN, MSN, BC, ANP
Jefferson College
Festus, Missouri

Rebecca Cappo, RN, MSN
Lenape Tech
Ford City, Pennsylvania

Brigitte Casteel, RN, BSN
Mountain Empire Community College
Big Stone Gap, Virginia

Virginia Christensen, RN
Tennessee Technology Center at Livingston
Livingston, Tennessee

Betty Coalmon, RN, BSN, MS, MEd
Bronx Community College
Bronx, New York

Danae Colbath, RN, BSN, CCRN
New Hampshire Community Technical College
Manchester, New Hampshire

Karen D. Danielson, RN, MSN
North Central State College
Mansfield, Ohio

Karen Davis, CPhT
Southeastern Technical College
Vidalia, Georgia

Connie Dempsey, RN, MSN
Stark State College of Technology
North Canton, Ohio

Gail Dunham, RN, MSN
Mid-Michigan Community College
Harrison, Michigan

Sally Flesch, RN, PhD
Black Hawk College
Moline, Illinois

Kimberly Friedmeyer, RN, BS
Erwin Technical Center
Tampa, Florida

Faith Garrett, ARNP-C, MSN
Lake Sumter Community College
Clermont, Florida

Pamela Gwin, RN, C
Brazosport College
Lake Jackson, Texas

Lutricia Harrison, RN, MSN
Kingwood College
Kingwood, Texas

Elizabeth A. Hoffman, MAEd, CMA
Baker College of Clinton Township
Clinton Township, Michigan

Beulah A. Hofmann, RN, MSN, CMA
Ivy Tech State College
Greencastle, Indiana

Melinda Huffman, RN, MSN, CCNS
Motlow College
Lynchburg, Tennessee

Robin Kern, RN, BSN
Moultrie Technical College
Moultrie, Georgia

Sylvia (Skippy) Klava, RN
Saint Paul College
St. Paul, Minnesota

Denise Way Lagueux, RN, MSN
Southeast Community College
Lincoln, Nebraska

Carolyn Levi, RN, MSN, WHNP
Grand Rapids Community College
Grand Rapids, Michigan

Patricia E. Lewin, RN
Mercer County Technical Schools
Trenton, New Jersey

Tina Lewis, MT (ASCP) (AMT)
Spencerian College
Louisville, Kentucky

David Martinez, RHE
International Business College
EI Paso, Texas

Alice McCutcheon, RN
Tennessee Technology Center at Paris
Paris, Tennessee

Perpetua (Pepper) McDonald, RN
Saint Paul College
St. Paul, Minnesota

Anna Meyers, RN, BSN, MS
Hamilton College, Omaha Campus, an affiliate of Kaplan University
Council Bluffs, Iowa

Frances D. Monahan, RN, PhD
SUNY Rockland Community College
Suffern, New York

Norma Moore, BS, MT (ASCP)
Laredo Community College
Laredo, Texas

Lisa Nagle, BSEd, CMA
Augusta Technical College
Augusta, Georgia

Sherry Nantroup, RN, MSN, FNP-C
Moorpark College
Moorpark, California

Mary Nifong, RN, MSN
Pikes Peak Community College
Colorado Springs, Colorado

Margaret Noirjean, RN, BSN
Dakota County Technical College
Rosemount, Minnesota

Elizabeth Peace, RN
Moultrie Technical College
Tifton, Georgia

Toni Phillips, RN, BSN
Santa Fe Community College
Gainesville, Florida

Jennifer Ponto, RN, BSN
South Plains College
Levelland, Texas

Diane Premeau, RHIT, RHIA
Chabot College
Fremont, California

Ruben Ramos, BS
Registered Healthcare Educator
International Business College
El Paso, Texas

Kim Rawson, RN, MSN
Bishop State Community College
Mobile, Alabama

Deborah Robinson, RN, MSN
Vermont Technical College
Randolph Center, Vermont

Elizabeth Rohan, AASN
Wharton County Junior College
Wharton, Texas

Terry Rudd, RN, MSN, CCRN
Mt. San Antonio College
Walnut, California

Jodene Scheller, RN, MSN
Lewis and Clark Community College
Godfrey, Illinois

Connie Schroeder, RN, MS
Danville Area Community College
Danville, Illinois

Brenda Sewell, RN, MS, HEd
North Texas Professional Career Institute
Dallas, Texas

Linda W. Shows, RN, BSN, MS
Jones County Junior College
Ellisville, Mississippi

Jackie Shrock, RN, BSN, MEd
Wayne Adult School of Practical Nursing
Smithville, Ohio

Cindy Smith, RN, AASN
Arkansas State University-Searcy
Searcy, Arkansas

Cindy Steury-Lattz, RN, MSN, APRN, BC
Kankakee Community College
Kankakee, Illinois

Karen Stevens, RN, MSN
Southeast Community College
Beatrice, Nebraska

Lucien L. Van Elsen, RPh, BS
Milwaukee Area Technical College
Milwaukee, Wisconsin

Lori Warren, RN, MA, CPC, CLNC
Spencerian College
Louisville, Kentucky

Muriel Zraunig, RN, MSN
Holyoke Community College
Holyoke, Massachusetts

Our thanks also go to Jeanine Brice, RN, MSN, who provided the **Nursing Process Focus charts** and the **Patients Need to Know** features; Paula Bostwick, RN, MSN, who provided the **Review Questions;** and Claudia Stoffel, RN, MSN who provided the answer rationales for the Review Questions. Their nursing experience, expertise, and dedication to the profession are very evident in these materials. Thanks to all!

BRIEF CONTENTS

GUIDE TO
CORE CONCEPTS IN PHARMACOLOGY

SECOND EDITION

A FOCUS ON CORE INFORMATION

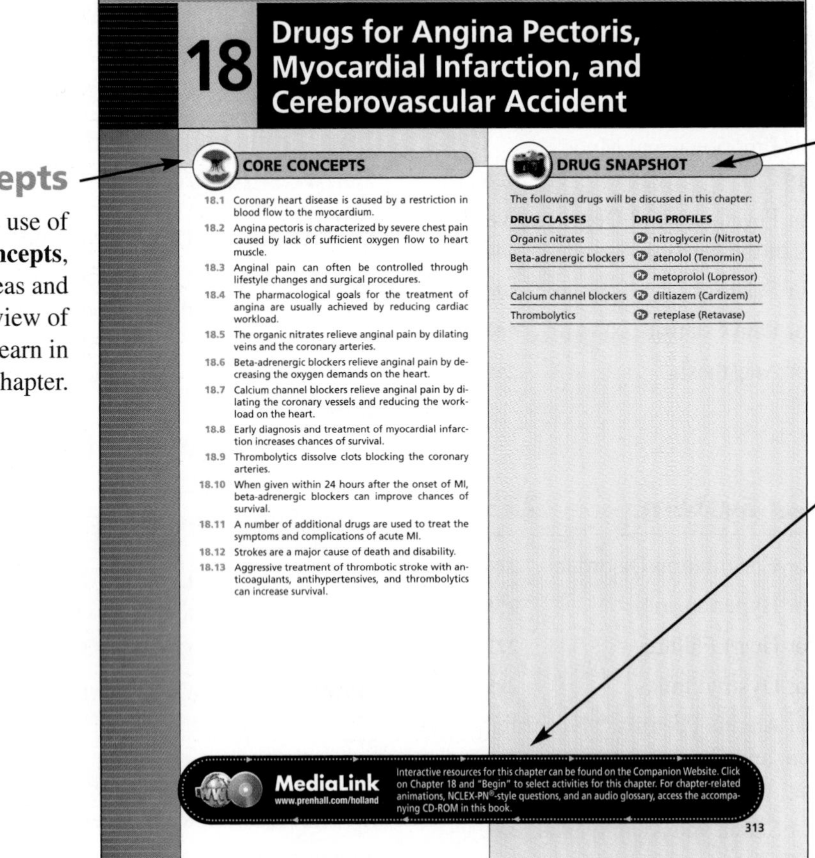

CHAPTER

18 Drugs for Angina Pectoris, Myocardial Infarction, and Cerebrovascular Accident

CORE CONCEPTS

18.1 Coronary heart disease is caused by a restriction in blood flow to the myocardium.
18.2 Angina pectoris is characterized by severe chest pain caused by lack of sufficient oxygen flow to heart muscle.
18.3 Anginal pain can often be controlled through lifestyle changes and surgical procedures.
18.4 The pharmacological goals for the treatment of angina are usually achieved by reducing cardiac workload.
18.5 The organic nitrates relieve anginal pain by dilating veins and the coronary arteries.
18.6 Beta-adrenergic blockers relieve anginal pain by decreasing the oxygen demands on the heart.
18.7 Calcium channel blockers relieve anginal pain by dilating the coronary vessels and reducing the workload on the heart.
18.8 Early diagnosis and treatment of myocardial infarction increases chances of survival.
18.9 Thrombolytics dissolve clots blocking the coronary arteries.
18.10 When given within 24 hours after the onset of MI, beta-adrenergic blockers can improve chances of survival.
18.11 A number of additional drugs are used to treat the symptoms and complications of acute MI.
18.12 Strokes are a major cause of death and disability.
18.13 Aggressive treatment of thrombotic stroke with anticoagulants, antihypertensives, and thrombolytics can increase survival.

DRUG SNAPSHOT

The following drugs will be discussed in this chapter:

DRUG CLASSES	DRUG PROFILES
Organic nitrates	nitroglycerin (Nitrostat)
Beta-adrenergic blockers	atenolol (Tenormin)
	metoprolol (Lopressor)
Calcium channel blockers	diltiazem (Cardizem)
Thrombolytics	reteplase (Retavase)

MediaLink www.prenhall.com/holland

Interactive resources for this chapter can be found on the Companion Website. Click on Chapter 18 and "Begin" to select activities for this chapter. For chapter-related animations, NCLEX-PN®-style questions, and an audio glossary, access the accompanying CD-ROM in this book.

313

Core Concepts

Through the use of numbered **Core Concepts**, students identify ideas and can get an overview of what they will learn in the chapter.

NEW—Drug Snapshot

This snapshot provides an at-a-glance list of the drug classes and related drug profiles covered in each chapter.

MediaLink

The **MediaLink** at the beginning of each chapter guides the student to resources, interactive exercises, and animations for that chapter on the Student CD-ROM and Companion Website. MediaLink serves as a gateway to additional learning and applications.

Concept Review 18.2

- How does decreasing the workload on the heart result in reduction in anginal pain?

Concept Reviews

Concept Reviews are questions placed strategically throughout the chapter to stimulate student comprehension and retention as they read.

NEW COVERAGE OF NURSING PROCESS

NEW—Nursing Focus

This edition provides focused nursing content, helping LPN/LVN students to provide safe and effective drug therapy. **Nursing Process Focus** flowcharts provide a succinct, easy-to-read view of the most important nursing actions for the commonly prescribed drug classes. Need-to-know nursing actions are presented in the nursing process which also include patient education and discharge planning. For more information, students can find Nursing Process Focus tables for every profile drug on the Companion Website at www.prenhall.com/holland.

NURSING PROCESS FOCUS

Patients Receiving Nitroglycerin

ASSESSMENT

Prior to administration:
- Obtain complete health history including allergies, drug history, and possible drug interactions
- Assess vital signs, ECG, frequency and severity of angina, and alcohol use
- Obtain history of cardiac disorders and blood testing including cardiac enzymes, CBC, BUN, creatinine, and liver function tests
- Assess if patient has taken sildenafil (Viagra) within last 24 hours

POTENTIAL NURSING DIAGNOSES

- Risk for Ineffective Tissue Perfusion, related to hypotension from drug
- Risk for Injury (dizziness or fainting), related to hypotension from drug
- Acute Pain (headache), related to adverse effects of drug
- Deficient Knowledge, related to drug therapy

PLANNING: Patient Goals and Expected Outcomes

The patient will:
- Experience relief or prevention of chest pain
- Report immediately any chest pain unrelieved by nitroglycerin
- Demonstrate an understanding of the drug's action by accurately describing drug side effects and precautions

IMPLEMENTATION

Interventions and (Rationales)	Patient Education/Discharge Planning
■ Ask patient to describe and rate pain prior to drug administration for description/documentation of anginal episode. ■ Obtain a 12-lead ECG to differentiate between angina and infarction. (Pharmacotherapy depends on which disorder is presenting.)	Instruct patient to: ■ Take 1 tablet every 5 min until pain is relieved or for up to 3 doses during an acute anginal attack ■ Call EMS if chest pain is not relieved after 3 doses ■ Place SL tablet under tongue or spray under tongue; do not inhale spray
■ Monitor blood pressure and pulse. Do not administer drug if patient is hypotensive. (Drug will further reduce blood pressure.) ■ Monitor alcohol use. (Extremely low blood pressure may result, which could cause death.) ■ Monitor for headache in response to use of nitrates.	■ Instruct patient to sit or lie down before taking medication and to avoid abrupt changes in position. ■ Emphasize the importance of avoiding alcohol while taking nitroglycerin. Instruct patient that: ■ Headache is a common side effect, that usually decreases over time ■ OTC medicines usually relieve the headache
■ Monitor for use of sildenafil (Viagra) concurrently with nitrates, because cardiovascular disease is a major cause of erectile dysfunction in men. (Life-threatening hypotension may result with concurrent use of sildenafil.)	Instruct patient to: ■ Not take Viagra within 24 hours after taking nitrates ■ Wait at least 24 hours after taking Viagra to resume nitrate therapy
■ Monitor need for prophylactic nitrates.	■ Advise patient to take medication prior to a stressful event or physical activity to prevent angina.

EVALUATION OF OUTCOME CRITERIA

Evaluate the effectiveness of drug therapy by confirming that patient goals and expected outcomes have been met (see "Planning").

See Table 18.2 for a list of drugs to which these nursing actions apply.

USING A PROTOTYPE APPROACH

Drug Profiles

The prototype approach introduces the one or two most representative drugs in each classification in detail. **Drug Profile** boxes highlight these important drugs. This edition now includes drug-drug and herb-drug interactions.

DRUG PROFILE: Anticoagulant: Pr *Warfarin (Coumadin)*

Actions and Uses:

Unlike heparin, the anticoagulant activity of warfarin can take several days to reach its maximum effect. This explains why heparin and warfarin therapy are overlapped. Warfarin inhibits the action of vitamin K that is essential for the synthesis of several clotting factors. Because these clotting factors are normally circulating in the blood, it takes several days for them to clear the plasma and for the anticoagulant effect of warfarin to appear. Another reason for the slow onset is that 99% of warfarin binds to plasma proteins and is unavailable to produce its effect. This high level of protein binding is responsible for a significant number of drug-drug interactions that may occur during warfarin therapy.

Adverse Effects and Interactions:

Like all anticoagulants, the most serious adverse effect of warfarin is abnormal bleeding. On discontinuation of therapy, the activity of warfarin can take up to 10 days to diminish. If life-threatening bleeding occurs during therapy, the anticoagulant effects of warfarin can be reduced in 6 hours through the IM or subcutaneous administration of its blocker, vitamin K. The therapeutic range of serum warfarin levels varies from 1 to 10 mcg/ml, to achieve an INR value of 2–3.

Extensive protein binding is responsible for numerous drug interactions, some of which include NSAIDs, diuretics, SSRIs, and other antidepressants, steroids, antibiotics and vaccines, and vitamins (for example, vitamin K). Use with NSAIDs may increase bleeding risk.

Use of warfarin with herbal supplements, such as feverfew, garlic, and ginger, may increase the risk of bleeding; use with arnica may increase the anticoagulant effect.

Mechanism in Action:

Many vitamin K–dependent clotting factors are essential for blood coagulation. The anticoagulant warfarin inhibits the amount of factors made available by the liver. Reducing vitamin K–dependent factors inhibits the formation of prothrombin, which is one of the final coagulation proteins in the clotting cascade. The result is slowed clot formation and increased bleeding time.

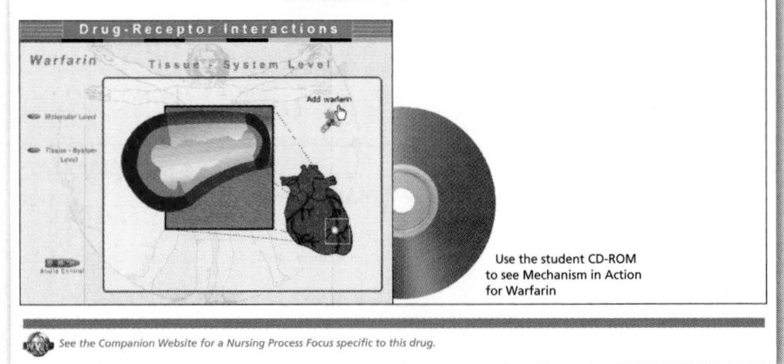

See the Companion Website for a Nursing Process Focus specific to this drug.

Mechanism in Action

Mechanism in Action encourages students to see how drugs act using computer animations on the Student CD-ROM.

TABLE 18.2 Organic Nitrates

DRUG	ROUTE AND ADULT DOSE	REMARKS
amyl nitrate (Vaporole)	Inhalation 1 ampule (0.18–0.3 ml) prn	Short acting; onset is 10–30 seconds; may be repeated in 3–5 minutes; also used as treatment for cyanide poisoning
isosorbide dinitrate (Dilatrate SR, Isordil, Sorbitrate)	PO 2.5–30 mg qid available;	For both acute attacks and long-term management; sublingual and chewable forms smaller dose is given to initiate therapy; extended-release form available
isosorbide mononitrate (Imdur, Ismo, Monoket)	PO 20 mg bid (max:240 mg/day with sustained release)	For the prevention of angina; a smaller dose is given to initiate therapy; extended-release form available
Pr nitroglycerin (Nitrostat, Nitrobid, Nitro-Dur, and others)	SL 1 tablet (0.3–0.6 mg) or 1 spray (0.4–0.8 mg) q 3–5 min (max: 3 doses in 15 min)	Dilates both arteries and veins; sublingual, oral, translingual, IV, transmucosal, transdermal, and topical forms available; extended-release form available
pentaerythrityl (Peritrate, Duotrate, Pentylan)	PO 10–20 mg tid or qid	Extended-release form available

Drug Tables

Drug tables provide the most important information for each drug in a user-friendly format. Drugs profiled within that chapter are also identified with a Profile icon. Pr

HIGHLIGHTS KEY INFORMATION FOR SAFE, EFFECTIVE NURSING CARE

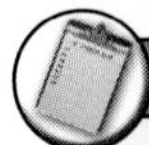

PATIENTS NEED TO KNOW

Patients treated for chest pain need to know the following:

Regarding Antianginals

1. Dissolve one nitroglycerin tablet under the tongue as soon as anginal pain is felt. If pain is not relieved in 5 minutes, use another. Many practitioners recommend a third nitroglycerin tablet for pain not relieved 5 minutes after the second dose. If chest pain/pressure is not relieved by 3 doses of nitroglycerin, call emergency medical services.
2. Rotate the application site of transdermal patches, and do not apply a new patch until after the old patch has been removed.
3. Change positions slowly. Postural hypotension may cause dizziness and even fainting.
4. Monitor blood pressure regularly, and report any consistent changes to a healthcare provider.

Regarding Anticoagulants

5. Do not eat large or inconsistent amounts of foods high in vitamin K while taking warfarin because this interferes with clotting time.
6. Do not take herbal supplements or OTC drugs before getting advice from a healthcare provider. Many drugs increase or decrease the effects of warfarin.
7. Report any symptoms of unusual bleeding or bruising to a healthcare provider. ■

Patient Teaching

The nursing student needs to learn how to teach drug administration to patients and families. To help the student, each drug chapter contains concise **Patients Need to Know** boxes that apply fundamental patient care principles to pharmacology.

Life Span Fact

Bleeding complications are more likely to occur in older adults. Prescribed doses of anticoagulants are generally lower for older patients, and this group receives more frequent assessments and laboratory testing to avoid serious complications.

NEW—Lifespan Content

Lifespan Facts provide important **pediatric** and **geriatric** considerations for drug therapy, so students understand variations in nursing care and drug actions due to age.

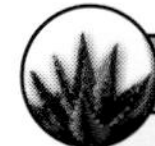

NATURAL ALTERNATIVES

Garlic for Cardiovascular Disease

Garlic (*Allium sativum*) is one of the best studied herbs. Indications for garlic are said to include arteriosclerosis, common cold, cough/bronchitis, high cholesterol, hypertension, tendency to infection, and many other conditions. It has been proven to be of value in only a few of these disorders.

A number of different substances, known as *alliaceous oils,* have been isolated from garlic and shown to have pharmacological activity. The supplement can be eaten as prepared garlic oil or fresh bulbs from the plant.

Garlic has been shown to decrease the aggregation or "stickiness" of platelets, thus producing an anticoagulant effect. Claims that garlic can reduce heart disease and the incidence of stroke may be related to this action. The healthcare provider may want to recommend that patients taking anticoagulant medications limit their intake of garlic to avoid bleeding complications. ■

Natural Alternatives

Natural Alternatives presents a popular herbal or dietary supplement that may be considered along with conventional drugs.

Fast Facts **Myocardial Infarction**

- About 1.1 million Americans experience a new or recurrent MI each year.
- About one third of patients experiencing an MI will die.
- About 250,000 Americans each year die of an acute MI within 1 hour of the onset of the symptoms.
- About 60% of patients who died suddenly of MI had no previous symptoms of the disease.
- Mortality from MI is slightly higher in men than women.
- Because women have MIs, at older ages, they are more likely to die from them within a few weeks.
- More than 20% of men and 40% of women will die from an MI within 1 year after being diagnosed.

Fast Facts

The **Fast Facts** feature puts the disease in a social and economic perspective.

NEW END OF CHAPTER REVIEW RESOURCES

Student practical and vocational nurses from around the country told us that they start their chapter reading from the end of the chapter. So to ensure students' success, in the classroom, on the NCLEX-PN® exam, and in the workplace, we put dynamite review resources at the end of each chapter.

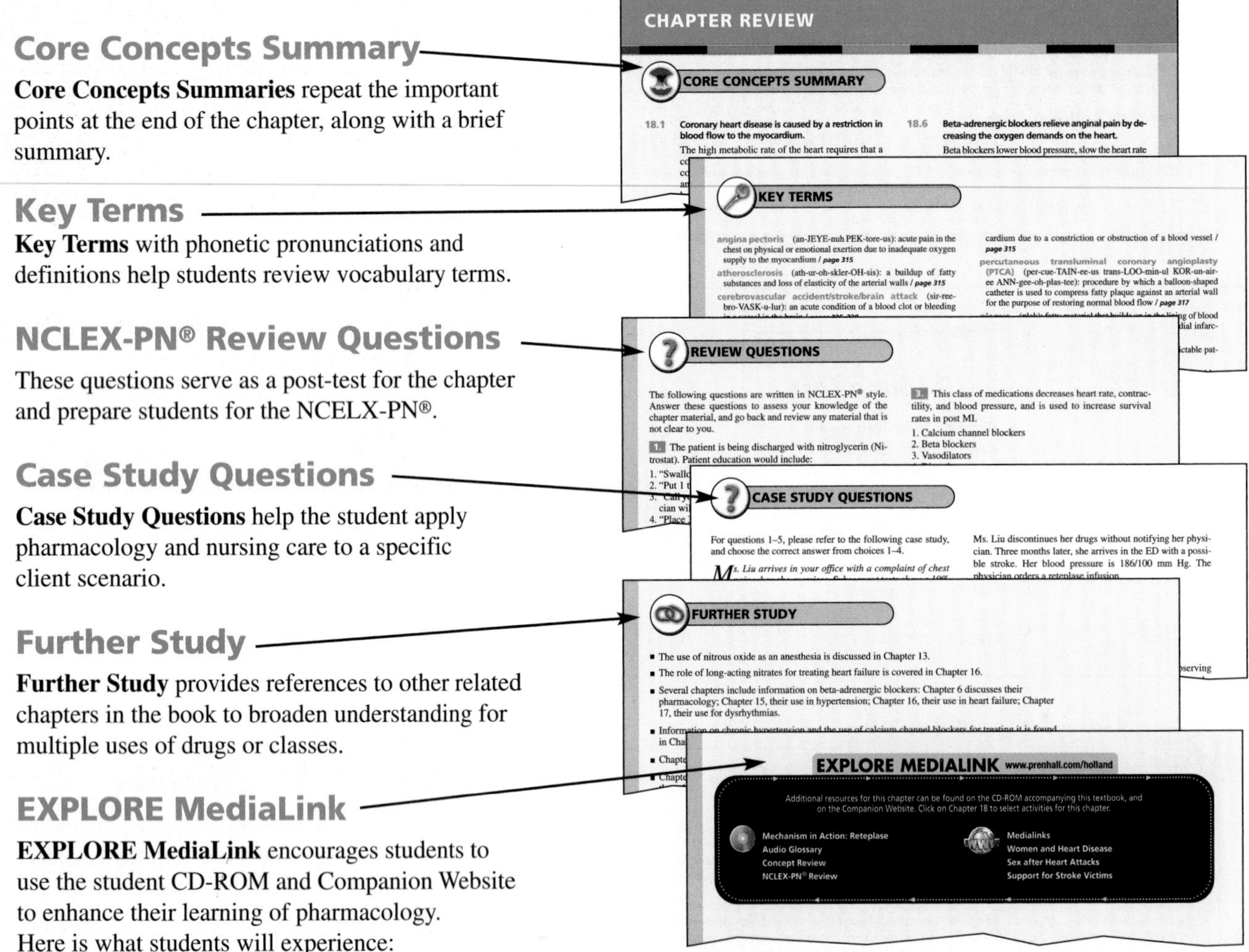

Core Concepts Summary

Core Concepts Summaries repeat the important points at the end of the chapter, along with a brief summary.

Key Terms

Key Terms with phonetic pronunciations and definitions help students review vocabulary terms.

NCLEX-PN® Review Questions

These questions serve as a post-test for the chapter and prepare students for the NCELX-PN®.

Case Study Questions

Case Study Questions help the student apply pharmacology and nursing care to a specific client scenario.

Further Study

Further Study provides references to other related chapters in the book to broaden understanding for multiple uses of drugs or classes.

EXPLORE MediaLink

EXPLORE MediaLink encourages students to use the student CD-ROM and Companion Website to enhance their learning of pharmacology. Here is what students will experience:

Student CD-ROM

- 37 animations showing Mechanism of Drug Actions
- NCLEX-PN® questions
- Audio Glossary of Key Terms and Prototype Drug Pronunciations
- Drug Dosage and Conversion Calculations
- Nursing in Action video exercises related to drug administration

Companion Website

- More NCLEX-PN® questions
- Case Studies
- Drug Matching exercises
- Dosage Calculation exercises
- Drug Review activities
- Care Plan activities
- Preventing Medication Errors Module
- Prototype and Classification Matching exercises

UNIT

1 2 3 4 5 6 7

1 BASIC CONCEPTS IN PHARMACOLOGY

UNIT CONTENTS

CHAPTER

1 Introduction to Pharmacology: Drug Regulation and Approval

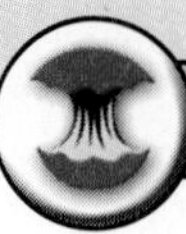

CORE CONCEPTS

1.1 Pharmacology is an expansive and challenging topic.

1.2 For healthcare professionals, the fields of pharmacology and therapeutics are connected.

1.3 Agents may be classified as traditional drugs, biologics, and natural alternatives.

1.4 Drugs are available by prescription or over the counter (OTC).

1.5 *Pharmaceutics* is the science of pharmacy.

1.6 Drug regulations were created to protect the public from drug misuse.

1.7 U.S. drug standards have become increasingly complex.

1.8 There are four stages of approval for therapeutic and biologic drugs.

1.9 Once criticized for being too slow, governmental agencies face new challenges for ensuring the safety of drugs.

1.10 Similar drug standards protect Canadian consumers.

1.11 Healthcare professionals must be prepared to deal with the threat of biologic and chemical attack.

OBJECTIVES

After reading this chapter, the student should be able to:

1. Explain the interdisciplinary nature of pharmacology and give examples of subject area expertise needed to learn the discipline well.
2. Identify groups of occupations in which a knowledge of pharmacology is important.
3. Explain how the disciplines of therapeutics and pharmacology are interconnected.
4. Distinguish between therapeutic drugs and agents such as foods, household products, and cosmetics.
5. Compare and contrast traditional drugs, biologics, and natural alternative therapies.
6. Identify the advantages and disadvantages of prescription and OTC drugs.
7. Distinguish between pharmaceutics and pharmacology.
8. Discuss the history of U.S. standards, acts, and organizations leading to the requirement that drug safety must be proven before marketing.
9. Discuss the role of the U.S. Food and Drug Administration in determining whether drugs may be used for therapy.
10. Discuss the roles and responsibilities of branches within the FDA in overseeing traditional therapeutic drugs, biologics, and natural alternative therapies.
11. Identify four stages of approval for therapeutic and biologic drugs.
12. Discuss current challenges facing the FDA in approving new drugs for market.
13. Explain the role of Health Canada in the management of Canadian health, drug, and safety issues.
14. Describe the Canadian drug approval process and explain points of similarity to the U.S. approval process.
15. Discuss the challenges facing healthcare professionals in view of modern-day bioterroist threats.

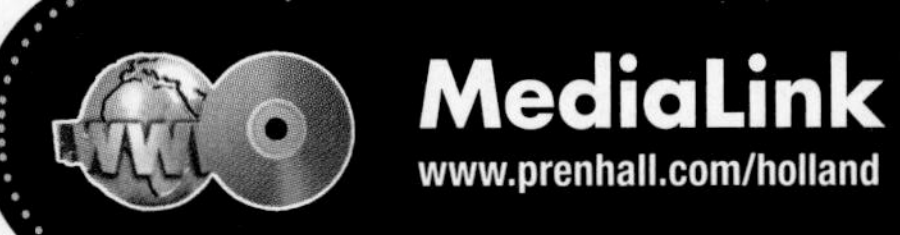

Interactive resources for this chapter can be found on the Companion Website. Click on Chapter 1 and "Begin" to select the activities for this chapter. For chapter-related animations, NCLEX-PN®-style questions, and an audio glossary, access the accompanying CD-ROM in this book.

Drugs are the most powerful weapon we have against diseases, worldwide epidemics, and bioterrorist threats. More drugs are being administered to consumers than ever before. Because of the number of new drugs becoming available for therapy, some experts are concerned that patients might be harmed if drugs are not thoroughly tested.

The purpose of this chapter is to introduce the subject of pharmacology and to emphasize the role of the government in ensuring drugs and natural alternatives are safe and effective for public use. The chapter also addresses the role that drug therapy has in fighting disease as governmental regulators, consumers, and healthcare professionals face new challenges in the years ahead.

Bioterrorist threats have led to widespread changes in emergency preparedness planning. This chapter also briefly introduces the role of pharmacology in the prevention and treatment of diseases or conditions that might develop because of biologic, chemical, or nuclear attack.

1.1 Pharmacology is an expansive and challenging topic

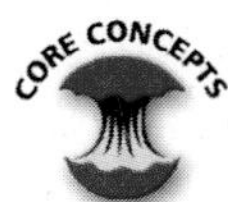

The word **pharmacology** is derived from two Greek words, *pharmakon,* which means "medicine," and *logos,* which means "study." Thus, *pharmacology* is defined as *"the study of medicine."*

pharmac = *medicine*
ology = *the study of*

Healthcare practitioners practice the discipline of pharmacology because it is the study of how drugs improve the health of the human body. If applied properly, drugs can dramatically improve our quality of life. If applied improperly, the consequences of drug action can be devastating.

The subject of pharmacology is an expansive topic ranging from a study of how drugs enter and travel throughout the body to the actual responses they produce. To learn the discipline well, students must master concepts from several interrelated areas including anatomy, physiology, chemistry, and **pathophysiology.** The useful application of drugs depends on knowledge from at least these areas.

patho = *disease*
physio = *the nature of*
ology = *the study of*

More than 10,000 brand and generic varieties of drugs with many different names, interactions, side effects, and complicated mechanisms of action are currently available. Keeping up with the numbers of drugs is a huge challenge. Many drugs may be prescribed for more than one disease, and most produce multiple effects in the body. Further complicating the study of pharmacology is the fact that drugs may cause different responses depending on factors such as gender, age, health status, body mass, and genetics.

1.2 For healthcare professionals, the fields of pharmacology and therapeutics are connected.

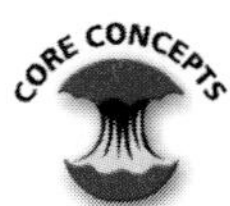

It is obvious that a thorough knowledge of pharmacology is important to those health professionals who prescribe drugs on a daily basis. This group includes physicians, physician's assistants, dentists, and advanced nurse practitioners. Depending on state or provincial law, other groups may also be permitted to prescribe medications. In this textbook, the group of occupations that is allowed to prescribe drugs will be referred to as *healthcare practitioners.*

A second group of occupations includes nursing, allied health and community service employees. These occupations have in common direct contact with patients or healthcare practitioners. Nurses and some other allied health workers are directly involved with drug administration as well as with issues related to drug education, management, and/or enforcement of drug laws. In this text, these occupations will be referred to as *healthcare providers.*

Some healthcare providers, such as nurses, may administer drugs on a daily basis while others may administer drugs occasionally. A strong knowledge of pharmacology is necessary to properly educate and advise patients regarding their healthcare needs. This knowledge is also essential to communicate effectively with healthcare practitioners, who rely heavily on nurses and allied health professionals to gather medical data from their patients and to follow up on results of therapy.

For healthcare providers studying pharmacology, it usually becomes apparent that the fields of pharmacology and therapeutics are connected. **Therapeutics** is the branch of medicine concerned with the treatment of disease and suffering. **Pharmacotherapeutics** is the use of medicine to treat disease.

TABLE 1.1	Characteristics of Traditional Therapeutic Drugs, Biologics, and Natural Alternative Therapies
Traditional Drug Therapies	■ Chemically produced in a laboratory ■ Routinely used by healthcare practitioners
Biologics	■ Naturally produced by the body itself, in animal cells, or in microorganisms ■ Includes hormones and vaccines ■ Routinely used by healthcare practitioners
Natural Alternative Therapies	■ Naturally produced ■ Includes herbs, extracts, vitamins, minerals, or dietary supplements

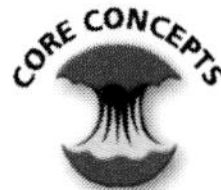

1.3 Agents may be classified as traditional drugs, biologics, and natural alternatives.

Drugs are chemical agents that produce biological responses within the body. From a broader perspective, drugs may be considered a part of the body's normal activities, from the essential gases that we breathe to the foods that we eat. Because drugs are defined so broadly, it is necessary to clearly separate them from other substances such as foods, household products, and cosmetics. Many agents, including antiperspirants, sunscreens, toothpastes, and shampoos, might alter the body's normal activities, but they are not considered to be medically therapeutic, as are drugs.

Therapeutic drugs are sometimes classified on the basis of how they are produced, either chemically or naturally. Most traditional drugs are chemically produced or synthesized in a laboratory. **Biologics** are agents naturally produced in animal cells, microorganisms, or by the body itself. **Natural alternative therapies** are herbs, natural extracts, vitamins, minerals, or dietary supplements. Table 1.1 contains a summary of characteristics associated with traditional drug therapies, biologics, and natural alternative therapies. Because drugs may be described in many ways, this text will limit its focus to agents used for therapy in a clinical or home setting. Traditional drugs and drug classes will be discussed more thoroughly in Chapter 2. Natural alternatives will be discussed more thoroughly in Chapter 5 ↔. In addition, most chapters include a feature called *Natural Alternatives* that highlights a specific herbal therapy or dietary supplement.

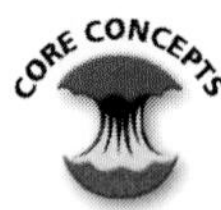

1.4 Drugs are available by prescription or over the counter (OTC).

Legal drugs are obtained either with a prescription or by purchasing them over the counter. There are differences between the two methods of dispensing. To obtain prescription drugs, patients must obtain a physician's order authorizing the patient to receive the drugs. The advantages to this are numerous. The practitioner has an opportunity to examine the patient and determine a specific diagnosis. The practitioner can maximize therapy by ordering the proper drug for the patient's condition and controlling the specific amount and frequency of the drug to be dispensed. The healthcare practitioner may give instructions on how to use the drug properly and what side effects to expect.

A drug's safety is related to its effectiveness. The difference between its usual effective dose and a dose that produces severe side effects is called its *margin of safety.* When drugs are used over long periods of time and demonstrate "wide" margins of safety—that is, they are very safe and effective—regulators often change them from being prescription drugs to being OTC drugs. Unlike prescription drugs, OTC drugs do not require a physician's order. Patients may treat themselves safely if they carefully follow instructions included with these OTC drugs. If patients do not follow these guidelines, OTC drugs can have serious side effects.

Patients often prefer to take OTC medications for many reasons. They may obtain OTC drugs more easily than prescription drugs. They do not have to make an appointment with a physician, which saves time and money. Without training, however, choosing the proper medication for a specific problem may be challenging. OTC drugs may react with foods, herbal products, and prescription or other OTC drugs. Patients may not be aware that some medications can impair their ability to function safely. Self-treatment is sometimes ineffective, and the potential for injury is much greater if the disease is allowed to progress without proper treatment.

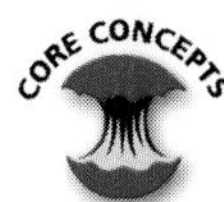

1.5 *Pharmaceutics* is the science of pharmacy.

Pharmaceutics is the science of preparing and dispensing drugs and is a very important part of pharmacotherapy. Often, the general public confuses the science of pharmaceutics with pharmacology. Generally, consumers recognize the root *pharm* and assume that *pharmacology* is the same as *pharmacy.* Correctly, *pharmaceutics* is the science of pharmacy. To describe it simply, pharmaceutics involves dispensing a drug to a patient after he or she has been examined by a licensed practitioner. Pharmacists are expert at cataloguing signs, symptoms, side effects, and drug interactions. They often act as drug advisors to patients making sure that they receive the proper medication and educating them about undesirable symptoms or interactions.

Concept Review 1.1

- Explain the meaning of this statement: "Pharmacotherapy involves the science of therapeutics and pharmaceutics."

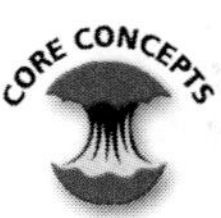

1.6 Drug regulations were created to protect the public from drug misuse.

For many years, there were no standards or guidelines to protect the public from drug misuse. Patients could not be assured that available medicines were not a form of quackery. The archives of drug regulatory agencies are filled with examples of early medicines, including rattlesnake oil for rheumatism; epilepsy treatment for spasms, hysteria, and alcoholism; and fat reducers for a slender, healthy figure. It became quite clear that drug regulations were needed to protect the public.

The first standards commonly used by pharmacists were early **formularies,** or lists of drugs and drug recipes. In 1820, the first comprehensive publication of drug standards, called the *U.S. Pharmacopoeia (USP),* was established. (See the timeline in Figure 1.1 ■.) A **pharmacopoeia** is a medical reference summary indicating standards of drug purity and strength and directions for synthesis. In 1852, a national professional society of pharmacists—the American Pharmaceutical Association (APhA)—was founded. From 1852 until 1975, two major sources maintained drug standards in the United States—the USP and the APhA's *National Formulary (NF).* All drug substances and products were covered in the USP; the NF focused on pharmaceutic ingredients. In 1975, the two organizations merged and created a single publication named the *U.S. Pharmacopoeia–National Formulary (USP-NF).* Official updates for the *USP-NF* are published regularly. Today, the USP label can be found on many medication vials verifying the exact ingredients found within the container, as shown in Figure 1.2 ■.

In the early 1900s, to protect the public, the government began to develop and enforce tougher drug legislation. In 1902, the Biologics Control Act was passed to standardize the quality of serums and other blood-related products. The Pure Food and Drug Act of 1906 gave the government power to control the labeling of medicines. In 1912, the Sherley Amendment prohibited the sale of drugs labeled with false therapeutic claims intended to cheat the consumer. In 1938, Congress passed the Food, Drug, and Cosmetic Act. This was the first law preventing the marketing of drugs that had not been thoroughly tested prior to marketing. According to the provisions of this law, drug companies were required to prove the safety and *efficacy* (that is, effectiveness) of any drug before it could be sold within the United States.

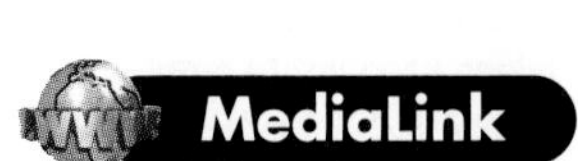

U.S. GOVERNMENTAL DRUG REGULATION

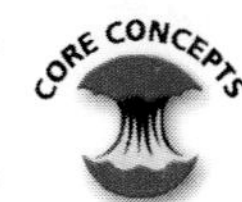

1.7 U.S. drug standards have become increasingly complex.

Much has changed in the regulation of drugs since 1938. In 1988, the Food and Drug Administration (FDA) was officially established as an agency of the U.S. Department of Health and Human Services. Today, the Center for Drug Evaluation and Research (CDER), a branch of the FDA,

FIGURE 1.1

TIMELINE	REGULATORY ACTS, STANDARDS, AND ORGANIZATIONS
1820	A group of physicians established the first comprehensive publication of drug standards called the **U.S. Pharmacopoeia (USP)**.
1852	A group of pharmacists founded a national professional society called the **American Pharmaceutical Association (APhA).** The APhA then established the **National Formulary (NF)**, a publication listing standardized pharmaceutical ingredients. The USP continued to catalogue all drug-related substances and products.
1862	This was the beginning of the **Federal Bureau of Chemistry,** established by President Lincoln. Over the years, duties were added, and it became the Food and Drug Administration (FDA).
1902	Congress passed the **Biologics Control Act** to control the quality of serums and other blood-related products.
1906	**The Pure Food and Drug Act** gave the government power to control the labeling of medicines.
1912	**The Sherley Amendment** made medicines safer by prohibiting the sale of drugs labeled with false therapeutic claims.
1938	Congress passed the **Food, Drug, and Cosmetic Act.** It was the first law preventing the marketing of drugs not thoroughly tested. This law now requires drug companies to submit a New Drug Application (NDA) to the Food and Drug Administration (FDA) before marketing the drug.
1944	Congress passed the **Public Health Service Act,** covering many health issues including biologic products and the control of communicable diseases.
1975	The U.S. Pharmacopoeia and National Formulary announced their union. The **USP-NF** became a single standardized publication.
1986	Congress passed the **Childhood Vaccine Act.** It authorized the FDA to acquire information about patients taking vaccines, to recall biologics, and to recommend civil penalties if guidelines were not followed.
1988	The **FDA** was officially established as an agency of the **U.S. Department of Health and Human Services.**
1992	Congress passed the **Prescription Drug User Fee Act.** It required that manufacturers of non-generic drugs and biologics pay fees to help improve the drug review process.
1997	**The FDA Modernization Act** was the largest reform effort of the drug review process since 1938.

Historical timeline of regulatory acts, standards, and organizations

has powerful control over whether prescription drugs and OTC drugs may be used for therapy. The CDER states its mission as "facilitating the availability of safe effective drugs, keeping unsafe or ineffective drugs off the market, improving the health of Americans, and providing clear, easily understandable drug information for safe and effective use." Any pharmaceutical laboratory, whether private, public, or academic, must obtain FDA approval before marketing any drug. Another branch of the FDA, the Center for Biologics Evaluation and Research (CBER), regulates the use of biologics including serums, vaccines, and products found in the bloodstream.

The FDA also oversees administration of herbal products and dietary supplements, but the Center for Food Safety and Applied Nutrition (CFSAN) regulates use of these substances. Herbal products and dietary supplements are regulated by the Dietary Supplement Health and Education Act of 1994. This act does not provide the same degree of protection as the Food, Drug, and Cosmetic Act of 1938. Herbal and dietary supplements may be marketed without prior approval from the FDA. This act is discussed in more detail in Chapter 5.

Life Span Fact

One historical achievement involving biologics is the 1986 Childhood Vaccine Act. This act authorized the FDA to acquire information about patients taking vaccines, to recall biologics, and to recommend civil penalties if guidelines regarding biologics were not followed.

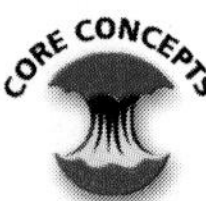

1.8 There are four stages of approval for therapeutic and biologic drugs.

The amount of time spent in the review and approval process, for both prescription and OTC drugs, depends on several checkpoints along a well-developed and organized plan. Most therapeutic drugs and biologics are reviewed in four stages, which are summarized in Figure 1.3 ■.

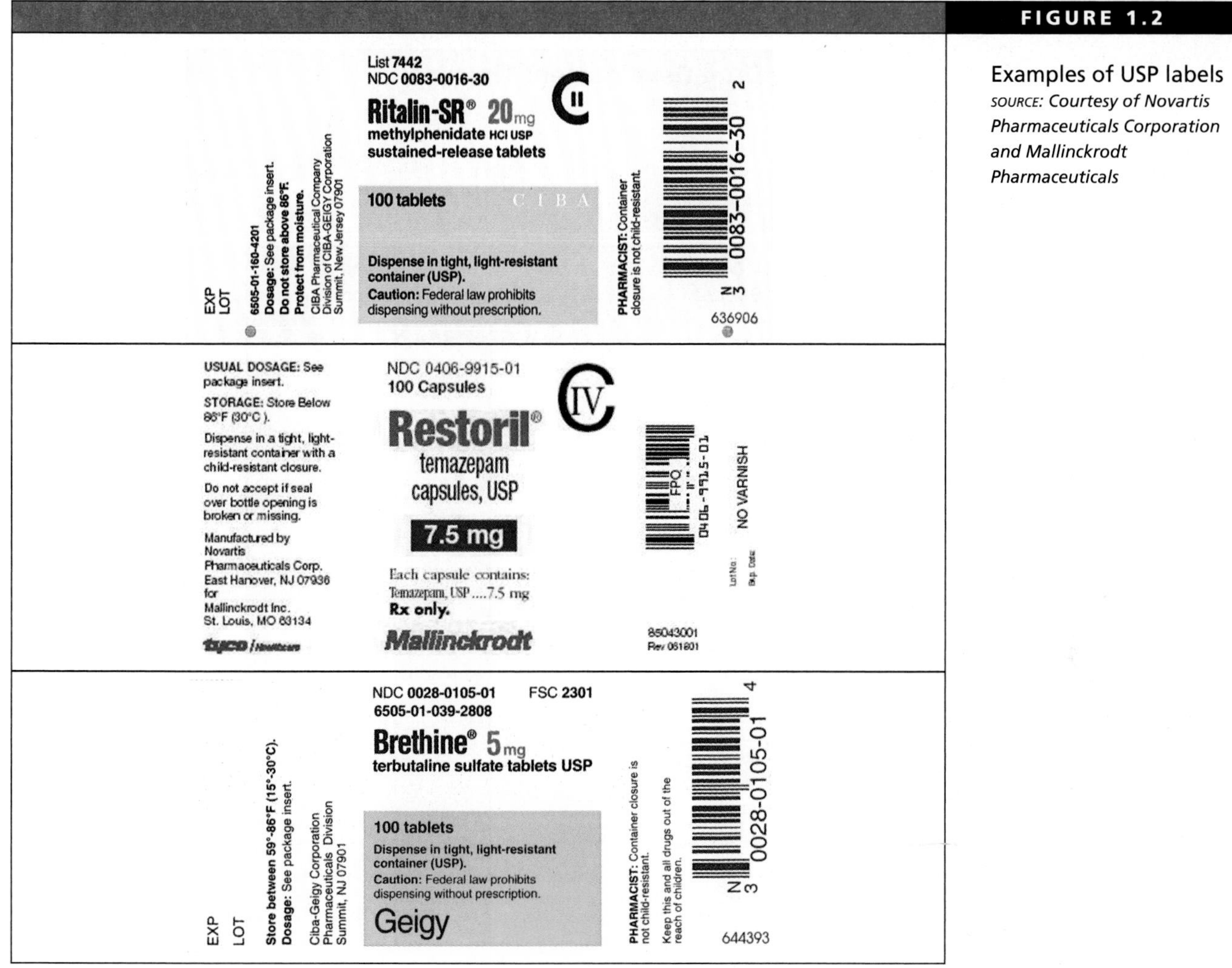

FIGURE 1.2

Examples of USP labels
SOURCE: Courtesy of Novartis Pharmaceuticals Corporation and Mallinckrodt Pharmaceuticals

These stages are (1) preclinical investigation, (2) clinical investigation, (3) submission of a new drug application (NDA) with review, and (4) postmarketing studies.

Preclinical Investigation

Preclinical investigation involves basic science research. Scientists perform many tests on cells grown in the laboratory (a process called *culture*) or on animals to examine the effectiveness of a range of drug doses and to look for any adverse effects. Laboratory tests on cells and animals are important because they assist in predicting whether drugs will cause harm in humans. Because laboratory tests do not always reflect the way a human responds, preclinical investigation results are always inconclusive.

Clinical Investigation

Clinical investigation is the second stage of drug approval that takes place in three different phases, termed *clinical phase trials*. This is the longest part of the drug approval process and involves **clinical pharmacology,** an area of medicine devoted to the evaluation of drugs used for human benefit. During these phases, clinical pharmacologists perform tests on volunteers and large groups of selected patients with certain diseases. Both scientists and healthcare practitioners establish drug doses and try to identify adverse effects. Clinical investigators address concerns such as whether the drug worsens other medical conditions, interacts unsafely with existing medications patients are taking, or affects one type of patient more than others.

Clinical Phase Trials. Clinical phase trials are essential because responses among patients vary. If a drug appears to be effective without causing serious side effects, approval for marketing may be accelerated, or the drug may be used for treatment immediately in special cases with

FIGURE 1.3

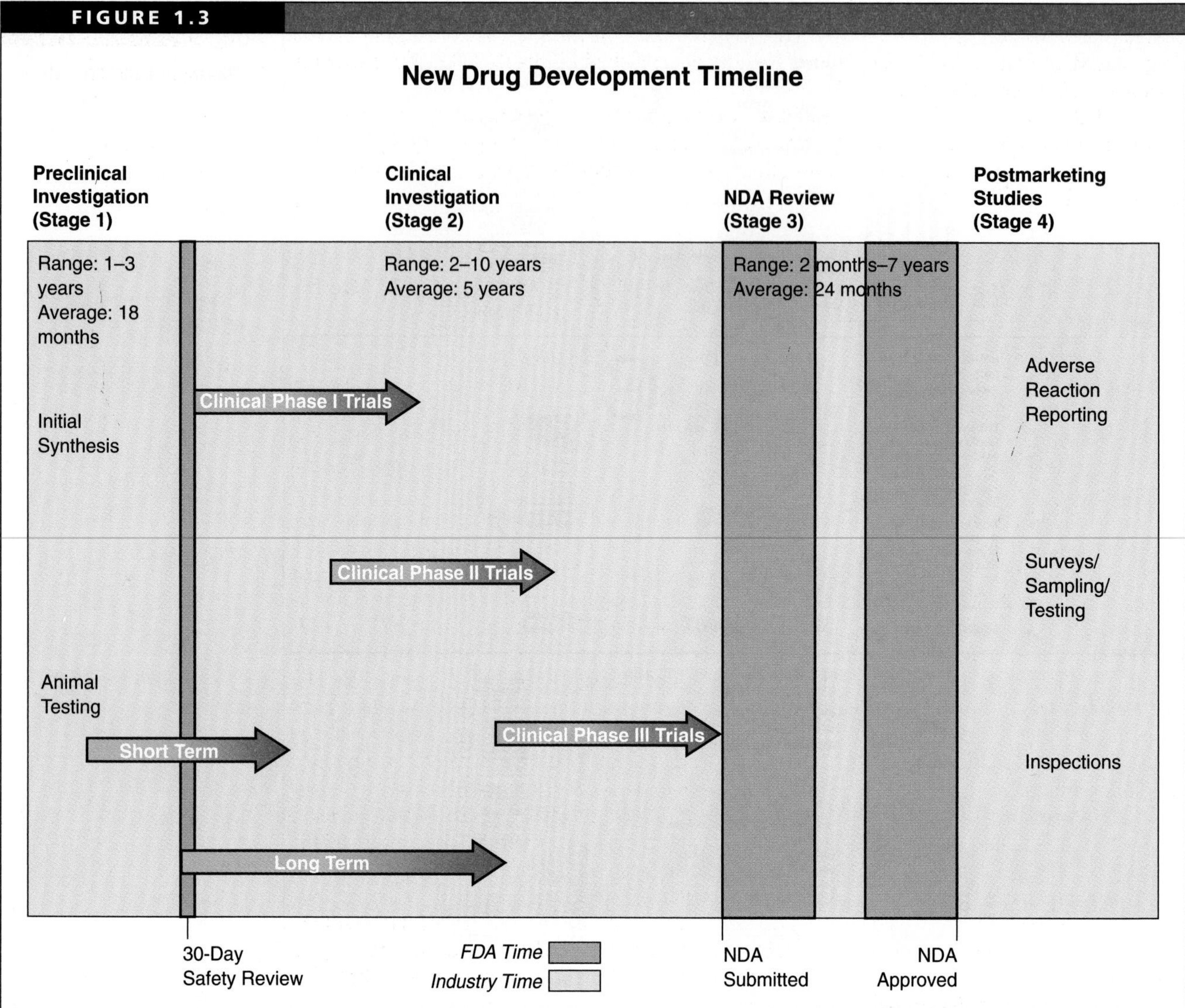

The approval of a new drug is a four-stage process: (1) preclinical investigation, (2) clinical investigation, (3) NDA submission and review, and (4) postmarketing studies. Within the second stage of clinical investigation, three phases of trials are conducted over 2 to 10 years. Postmarketing studies, also called *postmarketing surveillance,* continue in large patient groups during the fourth stage of drug development. *SOURCE: Pearson Education/PH College*

careful monitoring. If the drug shows promise but some minor problems are noted, the approval process is delayed until concerns are addressed. In any case, an NDA must be submitted before a drug is allowed to proceed to the next stage of the approval process.

Submission of a NDA with Review

A review of the NDA is the third stage of drug approval. During this stage, clinical phase III trials and animal testing may continue, depending on the results obtained from preclinical testing. If the NDA is approved, the process continues to the final stage. If the NDA is rejected, the process stops until concerns are addressed.

Postmarketing Studies

Postmarketing surveillance is the fourth stage of the drug approval process. It takes place after clinical trials and the NDA review process have been completed. Testing in humans is continued to check for any new harmful effects in larger and more diverse population. Some adverse effects take longer to appear and are not identified until a drug is used by large numbers of patients. One example is the diabetes drug troglitazone (Rezulin), which was placed on the market in 1997. In 1998, Great Britain banned its use after at least one death and several cases of liver failure were reported in diabetic patients taking the drug. The FDA became aware of a number of cases in the United States where Rezulin was linked with liver failure. Consumer advocates also claimed the drug caused several cases of heart failure. Rezulin was recalled in March 2000 after health professionals asked the FDA to reconsider its risks.

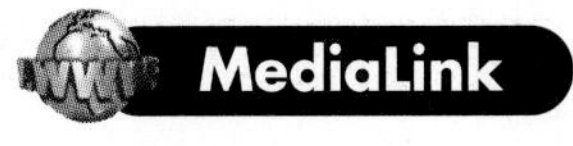

U.S. DRUG RECALLS

The FDA holds annual public meetings to hear comments from patients and professional and pharmaceutical organizations about the effectiveness and safety of new drug therapies. If the FDA discovers a serious problem, it will require that a drug be withdrawn from the market and its use discontinued.

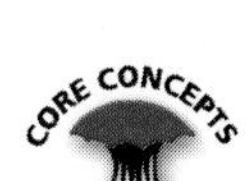

1.9 Once criticized for being too slow, governmental agencies face new challenges for ensuring the safety of drugs.

The public once criticized the FDA and other regulatory agencies for being too slow in bringing new, potentially lifesaving drugs to the consumer. In the early 1990s, organized consumer groups and drug manufacturers pressured governmental officials to speed up the drug review process. Reasons for delays in the FDA drug approval process were outdated guidelines, poor communication, and agency understaffing.

In 1992, FDA officials, members of Congress, and representatives from pharmaceutical companies negotiated the Prescription Drug User Fee Act on a 5-year trial basis. This act required drug and biologic manufacturers to provide yearly product user fees. With this extra income, the FDA hired more employees and restructured its organization to more efficiently handle the greater number of drug applications. Restructuring was a resounding success. From 1992 to 1996, the FDA approved double the number of drugs while cutting some review times by as much as half. In 1997, the FDA Modernization Act was passed, reauthorizing the Prescription Drug User Fee Act. It allowed drug companies to give healthcare practitioners information about *FDA-unapproved* uses of certain drugs. For example, sometimes drugs are approved to treat one condition, but not others; however, physicians may discover that the drug is useful in treating a different problem. When such a benefit is found frequently, a drug company is allowed to share accurate information with other physicians about the drug's "unapproved," but effective, use in treating another condition. The act also added nearly 700 employees to the FDA's drug and biologics program, and over $300 million was collected in user fees.

One concern now is that drugs are being developed at a faster rate than risks can be assessed. Officials are calling for patients, pharmacists, allied health workers, nurses, physicians, hospitals, and pharmaceutical companies to work together to minimize risks. Because of the higher numbers of drugs being approved for therapy, the potential for adverse drug-drug and drug-herbal interactions is greater than ever before.

Concept Review 1.2

- Can you recall the major U.S. acts, standards, and organizations leading up to the present time? When was the FDA established? What current U.S. laws regulate how drugs are approved for marketing?

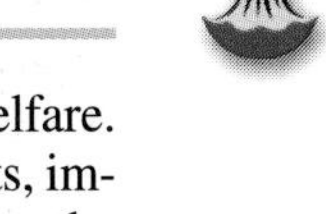

1.10 Similar drug standards protect Canadian consumers.

In Canada, the Health Protection Branch (HPB) is part of the Department of Health and Welfare. The HPB works to protect Canadians from the potential health hazards of marketed products, imported goods, and environmental agents. The Deputy Minister enforces regulations such as the Food and Drugs Act and the Tobacco Act.

Health Canada is the federal department working with provincial and territorial governments. It also works with other federal departments to ensure proper management of health and safety issues.

The Health Products and Food Branch (HPFB) of Health Canada regulates the use of therapeutic substances through several national programs: the Therapeutic Products Programme (TPP), the Office of Natural Health Products, and the Food Directorate. The TPP covers drugs including pharmaceuticals, narcotics, controlled and restricted drugs, and biologics. Some natural health products and food-based products called *nutraceuticals* are also regulated. The Office of

TABLE 1.2	Steps of Approval for Drugs Marketed Within Canada
Step 1	Preclinical studies or experiments performed in culture, living tissue, and small animals are performed, followed by extensive clinical trials or testing done in humans.
Step 2	A drug company completes a *drug submission* to Health Canada. This report details important safety and effectiveness information including how the drug product will be produced and packaged, expected therapeutic benefits, and adverse reactions.
Step 3	A committee of drug experts including medical and drug scientists reviews the drug submission to identify potential benefits and drug risks.
Step 4	Health Canada reviews information about the drug product and passes on important details to health practitioners and consumers.
Step 5	Health Canada issues a Notice of Compliance (NOC) and Drug Identification Number (DIN). Both permit the manufacturer to market the drug product.
Step 6	Health Canada monitors the effectiveness and concerns of the drug after it has been marketed. This is done by regular inspection, notices, newsletters, and feedback from consumers and healthcare professionals.

Natural Health Products focuses on natural substances—for example, homeopathic and herbal remedies. The Food Directorate regulates nutraceuticals.

The Food and Drugs Act is an important document because it specifies that drugs cannot be marketed without a Notice of Compliance (NOC) and Drug Identification Number (DIN) from Health Canada. Any drug that does not comply with standards established by recognized pharmacopoeias and formularies in the United States, Europe, Great Britain, or France cannot be labeled, packaged, sold, or advertised in Canada.

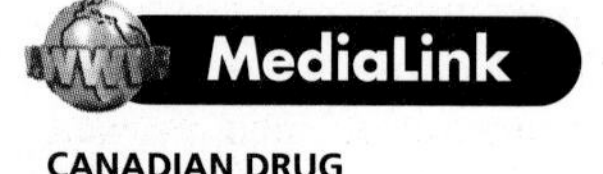

CANADIAN DRUG REGULATION

The basic outline for how drugs are approved in Canada is provided in Table 1.2. There are many similarities between how drugs are regulated in Canada and the United States. Both governments have realized a need to monitor newly developed traditional drugs, as well as natural products, minerals, vitamins, and herbs very carefully, because the potential for adverse effects is high. Canadian drugs may share the same names as their counterparts in the United States, or they may have unique names.

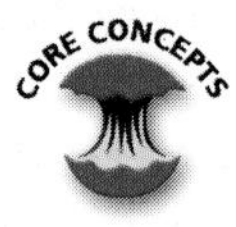

1.11 Healthcare professionals must be prepared to deal with the threat of biologic and chemical attack.

Prior to the September 11, 2001, terrorist attacks on the United States, concern about epidemic diseases was mainly focused on the possible spread of traditional infectious diseases such as influenza, tuberculosis, cholera, and human immunodeficiency virus (HIV). Healthcare providers were also concerned about widespread food poisoning and sexually transmitted diseases other than HIV, but because these diseases and conditions produced fewer fatalities, less attention was given to them.

Now, however, the healthcare community is more aware of the possibility of *bioterrorism*—the intentional use of infectious biologic agents, chemical substances, or radiation to cause widespread harm or illness. Such federal agencies as the Centers for Disease Control and Prevention (CDC) and the U.S. Department of Defense have increased efforts to inform, educate, and prepare the public for disease outbreaks caused by bioterrorism. In 2002, the U.S. Department of Homeland Security was organized to provide additional security and defense for the United States in a terrorist attack. The Department also prioritized the important issue of citizen prepardness educating families how to best prepare for natural emergencies and disasters.

bio = *microorganisms*
terrorism = *to induce fear*

The goals of a bioterrorist are to create widespread public panic and cause as many casualties as possible. The list of agents that can be used for this purpose is long. Some of these agents are easily obtainable and require little or no specialized knowledge to spread. The most worrisome are:

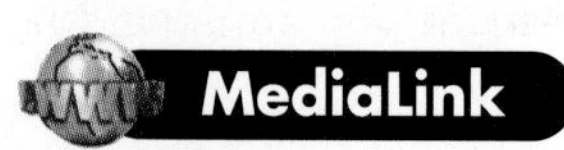

U.S. HOMELAND SECURITY

- Acutely infectious diseases such as anthrax, smallpox, plague, and hemorrhagic viruses

- Incapacitating chemicals such as nerve gas, cyanide, and chlorinated agents
- Nuclear and radiation emergencies

One can easily imagine what devastation would be caused if laboratories and healthcare professionals were not able to identify, isolate, and treat widespread disease caused by bioterrorism. The following chapters contain important information related to bioterrorism. Chapter 22 reviews the topic of antibiotics for the treatment of anthrax. The treatment of chemical warfare agents is discussed in Chapter 7. Chapter 29 includes discussion of the treatment of radiation exposure.

CHAPTER REVIEW

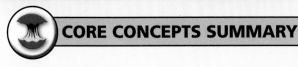

CORE CONCEPTS SUMMARY

1.1 Pharmacology is an expansive and challenging topic.

Pharmacology, the study of medicine, is a subject devoted to proper drug treatment and health of the human body. It is an expansive topic utilizing concepts from human biology, disease processes, and chemistry.

1.2 For healthcare professionals, the fields of pharmacology and therapeutics are connected.

Therapeutics is the science associated with the treatment of suffering and the prevention of disease. *Pharmacotherapeutics* is the useful application of drugs for the purpose of fighting disease. The study of pharmacology is important to health professionals from many different areas.

1.3 Agents may be classified as traditional drugs, biologics, and natural alternatives.

Drugs are chemical agents used to treat disease by producing biological responses within the body. Therapeutic drugs are classified as substances produced chemically or naturally. Biologics are natural agents produced by animal cells or microorganisms. Alternative therapies include natural herbs, plant extracts, or dietary supplements.

1.4 Drugs are available by prescription or over the counter (OTC).

There are two major methods of dispensing drugs. Prescription drugs require a physician's order; OTC drugs do not. There are advantages and disadvantages to both dispensing methods.

1.5 Pharmaceutics is the science of pharmacy.

Pharmaceutics involves the successful dispensation of drugs for therapeutic purposes. Dispensing medication safely is a major challenge for healthcare practitioners and patients.

1.6 Drug regulations were created to protect the public from drug misuse.

The first drug laws were acts created by Congress to protect patients from wrongful therapeutic claims. These and other standards form the basis of modern drug regulation agencies and organizations such as the Food and Drug Administration, and publications such as the *U.S. Pharmacopoeia-National Formulary.*

1.7 U.S. drug standards have become increasingly complex.

The Food and Drug Administration, a branch of the U.S. Department of Health and Human Services, is the primary agency regulating drug safety. Three branches of the FDA control policies regarding drug therapies: the Center for Drug Evaluation and Research (CDER), the Center for Biologics Evaluation and Research (CBER), and the Center for Food Safety and Applied Nutrition (CFSAN).

1.8 There are four stages of approval for therapeutic and biologic drugs.

Drug approval occurs in four stages: preclinical investigation, clinical investigation, submission of a new drug application (NDA) with review, and postmarketing studies. Clinical phase trials must be completed before drugs are approved for public use.

1.9 Once criticized for being too slow, governmental agencies face new challenges for ensuring the safety of drugs.

FDA officials, members of Congress, and pharmaceutical company representatives negotiated the

Prescription Drug User Fee Act and FDA Modernization Act. These acts have sped up the approval process and require drug and biologic manufacturers to provide yearly product user fees. The concern now is that drugs are being approved at a rate faster than risks can be assessed.

1.10 Similar drug standards protect Canadian consumers.

In Canada, the Health Protection Branch of the Department of Health and Welfare enforces regulations concerned with the Canadian Food and Drugs Act. The Health Products and Food Branch of Health Canada regulates the proper use of therapeutic drugs by issuing a Notice of Compliance (NOC) and Drug Identification Number (DIN) prior to drugs being marketed. Drugs in Canada are regulated in a manner similar to that used in the United States.

1.11 Healthcare professionals must be prepared to deal with the threat of biologic and chemical attack.

Drugs are among the most powerful weapons we have to combat bioterrorism. Federal agencies have taken an active role in educating and preparing the public and the healthcare community about disease outbreaks caused by bioterrorism.

KEY TERMS

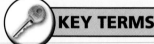

biologics (beye-oh-LOJ-iks): chemical agents that produce biological responses within the body; they are synthesized by cells of the human body, animal cells, or microorgansims / *page 4*

clinical pharmacology: an area of medicine devoted to the evaluation of drugs used for human therapeutic benefit / *page 7*

formularies (FOR-mew-LEH-reez): lists of drugs and drug recipes commonly used by pharmacists / *page 5*

natural alternative therapies: herbs, natural extracts, vitamins, minerals, or dietary supplements / *page 4*

pathophysiology (PATH-oh-fiz-ee-OL-oh-jee): the study of diseases and the functional changes occurring in the body as a result of diseases / *page 3*

pharmaceutics (far-mah-SOO-tiks): the science of preparing and dispensing drugs / *page 5*

pharmacology (far-mah-KOL-oh-jee): the study of medicines; the discipline pertaining to how drugs improve the health of the human body / *page 3*

pharmacopoeia (far-mah-KOH-pee-ah): medical reference summary indicating standards of drug purity, strength, and directions for synthesis / *page 5*

pharmacotherapeutics (far-mah-koh-THER-ah-PEW-tiks): treatment of diseases by the use of drugs / *page 3*

therapeutics (ther-ah-PEW-tiks): the branch of medicine concerned with the treatment of disease and suffering / *page 3*

REVIEW QUESTIONS

The following questions are written in NCLEX-PN® style. Answer these questions to assess your knowledge of the chapter material, and go back and review any material that is not clear to you.

1. Pathophysiology is defined as the study of:

1. How drugs enter and travel throughout the body
2. How drugs improve the health of the human body
3. Drugs and how they elicit different responses
4. Diseases and functional changes occurring as a result of disease

2. Biologics are:

1. Produced in nature such as herbs, natural extracts, vitamins, and minerals
2. Chemically produced in a laboratory
3. Naturally produced in animal cells, microorganisms, or by the body itself
4. Not used routinely by physicians

3. Antiperspirants, sunscreens, toothpaste, and shampoo alter the body's activities. Therefore, they are:

1. Considered to be medically therapeutic
2. Classified as traditional drugs because they are chemically produced and cause biologic responses in the body
3. Agents limited to therapy in a clinical or home setting
4. Commonly grouped as cosmetics, which are categorized separately from drugs

4. What are precautions patients need to know when taking OTC drugs?

1. Self-treatment is sometimes ineffective.
2. OTC drugs may react with foods, herbal products, and prescription or other OTC drugs.
3. The potential for injury is much greater if the disease is allowed to progress.
4. All of the above

5. Dispensing of drugs to patients after they have been examined by a licensed healthcare practitioner is:

1. Pharmacology
2. Pharmacy
3. Therapeutics
4. Healthcare

6. The act that abolished the long-standing ban on the distribution of drug information to the public regarding unapproved drug use and labeling is the:

1. Pure Food and Drug Act (1906)
2. Food, Drug, and Cosmetics Act (1938)
3. Prescription Drug User Fee Act (1992)
4. FDA Modernization Act (1997)

7. The longest part of the drug approval process is typically:

1. Preclinical investigation
2. Clinical investigation
3. NDA submission and review
4. Postmarketing studies

8. The legislation responsible for cutting new drug application review times as much as 50% is the:

1. Pure Food and Drug Act
2. Sherley Amendment
3. Public Health Services Act
4. Prescription Drug User Fee Act

9. One aspect of health protection standards that is clearly different in Canada compared with in the United States is:

1. Preclinical studies are performed followed by extensive clinical trials.
2. A committee of drug experts reviews the drugs submission to identify potential benefits and risks of the drug.
3. Drugs cannot be marketed without an NOC and a DIN.
4. The effectiveness and concerns of the drugs are monitored after they have been marketed.

10. Which of the following is considered a bioterrorist threat?

1. Anthrax contamination
2. Incapacitating chemicals
3. Radiation exposure
4. All of the above

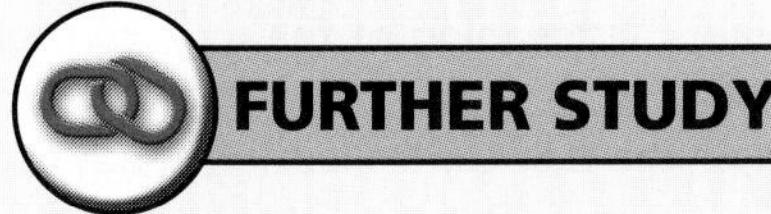

FURTHER STUDY

- Traditional drugs and drugs classes are discussed in Chapter 2.
- Chapter 5 covers natural alternatives and herbal and dietary supplements, including the Dietary Supplement Health and Education Act of 1994.
- Canadian drugs and their U.S. equivalents are listed in Appendix B.
- Chapter 22 reviews antibiotics for the treatment of anthrax.
- The treatment of chemical warfare agents is discussed in Chapter 7.
- Chapter 29 includes a discussion of the treatment of radiation exposure.

EXPLORE MEDIALINK www.prenhall.com/holland

Additional resources for this chapter can be found on the CD-ROM accompanying this textbook, and on the Companion Website. Click on Chapter 1 to select activities for this chapter.

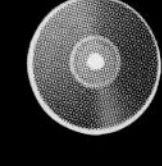

- Audio Glossary
- Concept Review
- NCLEX-PN® Review
- Nursing in Action
- Dosage Calculator

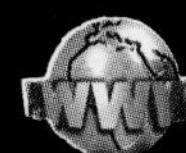

- U.S. Governmental Drug Regulation
- U.S. Drug Recalls
- Canadian Drug Regulation
- U.S. Homeland Security

CHAPTER

2 Drug Classes, Schedules, and Categories

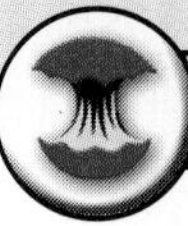

CORE CONCEPTS

2.1 Drugs may be organized by their therapeutic and pharmacological classifications.

2.2 Drugs have more than one name.

2.3 The differences between brand name drugs and their generic equivalents may include price, formulations, and, most important, bioavailability.

2.4 Drugs with a potential for abuse are categorized into schedules.

2.5 Canadian regulations restrict drugs of abuse.

2.6 All prescription drugs are classified according to safety in pregnancy categories to protect the unborn.

OBJECTIVES

After reading this chapter, the student should be able to:

1. Discuss the basis for placing drugs into therapeutic and pharmacological classes.
2. Explain the prototype approach to drug classification.
3. Describe what is meant by a drug's mechanism of action.
4. Distinguish between a drug's chemical name, generic name, and trade name.
5. Explain why generic drug names are preferred to other drug names.
6. Discuss why drugs are sometimes placed on a restrictive list and the controversy surrounding this issue.
7. Explain the meaning of the term *controlled substance.*
8. Explain the U.S. Controlled Substance Act of 1970 and the role of the U.S. Drug Enforcement Agency (DEA) in controlling drug abuse and misuse.
9. Identify the five drug schedules and examples of drugs at each level.
10. Explain how drugs are scheduled taking into account Parts III and IV of the Canadian Food and Drugs Act and the Narcotic Control Act.
11. Identify the five pregnancy categories and explain what each category represents.

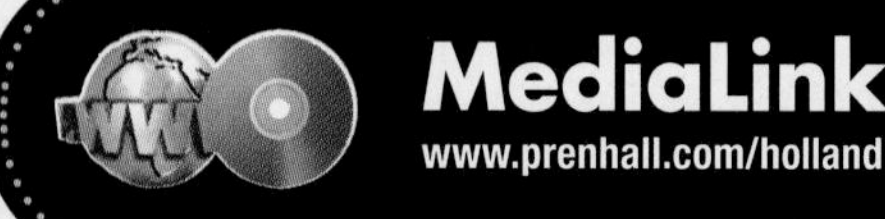

Interactive resources for this chapter can be found on the Companion Website. Click on Chapter 2 and "Begin" to select the activities for this chapter. For chapter-related animations, NCLEX-PN®-style questions, and an audio glossary, access the accompanying CD-ROM in this book.

Understanding drug classes can be very challenging. There are many ways that drugs can be classified, from a strict chemical group name to a trade name provided by the manufacturer. Because of the large number of drugs available, practitioners and consumers must have a system for identifying drugs and determining the limitations of their use. This chapter covers the various methods by which drugs may be organized, that is, by therapeutic or pharmacological classification. This chapter also discusses drug schedules and pregnancy categories because such information affects the routine use of many drugs.

2.1 Drugs may be organized by their therapeutic and pharmacological classifications.

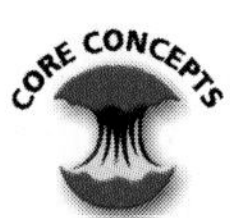

Medications may be classified in two major ways. Drugs may be organized by *therapeutic usefulness*. This is referred to as a **therapeutic classification.** Drugs also may be categorized by *how they work pharmacologically*. This is referred to as a **pharmacological classification.** Both methods are widely used in studying pharmacology. However, few practitioners make the distinction in a setting where the primary purpose of drug therapy is to improve the health of their patients.

MediaLink
THERAPEUTIC DRUG CLASSES

Table 2.1 shows the method of therapeutic classification, using cardiac care as an example. The cardiovascular system is concerned with the proper functioning of the heart and blood vessels. Many different types of drugs affect cardiovascular function. Some drugs influence blood clotting, while others lower blood cholesterol or prevent the onset of stroke. Drugs may be used to lower blood pressure, treat heart failure, correct abnormal heart rhythm, alleviate chest pain, and treat or prevent circulatory shock. Drugs that affect cardiac disorders may be placed in several therapeutic classes. For example, drugs that influence blood clotting are called *anticoagulants*. Medications that lower blood cholesterol are called *antihyperlipidemics*. Drugs that lower blood pressure are called *antihypertensives*.

A therapeutic classification need not be complicated. For example, it is appropriate to classify a medication simply as "a drug used for stroke" or "a drug used for shock." The key to therapeutic classification is to state clearly what a particular drug does clinically. A few examples of therapeutic classification are provided in Table 2.2.

A second way that drugs may be grouped is by pharmacological classification. Pharmacological classification addresses a drug's **mechanism of action,** or *how* a medication produces its effect in the body.

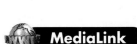

TABLE 2.1 Organizing Drugs by Therapeutic Classification

THERAPEUTIC FOCUS

Cardiac care / Drugs affecting cardiovascular function

THERAPEUTIC USEFULNESS	***THERAPEUTIC CLASSIFICATION***
influencing blood clotting	anticoagulants
lowering blood cholesterol	antihyperlipidemics
lowering blood pressure	antihypertensives
treating abnormal heartbeat	antidysrhythmics
treating chest pain (angina)	antianginal drugs

TABLE 2.2 Examples of Therapeutic Drug Classes*

anti-inflammatory drugs	antihypertensives
drugs that lower blood cholesterol	drugs for vomiting (emesis)
antipsychotic drugs	antidiarrheal drugs
antianxiety drugs	antacids
antidepressants	antibiotic drugs

**Note: While the names of some therapeutic categories may sound complicated, drug terminology will become more familiar as you begin to study drugs and drug classes. When studying this topic, always use a medical dictionary and reference drug guide.*

TABLE 2.3 Organizing Drugs by Pharmacological Classification

FOCUSING ON* HOW *A THERAPY MAY BE APPLIED

Therapy for high blood pressure may be achieved by:

MECHANISM OF ACTION	*PHARMACOLOGICAL CLASSIFICATION*
lowering plasma volume	diuretics
blocking heart calcium channels	calcium channel blockers
blocking hormonal activity	angiotensin-converting enzyme inhibitors
blocking stress-related activity	adrenergic blockers (drugs that inhibit actions of the sympathetic nervous system)
dilating peripheral blood vessels	vasodilators

Table 2.3 shows various types of pharmacological classifications using high blood pressure (hypertension) as an example. A *diuretic* is a class of drug used to treat hypertension by lowering plasma volume. Lowering plasma volume is the mechanism of action by which diuretics work. *Calcium channel blockers* treat hypertension by limiting the force of heart contractions. Other drugs, such as angiotensin-converting enzyme inhibitors, block components of a hormonal network called the *renin-angiotensin pathway,* thereby reducing hypertension. Notice that each example describes *how* hypertension may be controlled. A drug's pharmacological classification is more specific than a therapeutic classification and requires an understanding of human biochemical and physiological principles.

When studying a particular drug's mechanism of action, it is recommended that students first become comfortable with the broad drug classes and then gradually move to more specific examples.

Prototype drugs are an excellent place to start. A **prototype drug** is the original, well-understood drug model from which other medications in a pharmacological class have been developed. By learning the prototype drug, students may then predict the actions and adverse effects of other drugs in the same class. For example, by knowing the effects of penicillin V, students can apply this knowledge to the other drugs in the penicillin antibiotic class. *Students should be aware, however, that in many cases, the original drug prototype is not the most widely used drug in its class.* As new drugs are developed, features such as antibiotic resistance, fewer side effects, or a more precise sight of action might be factors that sway health practitioners away from using older drugs. Therefore, being familiar with the original drug prototypes and keeping up with newer and more popular drugs is an essential part of mastering the subject of pharmacology.

Concept Review 2.1

- What is the difference between a therapeutic classification and a pharmacological classification? What is a *prototype drug,* and is it different from any other drug within a pharmacological class?

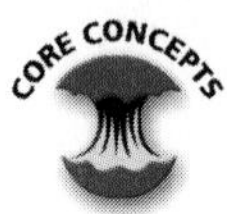

2.2 Drugs have more than one name.

A major challenge in studying pharmacology is learning thousands of drug names. Adding to this difficulty is the fact that most drugs have multiple names. The three basic types of drug names are chemical, generic, and trade names.

A **chemical name** is assigned, using standard nomenclature established by the International Union of Pure and Applied Chemistry (IUPAC). A drug has only one chemical name, which is sometimes helpful in predicting its physical and chemical properties. Although chemical names convey a clear and concise meaning about the nature of a drug, they are often complicated and difficult to remember or pronounce. For example, the chemical name of diazepam is 7-chloro-1, 3-ciphydro-1-methyl-5-phenyl-2H-1,4-benzodiazepin-2-one. In only a few cases, usually when the name is brief and easily remembered, are chemical names used. Examples of brief and therefore useful chemical names include lithium carbonate, calcium gluconate, and sodium chloride.

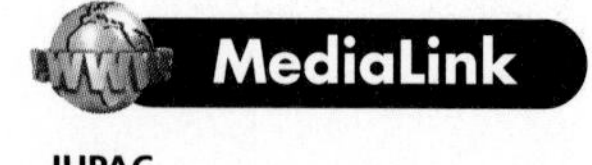

IUPAC

More practically, drugs are sometimes classified by *a portion* of their chemical structure, known as the chemical group name. Examples are antibiotics such as fluoroquinolones and

TABLE 2.4 Brand Name Products Containing Popular Generic Substances

GENERIC SUBSTANCES	BRAND NAMES
Aspirin	Acetylsalicylic acid, Acuprin, Anacin, Aspergum, Bayer, Bufferin, Ecotrin, Empirin, Excedrin, Maprin, Norgesic, Salatin, Salocol, Salsprin, Supac, Talwin, Triaphen-10, Vanquish, Verin, Zorprin
Diphenhydramine	Allerdryl, Benadryl, Benahist, Bendylate, Caladryl, Compoz, Diahist, Diphenadril, Eldadryl, Fenylhist, Fynex, Hydramine, Hydril, Insomnal, Noradryl, Nordryl, Nytol, Tussat, Wehdryl
Ibuprofen	Advil, Amersol, Apsifen, Brufen, Haltran, Medipren, Midol 200, Motrin, Neuvil, Novoprofen, Nuprin, Pamprin-IB, Rufen, Trendar

cephalosporins. Other common examples include phenothiazines, thiazides, and benzodiazepines. Although they may seem complicated when first encountered, familiarity with chemical group names may become helpful when communicating with fellow healthcare professionals.

The **generic name** of a drug is assigned by the U.S. Adopted Name Council. With few exceptions, generic names are less complicated and easier to remember than chemical names. Many organizations, including the FDA, the U.S. Pharmacopoeia, and the World Health Organization, routinely describe a medication by its generic name. Because there is only one generic name for each drug, healthcare providers often use this name, and students generally must memorize it.

A drug's **trade name** is assigned by the company marketing the drug. The name is usually selected to be short and easy to remember. The trade name is sometimes called the *proprietary, product,* or *brand* name. The term *proprietary* suggests ownership. In the United States, a drug developer is given exclusive rights to name and market a drug for 17 years after a new drug application (NDA) is submitted to the FDA. Because it takes several years for a drug to be approved, the amount of time spent in approval is usually subtracted from the 17 years. For example, if it takes 7 years for a drug to be approved, competing companies will not be allowed to market a generic equivalent drug for another 10 years. The rationale is that the developing company should be allowed sufficient time to recoup the millions of dollars in research and development costs it spent in designing the new drug. After 17 years, competing companies may sell a generic equivalent drug—sometimes using a different name, which the FDA must approve.

Trade names may be a challenge for students to learn because of the dozens of product names containing similar ingredients. In addition, some drugs—**combination drugs**—contain more than one active generic ingredient, making it more challenging to match one generic name with one product name. As an example, refer to Table 2.4 and consider the drug diphenhydramine (generic name), also called Benadryl (one of many trade names). Diphenhydramine is an antihistamine. Low doses of diphenhydramine can be purchased over the counter; higher doses require a prescription. When looking for diphenhydramine, healthcare providers may find it listed under many trade names, such as Allerdryl and Compoz, and provided alone or in combination with other active ingredients. Ibuprofen and aspirin are also examples of drugs with many different trade names. The rule of thumb is that the active ingredients in a drug are described by their generic name. When referring to a drug, the generic name is usually written in lowercase, whereas the trade name is capitalized.

Concept Review 2.2

- What are the major differences between a chemical, generic, and trade name? Which name is most often used to describe the active ingredients within a drug product?

2.3 The differences between brand name drugs and their generic equivalents may include price, formulations, and, most importantly, bioavailability.

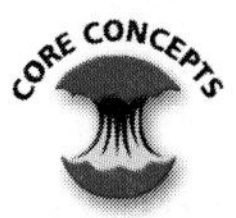

Usually generic drugs are less expensive than brand name drugs. The reason is a pharmaceutical company determines the price of a proprietary drug during its 17 years of exclusive rights to that new drug. Because there is no competition, the price can be kept quite high. A pharmaceutical company that developed a drug can sometimes use legal tactics to extend its exclusive rights to a drug, which can earn the company hundreds of millions of dollars per year in profits for a popular medicine. Once the exclusive rights end, competing companies market the generic drug for less money, and consumer savings may be considerable. In some states, pharmacists may routinely substitute a generic drug when the prescription calls for a brand name. In other states, the pharmacist must dispense drugs directly as written by a healthcare practitioner or obtain approval before providing a generic substitute.

The companies that market brand name drugs often fight aggressively against laws that might restrict the routine use of their brand name products. They claim that significant differences exist between a trade name drug and its generic equivalent and that switching to the generic drug may be harmful for the patient. Patient advocates, on the other hand, argue that generic substitutions should always be permitted because of the cost savings.

Are there really differences between a brand name drug and its generic equivalent? The answer is unclear. Despite the fact that the dosages may be identical, drug formulations are not always the same. The two drugs may have different *inert* ingredients. For example, in a tablet form, the active ingredients may be more tightly compressed in one of the preparations versus another, and this might affect how well the body can use the drug.

bio = *biological*
availability = *free to activate cellular targets*

The key to comparing brand name drugs and their generic equivalents lies in measuring the *bioavailability* of the two preparations. **Bioavailability** is the physiologic ability of the drug to reach its target cells and produce its effect. Bioavailability may be affected by inert ingredients and tablet compression. Anything that affects absorption of a drug, or its distribution to the target cells, can certainly affect drug action. Measuring how long a drug takes to exert its effect gives pharmacologists a crude measure of bioavailability. For example, if a patient is in circulatory shock and it takes a generic drug 5 minutes longer than the brand name drug to produce its effect, that difference would be significant. However, if a generic medication for arthritis pain relief takes 45 minutes to act, compared with the brand name drug which takes 40 minutes, it probably does not matter which drug is prescribed.

bio = *biological effect*
equivalence = *same*

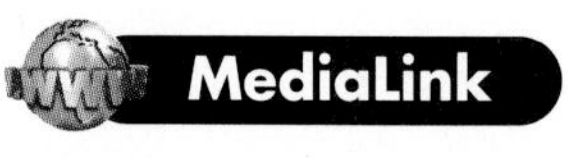

NEGATIVE DRUG FORMULARY LISTS

Some states (Florida, Kentucky, Minnesota, and Missouri, for example) have compiled a *negative* formulary list. A negative formulary is a list of trade name drugs that pharmacists may *not* dispense as generic drugs. These drugs must be dispensed exactly as written on the prescription, using the trade name drug the physician prescribed. In some cases, pharmacists must inform or notify patients of substitutions. Pharmaceutical companies and some healthcare practitioners have supported this action, claiming that generic drugs—even those which have small differences in bioavailability and bioequivalence—could adversely affect patient outcomes in those with critical conditions or illnesses. However, laws frequently change: In many instances, the efforts of consumer advocacy groups have led to changes in or elimination of negative formulary lists.

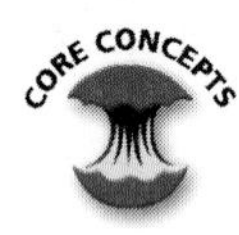

2.4 Drugs with a potential for abuse are categorized into schedules.

Some drugs are frequently abused or have a high potential for addiction. Technically, *addiction* refers to the overwhelming feeling that drives someone to use a drug repeatedly. *Dependence* is a related term, often defined as a physiologic or psychological need for a substance. *Physical dependence* refers to an altered physical condition caused by the nervous system adapting to repeated drug use. In this case, when the drug is no longer available, the individual experiences physical signs of discomfort known as *withdrawal.* In contrast, when an individual is *psychologically dependent,* there are few signs of physical discomfort when the drug is withdrawn; however, the individual feels an intense compelling desire to continue drug use. These concepts are discussed in detail in Chapter 6.

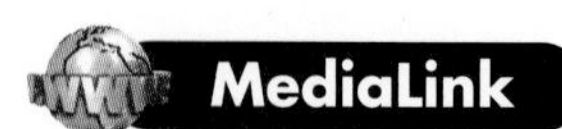

GUIDELINES FOR REFILLING SCHEDULED DRUGS

Drugs that cause dependency are restricted to use in situations of medical necessity, if they are allowed at all. According to law, drugs that have a significant potential for abuse are placed into five categories called *schedules.* These **scheduled drugs** are classified according to their potential for abuse: Schedule I drugs have the highest potential for abuse, and Schedule V drugs have the lowest. Schedule I drugs have little or no therapeutic value or are intended for research purposes only. Drugs in the other four schedules may be dispensed only in cases when therapeutic value has been determined. Schedule V is the only category in which some drugs may be dispensed without a prescription because the quantities of the controlled drug are so low that the possibility of causing dependence is extremely remote. Table 2.5 shows the five drug schedules with examples. Not all drugs with an abuse potential are regulated or placed into schedules. Tobacco, alcohol, and caffeine are significant examples.

TABLE 2.5 Drug Schedule and Examples

DRUG SCHEDULE	ABUSE POTENTIAL	DEPENDENCY POTENTIAL: PHYSICAL	DEPENDENCY POTENTIAL: PSYCHOLOGICAL	THERAPEUTIC USE (EXAMPLES*)
I	Highest	High	High	Limited or no therapeutic use (heroin, LSD, marijuana, and methaqualone)
II	High	High	High	Used therapeutically with prescription; some drugs no longer used (morphine, PCP, cocaine, methadone, and methamphetamine)
III	Moderate	Moderate	High	Used therapeutically with prescription (anabolic steroids, codeine and hydrocodone with aspirin or Tylenol, and some barbiturates)
IV	Lower	Lower	Lower	Used therapeutically with prescription (Darvon, Talwin, Equanil, Valium, and Xanax)
V	Lowest	Lowest	Lowest	Used therapeutically without prescription (OTC cough medicines with codeine)

*****All drugs developed for medicinal use in the United States must be approved by the FDA and the DEA. The FDA regulates human testing and the introduction of new drugs into the marketplace, whereas the DEA determines the schedule of and establishes production quotas for drugs with potential for abuse and to prevent their diversion to unlawful channels. The DEA also authorizes healthcare practitioners to prescribe controlled substances. The federal legislation that gives the DEA the right to control drugs of abuse (and thus impacts which drugs can be prescribed or not) is the Controlled Substances Act. See **http://www.dea.gov**.*

In the United States, a **controlled substance** is a drug restricted by the Controlled Substances Act of 1970 and later revisions. The Controlled Substances Act is also called the Comprehensive Drug Abuse Prevention and Control Act. Hospitals and pharmacies must register with the Drug Enforcement Administration (DEA) and use their assigned registration numbers to purchase scheduled drugs. They must maintain complete records of all quantities purchased and sold. Drugs with higher abuse potential have more restrictions. For example, a special order form must be used to obtain Schedule II drugs, and orders must be written and signed by the healthcare practitioner. Telephone orders to a pharmacy are not permitted. Refills for Schedule II drugs are not permitted; patients must visit their healthcare providers first. Those convicted of unlawful manufacturing, distributing, and dispensing of controlled substances face severe penalties.

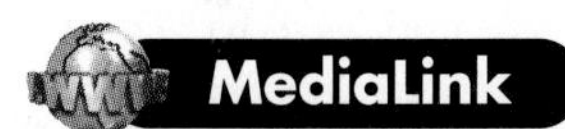

A–Z INDEX OF U.S. GOVERNMENT DEPARTMENTS AND AGENCIES DEALING WITH DRUGS

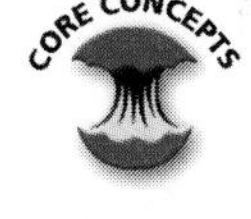

2.5 Canadian regulations restrict drugs of abuse.

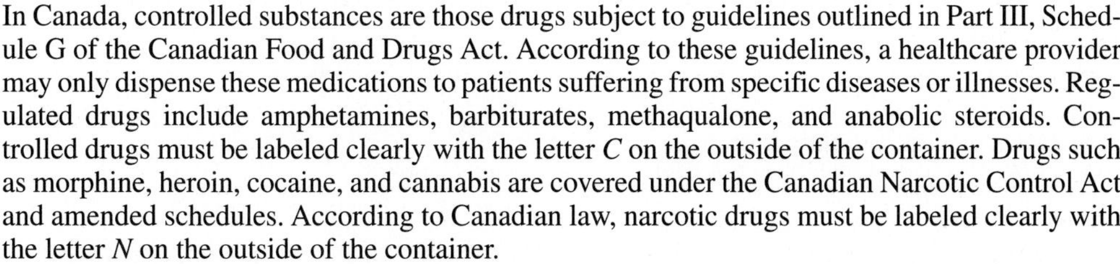

In Canada, controlled substances are those drugs subject to guidelines outlined in Part III, Schedule G of the Canadian Food and Drugs Act. According to these guidelines, a healthcare provider may only dispense these medications to patients suffering from specific diseases or illnesses. Regulated drugs include amphetamines, barbiturates, methaqualone, and anabolic steroids. Controlled drugs must be labeled clearly with the letter *C* on the outside of the container. Drugs such as morphine, heroin, cocaine, and cannabis are covered under the Canadian Narcotic Control Act and amended schedules. According to Canadian law, narcotic drugs must be labeled clearly with the letter *N* on the outside of the container.

Schedule F drugs are those drugs not controlled but requiring a prescription for their sale. Examples are methylphenidate (Ritalin), diazepam (Valium), and chlordiazepoxide (Librium).

Restricted drugs not intended for human use are covered in Part IV, Schedule H of the Canadian Food and Drugs Act. These are drugs used during a chemical or analytical procedure for medical, laboratory, industrial, educational, or research purposes. They include hallucinogens such as LSD (lysergic acid diethylamine) or MDMA (Ecstacy), and DOM (STP).

According to Canadian regulations, all prescription drugs (Schedule G drugs, narcotic drugs, and Schedule F drugs) are classified as Schedule I. All nonprescription drugs monitored for sale by pharmacists are classified as Schedule II. Nonprescription drugs that are not monitored by pharmacists are classified as Schedule III.

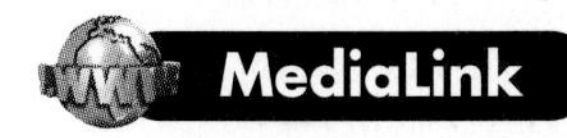

CANADIAN LAW AND DRUG CLASSIFICATION

Concept Review 2.3

- Are controlled drugs described the same way in Canada as in the United States? What about restricted drugs?

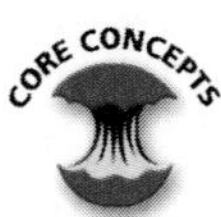

2.6 All prescription drugs are classified according to safety in pregnancy categories to protect the unborn.

Often a major concern that pregnant women have is whether a drug will harm their developing baby. Pregnant clients should never take any prescribed, illegal, or OTC drug or any herbal or dietary supplement without the advice of their healthcare practitioner. Any substance that will harm a developing fetus or embryo is referred to as a *teratogen.*

terato = *severe deformity*
gen = *something that produces*

To protect the unborn from the teratogenic effects of prescription drugs, the FDA has implemented a category system for classifying drugs based on how safe they are for pregnant women. According to this system, drugs are placed into one of five *pregnancy categories,* labeled as A, B, C, D, and X. These labels appear within package inserts and identify levels of risk to the fetus. The levels are based on degrees to which a drug has been proven to cause birth defects in laboratory animals or in human beings. These categories are summarized in Table 2.6.

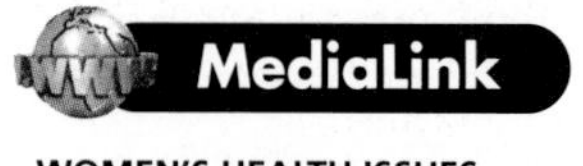

WOMEN'S HEALTH ISSUES

Consumers sometimes question whether the testing of laboratory animals is an effective way to predict harm to a developing human fetus or embryo. Results from animal testing are not always transferable to the human body. In fact, results from animal experimentation often vary from species to species. For this reason, consumers should always be cautious, even when there is reasonable assurance that a drug is extremely safe.

TABLE 2.6 Categories of Safety in Pregnancy

SAFETY CATEGORY	EXPLANATION	EXAMPLES
A Lowest Risk	Studies HAVE NOT shown a risk to women or to the fetus.	levothyroxine (Synthroid) thyroglobulin (Proloid) potassium chloride (K-Lor) potassium gluconate (Kaon Tablets) ferrous fumarate (Ferranol)
B	ANIMAL studies HAVE NOT shown a risk to the fetus or, if they have, studies in women have not confirmed this risk.	amoxicillin (Amoxil) insulin (Humulin R) fluoxetine (Prozac) loperamide (Imodium) penicillin V (Pen-Vee-K) ranitidine (Zantac)
C	ANIMAL studies HAVE shown a risk to the fetus, but controlled studies have not been performed in women.	acyclovir (Zovirax) mineral oil (Fleet Mineral Oil) senna (Senokot) hydrochlorothiazide (HydroDIURIL) furosemide (Lasix) iron dextran (K-FeRON) amitriptyline (Elavil)
D	Use of this drug category MAY cause harm to the fetus, but it may provide benefit to the mother in a life-threatening situation or if a safer therapy is not available.	tetracycline (Achromycin) cortisone acetate (Cortistan) warfarin (Coumadin)
X Highest Risk	Studies HAVE shown a significant risk to women and to the fetus.	iodinated glycerol (Organidin) castor oil (Purge) estrogen with progesterone (Ortho Novum) dienestrol (DV) norethindrone (Norlutin) oxymetholone (Anadrol)

CHAPTER REVIEW

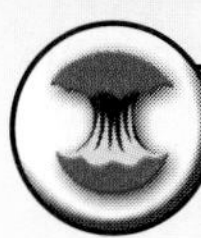

CORE CONCEPTS SUMMARY

2.1 **Drugs may be organized by their therapeutic and pharmacological classifications.**

Two common ways to classify drugs are by therapeutic classification and pharmacological classification. Therapeutic classes are based on a drug's clinical usefulness. Pharmacological classes are based on a drug's mechanism of action. Prototype drugs are used to compare drugs within the same classification.

2.2 **Drugs have more than one name.**

Drugs may be described by a chemical, generic, or trade name. There are advantages and disadvantages to each type of naming method.

2.3 **The differences between brand name drugs and their generic equivalents may include price, formulations, and, most important, bioavailability.**

In most states, generic drugs may be substituted for brand name products if the prescribing practitioner does not object. When generic drugs are substituted, differences in bioavailability may affect the safety and effectiveness of drug therapy.

2.4 **Drugs with a potential for abuse are categorized into schedules.**

Drugs that have a high potential for abuse or dependency are placed into one of five schedules (Schedule I through Schedule V). Schedule I is the most restrictive category. Schedule V is the least restrictive category. The U.S. Drug Enforcement Agency (DEA) handles drug misuse.

2.5 **Canadian regulations restrict drugs of abuse.**

In Canada, drug use is controlled by schedules outlined in the Canadian Food and Drugs Act. Schedule G drugs are referred to as controlled drugs. Controlled drugs, narcotics, and noncontrolled or Schedule F drugs are classified as Schedule I. All nonprescription drugs monitored for sale by pharmacists are classified as Schedule II. Nonprescription drugs not monitored by pharmacists are classified as Schedule III.

2.6 **All prescription drugs are classified according to safety in pregnancy categories to protect the unborn.**

All U.S. drugs are placed into one of five pregnancy categories, labeled as A, B, C, D, and X. Category A is the safest category. Category X is the most harmful.

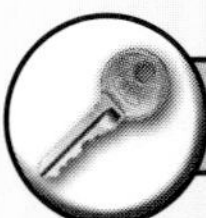

KEY TERMS

bioavailability (BEYE-oh-ah-VALE-ah-BILL-ih-TEE): the ability of a drug to reach its target cells and produce its effect / *page 18*

chemical name: strict chemical nomenclature used for naming drugs established by the International Union of Pure and Applied Chemistry (IUPAC) / *page 16*

combination drug: drug product with more than one active generic ingredient / *page 17*

controlled substance: in the United States a drug restricted by the Comprehensive Drug Abuse Prevention and Control Act. In Canada, a drug subject to guidelines outlined in Part III, Schedule G of the Canadian Food and Drugs Act / *page 19*

generic name (je-NARE-ik): nonproprietary name of a drug assigned by the government / *page 17*

mechanism of action: how a drug exerts its effects / *page 15*

pharmacological classification (FAR-mah-koh-LOJ-ik-ul): method for organizing drugs on the basis of their mechanism of action (how they work pharmacologically) / *page 15*

prototype drug (PRO-toh-type): an original, well-understood drug model from which other drugs in a pharmacological class have been developed / *page 16*

restricted drug: in Canada, a drug not intended for human use, covered in Part IV, Schedule H of the Canadian Food and Drugs Act / *page 19*

scheduled drugs: in the United States, a term describing a drug placed into one of five categories (I through V) based on its potential for misuse or abuse / *page 18*

therapeutic classification (ther-ah-PEW-tik): method for organizing drugs on the basis of their *therapeutic usefulness* / *page 15*

trade name: proprietary name of a drug assigned by the manufacturer; also called the *brand name* or *product name* / *page 17*

REVIEW QUESTIONS

The following questions are written in NCLEX-PN® style. Answer these questions to assess your knowledge of the chapter material, and go back and review any material that is not clear to you.

1. Which of the following types of drug classification focuses on what a drug does clinically?

1. Therapeutic
2. Pharmacological
3. Chemical
4. All of the above

2. *How* a medication produces its effects in the body is referred to as a drug's:

1. Therapeutic usefulness
2. Mechanism of action
3. Model for other drugs combating similar diseases
4. Clinical focus

3. In which of the following cases does a drug have only one name?

1. Chemical name
2. Generic name
3. Trade name
4. Both a and b

4. Which of the following statements is correct?

1. Because chemical drug names are often complicated and difficult to remember or pronounce, the chemical structure of a drug is rarely considered in pharmacotherapy.
2. Matching one active ingredient with one trade name product is not a particularly challenging job for the healthcare provider.
3. When referring to a drug, the generic name is usually capitalized, whereas the trade name is written in lowercase.
4. The drug trade name is sometimes called the *proprietary* name, suggesting ownership.

5. When examining the question, "Are there really differences between brand name drugs and their generic equivalents?" the answer that emerges from reading this chapter is:

1. Unclear.
2. Significant differences exist between a trade name drug and its generic equivalent.
3. Generic drugs are always best because they generally cost less.
4. Brand name drugs are preferred because of differences in bioavailability compared to generic equivalents.

6. An altered physical condition caused by the nervous system adapting to repeated drug use is:

1. Addiction
2. Physical dependence
3. Psychological dependence
4. Withdrawal

7. The Controlled Substances Act of 1970, and later revisions, enable the DEA to do which of the following?

1. Introduce drugs into the marketplace
2. Restrict the use of drugs that have a significant potential for abuse
3. Restrict the use of all drugs that have an abuse potential
4. Allow patients to obtain Schedule II drug refills without visiting their healthcare provider first

8. The drug schedule allowing therapeutic use of a drug with a prescription, but having relatively lower abuse and dependency potential than other scheduled drugs, is:

1. Schedule II
2. Schedule III
3. Schedule IV
4. Schedule V

9. In Canada, nonprescription drugs monitored for sale by pharmacists are classified as:

1. Schedule I
2. Schedule II
3. Schedule III
4. None of the above, because drugs in Canada are not placed into schedules

10. Pregnant patients:

1. Are without risk if they take drugs placed into pregnancy category X
2. Can take herbal or dietary supplements without fear of teratogenic effects to their developing baby
3. Are relatively safe if they take medications within pregnancy category B
4. Should never take drugs classified as pregnancy category D

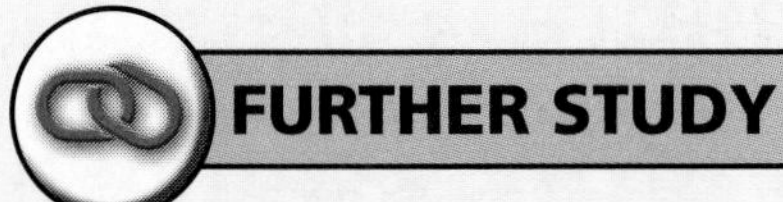

FURTHER STUDY

- Substance abuse is discussed in detail in Chapter 6.

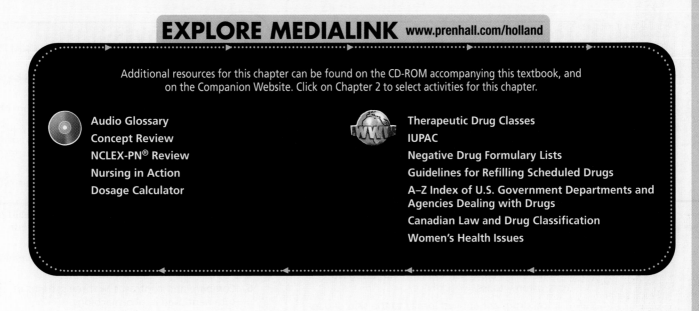

EXPLORE MEDIALINK www.prenhall.com/holland

Additional resources for this chapter can be found on the CD-ROM accompanying this textbook, and on the Companion Website. Click on Chapter 2 to select activities for this chapter.

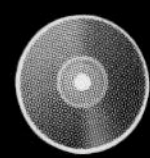

Audio Glossary
Concept Review
NCLEX-PN® Review
Nursing in Action
Dosage Calculator

Therapeutic Drug Classes
IUPAC
Negative Drug Formulary Lists
Guidelines for Refilling Scheduled Drugs
A–Z Index of U.S. Government Departments and Agencies Dealing with Drugs
Canadian Law and Drug Classification
Women's Health Issues

CHAPTER

3 Methods of Drug Administration

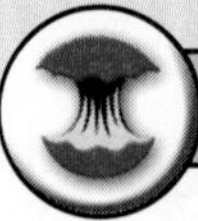

CORE CONCEPTS

3.1 A major goal in pharmacotherapy is to limit the number and severity of adverse drug events.

3.2 The rights of drug administration form the basis of proper drug delivery.

3.3 Successful pharmacotherapy depends on patient compliance.

3.4 Healthcare providers use accepted abbreviations to communicate the directions and times for drug administration.

3.5 Three systems of measurement are used in pharmacology: metric, apothecary, and household.

3.6 Certain protocols and techniques are common to all methods of drug administration.

3.7 Enteral drugs are given orally or via nasogastric or gastrostomy tubes.

3.8 Topical drugs are applied locally to the skin and associated membranes.

3.9 Parenteral administration refers to dispensing medications by routes other than oral or topical.

OBJECTIVES

After reading this chapter, the student should be able to:

1. Discuss drug administration as a component of safe and effective healthcare.
2. Describe the roles and responsibilities of the nurse, nursing assistants, therapists, and technicians regarding drug administration.
3. Explain how the six rights of drug administration impact patient safety.
4. Give specific examples of how the healthcare provider can increase patient compliance in taking medications.
5. Interpret abbreviations used in drug administration practices.
6. Compare and contrast the three systems of measurement used in pharmacology.
7. Explain the proper methods to administer enteral, topical, and parenteral drugs.
8. Compare and contrast the advantages and disadvantages of each route of drug administration.

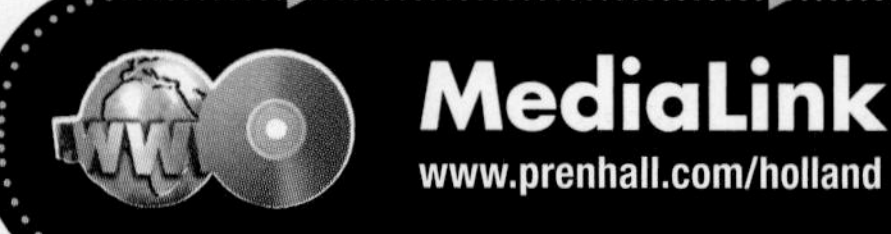

Interactive resources for this chapter can be found on the Companion Website. Click on Chapter 3 and "Begin" to select the activities for this chapter. For chapter-related animations, NCLEX-PN®-style questions, and an audio glossary, access the accompanying CD-ROM in this book.

Drug administration is an important part of providing comprehensive care to the patient. During drug administration, members of the healthcare team collaborate closely with pharmacists, physicians, each other, and their patients to ensure that prescribed medications are delivered safely. The purpose of this chapter is to introduce the roles and responsibilities of nurses and other healthcare professionals, to define the practice of safe and effective delivery of medications, and to provide a basic overview of the major routes of drug administration.

3.1 A major goal in pharmacotherapy is to limit the number and severity of adverse drug events.

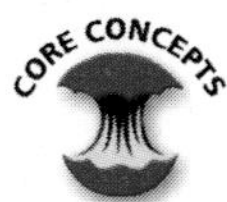

Whether administering drugs, supervising drug use, or providing assistance, the healthcare provider is expected to understand or at least be familiar with the general principles of drug delivery. The large number of different drugs and the potential consequences of medication errors make this an enormous task.

The nurse's main responsibilities include knowledge and understanding of the following:

- What drug is ordered
- Name (generic and trade) and drug classification
- Intended or proposed use
- Effects on the body
- Contraindications
- Special considerations (for example, the effect of age, weight, body fat distribution, and individual pathophysiological states on pharmacotherapeutic response)
- Side effects
- Why the medication has been prescribed for this particular patient
- How the medication is supplied by the pharmacy
- How the medication should be administered, including dosage ranges
- What nursing process considerations related to the medication apply to this patient

Nursing assistants, therapists, and technicians work closely with the nurses to provide care to the patients. Members of the health support staff, who do not administer medications but who have an equally important role in providing care to the patients, have a slightly different list of tasks. These tasks provide opportunity to monitor patients and make sure there are no unusual reactions or undesirable effects resulting from the medication. Tasks include:

- Monitoring blood pressure, pulse rate, and respiration rate
- Changing soiled or wet clothing, wraps, or bandages
- Dressing wounds, massaging, and caring for the skin's surface
- Preparing food trays or helping feed patients
- Observing patients and reporting significant symptoms, reactions, or changes in condition
- Reporting strange behaviors or habits
- Helping transport patients
- Monitoring special equipment

Before any drug is administered, healthcare staff must obtain, process, and communicate important information to one another about the patient's medical history, physical assessment, disease processes, learning needs, and capabilities. They must consider growth and developmental factors and remember that many variables can influence how a patient responds to medications. Understanding these variables can increase the success of pharmacotherapy. A major goal of pharmacotherapy is to limit the number and severity of adverse drug events. Many adverse effects are preventable. By applying their experience and knowledge of pharmacotherapeutics to clinical practice, healthcare providers can avoid many serious adverse drug reactions. Some adverse effects, however, are not preventable. It is vital that the healthcare team is prepared to recognize and respond to potential adverse medication effects. Allergic and anaphylactic reactions are particularly serious effects that must be carefully monitored and prevented, when possible. An **allergic**

reaction is an acquired hyperresponse of body defenses to a foreign substance (allergen). Signs of allergic reactions vary in severity and include skin rash with or without itching, edema, nausea, diarrhea, runny nose, or reddened eyes with tearing. On discovering that a patient is allergic to a product, it is the nurse's responsibility to first alert the charge nurse and patient's physician of the reaction in case it is necessary to give the patient medications to reverse the reaction. Next the nurse should document the allergy in the medical record and apply labels to the chart and medication administration record so that all healthcare personnel will be aware of the allergy. An agency-approved allergy bracelet should be placed on the patient. The pharmacist should also be told so that the medication can be checked for cross-sensitivity with other pharmacological products.

Anaphylaxis is a severe type of allergic reaction in which massive amounts of histamine and other chemical mediators of inflammation are released throughout the body. It can lead to life-threatening shock. Symptoms of anaphylaxis are severe shortness of breath, a sudden drop in blood pressure, and tachycardia. These symptoms require immediate attention. The pharmacotherapy of allergic reactions and anaphylaxis is covered in Chapter 21.

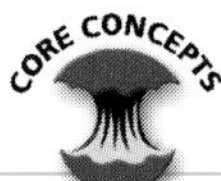

3.2 The rights of drug administration form the basis of proper drug delivery.

The traditional **six rights of drug administration** are the basis of safe delivery of medications. The six rights are simple and practical guidelines for nurses to use during drug preparation, delivery, and administration. The six rights are as follows:

- Right patient
- Right medication
- Right dose
- Right route of administration
- Right time of delivery
- Right documentation

Additional rights have been added over the years, depending on particular academic curricula or agency policies. Additions to the original six rights include the right to refuse medication, the right to receive drug education, and the right preparation.

The **three checks of drug administration** that nurses use with the six rights help to ensure patient safety and drug effectiveness. Traditionally these checks include the following:

- Checking the drug with the medication administration record (MAR) or medication information system when removing it from the medication drawer, refrigerator, or controlled substance locker
- Checking the drug when preparing it, pouring it, taking it out of the unit dose container, or connecting the IV tubing to the bag
- Checking the drug before administering it to the patient

Despite the use of these checks and rights to provide safe drug delivery, errors still occur, and some of them are fatal. Although the nurse is accountable for preparing and administering medications, many disciplines—including physicians, pharmacists, and other healthcare professionals—are responsible for safe drug practices.

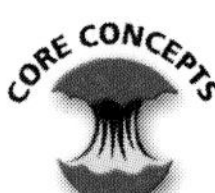

3.3 Successful pharmacotherapy depends on patient compliance.

Patient **compliance** is another major factor affecting the success of pharmacotherapy. Compliance means taking a medication in the way it was prescribed by the practitioner or, in the case of OTC drugs, following the instructions on the label. Patient noncompliance can include not taking the medication at all, taking it at the wrong time, or taking it in the wrong way.

Fast Facts Potentially Fatal Drug Reactions

Toxic Epidermal Necrolysis (TEN)

- Skin sloughing of 30% or more of the body (caused by skin cell breakdown)
- Severe and deadly allergic reaction caused by the drug
- Occurs when the liver fails to properly break down a drug, which then cannot be excreted normally
- Risk of death decreased if the drug is quickly withdrawn and supportive care is maintained

Stevens-Johnson Syndrome (SJS)

- Skin sloughing of 10% of the body
- Generalized blisterlike lesions following within a few days
- Nonspecific upper respiratory infection (URI) with chills, fever, and malaise usually signals the start of SJS

Even when healthcare providers conscientiously use all the principles of effective drug administration, patients may not agree that the prescribed drug regimen is worthwhile. Before administering the drug, the nurse should use the nursing process to develop a personalized care plan that will allow the patient to be an active participant in his or her care. Support staff can help ensure that the care plan works. It is important to remember that a responsible, well-informed adult always has the legal option to refuse any medication. This allows the patient to accept or reject the pharmacotherapy, based on accurate information that is presented in a way that the patient can understand.

In the plan of care, it is important to address information that the patient must know about the prescribed medications. This includes the name of the drug, why it was ordered, its expected actions, its possible side effects, and its potential interactions with other medications, foods, herbal supplements, or alcohol. Patients need to be reminded that they have an active role in ensuring their own medication effectiveness and safety.

Many factors influence whether patients comply with pharmacotherapy. The drug may be too expensive or may not be approved by the patient's health insurance plan. Patients sometimes forget doses of medications, especially when they must be taken three or four times per day. Patients often stop using drugs that have annoying side effects or that affect lifestyle. Adverse effects such as headache, dizziness, nausea, diarrhea, or impotence often cause noncompliance. Patients sometimes self-adjust their doses. Some patients believe that if one tablet is good, two must be better. Others believe they will become dependent on the medication if it is taken as prescribed, and so they take only half the required dose. Patients usually do not want to admit or report noncompliance to the nurse because they are embarrassed or fear being reprimanded. Because there are many reasons for noncompliance, the nurse must carefully question patients about their medications. When pharmacotherapy fails to produce the expected outcomes, noncompliance should be considered as a possible reason.

Life Span Fact

Many elderly patients take at least three different drugs each day, with some taking as many as eight. This leads to poor compliance among older patients. Noncompliance can be even greater for elderly patients with dementia or Alzheimer's disease.

Fast Facts Grapefruit Juice and Drug Interactions

- Grapefruit juice may not be safe for people who take certain medications.
- Chemicals in grapefruit juice lower the activity of specific enzymes in the intestinal tract that normally break down medications. This allows a larger amount of medication to reach the bloodstream, resulting in increased drug activity.
- Drugs that may be affected by grapefruit juice include certain sedative-hypnotic drugs, antibiotics, drugs that lower blood cholesterol, some antihistamines, and antifungal agents.
- Grapefruit juice should be consumed at least 2 hours before or 5 hours after taking a medication that may interact with it.
- Some drinks that are flavored with fruit juice could contain grapefruit juice, even if grapefruit is not part of the name of the drink. Check the ingredients label.

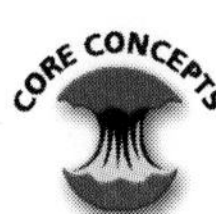

3.4 Healthcare providers use accepted abbreviations to communicate the directions and times for drug administration.

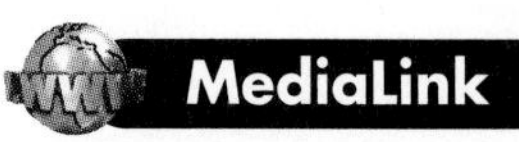

ABBREVIATIONS FOR SAFE MEDICATION ADMINISTRATION

Table 3.1 lists common abbreviations that are used to give directions about drug administration. A **STAT order** refers to a medication that should be given immediately and only once. This order is often used with emergency medications that are needed for life-threatening situations. The physician normally notifies the nurse of any STAT order, so it can be obtained from the pharmacy and administered immediately. Although not as urgent, an **ASAP** (as soon as possible) **order** should be available for administration to the patient within 30 minutes of the written order. (The exact time frame is usually defined by individual facilities.)

The **single order** is for a drug that is to be given only once and at a specific time. An example is a preoperative order. A **prn order** is administered as required by the patient's condition. The nurse makes the judgment, based on patient assessment, as to when the medication should be administered. Orders not written as STAT, ASAP, NOW, or prn are called **routine orders.** These are usually carried out within 2 hours of the time the order is written by the physician, but the exact timing is defined by each facility. A **standing order** is written in advance of a situation, and should be carried out under specific circumstances. An example of a standing order is a set of postoperative prn prescriptions that are written for all patients who have undergone a specific surgical procedure. A common standing order for patients who have had a tonsillectomy is "Tylenol elixir 325 mg PO q6h prn sore throat." Because of the legal implications of putting all patients into a single treatment category, standing orders are no longer permitted in some facilities.

Agency policies dictate that drug orders be reviewed by the attending physician within specific time frames, usually at least every 7 days. Prescriptions for narcotics and other scheduled drugs are often automatically stopped after 72 hours, unless specifically reordered by the physician. Automatic stop orders do not generally apply when the number of doses, or an exact period of time, is specified.

Some medications must be taken at specific times. If a drug causes stomach upset, it is usually administered with meals to prevent epigastric pain, nausea, or vomiting. Other medications should be administered between meals because food interferes with absorption. Some CNS drugs and antihypertensives are best administered at bedtime, because they may cause drowsiness. Sildenafil (Viagra) is unique in that it should be taken 30 to 60 minutes prior to expected sexual intercourse, to achieve an erection. The nurse must pay careful attention when educating patients about when and how to take their medications to increase compliance and therapeutic success.

TABLE 3.1 Drug Administration Abbreviations*

ABBREVIATION	MEANING	ABBREVIATION	MEANING
ac	before meals	q	every
ad lib	as desired/as directed	qh	every hour
AM	morning	qid	four times per day
bid	twice per day	q2h	every 2 hours (even)
cap	capsule	q4h	every 4 hours (even)
/d	per day	q6h	every 6 hours (even)
gtt	drop	q8h	every 8 hours (even)
h or hr	hour	q12h	every 12 hours
hs	hour of sleep/bedtime	Rx	take
no	number	SL	sublingual
pc	after meals; after eating	STAT	immediately; at once
PM	afternoon	tab	tablet
PO	by mouth	tid	three times per day
prn	when needed/necessary		

* *JCAHO recommends that some previously used abbreviations be spelled out to avoid medication errors: Use* daily *(not* qd*); use* every other day *(not* qod*).*

Once medications are administered, the nurse must correctly document that the medications have been given to the patient. It is necessary to write down the drug name, dosage, time administered, and any assessments, and to sign the documentation. If a medication is refused or not taken, this fact (along with the patient's reasons) must be recorded on the appropriate form within the medical record. Nursing assistants and healthcare staff can help verify patient compliance.

3.5 Three systems of measurement are used in pharmacology: metric, apothecary, and household.

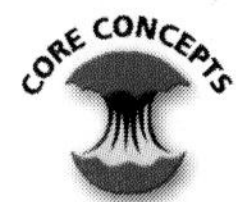

Dosages are labeled and dispensed according to their weight or volume. The most common system of drug measurement uses the **metric system.** The volume of a drug is expressed in terms of a liter (L) or a milliliter (ml). The abbreviation "cc" for cubic centimeter, a measurement of volume that is equivalent to 1 ml of fluid, is no longer recommended for use in medicine. The metric weight of a drug is stated in terms of kilograms (kg), grams (g), milligrams (mg), or micrograms (mcg). At one time, the abbreviation "µg" was used for micrograms, but this is no longer recommended.

The **apothecary** and **household systems** are older systems of measurement. Although most physicians and pharmacies use the metric system, these older systems may still be seen. Until the metric system totally replaces the other systems, the healthcare professional must recognize dosages based on all three systems of measurement. Approximate equivalents among metric, apothecary, and household units of volume and weight are listed in Table 3.2.

Because Americans are familiar with the teaspoon, tablespoon, and cup, it is important for the nurse to be able to convert between the household and metric systems of measurement. In the hospital, a glass of fluid is measured in milliliters—an 8 ounce glass of water is recorded as 240 ml. If a patient being discharged is ordered to drink 2400 ml of fluid per day, the nurse may instruct the patient to drink ten 8-ounce glasses or 10 cups of fluid per day. Likewise, when a child is to be given a drug that is administered in elixir form, the nurse should explain that 5 ml of the drug is the same as 1 teaspoon. The nurse should encourage the use of accurate medical dosing devices at home, such as oral dosing syringes, oral droppers, cylindrical spoons, and medication cups. These are preferred over the traditional household measuring spoon because they are more accurate. Eating utensils that are commonly referred to as teaspoons or tablespoons often do not hold the volume that their names imply.

TABLE 3.2 Metric, Apothecary, and Household Approximate Measurement Equivalents

METRIC	APOTHECARY	HOUSEHOLD
1 ml	15–16 minims	15–16 drops
4–5 ml (cc)	1 fluid dram	1 teaspoon or 60 drops
15 ml	4 fluid drams	1 Tablespoon or 3–4 teaspoons
30 ml	8 fluid drams or 1 fluid ounce	2 Tablespoons
240 ml	8 fluid ounces (½ pint)	1 glass or cup
500 ml	1 pint	2 glasses or 2 cups
1 L	32 fluid ounces or 1 quart	4 glasses or 4 cups or 1 quart
1 mg	1/60 grain	—
60–65 mg	1 grain	—
300–325 mg	5 grains	—
1 g	15–16 grains	—
1 kg	—	2.2 pounds

To convert grains to grams: Divide grains by 15 or 16.

To convert grams to grains: Multiply grams by 15 or 16.

To convert minims to milliliters: Divide minims by 15 or 16.

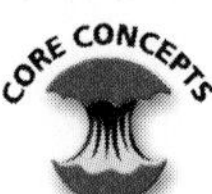

3.6 Certain protocols and techniques are common to all methods of drug administration.

The three general routes of drug administration are enteral, topical, and parenteral with subcategories among each general route. Each route has both advantages and disadvantages. Although some drugs are formulated to be given by several routes, others are made to be given by only one route. Pharmacokinetic considerations, such as how the route of administration affects drug absorption and distribution, are discussed in Chapter 4. Certain protocols and techniques are common to all methods of drug administration. The student should refer to the drug administration guidelines in the following list before reading about specific routes of administration.

- Review the medication order, and check for drug allergies.
- Wash hands and put on gloves, if indicated.
- Use aseptic technique when preparing and administering parenteral medications.
- Identify the patient by asking the person to state his or her full name (or by asking the parent or guardian if the patient is confused), checking the patient's identification band, and comparing this information with the MAR.
- Ask the patient about known allergies, and check to see if he or she is wearing an allergy identification band.
- Tell the patient what drug you are administering and how you will give it.
- Position the patient for the appropriate route of administration.
- For enteral drugs, assist the patient to a sitting position.
- If the drug is prepackaged as a unit dose, remove it from the packaging at the bedside when possible.
- Unless specifically instructed to do so in the orders, do not leave drugs at the patient's bedside.
- Document the medication administration and any important patient responses on the MAR.

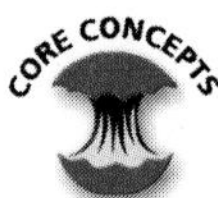

3.7 Enteral drugs are given orally or via nasogastric or gastrostomy tubes.

The **enteral route** includes drugs given orally and those administered through nasogastric (NG) or gastrostomy tubes. Oral drug administration (abbreviated PO, which refers to the Latin *per os,* meaning "by mouth") is the most common, most convenient, and usually the least costly of all routes. It is also considered the safest route because the skin's protective barrier is not broken. In cases of overdose, medications remaining in the stomach can be retrieved by causing vomiting. Oral preparations are available in tablet, capsule, caplet, and liquid forms. Medications administered by the enteral route take advantage of the large absorptive surfaces of the oral mucosa, stomach, or small intestine.

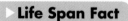

> **Life Span Fact**
>
> For children and elderly patients, as well as those who may have trouble swallowing, the nurse can crush tablets or open capsules and sprinkle the drug over food or mix it with juice to make it easier to swallow and to hide its taste.

Tablets and Capsules

Tablets and capsules are the most common forms of drugs. Patients prefer tablets or capsules over other routes and forms because they are easy to use. In some cases, tablets may be scored so they can easily be broken if the dose needs to be made smaller for a specific patient.

The nurse should always check the manufacturer's instructions for administering the medication to be sure that crushing or opening is allowed. Some tablets and capsules should not be crushed or opened because their ingredients are inactivated by doing so. Other medications can severely irritate the stomach mucosa and cause nausea or vomiting. Occasionally, drugs should not be crushed because they irritate the oral mucosa, are extremely bitter, or contain dyes that stain the teeth. Most drug guides provide lists of drugs that may not be crushed. Guidelines for administering tablets or capsules are given in Table 3.3A.

The strongly acidic contents within the stomach can destroy some medications. To overcome this problem, tablets may have a hard, waxy coating that protects the medicine from the acidity. These **enteric-coated** tablets are designed to dissolve in the alkaline environment of the small

TABLE 3.3 Enteral Drug Administration

DRUG FORM	ADMINISTRATION GUIDELINES
A. Tablet, capsule, or liquid	1. Check to be sure that the patient is alert and can swallow. 2. Place tablets or capsules into a medication cup. 3. If the medication is liquid, shake the bottle to mix the agent, and measure the dose into the cup at eye level. 4. Hand the patient the medication cup. 5. Offer a glass of water to facilitate swallowing the medication. Milk or juice may be offered (if not contraindicated). 6. Remain with the patient until all medication is swallowed.
B. Sublingual	1. Check that the patient is alert and can hold the medication under the tongue. 2. Instruct the patient not to chew or swallow the tablet, or move it around with the tongue. 3. Instruct the patient to allow the tablet to dissolve completely before swallowing saliva. 4. Place the sublingual tablet under the patient's tongue. 5. Remain with the patient to make sure that all of the medication has dissolved. 6. Offer the patient a glass of water.
C. Buccal	1. Check that the patient is alert and can hold the medication between the gums and the cheek. 2. Instruct the patient to allow the tablet to dissolve completely before swallowing saliva. 3. Instruct the patient not to chew or swallow the tablet or move it around with the tongue. 4. Place the buccal tablet between the gum line and the cheek. 5. Remain with the patient to be sure that all of the medication has dissolved. 6. Offer the patient a glass of water.
D. Nasogastric and gastrostomy	1. Administer liquid forms of the medication when possible to avoid clogging the tube. 2. If the medication is solid, crush it into a fine powder and mix it thoroughly with at least 30 ml of warm water until dissolved. 3. Verify the tube placement and make sure it is clear. 4. Turn off the feeding, if applicable. 5. Attach a syringe (30 or 60 ml) with plunger. Aspirate the patient's stomach contents and measure the volume. This is termed the *gastric residual volume.* If it is greater than 100 ml (for an adult), check the facility's policy. 6. Attach the syringe without plunger. Return the residual contents by allowing it to flow back into the tube via gravity. Flush the tube with about 10 ml (2 teaspoons) of tap water. 7. Pour the medication into the syringe barrel, also allowing it to flow into the tube by gravity. Give each medication separately, flushing between each with water. 8. Keep the head of the bed elevated 45 degrees for 1 hour to prevent aspiration. 9. Reestablish continual feeding, as scheduled.

intestine. It is important that the nurse not crush enteric-coated tablets because the medication would then be directly exposed to the stomach environment.

Studies have clearly shown that patients are less compliant when they must take more than one dose of medicine per day, particularly if the number is 3 doses or more. With this in mind, pharmacologists have tried to design new drugs that need to be administered only once or twice daily. **Sustained-release** tablets or capsules are designed to dissolve very slowly. They release medication over a longer time, which increases the drug's duration of action (or length of time the medication works). Also called *extended-release (XR), long-acting (LA),* or *slow-release (SR) medications,* these forms allow convenient once or twice daily dosing. These sustained-release medications must not be crushed or opened.

Giving medications by the oral route has some disadvantages. The patient must be conscious and able to swallow properly. Certain types of drugs, including proteins, are inactivated by digestive enzymes in the stomach and small intestine. Medications absorbed from the stomach and small intestine first travel to the liver, where they may be inactivated before they ever reach their target organs. This process, called *first-pass metabolism,* is discussed in Chapter 4. The significant variation in the motility of the GI tract among patients and in the tract's ability to absorb medications can create differences in bioavailability. In addition, children and some adults do not like to swallow large tablets and capsules or take oral medications that are distasteful.

Sublingual and Buccal Drug Administration

For sublingual and buccal administration, the patient does not swallow the tablet but instead keeps it in the mouth until it dissolves. The mucosa of the oral cavity contains a rich blood supply that provides an excellent absorptive surface for certain drugs. Medications given by this route are not destroyed by digestive enzymes, nor do they undergo first-pass metabolism in the liver.

For the **sublingual (SL) route,** the medication is placed under the tongue and allowed to dissolve slowly. The rich blood supply under the tongue results in a rapid onset of drug action. Sublingual dosage forms are most often formulated as rapidly disintegrating tablets or as soft gelatin capsules filled with liquid drug.

When multiple drugs have been ordered, the sublingual preparations should be administered after the oral medications have been swallowed. The patient should be instructed not to move the drug with the tongue, nor to eat or drink anything until the medication has completely dissolved. The sublingual mucosa is not suitable for extended-release formulations because it is a relatively small area and is constantly being bathed by saliva. Table 3.3B and Figure 3.1a ■ present important points about sublingual drug administration.

To administer by the **buccal route,** the tablet, capsule, lozenge, or troche is placed in the oral cavity between the gum and the cheek. The patient must be instructed not to touch the medication with the tongue, because it could get moved to the sublingual area where it would be more rapidly absorbed, or to the back of the throat where it could be swallowed. Medications are absorbed more slowly from the buccal mucosa than the sublingual area. The buccal route is preferred over the sublingual route for sustained-release delivery because of its greater mucosal surface area. Drugs formulated for buccal administration generally do not cause irritation and are small enough to not cause discomfort to the patient. Table 3.3C and Figure 3.1b ■ provide important guidelines for buccal drug administration.

Nasogastric and Gastrostomy Drug Administration

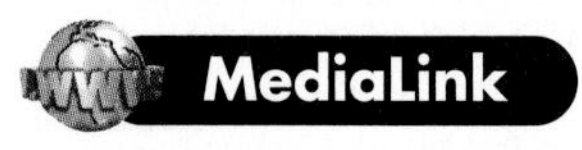

NASOGASTRIC/GASTROSTOMY THERAPY

Patients with a nasogastric (NG) tube or enteral feeding system such as a gastrostomy (G) tube may have their medications administered through these devices. The soft, flexible NG tube is inserted by way of the nasopharynx or oropharynx with the tip lying in the stomach. A G tube is surgically placed directly into the patient's stomach. Generally, the NG tube is used for short-term treatment, whereas the G tube is inserted for patients who require long-term care. Drugs administered through these tubes are usually in liquid form. Although solid drugs can be crushed or dissolved, they tend to clog the tubes. Sustained-release drugs should not be crushed and administered through NG or G tubes. Drugs administered by this route are exposed to the same physiological processes as those given orally. Table 3.3D gives important guidelines for administering drugs through NG or G tubes.

FIGURE 3.1

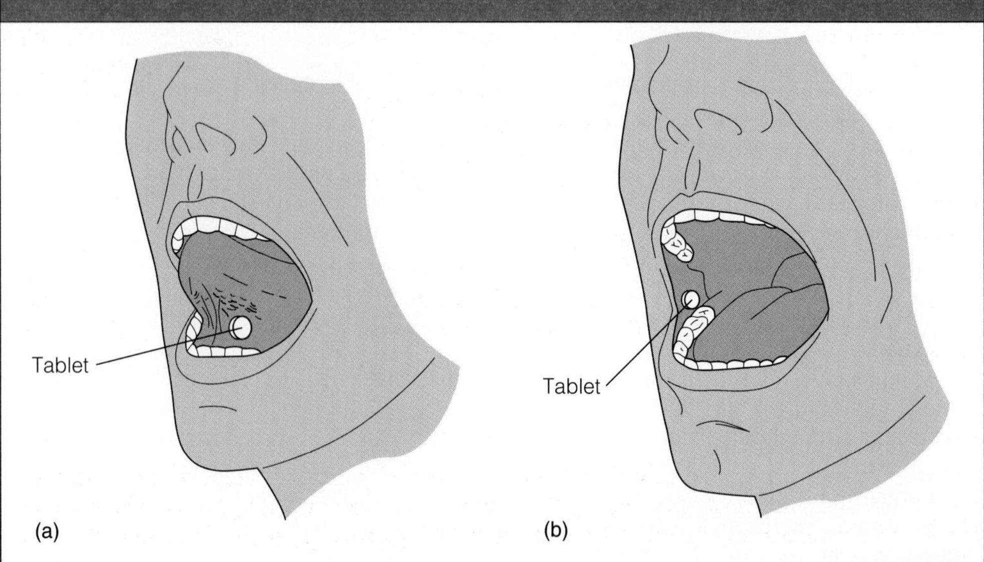

(a) Sublingual (under the tongue) drug administration;
(b) buccal (between the gums and cheek) drug administration

3.8 Topical drugs are applied locally to the skin and associated membranes.

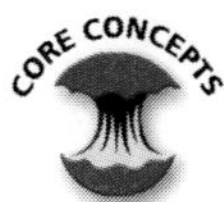

The **topical route** involves applying drugs locally to the skin or the membranous linings of the eye, ear, nose, respiratory tract, urinary tract, vagina, and rectum. These applications include the following:

- *Dermatologic preparations.* These drugs are applied to the skin using formulations that include creams, lotions, gels, powders, and sprays. This is the most common topical route.
- *Instillations and irrigations.* These drugs are applied into body cavities or orifices that include the eyes, ears, nose, urinary bladder, rectum, and vagina.
- *Inhalations.* Inhalers, nebulizers, or positive-pressure breathing apparatuses are used to apply these drugs to the respiratory tract. The most common indication for inhaled drugs is bronchoconstriction due to bronchitis or asthma. Many illegal, abused drugs are taken by this route because it provides a very rapid onset of drug action.

Drugs can be applied topically to produce a local or a systemic effect. Many drugs are applied topically to produce a local effect. For example, antibiotics may be applied to the skin to treat skin infections. Antineoplastic agents may be infused into the urinary bladder via catheter to treat tumors of the bladder mucosa. Corticosteroids are sprayed into the nostrils to reduce inflammation of the nasal mucosa due to allergic rhinitis. Local, topical delivery of these drugs produces fewer side effects compared with the same drugs given orally or parenterally. When these drugs are given topically, they are absorbed very slowly, and only small amounts reach the general circulation.

Other drugs are given topically to ensure slow release and absorption of the drug in the general circulation. These agents are given for their systemic (systemwide) effects. For example, a nitroglycerin patch is not applied to the skin to treat a local skin condition, but to treat the systemic condition of coronary artery disease. Likewise, prochlorperazine (Compazine) suppositories are inserted rectally not to treat a disease of the rectum but to alleviate nausea. The distinction between topical drugs given for local effects and those given for systemic effects is an important one for the nurse to know. In the case of local drugs, absorption is undesirable and may cause side effects. For systemic drugs, absorption is necessary for the therapeutic action of the drug. With either type of topical agent, drugs should not be applied to abraded or denuded skin, unless directed to do so.

Transdermal Delivery System

Transdermal patches are an effective means of delivering certain medications. Examples include nitroglycerin for angina pectoris and scopolamine (Transderm-Scop) for motion sickness. Although transdermal patches contain a specific amount of drug, the rate of delivery and the actual dose received may vary. Patches are changed on a regular basis, using a site rotation routine, which should be documented in the MAR. Before applying a transdermal patch, the nurse should verify that the previous patch has been removed and disposed of appropriately. Drugs to be administered by this route avoid the first-pass effect in the liver and bypass digestive enzymes. Table 3.4A and Figure 3.2 ■ illustrate the major points of transdermal drug delivery.

Ophthalmic Administration

The ophthalmic route is used to treat local conditions of the eye and surrounding structures. Common indications include excessive dryness, infections, glaucoma, and dilation of the pupil during eye examinations. Ophthalmic drugs are available in the form of eye irrigations, drops, ointments, and medicated disks. Figure 3.3 ■ and Table 3.4B give guidelines for adult administration.

Otic Administration

The otic route is used to treat local conditions of the ear, including infections and soft blockages of the auditory canal. Otic medications include eardrops and irrigations, which are usually ordered for cleaning. Figure 3.4 ■ and Table 3.4C present key points in administering otic medications.

Life Span Fact

Although the procedure for administering ophthalmic drugs is the same with a child as with an adult, it is advisable to enlist the help of an adult caregiver. In some cases, the infant or toddler may need to be immobilized with the arms wrapped to prevent accidental injury to the eye during administration. For the young child, demonstrating the procedure using a doll helps gain the child's cooperation and decreases the level of anxiety.

Life Span Fact

Administration of otic drugs to infants and young children must be performed carefully to avoid injury to sensitive structures of the ear. When giving otic drugs to children, gently pull the pinna down and back.

TABLE 3.4	Topical Drug Administration
DRUG FORM	**ADMINISTRATION GUIDELINES**
A. Transdermal	1. Obtain the transdermal patch, and read the manufacturer's guidelines. The application site and frequency of changing differ according to medication. 2. Apply gloves before handling the patch to avoid absorbing any medication. 3. Label the patch with the date, time, and your initials. 4. Remove the previous medication or patch, and cleanse the area. 5. If using a transdermal ointment, apply the ordered amount of medication in an even line directly on the premeasured paper that accompanies the medication tube. 6. Press the patch or apply the medicated paper to clean, dry, and hairless skin. 7. Rotate the sites to prevent skin irritation.
B. Ophthalmic	1. Instruct the patient to lie supine, or sit with the head slightly tilted back. 2. With your nondominant hand, pull the patient's lower lid down gently to expose the conjunctival sac, creating a pocket. 3. Ask the patient to look upward. 4. Hold the eyedropper 1/4 to 1/8 inch above the conjunctival sac. Do not hold the dropper over the patient's eye because this may stimulate the blink reflex. 5. Instill the prescribed number of drops into the center of the pocket. Avoid touching the eye or conjunctival sac with the tip of the eyedropper. 6. If applying ointment, apply a thin line of ointment evenly along the inner edge of the lower lid margin, from inner to outer canthus. 7. Instruct the patient to gently close the eye. Apply gentle pressure with your finger to the nasolacrimal duct at the inner canthus for 1–2 minutes to avoid overflow drainage into the nose and throat. This minimizes the risk of absorption into the systemic circulation. 8. With a tissue, remove the excess medication from around the patient's eye. 9. Replace the dropper. Do not rinse the eyedropper.
C. Otic	1. Instruct the patient to lie on his or her side or to sit with the head tilted so that the affected ear is facing up. 2. If necessary, use a clean washcloth to clean the pinna of the ear and the meatus to prevent any discharge from being washed into the ear canal during the instillation of the drops. 3. Hold the dropper 1/4 inch above the ear canal, and instill the prescribed number of drops into the side of the ear canal, allowing the drops to flow downward. Avoid placing the drops directly on the tympanic membrane. 4. Gently apply intermittent pressure to the tragus of the ear three or four times. 5. Instruct the patient to remain on his or her side for up to 10 minutes to prevent loss of medication. 6. If cotton ball is ordered, presoak with medication and insert it into the outermost part of ear canal. 7. Wipe any solution that may have dripped from the ear canal with a tissue.
D. Nasal drops	1. Ask the patient to blow his or her nose to clear the nasal passages. 2. Draw up the correct volume of drug into the dropper. 3. Instruct the patient to open and breathe through the mouth. 4. Hold the tip of the dropper just above the patient's nostril and, without touching the nose with the dropper, direct the solution laterally toward the midline of the superior concha of the ethmoid bone—not the base of the nasal cavity, where it will run down the throat and into the eustachian tube. 5. Ask the patient to remain in this position for 5 minutes. 6. Discard any remaining solution that is in the dropper.
E. Vaginal	1. Instruct the patient to assume a dorsal recumbent position with her knees bent and separated. 2. Place water-soluble lubricant into a medicine cup. 3. Apply gloves; open the suppository and lubricate the rounded end. 4. Expose the vaginal orifice by separating the labia with your nondominant hand. 5. Insert the rounded end of the suppository about 8–10 cm along the posterior wall of the vagina, or as far as it will pass. 6. If using a cream, jelly, or foam, gently insert applicator 5 cm along the posterior vaginal wall and slowly push the plunger until empty. Remove the applicator and place on a paper towel. 7. Ask the patient to lower her legs and remain lying in the dorsal recumbent position for 5–10 minutes following insertion. Offer the patient a perineal pad.

TABLE 3.4 Topical Drug Administration—*Continued*

DRUG FORM	ADMINISTRATION GUIDELINES
F. Rectal suppositories	1. Instruct the patient to lie on the left side (Sims' position). 2. Apply gloves; open the suppository and lubricate the rounded end. 3. Lubricate the gloved forefinger of your dominant hand with water-soluble lubricant. 4. Inform the patient when the suppository is to be inserted; instruct the patient to take slow, deep breaths and deeply exhale during insertion to relax the anal sphincter. 5. Gently insert the lubricated end of the suppository into the rectum, beyond the anal-rectal ridge to ensure retention. 6. Instruct the patient to remain in the Sims' position or lie supine to prevent expulsion of the suppository. 7. Instruct the patient to retain the suppository for at least 30 minutes to allow absorption, unless the suppository is administered to stimulate defecation.

FIGURE 3.2

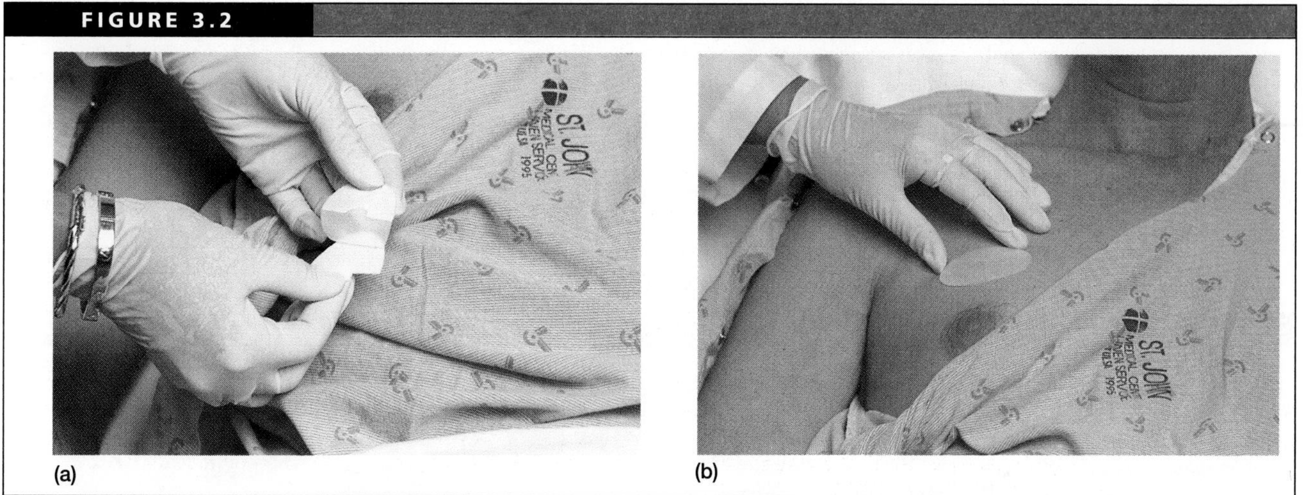

(a) (b)

Transdermal patch administration: Apply gloves before handling the patch and read the manufacturer's directions. Label the patch with the date and time and your initials. Remove any previous medication or patch, and cleanse the area. (a) Remove the protective coating from the patch and (b) apply the patch immediately to clean, dry, hairless skin.
SOURCE: Pearson Education/PH College

Nasal Administration

The nasal route, a **transmucosal** method of drug delivery is used for both local and systemic drug administration. The nasal mucosa provides an excellent absorptive surface for certain medications. Advantages of this route include ease of use and avoidance of the first-pass effect in the liver and the digestive enzymes. Nasal spray formulations of corticosteroids have revolutionized the treatment of allergic rhinitis because the medication is very safe when administered by this route.

Although the nasal mucosa provides an excellent surface for drug delivery, there is the potential for damage to the cilia within the nasal cavity, and mucosal irritation is common. In addition, unpredictable mucous secretion among some individuals may affect drug absorption from this site.

Drops or sprays are often used for their local **astringent effect,** which is to shrink swollen mucous membranes or to loosen secretions and facilitate drainage. This brings immediate relief from the nasal congestion caused by the common cold. The nose also provides the route to reach the nasal sinuses and the eustachian tube. Proper positioning of the patient prior to giving nose drops for sinus disorders depends on which sinuses are being treated. The same holds true for treatment of the eustachian tube. Table 3.4D and Figure 3.5 ■ illustrate important facts related to nasal drug administration.

FIGURE 3.3

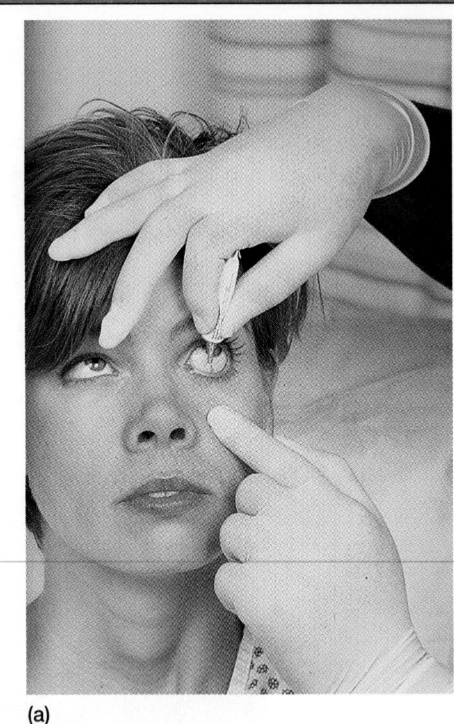

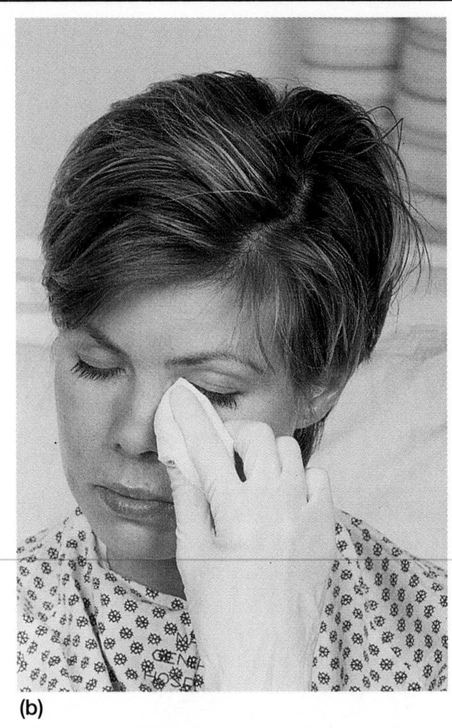

(a) (b)

Ophthalmic administration: (a) Pull the patient's lower lid down gently to expose the conjunctival sac. Have the patient look upward. Apply a thin line of eye ointment into the lower conjunctival sac. (b) Press gently on the nasolacrimal duct.
SOURCE: © Jenny Thomas Photography

FIGURE 3.4

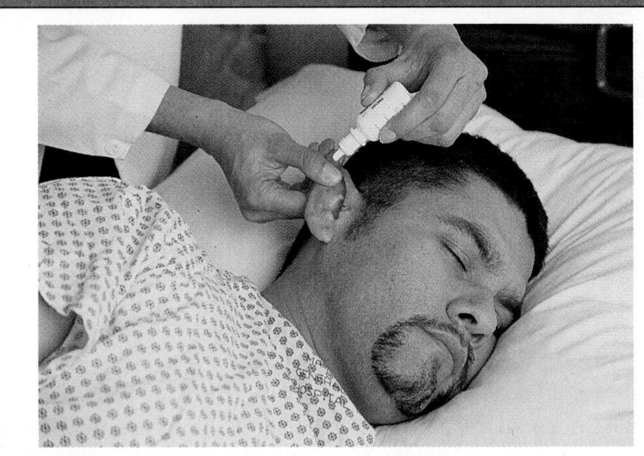

Otic drug administration: Instilling eardrops
SOURCE: © Elena Dorfman

Vaginal Administration

The vaginal route is used to deliver medications for treating local infections and to relieve vaginal pain and itching. Vaginal medications are inserted as suppositories, creams, jellies, or foams. It is important that the nurse explains the purpose of treatment and provides privacy for the patient. Before inserting vaginal drugs, the nurse should instruct the patient to empty her bladder. This lessens both the discomfort during treatment and the possibility of irritating or injuring the vaginal lining. The patient should be offered a perineal pad following administration. Table 3.4E and Figure 3.6 ■ provide guidelines regarding vaginal drug administration.

Rectal Administration

The rectal route may be used for either local or systemic drug administration. It is a safe and effective means of delivering drugs to patients who are comatose or who are experiencing nausea and vomiting. Rectal drugs are normally in suppository form, although a few laxatives and diagnostic agents are given via enema. Although absorption is slower than by other routes, it is steady

FIGURE 3.5

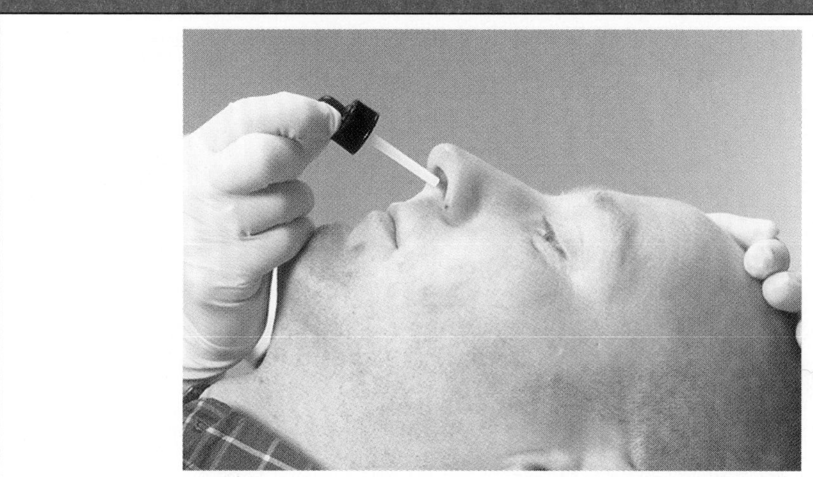

Nasal drug administration
SOURCE: Pearson Education/PH College

FIGURE 3.6

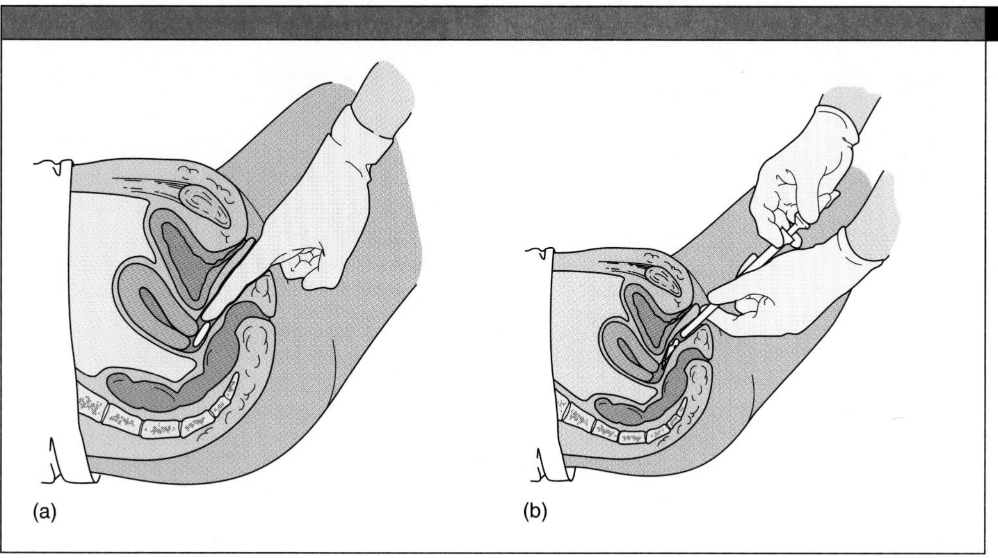

Vaginal drug administration: (a) instilling a vaginal suppository; (b) using an applicator to instill a vaginal cream
SOURCE: Pearson Education/PH College

and reliable as long as the medication can be retained by the patient. Venous blood from the lower rectum is not transported by way of the liver. Therefore, the first-pass effect is avoided, as are the digestive enzymes of the upper GI tract. Table 3.4F gives details about rectal drug administration.

3.9 Parenteral administration refers to dispensing medications by routes other than oral or topical.

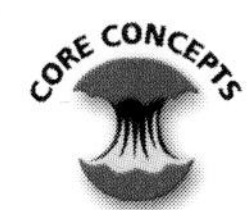

The **parenteral route** delivers drugs via a needle into the skin layers, subcutaneous tissue, muscles, or veins, with the needle angled at different degrees, depending on the type of injection, as shown in Figure 3.7 ■. More advanced parenteral delivery includes administration into arteries, body cavities (such as intrathecal), and organs (such as intracardiac). Parenteral drug administration is much more invasive (meaning that the delivery method "invades" the barrier that the skin provides to protect the body) than topical or enteral administration. Because of the possibility of introducing pathogenic microbes directly into the blood or body tissues, aseptic techniques must be strictly used. The nurse is expected to identify and use appropriate materials for parenteral drug delivery, including specialized equipment and techniques involved in the preparation and administration of injectable products. The nurse must know the correct anatomical locations for parenteral administration and safety procedures regarding hazardous equipment disposal.

FIGURE 3.7

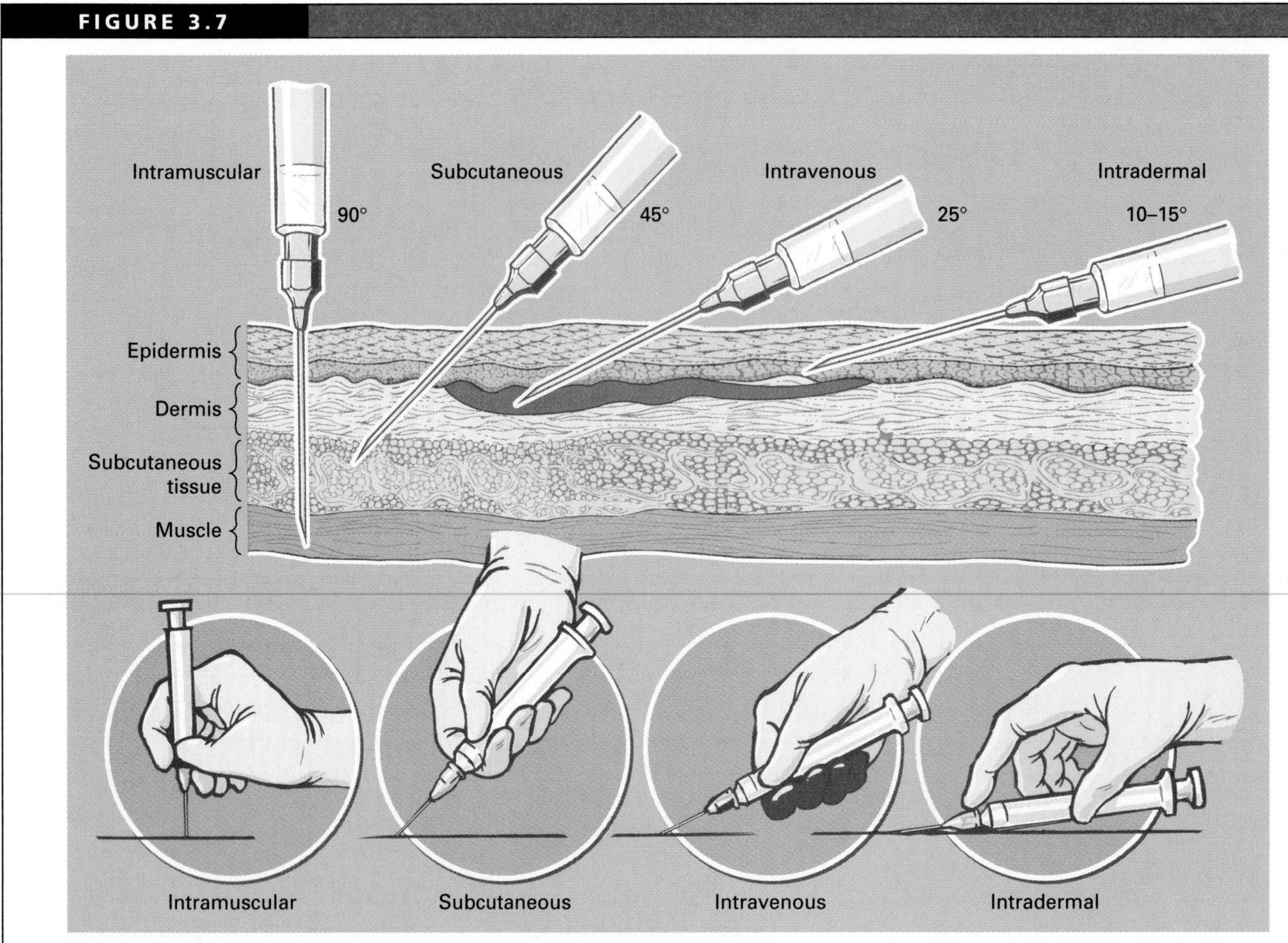

Parenteral drug administration: Gloves are worn for all parenteral drug administration. During intramuscular administration, a drug is injected into muscle at a 90° angle. Subcutaneous administration is into the subcutaneous tissue at a 45° angle. Intravenous administration is directly into the bloodstream and is done at a 25° angle. Intradermal administration is into the dermis at a 10°–15° angle. *SOURCE: Pearson Education/PH College.*

Intradermal and Subcutaneous Administration

Injection into the skin delivers drugs to the blood vessels that supply the layers of the skin. Drugs may be injected either intradermally or subcutaneously. The major difference between these methods is the depth of injection, which is controlled by the angle of needle placement (see Figure 3.7). An advantage of both methods is that they offer a means of administering drugs to patients who are unable to take them orally. Drugs administered by these routes avoid the first-pass effect in the liver and the digestive enzymes. Disadvantages are that only small volumes can be administered, and injections can cause pain and swelling at the injection site.

An **intradermal (ID) route** injection is administered into the dermis layer of the skin. Because the dermis contains more blood vessels than the deeper subcutaneous layer, drugs are more easily absorbed. This route is usually used for allergy and disease screening or for local anesthetic delivery prior to venous cannulation. Only very small volumes of drug, usually only 0.1 to 0.2 ml, can be given by ID injections. The usual sites for ID injections are the nonhairy skin surfaces of the upper back, over the scapulae, the high upper chest, and the anterior forearm. Guidelines for intradermal injections are given in Table 3.5A and Figure 3.8 ■.

A **subcutaneous (SC** or **SQ) route** injection is delivered to the deepest layers of the skin. Insulin, heparin, vitamins, some vaccines, and other medications are given in this area because the sites are easy to reach and provide rapid absorption. Body sites that are ideal for subcutaneous injections include the following:

- Posterior upper arm (above the triceps muscle)
- Middle two thirds of the anterior thigh area

- Subscapular areas of the upper back
- Upper dorsogluteal and ventrogluteal areas
- Abdominal areas, above the iliac crest and below the diaphragm, 2 inches out from the umbilicus

Subcutaneous doses are small in volume, usually ranging from 0.5 to 1 ml, and are given at a 45° (normal weight patient) to 90° angle (obese patient). The needle size varies with the patient's quantity of body fat but is usually 1/2 inch to 5/8 inch. The needle length is usually one half the size of a pinched/bunched skinfold that can be grasped between the thumb and forefinger. It is important to rotate injection sites in an orderly and documented manner, to promote absorption, minimize tissue damage, and alleviate discomfort. For insulin, however, rotation should be within an anatomical area that promotes reliable absorption and maintains consistent blood

TABLE 3.5 Parenteral Drug Administration

DRUG FORM	ADMINISTRATION GUIDELINES
A. Intradermal route	1. Prepare the medication in a tuberculin or 1 ml syringe, using a 25–27 gauge, 3/8–5/8 inch needle. 2. Apply gloves and cleanse the injection site with an antiseptic swab, using a circular motion. Allow the site to air dry. 3. With the thumb and index finger of your nondominant hand, spread the patient's skin taut. 4. Insert the needle, with the bevel facing upward, at a 10°–15° angle. 5. Advance the needle until the entire bevel is under the skin; do not aspirate. 6. Slowly inject the medication to form a small wheal or bleb (small raised area). 7. Withdraw the needle quickly, and pat the site gently with a sterile 2 × 2 gauze pad. Do not massage the area. 8. Instruct the patient not to rub or scratch the area.
B. Subcutaneous route	1. Prepare the medication in a 1–3 ml syringe using a 23–25 gauge, 1/2–5/8 inch needle. For heparin, the recommended needle is 3/8 inch and 25–26 gauge. 2. Choose the site, avoiding bony areas, major nerves, and blood vessels. For heparin, check your facility's policy for the preferred injection sites. 3. Check the previous rotation sites and select a new area for injection. 4. Apply gloves and cleanse the injection site with an antiseptic swab using a circular motion. 5. Allow the site to air dry. 6. Bunch the skin between the thumb and index finger of your nondominant hand. 7. Insert the needle at 45° or 90°, depending on the patient's body size and the length of the needle you are using: 90° for obese patients; 45° degrees for average-weight patients. 8. For nonheparin injections, aspirate by pulling back on the plunger. If blood appears, withdraw the needle, discard the syringe, and prepare a new injection. For heparin, do not aspirate, because aspiration can damage surrounding tissues and cause bruising. 9. Inject the medication slowly. 10. Remove the needle quickly. Gently massage the site with an antiseptic swab. *For heparin or insulin, do not massage the site, because bruising or bleeding may occur.*
C. Intramuscular route: ventrogluteal site	1. Prepare the medication using a 20–23 gauge, 1.5 inch needle. (Needle size may vary depending on the site and patient site.) 2. Apply gloves and cleanse the injection site with an antiseptic swab using a circular motion. Allow the site to air dry. 3. Locate the site by placing your hand with the heel on the greater trochanter and your thumb pointing toward the umbilicus. Point to the anterior iliac spine with your index finger, spreading your middle finger to point toward the iliac crest (forming a V). Injection of medication is given within the V-shaped area of the index and third finger. 4. Insert the needle with a smooth, dartlike movement at a 90° angle within the V-shaped area. 5. Aspirate, and observe for blood. If blood appears, withdraw the needle, discard the syringe, and prepare a new injection. 6. Inject the medication slowly and with smooth, even pressure on the plunger. 7. Remove the needle quickly. 8. Apply pressure to the site with a dry, sterile 2 × 2 gauze and gently massage to promote absorption of the medication into the muscle.

(continued)

TABLE 3.5	Parenteral Drug Administration—*Continued*
DRUG FORM	**ADMINISTRATION GUIDELINES**
D. Intravenous route	1. To add a drug to an IV fluid container: a. Verify the order and compatibility of the drug with the IV fluid. b. Prepare the medication in a 5–20 ml syringe using a 1–1.5 inch, 19–21 gauge needle. c. Apply your gloves and assess the injection site for signs and symptoms of inflammation or extravasation (oozing of tissue). d. Locate the medication port on the IV fluid container and cleanse it with an antiseptic swab. e. Carefully insert the needle or access device into the port and inject the medication. f. Withdraw the needle and mix the solution by rotating the container end to end. g. Hang the container and check the infusion rate. 2. To add drug to an IV bolus (IV push) using an existing IV line or IV lock (reseal): a. Verify the order and compatibility of the drug with the IV fluid. b. Determine the correct rate of infusion. c. Determine if IV fluids are infusing at the proper rate (IV line) and that the IV site is adequate. d. Prepare the drug in a syringe with a 19–21 gauge needle. e. Apply your gloves and assess the injection site for signs and symptoms of inflammation or extravasation (oozing of tissue). f. Select an injection port on the tubing that is closest to the insertion site (IV line). g. Cleanse the tubing or lock port with an antiseptic swab and insert the needle into the port. h. If administering medication through an existing IV line, occlude the tubing by pinching it just above the injection port. i. Slowly inject the medication over the designated time (which is not usually faster that 1 ml/min, unless otherwise specified). j. Withdraw the syringe. Release the tubing and ensure the proper IV infusion if using an existing IV line. k. If using an IV lock, check your facility's policy for use of saline flush before and after injecting medications.

glucose levels. When performing subcutaneous injections, it is not necessary to aspirate prior to the injection. Note that tuberculin syringes and insulin syringes are not interchangeable, and should not be substituted for each other. Table 3.5B and Figure 3.9 ■ include important information regarding subcutaneous drug administration.

Intramuscular Administration

An **intramuscular (IM) route** injection delivers medication into specific muscles. Because muscle tissue has a rich blood supply, medication moves quickly into blood vessels to produce a more rapid onset of action than with oral, ID, or SC administration. The anatomical structure of muscle permits this tissue to receive a larger volume of medication than the subcutaneous region. An adult with well-developed muscles can safely tolerate up to 5 ml of medication in a large muscle, although only 2 to 3 ml is recommended. The deltoid and triceps muscles should receive a maximum of 1 ml.

A major consideration for the nurse regarding IM drug administration is the selection of an appropriate injection site. Injection sites must be located away from bone, large blood vessels, and nerves. Both the size and length of the needle are determined by body size and muscle mass, the type of drug to be administered, the amount of adipose (fat) tissue overlying the muscle, and the age of the patient. Information regarding IM injections is given in Table 3.5C and Figure 3.10 ■. The four common sites for intramuscular injections are as follows:

Life Span Fact

The ventrogluteal site is a suitable site of IM injection for children and infants over 7 months of age.

- *Ventrogluteal site.* This area provides the greatest thickness of gluteal muscles, contains no large blood vessels or nerves, is sealed off by bone, and contains less fat than the buttock area, thus eliminating the need to determine the depth of subcutaneous fat.

(a) (b) (c) (d)

FIGURE 3.8

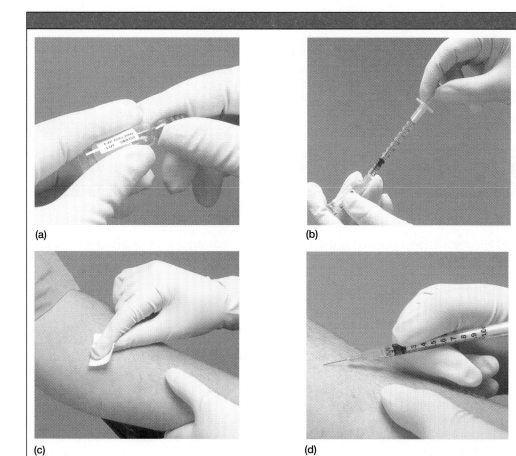

Intradermal administration: (a) The medication is checked. (b) The medication vial is held nearly vertical at eye level, and the drug is drawn into the syringe. (c) The administration site is prepared. (d) The needle is inserted, bevel up at 10°–15°. After administration, a 2 × 2 gauze pad is used to gently pat the site dry. *SOURCE: Pearson Education/PH College*

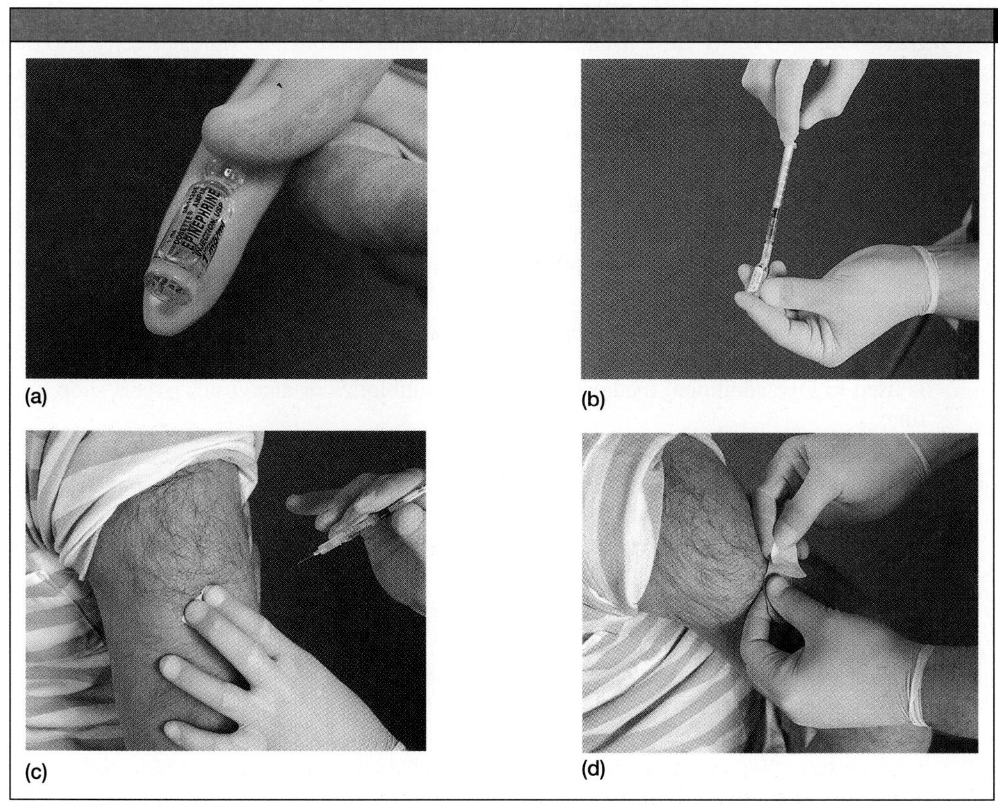

FIGURE 3.9

Subcutaneous administration: (a) The medication is checked. (b) With the vial held nearly vertical at eye level, the medication is drawn into the syringe. (c) The administration site is prepared and the needle is inserted at a 45° angle. (d) The needle is removed, and the puncture site is covered with an adhesive bandage. *SOURCE: Pearson Education/PH College*

FIGURE 3.10

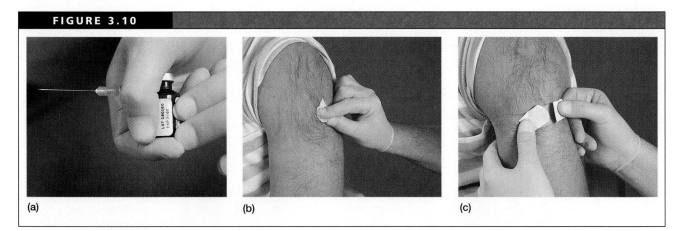

(a) (b) (c)

Intramuscular administration: (a) The medication is checked and drawn. (b) The administration site is prepared and the needle is inserted at a 90° angle. (c) The needle is removed and the puncture site is covered with an adhesive bandage.
SOURCE: Pearson Education/PH College

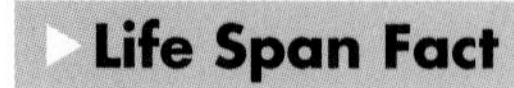

The vastus lateralis is the site of choice for IM injections in pediatric patients.

- *Deltoid site.* Used in well-developed teens and adults for volumes of medication not to exceed 1 ml.
- *Dorsogluteal site.* Used for adults and for children who have been walking for at least 6 months. The site is safe as long as the nurse appropriately locates the injection landmarks to avoid puncture or irritation of the sciatic nerve and blood vessels.
- *Vastus lateralis site.* Usually thick and well developed in both adults and children, the middle third of the muscle is the site for IM injections.

Intravenous Administration

The **intravenous (IV) route** involves administration of medications and fluids directly into the bloodstream and allows their immediate availability for use by the body. The IV route is used when a very rapid onset of action is desired. Like other parenteral routes, IV medications bypass the enzymes of the digestive system and the first-pass effect of the liver. The three basic types of IV administration are as follows:

- *Large-volume infusion.* This type of infusion is used for fluid maintenance, replacement, or supplementation. Compatible drugs may be mixed into a large-volume IV container with fluids such as normal saline or Ringer's lactate. Table 3.5D and Figure 3.11 ■ illustrate this technique.
- *Intermittent infusion.* A small amount of IV solution is "piggy-backed" (added) to the primary large-volume infusion. This type of infusion, illustrated in Figure 3.12 ■, is used to give additional medications such as antibiotics or analgesics over a short time.
- *IV bolus (push) administration.* A concentrated single dose of medication is delivered directly to the circulation via syringe. Bolus injections may be given through an intermittent injection port or by direct IV push. Details on the bolus administration technique are given in Table 3.5D and Figure 3.13 ■.

Although the IV route provides the fastest onset of drug action, it is also the most dangerous. Once injected, the medication cannot be retrieved. If the drug solution or the needle is contaminated, pathogens have a direct route to the bloodstream and body tissues. Patients who are receiving IV injections must be closely monitored for adverse reactions. Some adverse reactions occur immediately after injection; others may take hours or days to appear. Antidotes for drugs that can cause potentially dangerous or fatal reactions must always be readily available. Several types of needleless IV systems are also available and have been shown to greatly reduce the chance of needlestick injuries among healthcare professionals.

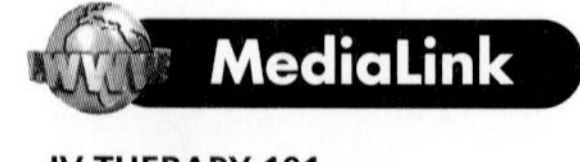

IV THERAPY 101

FIGURE 3.11

(a)

(b)

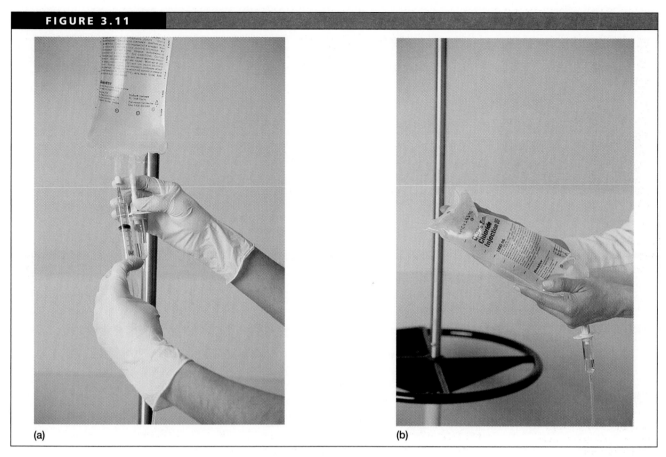

Adding a drug to an existing infusion: (a) inserting a drug through the injection port of an infusion container; (b) rotating the IV bag to distribute the drug *SOURCE: © Elena Dorfman*

FIGURE 3.12

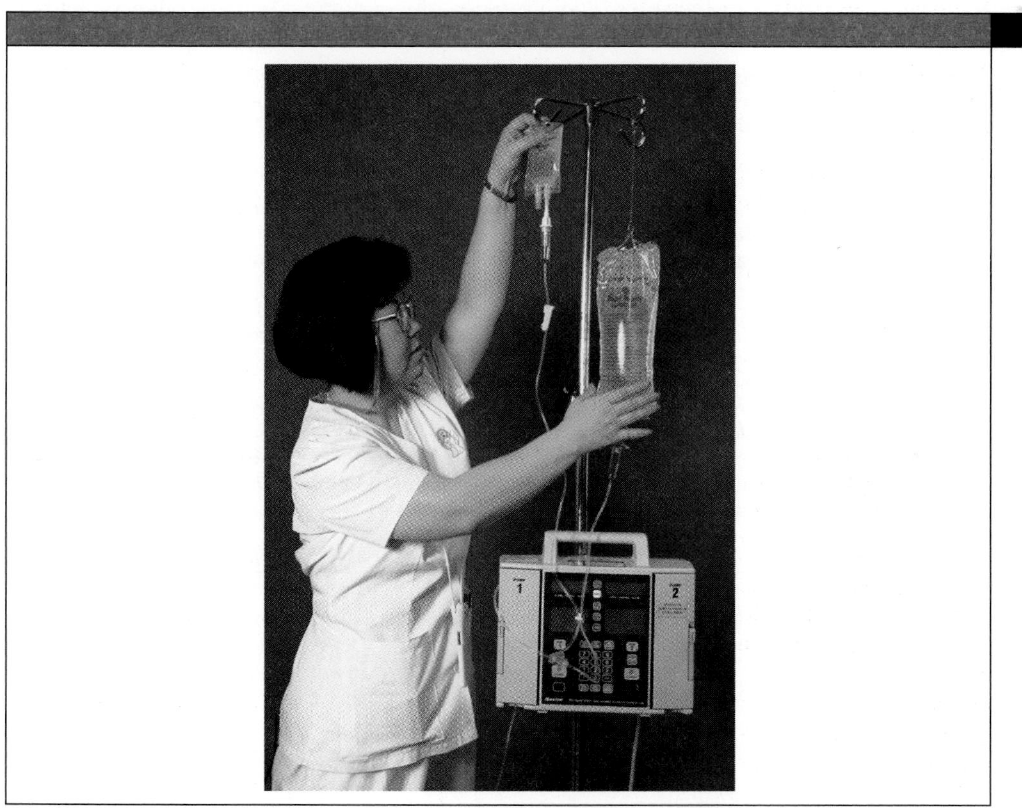

An intermittent IV infusion given piggyback to the primary infusion

SOURCE: Pearson Education/PH College

FIGURE 3.13

(a) (b) (c) (d)

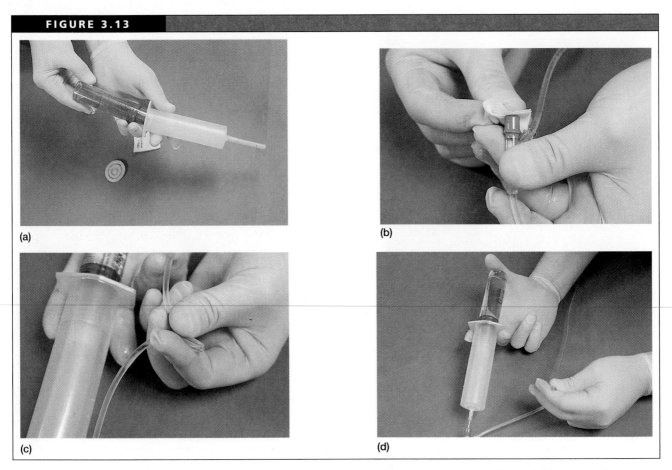

Intravenous bolus administration: (a) The drug is prepared. (b) The administration port is cleaned. (c) The line is pinched. (d) The drug is administered. *SOURCE: Pearson Education/PH College*

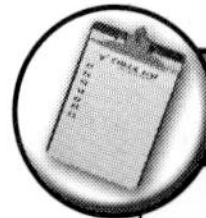

PATIENTS NEED TO KNOW

Patients need to know the following:

1. Always ask the healthcare practitioner or pharmacist which medication may be taken with food and water to reduce nausea and stomach irritation.
2. Do not crush, cut, or administer enteric-coated tablets with alkaline substances such as antacids.
3. Establish a routine for taking medications by selecting a familiar time of the day, usually at an hourly interval. Special organizers can be obtained to properly store medicines according to times, days, and dosages.
4. Follow the dosing times exactly. If a medication is missed, do not try to "catch up" on the next scheduled dose. If remembered soon, it is appropriate to take the medicine. Otherwise, wait until the next scheduled dose. An exception would be if the next dose is not scheduled until the next day. For answers to specific questions, consult a healthcare provider.
5. Store medications in a safe, dry place. Discard them if they become old or outdated.
6. Use the measuring device provided by the drug manufacturer to take medications. Do not rely on kitchen utensils to judge the exact recommended dose. ■

CHAPTER REVIEW

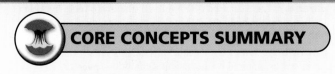

CORE CONCEPTS SUMMARY

3.1 **A major goal in pharmacotherapy is to limit the number and severity of adverse drug events.**

Healthcare staff must be familiar with the general principles of drug delivery. The nurse must have a comprehensive knowledge of the actions and side effects of drugs before they are administered, to limit the number and severity of adverse drugs events. Allergic and anaphylactic reactions are serious effects that must be carefully monitored and prevented, when possible.

3.2 **The rights of drug administration form the basis of proper drug delivery.**

The six rights and three checks are guidelines to safe drug administration, which is a collaborative effort among nurses, physicians, and other healthcare professionals. The six rights are right patient, right medication, right dose, right route of administration, right time of delivery, and right documentation. The three checks are checking the MAR, checking the drug during preparation, and checking the drug before administering it to the patient.

3.3 **Successful pharmacotherapy depends on patient compliance.**

For pharmacological compliance, the patient must understand and personally accept the value of the prescribed drug regimen. Understanding the reasons for noncompliance can help the healthcare team increase the success of pharmacotherapy.

3.4 **Healthcare providers use accepted abbreviations to communicate the directions and times for drug administration.**

There are established orders and time schedules by which medications are routinely administered. The single order (such as a preoperative order) is for a drug that is to be given only once and at a specific time. A prn order is administered as required by the patient's condition. Orders not written as STAT, ASAP, NOW, or prn are called routine orders. A standing order is written in advance of a situation and is to be carried out under specific circumstances. Documenting drug administration and reporting side effects are important responsibilities of the nurse.

3.5 **Three systems of measurement are used in pharmacology: metric, apothecary, and household.**

Healthcare professionals must recognize dosages based on all three systems of measurement: the metric, apothecary, and household systems. The nurse must be able to convert between household and metric systems of measurement.

3.6 **Certain protocols and techniques are common to all methods of drug administration.**

The student should understand drug administration guidelines before proceeding to a study of specific drug administration routes. The three general routes of drug administration are enteral, topical, and parenteral.

3.7 **Enteral drugs are given orally or via nasogastric or gastrostomy tubes.**

The enteral route includes drugs given orally and those administered through nasogastric (NG) or gastrostomy (G) tubes. The enteral route is the most effective way to administer drugs.

3.8 **Topical drugs are applied locally to the skin and associated membranes.**

Topical drugs are applied locally to the skin or membranous linings of the eye, ear, nose, respiratory tract, urinary tract, vagina, and rectum.

3.9 **Parenteral administration refers to dispensing medications by routes other than oral or topical.**

Parenteral administration is the dispensing of medications via a needle, usually into the skin layers (ID), subcutaneous tissue (SC or SQ), muscles (IM), or veins (IV).

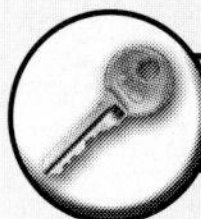

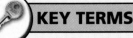

KEY TERMS

allergic reaction: a hyperresponse of body tissues to a foreign substance (allergen), in which patients experience uncomfortable and potentially serious symptoms including difficulty breathing, pain, swelling, skin rash, and other unfavorable signs / ***page 25***

anaphylaxis (ANN-ah-fah-LAX-iss): an acute allergic response to an antigen that results in severe hypotension and may cause death if untreated / ***page 26***

apothecary system of measurement (ah-POTH-eh-karee-ee): former system of weights and measures used by healthcare providers and pharmacists; replaced by the metric system / ***page 29***

ASAP order: means as soon as possible; a physician's order referring to the time frame that is often defined as less than 30 minutes / ***page 28***

astringent effect (ah-STRIN-jent): the skrinkage of swollen membranes or binding together of body surface material / ***page 35***

buccal route (BUCK-ahl): the administration of medications by the cheek or mouth / ***page 32***

compliance (kom-PLY-ans): taking a medication in the way it was prescribed by the practitioner; in the case of OTC drugs, following the instructions found on the label / ***page 26***

enteral route (EN-tur-ul): the major route by which drugs enter the body through the digestive tract / ***page 30***

enteric coated (in-TARE-ik): hard, waxy coating that enables drugs to resist the acidity of the stomach; these drug dissolve in the small intestine / ***page 30***

household system of measurement: older system of measurement involving teaspoons, tablespoons, cups, drops, pounds, etc. / ***page 29***

intradermal (ID) route (IN-trah-DERM-ul): method of parenteral drug delivery in which drugs are injected into the dermis of the skin / ***page 38***

intramuscular (IM) route (IN-trah-musk-u-lar): method of parenteral drug delivery in which drugs are injected into layers of muscle beneath the skin / ***page 40***

intravenous (IV) route (IN-trah-VEE-nus): method of parenteral drug delivery in which drugs are injected into the venous circulation / ***page 42***

metric system of measurement: the most common system of measurement involving kilograms (kg), grams (g), milligrams (mg), or micrograms (mcg), etc. / ***page 29***

parenteral route (pah-REN-tur-ul): the major route by which drugs enter the body other than the enteral or topical route / ***page 37***

prn order: Latin: *pro re nata;* physician's order; means to administer as required by the patient's condition / ***page 28***

routine order: standard order usually carried out within 2 hours of the time it was written by the physician / ***page 28***

single order: a physician's order for a drug that is to be given only once and at a specific time; an example is a preoperative order / ***page 28***

six rights of drug administration: practical guidelines for nurses to use during drug preparation, delivery, and administration of drugs / ***page 26***

standing order: a physician's order written in advance of a situation, which is to be carried out under specific circumstances / ***page 28***

STAT order: comes from *statim,* the Latin word meaning "immediately"; the time frame between writing the STAT order and administering the drug may be 5 minutes or less, depending on facility rules / ***page 28***

subcutaneous (SC or SQ) route (sub-kew-TAY-nee-us): method of parenteral drug delivery in which drugs are injected into the hypodermis of the skin / ***page 38***

sublingual (SL) route (sub-LIN-gwal): method of enteral drug delivery in which drugs are placed under the tongue / ***page 32***

sustained release: tablets or capsules that are designed to dissolve very slowly / ***page 31***

three checks of drug administration: nurses use these checks together with the six rights to help ensure patient safety and drug effectiveness / ***page 26***

topical route (TOP-ik-ul): the route by which drugs are placed directly onto the skin and associated membranes / ***page 33***

transdermal (trans-DER-mul): method of drug delivery, usually by a patch, in which drugs are absorbed across the layers of the skin for the purpose of entering the bloodstream / ***page 33***

transmucosal (trans-mew-KOH-sul): method of topical drug delivery in which drugs are applied directly to mucosal membranes, including the nasal and respiratory pathways and vagina / ***page 35***

REVIEW QUESTIONS

The following questions are written in NCLEX-PN® style. Answer these questions to assess your knowledge of the chapter material, and go back and review any material that is not clear to you.

1. A nurse enters the patient's room with an intravenous (IV) pole, special tubing, stethoscope, fairly large-looking syringe and plunger, and special container of formula. He explains that in the course of treatment, he will use all of these items. From your understanding of drug administration, which of the following therapies is he likely explaining?

1. Transdermal
2. Intravenous (parenteral)
3. Nasogastric (enteral)
4. Rectal

2. The main reason why extended-release medications must not be crushed is:

1. They are very distasteful, and this reduces patient compliance.
2. Crushing alters the rate of absorption and medication delivery.

3. Multiple drug pieces cause obstructive symptoms.
4. Crushed oral medications have reduced bioavailability.

3. One reason why it is necessary to aspirate the needle during an intramuscular injection is to:

1. Avoid placement of the needle into a blood vessel
2. Produce an air pocket for better drug distribution
3. Avoid nerve puncture
4. Remove air from the syringe

4. Which of the following routes of drug administration has the fastest onset of action?

1. Transdermal
2. Intramuscular
3. Intravenous
4. Ophthalmic

5. Which of the following orders should be carried out within 30 minutes (or per agency policy) of the written order?

1. STAT order
2. ASAP order
3. prn order
4. Standing order

6. It is often taught that the nurse should check the label three times during the course of administering a medication: before getting the medication out of the container or drawer, before placing it into the medication cup, and before administering the medication or when placing the stock bottle back on the shelf. Of the "six rights of drug administration," this example mainly refers to which "right"?

1. Right medication
2. Right dose
3. Right route of administration
4. Right time of delivery

7. Drug administration abbreviations shown in Table 3.1 mostly refer to which of the "six rights of drug administration"?

1. Right medication
2. Right dose
3. Right route of administration
4. Right time of delivery

8. The medication administration record (MAR) contains all of the following information EXCEPT:

1. Date of medication administration
2. Route of drug administration
3. Dose of medication
4. Apothecary system of drug measurement

In questions 9–12, match the abbreviation with the proper meaning in answers 1–4.

9. qh

10. qhs

11. qid

12. qod

1. This abbreviation should not be used. Instead write out "every other day."
2. Every hour.
3. The abbreviation should not be used. Instead, write out "nightly."
4. Four times per day.

FURTHER STUDY

- Chapter 19 discusses the pharmacotherapy of allergic reactions and anaphylaxis.
- Chapter 4 discusses how pharmacokinetic considerations, such as the route of administration, affect drug absorption and distribution.
- First-pass metabolism is discussed in Chapter 4.

EXPLORE MEDIALINK www.prenhall.com/holland

Additional resources for this chapter can be found on the CD-ROM accompanying this textbook, and on the Companion Website. Click on Chapter 3 to select activities for this chapter.

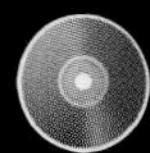

Audio Glossary
Concept Review
NCLEX-PN® Review
Nursing in Action
Dosage Calculator

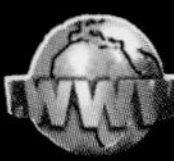

Abbreviations for Safe Medication Administration
Nasogastric/Gastrostomy Therapy
IV Therapy 101

CHAPTER

4 What Happens After a Drug Has Been Administered

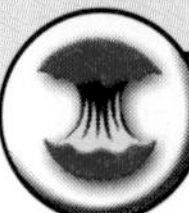

CORE CONCEPTS

4.1 Pharmacokinetics focuses on what the body does to the drugs.

4.2 Absorption is the first step in drug transport.

4.3 Distribution represents how drugs are transported throughout the body.

4.4 Metabolism is a process whereby drugs are made less or more active.

4.5 Excretion processes remove drugs from the body.

4.6 The rate of elimination and half-life characteristics influence drug responsiveness.

4.7 Pharmacodynamics focuses on what the drugs do to the body.

4.8 Drugs activate specific receptors to produce a response.

4.9 *Potency* and *efficacy* are terms often used to describe the success of drug therapy.

OBJECTIVES

After reading this chapter, the student should be able to:

1. Identify the four major processes of pharmacokinetics.
2. Discuss the factors affecting drug absorption.
3. Describe how plasma proteins affect drug distribution.
4. Explain the significance of the blood-brain barrier, blood-placental barrier, and blood-testicular barrier to drug therapy.
5. Explain the importance of the first-pass effect.
6. Describe how metabolic enzymes differ in younger and in older patients, and explain the significance of this difference to the success of drug therapy.
7. Explain how intermediate products of drug metabolism may produce a more intense response than the original drug.
8. Identify the major processes by which drugs are eliminated from the body.
9. Explain the importance of enterohepatic recirculation to drug therapy.
10. Explain how rate of elimination and plasma half-life ($t_{1/2}$) are related to the duration of drug action.
11. Discuss how successful pharmacotherapy depends on principles of pharmacodynamics.
12. Explain the significance of the receptor theory.
13. Describe how "blockers" of drug action work.
14. Compare and contrast the therapeutic terms *potency* and *efficacy.*

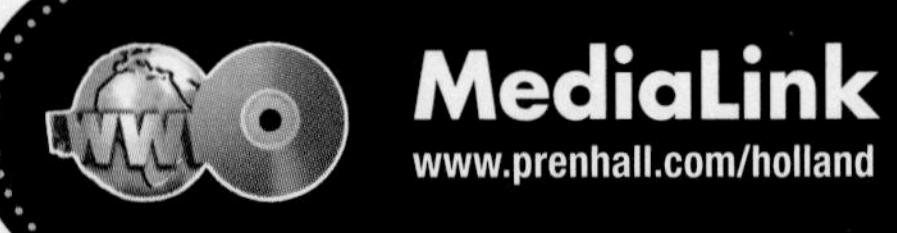

Interactive resources for this chapter can be found on the Companion Website. Click on Chapter 4 and "Begin" to select the activities for this chapter. For chapter-related animations, NCLEX-PN®-style questions, and an audio glossary, access the accompanying CD-ROM in this book.

Drugs do not affect all patients the same way. Whether a drug achieves or falls short of achieving a therapeutic response is an important concern to patients and healthcare professionals. Within a population, a dose of medication may produce a dramatic response in one patient while having no effect in another.

Many situations alter a drug's response. Patients sometimes take medications under conditions that interfere with drug activity. This interference is called a *drug interaction.* Well-known examples of food-drug interactions may occur when patients take their medication with food or beverages. Patients often take more than one medication at the same time. After drugs have been absorbed, the effectiveness of drug therapy may be altered by drug-drug interactions in the bloodstream.

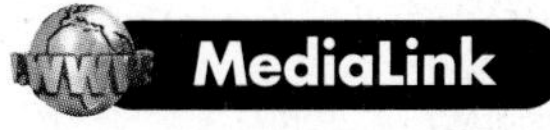

COUNCIL ON FAMILY HEALTH

To understand the impact that drug interactions have on drug safety and effectiveness, one must understand concepts from two important areas: pharmacokinetics and pharmacodynamics.

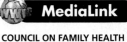

4.1 Pharmacokinetics focuses on what the body does to the drugs.

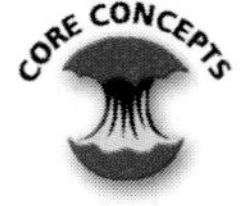

As the root words indicate, **pharmacokinetics** focuses on how drugs move within the body. Drug movement involves four processes: absorption, distribution, metabolism, and excretion, as shown in Figure 4.1 ■. A thorough knowledge of pharmacokinetics enables the healthcare provider to

pharmaco = *drug related*
kinetics = *movement*

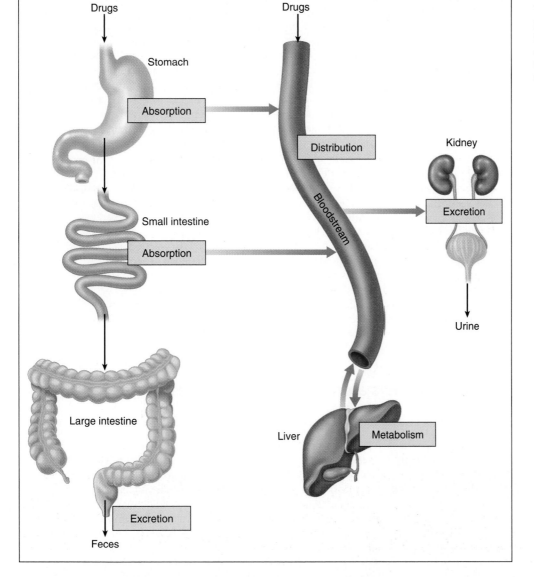

FIGURE 4.1

The four processes of pharmacokinetics (drug movement) are absorption, metabolism, distribution, and excretion.

understand the therapeutic effects of a drug, as well as to predict potential adverse effects of drug therapy.

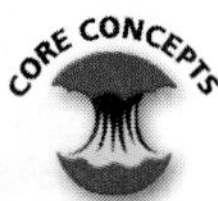

4.2 Absorption is the first step in drug transport.

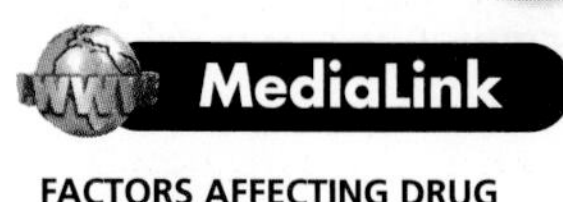

FACTORS AFFECTING DRUG ABSORPTION

Absorption is the first step in how the body handles a drug. Absorption is a process involving the movement of a substance from its site of administration across one or more body membranes. A drug may be absorbed locally and produce a biological effect at a remote site. Absorption may occur across the skin and associated mucous membranes, or drugs may move across membranes that line blood vessels. Ultimately most drugs move across many membranes to reach their target cells. Many basic science textbooks cover the ways that foods and drugs are absorbed including passive transport and energy-requiring transport processes. The presence of food in the digestive tract will slow the absorption of drugs.

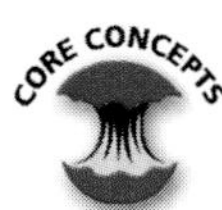

4.3 Distribution represents how drugs are transported throughout the body.

Distribution is the process by which drugs are transported after they have been absorbed or administered directly into the bloodstream. Between the site of drug administration and target tissue, there are many factors that affect drug movement. One important example is the *binding* that occurs between drugs and other substances, such as plasma proteins, already present in the bloodstream. When a drug binds with a plasma protein such as albumin, the drug is held by the plasma protein in the bloodstream where it is unable to reach its target cells. Often, a second drug will interfere with this binding by displacing the first drug from the plasma protein. In this case, the first drug's activity is intensified. The term *bioavailability* is often used to describe how much of a drug will be available after administration to produce a biological effect.

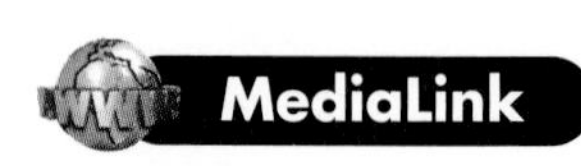

PREGNANCY

Even if a drug is not bound by plasma proteins, it still may not be able to reach all body tissues. Three important organs contain anatomical barriers that prevent some drugs from gaining access. These are the brain, the placenta, and the testes. Even though these organs have a larger blood supply compared to most other organs in the body, their cellular barriers only allow fat-soluble substances to cross. These special barriers are called the *blood-brain barrier, blood-placental barrier,* and *blood-testicular barrier.*

Some drugs are able to cross the blood-brain barrier without difficulty. These include antianxiety drugs, sedatives (sleep-inducing), and psychoactive (or mind-altering) drugs. Other medications, such as many antibiotics and anticancer medications, are absorbed easily from the intestinal tract, but they do not easily cross into the brain.

The blood-placental barrier serves an important protective function because it regulates which substances pass from the mother's bloodstream to the fetus. However, many potentially damaging agents such as cocaine and alcohol and even some prescription or OTC medications are not prevented from crossing this barrier. This is an extremely important issue: All food items and therapeutic drugs should be evaluated to assess their adverse effects on pregnant women and their unborn children, as discussed in Chapter 2 . The blood-testicular barrier prevents many drugs from reaching the male testes, making it difficult to treat testicular disorders.

4.4 Metabolism is a process whereby drugs are made less or more active.

Metabolism is the next step in pharmacokinetics. It is often described as the total of all chemical reactions in the body. Metabolism occurs in almost every cell and organ—including the intestinal tract and kidneys—but the liver is the primary site. The individual chemical reactions of metabolism are called **biotransformation** reactions: They are the chemical conversion of drugs from one form to another that may result in increased or decreased activity. Metabolism is important to drug therapy because these chemical reactions deactivate most drugs. Also, patients with liver disease usually receive much lower doses than normal because their liver is unable to metabolize the drug to a safe, active form.

bio = *biological*
transformation = *changing process*

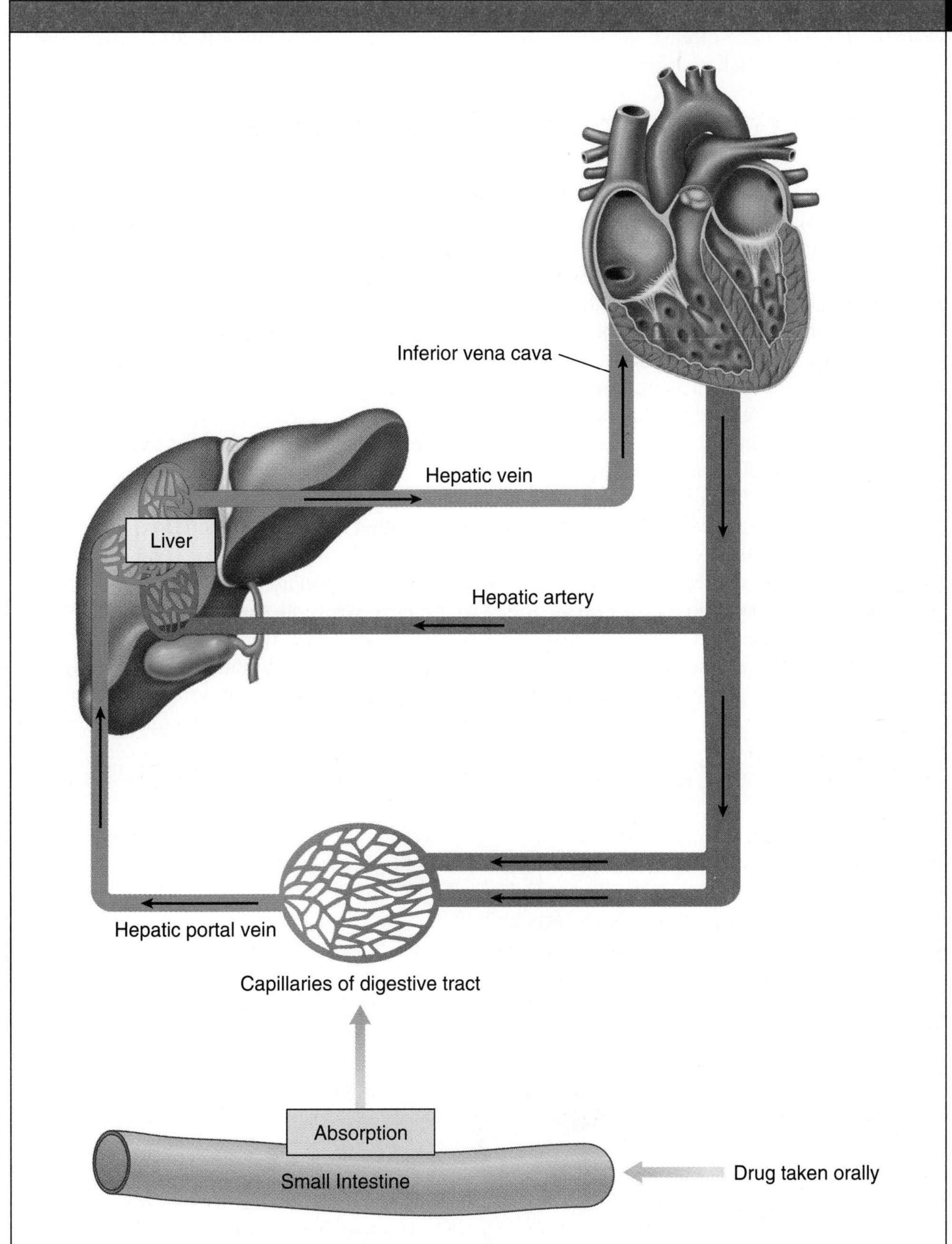

FIGURE 4.2

First-pass effect: Drugs given orally are absorbed through the intestinal wall and enter the hepatic portal circulation where they are taken directly to the liver for metabolism before reaching the heart and circulating throughout the rest of the body.

However, certain drugs called **prodrugs** require metabolism to make them active. In these cases, as the drug is broken down by chemical reactions of metabolism, the products formed by the breakdown produce a more intense response than does the original drug. An example of such a prodrug is sulfasalazine, which is not active in its original form taken by mouth. It is broken down by bacteria in the colon into two products that become active. However, such cases of prodrugs are infrequent. Usually, metabolism is affected by the use of other drugs or the presence of other diseases.

pro = *before*
drug = *medication form*

Another important mechanism that affects metabolism and drug action is the **first-pass effect.** Substances absorbed across the intestinal wall enter blood vessels known as the *hepatic portal circulation,* which carries blood directly to the liver (see Figure 4.2 ■). Drugs administered orally are absorbed into the hepatic portal circulation and are taken directly to the liver for metabolism. The liver may then metabolize the drug to a less active form before it is distributed to the rest of the body and target organs. In some cases, this first-pass effect can inactivate more than 90% of an orally administered drug before it can reach the general circulation.

Many patients differ in how efficiently their metabolic enzymes work to metabolize drugs. Age, kidney and liver disease, genetics, and other factors can dramatically affect metabolism. Some patients metabolize drugs very slowly; others, very quickly.

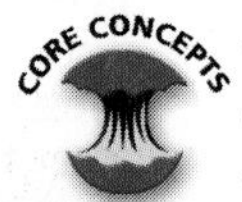

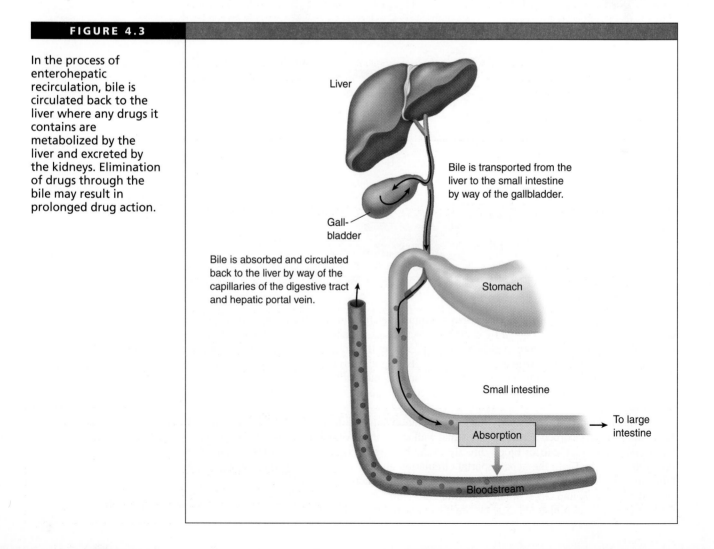

4.5 Excretion processes remove drugs from the body.

Life Span Fact

In general, metabolic enzyme activity is reduced in very young and in elderly patients. Therefore, pediatric and geriatric patients are usually more sensitive to medications than are other patients. Drug doses to the youngest and oldest age groups are often reduced to compensate for these differences.

The last step of pharmacokinetics is **excretion.** Most substances that enter the body are removed by urination, exhalation, defecation, and/or sweating. Drugs are normally removed from the body by the kidneys, the respiratory tract, bile, or glandular activity.

The main organ of excretion is the kidney. The major role of the kidneys is to remove all non-natural and harmful agents in the bloodstream while maintaining a balance of other natural substances. Most drugs are excreted by the kidneys. Therefore, kidney damage can significantly prolong drug action and is a common cause of adverse reactions. Drugs that affect the kidney and its filtration processes are presented in Chapter 28.

Drugs that are easily changed into a gaseous form are especially suited for excretion by the respiratory system. The rate of respiratory excretion is dependent on the many factors that affect gas exchange, including diffusion, gas solubility, and blood flow. The greater the blood flow into lung capillaries, the greater the excretion. In contrast to other methods of excretion, the lungs excrete most drugs in their original unmetabolized form.

Some drugs are excreted through bile. However, most components of bile are circulated back to the liver by a process known as **enterohepatic recirculation,** as shown in Figure 4.3 ■. Recirculating drugs are then metabolized by the liver and excreted by the kidneys. The fraction of drug that is not recirculated continues on its way to the feces. Elimination of drugs through bile may continue for several weeks after therapy has stopped and results in prolonged drug action.

FIGURE 4.3

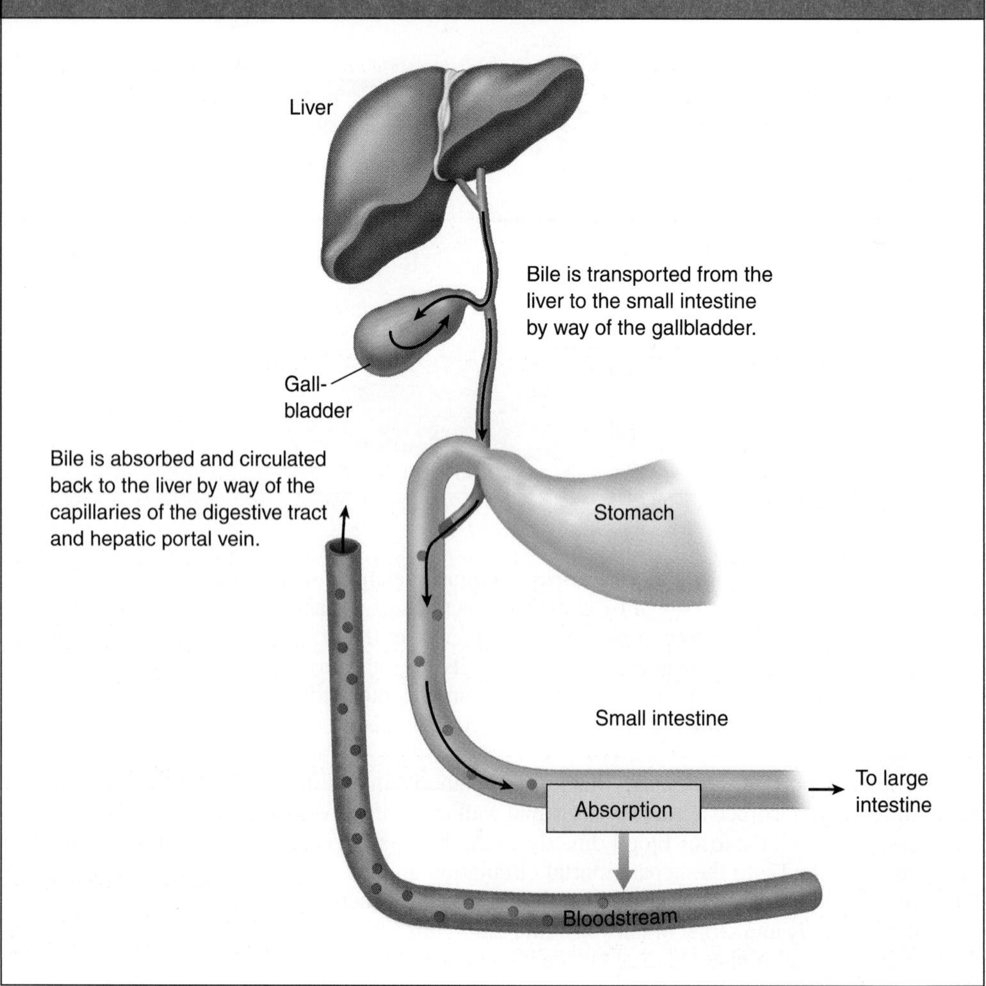

In the process of enterohepatic recirculation, bile is circulated back to the liver where any drugs it contains are metabolized by the liver and excreted by the kidneys. Elimination of drugs through the bile may result in prolonged drug action.

Glands (other than the breast glands) that produce body fluids such as saliva and sweat are less effective at excreting drugs. Most of the substances that are secreted in saliva and perspiration, such as urea or other waste products, are natural products. However, the breast glands can secrete any drug capable of crossing these membranes. Therefore, a breastfeeding mother should always check with her physician before taking any prescription drug, OTC drug, or natural alternative therapy.

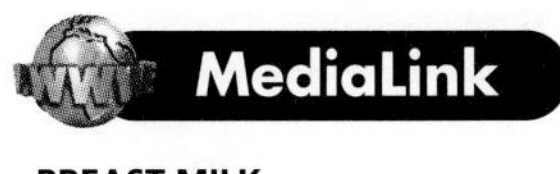

BREAST MILK

Concept Review 4.1

- What does the term *pharmacokinetics* mean? Can you describe the four major parts of pharmacokinetics?

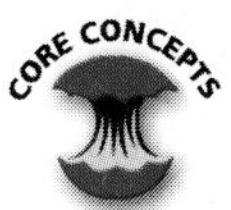

4.6 The rate of elimination and half-life characteristics influence drug responsiveness.

Elimination, which is another term for *excretion,* is often measured so that dosages of drugs can be determined more accurately. The term rate of elimination refers to the amount of drug removed per unit of time from the body by normal physiological processes. The rate of elimination is helpful in determining how long a particular drug will remain in the bloodstream and is thus an indicator of how long a drug will produce its effect.

The **half-life ($t_{1/2}$)** of a drug is a related measurement used to ensure that maximum therapeutic dosages are administered. Half-life is the length of time required for a drug's concentration in the plasma to decrease by one half. It is an indicator of how long a drug will produce its effect in the body. The larger the half-life value, the longer it takes for a drug to be eliminated. For example, a drug with a half-life of 10 hours will take longer to be eliminated from the body than a drug with a half-life of 5 hours. Drugs with longer half-lives may be given less frequently—for example, once per day.

When a patient has a renal or hepatic disease, the plasma half-life of a drug increases. This reflects the important relationship of half-life to metabolism and excretion. Some drugs have a half-life of just a few minutes, whereas others have a half-life of several hours or days.

Concept Review 4.2

- Why are rate of elimination and half-life ($t_{1/2}$) important to the healthcare practitioner?

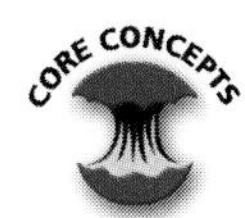

4.7 Pharmacodynamics focuses on what the drugs do to the body.

As discussed already, many variables influence the effectiveness of drug therapy, such as rate of administration, frequency of drug dosing, and a changing medical condition. Some of these factors are summarized in Table 4.1.

Successful pharmacotherapy depends on these variables as well as how effectively the body responds to drugs at specific target locations. This leads to another important core area of pharmacology: the field of pharmacodynamics. The field of pharmacodynamics is complex and requires extensive knowledge of physiology and biochemistry. **Pharmacodynamics** deals with the mechanisms of drug action, or how the drug exerts its effects. As the root words suggest, drugs

pharmaco = *drug related*
dynamics = *power*

TABLE 4.1 Factors That Influence the Effectiveness of Drug Therapy	
Concentration (dose) of administered drug	Metabolic rate (lower in children and elderly patients)
Frequency of drug dosing	Genetics
Food-drug interactions	Excretion rate (rate of elimination)
Drug-drug interactions	Half-life ($t_{1/2}$) of administered drug
Absorption rate (refer to Core Concept 4.1)	Changing medical condition (liver or kidney disease)

FIGURE 4.4

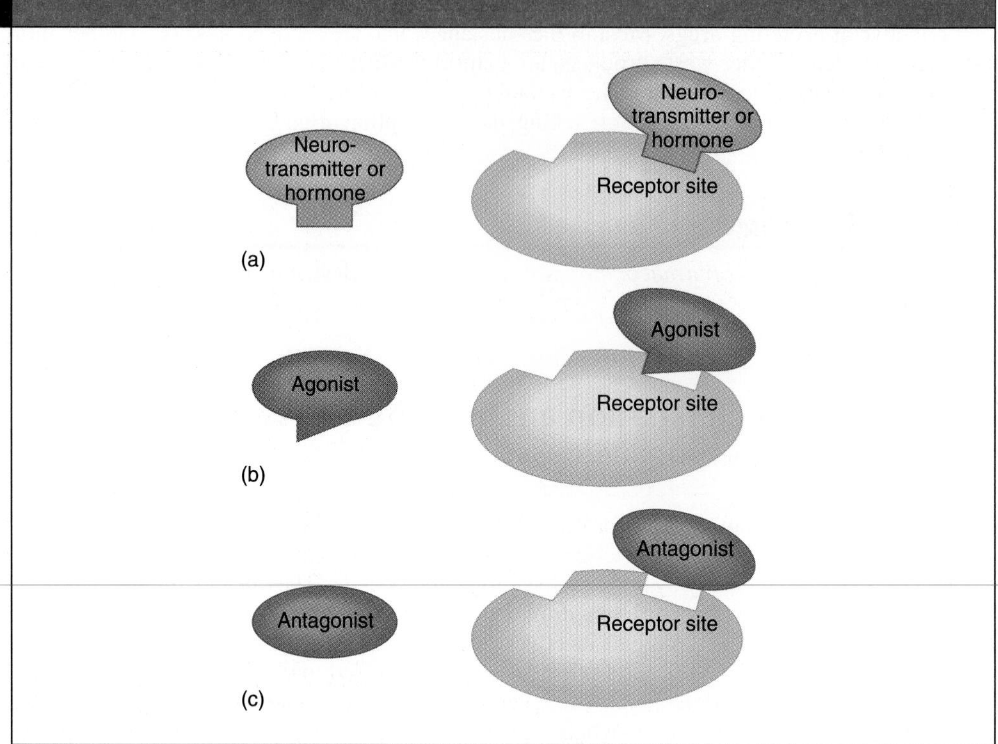

Cellular receptors: (a) A *neurotransmitter* or *hormone* has a specific shape to fit into a receptor site and cause a pharmacological response such as a nerve impulse being sent. A drug that is a close "mimic" of a neurotransmitter or hormone attaches to a receptor site and may either initiate a response (agonist) or prevent a response from occurring (antagonist). (b) An *agonist* is a drug that binds to the receptor (by fitting partially into the receptor) and produces a pharmacological response. (c) An *antagonist* is a drug that temporarily blocks or depresses the normal pharmacological response.

have a powerful influence on body processes. The remaining part of this chapter will be devoted to a few basic pharmacodynamic principles.

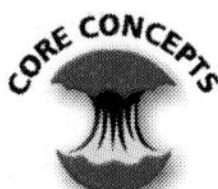

4.8 Drugs activate specific receptors to produce a response.

Successful pharmacotherapy is based on the principle that to treat a disorder, a drug must interact with specific receptors in its target tissue. The **receptor theory** is a classic theory referring to the cellular mechanism by which most drugs can change body processes. A **receptor** is any structural component of a cell to which a drug binds in a dose-related manner. Receptors can be located on the plasma cell membrane or in the cytoplasm or nucleus of the cell. The drug or natural body substance attaches to its receptor much like a lock and key (Figure 4.4 ■). Some drug actions are not linked to a receptor, but are connected directly with cell function, such as changing the membrane excitability or stability of a nerve or muscle cell.

The terms *agonist* and *antagonist* are often used to describe drug action at the receptor level. **Agonists** are drugs capable of binding with receptors and causing a cellular response; these are *facilitators* of cellular action. When they are present in the bloodstream, agonists cause the tissue to respond, resulting in a therapeutic action. **Antagonists** are drugs that inhibit or block the responses of agonists. Antagonists are also called *blockers.*

ant = *against*
agonist = *activator*

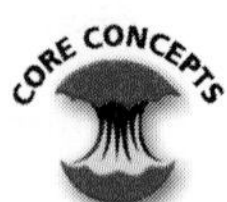

4.9 *Potency* and *efficacy* are terms often used to describe the success of drug therapy.

Potency refers to a drug's strength at a certain concentration or dose. As shown in Figure 4.5 ■, *dose-response curves* are used to compare potencies of different drugs. If drug A has a higher potency than drug B, it means that drug A will produce a more intense effect than drug B if both drugs are given at the same dose (Figure 4.5a). A higher potency also means that a much smaller dose of the medication will be needed to produce the same effect as another drug, as shown by the shift to the left of the dose-response curve for drug A in Figure 4.5a.

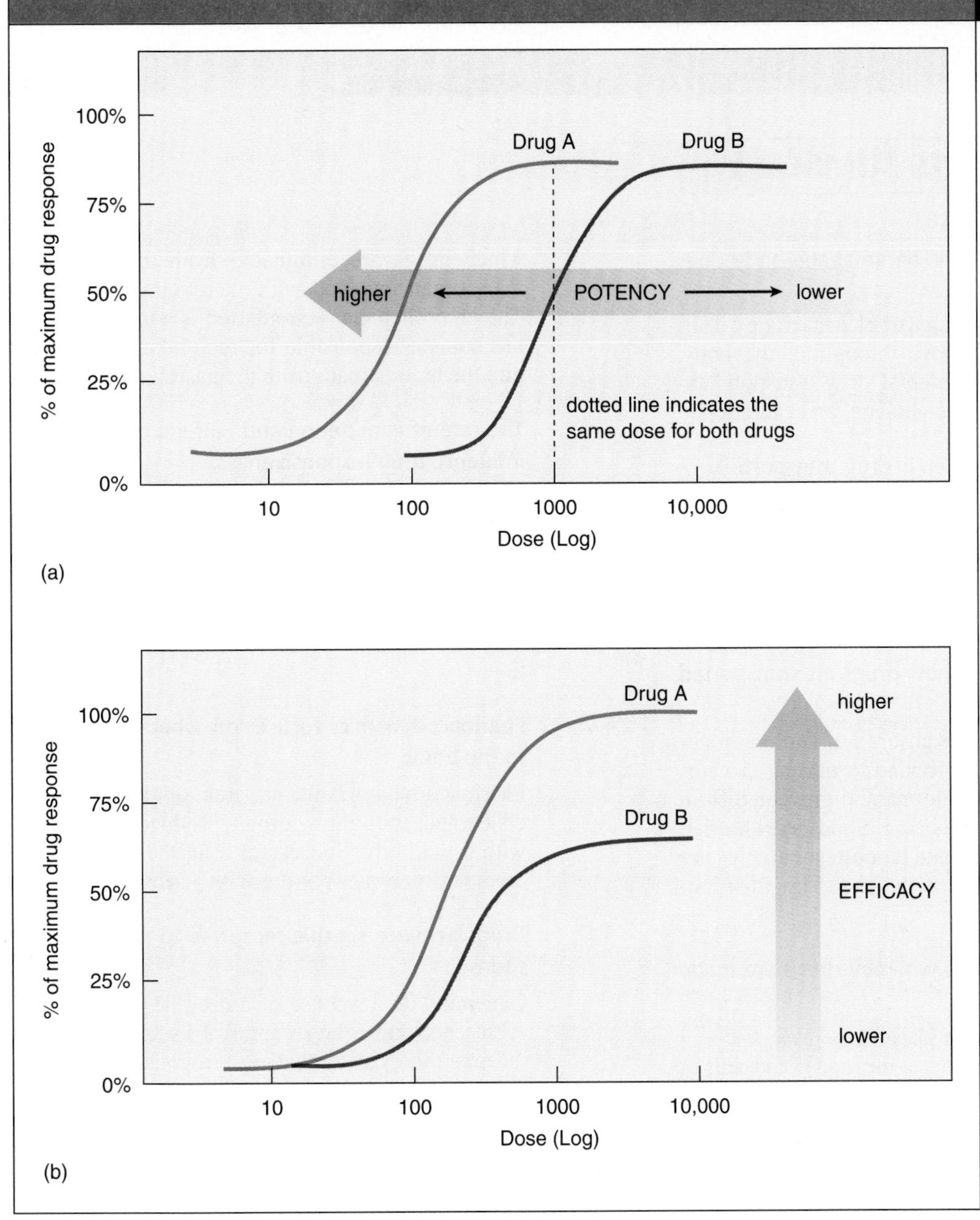

FIGURE 4.5

The curved lines are dose-response curves. The X-axis shows drug dose, which increases from left to right. The Y-axis shows the percent of maximum response for each drug, which increases from 0% at the bottom of the axis to 100% at the top. (a) Drug A has a higher *potency* than drug B because drug A's curve is to the left of drug B's curve. Therefore, a lesser dose of drug A is required for the same effect as a higher dose of drug B—indicating drug A's greater potency. (b) When the doses of both drugs are increased to the same amount, drug A's percent of maximum response reaches nearly 100%, whereas drug B's reaches only about 60%. As the doses are increased, drug A is more effective than drug B compared to drug A. In other words, drug A's *efficacy* is greater than drug B's efficacy.

Another core concept is **efficacy.** Efficacy refers to the ability of a drug to produce a more intense response as its concentration is increased. As an example, consider Figure 4.5b. If the doses of two similarly acting drugs (A and B) are increased, they will both produce a more intense effect, but drug B will have a maximum intensity that is lower than drug A. The drug reaching a lower maximum intensity compared to another drug is said to have a lower efficacy. In pharmacotherapeutics, it is generally more important to have a drug with higher efficacy than one with higher potency.

Concept Review 4.3

- What does the term *pharmacodynamics* mean? Identify the importance of receptors, agonists, and antagonists in how they influence drug action. What is the difference between a drug's potency and its efficacy?

CHAPTER REVIEW

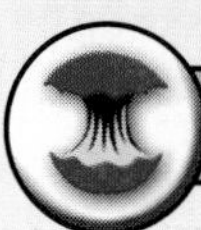

CORE CONCEPTS SUMMARY

4.1 Pharmacokinetics focuses on what the body does to the drugs.

Pharmacokinetics is an area of pharmacology dealing with how drugs move throughout the body. There are four components of drug transport: absorption, distribution, metabolism, and excretion.

4.2 Absorption is the first step in drug transport.

Absorption represents the first step in pharmacokinetics. It involves movement of a drug from its site of administration across body membranes. Drugs cross many membrances before reaching target organs. Drug absorption is affected by many factors.

4.3 Distribution represents how drugs are transported throughout the body.

Distribution begins after absorption and continues until drug action. Drugs bound to plasma proteins may be isolated in the plasma and prevented from reaching their target cells. The blood-brain barrier, blood-placental barrier, and blood-testicular barrier all represent areas in the body where drug distribution may be limited.

4.4 Metabolism is a process whereby drugs are made less or more active.

Metabolic processes take place in the liver, and to a lesser extent, in organs such as the kidney and cells of the gastrointestinal tract. The first-pass effect is an important phenomenon because many drugs absorbed across intestinal membranes are routed directly to the liver. Metabolic liver enzymes are usually less active in younger and in older patients; therefore, drug effects will most likely be greater in these age groups. Prodrugs are agents converted to a more active form when they are metabolically changed.

4.5 Excretion processes remove drugs from the body.

The kidneys, lungs, sweat glands, mammary glands, and gallbladder are the major routes by which drugs are eliminated from the body. The main organ involved with excretion is the kidney. The enterohepatic recirculation is a unique type of mechanism responsible for recirculating bile back into the bloodstream from the gastrointestinal tract.

4.6 The rate of elimination and half-life characteristics influence drug responsiveness.

The elimination rate of a drug is defined as the amount of drug removed from the body by normal physiological processes per unity of time. Plasma half-life is the amount of time it takes for the body to remove half of the drug from the general circulation. These factors affect the duration of drug action.

4.7 Pharmacodynamics focuses on what the drugs do to the body.

Pharmacodynamics is an area of pharmacology concerned with how drugs produce a response within the body. Successful drug therapy depends on the effectiveness of these responses.

4.8 Drugs activate specific receptors to produce a response.

Generally, the response of a drug begins when the agent encounters the receptor of its target cell. The receptor theory states that most responses in the body are caused by interactions of drugs with specific receptors. Receptors may be located on the plasma cell membrane, or they may be found in the cytoplasm or nucleus of the cell.

4.9 *Potency* and *efficacy* are terms often used to describe the success of drug therapy.

Potency relates to the concentration or amount of drug required to produce a maximum response. Efficacy refers to how great the maximal response of a drug is.

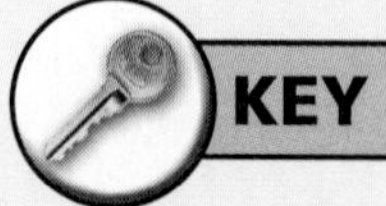

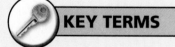

KEY TERMS

absorption (ab-SORP-shun): the process of moving a drug across body membranes / ***page 50***

agonists (AG-on-ists): drugs that are capable of binding with receptors in order to cause a cellular response / ***page 54***

antagonists (an-TAG-oh-nists): drugs that block the response of another drug / ***page 54***

biotransformation (BEYE-oh-trans-for-MAY-shun): the chemical conversion of drugs from one form to another that may result in increased or decreased activity / ***page 50***

distribution (dis-tree-BU-shun): the process of transporting drugs through the body / ***page 50***

efficacy (EFF-ik-ah-see): the effectiveness of a drug in producing a more intense response as its concentration is increased / ***page 55***

enterohepatic recirculation (EN-ter-oh-HEE-pah-tik): recycling of drugs and other substances by the circulation of bile through the intestine and liver / ***page 52***

excretion (eks-KREE-shun): the process of removing substances from the body / ***page 52***

first-pass effect: a mechanism whereby drugs are absorbed across the intestinal wall and enter into blood vessels, known as the hepatic portal circulation, which carries blood directly to the liver / ***page 51***

half-life ($t_{1/2}$): the length of time required for a drug to decrease its concentration in the plasma by one half of the original amount / ***page 53***

metabolism (meh-TAHB-oh-liz-ehm): the sum total of all chemical reactions in the body or an organ (for example, the liver) / ***page 50***

pharmacodynamics (FAR-mah-koh-deye-NAM-iks): the study of how the body responds to drugs and natural substances / ***page 53***

pharmacokinetics (FAR-mah-koh-kee-NET-iks): the study of what the body does to drugs / ***page 53***

potency (POH-ten-see): the power or strength of a drug at a specified concentration or dose / ***page 49***

prodrugs: drugs that become more active after they are metabolized / ***page 51***

receptor (ree-SEP-tor): the structural component of a cell to which a drug binds in a dose-related manner to produce a response / ***page 54***

receptor theory: a cellular mechanism by which most drugs produce their effects / ***page 54***

REVIEW QUESTIONS

The following questions are written in NCLEX-PN® style. Answer these questions to assess your knowledge of the chapter material, and go back and review any material that is not clear to you.

1. Patients with liver disorders would most likely have problems with which pharmacokinetic phase?

1. Absorption
2. Distribution
3. Metabolism
4. Excretion

2. The patient asks the nurse why she must take her medication twice a day instead of just once. The nurse's best response would be:

1. "Taking it once a day is fine as long as it is taken at the same time every day."
2. "Taking the medication twice a day ensures that maximum concentrations are maintained within the body."
3. "You will need to speak to your physician about this."
4. "The first dose of the medication is blocked by deactivation and the second dose is metabolized by the body."

3. Which of the following principals is true?

1. For a drug to be effective, it must be potent.
2. For drug efficacy to occur, a lower dose must be administered.
3. Antagonists bind to receptors and produce responses to block agonists.
4. The drug-receptor interaction must occur at its target tissue.

4. Drugs that bind with a receptor to produce a therapeutic response are called:

1. Antagonists
2. Facilitators
3. Agonists
4. Blockers

5. If a patient takes a medication on a full stomach, the nurse is aware the medication will be:

1. Absorbed more rapidly
2. Absorbed more slowly
3. Neutralized by gastric enzymes
4. Activated by gastric enzymes

6. Which of the following factors does not influence the effectiveness of drug therapy?

1. Temperature
2. Food-drug interactions
3. Route of administration
4. Time of administration

7. An antibiotic has been ordered for the patient with a brain abscess. The nurse identifies:

1. Antibiotics are not effective to treat brain abscesses.
2. Only fat-soluble substances will pass the blood-brain barrier.
3. The half-life of the antibiotic will be decreased.
4. The intestinal tract will prevent absorption from occurring.

8. When orally administered drugs are extensively metabolized by the liver with only part of the drug dose reaching target organs, this is known as:

1. Half-life
2. Potency
3. First-pass effect
4. Rate of elimination

9. These drugs inhibit cell function by preventing other drugs from binding with receptor sites and blocking cellular response.

1. Agonists
2. Antagonists
3. Facilitators
4. Anesthetics

10. Drug dosing in pediatric and elderly patients is often decreased due to:

1. Reduced enzyme activity
2. Enhanced enzyme activity
3. Decreased kidney function
4. Increased kidney function

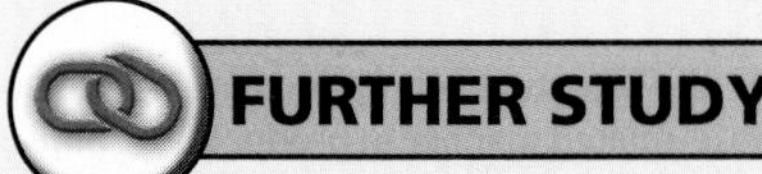

FURTHER STUDY

- Pregnant women need to be cautious about food and medications they take, as discussed in Chapter 2.
- Drugs that affect the kidney and its filtration processes are discussed in more detail in Chapter 28.

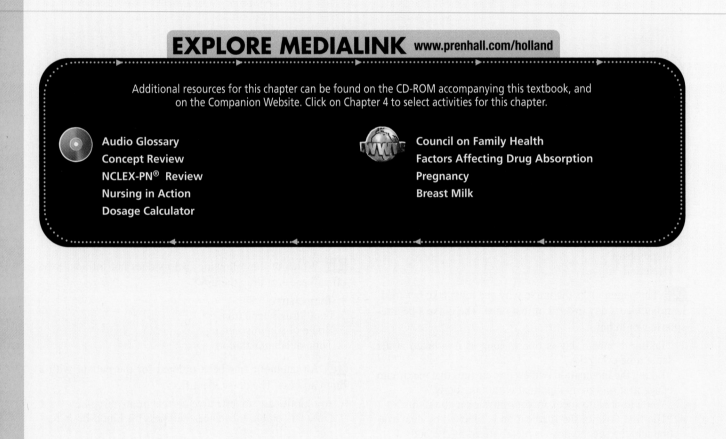

EXPLORE MEDIALINK www.prenhall.com/holland

Additional resources for this chapter can be found on the CD-ROM accompanying this textbook, and on the Companion Website. Click on Chapter 4 to select activities for this chapter.

Audio Glossary
Concept Review
NCLEX-PN® Review
Nursing in Action
Dosage Calculator

Council on Family Health
Factors Affecting Drug Absorption
Pregnancy
Breast Milk

CHAPTER

5 Herbs and Dietary Supplements

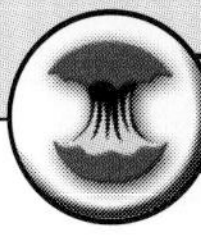

CORE CONCEPTS

5.1 Complementary and alternative therapies are used by a large number of people to prevent and treat disease.

5.2 Natural products from plants have been used as medicines for thousands of years.

5.3 Herbal products are standardized to a specific active ingredient.

5.4 Herbs can have significant pharmacological actions and can interact with conventional drugs, which may result in adverse effects.

5.5 Specialty supplements are widely used to promote wellness.

5.6 Dietary supplements are regulated by the Dietary Supplement Health and Education Act of 1994.

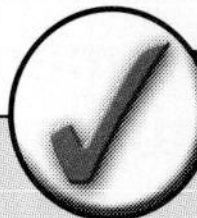

OBJECTIVES

After reading this chapter, the student should be able to:

1. Explain the role of complementary and alternative medicine in promoting patient wellness.
2. Discuss the reasons why herbal products and dietary supplements have increased in popularity in recent years.
3. Identify the parts of an herb that may contain active ingredients and the types of formulations made from these parts.
4. Describe the strengths and weaknesses of the Dietary Supplement Health and Education Act (DSHEA) of 1994.
5. Describe drug interactions and adverse effects that may be caused by herbal preparations.
6. Explain how herbal products are sometimes standardized based on specific active ingredients.

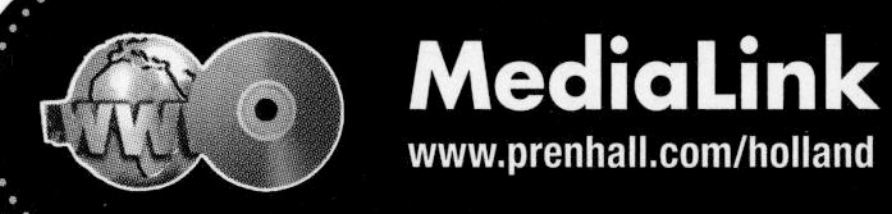

Interactive resources for this chapter can be found on the Companion Website. Click on Chapter 5 and "Begin" to select the activities for this chapter. For chapter-related animations, NCLEX-PN®-style questions, and an audio glossary, access the accompanying CD-ROM in this book.

Herbal and dietary supplements represent a multibillion dollar industry. Sales of these alternative therapies exceed $50 billion annually, with over 158 million consumers using them. Consumers have turned to these treatments for a wide variety of reasons. Many people have the impression that natural substances have more healing power than synthetic medications. The ready availability of OTC herbal supplements at a reasonable cost has convinced many to try them. This chapter examines the role of herbal and dietary supplements in the prevention and treatment of disease.

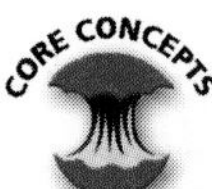

5.1 Complementary and alternative therapies are used by a large number of people to prevent and treat disease.

Complementary and alternative medicine (CAM) comprises an extremely diverse set of therapies and healing systems that are considered to be outside of mainstream healthcare. CAM systems have the following common characteristics.

- Focuses on treating each *individual* person
- Considers the health of the *whole* person
- Emphasizes the *integration of mind and body*
- Promotes disease *prevention, self-care,* and *self-healing*
- Recognizes the role of *spirituality* in health and healing

Because of its popularity, many have focused considerable attention on determining the effectiveness or lack of effectiveness of CAM. Although research into these alternative systems is currently underway, few CAM therapies have been subjected to rigorous clinical and scientific study. It is likely that some of these therapies will become mainstream treatments while others will be found ineffective. The line between what is defined as an alternative therapy and what is considered mainstream is constantly changing. Increasing numbers of practitioners are now accepting CAM therapies and recommending them to their patients. Table 5.1 describes some of these therapies.

TABLE 5.1 Complementary and Alternative Therapies

HEALING METHOD	EXAMPLES
Biological therapies	Herbal therapies Nutritional supplements Special diets
Alternate healthcare systems	Naturopathy Homeopathy Chiropractic Native American medicine (e.g., sweat lodges, medicine wheel) Chinese traditional medicine (e.g., acupuncture, Chinese herbs)
Manual healing	Massage Pressure-point therapies
Mind-body interventions	Yoga Meditation Hypnotherapy Guided imagery Biofeedback Movement-oriented therapies (e.g., music, dance)
Spiritual	Shamans Faith and prayer

Fast Facts Alternative Therapies in America

Possibly the largest nonscientific study of attitudes toward alternative therapies surveyed 45,000 people and was reported in *Consumer's Reports,* May 2000. Findings of this study include the following:

- Of those surveyed, 55% did not use alternative therapies, primarily because they were satisfied with standard medical treatments.
- To relieve symptoms that were not successfully treated with conventional therapies, 35% used alternative therapies.
- The most likely people trying alternatives were those in severe pain or with stress.
- For almost all medical conditions, respondents stated that prescription drugs were more effective than herbal therapies.
- For back pain and fibromyalgia, deep muscle massage was rated more effective than prescription drugs.
- Of those who tried alternatives, 25% did so at the recommendation of a doctor or nurse. Only 5% of doctors disapproved of alternative therapies.

Health professionals have long known the value of CAM therapies in preventing and treating disease. For example, prayer, meditation, massage, and yoga have been used for centuries to treat both body and mind. From a therapeutic perspective, much of the value of CAM therapies is their ability to reduce the need for medications. If a patient can find anxiety relief through massage or biofeedback therapy, for example, the use of anxiolytic drugs may be reduced or eliminated. Reduction of drug dose leads to fewer adverse effects and better compliance with drug therapy. Two of the CAM therapies are covered in detail here, **herbs** and **specialty supplements,** including vitamins and minerals, and their use as **dietary supplements.**

Concept Review 5.1

- How does the healing philosophy of complementary and alternative medicine differ from that of conventional mainstream medicine?

HERBAL PRODUCTS

In the past two decades, the number of people seeking herbal alternatives to conventional medical therapies has greatly increased. Many herbs are extensively used by patients as supplements to traditional pharmacotherapy.

5.2 Natural products from plants have been used as medicines for thousands of years.

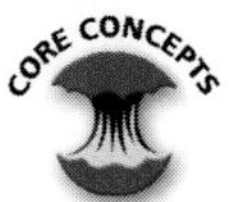

An herb is technically a **botanical** without woody tissue such as stems or bark. Over time, the terms *botanical* and *herb* have come to be used interchangeably to refer to any plant product with useful application, either as a food enhancer, such as flavoring, or as a medicine.

The use of botanicals in the treatment of disease has been recorded for thousands of years. One of the earliest recorded uses of plant products was a prescription for garlic in 3000 B.C. Eastern and Western medicine have recorded thousands of herbs and herb combinations claimed to have therapeutic value. Some of the most popular herbs and their primary uses are shown in Table 5.2.

The public's interest in herbal medicine began to decline when the pharmaceutical industry was born in the late 1800s. Drugs could be standardized and produced more cheaply than natural herbal products. In the early 1900s, regulatory agencies required that medicines be safe and effective. The focus of healthcare shifted to treating specific diseases, rather than promoting wellness and holistic care. Information about most herbal and alternative therapies was no longer taught in medical schools; these healing techniques were criticized as being unscientific relics of the past.

Beginning in the 1970s and continuing to the present day, herbal medicine has experienced a remarkable comeback. The majority of adult Americans are either currently taking herbal

TABLE 5.2 Popular Medicinal Herbs

COMMON NAME	MEDICINAL PART	PRIMARY USE(S)
Aloe	Juice from the leaves	Treat skin ailments (topical), constipation (oral)
Black cohosh	Roots	Relieve menopause symptoms
Cranberry	Berries/juice	Prevent urinary tract infection
Echinacea	Entire plant	Enhance immune system, as an anti-inflammatory
Garlic	Bulbs	Reduce blood cholesterol and blood pressure, as an anticoagulant
Ginger	Root	Relieve GI upset and motion sickness, as an anti-inflammatory
Ginkgo biloba	Leaves and seeds	Improve memory, reduce dizziness
Ginseng	Root	Relieve stress, enhance immune system, decrease fatigue
Kava kava	Rhizome	Reduce stress, promote sleep
Milk thistle	Seeds	As an antitoxin, protect against liver disease
Saw palmetto	Ripe fruit/berries	Relieve urinary problems related to prostate enlargement
Soy	Beans	As a source of protein, vitamins, and minerals; relieve menopausal symptoms; prevent cardiovascular disease; as an anticancer agent
St. John's wort	Flowers, leaves, stems	Reduce depression, reduce anxiety, as an anti-inflammatory
Valerian	Roots	Relieve stress, promote sleep

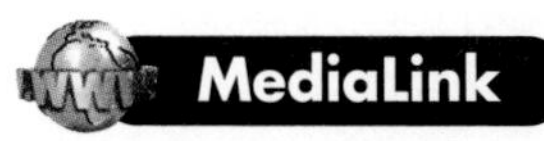

HERB RESEARCH FOUNDATION

Life Span Fact

Herbs and Dietary Supplements Can Help Elderly Patients

Dietary supplements such as herbs and other specialty products have the ability to positively influence the health of older patients. Nutritional deficiencies greatly increase with age, and supplements help to prevent or eliminate these deficiencies in seniors. The health practitioner should assess the need for such supplements in all elderly patients. Herbal remedies and specialty supplements have been successfully used to enhance the immune systems of older patients, reduce short-term memory loss, and improve overall health. There is research to suggest that herbal remedies such as gingko biloba may improve the symptoms of dementia in Alzheimer's disease.

products on a regular basis or have taken them in the past. This increase in popularity has been due to a number of factors, including increased availability of herbal products, aggressive marketing by the herbal industry, increased attention to natural alternatives, and renewed interest in preventive medicine. The gradual aging of the population has led to more patients seeking therapeutic alternatives for chronic conditions such as pain, arthritis, prostate difficulties, and the need for hormone replacement. In addition, the high cost of prescription medicines has driven many people to seek less expensive alternatives.

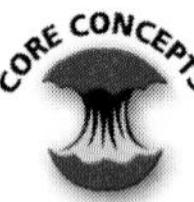

5.3 Herbal products are standardized to a specific active ingredient.

The active ingredients in an herbal product may be present in only one specific part of the plant or in all parts. For example, the active chemicals in chamomile are in the aboveground portion, such as the leaves, stems, berries, or flowers. For other herbs, such as ginger, the underground rhizomes and roots are used for their healing properties. When collecting or purchasing herbs for home use, it is important to know which portion of the plant contains the active chemicals.

Most modern drugs contain only one active ingredient. This chemical is standarized, accurately measured, and delivered to the patient in precise amounts. It is a common misconception that herbs also contain one active ingredient, which can be extracted and delivered to patients in exact amounts, like drugs. Each herb, however, may contain dozens of active chemicals, many of which have not yet been isolated, studied, or even identified. It is possible that some of these substances work together and may not have the same activity if isolated. Furthermore, the strength of an herbal preparation may vary depending on where the herb was grown and how it was collected, prepared, and stored.

Recent attempts have been made to standardize herbal products, using a marker substance such as the percent of flavones in ginkgo or the percent of lactones in kava kava. Some of these standardizations are shown in Table 5.3. Until science can better characterize these substances, however, it is best to view the active ingredient of an herb as being the entire herb. An example of the ingredients and standardization of ginkgo biloba is shown in Figure 5.1 ■.

TABLE 5.3 Standardization of Selected Herb Extracts

HERB	STANDARDIZATION	PERCENT
Black cohosh	Triterpene glycosides	2.5
Echinacea	Phenolics	4
Ginger	Pungent compounds	>10
Ginkgo	Flavoglycosides	24–25
	Lactones	5
Ginseng root	Ginseosides	20–30
Kava kava	Kavalactones	40–45
St. John's wort	Hypericins	0.3–0.5
	Hyperforin	3–5
Saw palmetto fruit	Total fatty acids	80–90

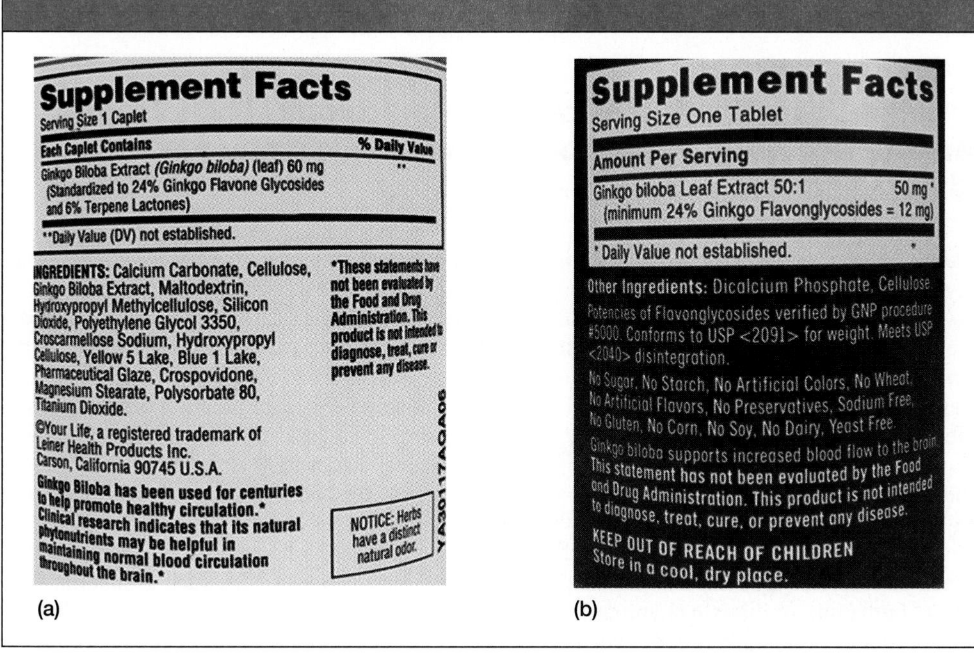

FIGURE 5.1

Note the lack of standardization of two ginkgo biloba labels: (a) 60 mg of extract, 24% Ginkgo Flavone Glycosides and 6% terpenes; and (b) 50:1 Ginkgo Leaf Extract, 24% Ginkgo Flavonglycosides.

The two basic formulations of herbal products are solid and liquid. Solid products include pills, tablets, and capsules made from dried herbs. Other solid products are salves and ointments that are administered topically. Liquid formulations are made by extracting the active chemicals from the plant using solvents such as water, alcohol, or glycerol. The liquids are then concentrated in various strengths. Liquid formulations of herbal preparations are described in Table 5.4. Some formulations of ginkgo biloba, one of the most popular herbals, are illustrated in Figure 5.2 ■.

TABLE 5.4 Liquid Formulations of Herbal Products

PRODUCT	DESCRIPTION
Tea	Fresh or dried herbs are soaked in hot water for 5–10 minutes before ingestion; convenient.
Infusion	Fresh or dried herbs are soaked in hot water for long periods, at least 15 minutes; stronger than teas.
Decoction	Fresh or dried herbs are boiled in water for 30–50 minutes until much of the liquid has boiled off; very concentrated.
Tincture	Active ingredients are extracted by soaking the herb in alcohol; alcohol remains as part of the liquid.
Extract	Active ingredients are extracted using organic solvents to form a highly concentrated liquid or solid form; solvent may be removed or be part of the final product.

FIGURE 5.2

Three different ginkgo formulations: tablets, tea bags, and liquid extract.

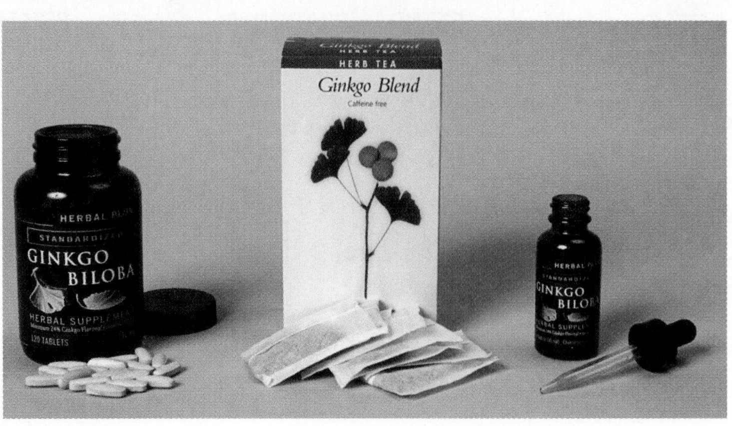

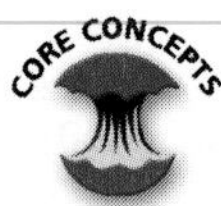

5.4 Herbs can have significant pharmacological actions and can interact with conventional drugs, which may result in adverse effects.

A key concept to remember when dealing with alternative therapies is that natural does not always mean better or safe. There is no question that some botanicals contain active chemicals as powerful as and perhaps more effective than currently approved medications. Thousands of years of experience, combined with current scientific research, have shown that some of these herbal remedies have therapeutic actions. Because a substance comes from a natural product, however, does not make it either safe or effective. For example, poison ivy is natural, but it certainly is not safe or therapeutic. Natural products may not offer an improvement over conventional therapy in treating certain disorders and, indeed, may be of no value whatsoever. Most importantly, a patient who substitutes an unproven alternative therapy for an established, effective medical treatment may delay healing, suffer harmful effects, and endanger his or her health.

Some herbal products contain ingredients that may interact with prescription drugs. For example, patients taking medications with potentially serious adverse effects, such as insulin, warfarin (Coumadin), or digoxin (Lanoxin), should be warned never to take any dietary supplement without first discussing their needs with a physician. Common herb-drug interactions are shown in Table 5.5.

Another warning that must be heeded with natural products is to beware of allergic reactions. Most herbal products contain a mixture of ingredients, and it is not unusual to find dozens of different chemicals in teas and infusions made from the flowers, leaves, or roots of a plant. Patients who have known allergies to certain foods or medicines should seek medical advice before taking an herbal product. It is always wise to take the smallest amount possible—less than the recommended dose—when starting herbal therapy to see if allergies or other adverse effects occur.

Health professionals have an obligation to seek the latest medical information on herbal products, since there is a good possibility that their patients are using them to supplement traditional medicines. Patients should be advised to be skeptical of claims on the labels of dietary supplements and to seek their health information from reputable sources. Health professionals must never condemn patients' use of alternative therapies, but instead be supportive and seek to understand their goals for taking the supplements. The healthcare provider will often need to educate patients on the role of alternative therapies in the treatment of their disorders and discuss which treatments or combination of treatments will best meet their health goals.

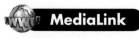

MEDLINE FOR HERBAL PRODUCTS

SPECIALTY SUPPLEMENTS

Specialty supplements are *nonherbal* dietary supplements that can come from plant and animal sources.

TABLE 5.5 Common Herb-Drug Interactions

COMMON NAME	INTERACTS WITH	COMMENTS
Echinacea	Amiodarone (Cordarone)	Possible increased liver toxicity
	Anabolic steroids	Possible increased liver toxicity
	Ketoconazole (Nizoral)	Possible increased liver toxicity
Garlic	Aspirin and NSAIDs	Increased bleeding potential
	Insulin and oral hypoglycemic agents	Additive hypoglycemic effects
	Warfarin (Coumadin)	Increased bleeding potential
Ginger	Aspirin and NSAIDs	Increased bleeding potential
	Heparin and warfarin	Increased bleeding potential
Ginkgo	Anticonvulsants	Possible decreased anticonvulsant effectiveness
	Aspirin and NSAIDs	Increased bleeding potential
	Heparin and warfarin	Increased bleeding potential
	Tricyclic antidepressants	Possible decreased seizure threshold
Ginseng	CNS depressants	Increased sedation
	Digoxin (Lanoxin)	Increased toxicity
	Diuretics	Possible weakened diuretic effects
	Insulin and oral hypoglycemic agents	Increased hypoglycemic effects
	Warfarin	Decreased anticoagulant effects
Kava kava	Barbiturates, benzodiazepines, and other CNS depressants	Increased sedation
	Levodopa/carbidopa (Dopar)	Worsened Parkinson's symptoms
	Phenothiazines	Increased risk and severity of dystonic reactions
St. John's wort	CNS depressants and opiates	Increased sedation
	Cyclosporine (Sandimmune)	Possible decreased cyclosporine levels
	Selective serotonin reuptake inhibitors (SSRIs)	Possible serotonin syndrome (headache, dizziness, sweating, agitation)
	Tricyclic antidepressants	Possible serotonin syndrome
	Warfarin (Coumadin)	Decreased anticoagulant effects
Valerian	Barbiturates, benzodiazepines, and other CNS depressants	Increased sedation

Data modified from **www.prenhall.com/drugguides**.

5.5 Specialty supplements are widely used to promote wellness.

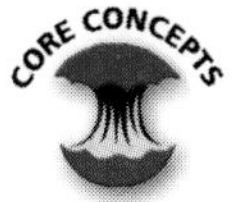

Specialty supplements are used to enhance a wide variety of body functions. Their actions are more specific than those of herbal products, and they are generally targeted for one or a small number of conditions. The most popular specialty supplements are shown in Table 5.6.

In general, the rationale for using specialty supplements is rational. For example, chondroitin and glucosamine are natural substances in the body necessary for cartilage growth and maintenance. Amino acids are natural building blocks of muscle protein. Flaxseed and fish oils contain omega fatty acids that have been shown to reduce the risk of heart disease in certain patients.

Unfortunately, the link between most specialty supplements and their benefits is unclear. In some cases, the body already has sufficient quantities of the substance; therefore, taking additional amounts may be of no benefit. In other cases, the supplement is marketed for conditions for which it has no proven effect. The good news is that these substances are generally not harmful, unless taken in large amounts. The bad news, however, is that they can give patients false hopes of an easy cure for a chronic condition such as heart disease or the pain of arthritis. As with herbal products, the health professional should advise patients to be skeptical about the health claims regarding the use of these supplements.

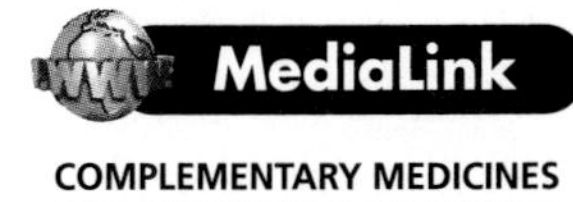

COMPLEMENTARY MEDICINES AND ALTERNATIVE THERAPIES

TABLE 5.6 Popular Specialty Supplements

NAME	COMMON USES
Acidophilus	Maintain intestinal health
Amino acids	Build protein, muscle strength, and endurance
Coenzyme Q10	Treat heart disease, as an antioxidant
Chondroitin	Treat arthritis and other joint problems
Dehydroepiandrosterone (DHEA)	Boost immune and memory functions
Fish oil	Reduce cholesterol, enhance brain function, increase visual acuity (due to presence of the omega-3 fatty acids)
Flaxseed oil	Reduce cholesterol, enhance brain function, increase visual acuity (due to presence of the omega-3 fatty acids)
Glucosamine	Treat arthritis and other joint problems
Methyl sulfonyl methane (MSM)	Reduce allergic reactions to pollen and foods, relieve pain and inflammation of arthritis and similar conditions
Soy isoflavone	Reduce the risk of certain types of cancer

Concept Review 5.2

- Explain the difference between an herb and a specialty dietary supplement.

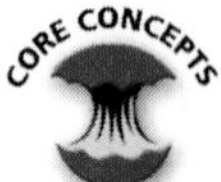

5.6 Dietary supplements are regulated by the Dietary Supplement Health and Education Act of 1994.

Since the passage of the Food, Drug and Cosmetic Act of 1935, Americans have come to expect that all prescription and OTC drugs have passed rigid standards of safety, prior to being marketed. Furthermore, it is assumed that the effectiveness of these drugs has been tested, and that they truly provide the therapeutic benefits claimed by the manufacturer. Indeed, most people would be outraged if they found out that the drug they purchased for pain relief or to cure an infectious disease was totally ineffective. Unfortunately, dietary supplements are regulated by a far less restrictive law, the **Dietary Supplement Health and Education Act (DSHEA) of 1994,** than are drugs. Therefore, Americans must be cautious.

According to the DSHEA. "dietary supplements" are exempted from the Food, Drug and Cosmetic Act. Dietary supplements are defined as products intended to enhance or supplement the diet not approved as drugs by the FDA. The DSHEA also requires these products to be clearly labeled as dietary supplements. An example of an herbal label for black cohosh is shown in Figure 5.3 ■.

One strength of the DSHEA is that it gives the FDA the power to remove from the market any product that poses a "significant or unreasonable" risk to the public. The FDA used this legislative guideline for the first time in 2004, when the dietary supplement ephedra was removed from the market because of reported serious side effects in some patients. It took 7 years from the time the FDA first warned consumers of the dangers of ephedra (1997) until it was removed in 2004.

Unfortunately, the DSHEA has significant weaknesses that allow a lack of standardization in the dietary supplement industry and lowered protection of the consumer. The following list describes these weaknesses.

- Dietary supplements do not have to be *tested* prior to marketing.
- The *effectiveness* of a dietary supplement does not have to be demonstrated by the manufacturer.
- The manufacturer does not have to prove the *safety* of the dietary supplement. It is the government's job to prove that the dietary supplement is *unsafe* and to take the necessary steps to remove it from the market.
- The label of a dietary supplement is not permitted to state that the product is intended to diagnose, treat, cure, or prevent any disease. However, claims may be stated about the product's effect on body structure and function, such as the following:

FIGURE 5.3

(a)

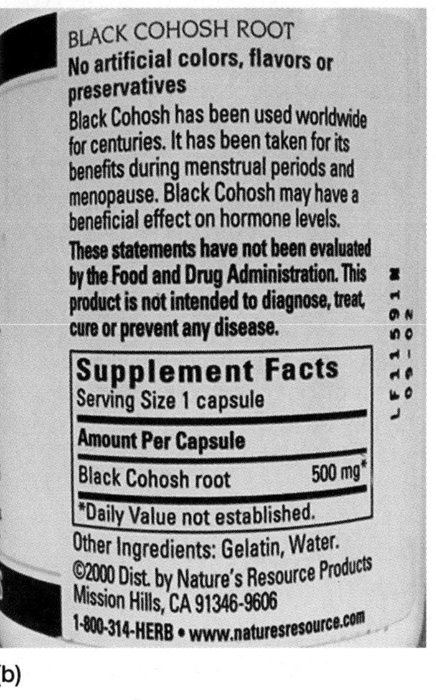

(b)

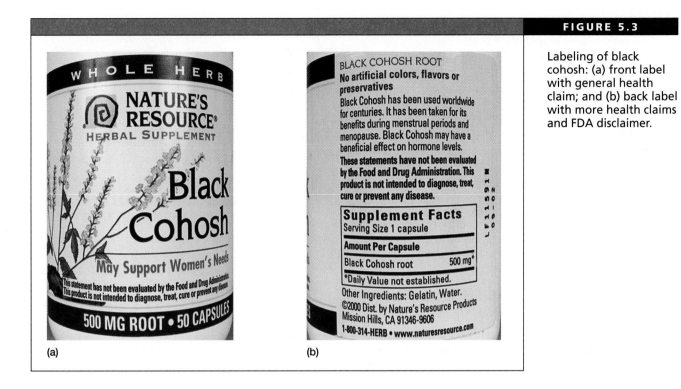

Labeling of black cohosh: (a) front label with general health claim; and (b) back label with more health claims and FDA disclaimer.

- Helps promote healthy immune systems
- Reduces anxiety and stress
- Helps to maintain cardiovascular function
- May reduce pain and inflammation

- If health claims are made, the label must include a disclaimer that states the FDA has not evaluated the claim and that the product is not intended to diagnose, treat, cure, or prevent any disease.
- The DSHEA does not regulate the *accuracy* of the label; the product may or may not contain the product listed in the amounts claimed.

Concept Review 5.3

- How does the federal regulation of an herb by the DSHEA differ from that of a prescription drug?

CHAPTER REVIEW

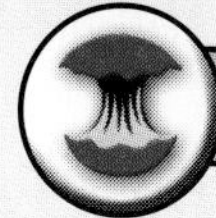

CORE CONCEPTS SUMMARY

5.1 Complementary and alternative therapies are used by a large number of people to prevent and treat disease.

Complementary and alternative medicine (CAM) is a set of different therapies and healing systems used by many patients for disease prevention and self-healing. Alternative therapies offer nonpharmacological ways to promote health and healing. They focus on the holistic treatment of each patient, integrate mind and body, and are often used in conjunction with conventional medical therapies.

5.2 Natural products from plants have been used as medicines for thousands of years.

Thousands of herbal therapies are recorded in Eastern and Western history. The popularity of alternative herbal remedies has increased in recent years.

5.3 Herbal products are standardized to a specific active ingredient.

Herbal products are marketed in a number of different formulations, some consisting of standardized extracts of specific chemicals, others containing whole herbs. Unlike drugs, herbs contain a large number of chemicals that may act in a coordinated manner, or *synergistically,* to produce a therapeutic effect. The active ingredients may be in the flowers, stems, or roots of an herb. Formulations include tablets, capsules, teas, or extracts.

5.4 Herbs can have significant pharmacological actions and can interact with conventional drugs, which may result in adverse effects.

Because a substance comes from a natural product does not make it safe or effective. Although botanicals may have therapeutic applications, they may not be the best product for the disease and may interact with prescription medicines.

5.5 Specialty supplements are widely used to promote wellness.

Specialty supplements include nonherbal therapies that are used to promote a specific aspect of wellness. These products usually have a rational basis for therapy, although their benefits have not always been proven.

5.6 Dietary supplements are regulated by the Dietary Supplement Health and Education Act of 1994.

The DSHEA loosely regulates herbal and dietary supplements. Dietary supplements and herbal products can be marketed without any proof that they are safe or effective. They do not have to be tested prior to marketing. The labels list ingredients but may contain statements that are inaccurate or unproven.

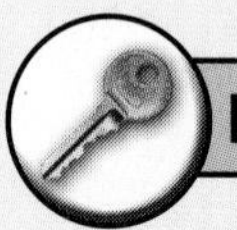

KEY TERMS

botanical (boh-TAN-ik-ul): a plant extract used to treat or prevent illness / *page 61*

complementary and alternative medicine (CAM): general term for treatments that consider the health of the whole person and promote disease prevention / *page 60*

dietary supplement: a nondrug substance regulated by the DSHEA / *page 61*

Dietary Supplement Health and Education Act (DSHEA) of 1994: primary law in the United States regulating herb and dietary supplements / *page 66*

herb: plant with a soft stem that is used in healing or as a seasoning / *page 61*

specialty supplement: a nonherbal dietary supplement used to enhance body functions / *page 61*

REVIEW QUESTIONS

The following questions are written in NCLEX-PN® style. Answer these questions to assess your knowledge of the chapter material, and go back and review any material that is not clear to you.

1. The patient is to be started on warfarin (Coumadin) therapy. It is important for the nurse to assess for the use of which herbs? (Select all that apply.)

1. Ginseng
2. Ginger
3. St. John's wort
4. Kava kava

2. Patients often use herbal therapies for which of the following reasons?

1. To prevent overuse of prescription medications
2. To increase feelings of wellness and promote holistic treatment
3. Because herbal therapies are much more regulated than prescription drugs
4. Because herbal therapies are so much safer than man-made drugs

3. It is important that patients receive education regarding herbal products because:

1. Herbal products are approved under strict FDA regulations.
2. Labeling is not always reliable and herbal products should be used with caution.
3. There are so few side effects, and they can be purchased without a prescription.
4. The manufacturer has repeatedly demonstrated effectiveness.

4. An example of a specialty supplement would be:

1. Acidophilus
2. Ginseng
3. Garlic
4. Ginkgo

5. It is important for the nurse to assess for the use of complementary and alternative medicine (CAM) because:

1. Patients must be warned that most CAM therapies are dangerous.
2. Additional treatment may not be needed.
3. CAM therapies could interact with prescription and OTC medications.
4. Most CAM therapies are totally ineffective.

6. The nurse understands specialty supplements are used:

1. For a diverse range of disease conditions
2. For treatment of a targeted condition
3. When prescriptive medications are no longer effective
4. When the body no longer makes sufficient quantities of the substance

7. The Dietary Supplement Health and Education Act (DHSEA) is responsible for:

1. Strict herbal product testing
2. Ensuring that herbal products are labeled as "dietary supplements"
3. Sending the herbal product to the FDA for evaluation
4. Ensuring safety of the product

8. The patient is admitted with digoxin (Lanoxin) toxicity. The nurse assesses for which of the following herbal products?

1. St. John's wort
2. Valerian
3. Fish oil
4. Ginseng

9. The patient requests information on alternative treatments for her arthritis. The nurse identifies which of the following supplements?

1. Garlic and soy
2. Fish oil
3. Chondroitin and glucosamine
4. DHEA

10. This herbal product is commonly used to enhance the immune system:

1. Soy
2. Saw palmetto
3. Cranberry
4. Echinacea

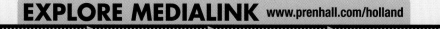

EXPLORE MEDIALINK www.prenhall.com/holland

Additional resources for this chapter can be found on the CD-ROM accompanying this textbook, and on the Companion Website. Click on Chapter 5 to select activities for this chapter.

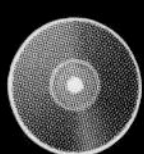

Audio Glossary
Concept Review
NCLEX-PN® Review
Nursing in Action
Dosage Calculator

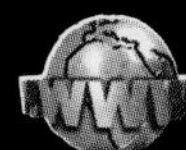

Herb Research Foundation
Medline for Herbal Products
Complementary Medicines and Alternative Therapies

CHAPTER

6 Substance Abuse

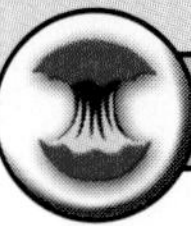

CORE CONCEPTS

6.1 Abused substances belong to many different chemical classes.

6.2 Addiction depends on multiple, complex, interacting variables.

6.3 Substance dependence is classified as physical dependence and psychological dependence.

6.4 Withdrawal results when an abused substance is no longer available.

6.5 Tolerance occurs when higher and higher doses of a drug are needed to achieve the initial response.

6.6 Central nervous system (CNS) depressants decrease the activity of the central nervous system.

6.7 Marijuana produces little physical dependence or tolerance.

6.8 Hallucinogens cause an altered state of thought and perception similar to that found in dreams.

6.9 CNS stimulants increase the activity of the central nervous system.

6.10 Nicotine is powerful and highly addictive.

OBJECTIVES

After reading this chapter, the student should be able to:

1. Discuss underlying causes of addiction.
2. Compare and contrast psychological and physical dependence.
3. Compare and contrast classic and conditioned withdrawal.
4. Explain the significance of drug tolerance to pharmacotherapy.
5. Explain the major characteristics of abuse, dependence, and tolerance resulting from the following substances:
   - **a.** Alcohol
   - **b.** Nicotine
   - **c.** Marijuana
   - **d.** Hallucinogens
   - **e.** CNS stimulants
   - **f.** Sedatives
   - **g.** Opioids

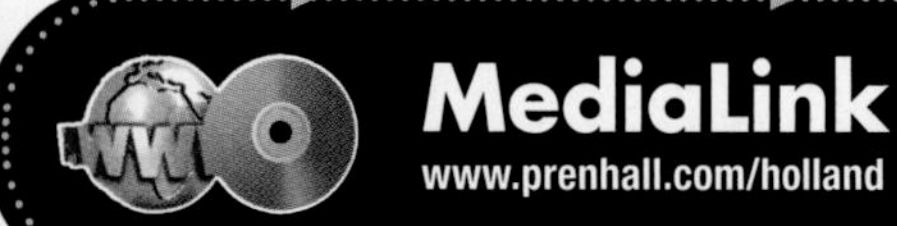

Interactive resources for this chapter can be found on the Companion Website. Click on Chapter 6 and "Begin" to select the activities for this chapter. For chapter-related animations, NCLEX-PN®-style questions, and an audio glossary, access the accompanying CD-ROM in this book.

Substance abuse is the self-administration of a drug in a way that one's culture or society views as abnormal and not acceptable. Throughout history, individuals have consumed both natural and prescription drugs to increase physical or mental performance, cause a relaxed feeling, change a psychological state, or simply fit in with the crowd. Substance abuse has a tremendous economic, social, and public health impact on society.

6.1 Abused substances belong to many different chemical classes.

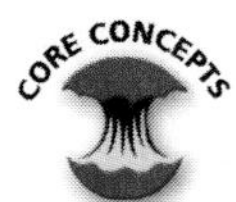

Substances from a wide variety of chemical classes are abused and can be taken by many different routes. Abused substances have in common an ability to affect the nervous system, particularly the brain. Some agents, such as opium, marijuana, cocaine, nicotine, caffeine, and alcohol, are obtained from natural sources. Others agents are synthetic or **designer drugs** that are created in illegal laboratories solely for making money in illegal drug trafficking.

Although the public often connects substance abuse with illegal drugs, this is not necessarily the case: Alcohol and nicotine are the two most commonly abused drugs. Legal prescription medications such as methylphenidate (Ritalin) and meperidine (Demerol) are sometimes abused. Volatile inhalants, found in common household products such as aerosols and paint thinners, are often abused. Illegal substances that are frequently abused include marijuana, **opioids** (which are *narcotic analgesics*), sedatives, and hallucinogens such as lysergic acid diethylamide (LSD) and phencyclidine (PCP).

Several drugs that were once used therapeutically are now illegal because of their high potential for abuse. Cocaine was once widely used as a local anesthetic, but today nearly all cocaine use and purchase is illegal. LSD is now illegal, although in the 1940s and 1950s, it was used in psychotherapy. Phencyclidine was popular in the early 1960s as an anesthetic, but was taken off

Fast Facts Substance Abuse in the United States

- Twenty-eight million Americans have used illicit drugs at least once.
- During the 2003–2004 school year, 25% of high school students used an illegal drug on a monthly or more frequent basis.
- An estimated 2.4 million Americans have used heroin during their lives.
- About one in five Americans has lived with an alcoholic while growing up. Children of alcoholic parents are four times more likely to become alcoholics than children of nonalcoholic parents.
- Alcohol is an important factor in 68% of manslaughters, 54% of murders, 48% of robberies, and 44% of burglaries.
- Among youth between the ages of 12 and 17, 7.2 million drank alcohol at least once in 2003. Girls were as likely as boys to drink alcohol.
- Barbiturate overdose is a factor in almost one third of all drug-related deaths.
- In 2003, 36% of 10th graders and 46% of 12th graders reported using marijuana and hashish.
- In 2003, 7.7% of high school seniors reported using cocaine, up from 5.9% in 1994.
- In 2002, 2 million Americans were currently using cocaine on a monthly basis; about 567,000 used crack cocaine.
- Approximately 70% of the cocaine entering the United States comes from Columbia and passes through southern Florida.
- In 2003, 16% of 8th graders and 11% of 12th graders reported using volatile inhalants.
- In 2002, 30% of all Americans were cigarette smokers, including 25% of those between the ages of 12 and 25.
- In 2003, 43% of 10th graders and 54% of 12th graders reported they had tried smoking cigarettes. Of the 12th graders, 8% consumed over half a pack or more each day.
- In 2003, 8% of 12th graders reported using ecstasy (MDMA).
- LSD is one of the most potent drugs known, with only 25–150 micrograms constituting a dose. In 2003, almost 9% of 12th graders reported using LSD.

TABLE 6.1 Commonly Abused Substances

	NATURAL SUBSTANCES	MEDICATIONS
LEGAL SUBSTANCES WITHOUT PRESCRIPTION		
Ethyl alcohol	✓ (drinking alcohol)	✓ (OTC drugs)
Methanol	✓ (solvents, varnishes)	
Caffeine	✓ (coffee)	✓ (OTC drugs)
Nicotine	✓ (tobacco)	✓ (smoking cessation)
LEGAL SUBSTANCES WITH PRESCRIPTION		
Barbiturates		✓ (sedative; CNS depressant)
Benzodiazepines		✓ (sedative; CNS depressant)
Opioids		✓ (pain therapy)
Ketamine		✓ (anesthetic)
Gamma hydroxybutyrate (GHB)		✓ (anesthetic)
Amphetamines, methamphetamines, and methylphenidate (Ritalin)		✓ (CNS stimulant)
Anabolic steroids		✓(weight gain; other uses)
ILLEGAL SUBSTANCES DISCONTINUED IN TRADITIONAL THERAPIES		
Opioids	✓ (opium)	✓ (heroin)
Cannabinoids (THC)*	✓ (marijuana)	✓ (glaucoma therapy)
LSD	✓ (rye/grain fungus)	✓ (psychiatric therapy)
Psilocybin	✓ (mushrooms)	
Mescaline	✓ (peyote)	
Phencyclidine (PCP)		✓ (anesthetic)
MDA*–designer drug–synthetic–no medicinal use		
MMDA* (Ecstasy or Ecstacy)–designer drug–synthetic–no medicinal use		
DOM* (STP)–designer drug–synthetic–no medicinal use		
Cocaine	✓ (coca plant)	✓ (local anesthetic)

**Chemical names are complicated and extensive; see Core Concepts 6.7 and 6.8 for more information.*

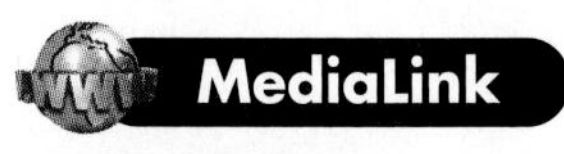

THE TEMPTATION OF ANABOLIC STEROIDS

the market in 1965 because patients reported hallucinations, delusions, and anxiety after recovering from anesthesia. The use of many of the amphetamines, once prescribed for bronchodilation, was stopped in the 1980s after psychotic episodes were reported. Commonly abused substances are summarized in Table 6.1.

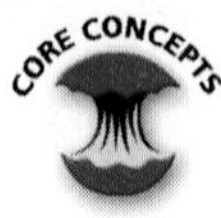

6.2 Addiction depends on multiple, complex, interacting variables.

addict = *given over*

Addiction, the progressive and chronic abuse of a substance, is an overwhelming feeling that drives someone to use a drug repeatedly, despite serious health and social consequences. It is impossible to predict accurately whether a person will become an addict. Scientists have used psychological profiles and investigated genetic links to attempt to predict a person's addictive tendency, but no firm connections have been found. Addiction depends on multiple, complex, interacting variables. These variables focus on the following categories:

- *Agent or drug of abuse* Cost, availability, dose, method of administration (e.g., oral, IV, inhalation), speed of onset/end of effect, and length of drug use
- *User factors* Genetic factors (e.g., metabolic enzymes, natural tolerance), tendency toward risk-taking behavior, prior experiences with drugs, disease that may require a scheduled drug
- *Environment* Social/community *norms* (normal behavior accepted within a community), role models, peer influences, educational opportunities

Addiction may begin with a real need for pharmacotherapy. For example, narcotic analgesics may be prescribed for pain or sedatives for a sleep disorder. A favorable experience of pain relief or being able to fall asleep may cause a patient to want to repeat these positive experiences.

It is a common misunderstanding, even among some health professionals, that the therapeutic use of scheduled drugs creates large numbers of addicted patients. In fact, prescription drugs rarely cause addiction, when used as prescribed. The risk of addiction for prescription medications is mostly a function of the dose and the length of therapy. For this reason, medications having a potential for abuse are usually prescribed at the lowest effective dose for the shortest time necessary to treat the medical problems (see Chapter 12 for more information on pain management). As mentioned in Chapters 1 and 2, numerous laws have been passed in an attempt to limit drug abuse and addiction.

6.3 Substance dependence is classified as physical dependence and psychological dependence.

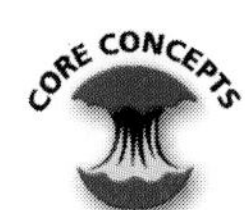

Whether a substance is addictive relates to how easily an individual can stop taking it repeatedly. When a person has an overwhelming desire to take a drug and cannot stop, it is referred to as *substance dependence.* Substance dependence is classified by two categories, physical and psychological dependence.

Physical dependence is an altered physical condition caused by the nervous system adapting to repeated substance use. Over time, the body's cells are tricked into believing that it is normal for the substance to continually be present. With physical dependence, uncomfortable symptoms, known as **withdrawal syndrome,** occur when the agent is stopped. Opioids, such as morphine and heroin, may produce physical dependence rather quickly with repeated doses, particularly when taken intravenously. Alcohol, sedatives, some stimulants, and nicotine are other examples of substances that may easily produce physical dependence with repeated use.

On the other hand, **psychological dependence** causes no signs of physical discomfort after the agent is stopped. The person, however, has an overwhelming desire to continue using the substance even if there are obvious negative economic, physical, or social consequences. This intense craving may be associated with the individual's home environment or social contacts. Strong psychological craving for a substance may continue for months or even years and is often responsible for relapses (a return to drug-seeking behavior) during substance abuse therapy. Psychological dependence usually occurs only after relatively high doses of the substance are used for a long time, such as with marijuana and antianxiety drugs. However, psychological dependence may develop quickly, perhaps after only one use, with crack—a potent, inexpensive form of cocaine.

6.4 Withdrawal results when an abused substance is no longer available.

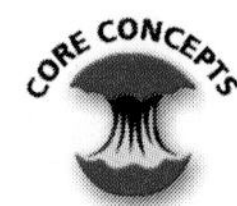

Once a patient becomes physically dependent and the substance is stopped, withdrawal syndrome will occur. Symptoms of withdrawal syndrome may be severe for patients who are physically dependent on alcohol and sedatives. Helping a patient withdraw from these agents is best done in a substance abuse treatment facility. Examples of withdrawal syndromes related to different abused substances are show in Table 6.2.

Prescription drugs may be used to reduce the severity of withdrawal symptoms. For example, alcohol withdrawal can be treated with a short-acting benzodiazepine such as oxazepam (Serax), and opioid withdrawal can be treated with methadone. Symptoms of nicotine withdrawal may be relieved by nicotine replacement therapy in the form of patches or chewing gum and the use of bupropion (Wellbutrin). No specific pharmacological treatments are indicated for withdrawal from CNS stimulants, hallucinogens, marijuana, or inhalants.

With chronic substance abuse, patients will often associate their conditions and surroundings—including social contacts with other users—with use of the drug. Users tend to return to drug-seeking behavior when they interact with other substance abusers. Counselors often encourage patients to stop associating with past social contacts or having relationships with other substance

TABLE 6.2 Withdrawal Symptoms of Selected Drugs of Abuse

DRUG	SYMPTOMS
Alcohol	Tremors, fatigue, anxiety, abdominal cramping, hallucinations, confusion, seizures, delirium
Barbiturates and other sedative-hypnotics	Insomnia, anxiety, weakness, abdominal cramps, tremor, anorexia, seizures, hallucinations, delirium
Benzodiazepines	Insomnia, restlessness, abdominal pain, nausea, sensitivity to light and sound, headache, fatigue, muscle twitches
Cocaine and amphetamines	Mental depression, anxiety, extreme fatigue, hunger
Hallucinogens	Rarely observed; dependent on specific drug
Marijuana	Irritability, restlessness, insomnia, tremor, chills, weight loss
Nicotine	Irritability, anxiety, restlessness, headaches, increased appetite, insomnia, inability to concentrate, decreased heart rate and blood pressure
Opioids	Excessive sweating, restlessness, dilated pupils, agitation, goosebumps, tremor, violent yawning, increased heart rate and blood pressure, nausea/vomiting, abdominal cramps and pain, muscle spasms with kicking movements, weight loss

abusers to lessen the possibility of relapse. With the assistance of self-help groups such as Alcoholics Anonymous, some patients are able to move to a drugfree lifestyle by making friends with new drug- and alcohol-free people.

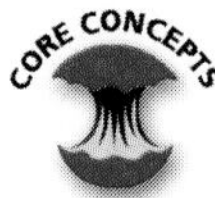

6.5 Tolerance occurs when higher and higher doses of a drug are needed to achieve the initial response.

Tolerance is a biological condition that occurs when the body adapts to a substance after it is repeatedly administered. Over time, higher doses of the agent are needed to produce the initial effect. For example, at the start of pharmacotherapy, a patient may find that 2 mg of a sedative is effective for causing sleep. After taking the medication for several months, the patient notices that it takes 4 mg or perhaps 6 mg to fall asleep. Development of drug tolerance is common for substances that affect the nervous system. Tolerance should be thought of as a natural consequence of continued drug use and not be considered evidence of addiction or substance abuse.

Tolerance does not develop at the same rate for all actions of a drug. For example, patients usually develop tolerance to the nausea and vomiting produced by narcotic analgesics after only a few doses. Tolerance to the mood-altering effects of these drugs and to their ability to reduce pain develops more slowly, but eventually may be complete. Tolerance never develops to the drug's ability to constrict the pupils. Patients will often put up with annoying side effects of drugs, such as the sleepiness caused by antihistamines, if they know that tolerance to these effects will develop quickly.

Once tolerance develops to one substance, it often also occurs with use of closely related drugs. This reaction is known as *cross-tolerance.* For example, a heroin addict will be tolerant to the analgesic effects of other opioids such as morphine or meperidine. Patients who have developed tolerance to alcohol will show tolerance to other CNS depressants such as barbiturates, benzodiazepines, and some general anesthetics. This is important to know because doses of related medications may need to be adjusted so that the patient receives maximum therapeutic benefit.

The terms *immunity* and *resistance* are often confused with *tolerance.* These terms more correctly refer to the immune system and infections, and they should not be used to mean tolerance. For example, microorganisms become *resistant* to the effects of an antibiotic; they do not become *tolerant.* Patients become tolerant to the effects of pain relievers; they do not become resistant. It is not acceptable to say that patients are immune to drug therapy.

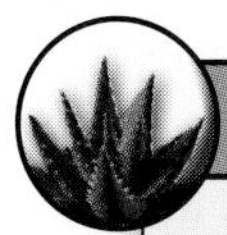

NATURAL ALTERNATIVES

Herbal Stimulants

Recovering from addiction may be a difficult experience. Some claim that discretionary use of some herbal stimulants may ease the symptoms associated with recovery. Examples include kola, damiana, Asiatic and Siberian ginseng, and gotu kola. These agents are thought to stimulate the central nervous system, providing just enough effect to reduce tension and the stresses associated with drug craving. ■

Concept Review 6.1

- What is the difference between physical dependence and psychological dependence? How do patients know when they are physically dependent on a substance?

6.6 Central nervous system (CNS) depressants decrease the activity of the central nervous system.

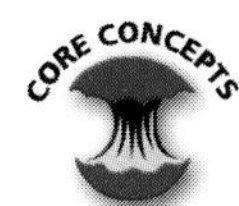

Central nervous system (CNS) depressants form a group of drugs that cause patients to feel sedated or relaxed. Drugs in this group include barbiturates, nonbarbiturate sedative-hypnotics, benzodiazepines, alcohol, and opioids. Although the majority of these are legal substances, they are controlled because of their abuse potential.

Sedatives

Sedatives, known as *tranquilizers,* are prescribed mostly for sleep disorders and some forms of epilepsy. The two primary classes of sedatives are the barbiturates (see Chapter 8 for their use in treating sleep disorders and Chapter 11 for their use in treating epilepsy) and the nonbarbiturate sedative-hypnotics ⊂⊃. Their actions, indications, safety profiles, and addictive potential are roughly the same. Physical dependence, psychological dependence, and tolerance develop when these agents are taken for long periods at high doses. Patients sometimes abuse these drugs by taking more doses than prescribed or by sharing their medication with friends. These drugs are frequently combined with other drugs of abuse such as CNS stimulators or alcohol. Addicts often alternate between amphetamines, which keep them awake for several days, and barbiturates, which help them to relax and fall asleep.

Many sedatives have a long duration of action. Effects may last an entire day, depending on the specific drug. Patients may appear dull or apathetic with slurred speech and lack of motor coordination. Four commonly abused barbiturates are pentobarbital (Nembutal), amobarbital (Amytal), secobarbital (Seconal), and a combination of secobarbital and amobarbital (Tuinal). The medical use of barbiturates and nonbarbiturate sedative-hypnotics has noticeably declined over the past 20 years.

Overdoses of barbiturates and nonbarbiturate sedative-hynotics are extremely dangerous. These drugs suppress the respiratory centers in the brain, and the user may stop breathing or enter a coma. Death may result from barbiturate overdose. Withdrawal symptoms from these drugs are similar to those of alcohol withdrawal and may be life threatening.

Benzodiazepines

Benzodiazepines are another group of CNS depressants that have a potential for abuse. They are one of the most widely prescribed classes of drugs and have largely replaced the barbiturates for certain disorders. Their primary indication is anxiety, thus they are called *anxiolytic* drugs (see Chapter 8 ⊂⊃). They are also used to prevent seizures (Chapter 11) and as muscle relaxants (Chapter 31) ⊂⊃. Popular benzodiazepines include alprazolam (Xanax), diazepam (Valium), temazepam (Restoril), triazolam (Halcion), and midazolam (Versed).

anxio = *anxiety/ restlessness*
lytic = *destruction*

Although benzodiazepines are the most frequently prescribed drug class, benzodiazepine abuse is not common. Those individuals who do abuse benzodiazepines may appear carefree, detached, sleepy, or disoriented. Death due to overdose is rare, even with high doses. Abusers may combine these agents with alcohol, cocaine, or heroin to increase their drug experience. If combined with other agents, however, overdose may cause death. The benzodiazepine withdrawal syndrome is less severe than that of barbiturates or alcohol.

Opioids

Opioids are prescribed for severe pain, persistent cough, and diarrhea. The opioid class includes natural substances found in the unripe seeds of the poppy plant, such as opium, morphine, and codeine, and synthetic drugs such as propoxyphene (Darvon), meperidine (Demerol), oxycodone (OxyContin), fentanyl (Duragesic, Sublimaze), methadone (Dolophine), and heroin. The therapeutic effects of the opioids are discussed in detail in Chapter 12.

eu = *healthy or well*
phoria = *bearing*

The effects of *oral* opioids begin within 30 minutes and may last over a day. *Parenteral* forms produce immediate effects, including the brief, intense rush of *euphoria* (pleasure) sought by heroin addicts. Individuals experience a range of CNS effects from extreme pleasure to slowed body activities and extreme sedation. Signs include constricted pupils, an increase in the ability to withstand pain, and respiratory depression.

Addiction to opioids can occur rapidly, and withdrawal can produce intense symptoms. While extremely unpleasant, withdrawal from opioids is not life threatening. Methadone is a narcotic sometimes used to treat opioid addiction. Although methadone has addictive properties of its own, it does not produce the same degree of euphoria as other opioids, and its effects are longer lasting. Heroin addicts are switched to methadone to prevent unpleasant withdrawal symptoms. Since methadone is taken orally, the serious risks associated with intravenous drug use, such as hepatitis and AIDS, are eliminated. Patients sometimes remain on methadone maintenance for their lifetimes. Withdrawal from methadone is more prolonged than from heroin or morphine, but the symptoms are less intense.

Ethyl Alcohol

Ethyl alcohol, commonly known as alcohol, is an often abused drug. Alcohol is a legal substance for adults and is available as beer, wine, and liquor. The economic, social, and health consequences of alcohol abuse are staggering. In contrast to the many negative consequences associated with long-term abuse of alcohol, drinking of small quantities of alcohol on a daily basis has been found to reduce the risk of stroke and heart attack.

Alcohol is classified as a CNS depressant, because it slows the actions of the region of the brain responsible for alertness and wakefulness. Alcohol easily crosses the blood-brain barrier and its effects can be noticed within 5 to 30 minutes. Effects of alcohol are directly related to the amount consumed within a certain time frame, and include relaxation, sedation, memory impairment, loss of motor coordination, reduced judgment, and decreased inhibition. **Alcohol intoxication** occurs when muscle coordination is lost and mental function is affected. It results in a characteristic odor to the breath and increased blood flow in certain areas of the skin, causing a flushed face, pink cheeks, or red nose. Although these symptoms are easily recognized, the nurse must be aware that other substances and disorders may cause similar effects. For example, many antianxiety agents, sedatives, and antidepressants can cause drowsiness, memory difficulties, and loss of motor coordination. Certain mouthwashes contain alcohol and cause the breath to smell alcoholic.

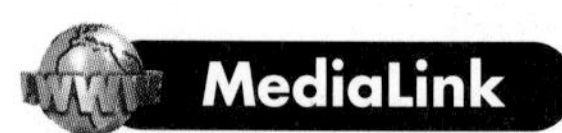

ALCOHOL POISONING AND TOXICITY

The presence of food in the stomach will slow the absorption of alcohol, thus delaying the onset of drug action. *Metabolism,* or detoxification of alcohol by the liver, occurs at a slow, constant rate, which is not affected by the presence of food. The average rate is about 15 ml per hour—equal to one alcoholic beverage per hour. If consumed at a higher rate, alcohol will accumulate in the blood and produce greater effects on the brain. An overdose of alcohol produces vomiting, severe hypotension, respiratory failure, and coma. Death due to alcohol poisoning is common.

cirr = *orange/yellow*
osis = *condition*

Chronic alcohol consumption produces both psychological and physiological dependence and results in a large number of adverse health effects. The organ most affected by chronic alcohol abuse is the liver. Alcoholism is a common cause of *cirrhosis,* a harmful and often fatal failure of the liver to perform its vital functions. Liver failure causes abnormalities in blood clotting and nutritional deficiencies, and sensitizes the patient to the effects of all medications metabolized by the liver.

Alcohol withdrawal syndrome is severe and may be life threatening. The use of anticonvulsants in the treatment of alcohol withdrawal is discussed in Chapter 11. Long-term treatment for alcohol abuse includes behavioral counseling and participation in self-help groups such as Alcoholics Anonymous. Disulfiram (Antabuse) may be given to discourage relapses. Disulfiram inhibits acetaldehyde dehydrogenase, the enzyme that metabolizes alcohol. If alcohol is consumed while taking disulfiram, the patient becomes violently ill within 5 to 10 minutes, with headache, shortness of breath, nausea/vomiting, and other unpleasant symptoms. Disulfiram is only effective in highly motivated patients, since the success of pharmacotherapy is entirely dependent on patient compliance. Alcohol sensitivity continues for up to 2 weeks after disulfiram has been discontinued. As a pregnancy category X drug, disulfiram should never be taken during pregnancy.

Concept Review 6.2

- Compare the potential for barbiturates or benzodiazepines to cause death or coma.

6.7 Marijuana produces little physical dependence or tolerance.

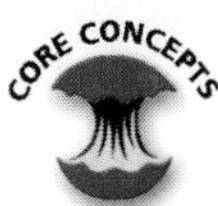

Cannabinoids are substances obtained from the hemp plant *Cannabis sativa,* which grows in tropical climates. Cannabinoid agents are usually smoked and include marijuana, hashish, and hash oil. Although more than 61 cannabinoid chemicals have been identified, the ingredient responsible for most of the psychoactive properties is delta-9-**tetrahydrocannabinol (THC).**

Marijuana (street names "grass," "pot," "weed," "reefer," or "dope") is a natural product obtained from *C. sativa.* It is the most commonly used illegal drug in the United States. Use of marijuana slows motor activity, decreases coordination, and causes disconnected thoughts, paranoia, and euphoria. It increases thirst and craving for food, particularly chocolate and other candies. One hallmark symptom of marijuana use is red or bloodshot eyes, caused by dilation of blood vessels. THC accumulates in the gonads.

para = *beside*
noia = *mind*

When inhaled, marijuana produces effects that occur within minutes and last up to 24 hours. Because marijuana smoke is inhaled more deeply and held within the lungs for a longer time than cigarette smoke, marijuana smoke introduces four times more tar into the lungs than tobacco smoke. Smoking marijuana on a daily basis may increase the risk of lung cancer and other respiratory disorders. Chronic use is associated with lack of motivation in achieving or pursuing life goals.

Unlike many abused substances, marijuana produces little physical dependence or tolerance. Withdrawal symptoms are mild, if they are experienced at all. Metabolites of THC, however, remain in the body for months to years, allowing laboratory specialists to determine easily whether someone has used marijuana. For several days after use, THC can also be detected in the urine. Despite numerous attempts by scientists to demonstrate therapeutic applications for marijuana, results have been controversial and the medical value of the drug remains to be proven.

Concept Review 6.3

- Name three legal substances often abused and also used in traditional therapies. Are these natural or synthetic substances? Compare ethyl alcohol and marijuana in terms of common use.

6.8 Hallucinogens cause an altered state of thought and perception similar to that found in dreams.

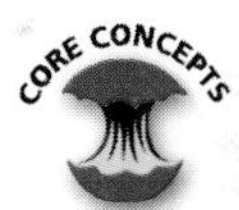

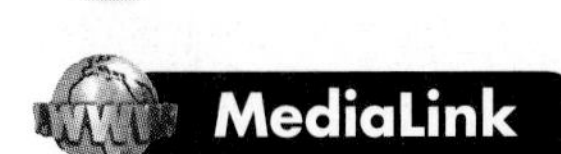

THE HISTORY OF LSD

Hallucinogens consist of an assorted class of chemicals that have in common the ability to produce an altered, dreamlike state of consciousness. Sometimes called **psychedelics,** the prototype substance for this class is *lysergic acid diethylamine (LSD).* All hallucinogens are Schedule I drugs and have no medical use.

For nearly all drugs of abuse, predictable symptoms occur in every user. Effects from hallucinogens, however, are highly variable and depend on the mood and expectations of the user and the surrounding environment in which the substance is used. Two patients taking the same agent will report completely different symptoms, and the same patient may report different symptoms with each use. Users who take LSD or *psilocybin* (a drug derived from a mushroom with the street names "magic mushrooms" and "shrooms") (Figure 6.1 ■) may experience symptoms such as laughter, visions, religious revelations, or deep personal insights. Common occurrences are hallucinations and afterimages (images that are projected onto people as they move). Users also report unusually bright lights and vivid colors. Some users hear voices; others report smells. Many experience a profound sense of truth and deep-directed thoughts. Unpleasant experiences can be terrifying and may include anxiety, panic attacks, confusion, severe depression, and paranoia.

LSD (street names "acid," "the beast," "blotter acid," "California sunshine") is made from a fungus that grows on rye and other grains. LSD is almost always used in an oral form. It can be manufactured in capsules, tablets, or liquids. A common and inexpensive method for distributing LSD is to place drops of the drug on small pieces of paper that often contain images of cartoon characters or graphics related to the drug culture. After drying, the paper containing the LSD is swallowed to produce the drug's effects.

LSD is distributed throughout the body immediately after use. Effects are experienced within an hour, and may last 6 to 12 hours. It affects the central and autonomic nervous systems,

FIGURE 6.1

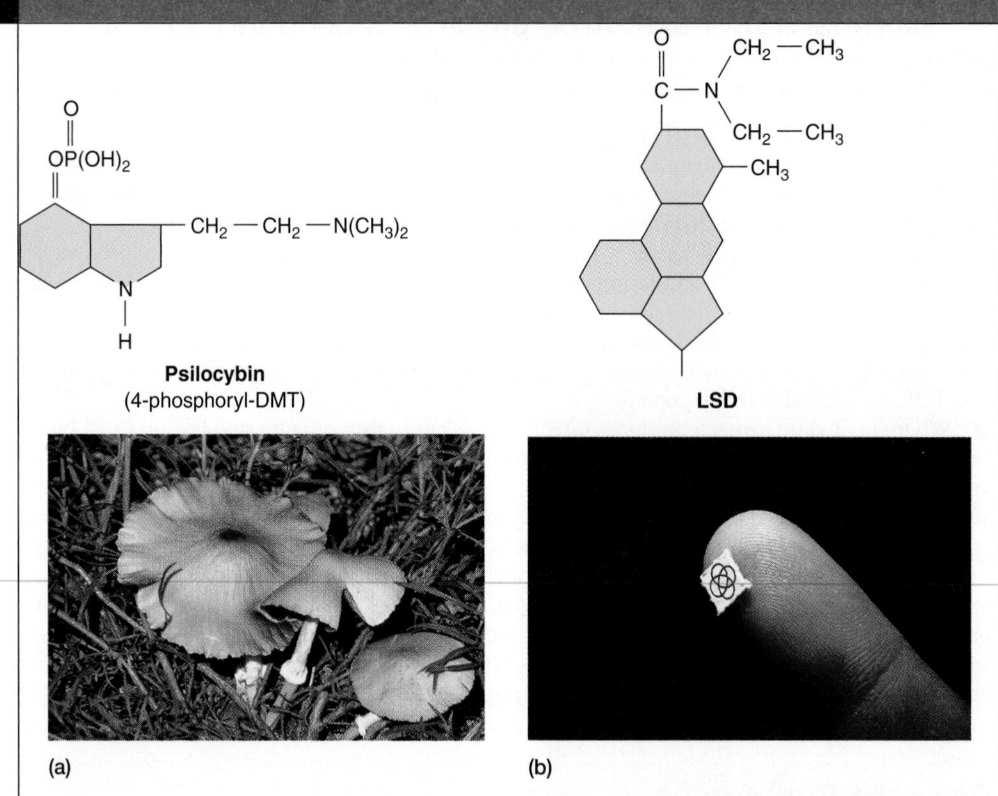

Comparison of the chemical structures of psilocybin and LSD. Psilocybin is derived from a mushroom, shown in (a); an LSD "blot" is shown in (b).
SOURCE: Pearson Education/PH College

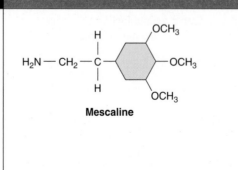

increasing blood pressure, elevating body temperature, dilating pupils, and increasing heart rate. Repeated use may cause memory loss and inability to reason. In extreme cases, patients may develop psychoses. One unusual adverse effect is flashbacks, in which the user experiences the effects of the drug again—sometimes weeks, months, or years after the drug was initially taken. Although users may experience tolerance, they have little or no dependence with hallucinogens.

Other hallucinogens that are abused include the following:

- *Mescaline:* found in the peyote cactus of Mexico and Central America (Figure 6.2 ■)
- *MDMA (3,4-methylenedioxymethamphetamine, "XTC," "Ecstasy," or "Ecstacy"):* an amphetamine originally created for research purposes, but now extremely popular as a drug of abuse
- *DOM (2,5 dimethoxy-4-methylamphetamine, "STP"):* a recreational drug often linked with rave parties
- *MDA (3,4-methylenedioxyamphetamine):* called the "love drug" because of a belief that it enhances sexual desires

FIGURE 6.2

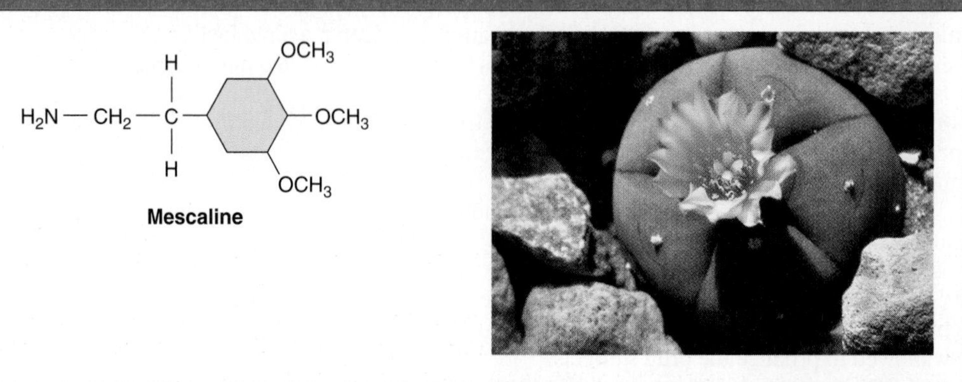

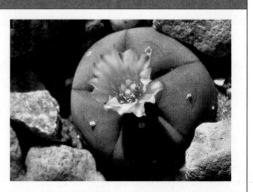

The chemical structure of mescaline, derived from the peyote plant (shown in photo)
SOURCE: Pearson Education/PH College

- *PCP (chemical name, phenylcyclohexylpiperadine; also called phencyclidine; street name "angel dust"):* produces a trancelike state that may last for days and results in severe brain damage; used as an animal tranquilizer
- *Ketamine ("date rape" drug or "special coke"):* produces unconsciousness and amnesia; primary legal use as an anesthetic

Concept Review 6.4

- In examining and interviewing a patient, how could you determine whether he or she is under the influence of marijuana or hallucinogens?

6.9 CNS stimulants increase the activity of the central nervous system.

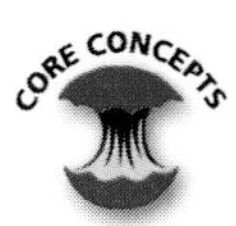

Stimulants include a varied family of drugs with the ability to increase the activity of the CNS. Some are available by prescription for use in the treatment of *narcolepsy* (a sleep disorder in which people fall asleep unexpectedly), obesity, and **attention deficit disorder (ADD)** (or attention deficit hyperactivity disorder [ADHD]). As drugs of abuse, CNS stimulants are taken to produce a sense of exhilaration, improve mental and physical performance, reduce appetite, prolong wakefulness, or simply "get high." Stimulants include amphetamines, cocaine, methylphenidate, and caffeine.

narco = *numbness or stupor*
lepsy = *seizure*

CNS stimulants have effects similar to the neurotransmitter norepinephrine, which is discussed in Chapter 7. Norepinephrine activates neurons in a part of the brain that affects awareness and wakefulness, called the *reticular formation* (see Chapter 8 for an in-depth discussion). High doses of amphetamines give the user a feeling of self-confidence, euphoria, alertness, and empowerment. Long-term use, however, often causes feelings of restlessness, anxiety, and fits of rage, especially when the user is coming down from a drug high.

Most CNS stimulants affect cardiovascular and respiratory activity, raising blood pressure and increasing respiration rate. Other symptoms include dilated pupils, sweating, and tremors. Overdoses of some stimulants lead to seizures and cardiac arrest.

Amphetamines and dextroamphetamines were once widely prescribed for depression, obesity, drowsiness, and congestion. In the 1960s, the healthcare profession realized that the risk for amphetamine dependence outweighed the drug's therapeutic usefulness. Because of the development of safer medications, the current therapeutic uses of these drugs are extremely limited. Most substance abusers get these agents from illegal laboratories, which can easily produce amphetamines and make tremendous profits.

Dextroamphetamine (Dexedrine) may be used to treat narcolepsy and for short-term weight loss when all other attempts to lose weight have been exhausted. Methamphetamine (street name "ice" or "crank") is often used as a recreational drug for those who like the rush that it provides. It usually is administered in powder or crystal form, but it also may be smoked. Methamphetamine is a Schedule II drug marketed under the trade name Desoxyn, although most abusers obtain it from illegal methamphetamine laboratories. A drug related to methamphetamine, called methcathinone (street name "cat"), is made illegally and snorted, taken orally, or injected intravenously. Methcathinone is a Schedule I agent.

Methylphenidate (Ritalin) is a CNS stimulant (Schedule II drug) that is widely prescribed for children diagnosed with ADD/ADHD (Chapter 9). Ritalin has a calming effect on children who are inattentive or hyperactive. It stimulates the alertness center in the brain and allows the child to focus on tasks for longer periods.

In adults, Ritalin usually produces the same effects as cocaine and amphetamines and is sometimes abused by adolescents and adults seeking euphoria. The tablets are crushed and used intranasally or dissolved in liquid and injected intravenously. Ritalin is also sometimes mixed with heroin (street name "speedball").

Cocaine is a natural substance obtained from leaves of the coca plant, which grows in the Andes Mountain region of South America. The plant has been used by Andean cultures since 2500 B.C. Natives of this region chew the coca leaves or make teas of the dried leaves. Because it is taken orally, its absorption is slow, and the leaves contain only 1% cocaine, users do not have the ill effects caused by chemically pure extracts from the plant. In the Andean culture, use of coca leaves is not considered substance abuse because it is part of that society's culture.

Cocaine is a Schedule II drug that produces actions similar to those of the amphetamines, although its effects are usually more rapid and intense. It is the second most commonly abused illegal drug in the United States. Routes of administration include snorting, smoking, and injecting. In smaller doses, cocaine produces feelings of intense euphoria, a decrease in hunger, analgesia, illusions of physical strength, and increased sensory perception. Larger doses will magnify these effects and also cause rapid heartbeat, sweating, dilation of the pupils, and elevated body temperature. After euphoria diminishes, the user often feels irritable, depressed, and distrustful, and usually has insomnia. Some users report the sensation that insects are crawling under their skin. Users who snort cocaine develop a chronic runny nose, a crusty redness around the nostrils, and deterioration of the nasal cartilage. Overdose can cause dysrhythmias, convulsions, stroke, or death due to respiratory arrest. The withdrawal syndrome for amphetamines and cocaine is much less intense than that from alcohol or barbiturates.

Caffeine is a natural substance found in the seeds, leaves, or fruits of more than 63 plant species throughout the world. Significant amounts of caffeine are consumed in chocolate, coffee, tea, soft drinks, and ice cream (Table 6.3). Sometimes caffeine is added to OTC pain relievers to help relieve migraines and other conditions. Caffeine travels to almost all parts of the body after ingestion, and several hours are needed for the body to metabolize and eliminate the drug. Caffeine has a pronounced diuretic effect.

Caffeine is considered a CNS stimulant because it produces increased mental alertness, restlessness, nervousness, irritability, and insomnia. The physical effects of caffeine include bronchodilation, increased blood pressure, increased production of stomach acid, and changes in blood glucose levels. Repeated use of caffeine may result in physical dependence and tolerance.

Concept Review 6.5

- Identify three groups of stimulants discussed in this section and give examples for each group. Identify major systems in the body affected by these stimulants.

TABLE 6.3 Caffeine Content of Common Food and Beverages

	SERVING SIZE	CAFFEINE (MG)
OTC DRUGS		
NoDoz, maximum strength; Vivarin	1 tablet	200
Excedrin	2 tablets	130
NoDoz, regular strength	1 tablet	100
Anacin (also available in caffeine-free formulation)	2 tablets	64
COFFEES		
Coffee, brewed and instant	8 ounces	95–135
Coffee, decaffeinated	8 ounces	5
TEAS		
Tea, leaf or bag	8 ounces	50
Tea, green	8 ounces	30
Tea, instant	8 ounces	15
SOFT DRINKS		
Mountain Dew	12 ounces	55.5
Diet Coke	12 ounces	46.5
Coca-Cola Classic	12 ounces	34.5
Pepsi-Cola	12 ounces	37.5
FROZEN DESSERTS AND YOGURTS		
Starbucks coffee ice cream, assorted flavors	1 cup	40–60
Dannon coffee yogurt	8 ounces	45
CHOCOLATES AND CANDIES		
Hershey's Special Dark chocolate bar	1 bar (1.5 ounces)	31
Hershey Bar (milk chocolate)	1 bar (1.5 ounces)	10
Cocoa or hot chocolate	8 ounces	85

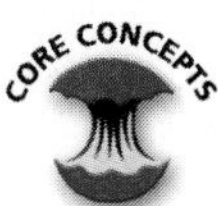

6.10 Nicotine is powerful and highly addictive.

Nicotine is sometimes considered a CNS stimulant because of its ability to increase alertness. However, its actions and long-term consequences place it into a class by itself. Nicotine is unique among abused substances in that it is legal, strongly addictive, and highly carcinogenic. Furthermore, use of tobacco can cause harmful effects from secondhand smoke to those in the immediate area of the smoker. Patients often do not consider tobacco use to be substance abuse.

The most common method by which nicotine enters the body is through the inhalation of cigarette, pipe, or cigar smoke. Tobacco smoke contains more than 1000 chemicals, many of which are carcinogens. The primary addictive substance in cigarette smoke is nicotine. Effects of inhaled nicotine may last from 30 minutes to several hours.

Nicotine affects many body systems, including the nervous, cardiovascular, and endocrine systems. Nicotine stimulates the CNS directly, causing increased alertness and ability to focus, feelings of relaxation, and lightheadedness. The cardiovascular effects of nicotine include accelerated heart rate and increased blood pressure, caused by activation of nicotinic receptors located within the autonomic nervous system (Chapter 7). These cardiovascular effects can be serious in patients taking oral contraceptives. The risk of a fatal heart attack is five times greater in smokers than in nonsmokers. Muscular tremors may occur with moderate doses of nicotine, and convulsions may result from very high doses. Nicotine affects the endocrine system by increasing the basal metabolic rate, leading to weight loss. Nicotine also reduces appetite. Chronic use leads to bronchitis, emphysema, and lung cancer.

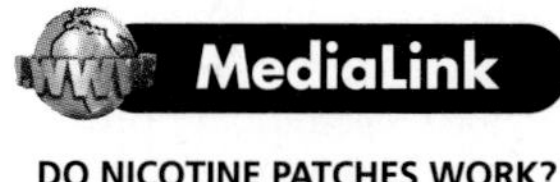

DO NICOTINE PATCHES WORK?

Both psychological and physical dependence occur relatively quickly with nicotine. Once started on tobacco, patients tend to continue their drug use for many years, despite overwhelming medical evidence that their quality of life will be adversely affected and their lifespan shortened. Discontinuation results in agitation, weight gain, anxiety, headache, and an extreme craving for the drug. Although nicotine replacement patches and gum and buproprion assist patients in dealing with the unpleasant withdrawal symptoms, only 25% of patients who attempt to stop smoking remain tobacco-free 1 year later.

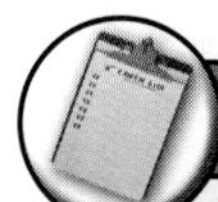

PATIENTS NEED TO KNOW

Patients taking medications with abuse potential need to know the following:

Regarding Alcohol

1. Limit alcoholic beverage intake to two drinks per day for men or one drink per day for women.
2. Avoid alcohol use entirely if liver disease, gastric reflux, peptic ulcers, or pregnancy exists.
3. Check with healthcare provider when combining alcohol and medications (prescription or over the counter). Alcohol is considered a CNS depressant, so never combine it with other CNS depressants.
4. Consuming more than one alcoholic drink per hour will usually result in blood alcohol levels above the legal limit for operating a vehicle.

Regarding CNS Stimulants

5. Avoid sources of caffeine such as OTC drugs with caffeine, chocolate, coffee, and tea if taking methylphenidate.
6. Always take methylphenidate (Ritalin) at least 6 hours prior to sleep to avoid insomnia.

Regarding CNS Depressants

7. Never take more CNS depressant medication than prescribed. If the prescribed dose is not providing sufficient relief, a healthcare provider should be notified, due to the possibility of a developed tolerance.
8. Never combine CNS depressants (including alcohol) unless advised to do so by a healthcare provider.

Regarding Tobacco

9. Secondhand smoke is dangerous, particularly to children and pregnant women. ▪

CHAPTER REVIEW

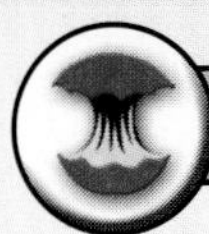

CORE CONCEPTS SUMMARY

6.1 **Abused substances belong to many different chemical classes.**

Abused substances come from many different chemical classes. Some abused substances, such as alcohol and nicotine, are available without a prescription. Others, such as barbiturates, benzodiazepines, and most opioids, have legitimate medical uses. Still others, such as LSD and heroin, are illegal, having no current medical applications.

6.2 **Addiction depends on multiple, complex, interacting variables.**

Addiction is an overwhelming feeling that causes someone to continue taking drugs. Although ideas have changed about addiction over the years, healthcare providers now recognize it as being dependent on drug factors, genetic factors, and environmental factors.

6.3 **Substance dependence is classified as physical dependence and psychological dependence.**

Dependence is an overwhelming need to take a drug on a continuous basis. Physical dependence occurs when the patient exhibits signs of withdrawal after the drug is discontinued. Psychological dependence is an intense craving for the drug.

6.4 **Withdrawal results when an abused substance is no longer available.**

When an abused drug is discontinued, patients may experience uncomfortable physical symptoms known as withdrawal syndrome. Symptoms vary depending on the specific drug of abuse and range from mild to life threatening.

6.5 **Tolerance occurs when higher and higher doses of a drug are needed to achieve the initial response.**

Tolerance occurs over time when patients adapt to continued drug use and require higher doses to produce the same effect.

6.6 **Central nervous system (CNS) depressants decrease the activity of the central nervous system.**

Substances that make patients feel relaxed and sleepy, and work by generally slowing neuronal activity in the brain include sedatives, opioids, and ethyl alcohol. Examples of sedatives are barbiturates and benzodiazepines. Because of their abuse potential, many of these substances are controlled. Ethyl alcohol is a legal substance.

6.7 **Marijuana produces little physical dependence or tolerance.**

The most commonly abused illegal substance is marijuana. Marijuana produces less physical dependence than most other drugs and produces less tolerance. The medical value of this drug remains controversial and unproven. The risks of using this substance are lung cancer, respiratory problems, and lack of motivation.

6.8 **Hallucinogens cause an altered state of thought and perception similar to that found in dreams.**

Hallucinogens, also called psychedelics, have the ability to produce altered states of consciousness and dreams. They include LSD, mescaline, MDMA (Ecstacy), DOM (STP), MDA (love drug), and ketamine, an anesthetic.

6.9 **CNS stimulants increase the activity of the central nervous system.**

Amphetamines, methylphenidate, cocaine, and caffeine increase alertness by stimulating the central nervous system. Some substances are available by prescription and are used for narcolepsy, obesity, and attention deficit disorder. Caffeine is available in many consumer products including chocolate, coffee, tea, soft drinks, and coffee ice cream. Cocaine is the second most commonly abused substance in America.

6.10 **Nicotine is powerful and highly addictive.**

Nicotine is a unique, legal, carcinogenic, highly addictive substance. The most common method of entry into the body is by inhalation of cigarette, pipe, or cigar smoke. Important effects of inhaled nicotine include stimulation of the CNS and increased cardiovascular effects.

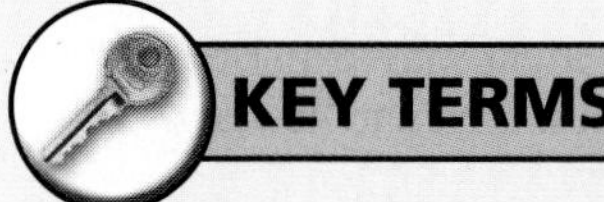

KEY TERMS

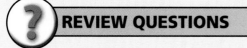

addiction (ah-DIK-shun): the continued use of a substance despite its negative health and social consequences / *page 72*

alcohol intoxication (AL-ku-hol in-tak-su-KA-shun): a condition of altered mental and physical function resulting from drinking more alcoholic beverages within a time frame than the body can tolerate / *page 76*

attention deficit disorder (ADD): consistent difficulty in focusing attention on a task for a sufficient length of time / *page 79*

designer drugs (de-ZEYE-ner drugs): drugs that are produced in a laboratory and are intended to mimic the effects of other psychoactive controlled substances / *page 71*

opioid (OH-pee-oyd): substance obtained from the unripe seeds of the poppy plant / *page 71*

physical dependence (FI-zi-kul dee-PEN-dens): the condition of experiencing unpleasant withdrawal symptoms when a substance is discontinued / *page 73*

psychedelics (seye-keh-DEL-iks): substances that alter perception and reality / *page 77*

psychological dependence (seye-koh-LOJ-i-kul dee-PEN-dens): an unpleasant, intense craving for a drug after it has been withdrawn / *page 73*

tetrahydrocannabinol (THC) (TEH-trah-HEYE-droh-cah-NAB-in-ol): the active chemical in marijuana / *page 77*

tolerance (TOL-er-ans): the process of adapting to a drug over time and requiring higher doses to achieve the same effect / *page 74*

withdrawal syndrome (with-DRAW-ul SIN-drom): unpleasant symptoms experienced when a physically dependent client discontinues the use of an abused drug/ *page 73*

REVIEW QUESTIONS

The following questions are written in NCLEX-PN® style. Answer these questions to assess your knowledge of the chapter material, and go back and review any material that is not clear to you.

1. The two most commonly abused drugs are:

1. Methylphenidate (Ritalin) and meperidine (Demerol)
2. Lysergic acid diethylamide (LSD) and phencyclidine (PCP)
3. Alcohol and nicotine
4. Opioids and inhalants

2. The patient has been diagnosed with a narcotic analgesic overdose. Which of the following symptoms are most likely associated with a narcotic analgesic overdose?

1. Irritability, restlessness, abdominal cramping
2. Excessive sweating, agitation, goosebumps, increased heart rate
3. Insomnia, hallucinations, tremors
4. Delirium, extreme fatigue, hunger, headaches

3. When the patient requires a higher dose of the substance to produce the initial effect, this is known as:

1. Toxicity
2. Resistance
3. Immunity
4. Tolerance

4. The patient has developed an opioid addiction. The nurse anticipates which of the following medications will be used for opioid withdrawal?

1. Methadone
2. Heroin
3. Diazepam (Valium)
4. Alprazolam (Xanax)

5. The nurse understands which of the following substances produces little physical dependence or tolerance:

1. Heroin
2. Marijuana
3. Alcohol
4. Cocaine

6. The nurse recognizes methylphenidate (Ritalin) is classified as a:

1. Schedule I drug
2. Schedule II drug
3. Schedule III drug
4. Schedule IV drug

7. The nurse assesses the patient and finds the following: increased heart rate, dilated pupils, elevated body temperature, and sweating. The nurse suspects:

1. Marijuana use
2. Heroin use
3. Cocaine use
4. Amphetamine use

8. Which of the following would the nurse find when assessing the patient for use of barbiturates?

1. Slurred speech, lack of muscle coordination, decreased respirations
2. Euphoria and irritability
3. Increased pain threshold and hallucinations
4. Increased blood pressure and respirations

9. Physical dependence differs from psychological dependence in that with physical dependence:

1. There is an intense craving for the drug.
2. There is an overwhelming need to take the drug.

3. The patient exhibits signs of withdrawal after the drug is discontinued.
4. Higher doses are required to produce the initial effect of the drug.

10. The nurse educates the client on disulfiram (Antabuse), saying that:

1. Only small amounts of alcohol may be ingested while on this drug.
2. If alcohol is ingested, the patient may experience shortness of breath, nausea and vomiting, and headache.
3. It is safe for use in pregnancy.
4. It enhances alcohol metabolism within the body.

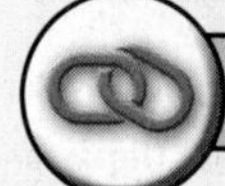

FURTHER STUDY

- The use of barbiturates is discussed in Chapter 8 (for treating sleep disorders) and in Chapter 11 (for treating epilepsy).
- Benzodiazepines are discussed in Chapter 8 (for treating anxiety), in Chapter 11 (for preventing seizures), and in Chapter 31 (for muscle relaxation).
- The therapeutic effects of opioids in managing pain are covered in detail in Chapter 12.
- The use of anticonvulsants in treating alcohol withdrawal is discussed in Chapter 11.
- Similarities between CNS stimulants and the neurotransmitter norepinephrine are covered in Chapter 7.
- An in-depth discussion of the reticular formation wakefulness and anxiety is in Chapter 8.
- The therapeutic applications of methylphenidate are discussed in Chapter 9.
- The cardiovascular effects of nicotine are discussed in Chapter 7.

EXPLORE MEDIALINK www.prenhall.com/holland

Additional resources for this chapter can be found on the CD-ROM accompanying this textbook, and on the Companion Website. Click on Chapter 6 to select activities for this chapter.

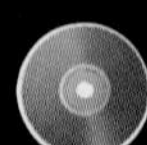

- Audio Glossary
- Concept Review
- NCLEX-PN® Review
- Nursing in Action
- Dosage Calculator

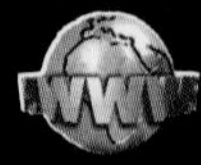

- The Temptation of Anabolic Steroids
- Alcohol Poisoning and Toxicity
- The History of LSD
- Do Nicotine Patches Work?

UNIT

1 2 3 4 5 6 7

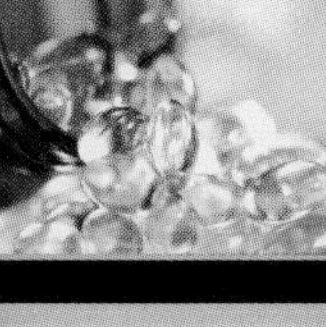

2 THE NERVOUS SYSTEM

UNIT CONTENTS

CHAPTER

7 Drugs Affecting Functions of the Autonomic Nervous System

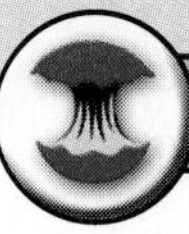

CORE CONCEPTS

7.1 The nervous system is divided into central and peripheral components.

7.2 The autonomic nervous system has sympathetic and parasympathetic branches.

7.3 Synapses are common sites of drug action.

7.4 Acetylcholine and norepinephrine are the two primary neurotransmitters in the autonomic nervous system.

7.5 Autonomic drugs are classified according to the receptors they stimulate or block.

7.6 Parasympathomimetics have few therapeutic uses because of their numerous side effects.

7.7 Anticholinergics are used to dry secretions and to treat asthma.

7.8 Sympathomimetics are primarily used for their effects on the heart, bronchial tree, and nasal passages.

7.9 Adrenergic blockers are primarily used to treat hypertension and are the most widely prescribed class of autonomic drugs.

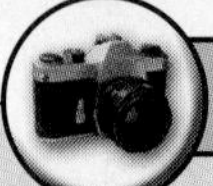

DRUG SNAPSHOT

The following drugs will be discussed in this chapter:

DRUG CLASSES		DRUG PROFILES
Parasympathomimetics	Pr	bethanechol (Urecholine)
Anticholinergics	Pr	atropine (Atropisol)
Sympathomimetics	Pr	phenylephrine (Neo-Synephrine)
Adrenergic blockers	Pr	prazosin (Minipress)

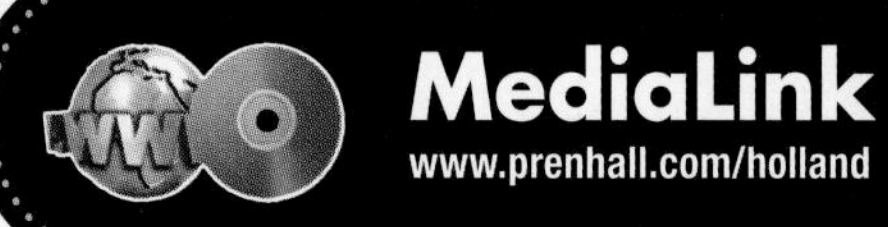

MediaLink
www.prenhall.com/holland

Interactive resources for this chapter can be found on the Companion Website. Click on Chapter 7 and "Begin" to select the activities for this chapter. For chapter-related animations, NCLEX-PN®-style questions, and an audio glossary, access the accompanying CD-ROM in this book.

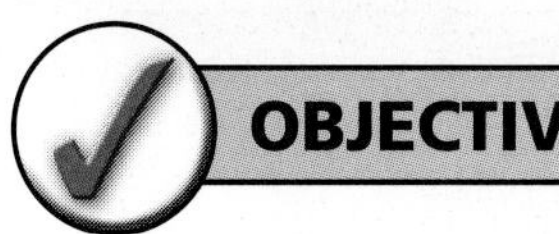

OBJECTIVES

After reading this chapter, the student should be able to:

1. Identify the two primary divisions of the nervous system.
2. Identify the three primary functions of the nervous system.
3. Compare and contrast the actions of the sympathetic and parasympathetic nervous systems.
4. Describe the three parts of a synapse.
5. Identify the neurotransmitters important to the autonomic nervous system and the types of nerves with which they are associated.
6. Compare and contrast nicotinic and muscarinic receptors.
7. Compare and contrast the types of effects when a drug stimulates alpha$_1$, alpha$_2$, beta$_1$, or beta$_2$-adrenergic receptors.
8. For each of the following classes, explain the mechanism of drug action, primary actions, and important adverse effects.
   a. Parasympathomimetics
   b. Anticholinergics
   c. Sympathomimetics
   d. Adrenergic blockers

Neuropharmacology represents one of the largest, most complicated, and least understood branches of pharmacology. Nervous system medications are used to treat a large and diverse set of conditions, including pain, anxiety, depression, schizophrenia, insomnia, and convulsions. Through their effects on nerves, medications are also used to treat many disorders that are considered diseases of other organ systems. Examples include abnormalities in heart rate and rhythm, high and low blood pressure, pressure within the eyeball, asthma, and even a runny nose.

The study of nervous system pharmacology includes the next seven chapters of this text. Traditionally, the study of neuropharmacology begins with the autonomic nervous system. A firm grasp of autonomic pharmacology is necessary to understand the pharmacology of other systems in the body.

7.1 The nervous system is divided into central and peripheral components.

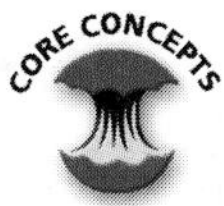

The nervous system has two major divisions: the *central nervous system (CNS)* and the *peripheral nervous system.* The CNS is made up of the brain and spinal cord. The peripheral nervous system consists of all nervous tissue outside the CNS. The basic functions of the nervous system are to:

- Recognize changes in the internal and external environments
- Process and integrate these environmental changes
- React to the environmental changes by producing an action or response

Figure 7.1 ■ shows the fundamental structural divisions of the peripheral nervous system. Nerves in the peripheral nervous system either recognize changes to the environment (sensory division) or respond to these changes by moving muscles or secreting chemicals (motor division). The *somatic nervous system* consists of nerves that provide voluntary control over skeletal muscle. Nerves of the *autonomic nervous system,* on the other hand, give involuntary control over smooth muscle, cardiac muscle, and glands. Organs and tissues regulated by nerves from the autonomic nervous system include the heart, digestive tract, respiratory tract, reproductive tracts, arteries, salivary glands, and portions of the eye.

auto = *self*
ic = *relating to*
soma = *body*

7.2 The autonomic nervous system has sympathetic and parasympathetic branches.

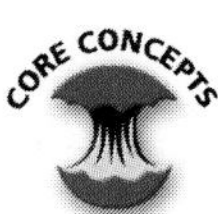

The autonomic nervous system has two subsystems called the **sympathetic nervous system** and the **parasympathetic nervous system.** Almost all organs and glands receive nerves from both branches of the autonomic nervous system.

FIGURE 7.1

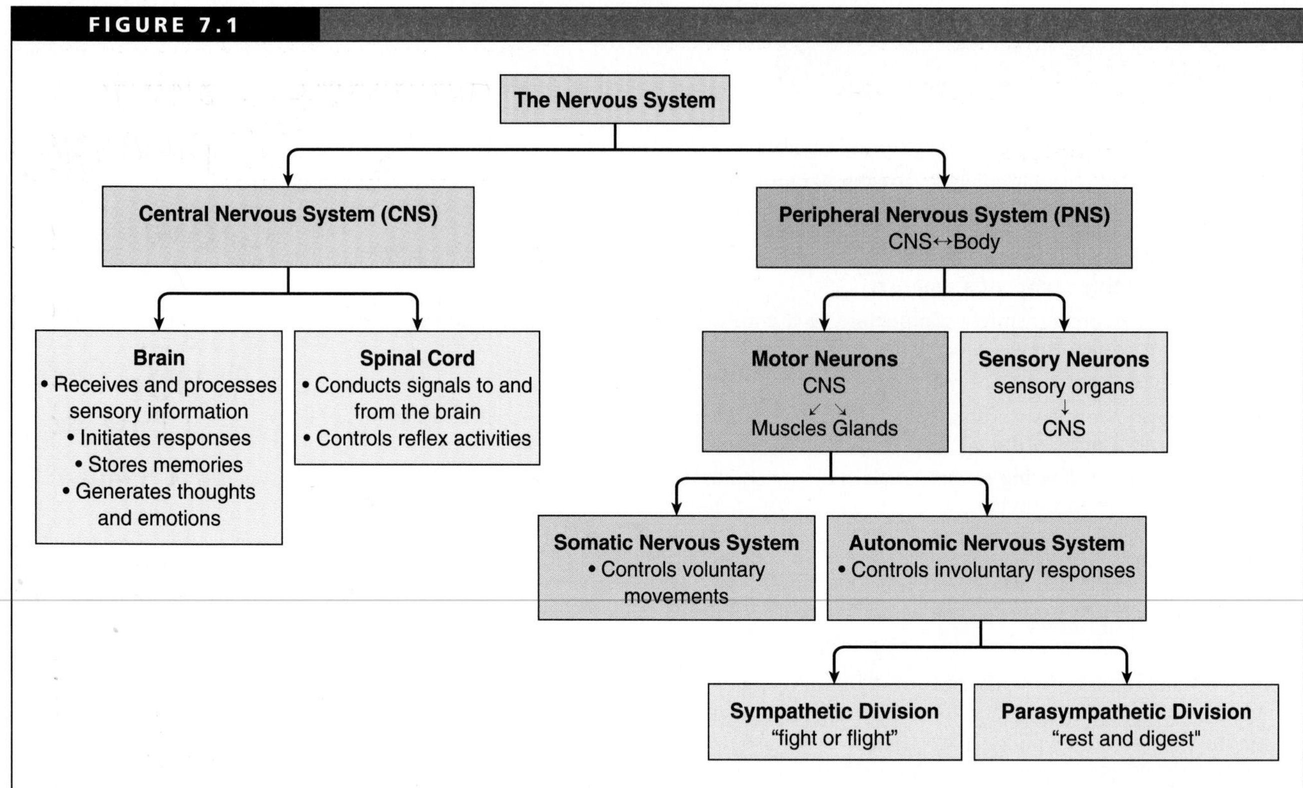

Functional divisions of the nervous system

The sympathetic nervous system is activated under conditions of stress, and produces a set of actions called the *fight-or-flight response.* On the other hand, the parasympathetic nervous system is activated under nonstressful conditions and produces symptoms called the *rest-and-digest response.* Most of the actions of the sympathetic branch are opposite to those of the parasympathetic branch. For example, activation of sympathetic nerves increases the heart rate, whereas activation of parasympathetic nerves decreases heart rate. The major actions of the two branches are shown in Figure 7.2 ■. It is essential to learn these actions early in the study of pharmacology because knowledge of autonomic effects is used to predict the actions and side effects of many drugs.

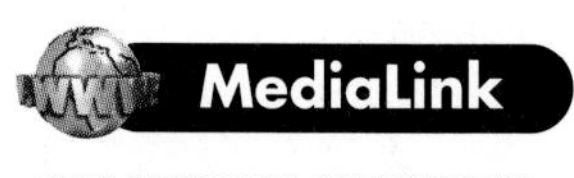

SELF-STUDY OF AUTONOMIC SYSTEM OF PHARMACOLOGY

Concept Review 7.1

- How would a person who is engaging in stressful or energetic activity benefit from the sympathetic effects of bronchodilation, slowed GI motility, and pupil dilation?

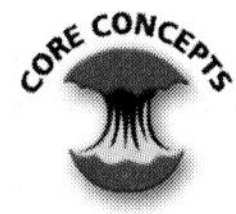

7.3 Synapses are common sites of drug action.

The basic functional cell of the nervous system is the *neuron.* For information to be transmitted throughout the nervous system, neurons must communicate with each other and with muscles and glands. A nerve impulse travels along a neuron to an, area at the end of the neuron called a *synapse.* The synapse contains a space called the *synaptic cleft,* which must be crossed for the impulse to reach the next neuron. The neuron generating the original impulse is called the *presynaptic neuron.* The nerve on the other side of the synapse, waiting to receive the impulse, is called the *postsynaptic neuron.* The basic structure of a synapse is shown in Figure 7.3 ■.

pre = *before*
post = *after*
synaptic = *relating to the synapse*

Chemicals called *neurotransmitters* allow nerve impulses to cross the synaptic cleft. Neurotransmitters are released into the synaptic cleft when a nerve impulse reaches the end of a presynaptic neuron. The neurotransmitter travels across the synaptic cleft to reach receptors on the postsynaptic neuron, which then regenerates the impulse. Many different types of neurotransmitters

FIGURE 7.2

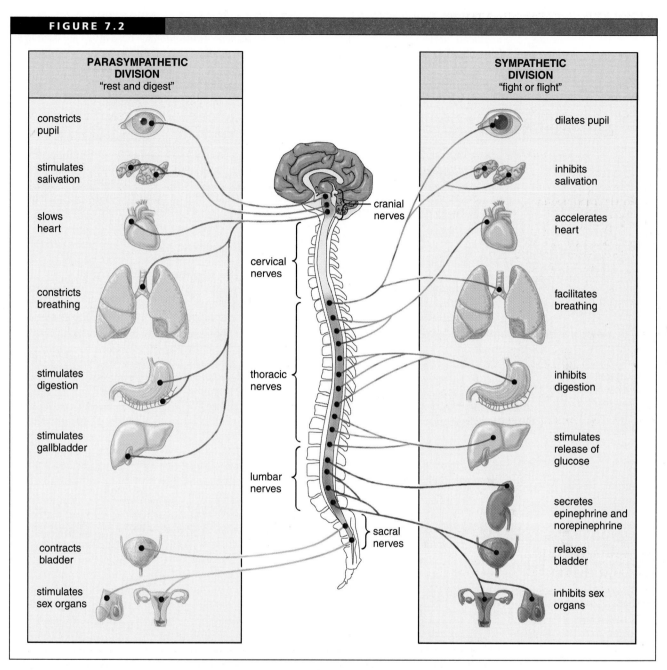

Effects of the sympathetic and parasympathetic nervous systems *SOURCE: Pearson Education/PH College*

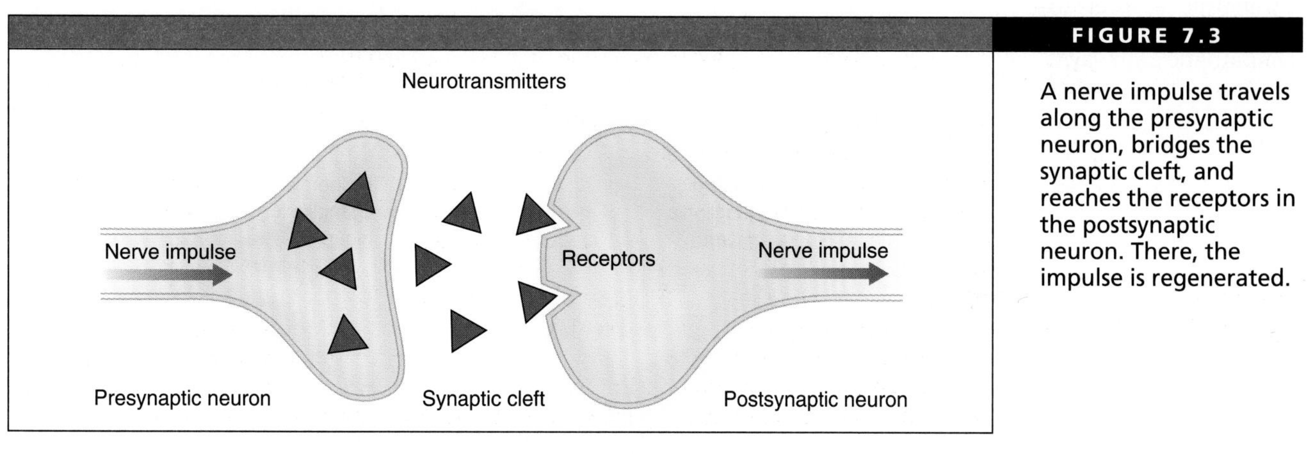

FIGURE 7.3

A nerve impulse travels along the presynaptic neuron, bridges the synaptic cleft, and reaches the receptors in the postsynaptic neuron. There, the impulse is regenerated.

are located throughout the nervous system, each connected with particular functions. *Many drugs are identical to or have the same general structure as neurotransmitters.* These drugs are used to affect autonomic functions by either blocking or enhancing the activity of these neurotransmitters.

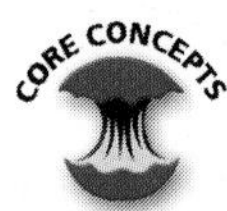

7.4 Acetylcholine and norepinephrine are the two primary neurotransmitters in the autonomic nervous system.

The two primary neurotransmitters of the autonomic nervous system are **norepinephrine (NE)** and **acetylcholine (Ach).** In the sympathetic nervous system, norepinephrine is released at the junction of the postsynaptic neuron and the organ or gland to be acted on. For example, sympathetic nerves in the heart release norepinephrine on cardiac muscle, which stimulates the heart to contract faster and with greater force. Sympathetic nerves also release norepinephrine in the smooth muscle lining the digestive tract, and its action is to slow contractions, or motility. Sympathetic nerves are sometimes called **adrenergic.** This term comes from the word *adrenaline,* which is a chemical closely related to norepinephrine.

adren = *adrenal gland (adrenaline)*

The physiology of acetylcholine is more complicated because it is released in several different locations. When released at the ends of parasympathetic neurons, it produces the opposite effects of norepinephrine, such as slowing the heart and increasing the motility of the digestive tract. Acetylcholine is also the neurotransmitter released at the end of all presynaptic neurons at sites called **ganglia,** which are collections of neuron cell bodies located outside of the spinal cord. In addition, acetylcholine is also a neurotransmitter of sympathetic neurons that activate sweat glands—this is a unique case in which acetylcholine is associated with sympathetic rather than parasympathetic activity. Neurons that release acetylcholine are often called **cholinergic.** The sites of acetylcholine and norepinephrine action are shown in Figure 7.4 ■.

cholin = *acetylcholine*
erg = *work*
ic = *relating to*

Because acetylcholine can stimulate receptors both in the ganglia and at the organ level, different names are assigned to these receptors. Acetylcholine receptors in the ganglia and in skeletal muscle are called **nicotinic** receptors, named after nicotine, the agent found in tobacco products. Acetylcholine receptors at the end of postsynaptic neurons in the parasympathetic nervous system are called **muscarinic** receptors, named after an extract of the mushroom *Amanita muscaria.* Nicotinic and muscarinic receptors are indicated in Figure 7.4.

Norepinephrine receptors are of two basic subtypes, **alpha** (α) and **beta** (β). *Alpha* and *beta*

FIGURE 7.4

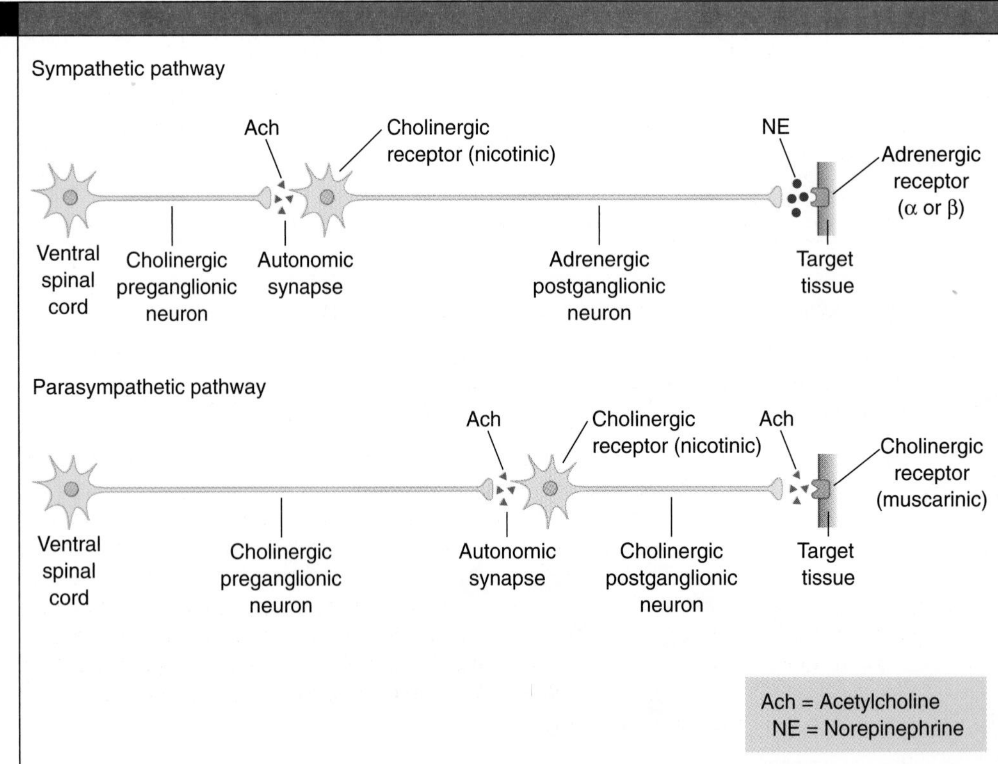

Acetylcholine (Ach) receptors in the ganglia and skeletal muscles are called *nicotinic.* Ach receptors at the ends of postganglionic neurons in the parasympathetic pathway are called *muscarinic.* Norepinephrine (NE) receptors are adrenergic receptors (α and β) in the sympathetic pathway.

TABLE 7.1 Types of Autonomic Receptors

NEUROTRANSMITTER	RECEPTOR	PRIMARY LOCATIONS	RESPONSES
acetylcholine (cholinergic)	muscarinic	parasympathetic target: organs other than the heart	stimulation of smooth muscle and gland secretions
		heart	decrease in heart rate and force of contraction
	nicotinic	cell bodies of postganglionic neurons (sympathetic and parasympathetic pathways)	stimulation of smooth muscle and gland secretions
norepinephrine (adrenergic)	$alpha_1$	all sympathetic target organs except the heart	constriction of blood vessels, dilation of pupils
	$alpha_2$	presynaptic adrenergic neuron terminals	inhibition of norepinephrine release
	$beta_1$	heart and kidneys	increase in heart rate and force of contraction; release of renin
	$beta_2$	all sympathetic target organs except the heart	inhibition of smooth muscle

are Greek letters commonly used in naming chemical and scientific compounds. These receptors are further subdivided into $beta_1$, $beta_2$, $alpha_1$, and $alpha_2$. Drugs may be selective and affect only one type of norepinephrine receptor, or they may affect all of them. The type of response depends on the specific type of receptor that is activated. Drugs may also affect one type of receptor at low doses and begin to affect other receptor subtypes when the dose is increased. Table 7.1 summarizes a list of receptors and expected responses to neurotransmitters.

7.5 Autonomic drugs are classified according to the receptors they stimulate or block.

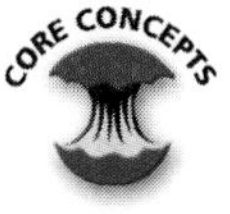

Because they can block or stimulate either the sympathetic or parasympathetic nervous systems, autonomic drugs are classified based on one of their four possible actions:

1. *Stimulation of the sympathetic nervous system.* These drugs are called **sympathomimetics** or **adrenergic agents** and produce the classic symptoms of the fight-or-flight response.
2. *Stimulation of the parasympathetic nervous system.* These drugs are called **parasympathomimetics** or **cholinergic agents** and produce the classic symptoms of the rest-and-digest response.
3. *Inhibition of the sympathetic nervous system.* These drugs are called **adrenergic blockers** and produce actions opposite to those of the sympathomimetics.
4. *Inhibition of the parasympathetic nervous system.* These drugs are called **anticholinergics** or **cholinergic blockers** and produce actions opposite to those of the parasympathomimetics.

Students beginning their study of pharmacology often have difficulty understanding the terminology and actions of autonomic drugs. It is really only necessary to learn one group because the others are logical extensions of the first. If the fight-or-flight symptoms of the sympathomimetics are learned, the actions of the other three groups can be remembered as being either the same or opposite. For example, both the sympathomimetics and the cholinergic blockers increase heart rate and dilate the pupil. The other two groups, the parasympathomimetics and the adrenergic blockers, have the opposite effects of slowing heart rate and constricting the pupils. Mastering the actions and terminology of autonomic drugs early in the study of pharmacology will reap rewards later in the course when these drugs are applied to various systems. See Table 7.2 for a quick review of the autonomic drugs.

TABLE 7.2 Review of Autonomic Drug Classes

	STIMULATION	INHIBITION
Parasympathetic Nervous System	Parasympathomimetics (cholinergic agents)	Anticholinergics (cholinergic blockers)
Sympathetic Nervous System	Sympathomimetics (adrenergic agents)	Sympatholytics (adrenergic blockers)

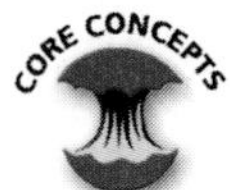

7.6 Parasympathomimetics have few therapeutic uses because of their numerous side effects.

Parasympathomimetics are drugs that mimic actions of the parasympathetic nervous system. These drugs are associated with rest-and-digest responses. Because of their high potential for serious adverse effects, direct-acting parasympathomimetics are used only in a clinical setting. For instance, in ophthalmology, they are used to reduce intraocular pressure in patients with glaucoma (Chapter 33 ⊂⊃). Others are used after anesthesia to stimulate the smooth muscles of the bowel or urinary tract.

Indirect-acting parasympathomimetic drugs, or drugs that inhibit the important enzyme acetylcholinesterase, have the same effect as direct-acting agents. These acetylcholinesterase inhibitors facilitate the effects of the natural neurotransmitter acetylcholine. Therefore, neostigmine (Prostigmin) and physostigmine (Antilirium) also cause actions associated with rest and digestion.

Several drugs in this class are used for their effects on acetylcholine receptors in skeletal muscle rather than for their parasympathetic action. For example, myasthenia gravis is an autoimmune disorder characterized by destruction of cholinergic receptors found in skeletal muscles. Administration of pyridostigmine (Mestinon) or neostigmine (Prostigmin) (Table 7.3) will stimulate skeletal muscle contraction and temporarily help to restore the severe muscle weakness found in this disease.

Nerve agents (see Chapter 1 ⊂⊃) such as Sarin and organophosphate insecticides are chemicals that inhibit acetylcholinesterase in the synaptic space. These agents can cause toxic parasympathomimetic effects. Symptoms are severe salivation, increased sweating, muscle twitching, involuntary urination and defecation, confusion, convulsions, and death. In an emergency, if a nerve agent were released, mark I injector kits containing the anticholinergic drug atropine or a related medication would be used to counteract the effects. Atropine blocks the attachment of acetylcholine to receptor sites and prevents the overstimulation caused by harmful nerve agents.

TABLE 7.3 Selected Parasympathomimetics

DRUG	CLINICAL USE
Pr bethanechol (Urecholine)	■ to contract bladder muscles (for treating urinary retention)
cevimeline HCl (Evoxac)	■ to increase salivation (for treating dry mouth)
neostigmine (Prostigmin)	■ to contract ureters (for treating urinary retention)
physostigmine (Antilirium)	■ to decrease intraocular pressure (for treating glaucoma); to counteract anticholinergic drug overdose
pilocarpine (Isopto Carpine; Salagen)	■ to decrease intraocular pressure (for treating glaucoma)
pyridostigmine (Mestinon)	■ treatment of myasthenia gravis

DRUG PROFILE: Parasympathomimetic: Pr *Bethanechol (Urecholine)*

Actions and Uses:

Bethanechol is a direct-acting parasympathomimetic that interacts with acetylcholine receptors to cause actions typical of parasympathetic stimulation. It affects mostly the digestive and urinary tracts, where it stimulates smooth muscle contraction. These actions are particularly useful in stimulating the return of normal GI and urinary tract function following general anesthesia.

Adverse Effects and Interactions:

The side effects of bethanechol are parasympathetic actions: increased salivation, sweating, abdominal cramping, and hypotension that can lead to fainting. It should not be given to patients with suspected urinary or intestinal obstruction or those with active asthma.

Do not use with ambenonium, neostigmine, and other cholinergic agents; mecamylamine (blocker of acetylcholine at the ganglia) may cause abdominal symptoms and hypotension. Procainamide, quinidine, atropine, and epinephrine reduce the effects of bethanechol.

See the Companion Website for a Nursing Process Focus specific to this drug.

NURSING PROCESS FOCUS

Patients Receiving Direct- and Indirect-Acting Parasympathomimetic Therapy

ASSESSMENT

Prior to administration:

- Obtain complete health history including vital signs, allergies, and drug history for possible drug interactions
- Assess reason for drug administration
- Assess for contraindications of drug administration
- Assess for urinary retention, urinary patterns initially and throughout therapy (direct acting)
- Assess muscle strength, and neuromuscular status, ptosis, diplopia, and chewing

POTENTIAL NURSING DIAGNOSES

- Urinary Incontinence (direct acting)
- Impaired Physical Mobility (indirect acting)
- Deficient Knowledge, related to drug therapy
- Risk for Injury, related to side effects

PLANNING: Patient Goals and Expected Outcomes

The patient will:

- Exhibit increased bowel and bladder function and tone by regaining normal pattern of elimination (direct acting)
- Exhibit a decrease in myasthenia gravis symptoms such as muscle weakness, ptosis, and diplopia (indirect acting)
- Demonstrate understanding of the drug's action by accurately describing drug side effects and precautions

IMPLEMENTATION

Interventions and (Rationales)	Patient Education/Discharge Planning
All Parasympathomimetics	
■ Monitor for adverse effects such as abdominal cramping, diarrhea, excessive salivation, increased sweating, difficulty breathing, muscle cramping, and hypotension. (These may indicate cholinergic crisis that requires atropine.)	■ Instruct patient to report nausea, vomiting, diarrhea, rash, jaundice, or change in color of stool, feeling faint, or any other adverse reactions to the drug.

continued...

(continued from page 93)

NURSING PROCESS FOCUS

Interventions and (Rationales)	Patient Education/Discharge Planning
■ Monitor liver enzymes at start of therapy and weekly for 6 weeks (for possible liver toxocity).	■ Instruct patient to adhere to laboratory testing regimen for serum blood level tests of liver enzymes as directed.
■ Assess and monitor for appropriate self-care administration to prevent complications.	Instruct patient to: ■ Take drug as directed on regular schedule to maintain serum levels and control symptoms ■ Not chew or crush sustained-release tablets ■ Take oral parasympathomimetics on empty stomach to lessen incidence of nausea and vomiting and to increase absorption
Direct Acting	
■ Monitor intake and output ratio. Palpate abdomen for bladder distention. (These drugs have an onset of action within 60 minutes because of binding of the drug to cholinergic receptors on the smooth muscle of the bladder, which relaxes the bladder to stimulate urination.)	■ Advise patient to be near bathroom facilities after taking these drugs.
■ Monitor for blurred vision (a cholinergic effect).	■ Advise patient that blurred vision is a possible side effect and to take appropriate precautions. ■ Instruct patient not to drive or engage in potentially hazardous activities until drug's effects are known.
■ Monitor for orthostatic hypotension.	■ Instruct patient to avoid abrupt position changes. Avoid prolonged standing in one place.
Indirect Acting	
■ Monitor muscle strength, and neuromuscular status, ptosis, diplopia, and chewing to determine if the therapeutic effect is achieved.	■ Instruct patient to report difficulty with vision or swallowing.
■ Schedule medication around meal times. (This will achieve therapeutic effect and aid in chewing and swallowing.)	■ Instruct patient to take medication about 30 minutes before meal.
■ Schedule activities to avoid fatigue.	Instruct patient to: ■ Plan activities according to muscle strength and fatigue ■ Take frequent rest periods to avoid fatigue
■ Monitor for muscle weakness. (This symptom, depending on time onset, indicates cholinergic crisis—overdose—OR myasthenic crisis—underdose.)	Instruct patient to: ■ Report any severe muscle weakness that occurs 1 hour after administration of medication ■ Report any muscle weakness that occurs 3 or more hours after medication administration, because this is a major symptom of myasthenic crisis

EVALUATION OF OUTCOME CRITERIA

Evaluate the effectiveness of drug therapy by confirming that patient goals and expected outcomes have been met (see "Planning").

See Table 7.3 for a list of drugs to which these nursing actions apply.

7.7 Anticholinergics are used to dry secretions and to treat asthma.

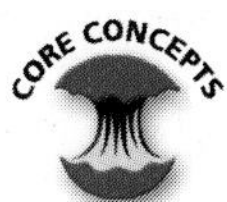

Anticholinergics are drugs that have actions opposite those of the parasympathetic branch. They mimic the fight-or-flight response. Although the term *anticholinergic* is commonly used, a better term for this class of drugs would be *muscarinic blockers,* which more accurately describes the location of their action. Most therapeutic uses of the anticholinergics relate to their autonomic actions: dilation of pupils, increase in heart rate, drying of secretions, and dilation of the bronchi. Anticholinergics have been widely used in medicine for many disorders. A relatively high incidence of side effects and the development of safer, and sometimes more effective, medications has limited the current use of anticholinergics. For example, anticholinergics were once drugs of choice in treating peptic ulcers, but they have been replaced by proton-pump inhibitors and H_2-receptor blockers (Chapter 26). Two important side effects that limit their usefulness include tachycardia (fast heart rate) and the tendency to cause urinary retention in men with prostate disorders. Some of the more common anticholinergics and their clinical uses are shown in Table 7.4.

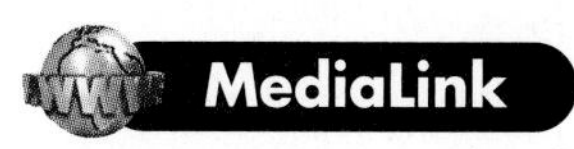

MOTION SICKNESS IN SPACE

TABLE 7.4 Selected Anticholinergics

DRUG	CLINICAL USE
Pr atropine	to dry secretions prior to anesthesia, increase heart rate, dilate pupils
cyclopentolate (Cyclogyl)	to dilate pupils
dicyclomine (Bentyl)	to treat irritable bowel syndrome
glycopyrrolate (Robinul)	to dry secretions prior to anesthesia, treat peptic ulcers
ipratropium (Atrovent)	to treat asthma
oxybutynin (Ditropan)	to treat urinary bladder urgency and incontinence
propantheline (Pro-banthine)	to treat irritable bowel syndrome, peptic ulcer
scopolamine (Hyoscine, Transderm-Scop)	to treat irritable bowel syndrome (autonomic effect); motion sickness (central effect)

DRUG PROFILE: Anticholinergic: Pr *Atropine*

Actions and Uses:

Atropine is a natural product found in the deadly nightshade plant, or Atropa belladonna. By blocking acetylcholine (muscarinic) receptors, atropine causes symptoms of the fight-or-flight response, such as increased heart rate, bronchodilation, decreased motility in the GI tract, mydriasis (pupil dilation), and decreased secretions from glands. Throughout history, atropine has been used for a variety of purposes, although its use has declined because of the development of safer, more effective medications. Atropine is used to treat hypermotility diseases of the GI tract such as irritable bowel syndrome, to suppress secretions during surgical procedures, to increase the heart rate in patients with a slow heart rate (or bradycardia), to dilate the pupil during eye examinations, and to cause bronchodilation in patients with asthma. Atropine is an antidote for poisoning with nerve gas agents and organophosphate insecticides.

Adverse Effects and Interactions:

The adverse effects of atropine limit its therapeutic usefulness. Side effects include dry mouth, constipation, urinary retention, and an increased heart rate. Atropine is usually contraindicated in patients with glaucoma because the drug may increase pressure within the eyeball.

Use of amantadine, antihistamines, tricyclic antidepressants, quinidine, disopyramide, and procainamide can increase the anticholinergic effects of atropine. Use with levodopa may decrease the effects of the latter. Use with methotrimeprazine may cause extrapyramidal effects. The antipsychotic effects of phenothiazines are decreased.

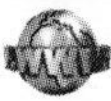
See the Companion Website for a Nursing Process Focus specific to this drug.

NURSING PROCESS FOCUS

Patients Receiving Anticholinergic Therapy

ASSESSMENT

Prior to administration:
- Obtain complete health history, including drug history to determine possible drug interactions and allergies
- Assess reason for drug administration
- Assess for heart rate, blood pressure, temperature, and elimination patterns (initially and throughout therapy)

POTENTIAL NURSING DIAGNOSES

- Deficient Knowledge, related to drug therapy
- Decreased Cardiac Output
- Risk for Imbalanced Body Temperature
- Impaired Oral Mucous Membranes
- Constipation
- Urinary Retention

PLANNING: Patient Goals and Expected Outcomes

The patient will:
- Exhibit a decrease in symptoms for which the medication is prescribed
- Demonstrate an understanding of drug's action by accurately describing drug side effects and precautions
- Verbalize techniques to avoid hazardous side effects associated with anticholinergic therapy

IMPLEMENTATION

Interventions and (Rationales)	Patient Education/Discharge Planning
■ Monitor for signs of anticholinergic crisis resulting from overdosage: fever, tachycardia, difficulty swallowing, ataxia, reduced urine output, psychomotor agitation, confusion, hallucinations.	■ Instruct patients to report side effects related to therapy such as shortness of breath, cough, dysphagia, syncope, fever, anxiety, right upper quadrant pain, extreme lethargy, or dizziness.
■ Report significant changes in heart rate or blood pressure, or development of dysrhythmias.	■ Instruct patient to monitor vital signs, ensuring proper use of home equipment.
■ Observe for side effects such as drowsiness, blurred vision, tachycardia, dry mouth, urinary hesitancy, and decreased sweating.	Instruct patient to: ■ Report side effects ■ Avoid driving and hazardous activities until effects of drugs are known ■ Wear sunglasses to decrease sensitivity to bright light
■ Provide comfort measures for dryness of mucous membranes such as apply lubricant to moisten lips and oral mucosa, assist in rinsing mouth. Use artificial tears for dry eyes, as needed.	Instruct patient to: ■ Use oral rinses, sugarless gum or candy, and frequent oral hygiene to help relieve dry mouth ■ Avoid alcohol-containing mouthwashes that can further dry oral tissue
■ Minimize exposure to heat or cold and strenuous exercise. (Anticholinergics can inhibit sweat gland secretions due to direct blockade of the muscarinic receptors on the sweat glands. Sweating is necessary for patients to cool down, so this inhibition of sweating can increase their risk for hyperthermia.)	■ Advise patient to limit activity outside when the temperature is hot. Strenuous activity in a hot environment may cause heat stroke.
■ Monitor intake and output ratio. Palpate abdomen for bladder distention.	■ Instruct patient to notify healthcare provider if difficulty in voiding occurs.
■ Monitor patients routinely for abdominal distention, and auscultate for bowel sounds.	■ Advise patient to increase fluid intake and add bulk to the diet, if constipation becomes a problem.

continued...

NURSING PROCESS FOCUS

EVALUATION OF OUTCOME CRITERIA

Evaluate the effectiveness of drug therapy by confirming that patient goals and expected outcomes have been met (see "Planning").

See Table 7.4 for a list of drugs to which these nursing actions apply.

7.8 Sympathomimetics are primarily used for their effects on the heart, bronchial tree, and nasal passages.

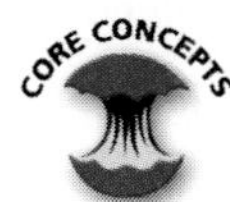

Sympathomimetics, or adrenergic agents have actions similar to activation of the sympathetic nervous system. They will produce responses characteristic of the fight-or-flight response. The sympathomimetics produce many of the same symptoms as the anticholinergics. However, because the sympathetic nervous system has alpha- and beta-subreceptors, the actions of many of the sympathomimetics are more specific and have wider therapeutic application.

Although most effects of sympathomimetics are predictable based on their autonomic actions, their primary effects depend on which adrenergic subreceptors are stimulated. Drugs such as phenylephrine (Neo-Synephrine) stimulate alpha$_1$-receptors and are often used to dry nasal secretions. Because beta$_1$-receptors are predominant in the heart, beta$_1$-agents such as dobutamine (Dobutrex) are used to stimulate the heart rate and increase its strength of contraction. Beta$_2$-agents such as albuterol (Proventil) cause bronchodilation and are useful in the treatment of asthma.

Some sympathomimetics are nonselective, stimulating more than one type of adrenergic receptor. For example, epinephrine stimulates all four types of adrenergic receptors and is used for cardiac arrest and asthma. Pseudoephedrine (Sudafed and others) stimulates both alpha$_1$- and beta$_2$-receptors and is used orally as a nasal decongestant. Isoproterenol (Isuprel) stimulates both beta$_1$- and beta$_2$-receptors and is used to increase the rate, force, and conduction speed of the heart, and occasionally to treat asthma. The nonselective drugs generally cause more autonomic-related side effects.

Some of the more commonly used sympathomimetics are shown in Table 7.5. Most drugs in this class are presented in other chapters of this text. For profiles of drugs in this class, see epinephrine (Adrenalin) and norepinephrine (Levophed) in Chapter 19, oxymetazoline (Afrin) in Chapter 21, and salmeterol (Serevent) in Chapter 25.

Concept Review 7.2

- Why do the sympathomimetics produce many of the same symptoms as the anticholinergics?

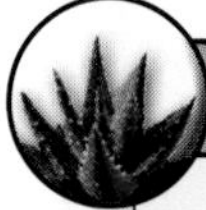

NATURAL ALTERNATIVES

Ma Huang or Ephedra as a Sympathomimetic

Ephedra is an herb that has been used in traditional Chinese medicine for ages. The primary plant species that contains ephedra is *Ephedra sinica,* also known as ma huang. Two active substances in ma huang are ephedrine and pseudoephedrine, both of which are available in OTC and prescription formulations. Dietary supplements of ephedra are usually standardized to contain 6–8% ephedrine alkaloids.

Ephedrine and pseudoephedrine are sympathomimetics and their actions are typical of sympathetic nervous system stimulation. The decongestant action of ephedra may benefit patients with allergies or the common cold. The bronchodilation effect may benefit those with asthma or chronic pulmonary disease. Many formulations of ephedra are marketed for use as energy enhancers and weight-loss products. Some of these products combine ephedra with caffeine. As a sympathomimetic, ephedra can have adverse effects on the cardiovascular system, such as increased blood pressure and rapid heart rate. Patients with hypertension, diabetes mellitus, heart disease, or enlarged prostate should not take ephedra without seeking medical advice. ■

TABLE 7.5 Selected Sympathomimetics

DRUG	PRIMARY RECEPTOR SUBTYPE	CLINICAL USE
albuterol (Proventil, Ventilin, Provax)	$beta_2$	to treat asthma
dobutamine (Dobutrex)	$beta_1$	to stimulate the heart
dopamine (Intropin)	$alpha_1$ and $beta_1$	to treat shock
epinephrine (Adrenalin, Primatene, Bronkaid)	alpha and beta	to treat asthma, cardiac arrest
isoproterenol (Isuprel)	$beta_1$ and $beta_2$	to treat asthma, dysrhythmias, heart failure
metaproterenol (Alupent)	$beta_2$	to treat asthma
metaraminol (Aramine)	$alpha_1$ and $beta_1$	to treat shock
norepinephrine (Levarterenol, Levophed)	$alpha_1$ and $beta_1$	to treat shock
oxymetazoline (Afrin)	alpha	to treat nasal congestion
Pr phenylephrine (Neo-Synephrine)	alpha	to treat nasal congestion
pseudoephedrine (Sudafed, Afrin, and others)	alpha and beta	to treat nasal congestion
ritodrine (Yutopar)	$beta_2$	to slow uterine contractions
salmeterol (Serevent)	$beta_2$	to treat nasal congestion
terbutaline (Brethine and others)	$beta_2$	to treat asthma

DRUG PROFILE: Sympathomimetic: Pr *Phenylephrine (Neo-Synephrine)*

Actions and Uses:

Phenylephrine is a selective alpha-adrenergic agent that is available in several different formulations, including intranasal, ophthalmic, IM, SC, and IV. All of its actions and indications result from sympathetic stimulation. When applied intranasally by spray or drops, it reduces nasal congestion by constricting small blood vessels in the nasal mucosa. Applied topically to the eye during ophthalmic examinations, phenylephrine can dilate the pupil, without causing significant paralysis of the eye muscles (cycloplegia). The parenteral administration of phenylephrine can reverse acute hypotension caused by spinal anesthesia or vascular shock. Because it lacks beta-adrenergic activity, it produces relatively few cardiac side effects at therapeutic doses. Its longer duration of activity and lack of significant cardiac effects gives phenylephrine some advantages over epinephrine or norepinephrine in treating acute hypotension.

Adverse Effects and Interactions:

When used topically or intranasally, side effects are uncommon. Prolonged intranasal use can cause burning of the mucosa and rebound congestion (Chapter 33). Ophthalmic preparations can cause narrow-angle glaucoma because of their mydriatic effect. High doses can cause reflex bradycardia due to the elevation of blood pressure caused by stimulation of $alpha_1$-receptors. When given parenterally, the drug should be used with caution in patients with advanced coronary artery disease or hypertension. Anxiety, restlessness, and tremor may occur due to the drug's stimulation effect on the CNS. Patients with hyperthyroidism may experience a severe increase in basal metabolic rate, resulting in increased blood pressure and tachycardia. Drug interactions may occur with MAO inhibitors, causing a hypertensive crisis. Increased effects may also occur with tricyclic antidepressants. This drug is incompatible with iron preparations (ferric salts).

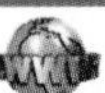

See the Companion Website for a Nursing Process Focus specific to this drug.

NURSING PROCESS FOCUS

Patients Receiving Sympathomimetic Therapy

ASSESSMENT

Prior to administration:

- Determine reason for drug administration
- Monitor vital signs, urinary output, and cardiac output (initially and throughout therapy).
- For treatment of nasal congestion, assess the nasal mucosa for changes such as excoriation or bleeding
- Obtain complete health history including allergies, drug history, and possible drug interactions

POTENTIAL NURSING DIAGNOSES

- Deficient Knowledge, related to drug therapy
- Decreased Cardiac Output
- Ineffective Cardiopulmonary Tissue Perfusion
- Risk for Injury, related to side effect of drug therapy
- Ineffective Breathing Pattern, related to nasal congestion
- Disturbed Sleep Pattern

PLANNING: Patient Goals and Expected Outcomes

The patient will:

- Exhibit a decrease in symptoms for which drug is being given
- Demonstrate understanding of drug's action by accurately describing drug side effects and precautions
- Return demonstrate proper nasal/ophthalmic medication instillation technique

IMPLEMENTATION

Interventions and (Rationales)	Patient Education/Discharge Planning
■ Closely monitor IV insertion sites for extravasation with IV administration. Use an infusion pump to deliver medication. ■ Use a tuberculin syringe when administering SC doses that are extremely small. ■ For metered-dose inhalation, shake container well, and wait at least 2 minutes between medications. ■ Instill only prescribed number of drops when using ophthalmic solutions.	Instruct patient to: ■ Use drug as prescribed, and not "double up" on doses ■ Take medication early in day to avoid insomnia
■ Monitor patient for side effects. (Side effects of sympathomimetics may be serious and limit therapy.)	Instruct patient to: ■ Immediately report shortness of breath, palpitations, dizziness, chest/arm pain or pressure, or other angina-like symptoms ■ Consult healthcare provider before attempting to use sympathomimetics to treat nasal congestion or eye irritation ■ Monitor blood pressure, pulse, and temperature to ensure proper use of home equipment
■ Monitor breathing patterns and observe for shortness of breath and/or audible wheezing. ■ Observe patient's responsiveness to light. (Some sympathomimetics cause photosensitivity by affecting the pupillary light accommodation/response.) ■ Provide eye comfort by reducing exposure to direct bright light in environment; shield eyes with a rolled washcloth or eye bandages for severe photosensitivity.	■ Instruct patient to immediately report any difficulty breathing. Instruct patient with a history of asthma to consult a healthcare provider before using OTC drugs to treat nasal stuffiness. ■ Instruct patients using ophthalmic sympathomimetics that transient stinging and blurred vision on instillation is normal. Headache and/or brow pain may also occur. ■ Instruct patient to avoid driving and other activities requiring visual acuity until blurring subsides.
■ For patients receiving nasal sympathomimetics, observe the nasal cavity. Monitor for rhinorrhea and epistaxis.	Instruct patient to: ■ Observe nasal cavity for signs of excoriation or bleeding before instilling nasal spray or drops; review procedure for safe instillation of nasal sprays or eye drops ■ Limit OTC usage of sympathomimetics; inform patient about rebound nasal congestion

EVALUATION OF OUTCOME CRITERIA

Evaluate the effectiveness of drug therapy by confirming that patient goals and expected outcomes have been met (see "Planning").

See Table 7.5 for a list of drugs to which these nursing actions apply.

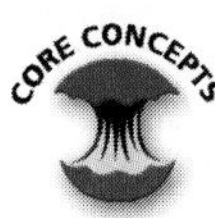

7.9 Adrenergic blockers are primarily used to treat hypertension and are the most widely prescribed class of autonomic drugs.

Adrenergic blockers inhibit the actions of the sympathetic nervous system. These agents produce many of the same responses as the parasympathomimetics, but they are more widely used. Because the sympathetic nervous system has alpha- and beta-subreceptors, the actions of adrenergic blockers are specific and have wide therapeutic application. In fact, they are the most widely prescribed class of autonomic drugs. Some of the adrenergic blockers are shown in Table 7.6.

Alpha-adrenergic blockers, or simply *alpha blockers,* are primarily used for their effects on vascular smooth muscle. By relaxing vascular smooth muscle in small arteries, alpha$_1$-blockers such as doxazosin (Cardura) cause vasodilation which results in decreased blood pressure. Their primary use is in the treatment of hypertension, either alone or in combination with other agents.

Some drugs in this class selectively block beta$_1$-receptors. Because beta$_1$-receptors are only present in the heart, the effects of drugs such as atenolol (Tenormin) are often called *cardioselective.* By slowing the heart rate, they lower blood pressure, which is their primary use.

Some beta blockers, such as propranolol (Inderal), are nonselective, blocking both beta$_1$- and beta$_2$-receptors. The nonselective beta blockers are used to treat hypertension, angina, and cardiac rhythm abnormalities. Their nonselective actions generally result in more side effects than the selective beta blockers. Profiles of adrenergic blockers can be found for doxazosin (Cardura) in Chapter 15, propranolol (Inderal) in Chapter 17, and atenolol (Tenormin) and metoprolol (Lopressor) in Chapter 18.

Concept Review 7.3

- Both parasympathomimetics and adrenergic blockers produce similar actions. Why are the adrenergic blockers used to treat hypertension, but the parasympathomimetics not used for this purpose?

TABLE 7.6 Selected Adrenergic Blockers

DRUG	PRIMARY RECEPTOR SUBTYPE	CLINICAL USE
acebutolol (Sectral)	beta$_1$	hypertension, dysrhythmias, angina
atenolol (Tenormin)	beta$_1$	hypertension and angina
carteolol (Cartrol)	beta$_1$ and beta$_2$	hypertension and glaucoma
carvedilol (Coreg)	alpha$_1$, beta$_1$, and beta$_2$	hypertension
doxazocin (Cardura)	alpha$_1$	hypertension
esmolol (Brevibloc)	beta$_1$	hypertension and dysrhythmias
metoprolol (Lopressor)	beta$_1$	hypertension, heart failure, MI
nadolol (Corgard)	beta$_1$ and beta$_2$	hypertension
phentolamine (Regitine)	alpha	severe hypertension
Pr prazosin (Minipress)	alpha$_1$	hypertension
propranolol (Inderal)	beta$_1$ and beta$_2$	dysrhythmias, hypertension, migraines, angina
sotalol (Betapace)	beta$_1$ and beta$_2$	dysrhythmias
terazosin (Hytrin)	alpha$_1$	hypertension
timolol (Blocadren, Timoptic)	beta$_1$ and beta$_2$	hypertension, angina, glaucoma

DRUG PROFILE: Adrenergic Blocker: *Prazosin (Minipress)*

Actions and Uses:

Prazosin is a selective alpha$_1$-adrenergic blocker that competes with norepinephrine at its receptors on vascular smooth muscle in arterioles and veins. Its major action is a rapid decrease in peripheral resistance that reduces blood pressure. It has little effect on cardiac output or heart rate, and it causes less reflex tachycardia than some other drugs in this class. Tolerance may occur to its antihypertensive effect. Its most common use is in combination with other agents, such as beta blockers or diuretics, in the pharmacotherapy of hypertension. Prazosin has a short half-life and is often taken two or three times per day.

Adverse Effects and Interactions:

Like other alpha blockers, prazosin has a tendency to cause orthostatic hypotension due to alpha$_1$-inhibition in vascular smooth muscle. In rare cases, this hypotension can be so severe as to cause unconsciousness about 30 minutes after the first dose. This is called the *first-dose phenomenon.* To avoid this situation, the first dose should be very low and given at bedtime. Dizziness, drowsiness, or lightheadedness may occur as a result of decreased blood flow to the brain due to the drug's hypotensive action. Reflex tachycardia may occur due to the rapid falls in blood pressure. The alpha blockade may also result in nasal congestion or inhibition of ejaculation.

Drug interactions include increased hypotensive effects with concurrent use of antihypertensives and diuretics.

See the Companion Website for a Nursing Process Focus specific to this drug.

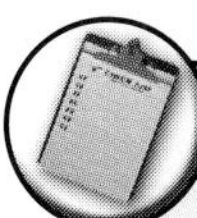

PATIENTS NEED TO KNOW

Patients treated with autonomic medications need to know the following:

In General

1. Do not take any OTC cold, cough, or sinus drugs without seeking medical advice because these likely contain autonomic agents.
2. Report any palpitations, shortness of breath, chest pain, or large changes in blood pressure immediately to a healthcare provider. Some of the most significant side effects of autonomic drugs relate to the cardiovascular system.
3. Notify a healthcare provider before taking autonomic drugs if the following conditions are present: thyroid disease, diabetes mellitus, dysrhythmias, or hypertension. Such medications have the potential to cause serious side effects in individuals with these conditions.
4. Move slowly when changing from a supine to an upright position to avoid dizziness and perhaps fainting. Many of the autonomic medications affect blood pressure.
5. Notify a healthcare provider if any significant change in bowel habits or abdominal cramping/constipation occurs after taking autonomic drugs.
6. Inform a healthcare provider before taking anticholinergic drugs if urinating difficulty is present or if the diagnosis of benign prostatic hypertrophy (BPH) has been made.
7. Chew gum or suck on hard candies if dry mouth is experienced when taking autonomic drugs. Proper oral hygiene is important to avoid dental caries.

Regarding Adrenergic Blockers

8. Do not discontinue the use of beta blockers abruptly because doing so can result in chest pain or rebound hypertension.
9. Alpha blockers can sometimes cause impotence as a side effect. If there are difficulties with ejaculation, notify a healthcare provider so that other drug options may be explored. ■

NURSING PROCESS FOCUS

Patients Receiving Adrenergic Blocker Therapy

ASSESSMENT

Prior to administration:

- Assess vital signs, urinary output, and cardiac output (initially and throughout therapy)
- Assess reason for drug administration
- Obtain complete health history including allergies, drug history, and possible drug interactions

POTENTIAL NURSING DIAGNOSES

- Deficient Knowledge, related to drug therapy
- Disturbed Sensory Perception
- Risk for Injury, related to dizziness, syncope
- Impaired Urinary Elimination
- Sexual Dysfunction

PLANNING: Patient Goals and Expected Outcomes

The patient will:

- Exhibit a decrease in blood pressure with fewer adverse effects
- Report a decrease in urinary symptoms such as hesitancy and difficulty voiding
- Demonstrate an understanding of drug's action by accurately describing drug side effects and precautions, and importance of follow-up care

IMPLEMENTATION

Interventions and (Rationales)	Patient Education/Discharge Planning
■ In patients with prostatic hypertrophy, monitor for urinary hesitancy/feeling of incomplete bladder emptying, and interrupted urinary stream.	■ Instruct patient to report increased difficulty with urination to healthcare provider.
■ Monitor for syncope. (Alpha-adrenergic blockers produce first-dose syncope phenomenon, and may cause loss of consciousness.)	Instruct patient to: ■ Take this medication at bedtime, and to take the first dose *immediately* before getting into bed ■ Avoid abrupt changes in position; warn patient about first-dose phenomenon and reassure that this effect diminishes with continued therapy
■ Monitor vital signs (especially blood pressure), level of consciousness, and mood. (Adrenergic blockers can exacerbate existing mental depression.)	■ Instruct patient to immediately report any feelings of dysphoria. ■ Interview patient regarding suicide potential; obtain a "no-self harm" verbal contract from the patient.
■ Monitor carefully for dizziness, drowsiness, or lightheadedness. (These are signs of decreased blood flow to the brain due to the drug's hypotensive action.)	Instruct patient: ■ To monitor vitals signs, especially blood pressure, ensuring proper use of home equipment ■ Regarding the normotensive range of blood pressure; instruct patient to consult the nurse regarding "reportable" blood pressure readings ■ To report dizziness or syncope that persists beyond the first dose, as well as paresthesia and other neurological changes
■ Observe for side effects that may include blurred vision, tinnitus, epistaxis, and edema.	Inform patient: ■ That nasal congestion may be a side effect ■ To report any adverse reactions to the healthcare provider ■ About the potential danger of concomitant use of OTC nasal decongestants

continued...

NURSING PROCESS FOCUS

Interventions and (Rationales)

- Monitor liver function (because of increased risk for liver toxicity).

Patient Education/Discharge Planning

Instruct patient to:

- Adhere to a regular schedule of laboratory testing for liver function as ordered by the healthcare provider
- Report signs and symptoms of liver toxicity: nausea, vomiting, diarrhea, rash, jaundice, abdominal pain, tenderness or distention, or change in color of stool
- About importance of ongoing medication compliance and follow-up

EVALUATION OF OUTCOME CRITERIA

Evaluate the effectiveness of drug therapy by confirming that patient goals and expected outcomes have been met (see "Planning").

See Table 7.6 for a list of drugs to which these nursing actions apply.

CHAPTER REVIEW

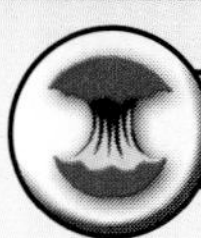

CORE CONCEPTS SUMMARY

7.1 **The nervous system is divided into central and peripheral components.**

The central nervous system consists of the brain and spinal cord. The peripheral nervous system consists of a sensory portion and a motor portion. Outgoing motor signals are characterized as voluntary (somatic) or involuntary (autonomic).

7.2 **The autonomic nervous system has sympathetic and parasympathetic branches.**

Stimulation of sympathetic nerves causes symptoms of the fight-or-flight response. Stimulation of parasympathetic nerves induces the rest-and-digest response. With few exceptions, the actions of the two divisions are opposite of each other.

7.3 **Synapses are common sites of drug action.**

Synapses consist of a presynaptic nerve and a postsynaptic nerve with a space between them called the synaptic cleft. Neurotransmitters cross this synaptic cleft to regenerate the nerve impulse.

7.4 **Acetylcholine and norepinephrine are the two primary neurotransmitters in the autonomic nervous system.**

Acetylcholine is the neurotransmitter at the end of all presynaptic nerves (ganglia), at sweat glands, and in skeletal muscle. Acetylcholine receptors may be nicotinic or muscarinic. Norepinephrine is the neurotransmitter at the organ level in the sympathetic nervous system. Norepinephrine receptors may be alpha or beta subtypes.

7.5 **Autonomic drugs are classified according to the receptors they stimulate or block.**

Sympathomimetics stimulate sympathetic nerves, and parasympathomimetics primarily stimulate parasympathetic nerves. Adrenergic blockers inhibit the sympathetic division, whereas cholinergic blockers mostly inhibit the parasympathetic branch.

7.6 **Parasympathomimetics have few therapeutic uses because of their numerous side effects.**

Parasympathomimetics are used to treat glaucoma and to stimulate the urinary or digestive tracts following general anesthesia. Toxic nerve agents are parasympathomimetics producing harmful effects in the body.

7.7 **Anticholinergics are used to dry secretions and to treat asthma.**

The use of cholinergic blockers has declined due to their numerous side effects. They are used to dry secretions, dilate the bronchi, and dilate the pupil.

7.8 Sympathomimetics are primarily used for their effects on the heart, bronchial tree, and nasal passages.

Sympathomimetics may stimulate one or several subtypes of adrenergic receptors. Uses include increasing the heart rate, dilating the bronchi, and drying excess secretions caused by colds.

7.9 Adrenergic blockers are primarily used to treat hypertension and are the most widely prescribed class of autonomic drugs.

Adrenergic blockers are the most commonly prescribed autonomic medications. They may be selective for only one receptor subtype such as the $beta_1$-blockers or inhibit several subtypes. Hypertension is their primary indication.

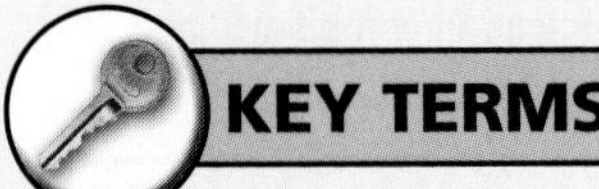

KEY TERMS

acetylcholine (ah-SEET-ul-KOH-leen): primary neurotransmitter of the parasympathetic nervous system; also present at somatic neuromuscular junctions and at sympathetic preganglionic nerves / *page 90*

adrenergic (add-rah-NUR-jik): a term relating to nerves that release norepinephrine or epinephrine / *page 90*

adrenergic agent (add-rah-NUR-jik A-jent): another name for a sympathomimetic drug / *page 91*

adrenergic blocker: drug that blocks the actions of the sympathetic nervous system / *page 91*

alpha receptor: type of subreceptor found in the sympathetic nervous system / *page 90*

anticholinergic: drug that inhibits the action of acetylcholine at its receptor / *page 91*

beta receptor: type of subreceptor found in the sympathetic nervous system / *page 90*

cholinergic (kol-in-UR-jik): a term relating to nerves that release acetylcholine / *page 90*

cholinergic agent: another name for a parasympathomimetic drug / *page 91*

cholinergic blocker: drug that blocks the actions of the parasympathetic nervous system / *page 91*

ganglia (GANG-lee-ah): collections of neuron cell bodies located outside the CNS / *page 90*

muscarinic (MUS-kah-RIN-ik): type of cholinergic receptor found in smooth muscle, cardiac muscle, and glands / *page 90*

nicotinic (NIK-oh-TIN-ik): type of cholinergic receptor found in ganglia of both the sympathetic and parasympathetic nervous systems / *page 90*

norepinephrine (nor-EH-pin-NEF-rin): primary neurotransmitter in the sympathetic nervous system / *page 90*

parasympathetic nervous system (PAIR-ah-SIM-pah-THET-ik): portion of the autonomic system that is active during periods of rest and digestion / *page 87*

parasympathomimetics (PAIR-ah-SIM-path-oh-mah-MET-iks): drugs that mimic the actions of the parasympathetic nervous system / *page 91*

sympathetic nervous system (SIM-pah-THET-ik): portion of the autonomic system that is active during periods of stress and which produces the fight-or-flight response / *page 87*

sympathomimetic (sim-PATH-oh-mih-MET-ik): drug that mimics the actions of the sympathetic nervous system / *page 91*

REVIEW QUESTIONS

The following questions are written in NCLEX-PN® style. Answer these questions to assess your knowledge of the chapter material, and go back and review any material that is not clear to you.

1. The nurse recognizes which of the following drugs is contraindicated in patients with glaucoma?

1. Sotalol (Betapace)
2. Betaxolol HCl (Betoptic)
3. Timolol (Timoptic)
4. Atropine

2. The patient diagnosed with glaucoma would most likely be prescribed which of the following drugs?

1. Adrenergic agents
2. Cholinergic agents
3. Adrenergic blockers
4. Cholinergic blockers

3. The nurse teaches the patient that rebound congestion can occur with long-term use of this sympathomimetic:

1. Albuterol (Proventil)
2. Ritodrine (Yutopar)
3. Slameterol (Serevent)
4. Phenylephrine (Neo-Synephrine)

4. The patient is diagnosed with urinary bladder urgency and incontinence. The nurse recognizes which of the following anticholinergics as being appropriate for this condition?

1. Dicyclomine (Bentyl)
2. Ipratropium (Atrovent)
3. Oxybutynin (Ditropan)
4. Scopolamine (Transderm-Scop)

5. Alpha-adrenergic blockers cause what to occur in the body?

1. Vasoconstriction and increased blood pressure
2. Vasodilation and decreased blood pressure
3. Bronchodilation
4. Increased heart rate and cardiac output

6. Metoprolol (Lopressor) is classified as a(n):

1. Alpha blocker
2. Beta blocker
3. Cholinergic
4. Anticholinergic

7. Prior to administering atenolol (Tenormin), the nurse should assess:

1. Respirations and blood pressure
2. Respirations and heart rate
3. Heart rate and blood pressure
4. Temperature and blood pressure

8. The body's response to stimulation of this autonomic receptor is increased heart rate and force of contraction, and release of renin:

1. Muscarinic
2. $Beta_1$
3. $Alpha_1$
4. $Beta_2$

9. The patient on bethanechol (Urecholine) must be assessed for:

1. Increased heart rate
2. Hypertension
3. Fluid overload
4. Dehydration

10. Anticholinergic drugs would be suspected for which of the following patient complaints?

1. Diaphoresis
2. Confusion
3. Dry mouth
4. Increased urination

CASE STUDY QUESTIONS

For questions 1–4, please refer to the following case studies, and choose the correct answer from choices 1–4.

Mr. Wheaton is an overweight patient with hypertension and seasonal allergies. He tells you he is taking an OTC natural remedy, ma huang, to help him lose weight.

1. Why should you be concerned about his use of ma huang?

1. Its parasympathomimetic actions may decrease his blood pressure, and he will faint.
2. It may have adverse effects on his allergies by causing increased nasal congestion.
3. Its sympathomimetic actions may increase his blood pressure.
4. Its anticholinergic actions may increase his heart rate.

2. What characteristic of ma huang may affect his seasonal allergies?

1. Its sympathetic actions include a decongestant action that may relieve nasal congestion.
2. Its bronchodilating effects may cause asthma.
3. The weight-loss effects will worsen his seasonal allergies.
4. Its anticholergic actions will counteract the drowsiness caused by his allergies.

Mrs. Lopez has been diagnosed with severe hypertension.

3. Which of the following drugs might she be prescribed?

1. Ipratropium (Atrovent)
2. Salmeterol (Serevent)
3. Prazosin (Minipress)
4. Phenylephrine (Neo-Synephrine)

4. Which class(es) of drugs could adversely affect Mrs. Lopez's hypertension?

1. Parasympathomimetics and anticholinergics
2. Sympathomimetics
3. Sympathomimetics and cholinergics
4. Adrenergic blockers

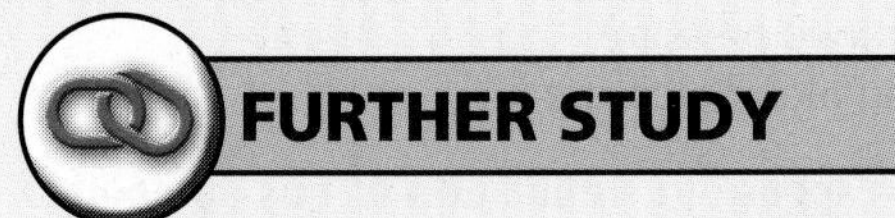

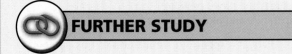

FURTHER STUDY

- Direct-acting parasympathomimetics that are used in ophthalmology are discussed in Chapter 33.
- See Chapter 26 for information on proton-pump inhibitors and H_2-receptor blockers.
- Additional information about several sympathomimetics is discussed in Chapter 19 (epinephrine and norepinephrine), Chapter 21 (oxymetazoline), and Chapter 25 (salmeterol).
- Certain adrenergic blockers are also featured in Chapter 15 (doxazosin), Chapter 17 (propranolol), and Chapter 18 (atenolol and metoprolol).

EXPLORE MEDIALINK www.prenhall.com/holland

Additional resources for this chapter can be found on the CD-ROM accompanying this textbook, and on the Companion Website. Click on Chapter 7 to select activities for this chapter.

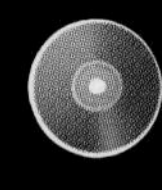

Audio Glossary
Concept Review
NCLEX-PN® Review
Nursing in Action
Dosage Calculator

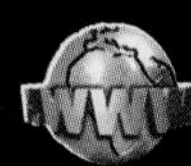

Self-Study of Autonomic System of Pharmacology
Motion Sickness in Space
Historical Use of Belladonna

CHAPTER

8 Drugs for Anxiety and Insomnia

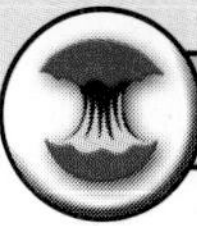

CORE CONCEPTS

8.1 Anxiety disorders fall into several categories.

8.2 Specific regions of the brain are responsible for anxiety and wakefulness.

8.3 Anxiety is managed with both pharmacological and nonpharmacological strategies.

8.4 An inability to sleep is linked with anxiety.

8.5 Anxiety and insomnia can be treated with many types of central nervous system (CNS) agents.

8.6 When taken properly, antidepressants can reduce symptoms of panic and anxiety.

8.7 Benzodiazepines are useful for the short-term treatment of anxiety and insomnia.

8.8 Barbiturates depress CNS function and cause drowsiness.

8.9 Additional drugs provide therapy for anxiety and anxiety-related symptoms.

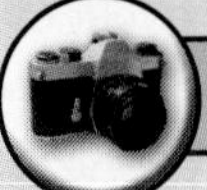

DRUG SNAPSHOT

The following drugs will be discussed in this chapter:

DRUG CLASSES	DRUG PROFILES
CENTRAL NERVOUS SYSTEM AGENTS	
Antidepressants	
Benzodiazepines	Pr lorazepam (Ativan)
Barbiturates	
OTHER DRUGS	
Nonbenzodiazepines, Nonbarbiturate CNS Depressants	Pr zolpidem (Ambien)

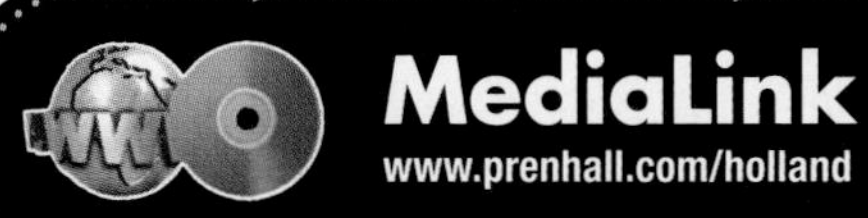

MediaLink
www.prenhall.com/holland

Interactive resources for this chapter can be found on the Companion Website. Click on Chapter 8 and "Begin" to select the activities for this chapter. For chapter-related animations, NCLEX-PN®-style questions, and an audio glossary, access the accompanying CD-ROM in this book.

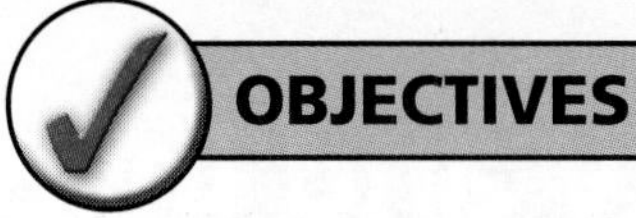

OBJECTIVES

After reading this chapter, the student should be able to:

1. Identify the major categories of anxiety disorders.
2. Discuss factors contributing to anxiety and explain some nonpharmacological therapies used to cope with this disorder.
3. Identify the four categories of CNS agents used to treat anxiety and sleep disorders.
4. Explain the pharmacological management of anxiety and insomnia.
5. Categorize drugs used for anxiety and insomnia based on their classification and mechanism of action.
6. For each of the classes listed in the Drug Snapshot, know representative drugs and explain their related clinical uses.

Patients experience nervousness and tension more often than any other symptoms. Seeking relief from these symptoms, patients often turn to a variety of pharmacological and alternative therapies. Most healthcare providers agree that even though drugs do not cure the underlying problem, they can provide short-term help to calm patients who are experiencing acute anxiety, or who have simple sleep disorders. This chapter deals with drugs that treat anxiety, cause sedation, or help patients sleep.

ANXIETY

According to the *International Classification of Diseases,* 10th edition (ICD-10), **anxiety** is a state of "apprehension, tension, or uneasiness that stems from the anticipation of danger, the source of which is largely unknown or unrecognized." Anxious individuals can often identify factors that bring on their symptoms. Most state that their feelings of anxiety are greater than what an actual event or circumstance should produce.

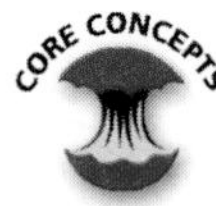

8.1 Anxiety disorders fall into several categories.

The anxiety experienced by people faced with a stressful environment or event is called *situational anxiety.* To a certain degree, situational anxiety is beneficial because it motivates people to accomplish tasks in a prompt manner—if for no other reason than to end the source of nervousness. Situational stress may be intense, but patients often learn to cope with the stress without seeking conventional medical intervention.

Generalized anxiety disorder (GAD) is difficult-to-control, excessive anxiety that lasts 6 months or more. It occurs in response to a variety of life events or activities, and it interferes with normal, day-to-day functions. It is by far the most common type of stress disorder and the one most frequently encountered by healthcare professionals. Symptoms include restlessness, fatigue, muscle tension, nervousness, inability to focus or concentrate, an overwhelming sense of dread, and sleep disturbances. Autonomic signs of sympathetic nervous system activation include blood pressure elevation, heart palpitations, varying degrees of respiratory change, dry mouth, and increased reflexes. Parasympathetic responses can include abdominal cramping, diarrhea, fatigue, urinary urgency, and numbness and tingling of the extremities. Females are slightly more likely to experience GAD, and its prevalence is highest in those ages 20 to 35.

A second category of anxiety, called **panic disorder,** is characterized by intense feelings of immediate apprehension, fearfulness, terror, or impending doom, accompanied by increased autonomic nervous system activity. Although panic attacks usually last less than 10 minutes, patients may describe them as seemingly endless. As many as 5% of the population will expe-

Fast Facts Anxiety Disorders

- About 19 million Americans experience anxiety every year.
- Other illnesses commonly coexist with anxiety, including depression, eating disorders, and substance abuse.
- The top five causes of anxiety (listed in order) affecting people between the ages of 18 and 54 are:
  Phobia (most common)
  Post-traumatic stress disorder
  Generalized anxiety
  Obsessive-compulsive disorder
  Panic
- For details, see the National Institutes of Mental Health website.

rience one or more panic attacks during their lifetimes, and women are affected about twice as often as men.

Other categories of anxiety disorders include phobias, obsessive-compulsive disorder, and post-traumatic stress disorder. **Phobias** are fearful feelings attached to specific situations or objects. Common phobias include fear of snakes, spiders, heights, or crowds. A fear of crowds is often termed *social anxiety.* Performers often experience feelings of dread and nervousness, or *performance anxiety.* Feeling anxious when in a crowd of strangers or during a performance may be expected, but feeling *extreme* fear in these situations may cause a person to avoid the fearful stimulus entirely—to the point that the person's behavior becomes unnatural and would be termed a *phobia.*

phobia = *fear*

Obsessive-compulsive disorder (OCD) describes recurrent, disturbing thoughts or repetitive behaviors that interfere with a person's normal activities or relationships. For example, a person may fear being exposed to germs. This fear may eventually lead the person to wash his or her hands over and over. After some time, this handwashing may be done so frequently that the person is unable to perform regular activities of life.

Post-traumatic stress disorder (PTSD) is a type of anxiety that develops in response to reexperiencing a previous traumatic life event such as combat experience, physical or sexual abuse, a natural disaster, or a murder. The person may dream about the event or be constantly reminded of the event by common everyday occurrences. This reexperiencing of the trauma leads to feelings of helplessness and anxiety that affect the person's ability to function normally.

8.2 Specific regions of the brain are responsible for anxiety and wakefulness.

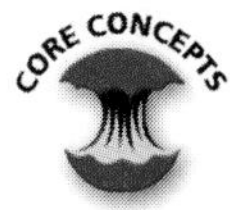

Anxiety and restlessness are associated with the limbic system and the reticular activating system. The **limbic system** is an area of the brain that is responsible for emotional expression, learning, and memory. Signals routed through the limbic system connect with the hypothalamus. Emotional states associated with this connection include anxiety, fear, anger, aggression, remorse, depression, sexual drive, and euphoria.

The hypothalamus is an important center that triggers unconscious responses to extreme stress such as increased blood pressure, elevated breathing rate, and dilated pupils. These are responses associated with the fight-or-flight response of the autonomic nervous system (see Chapter 7). The endocrine functions of the hypothalamus are discussed in Chapter 29.

The hypothalamus also connects with the **reticular formation,** a network of neurons found along the entire length of the brainstem. Stimulation of the reticular formation causes increased alertness and arousal; inhibition causes drowsiness and sleep.

The larger area in which the reticular formation is found is called the **reticular activating system (RAS).** The RAS controls sleeping and wakefulness and performs an alerting function for the cerebral cortex. It also helps a person focus attention on individual tasks by transmitting information to higher brain centers. The RAS is the neural mechanism thought to be responsible for emotions such as anxiety and fear. It is also the mechanism associated with restlessness and an interrupted sleeping pattern.

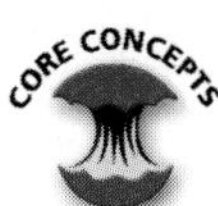

8.3 Anxiety is managed with both pharmacological and nonpharmacological strategies.

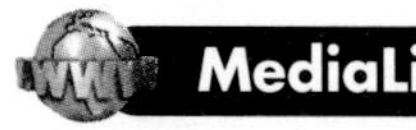

STRATEGIES FOR REDUCING STRESS

anxio = *anxiety*
lytic = *to dissolve away; break*

Although stress itself may be incapacitating, it is often only a symptom of an underlying disorder. Uncovering and addressing the cause of the anxiety is more productive than merely treating the symptoms with medications. Patients should be encouraged to explore and develop nonpharmacological coping strategies to deal with the underlying causes. Such strategies may include behavioral therapy, biofeedback techniques, meditation, and other complementary therapies. One model for anxiety management is shown in Figure 8.1 ■.

When anxiety becomes severe enough to significantly interfere with daily activities of life, pharmacotherapy is indicated. In most types of stress, **anxiolytics,** or drugs having the ability to relieve anxiety, are quite effective. These include medications in a number of therapeutic categories, including drugs for seizures (Chapter 11), depression (Chapter 9), and cardiovascular disorders (Chapter 15). Anxiolytics provide treatment for GAD, panic disorder, OCD, phobias, and PTSD.

Concept Review 8.1

- What does the term *anxiolytic* mean? What disorders do anxiolytic drugs treat?

INSOMNIA

Insomnia is a condition characterized by a patient's inability to fall asleep or remain asleep. Pharmacotherapy may be needed if the sleeplessness interferes with normal daily activities.

FIGURE 8.1

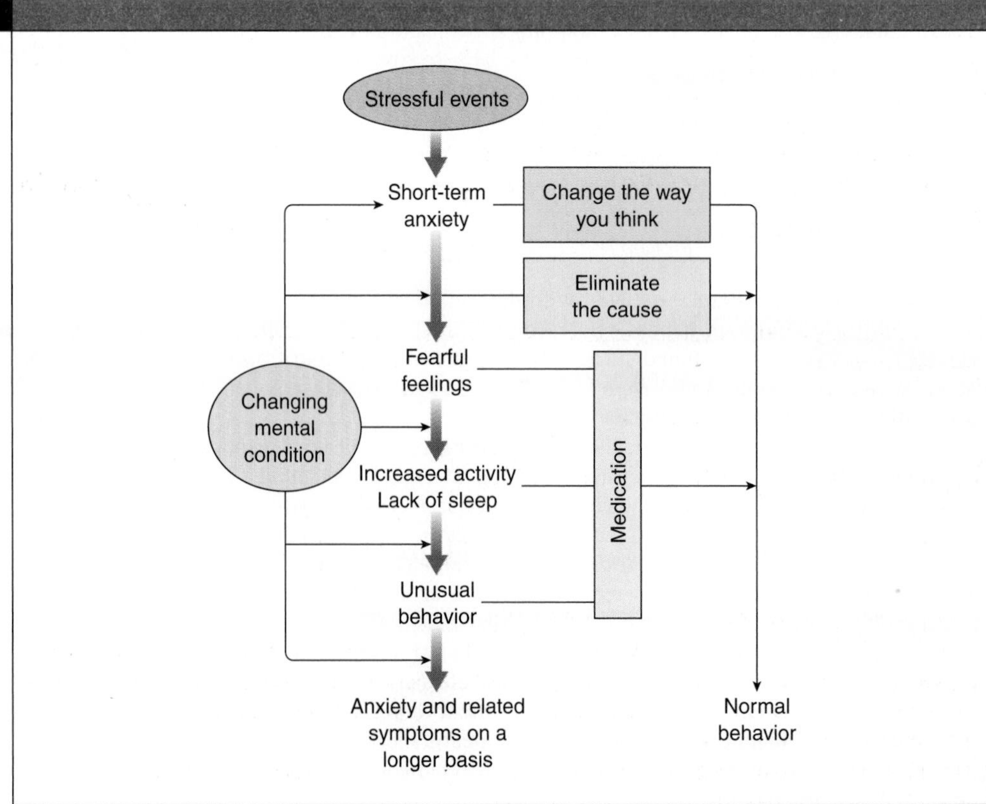

This model of anxiety shows how stressful events can cause short-term anxiety that may eventually change a person's mental condition, producing symptoms that last for a longer time. Nonpharmacologic coping strategies can often help eliminate short-term anxiety, whereas medication may be needed if anxiety lasts for longer periods or interferes with normal behavior.

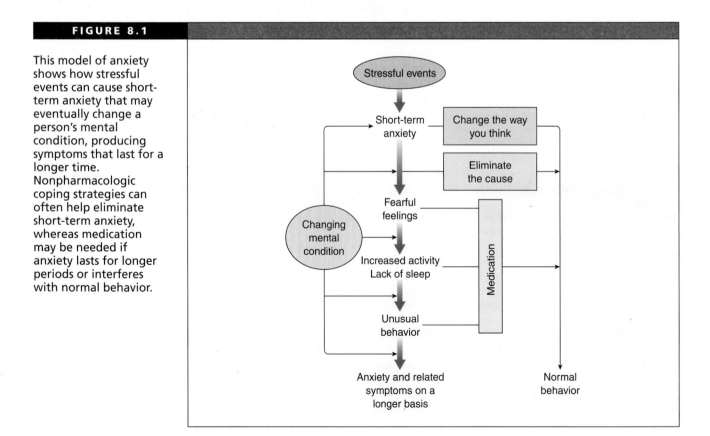

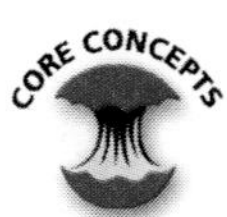

8.4 An inability to sleep is linked with anxiety.

Why is it that we need sleep? During an average lifetime, about 33% of our time is spent sleeping or trying to sleep. Insufficient sleep is associated with increased workplace and driving accidents. Although it is well established that sleep is essential for wellness, scientists are unsure of its function or how much is needed. Following are some theories:

- Inactivity during sleep gives the body time to repair itself.
- Sleep is a function that evolved as a protective mechanism. Throughout history, nighttime was the safest time of day.
- Sleep deals with "electrical" charging and discharging of the brain. The brain needs time for processing and filing new information collected throughout the day. When this is done without interference from the outside environment, these vast amounts of data can later be retrieved through memory.

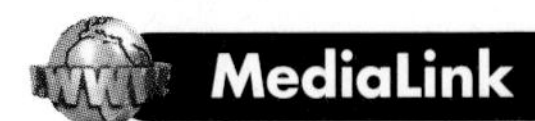

STAGES OF SLEEP

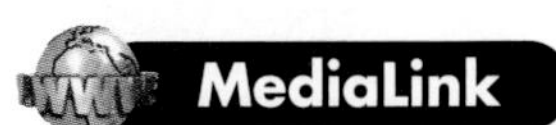

NATIONAL CENTER ON SLEEP DISORDERS RESEARCH

The acts of sleeping and waking are synchronized with many different bodily functions. Body temperature, blood pressure, hormone levels, and respiration fluctuate on a cycle throughout the 24-hour day. When this cycle is impaired, pharmacological and other interventions may be needed to readjust it. Increased levels of the neurotransmitter serotonin help initiate the various processes of sleep.

Insomnia, or sleeplessness, is a disorder sometimes associated with anxiety. There are several major types of insomnia. *Short-term* or *behavioral insomnia* may be attributed to stress caused by a hectic lifestyle or the inability to resolve day-to-day conflicts within the home or workplace. Worries about work, marriage, children, and health are common reasons for short-term sleep loss. When stress interrupts normal sleeping patterns, patients cannot sleep because their minds are too active. *Long-term insomnia* may be caused by depression, manic disorders, or chronic pain.

Foods or beverages containing stimulants such as caffeine may interrupt sleep. Patients may also find that using tobacco products makes them restless and edgy. Alcohol, while often enabling a person to fall asleep, may produce vivid dreams and frequent awakening that prevent restful sleep. Eating a large meal—especially one high in protein and fat—close to bedtime can interfere with sleep because metabolism increases to digest the food. Certain medications cause CNS stimulation, and these should not be taken immediately before bedtime. Stressful conditions—for example, too much light, an uncomfortable room temperature (especially one that is too warm), snoring, sleep apnea, and recurring nightmares—also interfere with sleep.

Nonpharmacological means of relieving insomnia are usually tried before drug therapy, because long-term use of sleep medications will likely worsen insomnia and may cause physical or psychological dependence. Some patients experience a phenomenon referred to as **rebound insomnia.** This effect occurs when a sedative drug is stopped abruptly or when it has been taken for a long time and drug dependence occurs. Alcohol abuse can also cause rebound insomnia.

Life Span Fact

Older patients are more likely to experience medication-related sleep problems. For the first night or two, drugs may seem to help the insomnia of an elderly patient, but as the medication accumulates in the system, it produces generalized brain dysfunction. The agitated patient may then be mistakenly overdosed with further medication.

Concept Review 8.2

- Why might a patient not be able to enjoy normal sleep? Why is long-term drug therapy for lack of sleep not a good idea?

Fast Facts Insomnia

- One third of the world's population has trouble sleeping during part of the year.
- Insomnia is more common in women than in men.
- Patients older than 65 sleep less than any other age group.
- Only about 70% of people with insomnia ever report this problem to their healthcare practitioner.
- People buy OTC sleep medications and combination drugs with sleep additives more than any other drug category. Trade name products include Anacin P. M., Exedrin P. M., Nytol, Quiet World, Sleep-Fez, Sominex, Tylenol P. M., and Unisom.
- As a natural alternative for sleep, some people take melatonin, kava kava, or valerian.

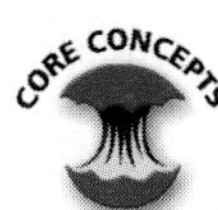

8.5 Anxiety and insomnia can be treated with many types of CNS agents.

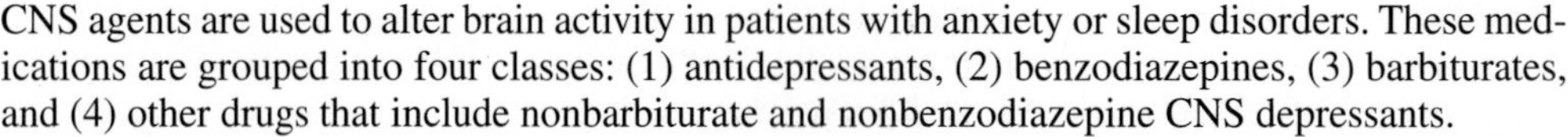

CNS agents are used to alter brain activity in patients with anxiety or sleep disorders. These medications are grouped into four classes: (1) antidepressants, (2) benzodiazepines, (3) barbiturates, and (4) other drugs that include nonbarbiturate and nonbenzodiazepine CNS depressants.

The use of antidepressants is one way to treat anxiety. **Antidepressants** have an ability to enhance mood by altering the levels of two important neurotransmitters in the brain—norepinephrine and serotonin. By restoring the balance of these neurotransmitters, antidepressants can reduce the symptoms associated with depression, panic, obsessive-compulsive behavior, and phobia. Typical antidepressants used to treat anxiety and insomnia include selective serotonin-reuptake inhibitors (SSRIs), tricyclic antidepressants (TCAs), and monoamine oxidase inhibitors (MAOIs). Use of the latter two types of drugs has declined in recent years. The mechanisms of action and important considerations of these drugs are covered in Chapter 9.

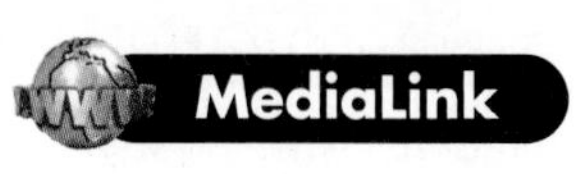

ANXIETY SELF-HELP WEBSITE

Another approach to relieving anxiety is the use of **CNS depressants** that slow neuronal activity in the brain. These drugs range from those that relax to those that sedate to those that cause sleep and anesthesia. Coma and death are the end stages of CNS depression. Some drug classes can produce the full range of CNS depression from relaxation to full anesthesia, whereas others are less effective across this range. Medications that depress the CNS are sometimes called **sedatives** because of their ability to sedate or relax a patient. At higher doses, some of these same drugs are called *hypnotics* because they can cause sleep. Therefore, the term **sedative-hypnotic** is often used to describe a drug with the ability to produce a calming effect at lower doses and to cause sleep at higher doses. *Tranquilizer* is an older term that is sometimes used to describe a drug that produces a calm or tranquil feeling.

CNS depressants used for anxiety and sleep disorders are categorized into two major classes—benzodiazepines and barbiturates. An additional category consists of miscellaneous drugs that are chemically unrelated to the benzodiazepines or barbiturates but have other important therapeutic usefulness in the treatment of anxiety. These other drugs include:

- Valproate (Depakote), an antiseizure medication
- Buspirone (BuSpar), a mild tranquilizer
- Atenolol (Tenormin) and propranolol (Inderal), beta blockers

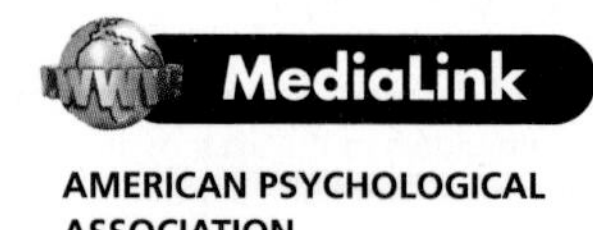

AMERICAN PSYCHOLOGICAL ASSOCIATION

Long-term use of many CNS depressants can lead to physical or psychological dependence, as discussed in Chapter 6. The withdrawal syndrome for some CNS depressants can cause life-threatening neurologic reactions, including fever, psychosis, and seizures. Other withdrawal symptoms include increased heart rate and lowered blood pressure; loss of appetite; muscle cramps; impaired memory, concentration, and orientation; abnormal sounds in the ears and blurred vision; and insomnia, agitation, anxiety, and panic. Noticeable withdrawal symptoms typically last 2 to 4 weeks. Subtle ones can last months.

Concept Review 8.3

- Describe what each of the following terms means in relation to anxiety and alertness: *CNS depressants, sedatives, hypnotics, sedative-hypnotics,* and *tranquilizers.*

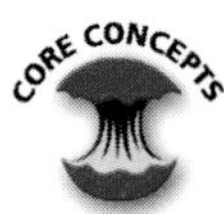

8.6 When taken properly, antidepressants can reduce symptoms of panic and anxiety.

In the 1960s, antidepressants were mainly used for the treatment of depression or depression that occurred with anxiety. Today, antidepressants are used to treat not only major depressive disorder (see Chapter 9), but also anxiety disorders such as panic disorder, OCD, social phobia, and PTSD. In the 21st century, the distinction between an antidepressant and an anxiolytic will probably disappear.

For most patients, panic symptoms come in two stages. The first stage is called *anticipatory anxiety* when the patient begins to think about an upcoming challenge and starts to feel dread. The second stage is when physical symptoms such as shortness of breath, rapid heart rate, and muscle tension begin. Many of the stressful symptoms are associated with activation of the autonomic

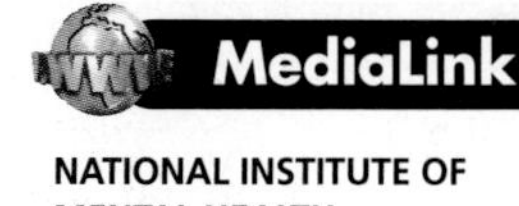

NATIONAL INSTITUTE OF MENTAL HEALTH

nervous system. The strategy in treating panic attacks is to help the patient face the fear and suppress symptoms during one or more of these stages. Drugs can lessen the negative thoughts associated with anticipating the panic, thereby reducing the stress. Drugs also decrease neuronal activity and suppress functions of the autonomic nervous system, helping the patient to remain calm. The patient can then use self-help skills to control behavior.

Antidepressants are often used to reduce symptoms of panic and anxiety. The medications that have been in use the longest for treating panic disorder are summarized in Table 8.1. The newer SSRIs and some atypical antidepressants not only treat panic symptoms but also treat symptoms of OCD and phobias and produce fewer side effects than the TCAs and MAOIs (Table 8.2).

As with all CNS agents, taking precautions helps to ensure that medications are taken properly. See Chapter 9 for important primary actions and adverse effects of these drugs. Following is a brief introduction of important considerations for each class of antidepressant.

- *TCAs*—These are not recommended in patients with a history of heart attack, heart block, or abnormal heart rhythm. Patients often have annoying anticholinergic effects (Chapter 7). Most TCAs are pregnancy category C or D. These drugs should not be used with alcohol or other CNS depressants. Patients with asthma, gastrointestinal disorders, alcoholism, schizophrenia, or bipolar disorder should use extreme caution with TCAs.
- *MAOIs*—Patients should strictly avoid foods containing tyramine (a form of the amino acid tyrosine) and caffeine. MAOIs intensify the effects of insulin and other diabetic drugs. Common side effects include orthostatic hypotension, headache, and diarrhea. MAOIs are rarely used due to serious side effects.
- *SSRIs*—These drugs are safer than other classes of antidepressants and less commonly cause sympathomimetic effects (increased heart rate and hypertension) and anticholinergic effects (dry mouth, blurred vision, urinary retention, and constipation) (Chapter 7). SSRIs can cause weight gain and sexual dysfunction. Too much of these medications can cause confusion, anxiety, restlessness, hypertension, tremors, sweating, fever, and muscle incoordination. SSRIs are often drugs of choice for anxiety.

TABLE 8.1 Older Antidepressants for Panic Disorder

DRUG	ROUTE AND ADULT DOSE	RELATED CLINICAL USES
TRICYCLIC ANTIDEPRESSANTS (TCAs)		
amitriptyline (Elavil)	PO 75–100 mg/day, may gradually increase to 150–300 mg/day (use lower doses in outpatients)	to treat depression
clomipramine (Anafranil)	PO 75–100 mg/day in divided doses	to treat OCD, depression
desipramine (Norpramin, Pertofrane, and others)	PO 75–100 mg/day at bedtime or in divided doses, may gradually increase to 150–300 mg/day (use lower doses in older adult patients)	to treat depression
doxepin (Sinequan or Adapin)	PO 30–150 mg/day at bedtime or in divided doses, may gradually increase to 300 mg/day (use lower doses in older adult patients)	to treat depression
imipramine (Tofranil) (see page 131 for the Profile Drug box)	PO 75–100 mg/day (max: 300 mg/day) in 1 or more divided doses	to treat depression, generalized anxiety
nortriptyline (Aventyl or Pamelor)	PO 25 mg three times/day or four times/day, gradually increased to 100–150 mg/day	to treat depression
MONOAMINE OXIDASE INHIBITOR (MAOIs)		
phenelzine (Nardil)	PO 15 mg three times/day, rapidly increase to at least 60 mg/day, may need up to 90 mg/day	to treat social anxiety, depression
tranylcypromine (Parnate)	PO 30 mg/day in 2 divided doses (20 mg in A.M., 10 mg in P.M.), may increase by 10 mg/day at 3-week intervals (max: 60 mg/day)	to treat depression

TABLE 8.2 Newer Antidepressants for Panic Disorder, Obsessive-Compulsive Disorder, and Phobias

DRUG	ROUTE AND ADULT DOSE	RELATED CLINICAL USES
SELECTIVE SEROTONIN-REUPTAKE INHIBITORS (SSRIs)		
citalopram (Celexa)	PO start at 20 mg/day, may increase to 40 mg/day if needed	to treat depression
escitalopram oxalate (Lexapro)	PO 10 mg/day, may increase to 20 mg/day if needed after 1 week	to treat depression, generalized anxiety, social anxiety
fluoxetine (Prozac) (see page 135 for the Profile Drug box)	20 mg/day in A.M., may increase by 20 mg/day at weekly intervals (max: 80 mg/day); 20 mg/day in A.M.; when stable may switch to 90 mg sustained-release capsule every week (max: 90 mg/week)	to treat depression, social anxiety
fluvoxamine (Luvox)	PO start with 50 mg/day, may increase slowly up to 300 mg/day given at bedtime or divided two times/day	to treat depression, social anxiety
paroxetine (Paxil)	PO 20–60 mg/day	to treat depression, social anxiety
sertraline (Zoloft)	PO begin with 50 mg/day, gradually increase every few weeks according to response (range: 50–200 mg)	to treat depression, social anxiety
ATYPICAL ANTIDEPRESSANTS		
trazodone (Desyrel)	PO 150 mg/day in divided doses, may increase by 50 mg/day every 3–4 days (max: 400–600 mg/day)	to treat depression, generalized anxiety
venlafaxine (Effexor)	Start with 37.5 mg sustained release every day and increase to 75–225 mg sustained release per day	to treat depression, social anxiety, generalized anxiety

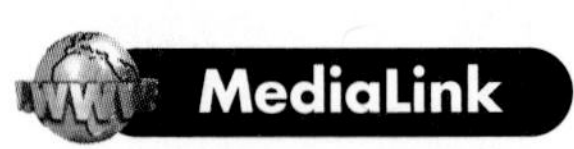

SOCIAL ANXIETY DISORDER AND HOW IT IS TREATED

- *Atypical antidepressants*—These drugs are chemically unrelated to the other antidepressants. Their side effects are similar to those of SSRIs. These drugs were the first effective alternatives to TCAs because of their more tolerable side effects, the most common of which include weight loss, anxiety, confusion, and nervousness.

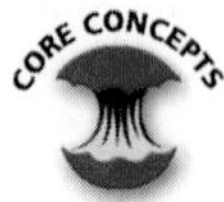

8.7 Benzodiazepines are useful for the short-term treatment of anxiety and insomnia.

benzo = *aromatic or ring structure*
di = *two*
azepine = *nitrogen containing*

The **benzodiazepines** are one of the most widely prescribed drug classes. The root word *benzo* refers to an aromatic compound, one having a carbon ring structure attached to different atoms or another carbon ring. Two nitrogen atoms incorporated into the ring structure are the reason for the *diazepine* portion of the name.

The benzodiazepines are used for panic disorder, generalized anxiety, phobias, and insomnia (Table 8.3). Since the introduction of the first benzodiazepines—chlordiazepoxide (Librium) and diazepam (Valium)—in the 1960s, the class has become one of the most widely prescribed in medicine. Although about 15 benzodiazepines are available, all have the same actions and adverse effects. They differ primarily in their onset and duration of action. Some, such as midazolam (Versed), have a rapid onset time of 15 to 30 minutes; others, such as halazepam (Paxipam), take 1 to 3 hours to reach peak blood levels. The benzodiazepines are categorized as Schedule IV drugs, although they produce considerably less physical dependence and result in less tolerance than the barbiturates.

TABLE 8.3 Benzodiazepines for Anxiety and Insomnia

DRUG	ROUTE AND ADULT DOSE	RELATED CLINICAL USES
PANIC DISORDER		
alprazolam (Xanax)	For panic attacks: PO 1–2 mg three times/day For anxiety: PO 0.25–0.5 mg three times/day	to treat generalized anxiety, phobias, social anxiety
clonazepam (Klonopin)	PO 1–2 mg/day in divided doses (max: 4 mg/day)	to treat phobias, social anxiety
ANXIETY		
chlordiazepoxide (Librium)	Mild anxiety: PO 5–10 mg three or four times/day Severe anxiety: PO 20–25 mg three or four times per day	to treat phobias
clorazepate (Tranxene)	PO 15 mg/day at bedtime (max: 4 mg/day)	
diazepam (Valium) (see page 182 for the Profile Drug box)	PO 2–10 mg two times/day	to treat panic
halazepam (Paxipam)	PO 20–40 mg three or four times/day	to treat phobias
Pr lorazepam (Ativan)	PO 2–6 mg/day in divided doses (max: 10 mg/day)	to treat panic, phobias
oxazepam (Serax)	PO 10–30 mg three or four times/day	to treat phobias
INSOMNIA		
estazolam (ProSom)	PO 1 mg at bedtime, may increase to 2 mg if necessary	
flurazepam (Dalmane)	PO 15–30 mg at bedtime	
quazepam (Doral)	PO 7.5–15 mg at bedtime	
temazepam (Restoril)	PO 7.5–30 mg at bedtime	
triazolam (Halcion)	PO 0.125–0.25 mg at bedtime (max: 0.5 mg/day)	

Benzodiazepines act by binding to the gamma-aminobutyric acid (GABA) receptor–chloride channel molecule (see Chapter 9). These drugs intensify the effect of GABA, which is a natural inhibitory neurotransmitter found throughout the brain. Most are metabolized in the liver to active metabolites and excreted primarily in urine. One major advantage of the benzodiazepines is that they do not produce life-threatening respiratory depression or coma if taken in excessive amounts. Death is unlikely, unless the benzodiazepines are taken in large quantities in combination with other CNS depressants, or the patient suffers from sleep apnea.

Most benzodiazepines are given orally. Those that can be given parenterally, such as diazepam (Valium) and lorazepam (Ativan), should be monitored carefully because of their rapid onset of CNS effects and possible respiratory depression.

Because of their greater safety, the benzodiazepines are preferred over the barbiturates for the short-term treatment of insomnia caused by anxiety. Benzodiazepines shorten the length of time it takes to fall asleep and reduce the frequency of interrupted sleep. Although most benzodiazepines increase total sleep time, some reduce stage IV sleep, and some affect REM sleep. In general, the benzodiazepines used to treat short-term insomnia are different from those used to treat generalized anxiety disorder (Table 8.3).

Benzodiazepines have a number of other important indications. Diazepam (Valium) is featured as a profile drug in Chapter 11 for its use in treating seizure disorders. Other uses include treatment of alcohol withdrawal symptoms (Chapter 6), central muscle relaxation (Chapter 31), and as induction agents in general anesthesia (Chapter 13).

NURSING PROCESS FOCUS

Patients Receiving Benzodiazepine and Nonbenzodiazepine Antianxiety Therapy

ASSESSMENT

Prior to administration:

- Obtain complete health history (both physical/mental), including allergies and drug history for possible drug interactions
- Identify factors that precipitate anxiety or insomnia
- Assess likelihood of drug abuse and dependence
- Establish baseline vital signs and level of consciousness

POTENTIAL NURSING DIAGNOSES

- Risk for Injury
- Anxiety
- Deficient Knowledge, related to drug therapy
- Ineffective Individual Coping
- Disturbed Sleep Pattern

PLANNING: Patient Goals and Expected Outcomes

The patient will:

- Experience an increase in psychological comfort
- Report absence of physical and behavioral manifestations of anxiety
- Demonstrate an understanding of the drug's action by accurately describing drug side effects and precautions

IMPLEMENTATION

Interventions and (Rationales)	Patient Education/Discharge Planning
■ Monitor vital signs. Observe respiratory patterns, especially during sleep, for evidence of apnea or shallow breathing. (Benzodiazepines can reduce the respiratory drive in susceptible patients.)	Instruct patient: ■ To consult the healthcare provider before taking this drug if snoring is a problem (Snoring may indicate an obstruction in the upper respiratory tract resulting in hypoxia.) ■ Regarding methods to monitor vital signs at home, especially respirations
■ Monitor neurological status, especially level of consciousness. (Confusion or lack of response may indicate overmedication.)	■ Instruct patient to report extreme lethargy, slurred speech, disorientation, or ataxia.
■ Ensure patient safety. (Drug may cause excessive drowsiness.)	Instruct patient: ■ To *not* drive or perform hazardous activities until effects of drug are known ■ To request assistance when getting out of bed and walking until effect of medication is known
■ Monitor patient's intake of stimulants, including caffeine (in beverages such as coffee, tea, cola and other soft drinks, and OTC analgesics such as Excedrin), and nicotine from tobacco products and nicotine patches. (These products can reduce the drug's effectiveness.)	Instruct patient to: ■ Avoid taking OTC sleep-inducing antihistamines such as diphenhydramine ■ Consult the healthcare provider before self-medicating with any OTC preparation
■ Monitor effect and emotional status. (Drug may increase risk of mental depression, especially in patients with suicidal tendencies.)	Instruct patient to: ■ Report significant mood changes, especially depression ■ Avoid consuming alcohol or taking other CNS depressants while on benzodiazepines because these increase depressant effect
■ Avoid abrupt discontinuation of therapy. (Withdrawal symptoms, including rebound anxiety and sleeplessness, are possible with abrupt discontinuation after long-term use.)	Instruct patient: ■ To take drug exactly as prescribed ■ To keep all follow-up appointments as directed by healthcare provider to monitor response to medication ■ About nonpharmacological methods for reestablishing sleep regimen

continued...

NURSING PROCESS FOCUS

EVALUATION OF OUTCOME CRITERIA

Evaluate effectiveness of drug therapy by confirming that patient goals and expected outcomes have been met (see "Planning").

See Table 8.3 for a list of drugs to which these nursing actions apply.

DRUG PROFILE: Benzodiazepines: Pr *Lorazepam (Ativan)*

Actions and Uses:

Lorazepam is a benzodiazepine that acts by increasing the effects of GABA, an inhibitory neurotransmitter, in the thalamic, hypothalamic, and limbic levels of the CNS. It is one of the most potent benzodiazepines. It has an extended half-life of 10 to 20 hours that allows for once or twice a day oral dosing. In addition to its use as an anxiolytic, lorazepam is used as a preanesthetic medication to provide sedation and for the management of status epilepticus.

Adverse Effects and Interactions:

The most common side effects of lorazepam are drowsiness and sedation, which may decrease with time. When given in higher doses or by the IV route, more severe effects may be observed, such as amnesia, weakness, disorientation, ataxia, sleep disturbance, blood pressure changes, blurred vision, double vision, nausea, and vomiting.

Lorazepam interacts with multiple drugs. For example, concurrent use of CNS depressants, including alcohol, increase sedation effects and the risk of respiratory depression and death. Lorazepam may contribute to digoxin toxicity by increasing the serum digoxin level. Symptoms include visual changes, nausea, vomiting, dizziness, and confusion.

Use with caution with herbal supplements. For example, sedation-producing herbs such as kava, valerian, chamomille, or hops may have an additive effect with medication. Stimulant herbs such as gotu-kola and ma huang may reduce the drug's effectiveness.

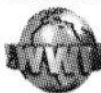
See the Companion Website for a Nursing Process Focus specific to this drug.

8.8 Barbiturates depress CNS function and cause drowsiness.

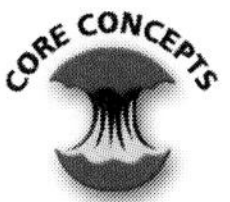

Barbiturates are drugs derived from barbituric acid. They are powerful CNS depressants that have been used in pharmacotherapy since the early 1900s for their sedative, hypnotic, and anti-seizure effects.

Until the discovery of the benzodiazepines, barbiturates were the drug of choice for treating anxiety and insomnia (Table 8.4). Although barbiturates are still indicated for several conditions, they are rarely, if ever, prescribed for treating anxiety or insomnia because of their significant side effects and the availability of more effective medications. The risk of psychological and physical dependence is high—several are Schedule II drugs. The withdrawal syndrome from barbiturates is extremely severe and can be fatal. Overdose results in profound respiratory depression, hypotension, and shock. People have used barbiturates to commit suicide, and death due to overdose is not uncommon.

TABLE 8.4 Barbiturates for Sedation and Insomnia

DRUG	ROUTE AND ADULT DOSE
SHORT ACTING	
pentobarbital sodium (Nembutal)	Sedative: PO 20–30 mg two or three times/day Hypnotic: PO 120–200 mg
secobarbital (Seconal)	Sedative: PO 100–300 mg/day in 3 divided doses Hypnotic: PO 100–200 mg
INTERMEDIATE ACTING	
amobarbital (Amytal)	Sedative: PO 30–50 mg two or three times/day Hypnotic: PO 65–200 mg (max: 500 mg)
aprobarbital (Alurate)	Sedative: PO 40 mg three times/day Hypnotic: PO 40–160 mg
butabarbital sodium (Butisol)	Sedative: PO 15–30 mg three or four times/day Hypnotic: PO 50–100 mg at bedtime
LONG ACTING	
mephobarbital (Mebaral)	Sedative: PO 32–100 mg three times/day
phenobarbital (Luminal)	Sedative: PO 30–120 mg/day

Barbiturates are capable of depressing CNS function at all levels. Like benzodiazepines, barbiturates act by binding to GABA receptor–chloride channel molecules, intensifying the effect of GABA throughout the brain. At low doses, they reduce anxiety and cause drowsiness. At moderate doses, they inhibit seizure activity (Chapter 9) and promote sleep, probably by inhibiting brain impulses traveling through the limbic system and the reticular activating system. At higher doses, some barbiturates can produce anesthesia (Chapter 13).

When taken for prolonged periods, barbiturates stimulate the microsomal enzymes in the liver that metabolize medications. This means that barbiturates can stimulate their own metabolism, as well as that of hundreds of other drugs that use these enzymes for their breakdown. With repeated use, tolerance develops to the sedative effects of these drugs, and cross-tolerance to other CNS depressants such as the opioids occurs. Tolerance does not develop, however, to the respiratory depressant effects.

Concept Review 8.4

- Identify the major drug classes used for sedation and insomnia. Why are CNS depressants especially dangerous if administered in high doses?

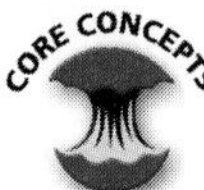

8.9 Additional drugs provide therapy for anxiety and anxiety-related symptoms.

The final group of CNS agents used for anxiety and sleep disorders consists of miscellaneous drugs that are chemically unrelated to either benzodiazepines or barbiturates.

Drugs for anxiety include the antiseizure medication valproate (Depakote), the CNS depressant buspirone (BuSpar), and the beta blockers atenolol (Tenormin) and propanolol (Inderal). Drugs for insomnia therapy include the newest of all nonbenzodiazepine CNS depressants, zaleplon (Sonata), and the relatively new drug, zolpidem (Ambien) (Table 8.5).

Buspirone (BuSpar) and zolpidem (Ambien) are commonly prescribed for their anxiolytic and hypnotic effects. The mechanism of action for buspirone (BuSpar) is unclear, but appears to be related to D_2 dopamine receptors in the brain. The drug triggers presynaptic dopamine receptors and has affinity for serotonin receptors. Buspirone is less likely than benzodiazepines to af-

TABLE 8.5 Additional Drugs for Anxiety and Insomnia

DRUG	ROUTE AND ADULT DOSE	RELATED CLINICAL USES
ANXIETY THERAPY		
Antiseizure Medication		
valproate (Depakote)	For mania: PO 250 mg three times/day (max: 60 mg/kg/day)	to treat panic
CNS Depressant (Mild Tranquilizer)		
buspirone (BuSpar)	PO 7.5–15 mg in divided doses, may increase by 5 mg/day every 2–3 days if needed (max: 60 mg/day)	to treat generalized anxiety, OCD
Beta Blockers		
atenolol (Tenormin) (see page 321 for the Profile Drug box)	PO 25–100 mg once/day	to treat performance anxiety, social anxiety
propranolol (Inderal) (see page 305 for the Profile Drug box)	For trembling: PO 40 mg two times/day (max: up to 320 mg/day)	to treat performance anxiety, social anxiety
INSOMNIA THERAPY		
Nonbenzodiazepines		
zaleplon (Sonata)	PO 10 mg at bedtime (max: 20 mg at bedtime)	
zolpidem (Ambien)	PO 5–10 mg at bedtime	

DRUG PROFILE: Nonbenzodiazepines, Nonbarbiturate CNS Depressants: *Zolpidem (Ambien)*

Actions and Uses:

Although it is a nonbenzodiazepine, zolpidem acts in a similar fashion to facilitate GABA-mediated CNS depression in the limbic, thalamic, and hypothalamic regions. The only indication for zolpidem is for short-term insomnia management (7–10 days). Zolpidem is pregnancy category B.

Adverse Effects and Interactions:

Side effects include daytime sedation, confusion, amnesia, dizziness, depression, nausea, and vomiting.

Drug interactions with zolpidem include an increase in sedation when used concurrently with other CNS depressants, including alcohol. When taken with food, absorption is slowed significantly and the onset of action may be delayed.

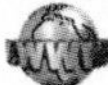
See the Companion Website for a Nursing Process Focus specific to this drug.

fect cognitive and motor performance and rarely interacts with other CNS depressants. Common side effects include dizziness, headache, and drowsiness. Dependence and withdrawal problems are less of a concern with buspirone. Therapy may take several weeks to achieve optimal results.

Zolpidem (Ambien) is a Schedule IV controlled substance limited to the short-term treatment of insomnia. It preserves deep sleep. Like other CNS depressants, it should be used cautiously in patients with respiratory impairment, in elderly patients, and when used with other CNS depressants. Lower dosages may be necessary in such cases. Also, because of the rapid onset of this drug (7 to 27 minutes), it should be taken just prior to expected sleep. Because zolpidem is metabolized in the liver and excreted by the kidneys, impaired liver or kidney function can increase blood drug levels.

Two drugs not listed in Table 8.5 are diphenhydramine (Benadryl) and hydroxyzine (Vistaril). These antihistamines produce drowsiness and may be beneficial in calming patients. They offer the advantage of not causing dependence, although their use is often limited by anticholinergic side effects. Diphenhydramine is a common component of OTC sleep aids (Chapter 21).

Concept Review 8.5

- What are the major drug classes used to treat generalized anxiety disorder and panic disorder?
- Name popular drugs within these classes.

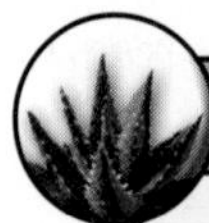

NATURAL ALTERNATIVES

Valerian

Valerian root (*Valeriana officinalis*) is a popular herbal product found in Europe and North America. It is an herbal choice for nervous tension and anxiety. It is said to promote rest without affecting REM sleep and has a reputation for calming an individual without causing side effects or discomfort. Its name comes from the Latin *valere,* which means "to be well." One thing that is *not well,* however, is its pungent odor, though many patients still claim that the smell is well worth the benefits. Valerian also is said to reduce pain and headaches without the worry of dependency. There is no drug hangover as is sometimes experienced with tranquilizers and sedatives. It is available as a tincture (alcohol mixture), tea, or extract. Sometimes it is placed in juice and consumed immediately before taking a nap or going to bed. ■

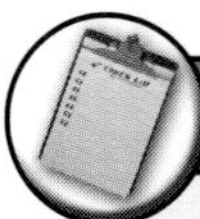

PATIENTS NEED TO KNOW

Patients taking anxiolytics and CNS depressants need to know the following:

1. Avoid stimulants such as coffee, tea, and chocolate because they counteract anxiolytics and sedatives and increase the symptoms of anxiety.
2. Exercise, progressive muscle relaxation, and slow, deep breathing can assist with anxiety relief.
3. Alcohol and other CNS depressants can increase the effects of anxiolytics. They should be avoided to decrease the risk of accidental depressant overdose and death.
4. Store anxiolytics and sedatives in a secure place to avoid accidental ingestion by children and animals. ■

CHAPTER REVIEW

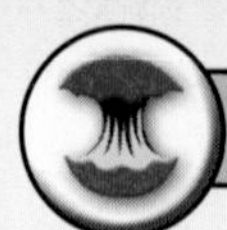

CORE CONCEPTS SUMMARY

8.1 **Anxiety disorders fall into several categories.**

There are at least five types of anxiety disorders: generalized anxiety, panic disorder, phobias, obsessive-compulsive disorder, and post-traumatic stress disorder.

8.2 **Specific regions of the brain are responsible for anxiety and wakefulness.**

The limbic system and the reticular activating system control anxiety and wakefulness. Neural signals passing between these two brain regions are responsible for anxiety, fear, restlessness, and an interrupted sleep pattern.

8.3 **Anxiety is managed with both pharmacological and nonpharmacological strategies.**

Patients should be encouraged to explore and develop coping strategies for dealing with stress. In cases when anxiety becomes too severe, anxiolytics are an effective treatment.

8.4 **An inability to sleep is linked with anxiety.**

There are many reasons why a patient might experience sleeplessness. Stress is one factor in short-term insomnia. Others include caffeine, nicotine, room temperature, light, snoring, and sleep apnea. In long-term insomnia, psychological and physiologic factors may be involved.

8.5 **Anxiety and insomnia can be treated with many types of CNS agents.**

Antidepressants treat stress and related symptoms by altering levels of norepinephrine and serotonin in the brain. Sedatives, sedative-hypnotics, and CNS depressants are terms used to describe benzodiazepines, barbiturates, and other drugs. These agents suppress impulses traveling through the limbic and reticular activating systems, thereby reducing symptoms of stress, producing drowsiness, and promoting sleep.

8.6 **When taken properly, antidepressants can reduce symptoms of panic and anxiety.**

Three classes of antidepressants treat panic and anxiety symptoms: tricyclic antidepressants (TCAs), monoamine oxidase inhibitors (MAOIs), and selective serotonin reuptake inhibitors (SSRIs). The new SSRIs are preferred since they produce fewer sympathomimetic and anticholinergic effects.

8.7 **Benzodiazepines are useful for the short-term treatment of anxiety and insomnia.**

Benzodiazepines are prescribed for certain types of insomnia. Several drugs are used; in general, they differ from the ones used to treat anxiety.

8.8 **Barbiturates depress CNS function and cause drowsiness.**

Barbiturates are rarely, if ever, prescribed for insomnia. The primary role of this class of drugs is sedation. They depress CNS function by binding to GABA receptors and causing drowsiness.

8.9 **Additional drugs provide therapy for anxiety and anxiety-related symptoms.**

Miscellaneous drugs provide relief from anxiety and anxiety-related symptoms. These include antiseizure medications, CNS depressants, and beta blockers. Antihistamines are often found in OTC medications.

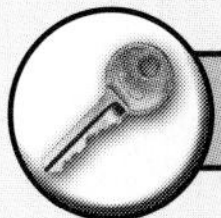

KEY TERMS

antidepressants (AN-tee-dee-PRESS-ahnts): drugs used for the treatment of depression and a range of anxiety disorders including panic, obsessive-compulsive, social phobia, and post-traumatic stress disorders / ***page 112***

anxiety: state of apprehension and autonomic nervous system activation resulting from exposure to a nonspecific or unknown cause / ***page 108***

anxiolytics (ANG-zee-oh-LIT-iks): drugs that relieve anxiety / ***page 110***

barbiturates (bar-bi-CHUR-ates): class of drugs derived from barbituric acid; they act as CNS depressants and are used for their sedative and antiseizure effects / ***page 117***

benzodiazepines (Ben-zo-di-AZ-eh-peenz): class of drugs used to treat anxiety and insomnia / ***page 114***

CNS depressants (dee-PRESS-ahnts): drugs that lower neuronal activity within the CNS / ***page 112***

generalized anxiety disorder (GAD): difficult-to-control, excessive anxiety that lasts 6 months or more / ***page 108***

insomnia (in-SOM-nee-uh): the inability to fall asleep or stay asleep / ***page 110***

limbic system (LIM-bik): area in the brain responsible for emotion, learning, memory, motivation, and mood / ***page 109***

obsessive-compulsive disorder (OCD): anxiety characterized by recurrent, intrusive thoughts or repetitive behaviors that interfere with normal activities or relationships / ***page 109***

panic disorder: anxiety characterized by intense feelings of immediate apprehension, fearfulness, terror, or impending doom / ***page 108***

phobias (FO-bee-ahs): fearful feelings attached to situations or objects / ***page 109***

post-traumatic stress disorder (PTSD): anxiety characterized by a sense of helplessness and the reexperiencing of a traumatic event, for example, war, physical or sexual abuse, natural disasters, or murder / ***page 109***

rebound insomnia: increased sleeplessness that occurs when long-term antianxiety or hypnotic medication is discontinued / ***page 111***

reticular formation (re-TIK-u-lurr): a network of neurons found along the entire length of the brainstem connected with the reticular activating system / ***page 109***

reticular activating system (RAS): the brain structure that projects from the brainstem and thalamus to the cerebral cortex; responsible for sleeping and wakefulness, and performs an alerting function / ***page 109***

sedatives (SED-ah-tivs): drugs that relax or calm the client / ***page 112***

sedative-hypnotic (SED-ah-tiv hip-NOT-ik): drug that, when given in lower doses, produces a calming effect and, when given in higher doses, produces sleep / ***page 112***

REVIEW QUESTIONS

The following questions are written in NCLEX-PN® style. Answer these questions to assess your knowledge of the chapter material, and go back and review any material that is not clear to you.

1. After 8 months of use, the patient abruptly discontinues his zaleplon (Sonata). The patient is now complaining of anxiety and inability to sleep. The nurses suspects:

1. A panic disorder
2. Long-term insomnia
3. Behavioral insomnia
4. Rebound insomnia

2. Your patient was started on buspirone (BuSpar) for his anxiety disorder 3 days ago. The patient now calls the physician's office stating that it "just isn't working." The nurse's best response would be:

1. "BuSpar should give you immediate relief. I will notify the physician this medication is not effective."
2. "It will take 3 to 4 weeks for the BuSpar to be fully effective."
3. "You may need an increased dose of BuSpar for it to work."
4. "You will need additional medications to ease your anxiety."

3. The patient is sleeping at the time the next sedative is ordered. The nurse should:

1. Wake the patient and administer the next dose of sedative
2. Notify the physician
3. Hold the dose and document the reason
4. Hold this dose and administer it with the next dose

4. The nurse educates the patient on zolpidem (Ambien) that it:

1. Will take a week for the medication to be effective
2. May be taken 2 to 3 hours before bedtime
3. Should be taken just prior to going to bed
4. Must be used long term to be effective

5. The patient has been taking barbiturates for the last few months for difficulty sleeping. The nurse's main concern for the patient that stopped taking the barbiturate would be:

1. Respiratory depression
2. Severe withdrawal
3. Hypotension
4. Shock

6. Which of the following nursing interventions would be most appropriate for a patient who has just been administered a sedative?

1. Orient to surroundings
2. Assess for respiratory dysfunction
3. Shut off the lights and close the door
4. Make sure the call light is within the patient's reach

7. The patient has been diagnosed with a panic disorder. The nurse recognizes symptoms of a panic disorder include:

1. Fatigue, muscle tension, nervousness
2. Dry mouth, diarrhea, restlessness
3. Feelings of immediate apprehension, terror, impending doom
4. Chronic insomnia, terror, nervousness

8. It is important to teach the patient to avoid __________, which can increase the effects of sedatives.

1. Nicotine
2. Alcohol
3. Chocolate
4. Tea

9. Which of the following is not used in the treatment of panic disorders?

1. Amitriptyline (Elavil)
2. Amobarbital (Amytal)
3. Diazepam (Valium)
4. Phenelzine (Nardil)

CASE STUDY QUESTIONS

For questions 1 and 2, please refer to the following case study and choose the correct answer from choices 1–4.

Ms. Reynolds is a 34-year-old interior designer who witnessed and was nearly involved in a fatal car accident on her way to a client's house about 6 months ago. Since that time, she has been having dreams about the accident and during the day, she often thinks about the events and the injured people she saw. She is fearful of driving and does all she can to avoid leaving her home-based office. When she hears a siren, she feels immediate anxiety and terror.

1. The disorder Ms. Reynolds is likely experiencing is called:

1. Obsessive-compulsive disorder (OCD)
2. Panic disorder
3. Phobia
4. Post-traumatic stress disorder (PTSD)

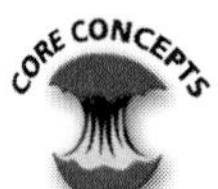

9.1 People suffer from depression for many reasons.

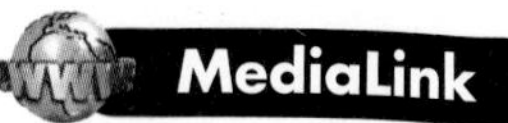

Depression is the most common mental health disorder of elderly patients, encompassing a variety of physical, emotional, cognitive, and social considerations.

MediaLink

DIET AND DEPRESSION

In some cases, depression may be situational or reactive, meaning that it results from challenging circumstances such as severe physical illness, loss of a job, death of a loved one, divorce, or financial difficulties coupled with inadequate psychosocial support. In other cases, the depression may be biological or organic in origin, associated with dysfunction of neurological processes leading to an imbalance of neurotransmitters. Family history of depression increases the risk of biological depression.

Most depressed patients are not found in psychiatric hospitals, but in mainstream everyday settings. Recognizing depression to properly diagnose and treat patients is a collaborative effort among healthcare providers, who should all be alert for signs and symptoms of depression in patients they treat. Often it is the pharmacist, working in a neighborhood pharmacy or supermarket, who recognizes that a person is depressed when the individual is self-medicating with remedies that enhance mood or using OTC sleep aids.

Some women experience intense mood shifts associated with hormonal changes during the menstrual cycle, pregnancy, childbirth, and menopause. For example, up to 80% of women experience depression 2 weeks to 6 months after the birth of a baby. Many women face additional stresses such as responsibilities both at work and home, single parenthood, and caring for children and aging parents. If mood is severely depressed and persists long enough, many women, including women with premenstrual distress disorder, postpartum depression, or menopausal distress, may benefit from medical treatment.

During the dark winter months, some patients experience a type of depression known as *seasonal affective disorder (SAD).* This type of depression is associated with a reduced release of the brain neurohormone, melatonin. Exposing patients on a regular basis to specific wavelengths of light may relieve SAD depression and prevent future episodes.

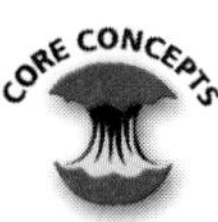

9.2 Treatment of severe depression requires both medication and psychotherapy for the best results.

The first step to treating depression is a complete health examination. Drugs, such as glucocorticoids, levodopa, and oral contraceptives can cause the same symptoms as depression, and the healthcare provider should rule out this possibility. Medical and neurological disorders, ranging from vitamin-B deficiencies to thyroid gland problems to early Alzheimer's disease, can mimic depression. If physical causes for depression are ruled out, a psychological evaluation is often performed by a psychiatrist or psychologist to confirm the diagnosis.

During the health examination, inquiries should be made about alcohol and drug use, and whether the patient has had thoughts about death or suicide. Further, a history should include questions about whether other family members have had a depressive illness and, if treated, what therapies they received and which of them were effective.

To determine a course of treatment, healthcare providers assess for well-accepted symptoms of depression. Patients diagnosed with **major depression** must show at least five of the following symptoms:

- Difficulty sleeping or sleeping too much
- Extreme fatigue; without energy
- Abnormal eating patterns (eating too much or not enough)
- Vague physical symptoms (GI pain, joint/muscle pain, or headaches)
- Inability to concentrate or make decisions
- Feelings of despair, lack of self-worth, guiltiness, and misery
- Obsession with death (a wish to die or to commit suicide)
- Avoidance of psychosocial and interpersonal interactions
- Lack of interest in personal appearance or sex
- Delusions or hallucinations

2. Not recognizing that she is experiencing a type of anxiety, Ms. Reynolds does not seek help. Instead, she finds that more and more she is compelled to perform a series of actions prior to driving anywhere in the car. She gets into her car, puts on her seat belt and pulls it tight, checks all her mirrors, and then takes her seat belt back off, and refastens it. Sometimes it takes her 20 to 30 minutes to repeatedly perform these actions before she leaves her driveway. Which of the following disorders might she also be experiencing?

1. Obsessive-compulsive disorder (OCD)
2. Panic disorder
3. Phobia
4. Generalized anxiety disorder

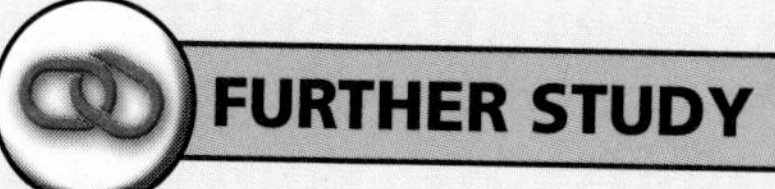

FURTHER STUDY

- Benzodiazepines are also discussed in Chapter 31 (for skeletal muscle spasms).
- Phenobarbital for the treatment of seizures is discussed in Chapter 11.
- Barbiturates can cause physical and psychological dependence, as discussed in Chapter 6.
- Valproic acid (Depakene) is also used to treat bipolar disorder, as discussed in Chapter 9.
- Phenytoin's antidysrhythmic properties are discussed in Chapter 17.
- Drugs for depression and hallucinations are also covered in Chapter 9.
- Drugs for alcohol abuse are discussed in Chapter 6.

EXPLORE MEDIALINK www.prenhall.com/holland

Additional resources for this chapter can be found on the CD-ROM accompanying this textbook, and on the Companion Website. Click on Chapter 8 to select activities for this chapter.

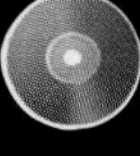

Audio Glossary
Concept Review
NCLEX-PN® Review
Nursing in Action
Dosage Calculator

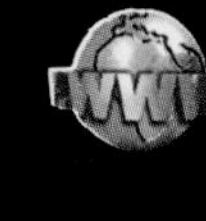

American Psychological Association
Strategies for Reducing Stress
National Institute of Mental Health
Stages of Sleep
National Center on Sleep Disorders Research
Anxiety Self-Help Website
Social Anxiety Disorder and How It Is Treated

CHAPTER

9 Drugs for Emotional and Mood Disorders

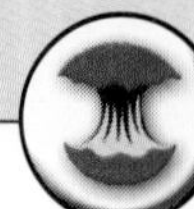

CORE CONCEPTS

9.1 People suffer from depression for many reasons.

9.2 Treatment of severe depression requires both medication and psychotherapy for the best results.

9.3 Antidepressants enhance mood by boosting the actions of neurotransmitters, including norepinephrine and serotonin.

9.4 Patients with bipolar disorder may experience emotions ranging from depression to extreme agitation.

9.5 Mood stabilization in bipolar patients is accomplished with lithium and other drugs.

9.6 Attention deficit–hyperactivity disorder presents challenges for children and adults.

9.7 CNS stimulants have been the main course of treatment for ADHD.

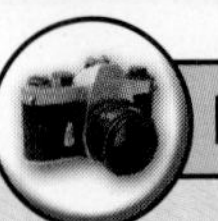

DRUG SNAPSHOT

The following drugs will be discussed in this chapter:

DRUG CLASSES	DRUG PROFILES
ANTIDEPRESSANTS	
Tricyclic antidepressants (TCAs)	Pr imipramine (Tofranil)
Selective serotonin-reuptake inhibitors (SSRIs)	Pr fluoxetine (Prozac)
Monoamine oxidase inhibitors (MAOIs)	Pr phenelzine (Nardil)
Atypical antidepressants	
DRUGS FOR BIPOLAR DISORDER	
Mood Stabilizers	Pr lithium (Eskalith)
Antiseizure drugs	
DRUGS FOR ATTENTION DEFICIT–HYPERACTIVITY DISORDER (ADHD)	
CNS stimulants	Pr methylphenidate (Ritalin)
Nonstimulant drugs for ADHD	

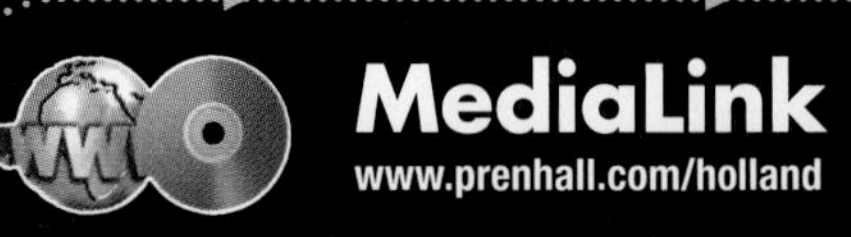

MediaLink
www.prenhall.com/holland

Interactive resources for this chapter can be found on the Companion Website. Click on Chapter 9 and "Begin" to select the activities for this chapter. For chapter-related animations, NCLEX-PN®-style questions, and an audio glossary, access the accompanying CD-ROM in this book.

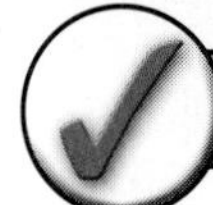

OBJECTIVES

After reading this chapter, the student should be able to:

1. Identify the two major categories of mood disorders and their symptoms.
2. Explain the causes of clinical depression.
3. Discuss the pharmacological management of patients with depression, bipolar disorder, and attention deficit–hyperactivity disorder (ADHD).
4. Identify symptoms of ADHD.
5. Know representative drug examples, and explain the mechanism of action, primary actions, and important adverse effects for each of the drug classes covered in this chapter.
6. Categorize drugs used for mood and emotional disorders based on their classifications and drug actions.

Inappropriate or unusually intense emotions are among the leading causes of mental health disorders. Although mood changes are a normal part of life, when those changes become severe and impair functioning within the family, work environment, or interpersonal relationships, an individual may be diagnosed as having a mood disorder. The two major categories of mood disorders are depression and bipolar disorder. A third emotional disorder, attention deficit–hyperactivity disorder (ADHD), is also included in this chapter.

DEPRESSION

Depression is a disorder characterized by many symptoms, some of which are depressed mood, lack of energy, sleep disturbances, abnormal eating patterns, and feelings of despair, guilt, and misery (Table 9.1).

TABLE 9.1 Situational and Biological Causes of Depression

SITUATIONAL CAUSES OF DEPRESSION

- Unpleasant life circumstances—grief from a lost loved one, divorce, loss of or dissatisfaction with a job, financial difficulty, excessive stress or responsibilities
- Negative thinking patterns—an environment that is likely to cause an individual to feel as if any attempts to escape or correct a situation are hopeless; poor self-image or lack of support from family or friends
- Substance abuse—substances that produce unpleasant side effects or withdrawal symptoms, such as opiates, alcohol, or other CNS depressants
- Medication intended for therapeutic use—unfavorable side effects from medication intended to treat a medical disorder, for example, some antihypertensive drugs and oral contraceptives

BIOLOGICAL (PHYSIOLOGICAL) CAUSES OF DEPRESSION

- Genetic—history of depression in one's family
- Hormonal changes in the body—fluctuations of reproductive or metabolic hormones
- Neurobiological dysfunction—chemical disturbances in the brain; usually related to abnormal functioning of the neurotransmitters or receptors for norepinephrine and/or serotonin
- Symptoms from a second disorder—almost any debilitating disorder, including head trauma, dementia, brain stroke or tumors, chronic pain, or thyroid dysfunction

In general, severe depressive illness, particularly that which reoccurs, requires treatment with both medication and psychotherapy to achieve the best response. Counseling therapies help patients gain insight into and resolve their problems through verbal give-and-take with the therapist. Behavioral therapies help patients learn how to obtain more satisfaction and rewards through their own actions and how to unlearn the behavioral patterns that contribute to or result from their depression.

Short-term psychotherapies that are helpful for some forms of depression are interpersonal and cognitive-behavioral therapies. Interpersonal therapy focuses on the patient's disturbed personal relationships that both cause and worsen the depression. Cognitive-behavioral therapy helps the patient change the negative style of thought and behavior that are often associated with depression. Psychodynamic therapies, often postponed until the depressive symptoms are significantly improved, focus on resolving the patient's internal conflicts.

In patients with serious and life-threatening **mood disorders** that are unresponsive to pharmacotherapy, *electroconvulsive therapy (ECT)* has been the traditional treatment. Although ECT has been found to be safe, there may be serious complications related to the anesthesia that is used and to seizure activity caused by ECT. Studies suggest that *repetitive transcranial magnetic stimulation (rTMS)* improves mood in major depression. In contrast to ECT, it has minimal effects on memory, does not require general anesthesia, and produces its effects without a generalized seizure.

trans = *across*
cranial = *head*

9.3 Antidepressants enhance mood by boosting the actions of neurotransmitters, including norepinephrine and serotonin.

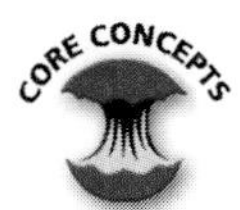

Antidepressants are medications that combat depression by enhancing mood. Depression is associated with an imbalance of neurotransmitters in certain regions of the brain. Although medication does not completely restore these chemical imbalances, it does help to reduce depressive symptoms while the patient develops effective means of coping.

Antidepressants work by increasing the action of certain neurotransmitters in the brain, including norepinephrine and serotonin (chemical name, 5-hydroxytryptamine, or 5-HT). There are two main ways in which most antidepressants work: (1) by blocking the enzymatic breakdown of norepinephrine, and (2) by slowing the reuptake of serotonin. The four primary classes of antidepressant drugs, also shown in Table 9.2, are as follows:

- Tricyclic antidepressants (TCAs)
- Selective serotonin-reuptake inhibitors (SSRIs)
- Monoamine oxidase inhibitors (MAOIs)
- Atypical antidepressants

tri = *three*
cyclic = *rings*

The atypical antidepressants include agents that do not fit into the first three categories. Agents such as bupropion (Wellbutrin) not only inhibit the reuptake of serotonin, but may also affect the activity of norepinephrine and dopamine, another neurotransmitter that plays a role in mood. Examples of atypical antidepressants are marprotiline (Ludiomil), mirtazapine (Remeron), nefazodone (Serzone), trazodone (Desyrel), and venlafaxine (Effexor).

Concept Review 9.1

- What are the major causes of depression? Identify symptoms of major depression. What is the name used to describe drugs that treat depression?

Tricyclic Antidepressants

Tricyclic antidepressants (TCAs) are drugs named for their three-ring chemical structure. They were the mainstay of depression pharmacotherapy from the early 1960s until the 1980s, and are still widely used.

TABLE 9.2 Antidepressants

DRUG	ROUTE AND ADULT DOSE	REMARKS
TRICYCLIC ANTIDEPRESSANTS (TCAs)		
amitriptyline (Elavil)	Adult: PO 75–100 mg/day(may gradually increase to 150–300 mg/day); geriatric: PO 10–25 mg at bedtime (may gradually increase to 25–150 mg/day)	For biological depression; inhibits gastric acid secretion by blocking histamine-2 receptors in the body
amoxapine (Asendin)	Adult: PO begin with 100 mg/day, may increase on day 3 to 300 mg/day; geriatric: PO 25 mg at bedtime, may increase every 3–7 days to 50–150 mg/day (max: 300 mg/day)	For situational and biological depression; not associated with cardiotoxicity; mild sedative
desipramine (Norpramin)	PO 75–100 mg/day, may increase to 150–300 mg/day	Active metabolite of imipramine
doxepin (Sinequan)	PO 30–150 mg/day at bedtime, may gradually increase to 300 mg/day	For depression accompanying anxiety or alcohol dependence
Pr imipramine (Tofranil)	PO 75–100 mg/day (max: 300 mg/day)	For biological depression or alcohol or cocaine dependence; may cause cardiac dysfunction and abnormal blood cell count; available IM; may control bedwetting in children
maprotiline (Ludiomil)	Mild to moderate depression: PO start at 75 mg/day and gradually increase every 2 weeks to 150 mg/day; severe depression: PO start at 100–150 mg/day and gradually increase to 300 mg/day	For a broad range of depression from mild to severe
nortriptyline (Aventyl, Pamelor)	PO 25 mg tid or qid; may increase to 100–150 mg/day	For biological depression; interactions similar to imipramine
protriptyline (Vivactil)	PO 15–40 mg/day in three to four divided doses (max: 60 mg/day)	For symptoms of depression; few sedative qualities; causes increased heart rate
trimipramine (Surmontil)	PO 75–100 mg/day (max: 300 mg/day)	For depression where there is a sleep disorder (has strong sedative effects)
SELECTIVE SEROTONIN-REUPTAKE INHIBITORS (SSRIs)		
citalopram (Celexa)	PO start at 20 mg/day (max: 40 mg/day)	Does not mimic the sympathetic response; has no acetylcholine blocking properties; does not inhibit MAOIs
escitalopram oxalate (Lexapro)	PO 10 mg daily, may increase to 20 mg after 1 week	May be used for generalized anxiety disorder; does not inhibit MAOIs
Pr fluoxetine (Prozac)	PO 20 mg/day in the A.M. (max: 80 mg/day)	May be used for obsessive-compulsive disorder and eating disorders
fluvoxamine (Luvox)	PO start with 50 mg/day (max: 300 mg/day)	May be used for obsessive-compulsive disorder; no severe cardiovascular side effects; fewer acetylcholine blocking effects
paroxetine (Paxil)	Depression: PO 10–50 mg/day (max: 80 mg/day); obsessive-compulsive disorder: PO 20–60 mg/day; panic attacks: PO 40 mg/day	May be used for obsessive-compulsive disorder and panic attacks
sertraline (Zoloft)	Adult: PO start with 50 mg/day, gradually increase every few weeks to a range of 50–200 mg; geriatric: start with 25 mg/day	Does not mimic sympathetic response; has no acetylcholine blocking properties; does not inhibit MAOIs
MONOAMINE OXIDASE INHIBITORS (MAOIs)		
isocarboxazid (Marplan)	PO 10–30 mg/day (max: 30 mg/day)	May cause peripheral edema and high blood pressure; used in cases where other approaches for treatment of depression are not successful

TABLE 9.2 Antidepressants

DRUG	ROUTE AND ADULT DOSE	REMARKS
MONOAMINE OXIDASE INHIBITORS (MAOIs) (continued)		
Pr phenelzine (Nardil)	PO 15 mg tid (max: 90 mg/day)	May cause a hypertensive crisis or respiratory depression; use cautiously in patients with epilepsy or diabetes, or who are likely to abuse drugs and alcohol
tranylcypromine (Parnate)	PO 30 mg/day (give 20 mg in A.M. and 10 mg in P.M.), may increase by 10 mg/day at 3-week intervals up to 60 mg/day	For severe depression in cases where patients have not responded to other medications
ATYPICAL ANTIDEPRESSANTS		
bupropion (Wellbutrin)	PO 75–100 mg tid (greater than 450 mg/day increases risk for adverse reactions)	For changing moods, schizoaffective disorders, and to quit smoking; increased risk for seizures; weaker blocker of serotonin and norepinephrine uptake
mirtazapine (Remeron)	PO 15 mg/day in a single dose at bedtime, may increase every 1–2 weeks (max: 45 mg/day)	Potent blocker of serotonin type 2 and 3 receptors; use caution in cases where patients have kidney or liver dysfunction
nefazodone (Serzone)	PO 50–100 mg bid, may increase up to 300–600 mg/day	Minimal cardiovascular effects; fewer effects in blocking acetylcholine; less sedation; less sexual dysfunction compared to other antidepressants
trazodone (Desyrel)	PO 150 mg/day, may increase by 50 mg/day every 3–4 days up to 400–600 mg/day	Increases total sleep time; reduces night awakenings; has anxiolytic effects
venlafaxine (Effexor)	PO 25–125 mg tid	Does not cause sedative or cardiovascular effects; does not block acetylcholine effects

TCAs act by inhibiting the reuptake of both norepinephrine and serotonin into presynaptic nerve terminals, as shown in Figure 9.1 ■. TCAs are used mainly for major depression and occasionally for milder situational depression. Clomipramine (Anafranil) is approved for treatment of obsessive-compulsive disorder, and other TCAs are sometimes used as unlabeled treatments for panic attacks (Chapter 8). One use for TCAs, not related to psychopharmacology, is to treat childhood enuresis (bedwetting).

pre = *before*
post = *after*
synaptic = *the synapse*

Although TCAs work well in depression, they have some unpleasant and serious side effects. The most common side effect is *orthostatic hypotension* (feeling dizzy when changing to an upright or standing position), which occurs due to vasoconstriction of blood vessels. Sedation is a frequently reported complaint at the beginning of therapy, but patients usually become tolerant to this effect after several weeks of treatment. Most TCAs have a long half-life, which increases the risk of side effects for patients with delayed excretion (Chapter 4). Anticholinergic effects, such as dry mouth, constipation, urinary retention, blurred vision, and tachycardia, are common (Chapter 4). Significant drug interactions can occur with CNS depressants, sympathomimetics, anticholinergics, and MAOIs. Now that newer antidepressants with fewer side effects are available, TCAs are less likely to be used as first-choice drugs in the treatment of depression.

Life Span Fact

TCAs can cause heart block and other cardiac side effects. They must be used cautiously in elderly patients or those with cardiac disease.

Selective Serotonin-Reuptake Inhibitors

Selective serotonin-reuptake inhibitors (SSRIs) are drugs that slow the reuptake of serotonin into presynaptic nerve terminals. They have become drugs of choice in the treatment of depression.

In the 1970s, it became increasingly clear that serotonin had a more substantial role in depression than once thought. Clinicians knew that the TCAs altered the sensitivity of serotonin to certain receptors in the brain, but they did not know how this was connected with depression. Ongoing efforts to find antidepressants with fewer side effects led to the development of the SSRIs.

FIGURE 9.1

TCAs inhibit the reuptake of both norepinephrine and serotonin.

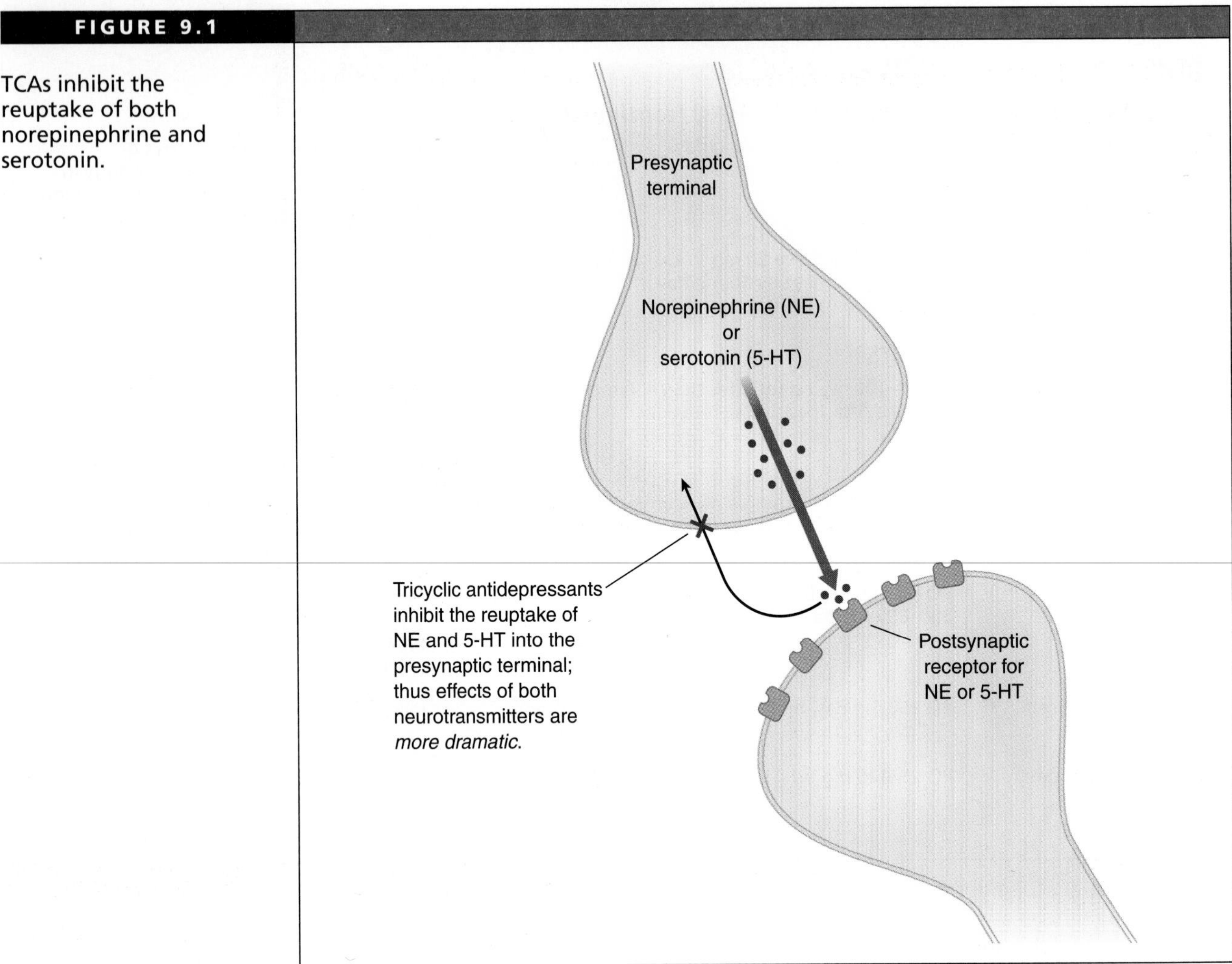

Serotonin (5-HT) is a natural neurotransmitter in the CNS and is found in high concentrations in neurons of the hypothalamus, limbic system, medulla, and spinal cord. Serotonin is important to several body activities, including the cycling between NREM and REM sleep, pain perception, and emotional states (Chapter 8). Lack of adequate serotonin in the CNS can lead to depression. Serotonin is metabolized to a less active substance by an enzyme located in presynaptic terminals called *monoamine oxidase (MAO).* A second enzyme, *catecholamine O-methyl transferase (COMT)* metabolizes serotonin in the synaptic cleft.

The TCAs inhibit the reuptake of both norepinephrine and serotonin into presynaptic nerve terminals, whereas the SSRIs are slective for just serotonin. Increased levels of serotonin in the synaptic gap cause complex neurotransmitter changes in presynaptic and postsynaptic neurons in the brain. Presynaptic receptors become less sensitive, whereas postsynaptic receptors become more sensitive. This concept is illustrated in Figure 9.2 ■.

SSRIs are about as effective as the TCAs for relieving depression. The major advantage of the SSRIs, and the one that makes them drugs of choice, is their greater safety. Sympathomimetic effects (increased heart rate and hypertension) and anticholinergic effects (dry mouth, blurred vision, urinary retention, and constipation) are less common with this drug class. Sedation is also experienced less frequently, and heart toxicity is not observed. All drugs in the SSRI class are equally effective and have similar side effects.

The most common side effects of SSRIs relate to sexual dysfunction. Up to 70% of both men and women may experience decreased libido and lack of ability to reach orgasm. In men, delayed ejaculation and impotence may occur. For patients who are sexally active, these side effects may result in noncompliance with pharmacotherapy. Other common side effects of SSRIs include nausea, headache, anxiety, and insomnia.

Serotonin syndrome (SES) is an adverse event that may occur when a patient is taking an SSRI and an additional medication that affects the metabolism, synthesis, or reuptake of serotonin.

DRUG PROFILE: Tricyclic Antidepressants: Pr *Imipramine (Tofranil)*

Actions and Uses:

Imipramine blocks the reupake of serotonin and norepinephrine into nerve terminals. It is mainly used for major depression, although it is occasionally used for the treatment of nocturnal enuresis in children. The nurse may find imipramine prescribed for a number of unlabeled uses including intractable pain, anxiety disorders, and withdrawal syndromes from alcohol and cocaine.

Adverse Effects and Interactions:

Side effects include sedation, drowsiness, blurred vision, dry mouth, and cardiovascular symptoms such as dysrhythmias, heart block, and extreme hypertension. Agents that mimic the action of noerpinephrine or serotonin should be avoided because imipramine inhibits their metabolism and may produce toxicity. Some patients may experience photosensitivity. Concurrent use of other CNS depressants, including alcohol, may cause sedation. Cimetidine (Tagamet) may inhibit the metabolism of imipramine, leading to increased serum levels and possible toxicity. Clonidine may decrease its antihypertensive effects, and increase risk for CNS depression. Use of oral contraceptives may increase or decrease imipramine levels. Disulfiram may lead to delirium and tachycardia.

Use with caution with herbal supplements, such as evening primrose oil or ginkgo, which may lower the seizure threshold. St. John's wort used with imipramine may cause serotonin syndrome.

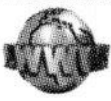

See the Companion Website for a Nursing Process Focus specific to this drug.

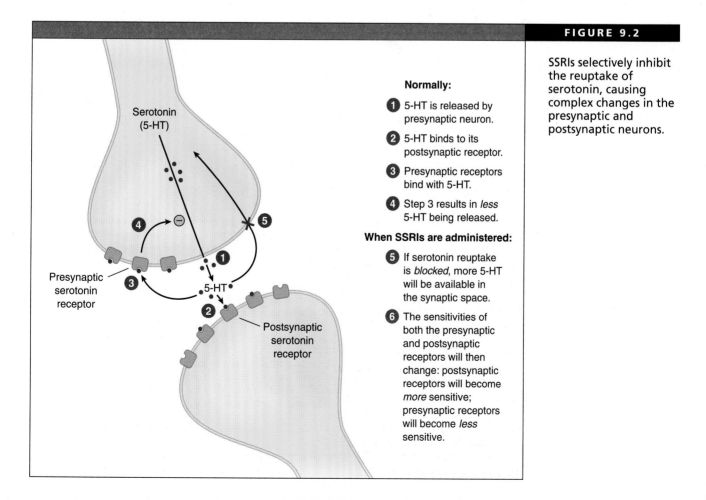

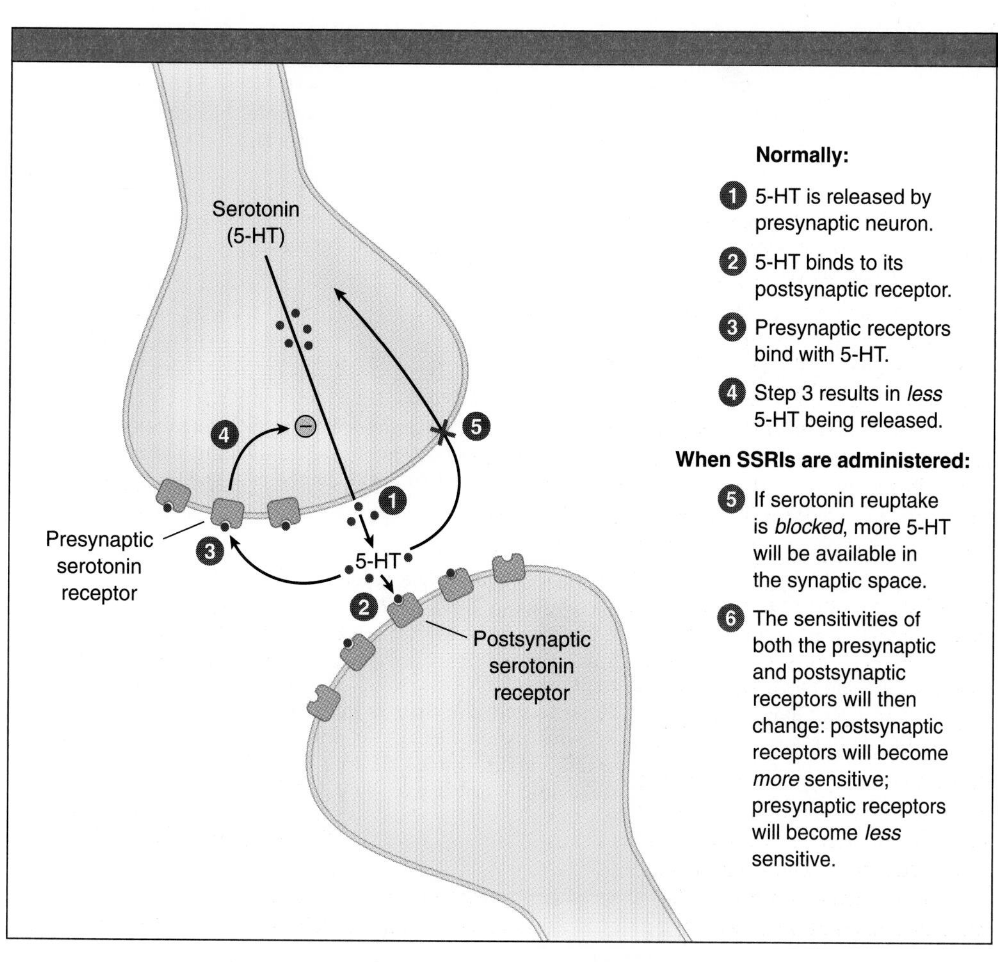

Serotonin (5-HT)
Presynaptic serotonin receptor
5-HT
Postsynaptic serotonin receptor
Normally:
1 5-HT is released by presynaptic neuron.
2 5-HT binds to its postsynaptic receptor.
3 Presynaptic receptors bind with 5-HT.
4 Step 3 results in *less* 5-HT being released.
When SSRIs are administered:
5 If serotonin reuptake is *blocked*, more 5-HT will be available in the synaptic space.
6 The sensitivities of both the presynaptic and postsynaptic receptors will then change: postsynaptic receptors will become *more* sensitive; presynaptic receptors will become *less* sensitive.

FIGURE 9.2

SSRIs selectively inhibit the reuptake of serotonin, causing complex changes in the presynaptic and postsynaptic neurons.

NURSING PROCESS FOCUS

Patients Receiving Antidepressant Therapy

ASSESSMENT

Prior to drug administration:

- Obtain complete health history including allergies, drug history, and possible drug interactions
- Obtain history or cardiac (including recent MI), renal, biliary, liver, and mental disorders including ECG and blood studies: CBC, platelets, glucose, BUN, creatinine, eletrolytes, liver function tests and enzymes, and urinalysis
- Assess neurological status, including seizure activity and identification of recent mood and behavior patterns

POTENTIAL NURSING DIAGNOSES

- Ineffective Coping
- Powerlessness
- Disturbed Thought Processes, related to side effects of drug, lack of positive coping skills
- Impaired Adjustment
- Deficient Knowlege, related to drug therapy
- Risk for Self-Directed Violence
- Urinary Retention, related to anticholinergic side effects of drug

PLANNING: Patient Goals and Expected Outcomes

The patient will:

- Report mood elevation and will effectively engage in activities of daily living
- Report an absence of suicidal ideations and improvement in thought processes
- Demonstrate a decrease in anxiety (e.g., ritual behaviors)
- Demonstrate an understanding of the drug's action by accurately describing drug effects and precautions

IMPLEMENTATION

Interventions and (Rationales)	Patient Teaching/Discharge Planning
▪ Monitor vital signs especially pulse and blood pressure. (Imipramine may cause orthostatic hypotension.)	Instruct patient to: ▪ Report any change in sensorium particularly impending syncope ▪ Avoid abrupt changes in position ▪ Monitor vital signs (especially blood pressure) ensuring proper use of home equipment ▪ Consult the nurse regarding "reportable" blood pressure readings (e.g., lower than 80/50 mm Hg)
▪ Observe for serotonin syndrome in SSRI use: confusion, mania, headache, respiratory problems, kidney failure, and possibly death (usually occurs with concurrent use of St. John's wort or MAOIs). ▪ If suspected, discontinue drug and initiate supportive care. Respond according to ICU/emergency department protocols.	▪ Inform patient that overdosage may result in serotonin syndrome, which can be life threatening.
▪ Monitor for paradoxical diaphoresis, which must be considered a significant sign, especially serious when coupled with nausea/vomiting or chest pain.	▪ Instruct patient to seek immediate medical attention for dizziness, headache, tremor, nausea/vomiting, anxiety, disorientation, hyperreflexia, diaphoresis, and fever.
▪ Monitor cardiovascular status. Observe for hypertension and signs of impending stroke or MI and heart failure.	▪ Instruct patient to immediately report severe headache, dizziness, paresthesias, bradycardia, chest pain, tachycardia, nausea/vomiting, or diaphoresis.
▪ Monitor neurological status. Observe for somnolence and seizures. (TCAs may cause somnolence related to CNS depression. May reduce the seizure threshold.)	Instruct patient to: ▪ Report significant changes in neurological status, such as seizures, extreme lethargy, slurred speech, disorientation, or ataxia and discontinue the drug ▪ Take dose at bedtime to avoid daytime sedation

continued...

NURSING PROCESS FOCUS

Interventions and (Rationales)	Patient Education/Discharge Planning
▪ Monitor mental and emotional status. Observe for suicidal ideation. (Therapeutic benefits may be delayed. Outpatients should have no more than a 7-day medication supply.) ▪ Monitor for underlying or concomitant psychoses such as schizophrenia or bipolar disorders. (May trigger manic states.)	Instruct patient: ▪ To immediately report dysphoria or suicidal impulses ▪ To commit to a "no-self harm" verbal contract ▪ That it may take 10–14 days before improvement is noticed, and about 1 month to achieve full therapeutic effect
▪ Monitor sleep–wake cycle. Observe for insomnia and/or daytime somnolence.	Instruct patient to: ▪ Take the drug very early in the morning to promote normal timing of sleep onset ▪ Avoid driving or potentially hazardous activities until effects of drug are known ▪ Take at bedtime if daytime drowsiness persists
▪ Monitor renal status and urinary output. (May cause urinary retention due to muscle relaxation in urinary tract. Imipramine is excreted through the kidneys. Fluoxetine is slowly metabolized and excreted, increasing the risk of organ damage. Urinary retention may exacerbate existing symptoms of prostatic hypertrophy.)	Instruct patient to: ▪ Monitor fluid intake and output ▪ Notify the healthcare provider of edema, dysuria (hesitancy, pain, diminished stream), changes in urine quantity or quality (e.g., cloudy, with sediment) ▪ Report fever or flank pain that may be indicative of a urinary tract infection related to urine retention
▪ Use cautiously with the elderly or young. (Diminished kidney and liver function related to aging can result in higher serum drug levels, and may require lower doses. Children, due to an immature CNS, respond paradoxically to CNS-active drugs.)	Instruct patient that: ▪ The elderly may be more prone to side effects such as hypertension and dysrhythmias ▪ Children on imipramine for nocturnal enuresis may experience mood alterations
▪ Monitor gastrointestinal status. Observe for abdominal distention. (Muscarinic blockade reduces tone and motility of intestinal smooth muscle, and may cause paralytic ileus.)	Instruct patient to: ▪ Exercise, drink adequate amounts of fluid, and add dietary fiber to promote stool passage ▪ Consult the nurse regarding a bulk laxative or stool softener if constipation becomes a problem
▪ Monitor liver function. Observe for signs and symptoms of hepatotoxicity. ▪ Monitor blood studies including CBC, differential, platelets, PT, PTT, and liver enzymes.	Instruct patient to: ▪ Report nausea, vomiting, diarrhea, rash, jaundice, epigastric or abdominal pain, tenderness, or change in color of stool ▪ Adhere to laboratory testing regimen for blood tests and urinalysis as directed
▪ Monitor hematologic status. Observe for signs of bleeding. (Imipramine may cause blood dyscrasias. Use with warfarin may increase bleeding time.)	▪ Instruct patient to report excessive bruising, fatigue, pallor, shortness of breath, frank bleeding, and/or tarry stools. ▪ Demonstrate guaiac testing on stool for occult blood.
▪ Monitor immune/metabolic status. Use with caution in patients with diabetes mellitus or hyperthyroidism. (If given in hyperthyroidism, can cause agranulocytosis. Imipramine may either increase or decrease serum glucose. Fluoxetine may cause initial anorexia and weight loss, but with prolonged therapy may result in weight gain of up to 20 pounds.)	▪ Instruct diabetics to monitor glucose level daily and consult nurse regarding reportable serum glucose levels. ▪ Instruct patient to monitor weight. Possible anorexia and weight loss will diminish with continued therapy.

continued...

(continued from page 133)

NURSING PROCESS FOCUS

Interventions and (Rationales)	Patient Education/Discharge Planning
▪ Observe for extrapyramidal and anticholinergic effects. In overdosage, 12 hours of anticholinergic activity is followed by CNS depression. ▪ Do not treat overdosage with quinidine, procainamide, atropine, or barbiturates. (Quinidine and procainamide can increase the possibility of dysrhythmia, atropine can lead to severe anticholinergic effects, and barbiturates can lead to excess sedation.)	Instruct patient to: ▪ Immediately report involuntary muscle movement of the face or upper body (e.g., tongue spasms), fever, anuria, lower abdominal pain, anxiety, hallucinations, psychomotor agitation, visual changes, dry mouth, and difficulty swallowing ▪ Relieve dry mouth with (sugar-free) hard candies, chewing gum, and drinking fluids ▪ Avoid alcohol-containing mouthwashes which can further dry oral mucous membranes
▪ Monitor visual acuity. Use with caution in narrow-angle glaucoma. (Imipramine may cause an increase in intraocular pressure. Anticholinergic effects may produce blurred vision.)	Instruct patient to: ▪ Report visual changes, headache, or eye pain ▪ Inform eye care professional of imipramine therapy
▪ Ensure patient safety. (Dizziness caused by postural hypotension increases the risk of fall injuries.)	Instruct patient to: ▪ Call for assistance before getting out of bed or attempting to ambulate alone ▪ Avoid driving or performing hazardous activities until blood pressure is stabilized and effects of the drug are known

EVALUATION OF OUTCOME CRITERIA

Evaluate the effectiveness of drug therapy by confirming that patient goals and expected outcomes have been met (see "Planning").

See Table 9.2 for a list of drugs to which these nursing actions apply.

The result is that serotonin accumulates in the body. Symptoms can begin as early as 2 hours or as late as several weeks after taking the first dose. SES can be produced by the administration of an SSRI with an MAOI, a TCA, lithium, or a number of other medications. Symptoms of SES include mental status changes (confusion, anxiety, restlessness), hypertension, tremors, sweating, fever, and lack of muscular coordination. Conservative treatment is to discontinue the SSRI and provide supportive care. In severe cases, mechanical ventilation and muscle relaxants may be necessary. If left untreated, death may occur.

Monoamine Oxidase Inhibitors

Monoamine oxidase inhibitors (MAOIs) are drugs that inhibit monoamine oxidase, an enzyme that stops the actions of neurotransmitters such as dopamine, norepinephrine, epinephrine, and serotonin. When these neurotransmitters are released from the nerve terminal, the body naturally regulates how long they act by breaking them down chemically with monoamine oxidase. MAOIs inhibit this breakdown of norepinephrine, dopamine, and serotonin in CNS neurons, allowing higher levels of these neurotransmitters in the brain (Figure 9.3 ■). Higher levels lead to intensified neurotransmission, which, in turn, lessens symptoms of depression.

In the 1950s, the monoamine oxidase inhibitors were the first drugs approved to treat depression. They are as effective as TCAs and SSRIs in treating depression, but they have a lower safety margin. Because of drug-drug and food-drug interactions, liver toxicity, and the development of safer antidepressants, MAOIs are now reserved for patients who are not responsive to other antidepressant classes.

DRUG PROFILE: Selective Serotonin-Reuptake Inhibitors (SSRIs): Pr *Fluoxetine (Prozac)*

Actions and Uses:

Fluoxetine acts by selectively inhibiting serotonin reuptake into presynaptic nerve terminals. Its main use is in major depression although it may be prescribed for obsessive-compulsive and eating disorders. Therapeutic actions include improved affect, mood enhancement, and increased appetite with maximum effects observed after several days to weeks. Fluoxetine is pregnancy category B.

Adverse Effects and Interactions:

Fluoxetine may cause headaches, nervousness, insomnia, nausea, and diarrhea. Foods high in the amino acid tryptophan should be avoided. Coadministration with selegiline may increase the risk of a hypertensive crisis. Tricyclic antidepressants administered with fluoxetine may produce serotonin syndrome. Symptoms of fluoxetine overdose include fever, confusion, shivering, sweating, and muscle spasms. Fluoxetine cannot be used if the patient took an MAOI within 14 days. Use with benzodiazepines may cause increased adverse CNS effects. Use with beta blockers can cause their decreased elimination, leading to hypotension or bradycardia. Use with phenytoin, clozapine, or theophylline may lead to decreased elimination of these drugs and toxicity. Use with warfarin may lead to increaed risk of bleeding due to competitive protein binding.

Fluoxetine should be used with caution with herbal supplements such as St. John's wort or L-tryptophan, which may cause serotonin syndrome, and kava, which may increase the effects of fluoxetine.

Mechanism in Action: 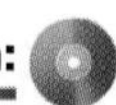

Fluoxetine (Prozac) is a selective serotonin-reuptake inhibitor (SSRI). It acts by blocking the recycling of the brain neurotransmitter serotonin into presynaptic nerve terminals. At the synaptic cleft, serotonin continually binds with postsynaptic receptors and activates excitatory postsynaptic potentials (EPSPs). This is thought to restore the mental state of a depressed patient to a normal level.

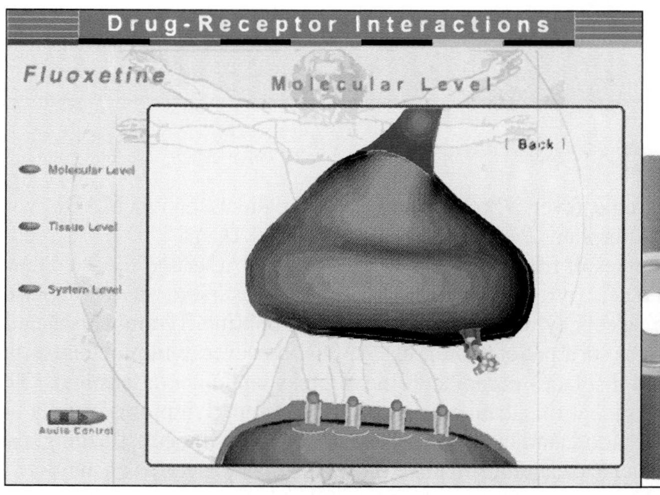

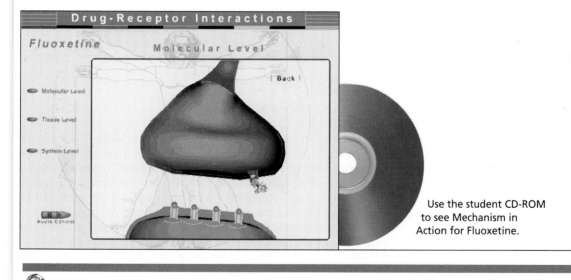

Use the student CD-ROM to see Mechanism in Action for Fluoxetine.

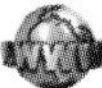 *See the Companion Website for a Nursing Process Focus specific to this drug.*

Common side effects of the MAOIs include orthostatic hypotension, headache, insomnia, and diarrhea. A primary concern is that these agents interact with a large number of foods and other medications, sometimes with serious effects. A hypertensive crisis can occur when an MAOI is used together with other antidepressants or sympathomimetic drugs. Combining an MAOI with an SSRI can produce serotonin syndrome. If given with antihypertensives, the patient can experience excessive hypotension. MAOIs also increase the hypoglycemic effects of insulin

FIGURE 9.3

MAOIs inhibit monoamine oxidase, an enzyme that stops the actions of neurotransmitters such as dopamine, norepinephrine, epinephrine, and serotonin.

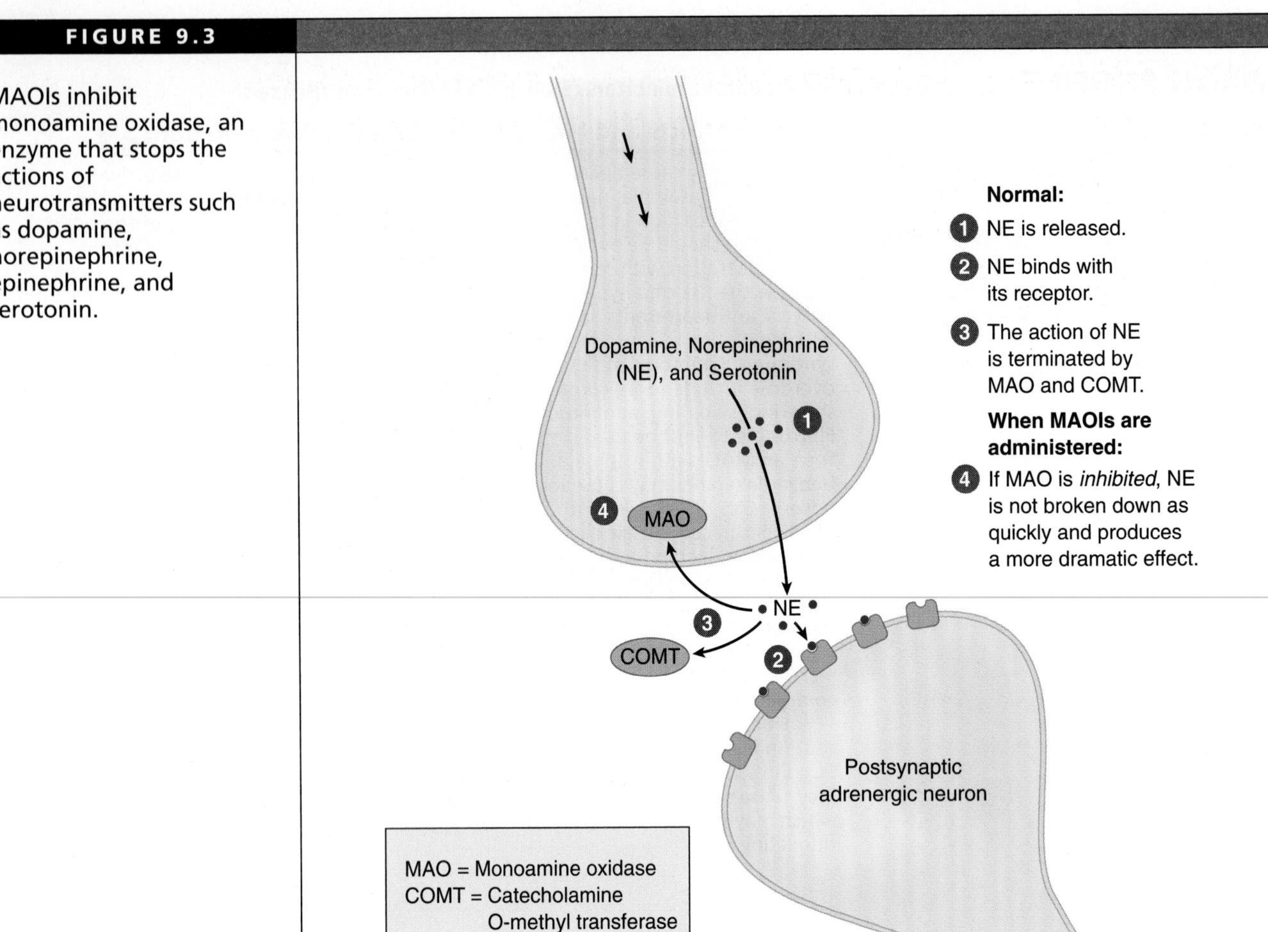
Normal:
1 NE is released.
2 NE binds with its receptor.
3 The action of NE is terminated by MAO and COMT.
When MAOIs are administered:
4 If MAO is inhibited, NE is not broken down as quickly and produces a more dramatic effect.
Dopamine, Norepinephrine (NE), and Serotonin
MAO
NE
COMT
Postsynaptic adrenergic neuron
MAO = Monoamine oxidase
COMT = Catecholamine O-methyl transferase

and oral antidiabetic drugs. Extreme fever is known to occur in patients taking MAOIs with meperidine (Demerol), dextromethorphan (Pedia Care and others), and TCAs.

A hypertensive crisis can also result from an interaction between MAOIs and foods containing tyramine, a form of the amino acid, tyrosine. In fact, tyrosine is a presursor to norepinephrine in the nervous system. In many respects, tyramine resembles norepinephrine. Tyramine is usually degraded by MAO in the intestines. If a patient is taking MAOIs, however, tyramine enters the bloodstream in high amounts and displaces norepinephrine in presynaptic nerve terminals. The result is a sudden increase in norepinephrine, causing acute hypertension. Symptoms usually occur within minutes of ingesting the food, and include occipital headache, stiff neck, flushing, palpitations, profuse sweating, and nausea. Calcium channel blockers may be given as an antidote to increased cardiovasular effects. Examples of foods containing tyramine are shown in Table 9.3.

Concept Review 9.2

- What are the three major classes of antidepressants? Name representative drugs within each class and describe how each drug works pharmacologically.

BIPOLAR DISORDER

Bipolar disorder is characterized by extreme and opposite moods. Patients may display signs of euphoria and depression or calmness and rage.

DRUG PROFILE: Monoamine Oxidase Inhibitors (MAOIs): Pr *Phenelzine (Nardil)*

Actions and Uses:

Phenelzine produces its effects by irreversible inhibition of monoamine oxidase; therefore, it intensifies the effects of norepinephrine in adrenergic synapses. It is used to manage symptoms of depression not responsive to other types of pharmacotherapy, and is occasionally used for panic disorder. Drug effects may continue for 2 to 3 weeks after therapy is discontinued.

Adverse Effects and Interactions:

Common side effects are constipation, dry mouth, orthostatic hypotension, insomnia, nausea, and loss of appetite. It may increase heart rate and neural activity leading to delirium, mania, anxiety, and convulsions. Severe hypertension may occur when ingesting foods containing tyramine. Seizures, respiratory depression, circulatory collapse, and coma may occur in cases of severe overdose. Many other drugs affect the action of phenelzine. Use with TCAs and SSRIs should be avoided, since the combination can cause temperature elevation and seizures. Opiates, including meperidine, should be avoided due to increased risk of respiratory failure or hypertensive crisis.

Phenelzine should be used with caution with herbal supplements, such as ginseng, which could cause headache, tremors, mania, insomnia, irritability, and visual hallucinations. Concurrent use of ephedra could cause hypertensive crisis.

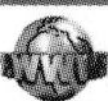
See the Companion Website for a Nursing Process Focus specific to this drug.

TABLE 9.3 Foods Containing Tyramine

FRUITS	DAIRY PRODUCTS	ALCOHOL	MEATS
Avocados	Cheese (cottage cheese is okay)	Beer	Beef or chicken liver
Bananas	Sour cream	Wines (especially red wines and Chianti)	Pate
Raisins	Yogurt		Meat extracts
Papaya products including meat tenderizers			Pickled or kippered herring
Canned figs			Pepperoni
			Salami
			Sausage
			Bologna/hot dogs
VEGETABLES	**SAUCES**	**YEAST**	**OTHER**
Pods of broad beans (fava beans)	Soy sauce	All yeast or yeast extracts	Chocolate

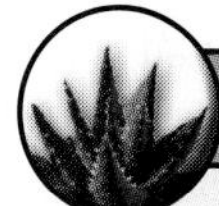

NATURAL ALTERNATIVES

St. John's Wort for Depression

St. John's Wort (*Hypericum perforatum*) is an herb found throughout Britain, Asia, Europe, and North America that is commonly used as an antidepressant. It gets its name from a legend that red spots once appeared on its leaves on the anniversary of St. John's beheading. *Wort* is a British term for "plant." Researchers once claimed that it produced its effects the same way as MAOIs do: by increasing the levels of serotonin, adrenaline, and dopamine in the brain. More recent evidence suggests that it may selectively inhibit serotonin reuptake. Some claim that it is more effective than fluoxetine (Prozac), paroxetine (Paxil), or sertraline (Zoloft) and produces fewer side effects. It has other uses including as an anti-infective agent for conditions such as staph and strep, for nerve pains such as neuralgia and sciatica, and for mental burnout. It is extremely important to avoid combinations of St. John's Wort and antidepressant medications unless prescribed by a healthcare practitioner. ■

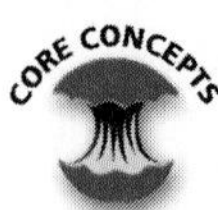

9.4 Patients with bipolar disorder may experience emotions ranging from depression to extreme agitation.

bi = *two*
polar = *extremes*

Bipolar disorder, also called *manic depression,* is characterized by extreme and opposite moods, such as euphoria and depression. Patients may oscillate rapidly between both extremes, or there may be prolonged periods in which mood is normal.

During the depressive stages of bipolar disorder, patients exhibit the symptoms of major depression described previously in this chapter. Patients with bipolar disorder also display signs of *mania,* an emotional state characterized by high psychomotor activity and irritability. Patients may shift quickly from emotions of extreme depression to extreme rage and agitation. Symptoms of mania, as shown in the following list, are generally the opposite of depressive symptoms.

- Insomnia
- Activity for days without rest and without appearing tired
- Easy agitation and aggression
- Feelings of exaggerated confidence
- Making choices without regard for a long-term plan or consequences of action
- Attention seeking
- Unusual interest in sex
- Drug abuse, including alcohol, cocaine, or sleeping medications
- Denial that the behavior is a problem

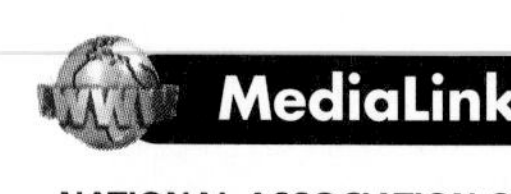

NATIONAL ASSOCIATION OF MENTAL ILLNESS

Concept Review 9.3

- Identify the symptoms of mania. How do manic symptoms generally compare with depressive symptoms?

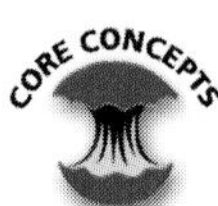

9.5 Mood stabilization in bipolar patients is accomplished with lithium and other drugs.

Drugs for bipolar disorder are called **mood stabilizers** because they have the ability to moderate extreme shifts in emotions between mania and depression. Some antiseizure drugs are also used for mood stabilization in bipolar patients.

The mainstay for the treatment of bipolar disorder is lithium (Eskalith and others) as monotherapy or in combination with other drugs. Lithium was approved in the United States in 1970. Before that time, its benefit in manic-depressive illness had been known; however, its therapeutic safety had not been proven. Other drugs that stabilize mood have multiple uses. For example, carbamazepine (Tegretol) and valproic acid (Depakene) are antiseizure drugs that have uses in bipolar disease (Chapter 11). Table 9.4 shows selected drugs used to treat bipolar disorder.

Lithium serum levels must be checked every 1 to 3 days when beginning therapy and every 2 to 3 months thereafter. To ensure therapeutic action, concentrations of lithium in the blood must remain within the range of 0.6 to 1.5 m/Eq/L. Close monitoring encourages compliance and helps to avoid toxicity. Lithium acts like sodium in the body, so conditions in which sodium is lost (e.g., excessive sweating or dehydration) can cause lithium toxicity. Lithium overdose may be treated with hemodialysis and supportive care.

It is not unusual for other drugs to be used in combination with lithium for the control of bipolar disorder. During the depressed stage, a TCA or an atypical antidepressant such as bupropion (Wellbutrin) may be necessary. During manic phases, a benzodiazepine will moderate manic symptoms (Chapter 8). In cases of extreme agitation, delusions, or hallucinations, an antipsychotic agent may be indicated (Chapter 10). Continued patient compliance is essential to achieving successful pharmacotherapy because some patients do not perceive their conditions as abnormal.

Concept Review 9.4

- Give the general name of drugs used to treat bipolar disorder. What is the main drug used to treat bipolar disorder, and how does it work pharmacologically? What other drugs treat bipolar disorder?

TABLE 9.4 Drugs for Bipolar Disorder: Mood Stabilizers

DRUG	ROUTE AND ADULT DOSE	REMARKS
Pr lithium (Eskalith)	PO initial 600 mg tid, maintenance 300 mg tid (max: 2.4 g/day)	For treatment of mania and depressive symptoms; must be used cautiously in epilepsy and in psychosis
ANTISEIZURE DRUGS		
carbamazepine (Tegretol)	PO 200 mg bid, gradually increased to 800–1200 mg/day in 3 to 4 divided doses	For treatment of manic depressive and schizoaffective symptoms; used as antiseizure medication
lamotrigine (Lamictal)	PO 50 mg/day for 2 weeks, then 50 mg bid for 2 weeks; may increase gradually up to 300–500 mg/day in 2 divided doses (max: 700 mg/day)	Used as antiseizure medication; fatal rash has been reported in children less than 16 years old
valproic acid (Depakene)	PO 250 mg tid (max: 60 mg/kg/day)	For treatment of mania and prevention of migraine headache; used as antiseizure medication

DRUG PROFILE: Mood Stabilizers: Pr *Lithium (Eskalith)*

Actions and Uses:

Although the exact mechanism of action is not clear, lithium is thought to alter the activity of neurons containing dopamine, norepinephrine, and serotonin by influencing their release, synthesis, and reuptake. Therapeutic actions are stabilization of mood during periods of mania and antidepressant effects during periods of depression. Lithium has neither antimanic nor antidepressant effects in individuals without bipolar disorder. After taking lithium for 2 to 3 weeks, patients are able to better concentrate and function in self-care.

Adverse Effects and Interactions:

Lithium may cause dizziness, fatigue short-term memory loss, increased urination, nausea, vomiting, loss of appetite, abdominal pain, diarrhea, dry mouth, muscular weakness, and slight tremors. Some drugs increase the rate at which the kidneys remove lithium from the bloodstream, including diuretics, sodium bicarbonate, and potassium citrate. Other drugs, such as methyldopa and probenecid, inhibit the rate of lithium excretion. Patients should not have a salt-free diet when taking this drug, because such a diet reduces lithium excretion. Diuretics enhance excretion of sodium and increase the risk of lithium toxicity. Use with anticholinergic drugs can cause urinary retention that, coupled with the polyuria effect of lithium, may cause a medical emergency. Alcohol can increase drug action.

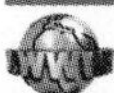
See Companion Website for a Nursing Process Focus specific to this drug.

ATTENTION DEFICIT–HYPERACTIVITY DISORDER

Attention deficit–hyperactivity disorder (ADHD) is a condition characterized by poor attention span, behavior control issues, and/or hyperactivity. Although usually diagnosed in childhood, symptoms of ADHD may extend into adulthood.

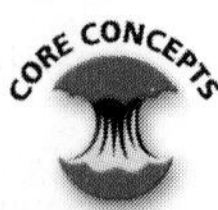

9.6 Attention deficit–hyperactivity disorder presents challenges for children and adults.

Life Span Fact

ADHD affects as many as 5% of all children. Most children diagnosed with this condition are between the ages of 3 and 7 years, and boys are four to eight times more likely to be diagnosed than girls.

ADHD is characterized by developmentally inappropriate behaviors involving difficulty in paying attention or focusing on tasks. ADHD may be diagnosed when a child's hyperactive behaviors significantly interfere with normal play, sleep, or learning activities. Hyperactive children usually have increased motor activity that is shown by a tendency to be fidgety and impulsive, and to interrupt and talk excessively during their developmental years; therefore, they may not be able to interact with others appropriately at home or school. In boys, the activity levels are usually more overt. Girls show less aggression and impulsiveness but more anxiety, mood swings, social withdrawal, and cognitive and language delays. Girls also tend to be older at the time of diagnosis, so problems and setbacks related to the disorder exist for a longer time before treatment interventions are undertaken. Symptoms of ADHD are shown in the following list.

- Easy distractability
- Failure to receive or follow instructions properly
- Inability to focus on one task at a time and tendency to jump from one activity to another
- Difficulty remembering
- Frequent loss or misplacing of personal items
- Excessive talking and interrupting other children in a group
- Inability to sit still when asked repeatedly
- Impulsiveness
- Sleep disturbances

Most children with ADHD have associated challenges. Many find it difficult to concentrate on tasks assigned in school. Even if they are gifted, their grades may suffer because they have difficulty following a conventional routine; discipline may also be a problem. Teachers are often the first to suggest that a child be examined for ADHD and receive medication when behaviors in the classroom escalate to the point of interfering with learning. A diagnosis is based on psychological and medical evaluations.

The cause of ADHD is not clear. Recent evidence suggests that hyperactivity may be related to a deficit or dysfunction of dopamine, norepinephrine, and serotonin in the reticular activating system of the brain (Chapter 8). ADHD was once thought to be caused by sugar, chocolate, high-carbohydrate foods and beverages, and certain food additives; but these have been disproved as causing or aggravating ADHD.

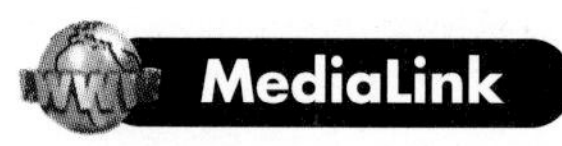

CHILDREN AND ADULTS WITH ADHD/ADD

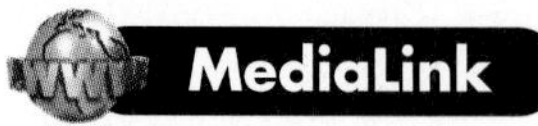

NATIONAL MENTAL HEALTH ASSOCIATION

One third to one half of children diagnosed with ADHD also experience symptoms of attention dysfunction in their adult years. Symptoms of *attention deficit disorder (ADD)* in adults appear similar to mood disorders and include anxiety, mania, restlessness, and depression, which can also cause difficulties in interpersonal relationships. Attention dysfunction in adults is often linked with poor self-esteem, diminished social success, and introverted behaviors. Patients may have mood swings similar to bipolar disorder.

CNS Stimulants

Traditional medications used to treat ADHD are central nervous system (CNS) stimulants. These drugs activate specific areas of the brain.

Fast Facts ADHD

- ADHD is the major reason why children are referred for mental health treatment.
- About one half are also diagnosed with oppositional defiant or conduct disorder.
- Anxiety disorder is diagnosed in 25%.
- About one third are also diagnosed with depression.
- Learning disabilities are present in about 20%.

9.7 CNS stimulants have been the main course of treatment for ADHD.

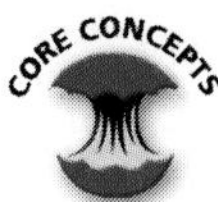

These drugs stimulate specific areas of the central nervous system that heighten alertness and increase focus. Recently, a non-CNS stimulant was approved to treat ADHD. Agents for treating ADHD are shown in Table 9.5.

Stimulants reverse many of the symptoms and help patients to focus on tasks. The most widely prescribed drug for ADHD is methylphenidate (Ritalin). Other CNS stimulants that are rarely prescribed include d- and l-amphetamine racemic mixture (Adderall), dextroamphetamine (Dexedrine), methamphetamine (Desoxyn), or pemoline (Cylert).

Patients taking CNS stimulants must be carefully monitored because the drugs may cause paradoxical hyperactivity. Adverse reactions include insomnia, nervousness, anorexia, and weight loss. Occasionally, a patient may suffer from dizziness, depression, irritability, nausea, or abdominal pain. These drugs are Schedule II controlled substances and pregnancy category C.

Non-CNS Stimulants

Non-CNS stimulants have been tried for ADHD; however, they are less effective. Clonidine (Catapres) is sometimes prescribed when patients are extremely aggressive, active, or have difficulty

TABLE 9.5 Drugs for Attention–Deficit/Hyperactivity Disorder

DRUG	ROUTE AND ADULT DOSE	REMARKS
CNS STIMULANTS		
d- and l-amphetamine racemic mixture (Adderall)	>6 years old: PO 5 mg daily to bid, may increase by 5 mg at weekly intervals (max: 40 mg/day); 3–5 years old: PO 2.5 mg one to two times/day, may increase by 2.5 mg at weekly intervals	May be used for daytime sleep disorder (narcolepsy); high potential for abuse; also called amphetamine sulfate
dextroamphetamine (Dexedrine)	3–5 years old: PO 2.5 mg daily to bid, may increase by 2.5 mg at weekly intervals; 6 years old: PO 5 mg daily to bid, increase by 5 mg at weekly intervals (max: 40 mg/day)	Potent appetite suppressant; should only be used for short-term treatment of ADHD; safety in children less than 3 years old has not been established
methamphetamine (Desoxyn)	≤6 years old: PO 2.5–5 mg daily to bid, may increase by 5 mg at weekly intervals (max: 20–25 mg/day)	Abuse potential high in adults
Pr methylphenidate (Ritalin)	PO 5–10 mg before breakfast and lunch, with gradual increase of 5–10 mg/week as needed (max: 60 mg/day)	Most widely used drug for ADHD patients; more dramatic effect on attention deficit than for hyperactivity
pemoline (Cylert)	>6 years old: PO 37.5 mg/day, may increase by 18.75 mg at weekly intervals (max: 112.5 mg/day)	Weak CNS stimulant; used in select cases as additional therapy; known hypersensitivity in children less than 6 years old
NONSTIMULANTS FOR ADD/ADHD		
atomoxetine (Strattera)	PO start with 40 mg in A.M., may increase after 3 days to target does of 80 mg/day given either once in the morning or divided morning or divided morning and late afternoon/early evening; may increase to max of 100 mg/day if needed	Inhibits reuptake of norepinephrine; safety and efficacy in children less than 6 years old has not been established
clonidine (Catapres)	PO 5 mcg/kg/day in 4 divided doses, average dose is 0.15–0.2 mg/day	Sometimes prescribed when patients are extremely aggressive, active, or have difficulty sleeping; stimulates alpha-2 receptors in the brain; available in transdermal patch

DRUG PROFILE: Drugs for ADHD, CNS Stimulants: Pr *Methylphenidate (Ritalin)*

Actions and Uses:

Methylphenidate activates the reticular activating system, causing heightened alertness in various regions of the brain, particularly those centers associated with focus and attention. Activation is partially achieved by the release of neurotransmitters such as norepinephrine, dopamine, and serotonin. Impulsiveness, hyperactivity, and disruptive behavior are usually reduced within a few weeks. These changes promote improved psychosocial interactions and academic performance.

Adverse Effects and Interactions:

In a non-ADHD patient, methylphenidate causes nervousness and insomnia. All patients are at risk for irregular heart beat, high blood pressure, and liver toxicity. Methylphenidate is a Schedule II drug, indicating its potential to cause dependence when used for extended periods. Periodic drug-free "holidays" are recommended to reduce drug dependence and to assess the patient's condition.

Methylphenidate interacts with many drugs. For example, it may decrease the effectiveness of anticonvulsants, anticoagulants, and guanethidine. Use with clonidine may increase adverse effects. Antihypertensives or other CNS stimulants could increase the vasoconstrictive action of methylphenidate. MAOIs may produce hypertensive crisis.

Mechanism in Action: 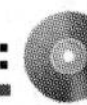

Methylphenidate (Ritalin) is a medication used for the treatment of attention deficit–hyperactivity disorder (ADHD) in children, and narcolepsy in adults. Methylphenidate increases norepinephrine (NE) release in ascending pathways of the reticular activating system (RAS), which maintains arousal and alertness. Methylphenidate also directly stimulates dopamine release in areas of the brain responsible for concentration.

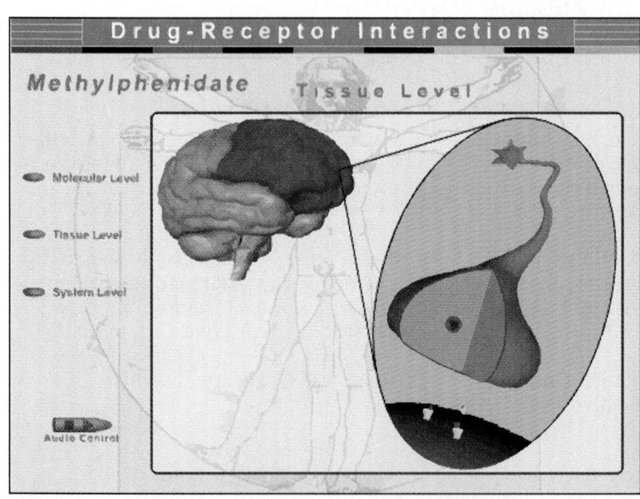

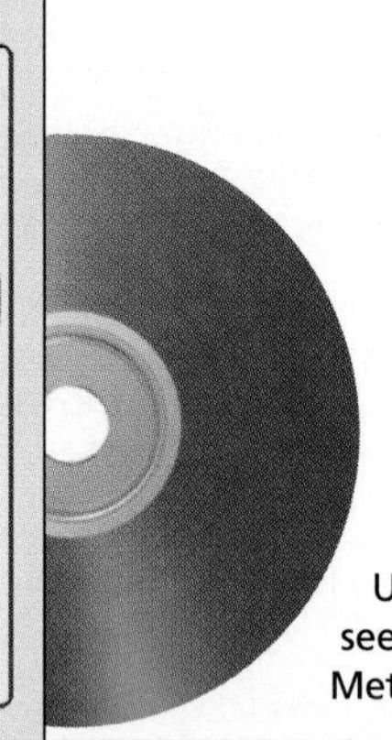

Use the student CD-ROM to see Mechanism in Action for Methylphenidate.

 *See the Companion Website for a Nursing Process Focus specific to this drug.*

falling asleep. Atypical antidepressants such as bupropion (Wellbutrin) and TCAs such as desipramine (Norpramin) and imipramine (Tofranil) are considered second-choice drugs for use when CNS stimulants fail to work or are contraindicated.

A recent addition to the treatment of ADHD in children and adults is atomoxetine (Strattera). Although its exact mechanism is not known, it is classified as a norepinephrine reuptake inhibitor. Patients on atomoxetine showed improved ability to focus on tasks and reduced hyperactivity. Efficacy appears to be equivalent to methylphenidate (Ritalin), although the drug is too new for long-term comparisons. Common side effects include headache, insomnia, upper abdominal pan, decreased appetite, and cough. Unlike methylphenidate, it is not a scheduled drug; thus, parents who are hesitant to place their child on stimulants now have a reasonable alternative.

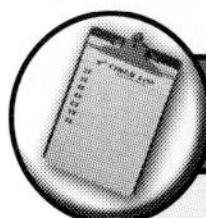

PATIENTS NEED TO KNOW

Patients taking antidepressants need to know the following:

In General

1. Avoid driving or operating machinery until you know your response to the medication. Its sedating effects can increase your risk for accidental injury.
2. Do not stop taking the medication without consulting your healthcare provider.
3. Antidepressants may take 1–4 weeks to become fully effective.

Regarding Tricyclics

4. Tricyclics may increase appetite, cause dizziness with rapid change of position, and be sedating. Report dry mouth, constipation, urinary retention, increase in heart rate and palpitations, or blurred vision if they occur.
5. Avoid the use of alcohol; it increases sedative effects.

Regarding MAOIs

6. MAO inhibitors may cause problems with sleep, agitation, dizziness when rapidly changing position, and dangerous interactions with other medications. Eating foods high in tyramine can cause a hypertensive crisis. Such foods include aged cheeses, wine, luncheon meats, and sausages.
7. Report any of the following side effects to a healthcare provider: increased heart rate or lightheadedness when changing positions.
8. Monitor weight; an increase or a decrease may occur.
9. A decrease in sexual interest or performance may occur. If this does, discuss a change in medication with a healthcare provider.

Regarding SSRIs

10. SSRIs may cause GI upset, dizziness, skin rash, and headache. Report these signs and symptoms to a healthcare provider.
11. Avoid foods containing large amounts of tryptophan, such as cottage cheese, poultry, peanuts, and sesame seeds.
12. Do not combine MAOIs and SSRIs. Do not take St. John's wort with any antidepressant. These combinations can cause serious side effects, termed serotonin syndrome: confusion, mania, headache, respiratory problems, kidney failure, and possibly death.
13. If insomnia is a problem, take the medication in the morning.
14. If nausea is a problem, take the medication with food, unless otherwise instructed.

For Attention Deficit–Hyperactivity Disorder (ADHD)

15. Many drugs used for the treatment of ADHD are controlled substances.
16. Dependence may occur due to the high abuse potential of CNS stimulants.
17. CNS stimulants often increase blood pressure. Monitor blood pressure closely.
18. Take drugs at least 6 hours before bedtime to avoid insomnia.
19. Avoid giving drinks containing caffeine to seizure-prone and diabetic children. (CNS stimulants lower the threshold in patients with seizure disorders and alter insulin needs in diabetic patients.)
20. Monitor height and weight in children with prolonged therapy.
21. Administer drugs after meals to reduce appetite-suppressive effects.
22. Do not take medication used to combat fatigue.
23. Even though atomoxetine (Strattera) is a nonstimulant ADHD medication, it still has many of the side effects of the other ADHD medications. ■

Concept Review 9.5

- What are the symptoms observed with ADHD patients? Which drug is most often used in the treatment of these symptoms? What are the common symptoms observed in adults with ADD?

CHAPTER REVIEW

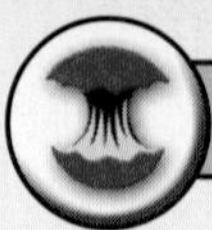

CORE CONCEPTS SUMMARY

9.1 People suffer from depression for many reasons.

The two major categories of mood disorders are depression and bipolar disorder. Depression may involve both situational and biological causes. The recognition of depression is a collaborative effort among healthcare providers. A third emotional disorder is attention deficit–hyperactivity disorder.

9.2 Treatment of severe depression requires both medication and psychotherapy for the best results.

After a health examination is performed to rule out physical causes of depression, a psychological evaluation may be performed. Patients diagnosed with a major depression have at least five symptoms of clinical depression. Treatment may include medication in addition to a number of other approaches including counseling and behavioral therapy, short-term psychotherapies, interpersonal therapy, psychodynamic therapies, and in extreme cases, electroconvulsive therapy (ECT) and repetitive transcranial magnetic stimulation (rTMS). Most therapeutic approaches involve a long-term commitment from patients, healthcare providers, and family.

9.3 Antidepressants enhance mood by boosting the actions of neurotransmitters, including norepinephrine and serotonin.

Drugs for depression are called antidepressants. The three major classes of antidepressants are tricyclic antidepressants (TCAs), selective serotonin-reuptake inhibitors (SSRIs), and monoamine oxidase inhibitors (MAOIs). All three drug classes work mainly by increasing the amount of norepinephrine, serotonin, and possibly other neurotransmitters in the nerve synapse and thereby intensifying neurotransmitter action and enhancing mood. Atypical antidepressants are a newer, fourth class of drugs for depression.

9.4 Patients with bipolar disorder may experience emotions ranging from depression to extreme agitation.

Bipolar disorder is characterized by sometimes extreme and opposite moods such as depression and euphoria. During the depressive stages, patients express signs of major depression. Patients may then change quickly to signs of mania or high psychomotor activity and irritability.

9.5 Mood stabilization in bipolar patients is accomplished with lithium and other drugs.

Drugs for bipolar disorder are called mood stabilizers. Lithium (Eskalith) is the mainstay treatment for bipolar disorder. Lithium is often used in combination with antidepressants, antianxiety, or antipsychotic agents. Antiseizure drugs are also used to treat bipolar disorder.

9.6 Attention deficit–hyperactivity disorder presents challenges for children and adults.

ADHD is a condition characterized by poor attention span, behavior control issues, and/or hyperactivity. ADHD is normally diagnosed in childhood, although one third to one half of children with symptoms of attention deficit experience signs into adulthood. As adults, patients with ADD have symptoms similar to mood disorders.

9.7 CNS stimulants have been the main course of treatment for ADHD.

The traditional drugs used to treat attention deficit in children have been CNS stimulants. Patients taking CNS stimulants must be carefully monitored to avoid adverse reactions. Recently, non-CNS stimulants, including the new drug atomoxetine (Strattera), have been used as a reasonable alternative to existing Schedule II controlled substances.

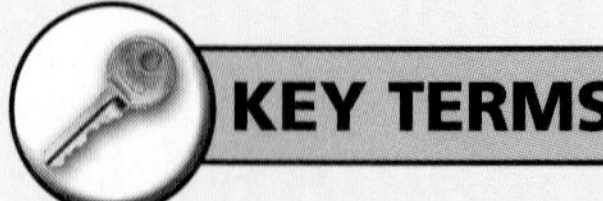

KEY TERMS

antidepressants (AN-tee-dee-PRESS-ahnts): drugs used for treatment of depression; mood enhancers / ***page 127***

attention deficit–hyperactivity disorder (ADHD): a disorder typically diagnosed in childhood and adolescence characterized by hyperactivity as well as attention, organization, and behavior control issues / ***page 139***

bipolar disorder (bi-PO-ler): a disorder characterized by extreme and opposite feelings, such as euphoria and depression or calmness and rage; also called *manic depression* / ***page 136***

major depression: a disorder characterized by at least five symptoms of depression / *page 126*

mood disorder: a disorder involving a change in behavior, such as clinical depression or bipolar disorder / *page 127*

mood stabilizers: drugs that level mood to treat bipolar disorder and mania / *page 138*

monoamine oxidase inhibitors (MAOIs) (mon-oh-AHM-een OK-se-daze): drugs inhibiting monoamine oxidase, an enzyme that terminates the actions of neurotransmitters such as dopamine, norepinephrine, epinephrine, and serotonin / *page 134*

selective serotonin-reuptake inhibitors (SSRIs) (sir-eh-TO-nin): drugs that selectively inhibit the reuptake of serotonin into nerve terminals / *page 129*

serotonin syndrome (SES): set of signs and symptoms associated with overmedication with antidepressants / *page 130*

tricyclic antidepressants (TCAs) (treye-SICK-lick): drugs with a three-ring chemical structure that inhibit the reuptake of norepinephrine and serotonin into nerve terminals / *page 127*

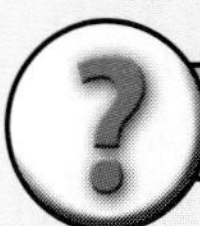

REVIEW QUESTIONS

The following questions are written in NCLEX-PN® style. Answer these questions to assess your knowledge of the chapter material, and go back and review any material that is not clear to you.

1. Patient education for the patient started on antidepressants would include:

1. The avoidance of tyramine-containing foods
2. The signs and symptoms of hypertension
3. That drowsiness is a common side effect
4. That it may take a combination of antidepressants for effectiveness to occur

2. If a patient taking MAOIs experiences a hypertensive crisis, what may be given as an antidote?

1. Meperidine (Demerol)
2. Dextromethorphan
3. Calcium channel blockers
4. Carbamazepine (Tegretol)

3. When the patient on lithium is dehydrated, this could lead to:

1. Lower serum lithium levels
2. Increased effectiveness
3. The need to increase the lithium dosage
4. Lithium toxicity

4. The patient on methlphenidate (Ritalin) should be assessed for:

1. Signs of weight loss
2. Hypotension
3. Renal toxicity
4. Extreme euphoria and insomnia

5. Which of the following symptoms would indicate to the nurse that a patient is experiencing lithium toxicity?

1. Increased urination, diarrhea, tremors
2. Dry mouth, vomiting, hypotension
3. Constipation, blurred vision, hypertension
4. Increased appetite, increased energy, memory loss

6. Imipramine (Tofranil) has been ordered in a patient experiencing depression. Patient teaching would include which of the following?

1. The use of alcohol is permitted with this drug.
2. Avoid standing up too quickly.
3. Effectiveness occurs within a few hours of administration.
4. If a dose is missed, double up on the next dose.

7. Your client is taking phenelzine (Nardil). The nurse teaches her to avoid eating:

1. Eggs
2. Aged cheeses
3. Onion
4. Apples

8. Which of the following antiseizure mediations may be used as a mood stabilizer?

1. Diazepam (Valium)
2. Phenytoin (Dilantin)
3. Valproic acid (Depakene)
4. Lorazepam (Ativan)

9. The patient has been started on an MAOI for depression and is now asking if she can add St. John's wort to increase the effectiveness of the antidepressant. The nurse's best response would be?

1. "St. John's wort is highly effective for depression. Adding it to your current medication will increase its effectiveness."
2. "Although St. John's wort has been found to be effective for depression, you should consult with your physician before adding it to your current medication routine."
3. "St. John's wort cannot be mixed with MAOIs because of drug interactions."
4. "Because St. John's wort is effective for depression, you will not need your medication."

10. Antidepressants improve mood by increasing levels of:

1. Epinephrine and norepinephrine
2. Reticular formation within the hypothalamus
3. Norepinephrine and serotonin
4. GABA and serotonin

CASE STUDY QUESTIONS

For questions 1–5, please refer to the following case study, and choose the correct answer from choices 1–4.

Mr. Coxilean, a 38-year-old man visits his family doctor and explains that lately he has been experiencing frequent headaches, disinterest in eating and sex, and a hard time "keeping focused." For the past 2 years, he has been taking OTC medication to help him sleep. Two times within the last year, he missed work because of extreme fatigue. Mr. Coxilean does not drink alcohol but admits, "The pressure is almost overwhelming sometimes."

1. Based on Mr. Coxilean's symptoms, and in the absence of laboratory test results, which of the following conditions would most likely be ruled out?

1. Bipolar disorder
2. Major depression
3. Thyroid condition
4. Vitamin-B deficiency

2. The main reason why Mr. Coxilean would not be treated with mood stabilizers is the lack of:

1. Complaints from patient suggesting attention deficit disorder
2. Toxicity concerns for this class of drug
3. Evidence that patient feels his condition is normal
4. Extreme shifts between mania and depression

3. If the lab values for Mr. Coxilean were normal, which of the following medications would be considered a drug of choice for his condition?

1. Doxepin (Sinequan)
2. Tranylcypromine (Parnate)
3. Sertraline (Zoloft)
4. Bupropion (Wellbutrin)

4. If phenelzine (Nardil) were prescribed for Mr. Coxilean, the healthcare provider would most likley tell him:

1. "Avoid reducing your salt intake. It increases excretion of this medication."
2. "Avoid chocolate and some other foods when taking this medication."
3. "You can take herbals, but avoid the use of St. John's wort."
4. "You can continue to take OTC medication for sleep, but monitor the frequency."

5. If SSRIs were prescribed for Mr. Coxilean, which of the following effects might still remain a problem?

1. Headaches
2. Loss of appetite
3. Poor sexual activity
4. Both a and c

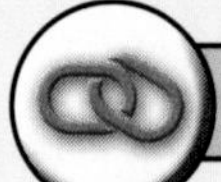

FURTHER STUDY

- Tricyclic antidepressants for panic attacks are covered in Chapter 8.
- Antiseizure drugs are discussed in Chapter 11.
- Benzodiazepines for treating anxiety are covered in Chapter 8.
- Antipsychotic agents are discussed in Chapter 10.
- The reticular activating system of the brain is further discussed in Chapter 8.

EXPLORE MEDIALINK www.prenhall.com/holland

Additional resources for this chapter can be found on the CD-ROM accompanying this textbook, and on the Companion Website. Click on Chapter 9 to select activities for this chapter.

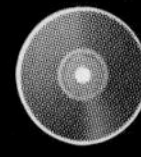

- Mechanism in Action:
  - Fluoxetine
  - Methylphenidate
- Audio Glossary
- Concept Review
- NCLEX-PN® Review
- Nursing in Action
- Dosage Calculator

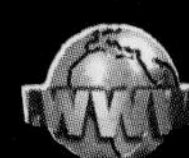

- Diet and Depression
- National Association of Mental Illness
- Children and Adults with ADHD/ADD
- National Mental Health Association

CHAPTER

10 Drugs for Psychoses and Degenerative Diseases of the Nervous System

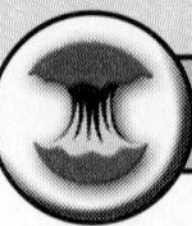

CORE CONCEPTS

10.1 Most psychoses have no identifiable cause and require long-term drug therapy.

10.2 Schizophrenic patients experience many different symptoms that may change over time.

10.3 The experience and skills of the healthcare provider are critical to the pharmacological management of psychoses.

10.4 Conventional antipsychotic agents include the phenothiazines, phenothiazine-like drugs, and nonphenothiazines.

10.5 Atypical antipsychotic agents and a newer drug class have been developed to better meet the needs of patients with psychoses.

10.6 Medication is unable to cure most degenerative diseases of the CNS.

10.7 Parkinson's disease is progressive, with the occurrence of full symptoms taking many years.

10.8 Parkinsonism drugs focus on restoring the balance between dopamine and acetylcholine in the brain.

10.9 Alzheimer's patients experience a dramatic loss of ability to perform tasks that require acetylcholine as a central neurotransmitter.

10.10 Alzheimer's disease is treated with acetylcholinesterase inhibitors.

10.11 Symptoms of multiple sclerosis result from demyelination of central nerve fibers.

10.12 Drugs for multiple sclerosis reduce immune attacks in the brain and treat unfavorable symptoms.

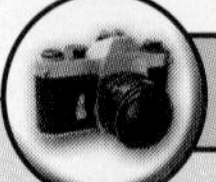

DRUG SNAPSHOT

The following drugs will be discussed in this chapter:

DRUG CLASSES	DRUG PROFILES
CONVENTIONAL (TYPICAL) ANTIPSYCHOTICS	
Phenothiazines	Pr chlorpromazine (Thorazine)
Nonphenothiazines	Pr haloperidol (Haldol)
ATYPICAL ANTIPSYCHOTICS	
	Pr clozapine (Clozaril)
DRUGS FOR PARKINSON'S DISEASE	
Dopaminergic agents	Pr levodopa (Larodopa)
Cholinergic blockers (anticholinergics)	Pr benztropine (Cogentin)
DRUGS FOR ALZHEIMER'S DISEASE	
Acetylcholine inhibitors	Pr donepezil (Aricept)
DRUGS FOR MULTIPLE SCLEROSIS	

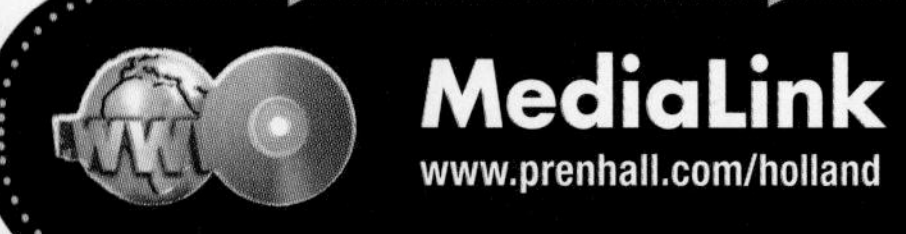

Interactive resources for this chapter can be found on the Companion Website. Click on Chapter 10 and "Begin" to select the activities for this chapter. For chapter-related animations, NCLEX-PN®-style questions, and an audio glossary, access the accompanying CD-ROM in this book.

OBJECTIVES

After reading this chapter, the student should be able to:

1. Explain theories for the cause of schizophrenia.
2. Compare and contrast the positive and negative symptoms of schizophrenia.
3. Explain the importance of patient drug compliance in the pharmacotherapy of schizophrenia.
4. Explain the symptoms associated with extrapyramidal side effects of antipsychotic drugs.
5. Identify the most common degenerative diseases of the CNS.
6. Describe symptoms of Parkinson's disease, Alzheimer's disease, and multiple sclerosis.
7. Explain the neurochemical basis for degenerative diseases of the CNS, focusing on the roles of important neurotransmitters in the brain.
8. For each of the drug classes, know representative drug examples and explain their mechanism of action, primary actions, and important adverse effects.
9. Explain the goals of pharmacotherapy and categorize drugs used in the treatment of psychosis and degenerative diseases based on their classification and drug action.

Severe mental illness can incapacitate a patient and intensely frustrate relatives and others who regularly interact or care for the patient. Before the 1950s, patients with acute mental dysfunction were put in institutions, often for their entire lives. In the 1950s, chlorpromazine (Thorazine) and other agents were introduced that revolutionized the treatment of mental illness. Today, healthcare providers struggle with the challenges of treating degenerative diseases of the CNS, such as Parkinson's disease, Alzheimer's disease, and multiple sclerosis (MS). Medications that are available today to treat these diseases provide relief for symptoms, but do not stop or reverse the ongoing degeneration that these conditions cause.

10.1 Most psychoses have no identifiable cause and require long-term drug therapy.

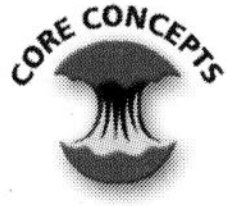

Patients with psychoses often cannot tell what is and is not real. They may have any of the following:

- *Delusions* (strong beliefs in something that is false or not based on reality); for example, the patient may believe that someone is planting thoughts in his or her head
- *Hallucinations* (seeing, hearing, or feeling something that is not there); for example, a patient may hear voices or see spiders crawling on walls that others around the patient do not see or hear
- *Illusions* (distorted or misleading perceptions of something that is actually real); for example, a patient may see a shadow and believe it is really a person
- *Disorganized behavior*
- *Difficulty relating to others*

Patients may be inactive or extremely agitated and combative. Some psychotic patients exhibit *paranoia,* a feeling that someone is "out to get them." Because these people are unable to distinguish what is real from what is illusion, they are often viewed as insane.

Psychoses can be acute or chronic. Acute psychotic episodes occur over hours or days, whereas chronic psychoses develop over months or years. Brain damage, overdoses of certain medications, extreme depression, chronic alcoholism, and drug addiction can cause psychoses, and genetic factors can play a role in some psychoses. Most psychoses, however, have no identifiable cause.

Fast Facts Psychosis

- Psychotic symptoms are the most disruptive kinds of behaviors in a daily routine.
- Symptoms of psychosis are most often associated with other mental health problems including substance abuse, depression, and dementia.
- Psychotic disorders are among the most misunderstood mental health disorders in North America.
- Over 2.5 million Americans have psychosis.
- Patients with psychosis often develop symptoms between age 13 and 25.

Source: National Mental Health Association (http://www.nmha.org/)

People with psychosis are usually unable to function normally in society without lifelong drug therapy and ongoing visits with a healthcare provider. Family members and social support groups are important sources of help for patients who cannot function without continuous drug therapy.

SCHIZOPHRENIA

schizo = *split*
phrenia = *mind*

Schizoprenia is the most common psychotic disorder, affecting 1% to 2% of the population. Symptoms generally begin to appear in early adulthood.

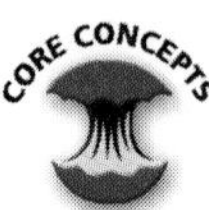

10.2 Schizophrenic patients experience many different symptoms that may change over time.

In men, symptoms most often begin between 15 and 24 years of age; in women, between 25 and 34 years. The following symptoms may appear quickly, take several months or years to develop, or may change over time:

- Hallucinations, delusions, or paranoia
- Strange behavior, such as talking in rambling statements or making up words
- Rapid changes from extreme hyperactivity to stupor
- Attitude of indifference toward or detachment from life activities
- Irrational behavior
- Neglect of personal hygiene, job, and school
- Noticeable withdrawal from social activities and relationships

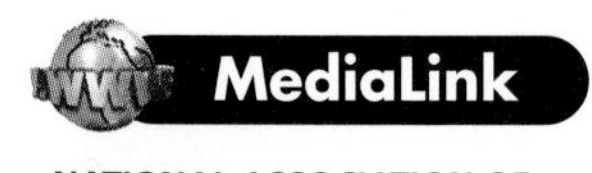

NATIONAL ASSOCIATION OF MENTAL ILLNESS

When observing patients with schizophrenia, healthcare workers should look for both positive and negative symptoms. **Positive symptoms** are those that *add on* to normal behavior. These include hallucinations, delusions, and disorganized thoughts or speech. **Negative symptoms** are those that *subtract from* normal behavior. These symptoms include lack of interest, motivation, responsiveness, or pleasure in daily activities. Proper diagnosis of positive and negative symptoms is important for selecting the most appropriate antipsychotic drug for treatment.

The cause of schizophrenia has not been determined, although several theories have been proposed. One is the genetic theory: Many patients with schizophrenia have family members with the same disorder. Another theory suggests that imbalances in neurotransmitters in specific areas of the brain cause the disorder. Symptoms of schizophrenia seem to be associated with dopamine type 2 (D_2) receptors that are located in specific areas of the brain. It is believed that these brain areas produce too much dopamine. Antipsychotic drugs act by attaching to D_2 receptors and prevent dopamine from attaching (Figure 10.1 ■). When about 65% of the D_2 receptors are blocked by antipsychotic drugs, psychotic behavior is reduced. However, this same area of the brain also controls motor activity (such as moving arms and legs together when walking). If an antipsychotic drug blocks too many of the D_2 receptors (for example, when too much drug is given), the patient may have difficulty coordinating walking.

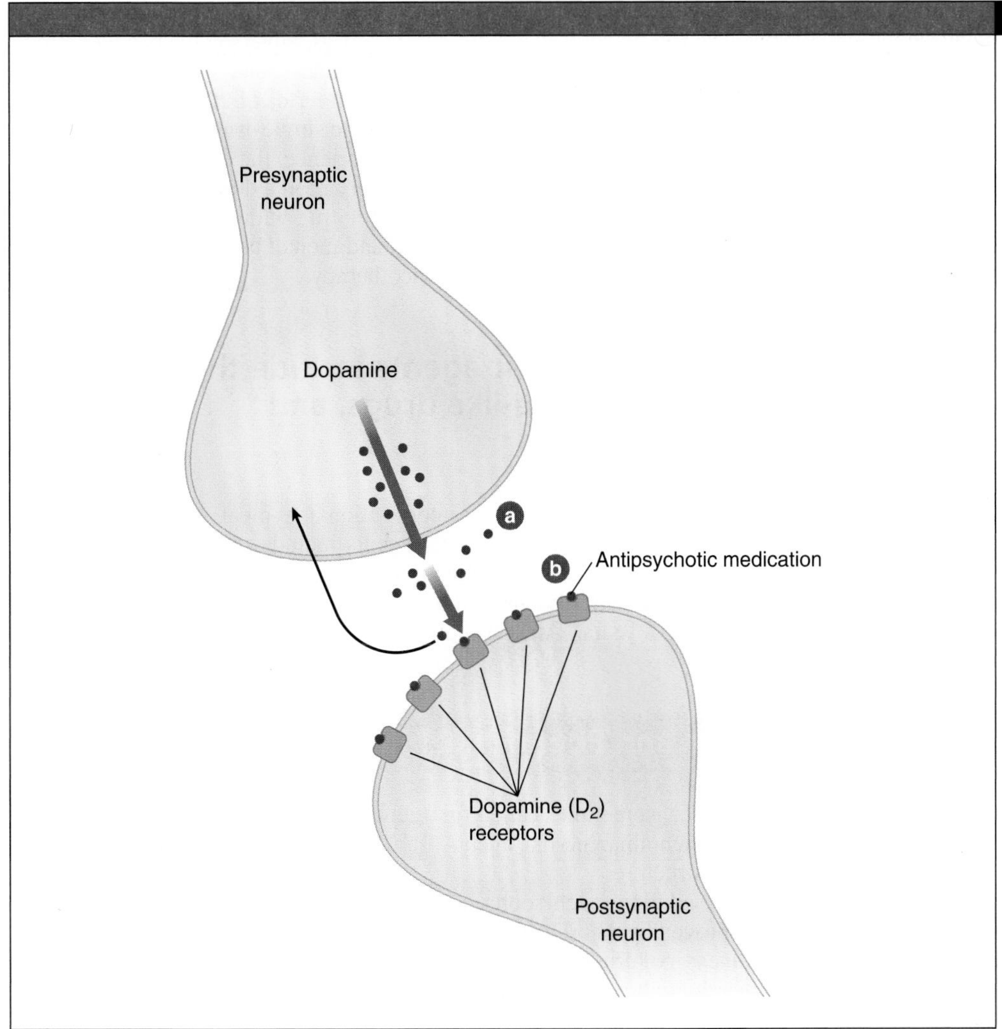

FIGURE 10.1

One theory of schizophrenia is that (a) too much dopamine is produced in a specific area of the brain. The extra dopamine overexcites the receptors.
(b) Antipsychotic drugs act by attaching to the receptors and preventing the extra dopamine from connecting to the receptors and causing overstimulation.

Schizoaffective disorder is a condition that includes symptoms of both schizophrenia and mood disorder. For example, a patient may have illusions, hallucinations, and delusions, followed by extreme depression. Over time, both positive and negative psychotic symptoms will appear.

schizo = *schizophrenia*
affective = *mood*

Many conditions can cause bizarre behavior, and these should be distinguished from schizophrenia. Repeated use of amphetamines or cocaine can create a paranoid syndrome. Certain complex partial seizures (Chapter 11) can cause unusual symptoms that are sometimes mistaken for psychoses. Brain tumors, infections, or hemorrhage can also cause bizarre, psychotic-like symptoms.

Concept Review 10.1

- What are the major types of psychoses? Describe major symptoms associated with each type. What distinguishes a positive symptom from a negative symptom?

10.3 The experience and skills of the healthcare provider are critical to the pharmacological management of psychoses.

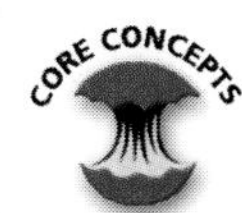

Management of severe mental illness is difficult. Many patients do not see themselves as abnormal and have difficulty understanding the need for medication. When that medication produces undesirable side effects, such as severe twitching or loss of sexual function, patients stop taking their medications and begin to have symptoms of their pretreatment illness. Agitation, distrust, and extreme frustration are common because patients cannot comprehend why others are unable to think and see the same way as they do.

From a pharmacological perspective, therapy has both a positive and negative side. Although many symptoms of psychosis can be controlled with current drugs, adverse effects are common and often severe. The antipsychotic agents do not cure mental illness, and symptoms remain in remission only as long as the patient chooses to take the drug. In terms of effectiveness, there is little difference among the various antipsychotic drugs; there is no single drug of choice for schizophrenia. Selection of a specific drug is based on clinician experience, the occurrence of side effects, and the needs of the patient. Those who operate machinery need a drug that does not cause sedation. Men and women who are sexually active may want a drug without negative effects on sexual behavior. The experience and skills of the physician and mental health nurse are particularly valuable to achieving successful psychiatric pharmacotherapy.

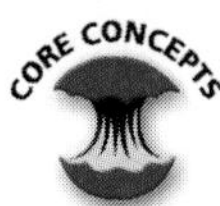

10.4 Conventional antipsychotic agents include the phenothiazines, phenothiazine-like drugs, and nonphenothiazines.

The two basic categories of drugs for psychoses are conventional (typical) antipsychotics and atypical antipsychotics. The conventional antipsychotic agents include the phenothiazines and phenothiazine-like drugs. Conventional antipsychotic agents are most effective for treating the positive signs of schizophrenia, such as hallucinations and delusions, and have been the treatment of choice for psychoses for 50 years. Antipsychotic drugs are sometimes referred to as **neuroleptics.**

neuro = *nervous*
leptic = *state of mind*

Phenothiazines and Phenothiazine-Type Drugs

The conventional antipsychotics, sometimes called first-generation or typical antipsychotics, include the phenothiazine and phenothiazine-like agents (Table 10.1). Within each category, agents are named by their chemical structure.

The first effective drug used to treat schizophrenia was the low-potency phenothiazine chlorpromazine (Thorazine), approved by the FDA for this use in 1954. Seven phenothiazines are now available to treat mental illness. All drugs are effective in blocking the excitement associated with the positive symptoms of schizophrenia, although they differ in their potency and side effects.

TABLE 10.1 Conventional Antipsychotic Drugs: Phenothiazines

DRUG	ROUTE AND ADULT DOSE	REMARKS
Pr chlorpromazine (Thorazine)	PO 25–100 mg tid or qid (max: 1000 mg/day) IM/IV 25–50 mg (max: 600 mg every 4–6 hours)	Strong sedative properties; controls nausea and vomiting, dementia, and hiccups not treated by any other means; for agitated patients
fluphenazine (Permitil, Prolixin)	PO 0.5–10 mg/day (max: 20 mg/day)	Also for dementia; available in IM or subcutaneous forms
mesoridazine besylate (Serentil)	PO 10–50 mg bid or tid (max: 400 mg/day)	Strong sedative properties; also for dementia, hyperactivity, alcohol dependence, and anxiety
perphenazine (Phenazine, Trilafon)	PO 4–16 mg bid to qid (max: 64 mg/day)	Also for dementia and nausea; available in IM and IV forms
promazine (Prozine, Sparine)	PO/IM 10–200 mg every 4–6 hours (max: 1000 mg/day)	For agitated and paranoid patients; useful for alcohol withdrawal
thioridazine (Mellaril)	PO 50–100 mg tid (max: 800 mg/day)	Strong sedative properties; for moderate to severe depression and dementia
trifluoperazine (Stelazine)	PO 1–2 mg bid (max 20 mg/day)	Also for dementia; use cautiously in patients with seizure disorders; available in IM form

False perceptions, such as hallucinations and delusions, often begin to diminish within days. Other symptoms, however, may require as long as 7 to 8 weeks of pharmacotherapy to show improvement. Phenothiazines are thought to act by preventing dopamine and serotonin from entering their receptor sites in certain regions of the brain.

The phenothiazines revolutionized the treatment of severe mental illness, but the numerous adverse effects they cause limit their usefulness. These are listed in Table 10.2.

Unlike many other drugs that primarily act on the CNS (e.g., amphetamines, barbiturates, anxiolytics, alcohol), antipsychotic drugs do not cause dependence. They also have a wide safety margin between a therapeutic and a lethal dose. Deaths due to overdoses of antipsychotic drugs are uncommon.

Particularly serious adverse reactions to antipsychotic drugs are **extrapyramidal symptoms (EPS).** These include acute dystonia, akathisia, Parkinsonism, and tardive dyskinesia. Acute *dystonias* are severe muscle spasms, particularly of the back, neck, tongue, and face that occur early in the course of pharmacotherapy. *Akathisia,* the most common EPS, is an inability to rest or relax. The patient paces, has trouble sitting or remaining still, and has difficulty sleeping. Symptoms of phenothiazine-induced *Parkinsonism* include tremor, muscle rigidity, stooped posture, and a shuffling gait. Long-term use of phenothiazines may lead to **tardive dyskinesia,** which is characterized by unusual tongue and face movements such as lip smacking and wormlike motions of the tongue. If EPS are reported early and the drug is withdrawn or the dosage is reduced, the side effects can be reversed. When higher doses are given for prolonged periods, EPS may become permanent.

tardive = *late*
dyskinesia = *abnormal movement*

With the conventional antipsychotics, it is not always possible to control the disabling symptoms of schizophrenia without producing some degree of EPS. In these patients, drug therapy may be warranted to treat these symptoms. Simultaneous treatment with an anticholinergic drug may prevent some EPS. For acute dystonia, benztropine (Cogentin) may be given parenterally. Levodopa (Dopar, Larodopa) is usually avoided. Beta-adrenergic blockers and benzodiazepines are sometimes given to reduce signs of akathisia.

Nonphenothiazine Drugs

The conventional, nonphenothiazine antipsychotic class consists of drugs whose chemical structures are dissimilar to the phenothiazines (see Table 10.3). Introduced shortly after the phenothiazines, initial expectations were that nonphenothiazines would produce fewer side effects. Unfortunately, this appears to not be the case. The side effects of nonphenothiazines are identical to those of phenothiazines, although the degree to which a particular effect occurs depends on the specific drugs. In general, the nonphenothiazine agents cause less sedation and fewer anticholinergic side effects than chlorpromazine (Thorazine), but cause an equal or even greater incidence of EPS. Simultaneous therapy with other CNS depressants must be carefully monitored due to the potential additive effects.

TABLE 10.2 Adverse Effects of Conventional Antipsychotic Agents

EFFECT	DESCRIPTION
Acute dystonia	Severe spasms, particularly the back muscles, tongue, and facial muscles; twitching movements
Akathisia	Constant pacing with repetitive, compulsive movements
Parkinsonism	Tremor, muscle rigidity, stooped posture, and shuffling gait
Tardive dyskinesia	Bizarre tongue and face movements such as lip smacking and wormlike motions of the tongue; puffing of cheeks, uncontrolled chewing movements
Anticholinergic effects	Dry mouth, tachycardia, blurred vision
Sedation	Usually diminishes with continued therapy
Hypotension	Particularly severe when quickly moving from a recumbent to an upright position
Sexual dysfunction	Impotence and diminished libido
Neuroleptic malignant syndrome	High fever, confusion, muscle rigidity, and high serum creatine kinase; can be fatal

TABLE 10.3 Conventional Antipsychotic Drugs: Nonphenothiazines

DRUG	ROUTE AND ADULT DOSE	REMARKS
chloroprothixene (Taractan)	PO 75–150 mg/day (max: 600 mg/day)	Prominent sedative effects; less hypotensive than phenothiazines; available in IV form
Pr haloperidol (Haldol)	PO 0.2–5 mg bid or tid	For severe psychosis, dementia, and Tourette's disorder; available in IM form
loxapine succinate (Loxitane)	PO start with 20 mg/day and rapidly increase to 60–100 mg/day in divided doses (max: 250 mg/day)	Also for dementia
molindone HCl (Moban)	PO 50–75 mg/day in 3–4 divided doses, may increase to 100 mg/day in 3–4 days (max: 225 mg/day)	May produce insomnia and drowsiness
pimozide (Orap)	PO 1–2 mg/day in divided doses; gradually increase every other day to 7–16 mg/day, whichever is less (max: 10 mg/day)	For Tourette's disorder; use cautiously in patients with seizure disorders
thiothixene HCl (Navane)	PO 2 mg tid; may increase up to 15 mg/day (max 60 mg/day)	Also for dementia; unlabeled use as an antidepressant

DRUG PROFILE: Antipsychotic; Phenothiazine: Pr *Chlorpromazine (Thorazine)*

Actions and Uses:

Chlorpromazine provides symptomatic relief of positive symptoms of schizophrenia and controls manic symptoms in patients with schizoaffective disorder. Many patients must take chlorpromazine for 7 or 8 weeks before they experience improvement. Extreme agitation may be treated with IM or IV injections, which begin to act within minutes. Chlorpromazine can also control severe nausea and vomiting.

Adverse Effects and Interactions:

Strong blockade of alpha-adrenergic receptors and weak blockade of cholinergic receptors explain some of chlorpromazine's adverse effects. Common side effects are dizziness, drowsiness, and orthostatic hypotension.

EPS occur mostly in elderly patients, women, and pediatric patients who are dehydrated. **Neurologic malignant syndrome** (NMS) may also occur. Patients taking chlorpromazine and exposed to warmer temperatures should be monitored more closely for symptoms of NMS.

Chlorpromazine interacts with several drugs. For example, use together with sedative medications such as phenobarbital should be avoided. Taking chlorpromazine with tricyclic antidepressants can elevate blood pressure. Use of chlorpromazine with antiseizure medication can lower the seizure threshold.

Use with caution with herbal supplements, such as kava and St. John's wort, which may increase the risk and severity of dystonia.

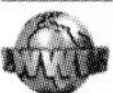
See the Companion Website for a Nursing Process Focus specific to this drug.

Drugs in the nonphenothiazine class have the same therapeutic effects and efficacy as the phenothiazines. They are also believed to act by the same mechanism as the phenothiazines, that is, by blocking postsynaptic D_2 receptors. As a class, they offer no significant advantages over the phenothiazines in the treatment of schizophrenia.

DRUG PROFILE: Antipsychotic; Nonphenothiazine: Pr *Haloperidol (Haldol)*

Actions and Uses:

Haloperidol is classified chemically as a butyrophenone. Its primary use is for the management of acute and chronic psychotic disorders. It may be used to treat patients with Tourette's syndrome and children with severe behavior problems such as unprovoked aggressiveness and explosive hyperexcitability. It is approximately 50 times more potent than chlorpromazine, but has equal efficacy in relieving symptoms of schizophrenia. Haldol LA is a long-acting preparation that lasts for approximately 3 weeks following IM or SC administration. This is particularly beneficial for patients who are uncooperative or unable to take oral medications.

Adverse Effects and Interaction:

Haloperidol produces less sedation and hypotension than chlorpromazine, but the incidence of EPS is high. Elderly patients are more likely to experience side effects and often are prescribed half the adult dose until the side effects of therapy can be determined. Although the incidence of NMS is rare, it can occur.

Haloperidol interacts with many drugs. For example, the following drugs decrease the effects/absorption of haloperidol: aluminum- and magnesium-containing antacids, levodopa (also increases chances of levodopa toxicity), lithium (increases chance of a severe neurological toxicity), phenobarbital, phenytoin (also increases chances of phenytoin toxicity), rifampin, and beta blockers (may increase blood levels of haloperidol thus leading to possible toxicity). Haloperidol inhibits the action of centrally acting antihypertensives.

Use with caution with herbal supplements, such as kava, which may increase the effect of haloperidol.

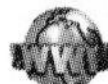
See the Companion Website for a Nursing Process Focus specific to this drug.

Concept Review 10.2

- What is a neuroleptic drug? What are the two major classes of drugs used to treat psychoses? How does each drug category generally affect positive and negative symptoms of schizophrenia?

10.5 Atypical antipsychotic agents and a newer drug class have been developed to better meet the needs of patients with psychoses.

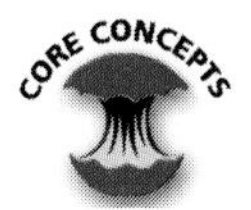

Atypical antipsychotics have become drugs of choice for treating psychoses. The approval of clozapine (Clozaril), the first atypical antipsychotic, marked the first major advance in the pharmacotherapy of psychoses since the discovery of chlorpromazine decades earlier. Clozapine, and the other drugs in this class, are called second generation, or atypical. Their broader spectrum of action controls both the positive and negative symptoms of schizophrenia (see Table 10.4). Furthermore, at therapeutic doses they do not produce EPS. Some drugs, such as clozapine, are especially useful for patients in whom other drugs have been unsuccessful. The mechanism of action of the atypical agents is unknown, but they are thought to act by blocking several different receptor types in the brain.

Although there are fewer side effects with atypical antipsychotics, adverse effects are still significant, and patients must be carefully monitored. Although most antipsychotics cause weight gain, the atypical agents are associated with obesity and its risk factors. Risperidone (Risperdal) and some of the other antipsychotic drugs may cause menstrual disorders and osteoporosis in women and decreased sex drive in both men and women. There is also concern that some atypical agents alter glucose metabolism, which could lead to type 2 diabetes.

NURSING PROCESS FOCUS

Patients Receiving Phenothiazines and Conventional Nonphenothiazine Therapy

ASSESSMENT

Prior to administration:

- Obtain complete health history (medical and psychological) including allergies, drug history, and possible drug interactions
- Obtain baseline lab studies (electrolytes, CBC, BUN, creatinine, WBC, liver enzymes, drug screens)
- Assess for hallucinations, level of consciousness, mental status
- Assess patient support system(s)

POTENTIAL NURSING DIAGNOSES

- Ineffective Therapeutic Regimen Management, related to noncompliance with medication regimen, presence of side effects, and need for long-term medication use
- Anxiety, related to symptoms of psychosis
- Risk For Injury, related to side effects of medication
- Noncompliance, related to length of time before medication reaches therapeutic levels, desire to use alcohol or illegal drugs
- Deficient Knowledge, related to no previous contact with psychosis or its treatment

PLANNING: Patient Goals and Expected Outcomes

The patient will:

- Report a reduction of psychotic symptoms, including delusions, paranoia, irrational behavior, hallucinations
- Demonstrate an understanding of the drug's action by accurately describing drug side effects, precautions, and measures to take to decrease any side effects
- Immediately report side effects or adverse reactions
- Adhere to recommended treatment regimen

IMPLEMENTATION

Interventions and (Rationales)	Patient Education/Discharge Planning
■ Monitor for decreased psychotic symptoms. (If patient continues to exhibit symptoms of psychosis, he or she may not be taking drug as ordered, may be taking an inadequate dose, or may not be affected by the drug; it may need to be discontinued and another antipsychotic begun.)	Instruct patient and caregiver to: ■ Notice increases or decreases of symptoms of psychosis, including hallucinations, abnormal sleep patterns, social withdrawal, delusions, or paranoia. ■ Contact physician if no decrease of symptoms occurs over a 6-week period.
■ Monitor for side effects such as drowsiness, dizziness, lethargy, headaches, blurred vision, skin rash, diaphoresis, nausea/vomiting, anorexia, diarrhea, menstrual irregularities, depression, hypotension, or hypertension.	■ Instruct patient and caregiver to report side effects. ■ Inform patient and caregiver that impotence, gynecomastia, amenorrhea, and anuresis may occur.
■ Monitor for anticholinergic side effects such as orthostatic hypotension, constipation, anorexia, genitourinary problems, respiratory changes, and visual disturbances.	Instruct patient to: ■ Avoid abrupt changes in position ■ Not drive or perform hazardous activities until effects of the drug are known ■ Report vision changes ■ Comply with required laboratory tests ■ Increase dietary fiber, fluids, and exercise to prevent constipation ■ Relieve symptoms of dry mouth with sugarless hard candy or gum and frequent drinks of water ■ Notify physician immediately if urinary retention occurs
■ Monitor for extrapyramidal (EPS) side effects such as the development of tremors, involuntary repetitive movements, decreased muscle tone, or increased restlessness. (Presence of EPS may be sufficient reason for patient to discontinue antipsychotic. Monitor for neuroleptic malignant syndrome [NMS], which is life threatening and must be reported and treated immediately.)	Instruct patient and caregiver to: ■ Recognize tardive dyskinesia, dystonia, akathisia, pseudoparkinsonism ■ Immediately seek treatment for elevated temperature, unstable blood pressure, profuse sweating, dyspnea, muscle rigidity, incontinence

continued...

NURSING PROCESS FOCUS

Interventions and (Rationales)	Patient Education/Discharge Planning
▪ Monitor for alcohol/illegal drug use. (Patient may decide to use alcohol or illegal drugs as a means of coping with symptoms of psychosis, so may stop taking the antipsychotic. Used concurrently, will cause increased CNS depressant effect.)	▪ Instruct patient to refrain from alcohol and illegal drug use. Refer patient to community support groups such as Alcoholics Anonymous or Narcotics Anonymous as appropriate.
▪ Monitor caffeine use. (Use of caffeine-containing substances will negate effects of antipsychotics.)	Instruct patient or caregiver to: ▪ Avoid caffeine ▪ Recognize common caffeine-containing products and assist in finding acceptable substitutes, such as decaffeinated coffee and tea, caffeine-free colas
▪ Monitor for cardiovascular changes, including hypotension, tachycardia, and ECG changes. (Haloperidol has fewer cardiotoxic effects than other antipsychotics, and may be preferred for patients with existing cardiovascular problems.)	▪ Instruct patient and caregiver that dizziness and falls, especially on sudden position changes, may indicate cardiovascular changes. Teach safety measures.
▪ Monitor for smoking. (Heavy smoking may decrease metabolism of haloperidol, leading to decreased effectiveness.)	▪ Instruct patient to stop or decrease smoking. Refer to smoking cessation programs, if indicated.
▪ Monitor elderly patients closely. (Elderly patients may need lower doses and a more gradual dosage increase. Elderly women are at greater risk for developing tardive dyskinesia.)	▪ Instruct caregiver to observe for unusual reactions such as confusion, depression, and hallucinations, and for symptoms of tardive dyskinesia, and to report them immediately. ▪ Instruct elderly patients or caregivers on ways to counteract anticholinergic effects of medication, while taking into account any other existing medical problems.
▪ Monitor lab results, including RBC and WBC counts, and drug levels.	▪ Advise patient and caregiver of necessity of having regular lab studies done.
▪ Monitor for use of medication. (All antipsychotics must be taken as ordered for therapeutic results to occur.)	▪ Instruct patient and caregiver that medication must be continued as ordered, even if no therapeutic benefits are felt, because it may take several months for full therapeutic benefits.
▪ Monitor for seizures. (Drug may lower seizure threshold.)	▪ Instruct patient and caregiver that seizures may occur and review appropriate safety precautions.
▪ Monitor patient's environment. (Drug may cause patient to perceive a brownish discoloration of objects or photophobia. Drug may also interfere with the ability to regulate body temperature.)	Instruct patient and caregiver to: ▪ Wear dark glasses to avoid discomfort from photophobia ▪ Avoid temperature extremes ▪ Be aware that perception of brownish discoloration of objects may appear, but it is not harmful

EVALUATION OF OUTCOME CRITERIA

Evaluate the effectiveness of drug therapy by confirming that patient goals and expected outcomes have been met (see "Planning").

See Tables 10.1 and 10.3 for lists of the drugs to which these nursing actions apply.

TABLE 10.4 Atypical Antipsychotic Drugs

DRUG	ROUTE AND ADULT DOSE	REMARKS
aripiprazole (Abilify)	PO 10–15 mg daily (max: 30 mg/day)	For schizophrenia; may cause loss of glycemic control in diabetic patients
Pr clozapine (Clozaril)	PO start at 25–50 mg/day and titrate to a target dose of 50–450 mg/day in 3 days, may increase further (max: 900 mg/day)	For schizophrenia (adults older than 16 years)
olanzapine (Zyprexa)	PO adult: start with 5–10 mg/day, may increase by 2.5–5 mg every week (range 10–15 mg/day (max: 20 mg/day); geriatric: start with 5 mg/day	Blocks alpha receptors and acetylcholine
quetiapine fumarate (Seroquel)	PO start with 25 mg bid, may increase to a target dose of 300–400 mg/day in divided doses	Patients may experience hypotension when changing positions; use cautiously in elderly patients
risperidone (Risperdal)	PO 1–6 mg bid, increase by 2 mg daily to an initial target dose of 6 mg/day	Unlabeled use in behavioral disturbances (patients with mental retardation)
ziprasidone (Geodon)	PO 20 mg bid (max: 80 mg bid)	Unlabeled use for Tourette's syndrome; patients may experience hypotension when changing positions

DRUG PROFILE: Atypical Antipsychotic: Pr *Clozapine (Clozaril)*

Actions and Uses:

Therapeutic effects of clozapine include remission of a range of psychotic symptoms including delusions, paranoia, and irrational behavior. Among severely ill patients, 25% show improvement within 6 weeks of starting clozapine; 60% show improvement within 6 months. Clozapine acts by interfering with the binding of dopamine to its receptors in the limbic system. Clozapine also binds to alpha-adrenergic, serotonergic, and cholinergic sites throughout the brain. This drug is pregnancy category B.

Adverse Effects and Interactions:

Because seizures and agranulocytosis are associated with clozapine use, a course of therapy with conventional antipsychotics is recommended before starting clozapine therapy. Common side effects are dizziness, drowsiness, headache, constipation, transient fever, salivation, flulike symptoms, and tachycardia. As with the conventional agents, elderly patients exhibit a higher incidence of orthostatic hypotension and anticholinergic side effects. Clozapine may also cause bone marrow suppression, which has been fatal in some cases.

Clozapine interacts with many drugs. For example, it should not be taken with alcohol, other CNS depressants, or with drugs that suppress bone marrow function, such as anticancer drugs.

Use together with antihypertensives may lead to hypotension. Benzodiazepines taken with clozapine may lead to severe hypotension and a risk for respiratory arrest. Use of digoxin or warfarin with clozapine may cause increased levels of those drugs, which could lead to increased cardiac problems or hemorrhage, respectively. If phenytoin is taken with clozapine, seizure threshold will be decreased.

Use with caution with herbal supplements such as kava, green tea, and milk thistle.

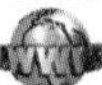
See the Companion Website for a Nursing Process Focus specific to this drug.

Due to side effects caused by conventional and atypical antipsychotic medications, a new drug category was developed to better meet the needs of patients with psychoses. This new category is called dopamine system stabilizers (DSSs). Aripiprazole (Abilify) is the first of these agents. It was approved by the FDA in November 2002 for the treatment of schizophrenia and

TABLE 10.5 Degenerative Diseases of the Central Nervous System

DISEASE	DESCRIPTION
Alzheimer's disease	Progressive loss of brain function characterized by memory loss, confusion, and dementia
Amyotrophic lateral sclerosis (ALS)	Progressive weakness and wasting of muscles caused by destruction of motor neurons
Huntington's chorea	Autosomal dominant genetic disorder resulting in progressive dementia and involuntary, spasmodic movements of limb and facial muscles
Multiple sclerosis (MS)	Demyelination of neurons in the CNS resulting in progressive weakness, visual disturbances, mood alterations, and cognitive deficits
Parkinson's disease	Progressive loss of dopamine in the CNS causing tremor, muscle rigidity, and abnormal movement and posture

schizoaffective disorder. Aripiprazole-treated patients appear to exhibit fewer EPS than patients treated with haloperidol (Haldol). Side effects include headache, nausea/vomiting, fever, constipation, and anxiety.

10.6 Medication is unable to cure most degenerative diseases of the CNS.

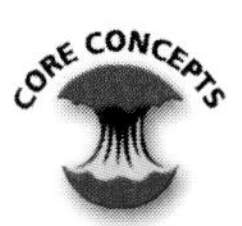

Degenerative diseases of the CNS include a variety of disorders with different causes and outcomes. Some, such as Huntington's disease, are quite rare, affect younger patients, and are caused by chromosomal defects. Others, such as Alzheimer's disease, affect millions of people, mostly elderly patients, and have a devastating economic and social impact. Table 10.5 lists the major degenerative disorders of the CNS.

The cause of most neurologic degenerative diseases is unknown. Most progress from hardly noticeable signs and symptoms early in the disease course to serious neurologic and cognitive deficits. In their early stages, these disorders may be difficult to diagnose. With the exception of Parkinson's disease, pharmacotherapy provides only minimal benefit. Currently, medication is unable to cure any of the degenerative diseases of the CNS.

Fast Facts Neurodegenerative Diseases

Parkinson's Disease

- Approximately 1.5 million Americans have Parkinson's disease.
- Most patients with Parkinson's disease are above the age of 50.
- Greater than 50% of Parkinson's patients who have difficulty with voluntary movement are less than 60 years of age.
- More men than women develop this disorder.

Dementia

- Approximately 4 million Americans have Alzheimer's disease.
- Alzheimer's disease mainly affects patients over the age of 65.
- Of all patients with dementia, 60% to 70% have Alzheimer's disease.

Multiple Sclerosis

- About 1.1 million people worldwide have MS.
- Onset of symptoms typically occurs between ages 15 and 40.
- Women are affected twice as often as men.
- MS occurs most often in Caucasian people of northern European origin.

SOURCE: THE NATIONAL PARKINSON'S FOUNDATION AND THE NATIONAL MENTAL HEALTH ASSOCIATION

PARKINSON'S DISEASE

Parkinson's disease is a degenerative disorder of the CNS caused by death of neurons that produce the brain neurotransmitter dopamine. It is the second most common degenerative disease of the nervous system, affecting over 1.5 million Americans. Pharmacotherapy is often successful in reducing some of the distressing symptoms of this disease.

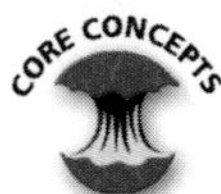

10.7 Parkinson's disease is progressive, with the occurrence of full symptoms taking many years.

Parkinson's disease primarily affects patients older than 50 years of age; however, even teenagers can develop the disorder. Men are affected slightly more often than women. The disease is progressive. The appearance of full symptoms often takes many years. The symptoms of Parkinson's disease, or **Parkinsonism,** are summarized as follows:

- *Tremors.* The hands and head develop a palsy-like motion or shakiness when at rest; pin-rolling, in which patients rub the thumb and forefinger together in a circular motion, is a common behavior in progressive states.
- *Muscle rigidity.* Stiffness may resemble symptoms of arthritis. Patients often have difficulty bending over or moving limbs. Some patients develop a rigid poker face. These symptoms may not be noticeable at first, but become more obvious as the disease progresses.
- *Bradykinesia.* This is the most noticeable of all symptoms. Patients may have difficulty chewing, swallowing, or speaking. Patients with Parkinson's disease have difficulties initiating movement and controlling fine muscle movements. Walking often becomes difficult, and patients shuffle their feet without taking normal strides.
- *Postural instability.* Patients may be hunched over slightly and may easily lose their balance. Stumbling results in frequent falls and injuries.

brady = *slow*
kinesia = *movement*

Although Parkinson's disease is a progressive, neurologic disorder primarily affecting muscle movement, other health problems often develop in these patients, including anxiety, depression, sleep disturbances, dementia, and disturbances of the autonomic nervous system such as difficulty urinating and performing sexually. Several theories have been proposed to explain the development of Parkinsonism. Because some patients with Parkinson's symptoms have a family history of this disorder, a genetic link is highly probable. Numerous environmental toxins, such as carbon monxide, cyanide, manganese, chlorine, and pesticides, also have been suggested as a cause, but results of studies have not proven the cause-effect link. Viral infections, head trauma, and stroke have also been proposed as causes of Parkinsonism.

Symptoms of Parkinsonism develop due to the degeneration and destruction of dopamine-producing neurons found within an area of the brain known as the *substantia nigra.* When not enough dopamine is released, this neurotransmitter cannot make contact with other critical areas of the brain.

substantia = *substance*
nigra = *black*

The most critical area for dopamine contact is the *corpus striatum,* an area responsible for controlling unconscious muscle movement. Patients with Parkinson's disease have a problem initiating movement and controlling movements. Balance, posture, muscle tone, and involuntary muscle movement depend on the proper balance of dopamine (inhibitory) and acetylcholine (stimulatory) in the corpus striatum. If dopamine is absent, acetylcholine is able to stimulate this area more. For this reason, drug therapy for Parkinsonism focuses not only on restoring dopamine function, but also on blocking the effect of acetylcholine within the corpus striatum.

corpus = *body*
striatum = *striped*

EPS develop in response to the same neurochemical actions that cause Parkinson's disease. Recall that antipsychotic drugs act by blocking dopamine receptors. Treatment with certain antipsychotic drugs may cause Parkinsonism-like symptoms, or EPS, by interfering with the same neural pathway and functions affected by the lack of dopamine.

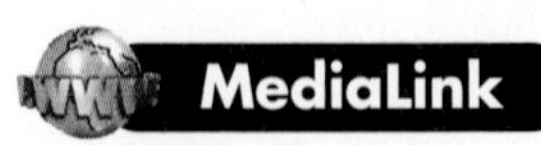

THE NATIONAL PARKINSON FOUNDATION

THE AMERICAN PARKINSON DISEASE ASSOCIATON

PARKINSON SOCIETY OF CANADA

EPS may occur suddenly, and become a medical emergency. With acute EPS, patients' muscles may spasm or lock up. Fever and confusion are other signs and symptoms of this reaction. If acute EPS occurs in a healthcare facility, short-term medical treatment can be provided by administering diphenhydramine (Benadryl). If the patient is not in a healthcare facility and these symptoms are recognized, the patient should immediately be taken to the emergency room. Untreated acute episodes of EPS can be fatal.

Concept Review 10.3

- Parkinson's disease primarily affects which body functions? What are the four major symptoms of this disorder?

10.8 Parkinsonism drugs focus on restoring the balance between dopamine and acetylcholine in the brain.

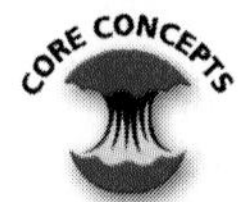

The goal of pharmacotherapy for Parkinson's disease is to increase the ability of the patient to perform normal daily activities such as eating, walking, dressing, and bathing. Although pharmacotherapy does not cure this disorder, it can dramatically reduce symptoms in some patients.

Antiparkinsonism agents are given to restore the balance of dopamine and acetylcholine in the corpus striatum of the brain. These drugs include dopaminergic agents and anticholinergics (cholinergic blockers).

Dopaminergic Agents

Dopaminergic drugs, shown in Table 10.6, are used to increase dopamine levels in the corpus striatum. The drug of choice for Parkinsonism is levodopa (Larodopa), a dopaminergic drug that

TABLE 10.6 Dopaminergic Drugs Used for Parkinsonism

DRUG	ROUTE AND ADULT DOSE	REMARKS
amantadine (Symmetrel)	PO 100 mg daily or bid	Also for infection with influenza A virus; for relief of drug-induced EPS; may cause release of dopamine from nerve terminals
bromocriptine (Parlodel)	PO 1.25–2.5 mg/day up to 100 mg/day in divided doses	Also for suppression of lactation, female infertility, and overproduction of growth hormone; activates the dopamine receptor directly
carbidopa-levodopa (Sinemet)	PO 1 tablet containing 10 mg carbidopa/100 mg levodopa or 25 mg carbidopa/100 mg levodopa tid (max: 6 tablets/day)	Prevents metabolism of levodopa, enhancing dopamine action
Pr levodopa (L-Dopa, Larodopa)	PO 500 mg–1 g/day, may be increased by 750 mg every 3–7 days	Chemical precursor to dopamine; dosage can be reduced by 70–80% if administered with carbidopa
pergolide (Permax)	PO start with 0.05 mg daily for 2 days, increase by 0.1 or 0.15 mg/day every 3 days for 12 days, then increase by 0.25 mg every third day (max: 5 mg/day)	Activates dopamine receptors
pramipexole (Mirapex)	PO start with 0.125 mg tid for 1 week, double this dose for the next week, continue to increase by 0.25 mg/dose tid every week to a target dose of 1.5 mg tid	Activates dopamine receptors
ropinirole hydrochloride (Requip)	PO start with 0.25 mg tid, may increase by 0.25 mg/dose tid every week to a target dose of 1 mg tid	Activates dopamine receptors
selegiline hydrochloride (L-Deprenyl, Eldepryl)	PO 5 mg/dose bid; doses greater than 10 mg/day are potentially toxic	Blocks MAO type B, the enzyme that degrades dopamine within nerve terminals
tolcapone (Tasmar)	PO 100 mg tid (max: 600 mg/day)	Blocks enzymes responsible for metabolizing dopamine

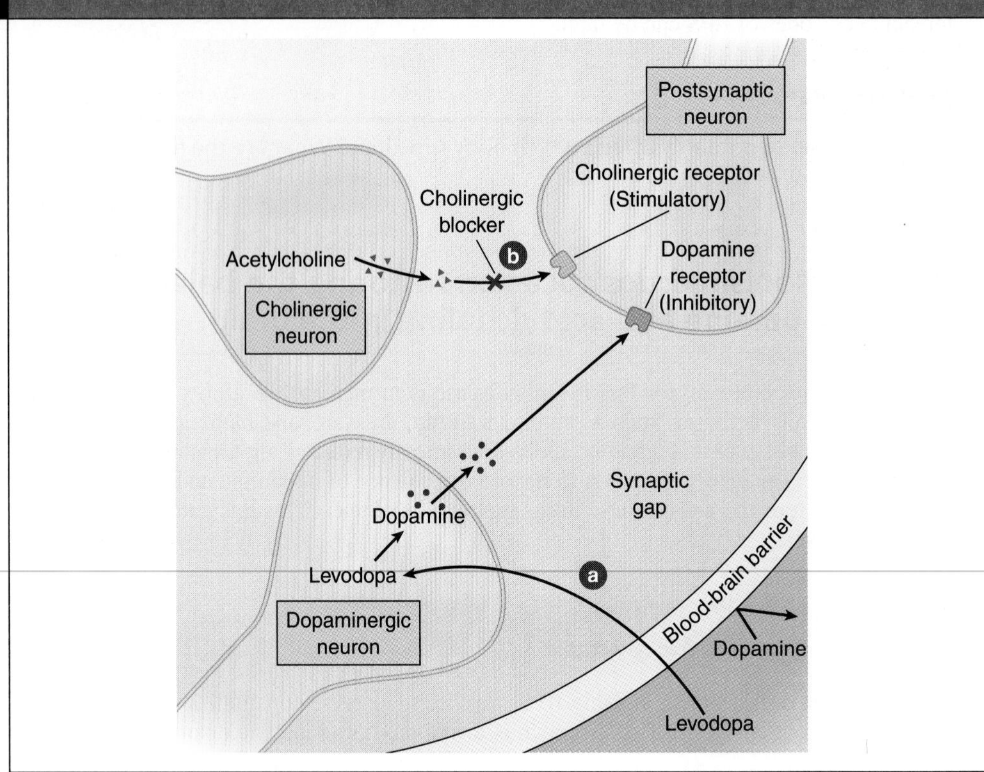

FIGURE 10.2 Dopamine cannot cross the blood-brain barrier. Levodopa, its precursor, can. Once levodopa crosses the blood-brain barrier, it is converted into dopamine, which normally inhibits firing of the next neuron. Natural acetylcholine in the brain stimulates the same postsynaptic neuron. Thus, to restore normal neuronal activity, drug therapy attempts to either (a) restore dopamine inhibitory action, or (b) block acetylcholine (cholinergic) stimulatory activity.

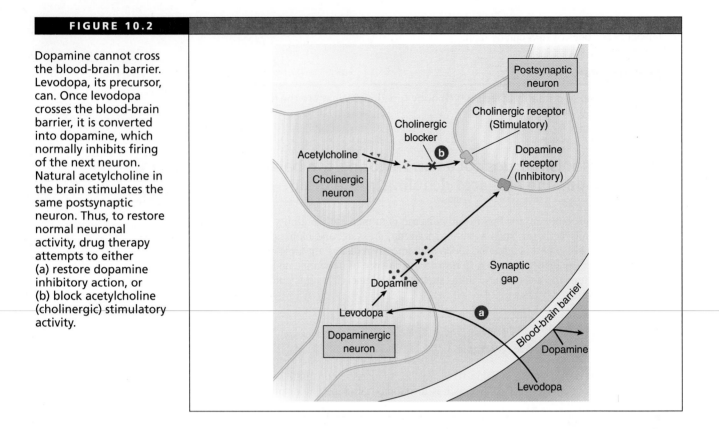

has been used more often than any other medication for this disorder. As shown in Figure 10.2 ■, levodopa is a precursor of (an agent that stimulates) dopamine synthesis. Supplying it directly with drug therapy leads to increased synthesis of dopamine within the nerve terminals. Levodopa can cross the blood-brain barrier, but dopamine cannot. Therefore, dopamine by itself is not used for therapy. The effectiveness of levodopa can be "boosted" by combining it with carbidopa. This combination, marketed as Sinemet, makes more levodopa available to enter the CNS.

Several additional approaches to enhancing dopamine are used in treating Parkinsonism. Tolcapone (Tasmar), entacapone (Comtan), and selegiline (Carbex, Eldepryl) inhibit enzymes that normally destroy levodopa and/or dopamine. Bromocriptine (Parlodel), pergolide (Permax), pramipexole (Mirapex), and ropinirole (Requip) directly activate the dopamine receptor. Amantadine (Symmetrel), an antiviral agent, causes the release of dopamine from its nerve terminals. All of these drugs are considered adjuncts (or additions) to the pharmacotherapy of Parkinsonism, because they are not as effective as levodopa.

Cholinergic Blockers (Anticholinergics)

A second approach to changing the balance between dopamine and acetylcholine in the brain is to give cholinergic blockers, or anticholinergics. By blocking the effect of acetylcholine, anticholinergics inhibit the overactivity of this neurotransmitter in the corpus striatum of the brain. These agents are shown in Table 10.7.

Anticholinergics such as atropine were the first agents used to treat Parkinsonism. The large number of side effects these agents cause has limited their use. The anticholinergics now used for Parkinsonism act on the CNS and produce fewer side effects. However, they still cause autonomic effects such as dry mouth, blurred vision, tachycardia, urinary retention, and constipation that are troublesome. The centrally acting anticholinergics are not as effective as levodopa in relieving severe symptoms of Parkinsonism. They are used early in the courses of the disease when symptoms are less severe, in patients who cannot tolerate levodopa, and in combination therapy with older antiparkinsonism drugs.

DRUG PROFILE: Dopaminergic Agent: Pr *Levodopa (Larodopa)*

Actions and Uses:

Levodopa restores the neurotransmitter dopamine in extrapyramidal areas of the brain, thus relieving some Parkinson's symptoms. To increase its effect, levodopa is often combined with other medications, such as carbidopa, which prevent its enzymatic breakdown. As long as 6 months may be needed to achieve maximum therapeutic effects.

Adverse Effects and Interactions:

Side effects of levodopa include uncontrolled and purposeless movements such as extending the fingers and shrugging the shoulders, involuntary movements, loss of appetite, nausea, and vomiting. Muscle twitching and spasmodic winking are easy signs of toxicity. Orthostatic hypotension is common in some patients. The drug should be discontinued gradually because abrupt withdrawal can produce acute Parkinsonism.

Levodopa interacts with many drugs. For example, tricyclic antidepressants decrease effects of levodopa, increase postural hypotension, may increase sympathetic activity, with hypertension and sinus tachycardia. Levodopa cannot be used if an MAOI was taken within 14 to 28 days because use together may cause hypertensive crisis. Haloperidol taken concurrently may antagonize therapeutic effects of levodopa. Methyldopa may increase toxicity. Antihypertensives may cause increased hypotensive effects. Anticonvulsants may decrease therapeutic effects of levodopa. Antacids containing magnesium, calcium, or sodium bicarbonate may increase levodopa absorption, which could lead to toxicity. Pyridoxine reverses antiparkinsonian effects of levodopa.

Use with caution with herbal supplements, such as kava, which may worsen symptoms of Parkinson's.

Mechanism in Action: 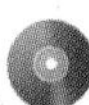

Clients with Parkinson's disease have a reduction of dopamine and an elevation of acetylcholine in specific regions of the brain. This imbalance is responsible for symptoms such as slow movements, tremor, muscle rigidity, shuffling gait, flat facial expression, speech impairment, and lack of fine psychomotor skills. Levodopa, a precursor to dopamine, crosses the blood-brain barrier and restores the imbalance between dopamine and acetylcholine, thereby treating Parkinson's symptoms.

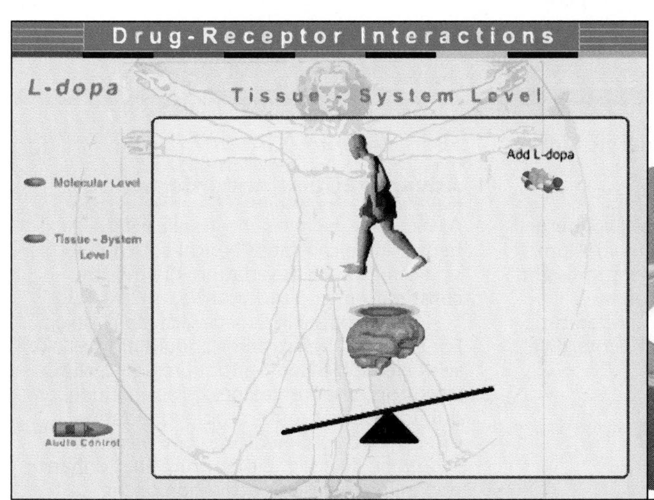

Use the student CD-ROM to see Mechanism in Action for Levodopa.

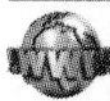 *See the Companion Website for a Nursing Process Focus specific to this drug.*

TABLE 10.7 Anticholinergic Drugs Used for Parkinsonism

DRUG	ROUTE AND ADULT DOSE	REMARKS
benztropine mesylate (Cogentin)	PO 0.5–1 mg/day, gradually increase as needed (max: 6 mg/day)	Also used to relieve EPS from neuroleptic drugs; does not lighten tardive dyskinesia
biperiden hydrochloride (Akineton)	PO 2 mg daily to qid	Blocks acetylcholine receptors; thus, actions associated with muscarinic blockade are observed (e.g., blurred vision, dry mouth); available in IM/IV forms.
diphenhydramine hydrochloride (Benadryl)	PO 25–50 mg tid or qid (max: 300/day)	Also for allergic reactions, motion sickness, sedation, and coughing; blocks cholinergic function even though it is an antihistamine; available in IM/IV forms.
procyclidine hydrochloride (Kemadrin)	PO 2.5 mg tid pc; may be increased to 5 mg tid if tolerated with an additional 5 mg at bedtime (max: 45–60 mg/day)	Blocks acetylcholine receptors in the brain
trihexyphenidyl (Artane)	PO 1 mg for day 1; double this for day 2; then increase by 2 mg every 3–5 days up to 6–10 mg/day (max: 15 mg/day)	Also used to relieve EPS; unlabeled use for Huntington's chorea and spasmodic torticollis

Concept Review 10.4

- Anti-Parkinson's drugs attempt to restore the balance of which two major central neurotransmitters?

ALZHEIMER'S DISEASE

Alzheimer's disease (AD) is a devastating, progressive, degenerative disease that generally begins after age 60. As many as 50% of people are affected by the age of 85. A patient generally

DRUG PROFILE: Cholinergic Blocker: Pr *Benztropine (Cogentin)*

Actions and Uses:

Benztropine acts by blocking excess cholinergic stimulation of neurons in the corpus striatum. It is used for relief of Parkinsonism symptoms and for the treatment of EPS brought on by antipsychotic pharmacotherapy. This medication suppresses tremors but does not affect tardive dyskinesia.

Adverse Effects and Interactions:

As expected from its autonomic action, benztropine can cause typical anticholinergic side effects such as sedation, dry mouth, constipation, and tachycardia.

Benztropine interacts with many drugs. For example, benztropine should not be taken with alcohol, tricyclic antidepressants, MAO inhibitors, phenothiazines, procainamide, or quinidine because of combined sedative effects. OTC cold medicines and alcohol should be avoided. Other drugs that enhance dopamine release or activation of the dopamine receptor may produce additive effects. Haloperidol will cause decreased effectiveness.

Antihistamines, phenothiazines, tricyclics, disopyramide quinidine may increase anticholinergic effects, and antidiarrheals may decrease absorption.

See the Companion Website for a Nursing Process Focus specific to this drug.

lives 5 to 10 years after being diagnosed with AD, which is the fourth leading cause of death. Pharmacotherapy has limited success in improving cognitive function in patients with AD.

AD is responsible for 70% of all dementia. **Dementia** is a degenerative disorder characterized by progressive memory loss, confusion, and inability to think or communicate effectively. Consciousness and perception are usually unaffected. Most causes of dementia are unknown, but atrophy (wasting away) or other structural changes within the brain are usual. Some of the known, but less frequent, causes of dementia include multiple strokes, severe infections, and toxins.

Despite extensive, ongoing research, the cause of Alzheimer's disease remains unknown. The early-onset form of AD that runs in families accounts for about 10% of cases and is caused by gene defects on chromosome 1, 14, or 21. Environmental, immunologic, and nutritional factors, as well as viruses, may be possible causes of brain damage that is seen in AD. Chronic inflammation and damage to cells from pollutants, radiation, administered drugs, or the body's own immune response may decrease the number and function of neurons in the brains of AD patients.

10.9 Alzheimer's patients experience a dramatic loss of ability to perform tasks that require acetylcholine as a central neurotransmitter.

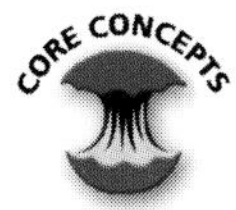

Alzheimer's patients experience a dramatic loss of ability to perform tasks that require acetylcholine as the neurotransmitter. Because acetylcholine is a major neurotransmitter within the *hippocampus* (an area of the brain responsible for learning and memory) and other parts of the cerebral cortex, neuronal function within these brain areas is especially affected. Thus, an inability to remember and to recall information is among the early symptoms of AD. Symptoms of AD include the following:

- Impaired memory and judgment
- Confusion or disorientation
- Inability to recognize family or friends
- Aggressive behavior
- Depression
- Psychoses, including paranoia and delusions
- Anxiety

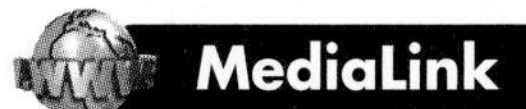

ALZHEIMER'S DISEASE INFORMATION PAGE

ALZHEIMER SOCIETY OF CANADA

10.10 Alzheimer's disease is treated with acetylcholinesterase inhibitors.

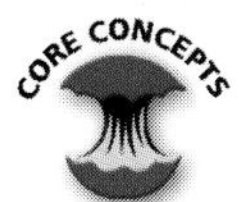

Drugs are used to slow memory loss and other progressive symptoms of dementia. Some drugs are given to treat associated symptoms such as depression, anxiety, or psychoses. The acetylcholinesterase inhibitors are the most widely used class of drugs for treating AD. These agents are shown in Table 10.8. Memantine (Namenda), the first of a new class of drugs called glutamergic inhibitors, was approved in October 2003.

Acetylcholinesterase Inhibitors

The FDA has approved only a few drugs for AD. The most effective of these medications acts by intensifying the effect of acetylcholine at the cholinergic receptor, as shown in Figure 10.3 ■. Acetylcholine is naturally degraded in the synapse by the enzyme **acetylcholinesterase (AchE).** When acetylcholinesterase is inhibited, acetylcholine levels increase and greatly affect the receptors. As described in Chapter 7, the acetylcholinesterase inhibitors are indirect-acting mimics of acetycholine.

TABLE 10.8 Acetylcholinesterase Inhibitors Used for Alzheimer's Disease

DRUG	ROUTE AND ADULT DOSE	REMARKS
Pr donepezil hydrochloride (Aricept)	PO 5–10 mg at bedtime	For mild to moderate dementia; may cause nausea, diarrhea, muscle cramps, and weight loss
galantamine (Reminyl)	PO start with 4 mg bid at least 4 weeks; if tolerated, may increase by 4 mg bid q4wk to target dose of 12 mg bid (max: 8–16 mg bid)	For mild to moderate dementia; may cause weight loss, dizziness, nausea, vomiting, and hypotension when changing positions
rivastigmine tartrate (Exelon)	PO start with 1.5 mg bid with food, may increase by 1.5 mg bid q2wk if tolerated; target dose 3–6 mg bid (max: 12 mg bid)	For mild to moderate dementia; may cause flulike symptoms, dizziness, weight loss
tacrine (Cognex)	PO 10 mg qid, increase in 40 mg/day increments not sooner than every 6 weeks (max: 160 mg/day)	For mild to moderate dementia; unlabeled used for severe dementia in patients with HIV infection; may cause nausea, vomiting, and liver toxicity

FIGURE 10.3

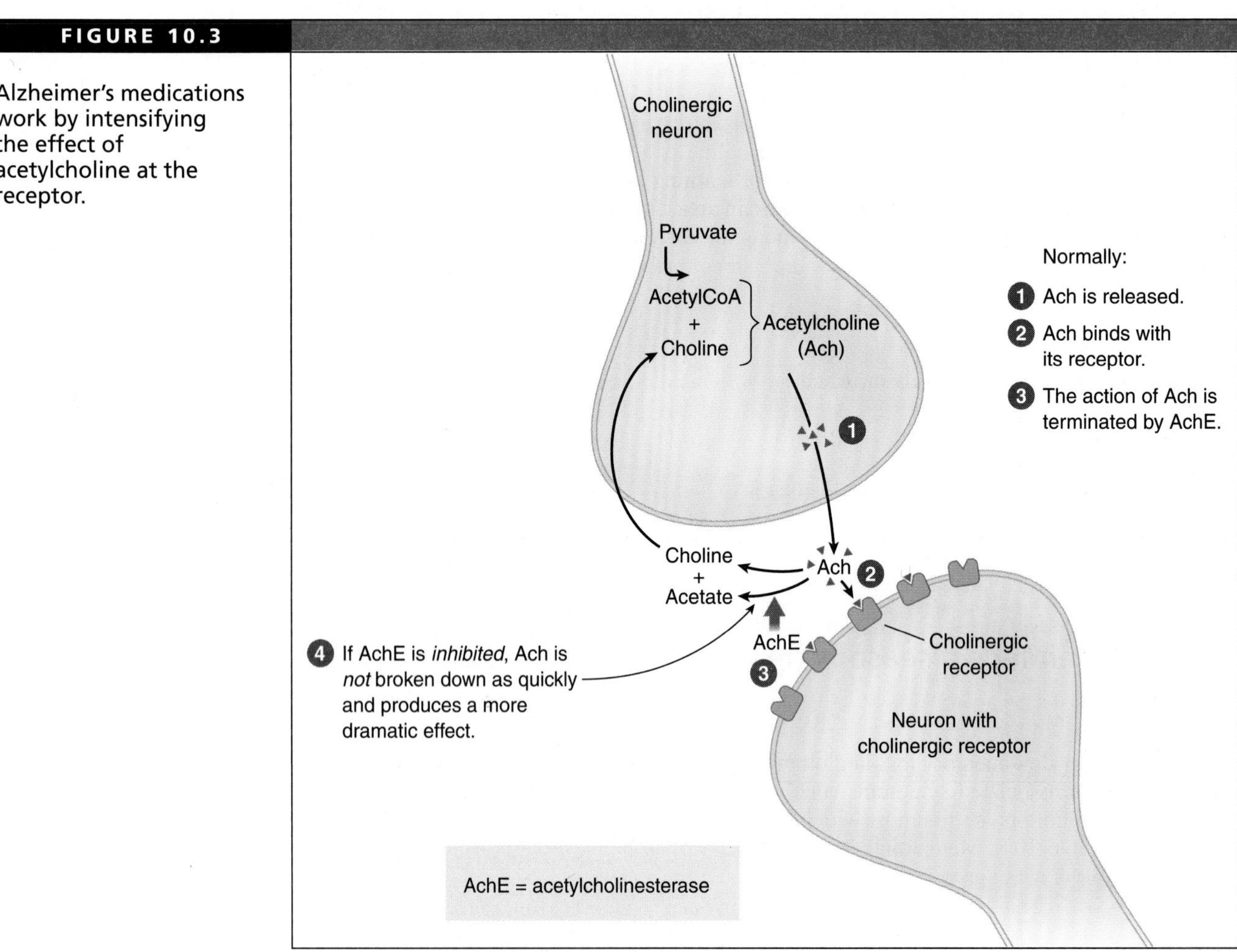

Alzheimer's medications work by intensifying the effect of acetylcholine at the receptor.

When treating AD, the goal of pharmacotherapy is to improve function in activities of daily living, behavior, and cognition. Although the acetylcholinesterase inhibitors improve all three functions, their effectiveness is limited, at best. These agents do not cure AD—they only slow its progression. Therapy is begun as soon as the diagnosis of AD is established. These agents are ineffective in treating the severe stages of this disorder, probably because so many neurons have died. Increasing the levels of acetylcholine is only effective if there are functioning neurons present. Therefore, as the disease progresses, the acetylcholinesterase inhibitors are often discontinued. Their therapeutic benefit is not great enough to outweigh their expense or the side effects they may cause.

All acetylcholinesterase inhibitors used to treat AD are equally effective. Their side effects are those expected of drugs that enhance the parasympathetic nervous system (Chapter 7), and include nausea, vomiting, and diarrhea. Of the agents available for AD, tacrine (Cognex) is associated with liver toxicity. Rivastigmine (Exelon) is associated with weight loss, a potentially serious side effect in some elderly patients. When discontinuing therapy, doses of the acetylcholinesterase inhibitors should be lowered gradually.

Although acetylcholinesterase inhibitors are the mainstay of treatment for AD dementia, several other agents are being investigated for their possible benefit in delaying the progression of AD. Because at least some of the neuronal changes in AD are caused by oxidative cellular damage, antioxidants such as vitamin E are being examined for their effects in AD patients. Other agents currently being examined are anti-inflammatory agents, estrogen, and ginkgo biloba.

Agitation occurs in most patients with AD. This may be accompanied by delusion, paranoia, hallucinations, or other psychotic symptoms. Atypical antipsychotic agents such as risperidone (Risperdal) and olanzapine (Zyprexa) may be used to control these episodes. Conventional antipsychotics such as haloperidol (Haldol) are occasionally prescribed, though EPS often limit their use.

Although not as common as agitation, anxiety and depression may also occur in AD patients. Anxiolytics such as buspirone (BuSpar) or some of the benzodiazepines are used to control excessive anxiety (Chapter 8). Mood stabilizers such as sertraline (Zoloft), citalopram (Celexa), or fluoxetine (Prozac) are given when major depression interferes with daily activities (Chapter 9).

Concept Review 10.5

- Alzheimer's disease is a dysfunction of which brain neurotransmitters? How do drugs for Alzheimer's disease restore neurotransmitter function and improve symptoms of dementia?

DRUG PROFILE: Acetylcholinesterase Inhibitor: Pr *Donepezil (Aricept)*

Actions and Uses:

Donepezil is an AchE inhibitor that improves memory in cases of mild to moderate Alzheimer's dementia by enhancing the effects of acetylcholine in neurons in the cerebral cortex that have not yet been damaged. Patients should receive pharmacotherapy for at least 6 months prior to assessing maximum benefits of drug therapy. Improvement in memory may be observed as early as 1 to 4 weeks following medication. The therapeutic effects of donepezil are often short-lived, and the degree of improvement is modest, at best. An advantage of donepezil over other drugs in its class is that its long half-life permits it to be given once daily.

Adverse Effects and Interactions:

Common side effects of donepezil are vomiting, diarrhea, and darkened urine. CNS side effects include insomnia, syncope, depression, headache, and irritability. Musculoskeletal side effects include muscle cramps, arthritis, and bone fractures. Generalized side effects include headache, fatigue, chest pain, increased libido, hot flashes, urinary incontinence, dehydration, and blurred vision. Unlike tacrine, hepatotoxicity has not been observed. Patients with bradycardia, hypotension, asthma, hyperthyroidism, or active peptic ulcer disease should be monitored carefully. Anticholinergics will be less effective. Donepezil interacts with several other drugs. For example, bethanechol causes a synergistic effect. Phenobarbital, phenytoin, dexamethasone, and rifampin may speed elimination of donepezil. Quinidine or ketoconazole may inhibit metabolism of donepezil. Because donepezil acts by increasing cholinergic activity, two parasympathomimetics should not be administered at the same time.

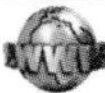
See the Companion Website for a Nursing Process Focus specific to this drug.

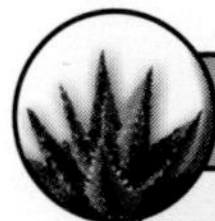

NATURAL ALTERNATIVES

Ginkgo Biloba for Treatment of Dementia

Ginkgo biloba has been used for many years to improve memory. In Europe, an extract of this herb is already approved for the treatment of dementia. In one of the first U.S. studies, 120 mg of ginkgo taken daily was shown to improve mental functioning and stabilize Alzheimer's disease. In other studies, clinical results were seen between 4 weeks and 6 months of treatment and were found to be relevant. Patients need to speak with their healthcare providers before taking this herb. Although most patients can take ginkgo without problems, those on anticoagulants may have an increased risk of bleeding. ▪

MULTIPLE SCLEROSIS

Multiple sclerosis (MS) is an autoimmune disorder of the CNS. This is a condition in which antibodies target and slowly destroy tissues in the brain and spinal cord. As tissues are damaged, inflammation of nervous tissue causes *demyelination,* or the loss of myelin, a fatty material that acts as a protective insulator of nerve fibers. The loss of myelin leaves multiple areas of hard scarred tissue (plaques) along the covering of nerve cells. Axons are gradually destroyed, disrupting the ability of the nerves to conduct electrical impulses to and from the brain.

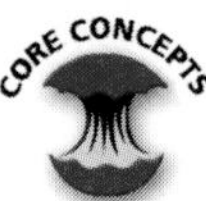

10.11 Symptoms of multiple sclerosis result from demyelination of central nerve fibers.

Over time, as demyelination continues, various symptoms of MS occur. Some of the more common symptoms include fatigue, heat sensitivity, pain, spasticity (muscle cramps and spasms), cognitive problems, balance and coordination problems, and bowel and bladder symptoms. The course of MS is unpredictable, and each patient will experience a variety of symptoms.

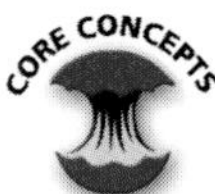

10.12 Drugs for multiple sclerosis reduce immune attacks in the brain and treat unfavorable symptoms.

The two basic strategies for treating MS are shown in Table 10.9. One approach attempts to reduce inflammation and prevent attacks on the nervous system. The other strategy emphasizes treatments to relieve symptoms.

The most treatable form of this disorder is *relapsing-remitting MS (RRMS).* This condition involves unpredictable relapses (attacks) during which time new symptoms appear or existing symptoms become more severe. These symptoms can last for varying periods (days or months), followed by partial or total remission (recovery). In RRMS, the disease may be inactive for months or years. On average, people with RRMS have one or two attacks a year.

Interferon beta-1a (Avonex, Rebif) and interferon beta-1b (Betaseron) are the only clinically proven drugs for treating the underlying causes of MS and for decreasing the overall relapse rate. One type of treatment, immunostimulants, are discussed in Chapter 21.

Another drug treatment, glatiramer acetate (Copaxone), formerly known as *copolymer-1,* is a synthetic protein that simulates myelin basic protein, an essential part of the nerve's myelin coating. Since glatiramer acetate resembles myelin, it is thought to curb the body's attack on the myelin covering and reduce the creation of new brain lesions. Copaxone is available in prefilled syringes that can be stored at room temperature for several days. However, patients often complain of side effects and having to inject themselves. Side effects include redness, pain, swelling, itching or a lump at the site of injection. Flushing, chest pain, weakness, infection, pain, nausea, joint pain, anxiety, and muscle stiffness are common adverse effects.

Miscellaneous drugs used for MS include modafinil (Provigil) and amantadine (Symmetrel) for treating fatigue, memory loss, and progressive weakness symptoms. Modafinil is an

TABLE 10.9 Drugs Used for Multiple Sclerosis

DRUG	DRUG CLASSIFICATION	
FOR IMMUNE ATTACKS AGAINST THE CNS		
interferon beta-1a (Avonex, Rebif)	Immunostimulant	
interferon beta-1b (Betaseron)	Immunostimulant	
glatiramer acetate (Copaxone)	Myelin protein builder	
FOR THE RELIEF OF MS SYMPTOMS		**SYMPTOMS**
modafinil (Provigil)	Alpha-adrenergic stimulant	Fatigue, memory loss, weakness
amantadine (Symmetrel)	Dopaminergic drug	Fatigue, memory loss, weakness
gabapentin (Neurontin)	Antiseizure drug	Anxiety, insomnia, neuropathic pain
methylprednisolone (Solu-Medrol)	Glucocorticoid	Myelin swelling and inflammation

$alpha_1$-adrenergic agent that is thought to activate receptors that respond to the neurotransmitter norepinephrine in the brain. This agent increases alertness and energy and improves memory. Gabapentin (Neurontin) is an antiseizure drug that is used for treating mood disturbances including depression and sensitivity to pain. Methylprednisolone (Solu-Medrol), a steroidal anti-inflammatory agent, may be administered IV to treat symptoms of swelling and inflammation in the CNS.

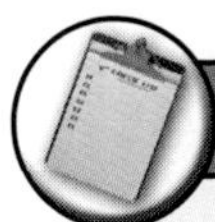

PATIENTS NEED TO KNOW

Patients being treated for psychoses and degenerative diseases of the nervous system need to know the following:

Regarding Antipsychotics

1. It is important to report the development of tremors, involuntary repetitive movements, decreased muscle tone, or increased restlessness to your healthcare practitioner. These symptoms may indicate serious side effects that can be reversed if medication is changed soon after they start.
2. Consult a healthcare provider if dry mouth, rapid heart rate, constipation, or urinary retention occurs. An additional medication may be prescribed to relieve these signs and symptoms.
3. Avoid taking antacids with antipsychotics because they delay or decrease antipsychotic absorption.
4. Avoid alcohol while taking antipsychotics; it increases the depressant effects.
5. Extra protection from the sun is necessary; wear a hat and sunscreen.
6. Avoid driving or operating machinery until response to the medication is known. Its sedating effects can increase the risk for accidental injury.
7. Contact a healthcare provider for guidance if symptoms get worse or are not relieved by the medication. Do not stop the medication unless directed to do so.

Regarding Drugs for Parkinson's Disease or Dementia

8. Do not eat high-protein foods or foods high in vitamin B_6 (such as wheat germ, liver, green leafy vegetables, bananas, and fish) if you are taking levodopa. These foods interfere with drug effectiveness.
9. Be extremely careful about getting up quickly from a seated position. Many dementia drugs cause dizziness, lightheadedness, blurred vision, and difficulty in concentrating.
10. Do not skip taking the medications, and do not take OTC preparations (especially cold or cough medicines) without checking with a healthcare provider.
11. Urine may become a little dark. This is a normal side effect of dopamine-like drugs.
12. Do not drink alcoholic beverages or take sedatives. Combined effects may be harmful.
13. Be familiar with adverse effects specific for the drugs being taken. Drugs used for Parkinson's may produce nausea, dry mouth, and diminished sweating in some cases. Drugs used for dementia may cause nausea, diarrhea, muscle cramps, weight loss, and change in urine color. ■

CHAPTER REVIEW

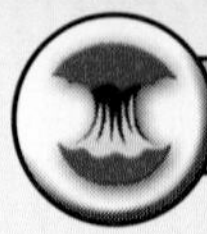

CORE CONCEPTS SUMMARY

10.1 Most psychoses have no identifiable cause and require long-term drug therapy.

Psychosis is characterized by delusions, hallucinations, and illusions. Some psychotic patients exhibit paranoia. Psychoses are classified as acute or chronic. Sometimes a cause can be found for the psychosis, but the vast majority of cases have no identifiable cause. Most patients are not able to function normally in society without long-term drug therapy.

10.2 Schizophrenic patients experience many different symptoms that may change over time.

Schizophrenia is the most common psychiatric disorder characterized by abnormal thoughts, disordered communication, withdrawal, and suicidal risk. Patients with schizophrenia exhibit positive or negative symptoms. Proper diagnosis of these symptoms is important for selecting the appropriate antipsychotic drug. The cause of schizophrenia has not been determined. Symptoms seem to be associated with the *dopamine type 2 (D_2) receptor* located in a specific area of the brain. Schizoaffective disorder is a condition in which patients exhibit symptoms of both schizophrenia and mood disorder.

10.3 The experience and skills of the healthcare provider are critical to the pharmacological management of psychoses.

Management of severe mental illness is difficult. Many patients do not see themselves as abnormal and have difficulty understanding the need for medication. Although many symptoms of psychosis can be controlled with current drug therapy, adverse effects are common and often severe. Skills of the healthcare team are particularly valuable to achieving successful psychiatric drug treatment.

10.4 Conventional antipsychotic agents include the phenothiazines, phenothiazine-like drugs, and nonphenothiazines.

Antipsychotic drugs are sometimes called *neuroleptics.* The two basic categories of drugs for psychosis are conventional (typical) antipsychotics and atypical antipsychotics. With conventional antipsychotics, it is not always possible to control *extrapyramidal symptoms (EPS)* that include muscle spasms (*dystonia*), inability to sit down (*akathisia*), and unusual tongue and facial movements (*tardive dyskinesia*). Phenothiazines, phenothiazine-like drugs, and nonphenothiazines treat positive signs of schizophrenia, but all have unpleasant side effects.

10.5 Atypical antipsychotic agents and a newer drug class have been developed to better meet the needs of patients with psychoses.

Atypical antipsychotic drugs treat both positive and negative signs of schizophrenia, and have become the drugs of choice for treating psychoses. Like the phenothiazine drugs, atypical agents block D_2 receptors. Although there are fewer side effects with atypical agents, adverse effects are still significant and patients must be carefully monitored. Dopamine system stabilizers (DSSs) represent a newer drug category developed to better meet the needs of psychotic patients.

10.6 Medication is unable to cure most degenerative diseases of the CNS.

Degenerative diseases of the CNS include Alzheimer's disease, multiple sclerosis, and Parkinson's disease. The cause of most neurological degenerative disorders is unknown. With the exception of Parkinson's disease, drug therapy provides only minimal benefit.

10.7 Parkinson's disease is progressive, with the occurrence of full symptoms taking many years.

Parkinson's disease, or *Parkinsonism,* is a degenerative disorder caused by death of neurons that produce the brain neurotransmitter dopamine. Dopamine-producing neurons in the substantia nigra supply nerve signals to the corpus striatum. When dopamine is depleted, symptoms of Parkinsonism including tremors, muscle rigidity, bradykinesia (slow movement), and postural instability occur. These symptoms are the same EPS effects caused by prolonged antipsychotic drug treatment.

10.8 Parkinsonism drugs focus on restoring the balance between dopamine and acetylcholine in the brain.

Balance, posture, muscle tone, and involuntary muscle movement depend on the proper balance of the neurotransmitter dopamine (inhibitory) and acetylcholine (stimulatory) in the corpus striatum. Drug therapy for Parkinsonim focuses on restoring dopamine function (dopaminergic agents) and blocking the effect of acetylcholine overactivity (cholinergic blockers).

10.9 Alzheimer's patients experience a dramatic loss of ability to perform tasks that require acetylcholine as a central neurotransmitter.

Alzheimer's disease (AD) is a devastating, progressive, degenerative disease characterized by impaired memory, confusion or disorientation, inability to recognize family or friends, aggressive behavior, depression, psychoses, and anxiety. AD is responsible for 70% of all *dementia.* Although the cause of AD may be unknown, structural brain damage and a dramatic loss of ability to perform tasks that require acetylcholine as the neurotransmitter has been documented.

10.10 Alzheimer's disease is treated with acetylcholinesterase inhibitors.

Only a few drugs for AD have been approved. Most drugs act by intensifying the effect of acetylcholine at the cholinergic receptor. Acetylcholine is naturally degraded in the synapse by the enzyme acetylcholinesterase. When acetylcholinesterase is inhibited, acetylcholine levels increase and produce a greater effect on the receptor. This treatment improves function in activities of daily living, behavior, and cognition.

10.11 Symptoms of multiple sclerosis result from demyelination of central nerve fibers.

Multiple sclerosis is an autoimmune disorder of the CNS. Antibodies slowly destroy tissues (myelin) in the brain and spinal cord, disrupting the ability of nerves to conduct electrical impulses. Over time, debilitating symptoms appear including fatigue, heat sensitivity, pain, muscle cramps and spasms, impaired ability to think and reason, balance and coordination problems, and bowel and bladder symptoms.

10.12 Drugs for multiple sclerosis reduce immune attacks in the brain and treat unfavorable symptoms.

Two strategies for treating MS are reducing the impaired immune response and relieving the symptoms. The most treatable form of MS is *relapsing-remitting MS (RRMS),* in which unpredictable relapses occur. Drug treatments include immunostimulants, myelin-building protein, and miscellaneous drugs traditionally used for treating inflammation, pain, fatigue, memory loss, and progressive weakness.

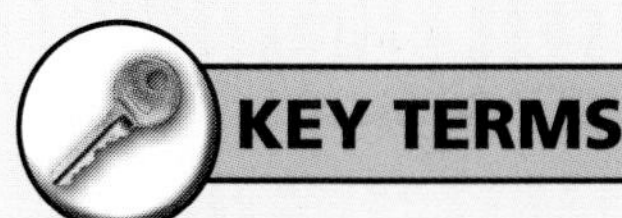

KEY TERMS

acetylcholinesterase (AchE) (AS-ee-til-KOH-lin-ES-ter-ays): an enzyme that degrades acetylcholine within the synapse, enhancing effects of the neurotransmitter / ***page 165***

Alzheimer's disease (AD) (ALLZ-heye-mers): most common dementia characterized by loss of memory, confusion, disorientation, and loss of judgment; hallucinations and delusions may also occur / ***page 164***

dementia (dee-MEN-she-ah): degenerative disorder characterized by progressive memory loss, confusion, and the inability to think or communicate effectively / ***page 165***

extrapyramidal–symptoms (EPS) (peh-RAM-ed-el): symptoms where muscles become very rigid because of overmedication with antipsychotics or by lack of dopamine function in the corpus striatum / ***page 153***

multiple sclerosis (MS) (skle-ROH-sis): autoimmune disorder of the central nervous system; a condition where antibodies slowly destroy tissues in the brain and spinal cord / ***page 168***

negative symptoms: symptoms that subtract from normal behavior; signs that are used to assist with the diagnosis of schizophrenia / ***page 150***

neuroleptic malignant syndrome (NMS) (noo-roh-LEP-tik): a potentially fatal condition caused by some antipsychotic medications; symptoms include an extremely high body temperature, drowsiness, changing blood pressure, irregular heartbeat, and muscle rigidity / ***page 154***

neuroleptics (noo-roh-LEP-ticks): drugs used to treat psychoses / ***page 152***

Parkinsonism: degenerative disorder of the nervous system caused by a deficiency of the brain neurotransmitter dopamine; this deficiency results in disturbances of muscle movement / ***page 160***

positive symptoms: symptoms that add on to normal behavior; signs that are used to assist with the diagnosis of schizophrenia / ***page 150***

schizoaffective disorder (SKIT-soh-ah-FEK-tiv): disorder with symptoms similar to schizophrenia and mood disorders / ***page 151***

schizophrenia (SKIT-soh-FREN-ee-uh): type of psychosis characterized by abnormal thoughts and thought processes, withdrawal from other people and the outside environment, and apparent preoccupation with one's own mental state / ***page 150***

tardive dyskinesia (TAR-div dis-ki-NEE-zee-uh): involuntary movements of facial muscles and the tongue that occur due to long-term antipsychotic therapy / ***page 153***

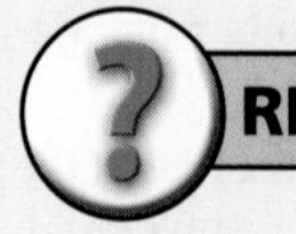

REVIEW QUESTIONS

The following questions are written in NCLEX-PN® style. Answer these questions to assess your knowledge of the chapter material, and go back and review any material that is not clear to you.

1. Which of the following statements is true?

1. Antipsychotic medications cure mental illnesses.
2. The severe side effects of antipsychotic drugs can lead to noncompliance.
3. Antipsychotic medications are only administered when the patient is symptomatic.
4. Antipsychotic drugs improve symptoms within hours of administration.

2. The patient taking levodopa must avoid foods high in:

1. Vitamin A
2. Vitamin B_{12}
3. Folic acid
4. Vitamin B_6

3. Which of the following symptoms does the nurse recognize as an anticholinergic effect of chlorpromazine (Thorazine)?

1. Hallucinations, illusions, paranoia
2. Hypertension, polyuria, increased salvation
3. Dry mouth, postural hypotension, urinary retention
4. Fever, flulike symptoms, decreased WBC count

4. The patient is on thioridazine (Mellaril) and has developed muscle spasms, difficulty sleeping, and a shuffling gait. The nurse recognizes this as:

1. Anticholinergic effects
2. Cholinergic effects
3. Extrapyramidal side effects
4. Parkinson's disease

5. The patient has developed which of the following degenerative CNS diseases that is exhibited by progressive dementia and involuntary muscle spasms?

1. Parkinson's disease
2. Huntington's chorea
3. Multiple sclerosis
4. Alzheimer's disease

6. Drug therapy for the Parkinson's patient focuses on:

1. Increasing cholinergic stimulation within the brain
2. Restoring acetylcholine and blocking dopamine within the brain
3. Restoring dopamine function and blocking acetylcholine within the brain
4. Destroying dopamine receptors within the brain

7. The Alzheimer's patient has been started on rivastigmine (Exelon). The nurse assesses the patient for:

1. Liver toxicity
2. Weight loss
3. Renal failure
4. Extrapyramidal side effects

8. The patient taking gingko biloba must be assessed for use of which of the following drugs?

1. Lanoxin
2. Coumadin
3. Lasix
4. Dilantin

9. Which of the following patients would be most likely to experience akathisia?

1. A 45-year-old man who is taking lithium
2. A 67-year-old woman who is taking levodopa
3. A 57-year-old man who is taking benztropine (Cogentin)
4. A 73-year-old woman who is taking chlorpromazine (Thorazine)

10. The patient on haloperidol (Haldol) is experiencing tardive dyskinesia. Which of the following drugs would the nurse anticipate being ordered?

1. Levodopa
2. Risperidone (Risperdal)
3. Benztropine (Cogentin)
4. Chlorpromazine (Thorazine)

CASE STUDY QUESTIONS

For questions 1–3, please read the following case study, and choose the correct answer from choices 1–4.

Mr. Wayne, age 38, has been diagnosed with a psychosis characterized by the following symptoms: reports of seeing people that are not there, talking about government agents who are trying to kill him, and communicating with "double agents" about suspicious behavior. This patient has been in and out of the hospital for the last 4 weeks. Mr. Wayne's family reports difficulty in controlling him since he has not been taking his medication. Members in the community have seen Mr. Wayne pacing up and down the highway for several weeks. It becomes necessary to temporarily confine Mr. Wayne for medical treatment. He has had this disorder for 10 years and has a strong, supportive family (mother and father).

1. The symptoms described for Mr. Wayne are called __________ symptoms and respond best to treatment with which class of antipsychotic medication?

1. Positive; conventional or typical antipsychotics
2. Negative; conventional or typical antipsychotics
3. Positive; atypical antipsychotics
4. Negative; atypical antipsychotics

2. Assume Mr. Wayne has been taking chlorpromazine (Thorazine) for most of the 10 years he has been experiencing psychotic episodes. Which of the following medications would have been given to him to reduce the incidence of extrapyramidal side effects (EPS)—particularly dystonia?

1. Levodopa (Dopar, Larodopa)
2. Benztropine (Cogentin)
3. Thioridazine (Mellaril)
4. Trifluoperazine (Stelazine)

3. Extrapyramidal side effects (EPS) develop for the same neurochemical reasons as which of the following disorders?

1. Schizoaffective disorder
2. Parkinson's disease
3. Alzheimer's disease
4. Multiple sclerosis

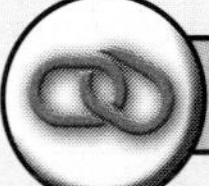

FURTHER STUDY

- A discussion of complex partial seizures, some of which are mistaken for psychosis, is included in Chapter 11.
- Chapter 7 includes more information on acetylcholinesterase inhibitors and their effects on the parasympathetic nervous system.
- More information on anxiolytics can be found in Chapter 8.
- Mood stabilizers are discussed in greater detail in Chapter 9.
- Chapter 21 discusses immunostimulants.
- In addition to its use in Parkinsonism, diphenhydramine is a drug profile for allergies in Chapter 21.
- Amantadine is also an antiviral drug, and is discussed in Chapter 23.

EXPLORE MEDIALINK www.prenhall.com/holland

Additional resources for this chapter can be found on the CD-ROM accompanying this textbook, and on the Companion Website. Click on Chapter 10 to select activities for this chapter.

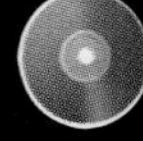

- Mechanism in Action
- Audio Glossary
- Concept Review
- NCLEX-PN® Review
- Nursing in Action
- Dosage Calculator

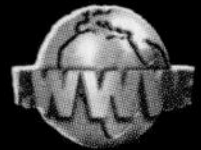

- National Association of Mental Illness
- The National Parkinson Foundation
- The American Parkinson Disease Association
- Parkinson Society of Canada
- Alzheimer's Disease Information Page
- Alzheimer Society of Canada

CHAPTER

11 Drugs for Seizures

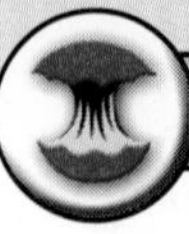

CORE CONCEPTS

11.1 All convulsions are seizures, but not all seizures are convulsions.

11.2 Many causes of seizure activity are known; a few are not.

11.3 Epileptic seizures are typically identified as partial, generalized, and special epileptic syndromes.

11.4 Effective seizure management involves strict adherence to drug therapy.

11.5 The goal of antiseizure drug therapy is to suppress neuronal activity just enough to prevent abnormal or repetitive firing.

11.6 By increasing the effects of GABA in the brain, drugs reduce a wide range of seizure types.

11.7 Hydantoin and phenytoin-like drugs are generally effective in treating partial seizures and tonic-clonic seizures.

11.8 Succinimides generally treat absence seizures.

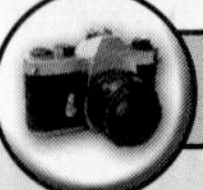

DRUG SNAPSHOT

The following drugs will be discussed in this chapter:

DRUG CLASSES	DRUG PROFILES
DRUGS THAT POTENTIATE GABA ACTION	
Barbiturates	Pr phenobarbital (Luminal)
Benzodiazepines	Pr diazepam (Valium)
Miscellaneous GABA Agents	
HYDANTOINS AND PHENYTOIN-LIKE DRUGS	
Hydantoin	Pr phenytoin (Dilantin)
Phenytoin-like drugs	Pr valproic acid (Depakene)
SUCCINIMIDES	Pr ethosuximide (Zarontin)

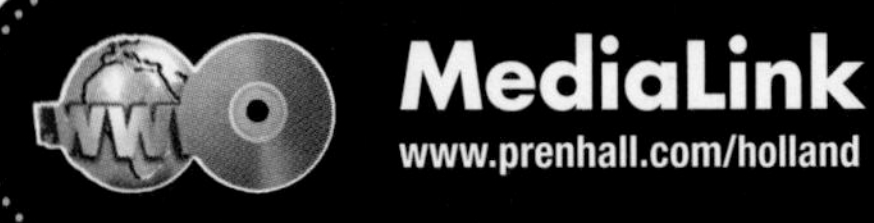

Interactive resources for this chapter can be found on the Companion Website. Click on Chapter 11 and "Begin" to select the activities for this chapter. For chapter-related animations, NCLEX-PN®-style questions, and an audio glossary, access the accompanying CD-ROM in this book.

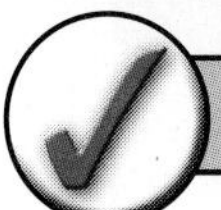

OBJECTIVES

After reading this chapter, the student should be able to:

1. Compare and contrast the terms *epilepsy, seizures,* and *convulsions.*
2. Recognize the causes of epilepsy.
3. Relate signs and symptoms to specific types of seizures.
4. Describe the pharmacological management of epilepsy.
5. Explain the importance of patient drug compliance in the pharmacotherapy of epilepsy.
6. For each of the drug classes, know representative drug examples and explain their mechanisms of drug action, primary actions, and important adverse effects.
7. Categorize drugs used in the treatment of epilepsy based on their classifications and mechanisms of action.

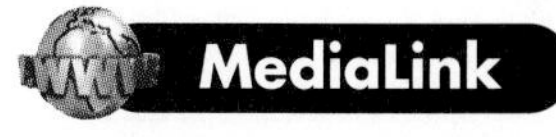

THE EPILEPSY FOUNDATION OF AMERICA (EFA)

NATIONAL INSTITUTE OF NEUROLOGICAL DISORDERS AND STROKE (NINDS)

EPILEPSY CANADA

Epilepsy is defined as any disorder characterized by recurrent seizures. The symptoms of epilepsy depend on the type of seizure and may include blackout, fainting spells, sensory disturbances, jerking body movements, and temporary loss of memory. More than 2 million Americans have epilepsy, the most common neurological disease. This chapter will examine the pharmacotherapy of the different types of seizures.

SEIZURES

A **seizure** is a disturbance of electrical activity in the brain that may affect consciousness, motor activity, and sensation. The symptoms of seizure are caused by abnormal or uncontrollable neuronal discharges within the brain. These abnormal discharges can be measured using an electroencephalogram (EEG), a valuable tool in diagnosing seizure disorders. Figure 11.1 ■ compares normal and abnormal EEG recordings.

11.1 All convulsions are seizures, but not all seizures are convulsions.

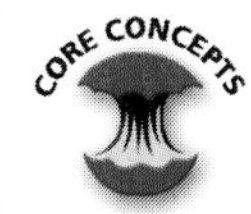

The terms *convulsion* and *seizure* are not the same. **Convulsions** specifically refer to involuntary, violent spasms of the large skeletal muscles of the face, neck, arms, and legs. Although some types of seizures do indeed involve convulsions, other seizures do not. Thus, it may be stated that all convulsions are seizures, but not all seizures are convulsions. Because of this difference, agents used to treat epilepsy are often referred to as antiseizure medications, rather than anticonvulsants.

Fast Facts Disorders Associated with Seizures

- Close to 2 million Americans have epilepsy.
- Most patients with epilepsy are younger than age 45.
- One of every 100 teenagers has epilepsy.
- Of the U.S. population, 10% will have a seizure within their lifetimes.
- About 10% of Patients with alcohol dependency have problems with seizures.
- About 400,000 of adult alcoholics going to the emergency room with withdrawal complaints, 60% have seizures within 6 hours after arrival.

FIGURE 11.1

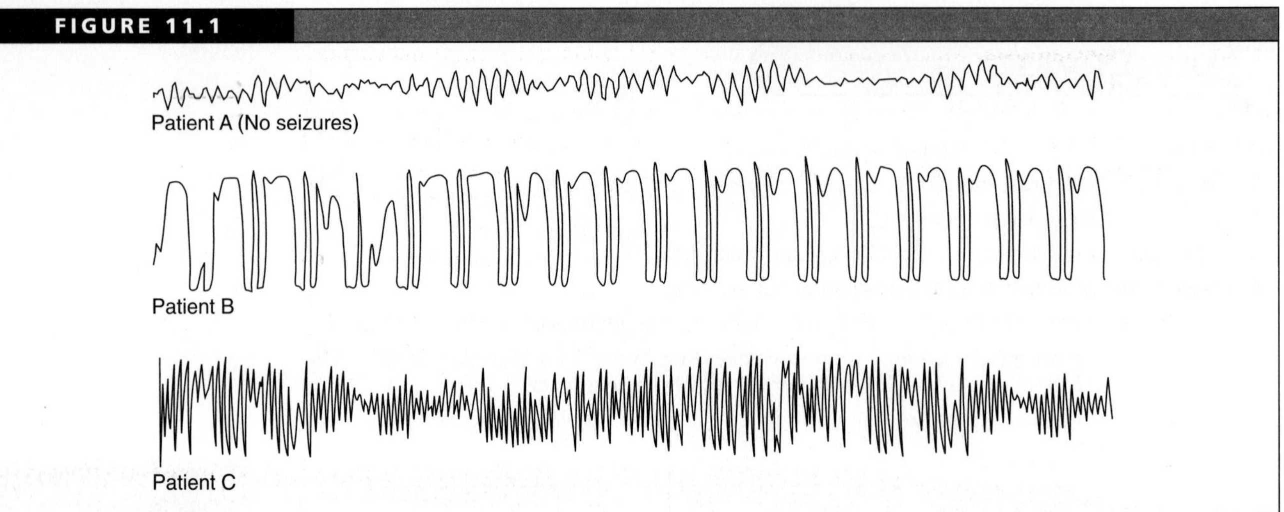

Neurons produce tiny impulses when they communicate. These impulses may be detected by an electroencephalogram (EEG), a device that captures brain-wave activity. Brain waves have characteristic patterns termed *alpha, beta, delta,* and *theta.* Although interpretation of brain waves is a complex art, you can see from these examples that the EEG tracings of patients B and C are dramatically different from those of patient A, who has no seizures. Alpha waves are the predominant waveform observed in patients with normal brain activity.

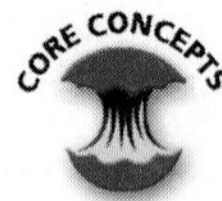

11.2 Many causes of seizure activity are known; a few are not.

A seizure is considered a symptom of an underlying disorder, rather than a disease in itself. There are many different causes of seizure activity. Seizures can result from acute situations or occur on a chronic basis, as with epilepsy. In some cases, the exact cause may not be identified.

The following are known causes of seizures:

- *Infectious diseases.* Acute infections such as meningitis and encephalitis can cause inflammation in the brain.
- *Trauma.* Physical trauma, such as direct blows to the skull, may increase intracranial pressure; chemical trauma, such as the presence of toxic substances or the ingestion of poisons, may cause brain injury.
- *Metabolic disorders.* Changes in fluid and electrolytes such as hypoglycemia, hyponatremia, and water intoxication may cause seizures by altering electrical impulse transmission at the cellular level.
- *Vascular diseases.* Changes in oxygenation—for example, caused by respiratory hypoxia and carbon monoxide poisoning—and changes in perfusion such as that caused by hypotension, cerebral vascular accidents, shock, and cardiac dysrhythmias may be causes.
- *Pediatric disorders.* Rapid increase in body temperature may result in a febrile (occuring during fever) seizure.
- *Neoplastic disease.* Tumors, especially rapidly growing ones, may occupy space, increase intracranial pressure, and damage brain tissue by disrupting blood flow.

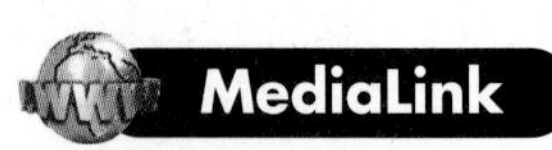

NATIONAL INSTITUTE ON ALCOHOL ABUSE AND ALCOHOLISM (NIAAA)

When given in high doses, certain medications for mood disorders, psychoses, and local anesthesia may cause seizures because of altered levels of neurotransmitters. Seizures may also occur from drug abuse, as with cocaine, or during withdrawal syndromes from alcohol or sedative-hypnotic drugs.

Pregnancy is a major concern for patients with epilepsy. Additional barrier methods of birth control might be considered to avoid unintended pregnancy because some antiseizure medications decrease the effectiveness of oral contraceptives. Most antiseizure drugs are pregnancy category D. Women should consult with their healthcare provider prior to pregnancy to determine the most appropriate plan of action for seizure control, given their seizure history. Because some antiseizure drugs may cause folate (vitamin-B complex) deficiency—a condition linked to increased risks of neural tube defects—vitamin supplements may be necessary. Pregnant women may experience coma and convulsive seizures with **eclampsia,** a pregnancy-caused disorder resulting from **pre-eclampsia,** which is characterized by hypertension, headaches, and edema of the lower extremities.

pre = *before*
ec = *out*
lamp(s) = *to shine*
ia = *condition of*

In some cases, the cause of seizure activity cannot be found. Patients may have a low tolerance to environmental triggers, and seizures may occur when they are sleep deprived, exposed to strobe or flickering lights, or when small fluid and electrolyte imbalances occur. Seizures represent the most common serious neurological problem affecting children, with an overall incidence approaching 2% for febrile seizures and 1% for epilepsy with a clear cause. Seizures resulting from one-time serious events generally do not reoccur after the situation has been resolved. However, if a brain abnormality exists after such a situation resolves, then continuing seizures are likely.

Seizures can have a significant impact on quality of life. They may cause serious injury if they occur while a person is driving a vehicle or performing a dangerous activity. Without pharmacotherapy, epilepsy can severely limit participation in school, employment, and social activities and affect self-esteem. Chronic depression may accompany poorly controlled seizures. Proper treatment, however, can eliminate seizures completely in many patients. Important considerations include identifying patients at risk for seizures, documenting the pattern and type of seizure activity, and implementing safety precautions. In collaboration with the patient, healthcare provider, and pharmacist, the healthcare worker is instrumental in achieving positive therapeutic outcomes. Through a combination of pharmacotherapy, patient-family support, and education, effective seizure control can be achieved by most patients.

11.3 Epileptic seizures are typically identified as partial, generalized, and special epileptic syndromes.

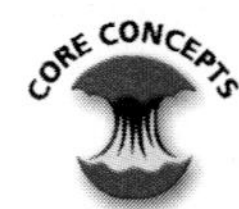

Seizure symptoms vary depending on the areas of the brain affected by the abnormal electrical activity. These symptoms can range from sudden, violent shaking and total loss of consciousness to muscle twitching or slight tremor (shaking) of a limb. Staring into space, altered vision, and difficult speech are other behaviors a person may exhibit during a seizure. Determining the cause of recurrent seizures is important to plan for appropriate treatment options.

Life Span Fact

Onset of epilepsy is most common among the youngest and oldest age groups. About 50% of children have a generalized epilepsy syndrome compared with about 20% of adults. The incidence of epilepsy in elderly adults is greater than among the general population, perhaps because of the greater prevalence of mild strokes and cardiac arrest in this age group.

Methods of classifying epilepsy have evolved over time. The terms *grand mal* and *petit mal* epilepsy, for the most part, have been replaced by more descriptive and detailed categorization. Epilepsies are typically identified using the International Classification of Epileptic Seizures nomenclature, as *partial (focal), generalized,* and *special epileptic syndromes.* Types of partial or generalized seizures may be recognized based on symptoms observed during a seizure episode. Some symptoms are hard to notice and reflect the simple nature of neuronal misfiring in specific areas of the brain; others are more complex.

Partial Seizures

Partial (focal) seizures involve a limited portion of the brain. They may start on one side and travel only a short distance before they stop. The area where the abnormal electrical activity starts is known as an abnormal *focus* (plural, *foci*).

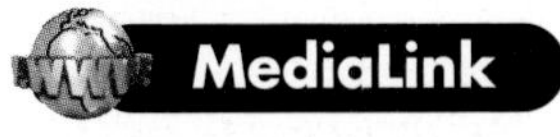

SEIZURE TYPES BY AGE GROUP

Simple partial seizures have an onset that may begin as a small, limited focus, that progress to a generalized seizure. Patients with simple partial seizures may feel for a brief moment that their precise location is vague, and they may hear and see things that are not there. Some patients smell and taste things that are not present, or have an upset stomach. Others may become emotional and experience a sense of joy, sorrow, or grief. The arms, legs, or face may twitch.

Complex partial seizures (formerly known as *psychomotor* or *temporal lobe seizures*) show sensory, motor, or autonomic symptoms, with some degree of altered or impaired consciousness. Total loss of consciousness may not occur during a complex partial seizure, but a brief period of somnolence or confusion may follow the seizure. Such seizures are often preceded by an *aura* that is sometimes described as an unpleasant odor or taste. Seizures may start with a blank stare, and patients may begin to chew or swallow repetitively. Some patients fumble with clothing; others may try to take off their clothes. Most patients will not pay attention to verbal commands and will act as if they are having a psychotic episode. After a seizure, patients do not remember the seizure incident.

Generalized Seizures

As the name suggests, **generalized seizures** are not localized to one area but travel throughout the entire brain on both sides. The seizure is thought to originate bilaterally and symmetrically within the brain.

bi = *two*
lateral = *sides*

sym = *same*
metrically = *measurement*

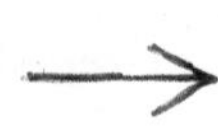

Absence seizures (formerly known as *petit mal seizures*) most often occur in children and last only a few seconds. Absence seizures involve a loss or reduction of normal activity. Staring and temporary loss of responsiveness are the most common signs, but there may be slight motor activity with eyelid fluttering or myoclonic jerks. Because these episodes are hard to detect and only last a few seconds, absence epilepsy may go unrecognized for a long time or be mistaken for daydreaming or attention deficit disorder.

a = *without*
tonic = *tension*

Atonic seizures are sometimes called *drop attacks,* because patients often stumble and fall for no apparent reason. Episodes are very short, lasting only a matter of seconds.

Tonic-clonic seizures (formerly known as *grand mal seizures*) are the most common type of seizure in all age groups. Seizures may be preceded by an aura, a warning that some patients describe as a spiritual feeling, a flash of light, or a special noise. Intense muscle contractions indicate the tonic phase. A hoarse cry may occur at the onset of the seizure due to air being forced out of the lungs, and patients may temporarily lose bladder or bowel control. Breathing may become shallow and even stop momentarily. The clonic phase is characterized by alternating contraction and relaxation of muscles. The seizure usually lasts 1 to 2 minutes, after which the patient becomes drowsy, disoriented, and sleeps deeply.

Life Span Fact

Preventing the onset of high fever is the best way to control febrile seizures in children.

Special Epileptic Syndromes

Special epileptic seizures include the febrile seizures of infancy, reflex epilepsies, and other forms of myoclonic epilepsies. Myoclonic epilepsies often go along with other neurological abnormalities or progressively debilitating symptoms.

febrile = *fever*

Febrile seizures typically cause tonic-clonic motor activity lasting 1 or 2 minutes with rapid return of consciousness. These occur together with a rapid rise in body temperature and usually occur only once during any given illness. Febrile seizures are most likely to occur in the 3-month to 5-year age group. As many as 5% of all children experience febrile seizures.

myo = *muscle*
clonic = *jerking motion*

Myoclonic seizures are characterized by large, jerking body movements. Major muscle groups contract quickly, and patients appear unsteady and clumsy. They may fall from a sitting position or drop whatever they are holding. *Infantile spasms* are an example of a type of generalized, myoclonic seizure and are distinguished by short-lasting muscle spasms in the trunk and extremities. Such spasms are often not identified as seizures by parents or healthcare providers because the movements are much like the normal infantile startle reflex.

status = *state of*
epilepticus = *seizure activity*

Status epilepticus is a medical emergency that occurs when a seizure is repeated continuously. It could occur with any type of seizure, but usually generalized tonic-clonic seizures are seen. When generalized tonic-clonic seizures last long or are continuous, the time in which breathing is affected by muscle contraction is lengthened and hypoxia may develop. The continuous muscle contraction also can lead to hypoglycemia, acidosis, and hypothermia due to increased metabolic needs, lactic acid production, and heat loss during contraction. Carbon dioxide retention also leads to acidosis. If not treated, status epilepticus could lead to brain damage and death. Medical treatment involves the IV administration of antiseizure medications. Steps must also be taken to ensure that the airway remains open.

Concept Review 11.1

- What is epilepsy? What is the difference between a seizure and a convulsion? Name and identify signs of the more common types of seizures.

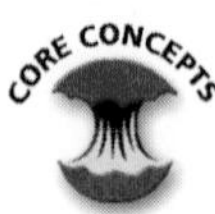

11.4 Effective seizure management involves strict adherence to drug therapy.

The choice of drug for epilepsy pharmacotherapy depends on the type of seizures the patient is experiencing, the patient's previous medical history, diagnostic studies, and the pathological processes causing the seizures. Once a medication is selected, the patient is placed on a low initial dose. The amount is gradually increased until seizure control is achieved, or the side effects of the drug prevent additional increases in dose. Blood levels of the drug may be checked to assist the healthcare provider in determining the most effective drug concentration. If seizure activity continues, a different medication is added in small doses while the dose of the first drug is slowly reduced. Because seizures are likely to occur with abrupt withdrawal, antiseizure medication is withdrawn over a period of 6 to 12 weeks.

TABLE 11.1 Drugs Used for the Management of Specific Types of Seizures

		GENERALIZED SEIZURES			
		Absence, Atonic			Tonic-clonic
	Partial Seizures		Special Epileptic Syndromes		
	Simple or Complex		Febrile Seizures	Myoclonic Seizures	Status Epilepticus
BARBITURATE					
phenobarbital (Luminal)	✓		✓	✓	✓
BENZODIAZEPINES					
diazepam (Valium)	✓		✓	✓	✓
lorazepam (Ativan)	✓			✓	✓
HYDANTOINS (PHENYTOIN-LIKE)					
phenytoin (Dilantin)	✓				✓
carbamazepine (Tegretol)	✓				✓
valproic acid (Depakene)	✓	✓	✓	✓	✓
SUCCINIMIDE					
ethosuximide (Zarontin)		✓		✓	

In most cases, a single drug effectively manages seizures. In some patients, two antiseizure medications may be needed to control seizure activity, although additional side effects may then occur. Some antiseizure drug combinations may actually increase the incidence of seizures.

Once seizures have been controlled, patients are continued indefinitely on the antiseizure drug. After several years of being seizure free, patients may question the need for their medication. In general, withdrawal of antiseizure drugs should only be attempted after at least 3 years of being seizure free, and only under the close observation and direction of the healthcare provider. Doses of medications are reduced slowly, one at a time, over a period of several months. If seizures reoccur during the withdrawal process, pharmacotherapy is resumed, usually with the same drug. Table 11.1 (above) shows common antiseizure drugs, based on the type of seizure.

Concept Review 11.2

- Give the names of seven traditional drugs used for the management of specific seizure types. Match the drugs with the types of seizures they best control. Which one of these drugs is used for a broader range of seizures than the others?

11.5 The goal of antiseizure drug therapy is to suppress neuronal activity just enough to prevent abnormal or repetitive firing.

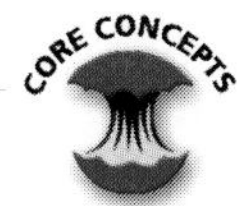

Antiseizure pharmacotherapy is designed to control the movement of electrolytes across neuronal membranes or affect neurotransmitter balance. In a resting state, neurons are normally surrounded by a higher concentration of sodium, calcium, and chloride ion. Potassium levels are higher inside the cell. An influx (flowing inward) of sodium or calcium into the neuron *enhances* neuronal activity, whereas an influx of chloride ion *suppresses* neuronal activity.

The goal of antiseizure pharmacotherapy is to suppress neuronal activity just enough to prevent abnormal or repetitive firing. To this end, there are three general mechanisms by which antiseizure drugs act:

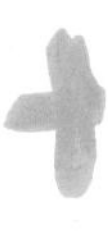

1. Stimulating an influx of chloride ions, an effect associated with the neurotransmitter *gamma-aminobutyric acid (GABA)*

2. Delaying an influx of sodium
3. Delaying an influx of calcium

Within these three *pharmacological* classes are at least four major *chemical* classes: benzodiazepines, barbiturates, hydantoins, and succinimides. A fifth category consists of miscellaneous drug types not related chemically to the four major classes. Because of the complexity of drug classification, it is best to cover antiseizure drugs as "drugs that increase GABA action," hydantoins and phenytoin-like drugs, and succinimides. (See Drug Snapshot at the beginning of this chapter.)

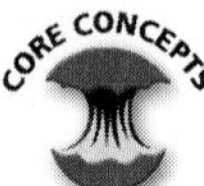

11.6 By increasing the effects of GABA in the brain, drugs reduce a wide range of seizure types.

Several important antiseizure drugs act by changing the action of GABA, the primary inhibitory neurotransmitter in the brain. These agents mimic the effects of GABA by stimulating an influx of chloride ions that interact with the GABA receptor–chloride channel molecule. A model of this receptor is shown in Figure 11.2 ■. When the receptor is stimulated, chloride ions move into the cell, thus suppressing the ability of neurons to fire.

Barbiturates, benzodiazepines, and several miscellaneous drugs reduce seizure activity by intensifying GABA action. The major effect of enhancing GABA activity is CNS depression. These agents are shown in Table 11.2.

As a class, barbiturates have a low margin of safety, cause serious CNS depression, and have a high potential for dependence. Phenobarbital, however, is able to suppress abnormal neuronal discharges without causing sedation. It is inexpensive, long acting, and usually produces few adverse effects. When given orally, it may take several weeks to achieve optimum antiseizure activity. The antiseizure properties of phenobarbital were discovered in 1912, and the drug is still one of the most commonly prescribed for epilepsy.

Other barbiturates are occasionally used for epilepsy. Mephobarbital (Mebaral) is converted to phenobarbital in the liver, and offers no significant advantages over phenobarbital. Amobarbital (Amytal) is an intermediate-acting barbiturate that is given IM or IV to terminate status epilepticus. Unlike phenobarbital, which is a Schedule IV drug, amobarbital is a Schedule II drug and has a higher risk for dependence; it is not given orally as an antiseizure drug.

Like barbiturates, benzodiazepines intensify the effect of GABA in the brain. The benzodiazepines bind to the GABA receptor directly, suppressing abnormal neuronal foci. Benzodiazepines

FIGURE 11.2

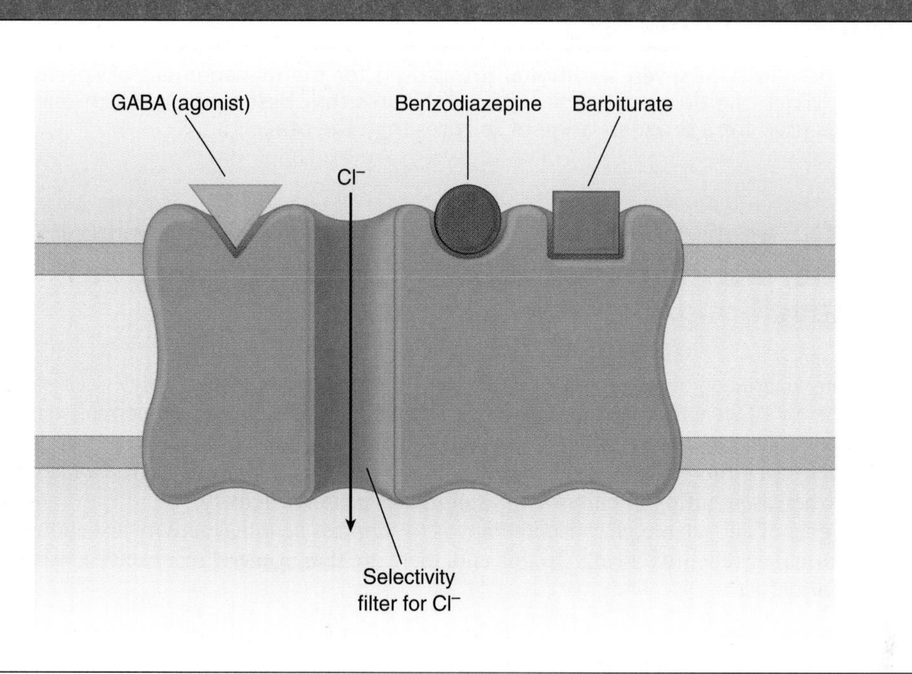

Model of the GABA receptor channel. The chloride selectivity filter allows the channel to open exclusively to chloride ions when GABA agents, benzodiazepines, or barbiturates bind to the cellular receptor (shown in blue). After the influx of chloride ions, the net result is inhibition of the nervous impulse or action potential.

TABLE 11.2 Antiseizure Drugs that Potentiate GABA Action

DRUG	ROUTE AND ADULT DOSE	REMARKS
BARBITURATES		
amobarbital (Amytal)	IV 65–500 mg (max: 1 g)	For control of status epilepticus or acute convulsive episodes; also for insomnia and preoperative sedation; Schedule IV drug
pentobarbital (Nembutal)	PO/IM 150–200 mg in 2 divided doses; IV 100 mg, may increase to 500 mg if necessary	For emergency control of general seizure activity; also for insomnia and preoperative sedation; Schedule II drug
Pr phenobarbital (Luminal)	For seizures: PO 100–300 mg/day, IV/IM 200–600 mg up to 20 mg/kg For status epilepticus: IV 15–18 mg/kg in single or divided doses (max: 20 mg/kg)	For the management of tonic-clonic seizures, partial seizures, status epilepticus, and eclampsia; also for sedation; Schedule IV drug
secobarbital (Seconal)	IM/IV 5.5 mg/kg repeated q3–4h if necessary (IV infusion at less than 50 mg/15 sec)	For emergency control of seizure activity caused by conditions such as tetanus or poisons; also for insomnia and preoperative sedation; Schedule II drug
BENZODIAZEPINES		
clonazepam (Klonopin)	PO 1.5 mg/day in 3 divided doses, increased by 0.5–1 mg every 3 days until seizures are controlled	For absence (petit mal) seizures and minor motor seizures; also for panic disorder; Schedule IV drug
clorazepate dipotassium (Tranxene)	PO 7.5 mg tid	For partial seizures; also for anxiety; Schedule IV drug
Pr diazepam (Valium)	IM/IV 5–10 mg (repeat as needed at 10–15 min intervals up to 30 mg; repeat again as needed every 2–4 hr); IV push, administer emulsion at 5 mg/min	Drug of choice for status epilepticus; also for anxiety and muscle spasms
lorazepam (Ativan)	IV 4 mg injected slowly at 2 mg/min; if inadequate response after 10 min, may repeat once	Most potent of the available benzodiazepines; for management of status epilepticus; also for nausea and vomiting, preoperative sedation, anxiety, and insomnia; Schedule IV drug
MISCELLANEOUS		
gabapentin (Neurontin)	For additional therapy: PO start with 300 mg on day 1, 300 mg bid on day 2, 300 mg tid on day 3, continue to increase over 1 week to a dose of 1200 mg/day (400 mg tid); may increase to 1800–2400 mg/day	Chemical structure similar to GABA; speeds up the release of GABA from brain neurons; used for partial seizures or seizures that could become generalized
primidone (Mysoline)	PO 250 mg/day, increase by 250 mg/week up to max of 2 g in 2–4 divided doses	Produces an action similar to barbiturates; used in combination with other anticonvulsant agents; for complex partial and generalized tonic-clonic seizures
tiagabine (Gabatril)	PO start with 4 mg/day, may increase by 4–8 mg/day every week up to 56 mg/day in 2–4 divided doses	Inhibits uptake of GABA into presynaptic neurons, prolonging GABA action; for the treatment of partial seizures
topiramate (Topamax)	PO start with 50 mg/day, increase by 50 mg/week to effectiveness (max: 1600 mg/day)	Sugarlike chemical molecule; enhances the action of GABA; for partial seizures
trimethadione (Tridone)	PO start with 300 mg tid, may increase by 300 mg every week until seizures are controlled (max: 2400 mg/day taken in 3–4 doses)	Used to treat absence (petit mal) seizures when other antiseizure medications are not effective

DRUG PROFILE: Barbiturate: Pr *Phenobarbital (Luminal)*

Actions and Uses:

Phenobarbital is a long-acting barbiturate, used for the management of a variety of seizures. It is also used for insomnia. Phenobarbital should not be used for pain relief, as it may increase a patient's sensitivity to pain.

Phenobarbital acts biochemically in the brain by enhancing the action of the neurotransmitter GABA, which is responsible for suppressing abnormal neuronal discharges that can cause epilepsy.

Adverse Effects and Interactions:

Phenobarbital is a Schedule IV drug that may cause dependence. Common side effects include drowsiness, vitamin deficiencies (vitamin D, folate, B_9 and B_{12}), and laryngospasms. With overdose, phenobarbital may cause severe respiratory depression, CNS depression, coma, and death. Phenobarbital is a pregnancy category D drug.

Phenobarbital interacts with many other drugs. For example, it should not be taken with alcohol or other CNS depressants. These substances potentiate the action of barbiturates, increasing the risk of life-threatening respiratory depression or cardiac arrest. Phenobarbital increases the metabolism of many other drugs, reducing their effectiveness.

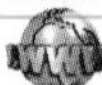
See the Companion Website for a Nursing Process Focus specific to this drug.

DRUG PROFILE: Benzodiazepine: Pr *Diazepam (Valium)*

Actions and Uses:

Diazepam binds to the GABA receptor–chloride channels throughout the CNS. It produces its effects by suppressing neuronal activity in the limbic system and subsequent impulses that might be transmitted to the reticular activating system. Effects of this drug are suppression of abnormal neuronal foci that may cause seizures, calming without strong sedation, and skeletal muscle relaxation. When used orally, maximum therapeutic effects may take from 1 to 2 weeks. Tolerance may develop after about 4 weeks. When given IV, effects occur in minutes and its anticonvulsant effects last about 20 minutes.

Adverse Effects and Interactions:

Diazepam should not be taken with alcohol or other CNS depressants because of combined sedation effects. Other drug interactions include cimetidine, oral contraceptives, valproic acid, and metoprolol, which potentiate diazepam's action; and levodopa and barbiturates, which decrease diazepam's action. Diazepam increases the levels of phenytoin in the bloodstream, and may cause phenytoin toxicity. When given IV, hypotension, muscular weakness, tachycardia, and respiratory depression and are common. Because of tolerance and dependency, use of diazepam is reserved for short-term seizure control, or for status epilepticus.

Use with caution with herbal supplements, such as kava and chamomile, which may cause an increased effect.

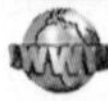
See the Companion Website for a Nursing Process Focus specific to this drug.

used in treating epilepsy include clonazepam (Klonopin), clorazepate (Tranxene), lorazepam (Ativan), and diazepam (Valium). Indications include absence seizures and myoclonic seizures. Parenteral diazepam is used to terminate status epilepticus. Because tolerance may begin to develop after only a few months of therapy with benzodiazepines, seizures may reoccur unless the dose is periodically adjusted. These agents are generally not used alone in seizure pharmacotherapy but instead serve as add-ons to other antiseizure drugs for short-term seizure control.

The benzodiazepines are one of the most widely prescribed classes of drugs, used not only to control seizures but also for the treatment of anxiety, skeletal muscle spasms, and alcohol withdrawal symptoms.

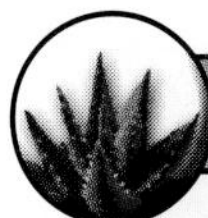

NATURAL ALTERNATIVES

Scullcap (Skullcap) for Epilepsy

Scullcap (Skullcap), also called *mad-dog weed, helmet flower,* or *madweed,* is a wet ground herb of swampy origin found in the eastern part of North America, from Florida to British Columbia to Ontario. Its scientific name is *Sculellaria laterifolia;* a closely related species called *Sculellaria glaericulata* may be found in temperate zones of Britain and most of Europe.

This herb has been used centuries as a nervous system relaxant. It has many of the antianxiety effects of the benzodiazepines and the sedative properties of the barbiturates. Chemical elements of this herb bind to the GABA receptor–chloride channel molecule. Scullcap is known for its treatment of epilepsy and for its ability to soothe nervous excitement or to cause sleep. It may also produce a calming effect in disorders such as depression, bipolar disorder, muscle pain, and inflammation. ▪

Several nonbenzodiazepine, nonbarbiturate agents act to suppress seizure activity by either directly activating the GABA receptor or enhancing the effect of the naturally occurring GABA neurotransmitter. Examples of these newer drugs, first approved by the FDA in the 1990s, are gabapentin (Neurontin) and tiagabine (Gabatril).

Although it is technically classified an *oxazolidinedione,* trimethadione (Tridone) is placed in this section because of its miscellaneous nature. It is the only drug in its class and is occasionally used for the treatment of absence seizures.

11.7 Hydantoin and phenytoin-like drugs are generally effective in treating partial seizures and tonic-clonic seizures.

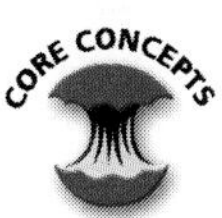

Hydantoins and phenytoin-like drugs dampen CNS activity by delaying an influx of sodium ions across neuronal membranes. Hydantoins and several other related antiseizure drugs act by this mechanism.

Sodium channels guide the movement of sodium across neuronal membranes into the intracellular space. Sodium movement is the major factor that determines whether a neuron will undergo an **action potential.** If these channels are temporarily inactivated, neuronal activity will be suppressed. With hydantoin and phenytoin-like drugs (Table 11.3), sodium channels are not blocked; they are just made to be less sensitive. If channels are blocked, neuronal activity completely stops, as occurs with local anesthetic drugs (see Chapter 12).

The oldest and most prescribed hydantoin is phenytoin (Dilantin). Approved in the 1930s, phenytoin is a broad-spectrum drug that is useful in treating all types of epilepsy except absence seizures. It is able to provide effective seizure suppression, without the CNS depression or potential for abuse associated with barbiturates. Patients vary significantly in their ability to metabolize phenytoin; therefore, dosages must be individualized. Phenytoin has a *narrow therapeutic range,* or *index*—meaning that the difference between a therapeutic and a toxic dose is very small. Therefore, patients taking phenytoin must be carefully monitored. The other hydantoins are used much less frequently than phenytoin.

Several widely used drugs share a mechanism of action similar to the hydantoins, including carbamezepine (Tegretol) and valproic acid (Depakene, Depakote, Epivil), which is also available as divalproex sodium or valproate. Carbamazepine is a drug of choice for tonic-clonic and partial seizures because it produces fewer adverse effects than phenytoin or phenobarbital. Valproic acid is a drug of choice for absence seizures. Both carbamazepine and valproic acid are also used for bipolar disorder (see Chapter 9). Newer antiseizure drugs, which have more limited uses, include zonisamide (Zonegran), felbamate (Felbatol), and lamotrigine (Lamictal).

11.8 Succinimides generally treat absence seizures.

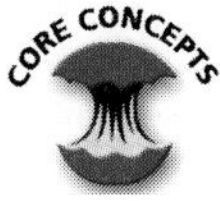

Several types of calcium channels guide the movement of calcium into and out of cells. Many factors determine calcium movement, including a change in voltage across cellular membranes, the binding of natural neurotransmitters, hormones, and drugs. Calcium influx is necessary for neuronal impulse transmission.

TABLE 11.3 Hydantoins and Phenytoin-like Drugs

DRUG	ROUTE AND ADULT DOSE	REMARKS
HYDANTOINS		
fosphenytoin sodium (Cerebyx)	IV initial dose 15–20 mg PE/kg at 100–150 mg PE/min followed by 4–6 mg PE/kg/d (PE = phenytoin equivalents)	Converted to phenytoin in the body; for control of status epilepticus; short-term substitute for oral phenytoin
Pr phenytoin (Dilantin)	PO 15–18 mg/kg or 1 g initial dose, then 300 mg/day in 1–3 divided doses; may be gradually increased 100 mg/week	For tonic-clonic seizures, psychomotor seizures, and seizures after head trauma
PHENYTOIN-LIKE AGENTS		
carbamazepine (Tegretol)	PO 200 mg bid, gradually increased to 800–1200 mg/day in 3–4 divided doses	For grand mal and psychomotor seizures; useful in trigeminal neuralgia (condition characterized by intense pain along the angle of the jaw); also for manic-depressive disorder
felbamate (Felbatol)	Lennox-Gastaut syndrome: PO start at 15 mg/kg/day in 3–4 divided doses; may increase 15 mg/kg at weekly intervals to max of 45 mg/kg/day Partial seizures: PO start with 1200 mg/day in 3–4 divided doses; may increase by 600 mg/day every 2 weeks (max: 3600 mg/day)	For use in Lennox-Gastaut syndrome and partial seizures
lamotrigine (Lamictal)	PO 50 mg/day for 2 weeks, then 50 mg bid for 2 weeks; may increase gradually up to 300–500 mg/day in 2 divided doses (max: 700 mg/day)	For partial seizures, generalized tonic-clonic seizures, and myoclonic seizures
Pr valproic acid (Depakene)	PO/IV 15 mg/kg/day in divided doses when total daily dose is greater than 250 mg; increase 5–10 mg every week until seizures are controlled (max: 60 mg/kg/day)	Unrelated to most other antiseizure drugs; for absence seizures and mixed generalized types of seizures
zonisamide (Zonegran)	PO 100–400 mg/day	Broad-spectrum medication; newer drug for partial seizures; it is a sulfonamide, which means that it may cause an allergic reaction in some clients

succin = *chemical with two –CO groups*
imide = *chemical with one = NH group*

Succinimides delay the entry of calcium into neurons by blocking calcium channels. Simply, antiseizure drugs of this group increase the *electrical threshold*—that is, the excitable level at which there is no turning back: The neuron must fire. If the electrical threshold is increased, the possibility of abnormal firing decreases and seizures are less likely to occur.

Ethosuximide (Zarontin) is the most commonly prescribed drug in this class (Table 11.4). It remains a drug of choice for absence seizures. Valproic acid is also effective for these types of seizures. Some of the newer antiseizure agents, such as lamotrigine (Lamictal) and zonisamide (Zonegran), are being investigated for their roles in treating absence seizures.

TABLE 11.4 Succinimides

DRUG	ROUTE AND ADULT DOSE	REMARKS
Pr ethosuximide (Zarontin)	PO 250 mg bid, increased every 4–7 days (max: 1.5 g/day)	For absence seizures, myoclonic seizures, and akinetic epilepsy
methsuximide (Celontin)	PO 300 mg/day, may increase every 4–7 days (max: 1.2 g/day in divided doses)	For absence seizures; may be used in combination with other anticonvulsants in mixed types of seizure activity
phensuximide (Milontin)	PO 0.5–1 g bid or tid	For absence seizures; similar characteristics to methsuximide

DRUG PROFILE: Hydantoin: Pr *Phenytoin (Dilantin)*

Actions and Uses:

Phenytoin acts by desensitizing sodium channels in the CNS responsible for neuronal responsivity. Desensitization prevents the spread of disruptive electrical charges in the brain that produce seizures. It is effective against most types of seizures except absence seizures. Phenytoin has antidysrhythmic activity similar to lidocaine (class IB). An unlabeled use is for digitalis-induced dysrhythmias.

Adverse Effects and Interactions:

Phenytoin may cause dysrhythmias, such as bradycardia or ventricular fibrillation, severe hypotension and hyperglycemia. Severe CNS reactions include headache, nystagmus, ataxia, confusion and slurred speech, paradoxical nervousness, twitching, and insomnia. Peripheral neuropathy may occur with long-term use. Phenytoin can cause multiple blood dyscrasias, including agranulocytosis and aplastic anemia. It may cause severe skin reactions, such as rashes, including exfoliative dermatitis, and Stevens-Johnson syndrome. Connective tissue reactions include lupus erythematosa, hypertrichosis, hirsutism, and gingival hypertrophy.

Phenytoin interacts with many other drugs, including oral anticoagulants, glucocorticoids, H_2 antagonists, antituberculin agents, and food supplements such as folic acid, calcium, and vitamin D. It impairs the effectiveness of drugs such as digitoxin, doxycycline, furosemide, estrogens and oral contraceptives, and theophylline. Phenytoin, when combined with tricyclic antidepressants, can trigger seizures.

Use with caution with herbal supplements, such as herbal laxatives (buckthorn, cascara sagrada, and senna), which may increase potassium loss.

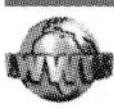
See the Companion Website for a Nursing Process Focus specific to this drug.

DRUG PROFILE: Phenytoin-Like Drug: Pr *Valproic Acid (Depakene)*

Actions and Uses:

The mechanism of action of valproic acid is the same as phenytoin, although effects on GABA and calcium channels may cause some additional actions. It is useful for a wide range of seizure types, including absence seizures and mixed types of seizures. Other uses include prevention of migraine headaches and treatment of bipolar disorder.

Adverse Effects and Interactions:

Side effects include sedation, drowsiness, GI upset, and prolonged bleeding time. Other effects include visual disturbances, muscle weakness, tremor, psychomotor agitation, bone marrow suppression, weight gain, abdominal cramps, rash, alopecia, pruritus, photosensitivity, erythema multiforme, and fatal hepatotoxicity.

Valproic acid interacts with many drugs. For example, aspirin, cimetidine, chlorpromazine, erythromycin, and felbamate may increase valproic acid toxicity. Concomitant warfarin, aspirin, or alcohol use can cause severe bleeding. Alcohol, benzodiazepines, and other CNS depressants potentiate CNS depressant action. Lamotrigine, phenytoin, and rifampin lower valproic acid levels. Valproic acid increases serum phenobarbital and phenytoin levels. Use of clonazepam concurrently with valproic acid may induce absence seizures.

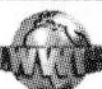
See the Companion Website for a Nursing Process Focus specific to this drug.

Concept Review 11.3

- Name three major pharmacological categories and at least four chemical categories of antiseizure medication. Which drug examples do not conveniently fit into only one drug class, and why not?

DRUG PROFILE: Succinimide: 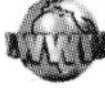 *Ethosuximide (Zarontin)*

Actions and Uses:

Ethosuximide is a drug of choice for absence (petit mal) seizures. It depresses the activity of neurons in the motor cortex by elevating the neuronal threshold. It is usually ineffective against psychomotor or tonic-clonic seizures; however, it may be given in combination with other medications, which better treat these conditions. It is available in tablet and flavored syrup formulations.

Adverse Effects and Interactions:

Ethosuximide may impair mental and physical abilities. Psychosis or extreme mood swings, including depression with suicidal intent, can occur. Behavioral changes are more prominent in patients with a history of psychiatric illness. Central nervous system effects include dizziness, headache, lethargy, fatigue, ataxia, sleep pattern disturbances, attention difficulty, and hiccups. Bone marrow suppression and blood dyscrasias are possible, as is systemic lupus erythematosus.

Other reactions include gingival hypertrophy and tongue swelling. Common side effects are abdominal distress and weight loss.

Drug interactions include ethosuximide, which increases phenytoin serum levels. Valproic acid causes ethosuximide serum levels to fluctuate (increase or decrease).

See the Companion Website for a Nursing Process Focus specific to this drug.

NURSING PROCESS FOCUS

Patients Receiving Antiseizure Drug Therapy

ASSESSMENT

Prior to administration:

- Obtain complete health history including allergies and drug history, to determine possible drug interactions
- Assess neurological status, including identification of recent seizure activity
- Assess growth and development

POTENTIAL NURSING DIAGNOSES

- Risk for Injury, related to drug side effects
- Deficient Knowledge, related to drug therapy
- Noncompliance

PLANNING: Patient Goals and Outcomes

The patient will:

- Experience the absence of, or a reduction in the number or severity of, seizures
- Avoid physical injury related to seizure activity or medication-induced sensory changes
- Demonstrate an understanding of the drug's action by accurately describing drug effects and precautions

continued...

NURSING PROCESS FOCUS

IMPLEMENTATION

Interventions and (Rationales)	Patient Education/Discharge Planning
■ Monitor neurological status, especially changes in level of consciousness and/or mental status. (Sedation may indicate impending toxicity.)	Instruct the patient to: ■ Report any significant change in sensorium, such as slurred speech, confusion, hallucinations, or lethargy ■ Report any changes in seizure quality or unexpected involuntary muscle movement such as twitching, tremor, or unusual eye movement
■ Protect the patient from injury during seizure events until therapeutic effects of drugs are achieved.	■ Instruct patient to avoid driving and other hazardous activities until effects of the drug are known.
■ Monitor effectiveness of drug therapy. Observe for developmental changes, which may indicate a need for dose adjustment.	Instruct patient to: ■ Keep a seizure diary to chronicle symptoms phase, or during dose adjustment ■ Take the medication exactly as ordered, including the same manufacturer's drug each time the prescription is refilled (Switching brands may result in alterations in seizure control.) ■ Take a missed dose as soon as remembered, but do not take double doses (Doubling doses could result in toxic serum level.)
■ Monitor for adverse effects. Observe for hypersensitivity, nephrotoxicity, and hepatotoxicity.	■ Instruct patient to report side effects specific to drug regimen.
■ Monitor oral health. Observe for signs of gingival hypertrophy, bleeding, or inflammation (phenytoin-specific).	Instruct patient to: ■ Use a soft toothbrush and oral rinses as prescribed by the dentist ■ Avoid mouthwashes containing alcohol ■ Report changes in oral health such as excessive bleeding or inflammation of the gums ■ Maintain a regular schedule of dental visits
■ Monitor gastrointestinal status. (Valproic acid is a GI irritant and anticoagulant.) ■ Conduct guaiac stool testing for occult blood. (Phenytoin's CNS depressant effects decrease GI motility, producing constipation.)	Instruct patient to: ■ Take the drug with food to reduce GI upset ■ Immediately report any severe or persistent heartburn, upper GI pain, nausea, or vomiting ■ Increase exercise, fluid, and fiber intake to facilitate stool passage
■ Monitor nutritional status. (Phenytoin's action on electrolytes may cause decreased absorption of folic acid, vitamin D, magnesium, and calcium. Deficiencies in these vitamins and minerals lead to anemia and osteoporosis. Valproic acid may cause an increase in appetite and weight.)	■ Instruct patient in dietary or drug administration techniques specific to prescribed medications. ■ Instruct patient to report significant changes in appetite or weight gain.
■ Obtain information and monitor use of other medications. Antiseizure medications should not be used with CNS depressants or alcohol.	■ Instruct patient to report use of any medication to healthcare provider. ■ Inform patient not to drink alcohol while taking these medications.

EVALUATION OF OUTCOME CRITERIA

Evaluate effectiveness of drug therapy by confirming that patient goals and expected outcomes have been met (see "Planning").

See Table 11.4 for a list of drugs to which these nursing actions apply.

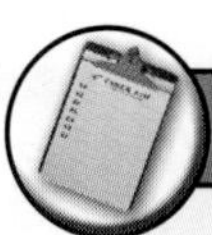

PATIENTS NEED TO KNOW

Patients taking antiseizure medications need to know the following:

In General

1. Never abruptly stop taking antiseizure medication; doing so can cause seizures.
2. Avoid alcohol and other CNS depressants because they can increase sedation.
3. Antiseizure medications may cause drowsiness; avoid driving and the use of machinery that could lead to injury.
4. It may require several dosage adjustments over many months to find the dosage that allows performance of normal daily activities while controlling seizures.
5. It is important to keep laboratory appointments because many antiseizure medications require blood testing to ensure that the drug is at a safe and effective level in the blood.
6. Consult a healthcare provider before trying to become pregnant; some antiseizure medications are not safe to use during pregnancy.
7. Report excess fatigue, drowsiness, agitation, or confusion to a healthcare practitioner.

Regarding Hydantoins

8. Report the following side effects to a healthcare provider: gum overgrowth (gingival hyperplasia) or skin rash, tremors, weight gain, diarrhea, irregular menses, dizziness, nausea, or oversedation.
9. Hydantoins interact with many other drugs; do not add any other prescription, OTC drugs, or herbal supplements until a healthcare provider is consulted. Do not consume alcohol while taking these medications.

Regarding Succinimides

10. Report the following side effects to a healthcare provider: hiccups or epigastric pain with ethosuximide (Zarontin), drowsiness, or increased bleeding time. ▪

CHAPTER REVIEW

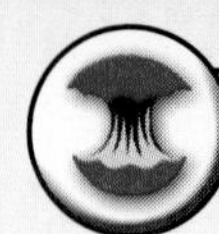

CORE CONCEPTS SUMMARY

11.1 All convulsions are seizures, but not all seizures are convulsions.

Epilepsy is any disorder characterized by recurrent seizures. *Seizures* are abnormal and uncontrolled neuronal brain discharges. *Convulsions* are uncontrolled muscle contractions that accompany some major seizures. Drugs used to treat epilepsy are often referred to as *antiseizure* medications, rather than anticonvulsants.

11.2 Many causes of seizure activity are known; a few are not.

A seizure is considered a symptom of epilepsy rather than a disorder itself. In some cases, the exact cause of seizures is not known; however, there are many known causes. Seizures are the most common neurological problem. Through a combination of pharmacotherapy, patient-family support, and education, effective seizure control can be achieved by most patients.

11.3 Epileptic seizures are typically identified as partial, generalized, and special epileptic syndromes.

Epilepsies are identified using the International Classification of Epileptic Seizures nomenclature, as partial (focal), generalized, and special epileptic syndromes. Partial seizures are further described as simple or complex seizures. Generalized seizures are described as absence seizures, atonic seizures, and tonic-clonic seizures. Special epileptic syndromes include febrile seizures, myoclonic seizures, and status epilepticus.

11.4 Effective seizure management involves strict adherence to drug therapy.

The choice of drug for epilepsy pharmacotherapy depends on the type of seizures the patient is experiencing, the patient's previous medical history, diagnostic studies, and the pathological processes causing the seizures. In most cases, a single drug can effectively manage seizures. In some patients, two antiseizure medications may be necessary.

11.5 The goal of antiseizure drug therapy is to suppress neuronal activity just enough to prevent abnormal or repetitive firing.

There are three general mechanisms by which antiseizure drugs act: stimulating an influx of chloride ion (an effect associated with the neurotransmitter GABA), delaying an influx of sodium, and delaying an influx of calcium. Antiseizure drugs are represented by at least four major chemical classes.

11.6 By increasing the effects of GABA in the brain, drugs reduce a wide range of seizure types.

Many antiseizure drugs mimic the effects of GABA by stimulating an influx of chloride ions that interact with the GABA receptor—chloride channel molecule. Barbiturates, benzodiazepines, and several miscellaneous drugs reduce seizure activity by intensifying GABA action.

11.7 Hydantoin and phenytoin-like drugs are generally effective in treating partial seizures and tonic-clonic seizures.

This class of drugs depresses CNS activity by delaying an influx of sodium ions across neuronal membranes. Several widely used drugs include phenytoin (Dilantin), carbamazepine (Tegretol), and valproic acid (Depakene, Depakote, Epivil).

11.8 Succinimides generally treat absence seizures.

Succinimides delay entry of calcium into neurons by blocking calcium channels, increasing the electrical threshold, and reducing the likelihood that an action potential will be generated. Ethosuximide (Zarontin) is the most commonly prescribed drug in this class.

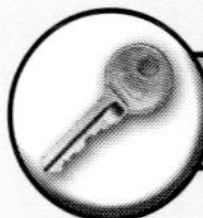

KEY TERMS

action potential (poh-TEN-shial): an electrical signal of a single cell (muscle or nerve) generated by the opening and closing of special ion channels located on the cell's membrane / ***page 183***

convulsions (kon-VULL-shuns): uncontrolled muscle contractions or spasms that occur in the face, torso, arms, or legs / ***page 175***

eclampsia (ee-KLAMP-see-uh): condition in which seizures and/or a coma develop in a patient with pre-eclampsia / ***page 177***

epilepsy (EPP-ih-lepp-see): disorder of the CNS characterized by seizures and/or convulsions / ***page 175***

generalized seizures: seizures that travel throughout the entire brain on both side / ***page 177***

partial (focal) seizures: seizures that start on one side of the brain and travel a short distance before stopping / ***page 177***

pre-eclampsia (pree-ee-KLAMP-see-uh): condition in which hypertension develops because of pregnancy or recent pregnancy. Hypertension is accompanied by proteinuria and/or edema / ***page 177***

seizure (SEE-zhurr): symptom of epilepsy characterized by abnormal neuronal discharges within the brain / ***page 175***

status epilepticus (ep-ih-LEP-tih-kus): condition characterized by repeated seizures / ***page 178***

REVIEW QUESTIONS

The following questions are written in NCLEX-PN® style. Answer these questions to assess your knowledge of the chapter material, and go back and review any material that is not clear to you.

1. Most antiseizure medications fall under which pregnancy category?

1. A
2. B
3. C
4. D

2. The patient on phenytoin (Dilantin) asks why he must have his labs checked. The nurse's best response would be:

1. "Dilantin can cause blood disorders."
2. "You will need to ask your doctor."
3. "We are checking to make sure you are getting enough but not too much medication."
4. "We must see if you are developing any side effects of the medication."

3. The patient on antiseizure medication wants to know how long he must take his medication before he is cured. The nurse's best response would be:

1. "You should be totally seizure free in 1 to 3 weeks."
2. "We may need to add additional medications before you are cured."
3. "It may take up to 3 years before you are cured."
4. "Seizures are not curable. The goal of therapy is to control seizure activity."

4. This drug, given parentally, is used to terminate status epilepticus.

1. Diazepam (Valium)
2. Gabapentin (Neurontin)
3. Clorazepate (Tranxene)
4. Clonazepam (Klonopin)

5. This phase of a seizure is characterized by alternating contractions and relaxation of the muscles.

1. Absence
2. Clonic
3. Febrile
4. Myoclonic

6. One of the most common side effects of antiseizure drugs is:

1. GI upset
2. Spasms
3. Drowsiness
4. Dry mouth

7. An overdose of this antiseizure drug may cause severe respiratory depression, CNS depression, coma, and death.

1. Clonazepam (Klonopin)
2. Lorazepam (Ativan)
3. Diazepam (Valium)
4. Phenobarbital (Luminal)

8. The nurse should assess the patient on ethosuximide (Zarontin) for which of the following?

1. Urinary dysfunction
2. Gingival hyperplasia
3. Tremors
4. Depression

9. The nurse must assess for gingival hyperplasia with this antiseizure medication.

1. Valproic acid (Depakene)
2. Carbamazepine (Tegretol)
3. Phenytoin (Dilantin)
4. Amobarbital (Amytal)

10. This antiseizure medication increases phenytoin serum levels.

1. Ethosuximide (Zarontin)
2. Phenobarbital (Luminal)
3. Carbamazepine (Tegretol)
4. Valproic acid (Depakene)

CASE STUDY QUESTIONS

For questions 1–4, please refer to the following case study, and choose the correct answer from choices 1–4.

Ms. Anthonia and her 9-year-old daughter, Leslie, recently visited the family physician. Ms. Anthonia was concerned that Leslie's development might be stunted. Several complaints were noted: "Leslie sometimes acts very unusual, like she is not paying attention . . . on occasion she is unresponsive and bats her eyes . . . this sometimes lasts for a few seconds and everything appears normal again . . . lately she has been waking up a lot during the night." During the interview, the physician discovered that Ms. Anthonia was taking medication for bipolar disorder. After a complete neurological exam and set of laboratory tests, the family physician prescribed ethosuximide (Zarontin) for Leslie to be taken in gradually increased doses over 7 days and then for a sustained period at the same dose. The physician then scheduled a return visit to the clinic in 7 days.

1. Which of the following is the most likely diagnosis for Leslie?

1. Bipolar disorder
2. Partial seizures
3. Absence seizures
4. Tonic-clonic seizures

2. The mechanism by which ethosuximide (Zarontin) will treat Leslie's condition is:

1. Enhanced release of GABA neurotransmitter
2. Desensitization of sodium channels located along neuronal membranes
3. Delayed entry of calcium into cortical neurons
4. Activation of the GABA receptor

3. Which of the following is the most likely reason for Leslie's return visit to the clinic?

1. Her medication has a high potential for dependence; Leslie's physician wants to reexamine her.
2. One of the adverse effects of Leslie's medication is anemia; this adverse effect will need to be determined.
3. Serum drug levels will be necessary to determine the most effective drug concentration.
4. Her medication has a low margin of safety; Leslie's physician just wants to be sure.

4. If one of the following medications were prescribed for Leslie as a second medication, which one would cause ethosuximide (Zarontin) serum levels to fluctuate?

1. Phenobarbital (Luminal)
2. Diazepam (Valium)
3. Phenytoin (Dilantin)
4. Valproic acid (Depakene)

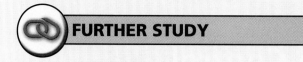

FURTHER STUDY

- Local anesthesia is discussed in Chapter 12.
- The use of the antiseizure medications carbamazepine and valproic acid for bipolar disorder is discussed in Chapter 9.

EXPLORE MEDIALINK www.prenhall.com/holland

Additional resources for this chapter can be found on the CD-ROM accompanying this textbook, and on the Companion Website. Click on Chapter 11 to select activities for this chapter.

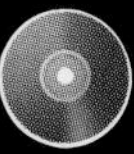

Audio Glossary
Concept Review
NCLEX-PN® Review
Nursing in Action
Dosage Calculator

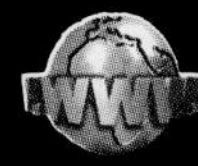

The Epilepsy Foundation of America (EFA)
National Institute of Neurological Disorders and Stroke (NINDS)
Epilepsy Canada
National Institute on Alcohol Abuse and Alcoholism (NIAAA)
Seizure Type by Age Group

CHAPTER

12 Drugs for Pain Control

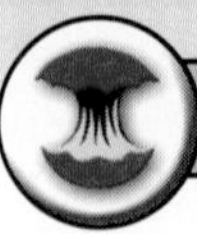

CORE CONCEPTS

12.1 Pain assessment is the first step to pain management.

12.2 Nonpharmacological techniques assist patients in obtaining adequate pain relief.

12.3 Pain transmission processes allow several targets for pharmacological intervention.

12.4 Opioid analgesic medications exert their effects by interacting with specific receptors.

12.5 Narcotic opioids have multiple therapeutic effects including relief of severe pain.

12.6 Nonsteroidal anti-inflammatory drugs are the drugs of choice for inflammatory pain.

12.7 Headaches can be effectively treated with a variety of drug classes.

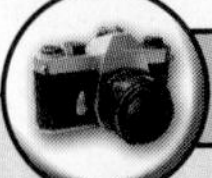

DRUG SNAPSHOT

The following drugs will be discussed in this chapter:

DRUG CLASSES	DRUG PROFILES
OPIOID (NARCOTIC) ANALGESICS	
Opioid agonists	Pr morphine (Astramorph, others)
Opioid antagonists	Pr naloxone (Narcan)
Opioids with mixed agonist–antagonist activity	
NONOPIOID ANALGESICS	
Nonsteroidal anti-inflammatory drugs (NSAIDs)	
Aspirin and other salicylates	Pr aspirin (Acetylsalicylic acid, ASA)
Ibuprofen and ibuprofen-like drugs	
Selective COX-2 inhibitors	
Acetaminophen	
Centrally acting drugs	
ANTIMIGRAINE AGENTS	
Triptans	Pr sumatriptan (Imitrex)
Ergot alkaloids	
Other antimigraine agents	

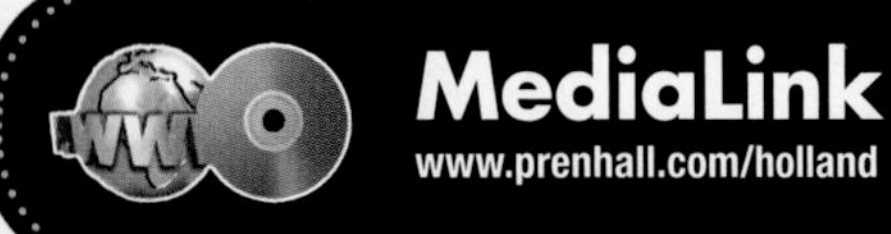

Interactive resources for this chapter can be found on the Companion Website. Click on Chapter 12 and "Begin" to select the activities for this chapter. For chapter-related animations, NCLEX-PN®-style questions, and an audio glossary, access the accompanying CD-ROM in this book.

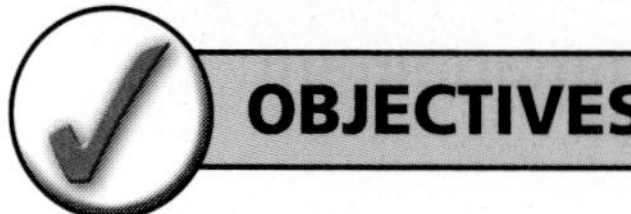

OBJECTIVES

After reading this chapter, the student should be able to:

1. Relate the importance of pain assessment to effective pharmacotherapy.
2. Explain the neural mechanism for pain at the level of the spinal cord.
3. Explain how pain can be controlled by inhibiting the release of spinal neurotransmitters.
4. Describe the role of nonpharmacological therapies in pain management.
5. Compare and contrast the types of opioid receptors and their importance to pharmacology.
6. Explain the role of opioid antagonists in the diagnosis and treatment of acute opioid toxicity.
7. Describe the long-term treatment of opioid dependence.
8. Compare the pharmacotherapeutic approaches of preventing migraines to those of aborting migraines.
9. For each of the major drug classes, know representative drug examples, and explain the mechanisms of drug action, primary actions, and important adverse effects for each.
10. Categorize drugs used in the treatment of pain based on their classifications and mechanisms of action.

Pain is physiological and emotional experience characterized by unpleasant feelings, usually associated with trauma and disease. On a simple level, pain may be viewed as a defense mechanism that helps people to avoid potentially damaging situations and encourages them to seek medical help. Although the neural and chemical mechanisms for pain are fairly straightforward, many psychological and emotional processes modify this sensation. Anxiety, fatigue, and depression can increase the perception of pain. Positive attitudes and support from caregivers may reduce the perception of pain. Patients are more likely to tolerate their pain if they know the source of the sensation and the medical course of treatment designed to manage the pain. For example, if patients know that the pain is temporary, such as during labor or after surgery, they are more likely to be accepting of the pain.

ACUTE OR CHRONIC PAIN

Pain can be classified as either acute or chronic. Acute pain is an intense pain occurring over a defined time, usually from injury to recovery. Chronic pain persisting longer than 6 months, can interfere with daily activities, and is associated with feelings of helplessness or hopelessness.

Fast Facts Pain

- Pain is a common symptom.

  Approximately 16 million people experience chronic arthritic pain.
  At least 31 million adults report low back pain, with 19 million people experiencing this on a chronic basis.
  Currently, 50 million people are fully or partially disabled as a result of pain.
  Over 50% of adults experience muscle pain each year.
  Up to 40% of people with cancer report moderate to severe pain.

- About 28 million Americans suffer from headaches and migraines.

  Use of drug therapy and other measures controls 95% of migraines.
  After puberty, women have four to eight times more migraines than men.
  Before puberty, more boys have migraines than girls.
  Headaches and migraines appear mostly among people age 20 to 40.
  Persons with a family history of headache or migraine have a higher chance of developing these disorders.

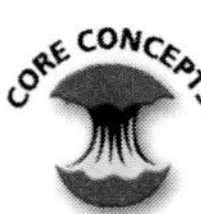

12.1 Pain assessment is the first step to pain management.

The psychological reaction to pain is a subjective experience. The same degree and type of pain may be described as excruciating and unbearable by one patient, while not mentioned by another. Several numerical scales and survey instruments are available to help healthcare providers standardize pain assessment and measure the progress of drug therapy. Successful pain management depends on an accurate assessment of both the degree of pain experienced by the patient and the potential disorders that may be causing the pain. Selection of the correct therapy is dependent on the nature and character of the pain.

Pain is termed *acute* or *chronic* and can also be classified by its source. Injury to *tissues* produces *nociceptor pain.* This type of pain may be further subdivided into *somatic pain,* which produces sharp, localized sensations, or *visceral pain,* which is described as a generalized dull, throbbing, or aching pain. The term **nociceptor** refers to activation of receptor nerve endings that receive and transmit pain signals to the spinal cord and brain. In contrast, *neuropathic pain* is caused by direct injury to the *nerves* and typically is described as burning, shooting, or numb pain. Whereas nociceptor pain responds quite well to conventional pain relief medications, neuropathic pain responds less successfully.

noci = *pain or injury*
ceptor = *receiver*

Concept Review 12.1

- What questions would you ask to identify a patient's type of pain? How would you distinguish between acute pain and chronic pain? Which is the most difficult type of pain to treat?

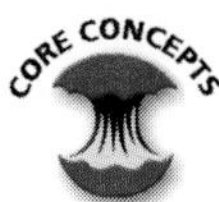

12.2 Nonpharmacological techniques assist patients in obtaining adequate pain relief.

Although drugs are quite effective at relieving pain in most patients, they can have significant side effects. For example, at high doses, aspirin causes gastrointestinal (GI) bleeding, and the opioids causes significant drowsiness and have the potential for dependence.

Nonpharmacological techniques may be used in place of drugs or in addition to pharmacotherapy to help patients obtain adequate pain relief. When used together with medication, nonpharmacological techniques may allow medication doses to be lowered. Lower doses may mean fewer drug-related adverse effects. Some nonpharmacological techniques used for reducing pain are as follows:

- Acupuncture
- Biofeedback therapy
- Massage
- Heat or cold packs
- Meditation
- Relaxation therapy
- Art or music therapy
- Imagery
- Chiropractic manipulation
- Hypnosis
- Therapeutic touch
- Transcutaneous electrical nerve stimulation (TENS)
- Energy therapies such as reiki and qi gong

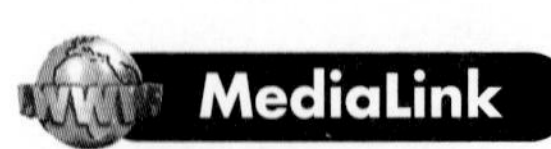

THE AMERICAN HOLISTIC NURSES ASSOCIATION

in = *opposite of*
tractable = *control*

invasive = *tending to spread*

Patients with *intractable* (meaning "not easy to relieve") cancer pain sometime require more *invasive* techniques if rapidly growing tumors press on vital tissues and nerves. Furthermore, chemotherapy and surgical treatments for cancer can cause severe pain. Radiation therapy may provide pain relief by shrinking solid tumors that may be pressing on nerves. Surgery may be used to reduce pain by removing part of or the entire tumor. Injection of alcohol or other neurotoxic substance into neurons is occasionally performed to cause nerve blocks. Nerve blocks irreversibly stop impulse transmission along the treated nerves, and have the potential to provide total pain relief.

12.3 Pain transmission processes allow several targets for pharmacological intervention.

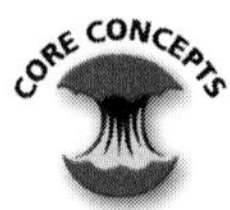

The process of pain transmission begins when nociceptors are stimulated. These receptors are free nerve endings strategically located throughout the body. The nerve impulse signaling the pain is sent to the spinal cord along two types of sensory neurons, called Aδ and C fibers. **Aδ fibers** are wrapped thinly in myelin, a fatty substance that speeds nerve transmission. **C fibers** are *unmyelinated;* thus, they carry nerve transmissions more slowly. The Aδ fibers signal sharp, well-defined pain, whereas the C fibers conduct dull, poorly localized pain.

Once pain impulses reach the spinal cord, neurotransmitters pass the message along to the next neuron. Here, a neurotransmitter called **substance P** is thought to be responsible for continuing the pain message, although other neurotransmitter candidates have been proposed. Spinal substance P is critical because it controls whether pain signals will continue to the brain. The activity of substance P may be affected by other neurotransmitters released from neurons in the CNS. One group of neurotransmitters, called **endogenous opioids,** includes endorphins, dynorphins, and enkephalins. Figure 12.1 ■ shows one point of contact where endogenous opioids modify, or change, sensory information at the level of the spinal cord. If the pain impulse reaches the brain, it may respond with many possible actions. For instance, the brain may signal the skeletal muscles to jerk away from a sharp object. In other instances, such as in those suffering from chronic pain, the impulses reaching the brain may result in mental depression brought on by thoughts of death or disability.

endo = *within*
genous = *coming from*

Because pain signals begin at nociceptors located within peripheral body tissues and then proceed through the CNS, there are several targets where medications can work to stop pain transmission. In general, the two main classes of pain medications act at different locations: the nonsteroidal anti-inflammatory drugs (NSAIDs) act at the peripheral level, whereas the opioids act within the CNS.

Concept Review 12.2

- What is a nociceptor? Consider substance P and endogenous opioids, and describe how pain can be regulated.

12.4 Opioid analgesic medications exert their effects by interacting with specific receptors.

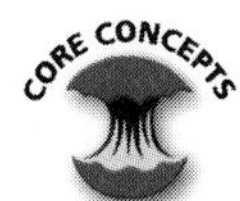

Analgesics are medications used to relieve pain. The two basic categories of analgesics are the opioids and the nonopioids. An **opioid** analgesic is a natural or synthetic morphine-like substance responsible for reducing severe pain. Opioids are *narcotic* substances, meaning that they produce numbness or stuporlike symptoms.

an = *without*
algesia = *pain*

opi = *opium*
oid = *shape or form*

Terminology associated with the narcotic analgesic medications is often confusing. Several of these drugs are obtained from opium, a milky extract from the unripe seeds of the poppy plant, which contains over 20 different chemicals having pharmacological activity. Opium consists of 9% to 14% morphine and 0.8% to 2.5% codeine. These natural substances are called **opiates.** In a search for safer analgesics, chemists have created several dozen synthetic drugs with activity similar to that of the opiates. *Opioid* is a general term referring to any of these substances, natural or synthetic, and is often used interchangeably with the term *opiate.*

Narcotic is a general term used to describe morphine-like drugs that produce analgesia and CNS depression. Narcotics may be natural, such as morphine, or synthetic such as meperidine (Demerol). In common usage, a narcotic analgesic is the same as an opioid, and the terms are often used interchangeably. In the context of drug enforcement, however, the term *narcotic* is often used to describe a much broader range of abused illegal drugs such as hallucinogens, heroin, amphetamines, and marijuana.

narc = *numbness or stupor*
otic = *like*

FIGURE 12.1

Neural pathways for pain

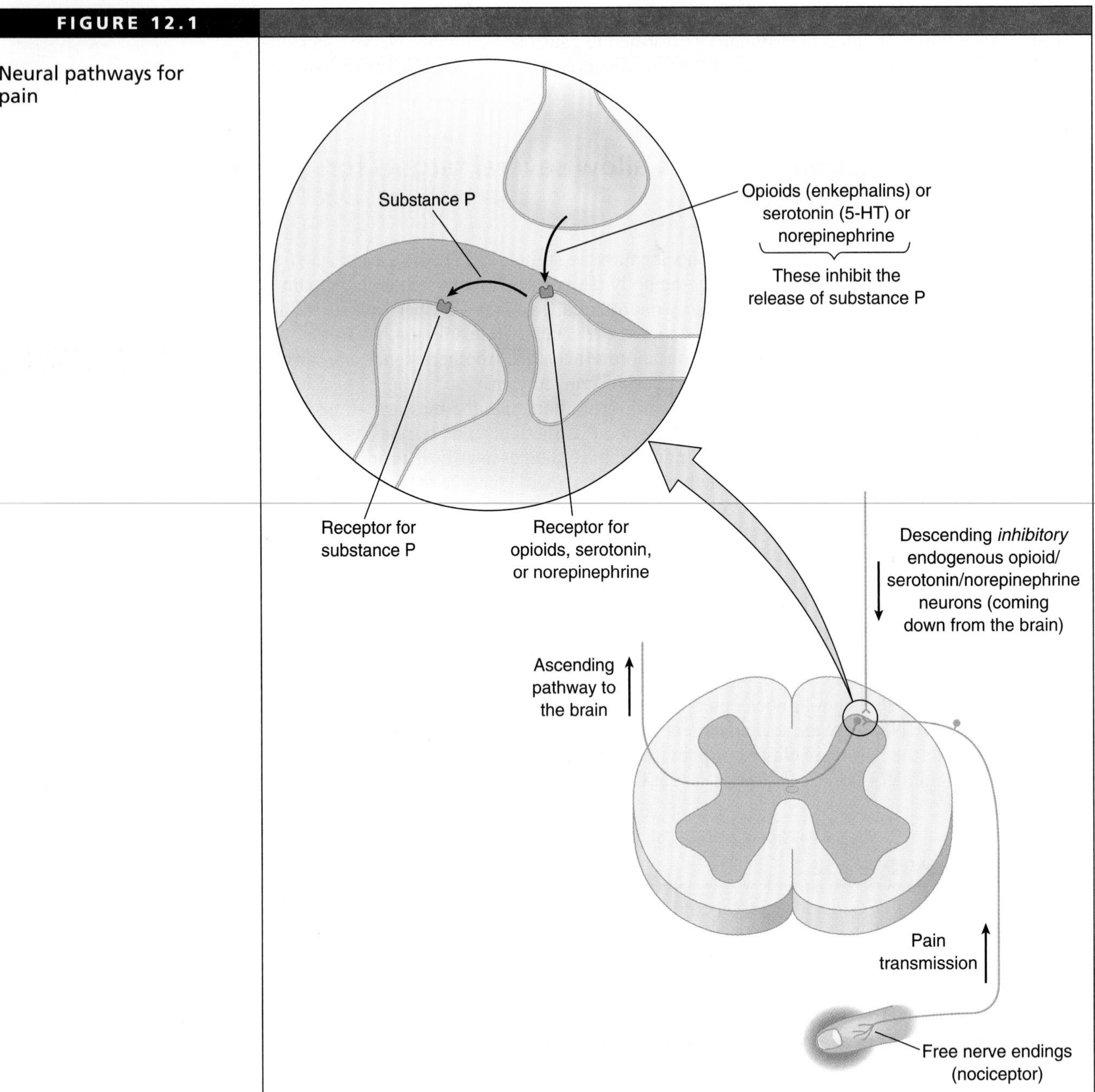

Opioids interact with at least six types of receptors: mu (types one and two), kappa, sigma, delta, and epsilon. From the perspective of pain management, the *mu* and *kappa receptors* are the most important. Some opioids stimulate a particular receptor; others block a receptor. The types of actions produced by activating mu and kappa receptors are shown in Table 12.1.

Some opioids, such as morphine, activate both mu and kappa receptors. Other opioids such as pentazocine (Talwin) exert mixed opioid stimulating-blocking effects by activating the kappa receptor but blocking the mu receptor. Opioid blockers such as naloxone (Narcan) inhibit both the mu and kappa receptors. This is the body's natural way of providing the mechanism for different body responses from one substance. Figure 12.2 ■ illustrates opioid actions on the mu and kappa receptors.

Opioids are drugs of choice for moderate to severe pain that cannot be controlled with other classes of analgesics. More than 20 different opioids are available as medications, and they can be classified by similarities in their chemical structures, by their mechanisms of action, or by their effectiveness (Table 12.2). The most useful method is by effectiveness, which places opiates into categories of strong or moderate narcotic activity.

TABLE 12.1	Responses Produced by Activation of Specific Opioid Receptors	
RESPONSE	**MU RECEPTOR**	**KAPPA RECEPTOR**
Analgesia	x	x
Decreased GI motility	x	x
Euphoria	x	
Miosis (constricted pupils)		x
Physical dependence	x	
Respiratory depression	x	
Sedation	x	x

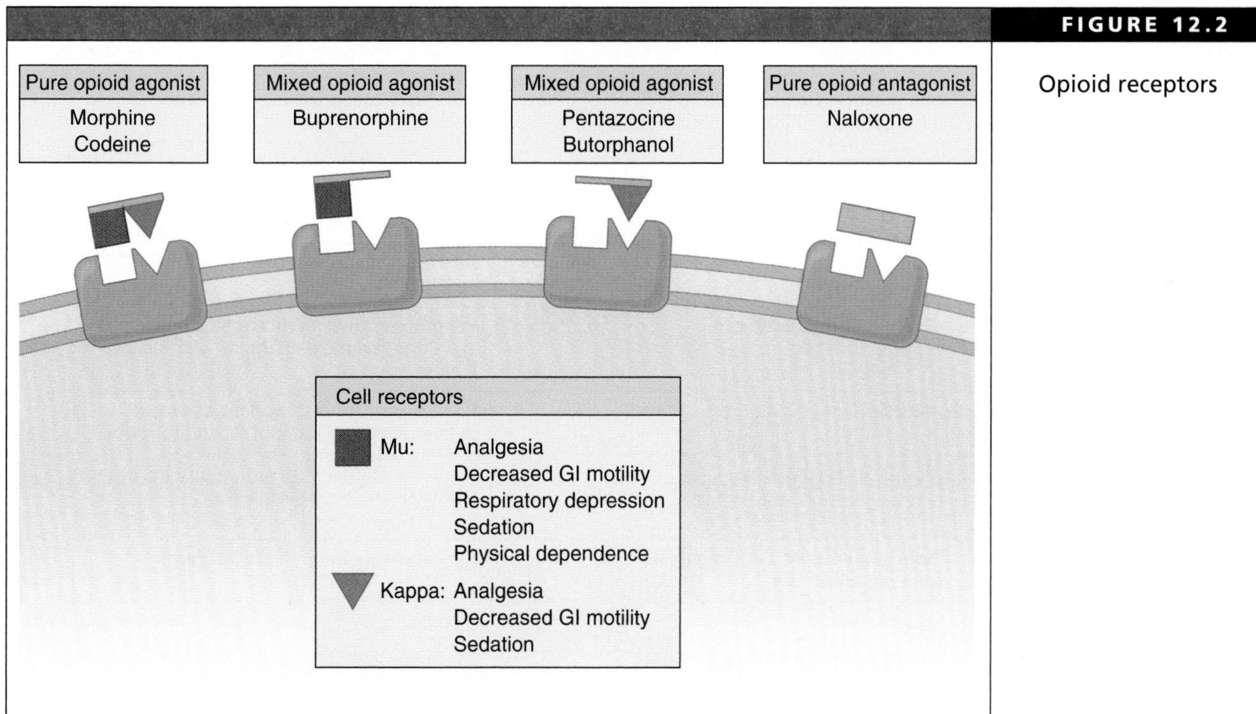

FIGURE 12.2

Opioid receptors

Concept Review 12.3

- Distinguish between the following terms: *opioid, opiate,* and *narcotic.* Name six classes of opioid receptors and identify those that are connected with analgesia.

Opioid Agonists

Narcotic opioid agonists bind to opioid receptors and produce multiple responses throughout the body. Morphine is the "representative" drug used to treat severe pain. It is the standard against which the effectiveness of every other opioid is compared.

12.5 Narcotic opioids have multiple therapeutic effects including relief of severe pain.

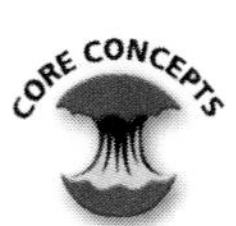

Opiates produce many important effects other than analgesia. They are effective at suppressing the cough reflex and at slowing the *motility,* or movement, of the GI tract for cases of severe diarrhea. As powerful CNS depressants, opioids can cause sedation, which may be either

TABLE 12.2 Opioids for Pain Management

DRUG	ROUTE AND ADULT DOSE	REMARKS
OPIOID AGONISTS WITH MODERATE EFFECTIVENESS		
codeine	PO 15–60 mg qid	Also for cough; available in IM and subcutaneous forms; combination drug with aspirin is called Empirin with codeine and with acetaminophen, Tylenol with codeine
hydrocodone bitartrate (Hycodan)	PO 5–10 mg q4–6h prn (max:15 mg/dose)	Also for cough; combination drug with acetaminophen is called Amacodone C, Co-Gesic, Vicodin, Dolacet, Norcet, and Norco
oxycodone hydrochloride (OxyContin) oxycodone terephthalate (Percocet-5, Roxicet, others)	PO 5–10 mg qid prn	Combination drug with acetaminophen is called Percocet or Tylox; with aspirin is called Percodan or Roxiprin
propoxyphene hydrochloride (Darvon) propoxyphene napsylate (Darvon-N)	PO 65 mg (HCl form) or 100 mg (napsylate form) q4h prn (max: 390 HCl/day; max: 600 mg napsylate/day)	Combination drug with acetaminophen is called Darvocet or Propacet and with aspirin and caffeine is called Darvon or Dolene
OPIOID AGONISTS WITH HIGH EFFECTIVENESS		
hydromorphone hydrochloride (Dilaudid)	PO 1–4 mg q4–6h prn	Also for cough; available in IM, IV, subcutaneous, and rectal forms
levorphanol tartrate (Levo-Dromoran)	PO 2–3 mg tid to qid prn	Also available in subcutaneous form
meperidine hydrochloride (Demerol)	PO 50–150 mg q3–4h prn	For preoperative medication or obstetric analgesia; available in IM, IV, and subcutaneous forms
methadone hydrochloride (Dolophine)	PO 2.5–10 mg q3–4h prn	For detoxification treatment of opioid dependency; available in IM and IV forms
Pr morphine sulfate (Astramorph PF, Duramorph, others)	PO 10–30 mg q4h prn	Available in IM, IV, subcutaneous, intrathecal, epidural, and rectal forms
oxymorphone hydrochloride (Numorphan)	Subcutaneous/IM 1–1.5 mg q4–6h prn; pr 5 mg q4–6h prn	Also available in IV and rectal forms
OPIOID ANTAGONISTS		
nalmefene hydrochloride (Revex)	Subcutaneous/IM/IV use 1 mg/mL concentration; nonopioid dependent: 0.5 mg/70 kg; opioid dependent: 0.1 mg/70 kg	For opioid overdose and postoperative opioid depression
Pr naloxone hydrochloride (Narcan)	IV 0.4–2 mg, may be repeated every 2–3 min up to 10 mg if necessary	For opioid overdose and postoperative opioid depression
naltrexone hydrochloride (Trexan, ReVia)	PO 25 mg followed by another 25 mg in 1 hour if no withdrawal response (max: 800 mg/day)	For management of opiate or alcohol dependence; longer lasting effect than naloxone
OPIOIDS WITH MIXED AGONIST–ANTAGONIST EFFECTS		
buprenorphine hydrochloride (Buprenex)	IM/IV 0.3 mg q6h (max: 0.6 mg q4h)	For moderate to severe pain; also available in subcutaneous, epidural, and rectal forms
butorphanol tartrate (Stadol)	IM 1–4 mg q3–4h prn (max: 4 mg/dose)	For obstetrical analgesia during labor, cancer pain, renal colic, and burns; available in IV and intranasal forms
dezocine (Dalgan)	IV 2.5–10 mg (usually 5 mg) q2–4h; IM 5–10 mg (usually 10 mg) q3–4h	Causes less respiratory depression than morphine sulfate
nalbuphine hydrochloride (Nubain)	Subcutaneous/IM/IV 10–20 mg q3–6h prn (max: 160 mg/day)	For moderate to severe pain
pentazocine hydrochloride (Talwin)	PO 50–100 mg q3–4h (max: 600 mg/day); subcutaneous/IM/IV 30 mg q3–4h (max: 360 mg/day)	For moderate to severe pain (much lower dose for women in labor)

DRUG PROFILE: Opioid Agonist: Pr *Morphine (Astramorph PF, Duramorph, others)*

Actions and Uses:

Morphine binds with both mu and kappa receptor sites to produce strong, analgesia. It causes euphoria, constriction of the pupils, and stimulation of cardiac muscle. It is used for relief or serious acute and chronic pain after nonnarcotic analgesics have failed, as preanesthetic medication, to relieve shortness of breath associated with heart failure and pulmonary edema, and for acute chest pain connected with MI.

Adverse Effects and Interactions:

Morphine may cause dysphoria (restlessness, depression, and anxiety), hallucinations, nausea, constipation, dizziness, and an itching sensation. Overdose may result in severe respiratory depression or cardiac arrest. Tolerance develops to the analgesic, sedative, and euphoric effects of the drug. Cross-tolerance also develops between morphine and other opioids such as heroin, methadone, and meperidine. Physical and psychological dependence develop when high doses are taken for prolonged periods. Morphine may intensify or mask the pain of gallbladder disease, due to biliary tract spasms.

Morphine interacts with several drugs. For example, use with CNS depressants, such as alcohol, other opioids, general anesthetics, sedatives, and antidepressants such as MAO inhibitors and tricyclics, increases the action of opiates, and thereby raises the risk of severe respiratory depression and death.

Use with caution with herbal supplements, such as yohimbe, which may increase the effect of morphine.

Mechanism in Action: 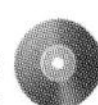

Morphine is an opioid that produces many actions throughout the central nervous system. One important action occurs at the level of the dorsal horn spinal cord. Here, morphine binds presynaptically to primary afferent neurons reducing the amount of released pain neurotransmitter. Simultaneously, morphine binds postsynaptically to second-order neurons responsible for transmitting ascending pain impulses to the brain.

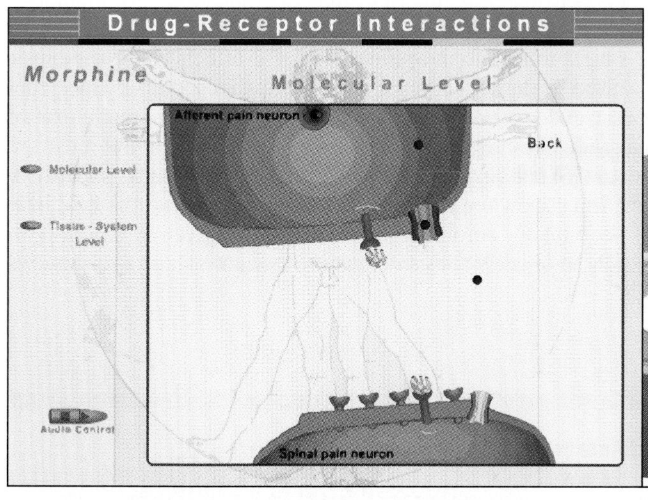

Use the student CD-ROM to see Mechanism in Action for Morphine.

See the Companion Website for a Nursing Process Focus specific to this drug.

a therapeutic effect or a side effect, depending on the patient's disease state. Some patients experience euphoria and intense relaxation, which are reasons why opiates are sometimes abused. There are many adverse effects, including respiratory depression, sedation, nausea, and vomiting.

All of the narcotic analgesics have the potential to cause physical and psychological dependence, as discussed in Chapter 6. Many healthcare providers and nurses are hesitant to administer the proper amount of opioid analgesics for fear of causing patient dependence or of producing serious adverse effects such as sedation or respiratory depression. Because of this

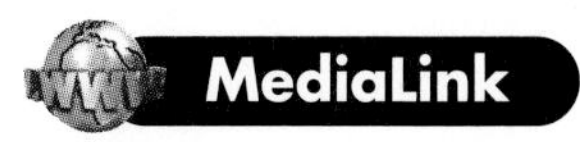

JCAHO STANDARDS ON PAIN MANAGEMENT

tendency to undermedicate, patients may not receive complete pain relief. When used according to accepted medical practice, patients can, and indeed should, receive the pain relief they need without fear of addiction or adverse effects.

syn = *together*
erg = *work*
istically = *ability to*

It is common practice to combine opioids and nonnarcotic analgesics into a single tablet or capsule. The two classes of analgesics work *synergistically* to relieve pain, and the dose of narcotic can be kept small to avoid dependence and opioid-related side effects. Five common combination analgesics are as follows:

- Vicodin (hydrocodone, 5 mg; acetaminophen, 500 mg)
- Percocet (oxycodone HCl, 5 mg; acetaminophen, 325 mg)
- Percodan (oxycodone HCl, 4.5 mg; oxycodone terephthalate, 0.38 mg; aspirin, 325 mg)
- Darvocet-N 50 (propoxyphene napsylate, 50 mg; acetaminophen, 325 mg)
- Empirin with Codeine No. 2 (codeine phosphate, 15 mg; aspirin, 325 mg)

Some opioids are used primarily for conditions other than pain. For example, alfentanil (Alfenta), fentanyl (Sublimaze), remifentanil (Ultiva), and sufentanil (Sufenta) are used for general anesthesia; these are discussed in Chapter 13. Codeine is most often prescribed as a cough suppressant and is covered in Chapter 25. Opiates used in treating diarrhea are presented in Chapter 26.

Opioid Antagonists

Opioid antagonists are substances that prevent the effects of opioid agonists. These agents are sometimes called "competitive antagonists" because they compete with opioid agonists for access to the opioid receptor site.

Opioid overdose can occur as a result of overly aggressive pain therapy or as a result of substance abuse. Any opioid may be abused for its psychoactive effects; however, morphine, meperidine, and heroin are preferred because of their potency. Although heroin is currently available as a legal analgesic in many countries, it is considered by the FDA to be too dangerous for therapeutic use. It is a major drug of abuse. Once injected or inhaled, heroin rapidly crosses the blood-brain barrier to enter the brain, where it is metabolized to morphine. Thus, the effects and symptoms of heroin administration are actually caused by the activation of mu and kappa receptors by morphine. The initial effect is an intense euphoria, called a *rush,* followed by several hours of deep relaxation.

Acute opioid intoxication is a medical emergency. Respiratory depression is the most serious problem. The opioid antangonist naloxone (Narcan) may be infused to reverse respiratory depression and other acute symptoms. In cases when the patient is unconscious and the healthcare provider is unclear what drug has been taken, opioid antagonists may be given to diagnose the overdose. If the opioid antagonist fails to quickly reverse the acute symptoms, the overdose was likely due to a nonopioid substance.

DRUG PROFILE: Opioid Antagonist: Pr *Naloxone (Narcan)*

Actions and Uses:

Naloxone is a pure opioid antagonist, blocking both mu and kappa receptors. It is used for complete or partial reversal of opioid effects in emergency situations when acute opioid overdose is suspected. Given intravenously, it begins to reverse opioid-initiated CNS and respiratory depression within minutes. It will immediately cause opioid withdrawal symptoms in patients physically dependent on opioids. It is also used to treat postoperative opioid depression. It is occasionally given as adjunctive therapy to reverse hypotension caused by septic shock. Naloxone is pregnancy category B.

Adverse Effects and Interactions:

Naloxone itself has minimal toxicity. However, in reversing the effects of opioids, the patient may experience rapid loss of analgesia, increased blood pressure, tremors, hyperventilation, nausea/vomiting, and drowsiness. It should not be used for respiratory depression caused by nonopioid medications.

Drug interactions include a reversal of the analgesic effects of narcotic agonists and agonist–antagonists.

See the Companion Website for a Nursing Process Focus specific to this drug.

Opioids with Mixed Agonist–Antagonist Activity

Narcotic opioids that have mixed agonist–antagonist activity stimulate the opioid receptor; thus, they cause analgesia. However, the withdrawal symptoms or side effects are not as intense due to partial activity of receptor subtypes.

Although effective at relieving pain, the opioids have a greater risk for dependence than almost any other class of medications. Tolerance develops relatively quickly to the euphoric effects of opioids, causing users to increase their doses and take the drug more frequently. The higher and more frequent doses rapidly cause physical dependence in opioid abusers.

When physically dependent patients attempt to discontinue drug use, they experience extremely uncomfortable symptoms that lead many to continue their drug-taking behavior. As long as the drug is continued, they feel "normal," and many can continue work or social activities. If a person abruptly discontinues the drug, he or she will experience withdrawal symptoms for about 7 days before overcoming the physical dependence.

The intense craving that characterizes psychological dependence may occur for many months, and even years, following discontinuation of opioids. This often results in a return to drug-seeking behavior unless significant support is available.

One common method of treating opioid dependence is to switch the patient from IV and inhalation forms of illegal drugs to methadone (Dolophine). Although it is an opioid, oral methadone does not cause the euphoria of the injectable opioids. Methadone also does not cure the dependence, and the patient must continue taking the drug to avoid withdrawal symptoms. This therapy, called *methadone maintenance,* may continue for many months or years, until the patient decides to enter a total withdrawal treatment program. Methadone maintenance allows patients to return to productive work and social relationships without the physical, emotional, and criminal risks of illegal drug use.

A newer treatment option is to administer buprenorphine (Subutex), a mixed opioid agonist–antagonist, by the sublingual route. Subutex is used early in opioid abuse therapy to prevent opioid withdrawal symptoms. Another combination agent, Suboxone, contains both buprenorphine and naloxone, and is used later in the maintenance of opioid addiction.

Practitioners must be aware when administering opioids with mixed agonist–antagonist activity that in some ways they act similarly to pure opioid agonists; however, when mixed agents are administered in combination with opioid agonists, their pain-blocking properties will be reduced. Thus, there is a tendency to overprescribe mixed opioids thereby promoting drug misuse. This is true even though the potential for causing opioid addiction in most cases is lower than with pure opioid agonists.

NURSING PROCESS FOCUS

Patients Receiving Opioids

ASSESSMENT

Prior to administration:

- Obtain complete health history including allergies, drug history, and possible drug interactions
- Assess pain (quality, intensity, location, duration)
- Assess respiratory function
- Assess level of consciousness before and after administration
- Obtain vital signs

POTENTIAL NURSING DIAGNOSES

- Deficient Knowledge, related to drug therapy
- Acute Pain, related to injury, disease, or surgical procedure
- Ineffective Breathing Pattern, related to action of medication
- Constipation
- Disturbed Sleep Pattern, related to surgical pain

PLANNING: Patient Goals and Expected Outcomes

The patient will:

- Report pain relief or a reduction in pain intensity
- Demonstrate an understanding of the drug's action by accurately describing drug side effects and precautions
- Immediately report effects such as untoward or rebound pain, restlessness, anxiety, depression, hallucination, nausea, dizziness, and itching

continued...

(continued from page 201)

NURSING PROCESS FOCUS

IMPLEMENTATION

Interventions and (Rationales)	Patient Education/Discharge Planning
▪ Opioids may be administered PO, subcutaneously, IM, IV, or PR. ▪ Opioids are Schedule II controlled substances. (Opioids produce both physical and psychological dependence.)	Instruct patient: ▪ To take necessary steps to safeguard drug supply; avoid sharing medications with others ▪ That oral *capsules* may be opened and mixed with cool foods; extended-release *tablets,* however, may not be chewed, crushed, or broken ▪ That oral solution ordered sublingually may be in a higher concentration than solution for swallowing
▪ Monitor liver function via laboratory tests. (Opioids are metabolized in the liver. Hepatic disease can increase blood levels of opioids to toxic levels.)	Instruct patient to: ▪ Report nausea, vomiting, diarrhea, rash, jaundice, abdominal pain, tenderness or distention, or change in color of stool ▪ Adhere to laboratory testing regimen for liver function as ordered by the healthcare provider
▪ Monitor vital signs, especially depth and rate of respirations/pulse oximetry. ▪ Withhold the drug if the patient's respiratory rate is below 12, and notify the healthcare provider. ▪ Keep resuscitative equipment and a narcotic-antagonist such as naloxone (Narcan) accessible. (Opioid antagonists may reverse respiratory depression, decrease level of consciousness, and initiate other symptoms of narcotic overdose.)	Instruct patient or caregiver to: ▪ Monitor vital signs regularly, particularly respirations ▪ Withhold medication for any difficulty in breathing or respirations below 12 breaths per minute; report symptoms to the healthcare provider
▪ Monitor neurological status; perform neuro checks regularly. ▪ Monitor changes in level of consciousness. (Decreased LOC and sluggish pupillary response may occur with high doses.) ▪ Observe for seizures. (Drug may increase intracranial pressure.)	Instruct patient to: ▪ Report headache or any significant change in sensorium, such as an aura or other visual effects that may indicate an impending seizure ▪ Recognize seizures and methods to ensure personal safety during a seizure ▪ Report any seizure activity immediately
▪ If ordered prn, administer medication upon patient request or when nursing observations indicate patient expressions of pain.	Instruct patient to: ▪ Alert the nurse immediately upon the return or increase of pain ▪ Notify the nurse regarding the drug's effectiveness
▪ Monitor renal status and urinary output. (May cause urinary retention, which may exacerbate existing symptoms of prostatic hypertrophy.)	Instruct patient or caregiver to: ▪ Measure and monitor fluid intake and output ▪ Report symptoms of dysuria (hesitancy, pain, diminished stream), changes in urine quality or scanty urine output ▪ Report fever or flank pain that may be indicative of a urinary tract infection
▪ Monitor for other side effects such as restlessness, dizziness, anxiety, depression, hallucinations, nausea, and vomiting. (Hives or itching may indicate an allergic reaction due to the production of histamine.)	Instruct patient or caregiver to: ▪ Recognize side effects and symptoms of an allergic or anaphylactic reaction ▪ Immediately report any shortness of breath, tight feeling in the throat, itching, hives or other rash, feelings of dysphoria, nausea, or vomiting ▪ Avoid the use of sleep-inducing OTC antihistamines, without first consulting the healthcare provider

continued...

NURSING PROCESS FOCUS

Interventions and (Rationales)	Patient Education/Discharge Planning
■ Monitor for constipation. (Drug slows peristalsis.)	Instruct patient to: ■ Maintain an adequate fluid and fiber intake to facilitate stool passage ■ Use a stool softener or laxative as recommended by the healthcare provider
■ Ensure patient safety. ■ Monitor ambulation until response to drug is known. (Drug can cause sedation and dizziness.)	Instruct patient to: ■ Request assistance when getting out of bed ■ Avoid driving or performing hazardous activities until effect of drug is known
■ Monitor frequency of requests and stated effectiveness of narcotic administered. (Opioids cause tolerance and dependence.)	Instruct patient and caregiver: ■ Regarding cross-tolerance issues ■ To monitor medication supply to observe for hoarding, which may signal an impending suicide attempt ■ When educating patients suffering from terminal illnesses, address the issue of drug dependence from the perspective of reduced life expectancy

EVALUATION OF OUTCOME CRITERIA

Evaluate the effectiveness of drug therapy by confirming that patient goals and expected outcomes have been met (see "Planning").

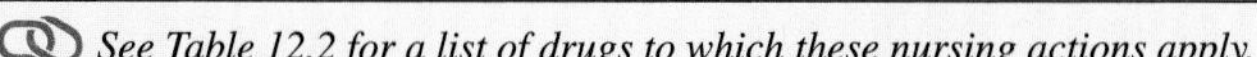

See Table 12.2 for a list of drugs to which these nursing actions apply.

12.6 Nonsteroidal anti-inflammatory drugs are the drugs of choice for inflammatory pain.

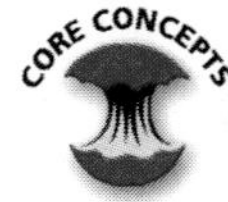

The NSAIDs have antipyretic (antifever) and anti-inflammatory activity, as well as analgesic (pain-reducing) properties. Some of the NSAIDs, such as the selective COX-2 inhibitors, are used primarily for their anti-inflammatory properties. Celecoxib (Celebrex) and rofecoxib (Vioxx), once top-selling arthritis medications, have been linked to the risk of heart attack and stroke. Vioxx was removed from the market on September 30, 2004, after a study revealed that this drug was linked to heart attacks, strokes, blood clots, and cardiovascular injuries. NSAIDs are also used in the treatment of fever (see Chapter 21). Table 12.3 highlights the common nonopioid analgesics.

Nonsteroidal Anti-inflammatory Drugs

The nonopioid analgesics include the nonsteroidal anti-inflammatory drugs (NSAIDs), acetaminophen, and a few centrally acting agents. The NSAIDs inhibit **cyclooxygenase,** an enzyme responsible for the formation of prostaglandins. When cyclooxygenase is inhibited, inflammation and pain are reduced.

NSAIDs are the drugs of choice for mild to moderate pain, especially for pain associated with inflammation. These drugs have many advantages over the opioids. Aspirin and ibuprofen are available as OTC drugs and are inexpensive. Ibuprofen is available in many different formulations, including those designed for children. Many are safe and produce adverse effects only at high doses. Other NSAIDs such as the COX-2 inhibitors are being investigated for possible adverse effects.

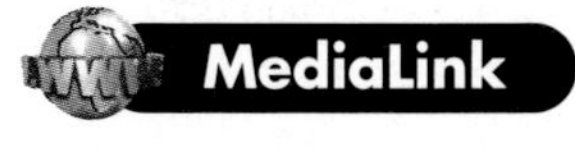

THE OXFORD PAIN INTERNET SITE

DRUG PROFILE: NSAIDs: *Aspirin (Acetylsalicylic Acid, ASA)*

Actions and Uses:

Aspirin inhibits prostaglandin synthesis involved in the processes of pain and inflammation and produces mild to moderate relief of fever. It has limited effects on peripheral blood vessels, causing vasodilation and sweating. Aspirin has significant anticoagulant activity and this property is reposnsible for its ability to reduce the risk of mortality following MI, and to reduce the incidence of strokes. Aspirin has also been found to reduce the risk of colorectal cancer, although the mechanism by which it affords this protective effect is unknown.

Adverse Effects and Interactions:

At high doses, such as those used to treat severe inflammatory disorders, aspirin may cause gastric discomfort and bleeding because of its antiplatelet effects. Enteric-coated tablets and buffered preparations are available for patients who experience GI side effects.

Because aspirin increases bleeding time, it should not be given to patients receiving anticoagulant therapy such as warfarin, heparin, and plicamycin. ASA may increase the action of oral hypoglycemic agents. Effects of NSAIDs, uricosuric agents such as probenecid, beta blockers, spironolactone, and sulfa drugs may be decreased when combined with ASA.

Use with phenobarbital, antacids, and glucocorticoids may decrease ASA effects. Insulin, methotrexate, phenytoin, sulfonamides, and penicillin may increase effects. When taken with alcohol, pyrazolone derivatives, steroids, or other NSAIDs, there is an increased risk for gastric ulcers.

Use with caution with herbal supplements, such as feverfew, which may increase the risk of bleeding.

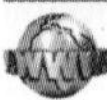
See the Companion Website for a Nursing Process Focus specific to this drug.

mediators = *middle agents*

brady = *slow*
kinin = *movement*

syn = *together*
thesis = *put*

The NSAIDs act by inhibiting pain mediators at the nociceptor level. When tissue is damaged, chemical mediators are released locally, including histamine, potassium ion, hydrogen ion, bradykinin, and prostaglandins. **Bradykinin** is associated with the sensory impulse of pain. **Prostaglandins** can cause pain through the formation of proinflammatory substances.

Prostaglandins are formed with the help of two enzymes—cyclooxygenase type one (COX-1) and cyclooxygenase type two (COX-2). Aspirin inhibits both COX-1 and COX-2. Because the COX-2 enzyme is more specific for the *synthesis* of those prostaglandins that cause pain and inflammation, the selective COX-2 inhibitors were developed to provide more specific pain relief. Figure 12.3 ▪ illustrates the mechanisms involved in pain at the nociceptor level.

Acetaminophen

Several important nonopioid analgesics are not classified as NSAIDs. Acetaminophen is a nonopioid analgesic that is as equally effective as aspirin and ibuprofen for relieving pain. Acetaminophen is featured as a representative medication also used to reduce fever.

Centrally Acting Drugs

Clonidine (Catapres) and tramadol (Ultram) are centrally acting analgesics. Tramadol has weak opioid activity, though it is not thought to relieve pain by this mechanism.

Concept Review 12.4

- Think about cyclooxygenase inhibitors (NSAIDs) and prostaglandins, and then describe how pain might be regulated at the nociceptor.

TABLE 12.3 Nonopioid Analgesics

DRUG	ROUTE AND ADULT DOSE	REMARKS
Pr acetaminophen (Tylenol)	PO 325–650 mg q4–6h	Also for fever; available in rectal form
NSAIDS		
Selective COX-2 Inhibitors		
celecoxib (Celebrex)	PO 100–200 mg bid or 200 mg/daily	Also for inflammation
Ibuprofen and Ibuprofen-like: Nonsalicylates		
diclofenac (Cataflam, Voltaren)	PO 50 mg bid to qid (max: 200 mg/day)	Also for inflammation
diflunisal (Dolobid)	PO 1000 mg followed by 500 mg bid to tid	Also for inflammation
etodolac (Lodine)	PO 200–400 mg tid to qid	Also for inflammation
fenoprofen calcium (Nalfon)	PO 200 mg tid to qid	Also for inflammation
flurbiprofen (Ansaid)	PO 50–100 mg tid to qid (max: 300 mg/day)	Similar to ibuprofen
ibuprofen (Advil, Motrin)	PO 400 mg tid to qid (max: 1200 mg/day)	Also for fever and inflammation
indomethacin (Indocin)	PO 25–50 mg bid or tid (max: 200 mg/day) or 75 mg sustained release one to two times/day	Also used for moderate to severe rheumatoid arthritis and acute gouty arthritis
ketoprofen (Actron, Orudis)	PO 12.5–50 mg tid to qid	Also for inflammation
ketorolac tromethamine (Toradol)	PO 10 mg qid prn (max:40 mg/day)	Also for allergic conjunctivitis, available in IM/IV forms
mefanamic acid (Ponstel)	PO loading dose 500 mg, maintenance dose 250 mg q6h prn	Used for short-term relief of mild to moderate pain, including menstrual cramps
meloxicam (Mobic)	PO 7.5 mg daily (max: 15 mg/day)	Used for osteoarthritis
nabumetone (Relafen)	PO 1000 mg daily (max: 2000 mg/day)	Inhibits COX-2 more than COX-1
Pr naproxen (Naprosyn, Naprelan)	PO 500 mg followed by 200–250 mg tid to qid (max: 1000 mg/day)	Also for inflammation
Pr naproxen sodium (Aleve, Anaprox, others)	PO 250–500 mg bid (max: 1000 mg/day naproxen)	Also for dysmenorrhea
oxaprozine (Daypro)	PO 600–1200 mg daily (max: 1800 mg/day)	Similar to naproxen; once-a-day dosage
piroxicam (Feldene)	PO 10–20 mg daily to bid (max: 20 mg/day)	Has prolonged half-life
sulindac (Clinoril)	PO 150–200 mg bid (max: 400 mg/day)	Also for inflammation
tolmetin (Tolectin)	PO 400 mg tid (max: 2 g/day)	Also for inflammation
Salicylates		
Pr aspirin (Acetylsalicylic acid, ASA)	PO 350–650 mg q4h (max: 4 g/day)	Also for fever, inflammation, and thromboembolic disorders, prevention of transient ischemic attacks and heart attacks; rectal form available
choline salicylate (Arthropan)	PO 435–870 mg (2.5–5 mL) q4h	Also for inflammation; may be indicated for patients who have difficulty swallowing tablets or capsules
salsalate (Disalcid)	PO 325–3000 mg daily in divided doses (max: 4 g/day)	Also for fever, inflammation
CENTRALLY ACTING AGENTS		
clonidine (Catapres)	PO 0.1 mg bid to tid (max: 0.8 mg/day)	Also used for hypertension
tramadol (Ultram)	PO 50–100 mg q4–6h prn (max: 400 mg/day), may start with 25 mg/day and increase by 25 mg every 3 days up to 200 mg/day	Causes less respiratory depression than morphine

FIGURE 12.3

Mechanisms of pain at the nociceptor level

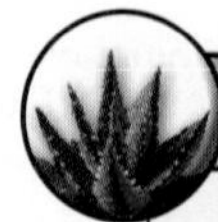

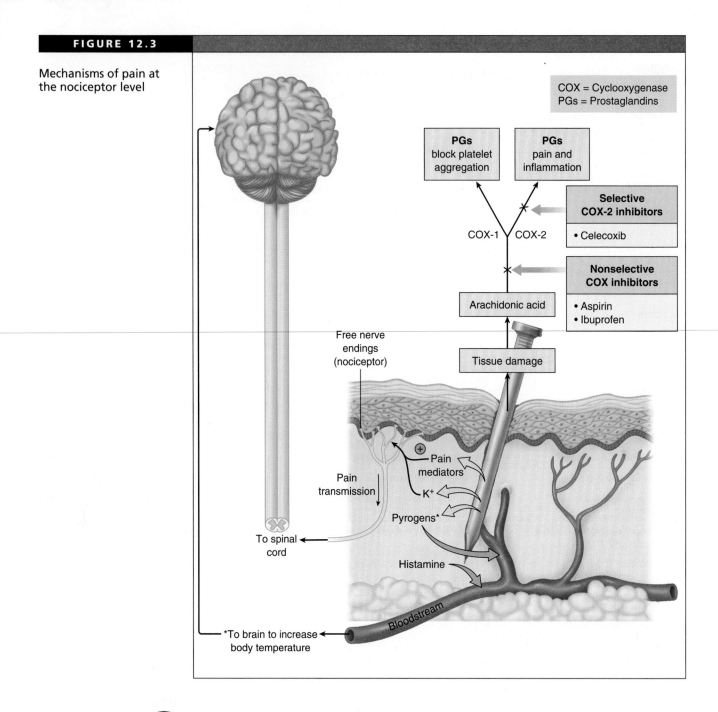

NATURAL ALTERNATIVES

Evening Primrose for Pain

Evening primrose (*Primula vulgaris*) was once considered a medicinal herb for rheumatism, gout, and paralysis. Among modern herbalists, it has several uses depending on which part of the flower is collected. Interestingly, one can find reports of many illnesses where primrose may be helpful, including arthritis, anxiety, high cholesterol levels, irritability, ADHD disorder, and fibromyalgia. Oil of primrose contains an essential fatty acid called *linoleic acid,* which is a natural precursor to gamma linolenic acid, a substance having a reputation for reducing breast tenderness and improving headaches resulting from premenstrual syndrome. Thus, evening primrose oil is sometimes suggested as a natural remedy for primary dysmenorrhea. Although some scientific reports are skeptical, other studies suggest that women with premenstrual syndrome are deficient in gamma linolenic acid. It may be that replacing this deficiency somehow blocks natural mechanisms for the transmission of pain. ▪

DRUG PROFILE: Nonopioid Analgesic: Pr *Acetaminophen (Tylenol)*

Actions and Uses:

Acetaminophen reduces fever by direct action at the level of the hypothalamus and causes dilation of peripheral blood vessels enabling sweating and dissipation of heat. Acetaminophen and aspirin have equal efficacy in relieving pain and reducing fever.

Acetaminophen has no anti-inflammatory action; therefore, it is not effective in treating arthritis or pain caused by tissue swelling following injury. The primary therapeutic usefulness of acetaminophen is for the treatment of fever in children and for relief of mild to moderate pain when aspirin is contraindicated. Acetaminophen is pregnancy category B.

Adverse Effects and Interactions:

Acetaminophen is quite safe and adverse effects are uncommon at therapeutic doses. Unlike aspirin, acetaminophen has no direct anti-inflammatory effect and does not affect blood coagulation or cause gastric irritation. It is not recommended in patients who are malnourished. In such cases, acute toxicity may result leading to renal failure, which can be fatal. Other signs of acute toxicity include nausea, vomiting, chills, and abdominal discomfort.

Acetaminophen inhibits warfarin metabolism, causing warfarin to accumulate to toxic levels. High-dose or long-term acetaminophen usage may result in elevated warfarin levels and bleeding. Ingestion of this drug with alcohol is not recommended due to the possibility of liver failure from hepatic necrosis.

The patient should avoid taking herbs that have the potential for liver toxicity, including comfrey, coltsfoot, and chaparral.

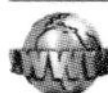
See the Companion Website for a Nursing Process Focus specific to this drug.

NURSING PROCESS FOCUS

Patients Receiving Antipyretic Therapy

ASSESSMENT

Prior to administration:

- Obtain complete health history (mental and physical), including data on origin of fever, recent surgeries, or trauma
- Obtain vital signs; assess in context of patient's baseline values
- Obtain patient's complete medication history, including nicotine and alcohol consumption, to determine possible drug allergies and/or interactions

POTENTIAL NURSING DIAGNOSES

- Pain
- Hyperthermia
- Risk for Injury (hepatic toxicity), related to adverse effects of drug therapy

PLANNING: Patient Goals and Expected Outcomes

The patient will:

- Experience a reduction in body temperature
- Demonstrate an understanding of the drug's action by accurately describing drug side effects and precautions

IMPLEMENTATION

Interventions and (Rationales)	Patient Education/Discharge Planning
■ Assess for intolerance to ASA for possible cross-hypersensitivity to other NSAIDs or acetaminophen.	■ Inform patient to immediately report any difficulty breathing, itching, or skin rash.

continued...

(continued from page 207)

NURSING PROCESS FOCUS

Interventions and (Rationales)	Patient Education/Discharge Planning
■ Monitor hepatic and renal function. (Antipyretics are metabolized in the liver and excreted by the kidneys.)	Instruct patient: ■ To report signs of liver toxicity: nausea, vomiting, anorexia, bleeding, severe upper or lower abdominal pain, heartburn, jaundice, or a change in the color or character of stools ■ To adhere to laboratory testing regimen for serum blood tests as directed
■ Use with caution in patients with a history of excessive alcohol consumption. (Alcohol increases the risk of liver damage associated with acetaminophen or NSAID administration.)	■ Advise patient to abstain from alcohol while taking this medication.
■ Use with caution in diabetics. Observe for signs of hypoglycemia which may occur with acetaminophen usage.	Instruct patient to immediately report: ■ Excessive thirst ■ Large increase or decrease in urine output ■ Advise patients with diabetes mellitus that acetaminophen may cause low blood sugar and require insulin dose adjustments

EVALUATION OF OUTCOME CRITERIA

Evaluate the effectiveness of drug therapy by confirming that patient goals and expected outcomes have been met (see "Planning").

See Table 12.3 for a list of drugs to which these nursing actions apply.

TENSION HEADACHE AND MIGRAINE

Headache is one of the most common complaints of patients. Living with headache can interfere with activities of daily life, thus causing great distress. The pain and difficulty of focusing and concentrating results in work-related absences and neglect of home and family. When headaches are persistent, or occur as migraines, drug therapy is needed.

Of the many types of headaches, the most common is the **tension headache.** It occurs when muscles of the head and neck tighten in response to stress. The tightness causes a steady and lingering pain. Although quite painful, tension headaches usually end when the stress is resolved. They are generally considered an annoyance rather than a medical emergency. Tension headaches can usually be effectively treated with OTC analgesics such as aspirin, acetaminophen, or ibuprofen.

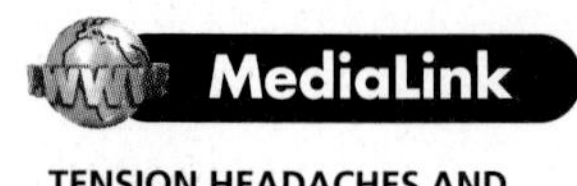

TENSION HEADACHES AND MIGRAINE

The most painful type of headache is the **migraine,** which is characterized by throbbing or pulsating pain, sometimes preceded by an aura, similar to those that warn of a seizure (see Chapter 11). The **auras** of migraine are sensory cues—such as seeing jagged lines or flashing lights, smelling, tasting, or hearing something strange—that let the patient know that a migraine attack is coming soon. Most patients with migraines also have nausea and vomiting. Triggers for migraines include nitrates and monosodium glutamate (MSG) found in many Asian foods, red wine, perfumes, food additives, caffeine, chocolate, and aspartame (a sugar substitute). By avoiding these substances, some patients can prevent the onset of a migraine attack.

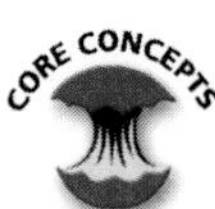

12.7 Headaches can be effectively treated with a variety of drug classes.

There are two primary goals for the pharmacological therapy of migraines (see Table 12.4). The first is to stop migraines in progress, and the second is to prevent migraines from occurring. For the most part, the drugs used to stop migraines are different than those used for *prophylaxis* (that is, *prevention*). Drug therapy is most effective if begun before a migraine has reached a severe level.

pro = *before*
phylaxis = *guarding*

TABLE 12.4 Antimigraine Drugs

DRUG	ROUTE AND ADULT DOSE	REMARKS
DRUGS FOR TERMINATING MIGRAINES		
Ergotamine Alkaloids		
dihydroergotamine mesylate (D.H.E. 45, Migranal)	IM 1 mg, may be repeated at 1-hour intervals to a total of 3 mg (max: 6 mg/week)	Also available as nasal spray; pregnancy category X; for migraine termination; may be used in combination with low-dose heparin to prevent postop deep vein thrombosis
ergotamine tartrate (Ergostat)	PO 1–2 mg followed by 1–2 mg every 30 minutes until headache stops (max: 6 mg/day or 10 mg/week)	Also available in sublingual, inhalant, or rectal forms; may cause physical dependence; pregnancy category X; for migraine termination
Triptans		
almotriptan (Axert)	PO 6.25–12.5 mg, may repeat in 2 hours if necessary (max: 2 tablets/day)	May cause heart palpitations and rapid heartbeat.
eletriptan (Relpax)	PO 20–40 mg, may repeat in 2 hours if necessary (max: 80 mg/day)	May cause hypotension in elderly patients
frovatriptan (Frova)	PO 2.5 mg, may repeat in 2 hours if necessary (max: 7.5 mg/day)	May cause chest pains and heart palpitations
naratriptan (Amerge)	PO 1–2.5 mg, may repeat in 4 hours if necessary (max: 5 mg/day)	Serotonin stimulator; for migraine termination
rizatriptan (Maxalt)	PO 5–10 mg, may repeat in 2 hours if necessary (max: 30 mg/day); 5 mg with concurrent propranolol (max: 15 mg/day)	May cause myocardial infarction
Pr sumatriptan (Imitrex)	PO 25 mg for 1 dose (max: 100 mg)	Serotonin stimulator; subcutaneous and intranasal forms available; for migraine termination
zolmitriptan (Zomig)	PO 2.5–5 mg, may repeat in 2 hours if necessary (max: 10 mg/day)	Serotonin stimulator; for migraine termination
DRUGS FOR PREVENTING MIGRAINES		
Triptans		
almotriptan (Axert)	PO 6.25–12.5 mg, may repeat in 2 hours if necessary (max: 2 tablets/day)	May cause heart palpitations and rapid heartbeat
eletriptan (Relpax)	PO 20–40 mg, may repeat in 2 hours if necessary (max: 80 mg/day)	May cause myocardial infarction
frovatriptan (Frova)	PO 2.5 mg, may repeat in 2 hours if necessary (max: 7.5 mg/day)	May cause chest pain and heart palpitations
Beta-Adrenergic Blockers		
atenolol (Tenormin)	PO 25–50 mg daily (max: 100 mg/day)	Also used for hypertension and angina
metoprolol (Lopressor)	PO 50–100 mg daily bid (max: 450 mg/day)	Also for angina and MI; sustained-release and IV forms available
propranolol hydrochloride (Inderal)	PO 80–240 mg/day in divided doses, may need 160–240 mg/day	Beta-adrenergic blocker for migraine prevention
timolol (Blocadren)	PO 10 mg bid, may increase to 60 mg/day in 2 divided doses	Also for hypertension, angina, and glaucoma
Calcium Channel Blockers		
nifedipine (Procardia)	PO 10–20 mg tid (max: 180 mg/day)	Selective for calcium channels in blood vessels; decreases peripheral vascular resistance and increases cardiac output; also for hypertension and angina; sustained-release form available
nimodipine (Nimotop)	PO 60 mg q4h for 21 days; start therapy within 96 hours of subarachnoid hemorrhage	Use in migraines is an unlabeled use; primary use is for improvement of neurological symptoms following a stroke
Pr verapamil hydrochloride (Calan)	PO 40–80 mg tid	Unlabeled use for migraine prevention

continued...

TABLE 12.4 Antimigraine Drugs—*Continued*

DRUG	ROUTE AND ADULT DOSE	REMARKS
***DRUGS FOR PREVENTING MIGRAINES*—Continued**		
Tricyclic Antidepressants		
amitriptyline hydrochloride (Elavil)	PO 75–100 mg/day	Unlabeled use for migraine prevention
imipramine (Tofranil)	PO 75–100 mg/day (max: 300 mg/day)	May cause cardiac dysfunction and abnormal blood cell count; also for alcohol or cocaine dependence; may control bedwetting in children; available IM
Miscellaneous Agents		
valproic acid (Depakene, Depakote)	PO 250 mg bid (max: 100 mg/day)	Also for absence seizures and mixed generalized types of seizures and mania
methysergide (Sansert)	PO 4–8 mg/day in divided doses	Similar to ergotamine; for migraine prevention
riboflavin (vitamin B_2)	PO as a supplement: 5–10 mg/day; for deficiency: 5–30 mg/day in divided doses	Deficiency caused by chronic diarrhea, liver disease, alcoholism, or inadequate consumption of milk or animal products

DRUG PROFILE: Antimigraine Agent; Triptan: Pr *Sumatriptan (Imitrex)*

Actions and Uses:

Sumatriptan belongs to a relatively new group of antimigraine drugs known as the triptans. The triptans act by causing vasoconstriction of cranial arteries; this vasoconstriction is moderately selective and does not usually affect overall blood pressure. This medication is available in oral, intranasal, and subcutaneous forms. Subcutaneous administration ends migraine attacks in 10 to 20 minutes; the dose may be repeated 60 minutes after the first injection, to a maximum of 2 doses per day. If taken orally, sumatriptan should be administered as soon as possible after the migraine is suspected or has begun.

Adverse Effects and Interactions:

Some dizziness, drowsiness, or a warming sensation may be experienced after taking sumatriptan; however, these effects are not normally severe enough to warrant stopping therapy. Because of its vasconstricting action, the drug should be used cautiously, if at all, in patients with recent MI, or with a history of angina pectoris, hypertension, or diabetes.

Sumatriptan interacts with several drugs. For example, an increased effect may occur when taken with MAOIs and SSRIs. Further vasoconstriction can occur when taken with ergot alkaloids and other triptans.

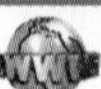

See the Companion Website for a Nursing Process Focus specific to this drug.

Triptans

The two major drug classes used as antimigraine agents, the triptans and the ergot alkaloids, both stimulate serotonin (5-HT). Serotonin receptors are found throughout the CNS, and in the cardiovascular and GI systems. At least five receptor subtypes have been identified. In addition to the triptans, other drugs acting as serotonin receptors include the popular antianxiety agents fluoxetine (Prozac) and buspirone (BuSpar).

Pharmacotherapy to stop migraines usually begins with acetaminophen or NSAIDs. If OTC analgesics are unable to stop the migraine, the drugs of choice are often the triptans. The first of the triptans, sumatriptan (Imitrex), was marketed in the United States in 1993. These agents are selective for the 5-HT_1 receptor subtype, and they are thought to act by constricting certain vessels within the brain. They are effective in stopping migraines with or without auras. Although oral forms of the triptans are the most convenient, patients who experience nausea and vomiting during a migraine may require an alternate dosage form. Intranasal formulation and prefilled syringes of triptans are available for patients who are able to self-administer the medication.

Ergot Alkaloids

For patients who are unresponsive to triptans, the ergot alkaloids may be used to stop migraines. The actions of the ergot alkaloids have been known for thousands of years. The first purified alkaloid, ergotamine (Ergostat), was isolated from the ergot fungus in 1920. Ergotamine is an inexpensive drug that is available in oral, sublingual, and suppository forms. Modification of the original molecule has produced a number of other pharmacologically useful drugs, such as dihydroergotamine (Migranal). Dihydroergotamine is given parenterally and as a nasal spray. Because the ergot alkaloids interact with adrenergic and dopaminergic receptors, as well as serotonin receptors, they produce multiple actions and side effects. Many ergot alkaloids are pregnancy category X drugs.

Other Antimigraine Agents

Drugs for migraine prophylaxis include many classes of drugs that are discussed in other chapters of this textbook. They include beta-adrenergic blockers (Chapter 17), calcium channel blockers (Chapter 15), antidepressants (Chapter 9), and antiseizure drugs (Chapter 11). Because these drugs have the potential to produce side effects, prophylaxis is only started if the number of migraines is high and the patient does not respond to the drugs used to stop migraines. Of the various drugs, propranolol (Inderal) is one of the most commonly prescribed. Amitriptyline (Elavil) is preferred for patients who may have a mood disorder or suffer from insomnia in addition to their migraines.

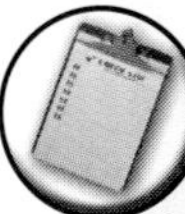

PATIENTS NEED TO KNOW

Patients taking pain medication need to know the following:

In General

1. Carefully describe pain to your healthcare provider so that the analgesic medication being taken is suited to the complaint.
2. Report any OTC medication taken for pain to your healthcare provider to minimize adverse effects and interactions.
3. Aspirin has many undesirable side effects, mainly related to gastric upset and bleeding. Follow instructions carefully and watch for drug interactions or contraindications.

Regarding Opiates

4. Avoid combining pain medications with alcohol and other CNS depressants (especially opioids).
5. Vital signs will be monitored with all opioid medications because of their CNS depressant effects.
6. Get up slowly from seated positions because certain pain medications cause lightheadedness.
7. Avoid operating machinery or driving a car if taking opiates because of symptoms of dizziness, blurred vision, and drowsiness.
8. Do not abruptly stop taking opioids; this could result in withdrawal. Signs include chills, abdominal and muscle cramps, severe itching, sweating, restlessness, anxiety, yawning, and drug-seeking behavior. ■

CHAPTER REVIEW

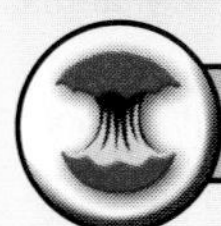

CORE CONCEPTS SUMMARY

12.1 Pain assessment is the first step to pain management.

Pain is a subjective experience where many patients describe discomfort differently. Pain may be classified as acute (from injury to recovery) or chronic (longer than 6 months). Pain may be classified as nociceptor pain and further divided into somatic or visceral pain and neuropathic pain.

12.2 **Nonpharmacological techniques assist patients in obtaining adequate pain relief.**

Nonpharmacological techniques may be used in place of drugs or as an adjunct to drug therapy. When used along with medication, nonpharmacological techniques may allow lower doses to be given with possibly fewer drug-related adverse effects. More invasive techniques in patients with intractable pain may include chemotherapy, surgery, radiation therapy, and injection of alcohol or neurotoxic substances for nerve blocks.

12.3 **Pain transmission processes allow several targets for pharmocological intervention.**

Pain signals involve nerve impulses along two types of sensory neurons, Aδ and C fibers. Once impulses reach the spinal cord, substance P is thought to transmit pain at the spinal level. The release of substance P is controlled by descending neurons that release neurotransmitters called *endogenous opioids.* If not blocked, the impulse travels to the brain where pain information is sensed and a response to the sensation is initiated. Opioids act at the level of the central nervous system (CNS); nonsteroidal anti-inflammatory drugs (NSAIDs) act at the level of the peripheral nervous system (PNS).

12.4 **Opioid analgesic medications exert their effects by interacting with specific receptors.**

Two types of receptors mediate analgesia (pain relief)—mu receptors and kappa receptors. Both are opioid receptors that respond to natural or synthetic morphine-like substances. Natural substances extracted from unripe seeds of the poppy plant are called *opiates. Narcotic* is a general term referring to morphine-like drugs. In the context of drug enforcement, the term *narcotic* includes a much broader classification of abused illegal drugs.

12.5 **Narcotic opioids have multiple therapeutic effects including relief of severe pain.**

Opioids produce many effects including analgesia for intense pain, cough suppression, suppression of GI motility in diarrhea treatment, sedation, and euphoria. It is common practice to place opioids and nonnarcotic analgesics in a single tablet or capsule. Acute opioid intoxication is treated with the opioid antagonist naloxone. All of the narcotic analgesics have the potential to cause physical and psychological dependence. The opioids have a greater risk of dependency than most any of the other classes of medications. In treating opioid dependence, medication is often switched to another narcotic drug with less intense withdrawal symptoms.

12.6 **Nonsteroidal anti-inflammatory drugs are the drugs of choice for inflammatory pain.**

NSAIDs are used to treat less severe pain associated with inflammation. NSAIDs have antifever as well as pain-reducing properties. These effects are achieved by inhibition of enzymes called cyclooxygenase type one (COX-1) and cyclooxygenase type two (COX-2). When cyclooxygenase (COX) is inhibited, prostaglandin synthesis is prevented. Some medications are selective for the COX-2 receptor. Other antifever and pain-reducing medictions including acetaminophen and centrally acting agents do not have anti-inflammatory or COX-inhibiting properties.

12.7 **Headaches can be effectively treated with a variety of drug classes.**

Headaches in two categories—tension headaches and migraines—are the most common complaints of patients. The two primary goals of migraine therapy are migraine termination and migraine prevention. The two major classes of antimigraine agents are ergot alkaloids and triptans. Drugs for migraine prophylaxis include beta-adrenergic blockers, calcium channel blockers, antidepressants, and antiseizure drugs.

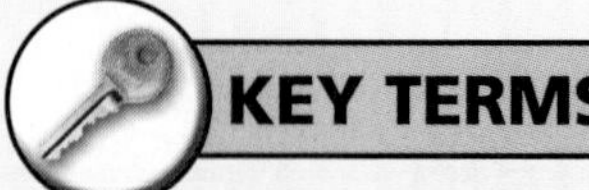

KEY TERMS

Aδ fibers: nerves that transmit sensations of sharp pain / *page 195*

analgesic (an-ul-JEE-zik): drug used to reduce or eliminate pain / *page 195*

aura (AUR-uh): sensory cue such as bright lights, smells, or tastes that precede a migraine / *page 208*

bradykinin (bray-dee-KYE-nin): chemical mediator of pain released following tissue damage / *page 204*

C fibers: nerves that transmit dull, poorly localized pain / *page 195*

cyclooxygenase (sye-klo-OK-sah-jen-ays): enzyme involved in the synthesis of prostaglandins / *page 203*

endogenous opioids (en-DAHJ-en-nuss O-pee-oyds): chemicals produced naturally within the body that decrease or eliminate pain; they closely resemble the actions of morphine / *page 195*

migraine (MYE-grayne): severe headache preceded by auras that may include nausea and vomiting / *page 208*

narcotic (nar-KOT-ik): natural or synthetic drug related to morphine; may be used as a broader legal term referring to hallucinogens (LSD), CNS stimulants, marijuana, and other illegal drugs / *page 195*

nociceptor (no-si-SEPP-ter): receptor connected with nerves that receive and transmit pain signals to the spinal cord and brain / *page 194*

opiate (OH-pee-aht): natural substance extracted from the poppy plant / *page 195*

opioid (OH-pee-oyd): natural or synthetic morphine-like substance / ***page 195***

prostaglandins (pros-tah-GLAN-dins): chemicals released after tissue damage, leading to pain, inflammation, and other body reactions / ***page 204***

substance P: neurotransmitter within the spinal cord involved in the neural transmission of pain / ***page 195***

tension headache: common type of head pain caused by stress and relieved by nonnarcotic analgesics / ***page 208***

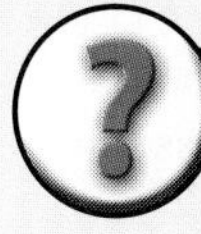

REVIEW QUESTIONS

The following questions are written in NCLEX-PN® style. Answer these questions to assess your knowledge of the chapter material, and go back and review any material that is not clear to you.

1. Your patient has osteoarthritis. Which of the following drugs would the nurse anticipate being ordered?

1. Sumatriptan (Imitrex)
2. Acetaminophen (Tylenol)
3. Fentanyl (Sublimaze)
4. Etodolac (Lodine)

2. The patient is no sumatriptan (Imitrex) for migraines. For which of the following should the nurse instruct the patient to notify his physician immediately?

1. Chest pain
2. GI upset
3. Bleeding
4. Lethargy

3. When a patient is receiving a NSAID, the nurse must assess the patient for:

1. GI upset and bleeding
2. Urinary retention
3. Blurred vision
4. Anorexia, headache

4. The patient is experiencing opioid dependency. Which drug is used to treat opioid dependence?

1. Oxycodone hydrochloride (OxyContin)
2. Propoxyphene hydrochloride (Darvon)
3. Hydromorphone hydrochloride (Dilaudid)
4. Methadone (Dolophine)

5. The nurse understands that pain signals begin at the __________ and proceed through the central nervous system.

1. Spinal cord
2. Viscera
3. Nociceptors
4. Substance P

6. Prior to administering pain medication, what must be assessed?

1. The patient's diagnosis
2. The location, severity, and quality of pain
3. When the patient last had a meal
4. The patient's ability to become addicted

7. The patient has been receiving morphine sulfate for pain control. Assessment reveals a decreased level of consciousness and shallow respirations at a rate of 8 per minute. The nurse anticipates what opioid antagonist being ordered?

1. Butorphanol (Stadol)
2. Hydrocodone bitartrate (Hycodan)
3. Naloxone hydrochloride (Narcan)
4. Oxycodone hydrochloride (OxyContin)

8. The patient is allergic to aspirin. Which of the following drugs may be an alternative for mild relief?

1. Acetaminophen
2. Morphine sulfate
3. Etodolac (Lodine)
4. Fentanyl (Sublimaze)

9. Side effects of ergotamine (Ergostate) include:

1. Bradycardia, chest pain, and hypertension
2. Nausea, vomiting, chest pain, and tachycardia
3. Urinary retention, hypertension, and peripheral dilation
4. Peripheral constriction, bradycardia, and chest pain

10. Chronic pain is:

1. Intense and lasts less than 3 months
2. Persistent, interferes with daily activities, and lasts longer than 6 months
3. Somatic in nature, which makes it difficult to treat
4. Neuropathic in nature, which makes it difficult to treat

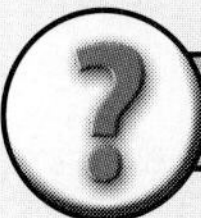

CASE STUDY QUESTIONS

For questions 1–5, please refer to the following case study, and choose the correct response from choices 1–4.

Ms. Coidiuf, age 42, sustained a back injury 3 years ago, which responded well to treatment with nonsteroidal anti-inflammatory medication. Over the last 6 months, Ms. Coidiuf has been seeing her physician again with complaints of painful sensations "shooting" down her right hip. Despite careful attention, it appears that Ms. Coidiuf's pain is no longer responding to anti-inflammatory medication. Her physician prescribes a narcotic analgesic (moderate effectiveness) with acetaminophen, hoping this treatment might provide relief. Following three physical therapy sessions, the patient continues to report that she is "still miserable," leading her physician to believe that her condition is worsening. Heat packs, massage, and relaxation therapy have not been successful.

1. Based on Ms. Coidiuf's complaints over the last 6 months, her pain can be classified as:

1. Nociceptor pain
2. Visceral pain
3. Neuropathic pain
4. Both a and b

2. Which of the following symptoms has Ms. Coidiuf likely avoided by her physician switching to narcotic therapy?

1. Decreased GI motility
2. GI bleeding
3. Drowsiness
4. Vomiting

3. The most likely target of pharmacological intervention for Ms. Coidiuf 3 years ago was:

1. Inhibition of spinal substance P release
2. Release of endorphin neurotransmitters in the central nervous system (CNS)
3. Inhibition of pain transmitted by Aδ fibers
4. Inhibition of cyclooxygenase (COX) enzyme

4. Which of the following narcotic analgesics was probably given to Ms.Coidiuf?

1. Percocet
2. Talwin
3. Dilaudid
4. Demerol

5. With continued pharmacological intervention, which of the following would be less of a concern for Ms. Coidiuf?

1. Tolerance to the medication
2. Withdrawal symptoms
3. Sedation
4. Respiratory depression

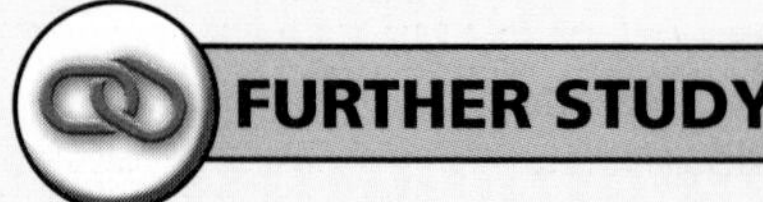

FURTHER STUDY

- More information on the following classes of drugs can be found in these chapters: beta-adrenergic blockers (Chapter 7), calcium channel blockers (Chapter 15), antidepressants (Chapter 9), and antiseizure drugs (Chapter 11).
- NSAIDs used for inflammation are presented in Chapter 21.
- The use of acetylcysteine as an antidote for acetaminophen overdose is discussed in Chapter 25.
- Opioids used to treat diarrhea are covered in Chapter 26.

EXPLORE MEDIALINK www.prenhall.com/holland

Additional resources for this chapter can be found on the CD-ROM accompanying this textbook, and on the Companion Website. Click on Chapter 12 to select activities for this chapter.

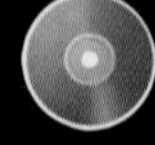

Mechanism in Action: Morphine
Audio Glossary
Concept Review
NCLEX-PN® Review
Nursing in Action
Dosage Calculator

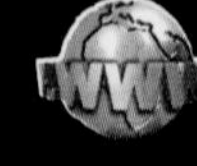

The American Holistic Nurses Association
JCAHO Standards on Pain Management
The Oxford Pain Internet Site
Tension Headaches and Migraine

CHAPTER

13 Drugs for Anesthesia

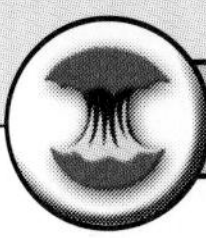

CORE CONCEPTS

13.1 Local anesthesia causes a rapid loss of sensation to a limited part of the body.

13.2 Local anesthetics produce their therapeutic effect by blocking the entry of sodium ions into neurons.

13.3 Local anesthetics are classified by their chemical structures.

13.4 General anesthesia is a loss of sensation occurring throughout the entire body, accompanied by a loss of consciousness.

13.5 General anesthetics are usually administered by the IV or inhalation routes.

13.6 Intravenous anesthetics are important supplements to general anesthesia and include barbiturates, opioids, and benzodiazepines.

13.7 Nonanesthetic drugs are used as adjuncts to anesthesia and include barbiturates, barbiturate-like drugs, opioids, neuromuscular blocking agents, and other miscellaneous drugs.

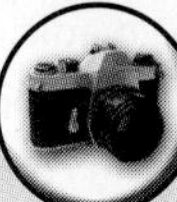

DRUG SNAPSHOT

The following drugs will be discussed in this chapter:

DRUG CLASSES	DRUG PROFILES
LOCAL ANESTHESIA	
Amides	Pr lidocaine (Xylocaine)
Esters	
Miscellaneous agents	
GENERAL ANESTHESIA	
Inhalation agents	
Gases	Pr nitrous oxide
Volatile liquids	Pr halothane (Fluothane)
Intravenous agents	Pr thiopental (Pentothal)
ADJUNCTS TO ANESTHESIA	
Neuromuscular blocker	Pr succinylcholine (Anectine)

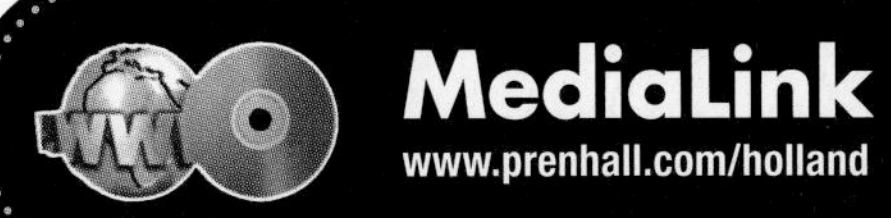

MediaLink
www.prenhall.com/holland

Interactive resources for this chapter can be found on the Companion Website. Click on Chapter 13 and "Begin" to select the activities for this chapter. For chapter-related animations, NCLEX-PN®-style questions, and an audio glossary, access the accompanying CD-ROM in this book.

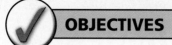

OBJECTIVES

After reading this chapter, the student should be able to:

1. Compare and contrast the five major routes for administering local anesthetics.
2. Describe differences between the two major chemical classes of local anesthetics.
3. Explain why epinephrine and sodium hydroxide are sometimes found as part of the local anesthetic medicine.
4. Identify the actions of general anesthetics within the CNS.
5. Compare and contrast the two primary ways that general anesthesia may be induced.
6. Identify the four stages of general anesthesia.
7. For each of the drug classes listed, know representative drugs and be able to explain their mechanisms of action, primary actions, and important adverse effects.
8. Categorize drugs used for anesthesia based on their classifications and actions in the body.

an = *without*
thesia = *sensation*

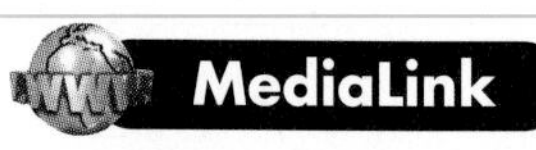

VIRTUAL ANESTHESIA TEXTBOOK

Anesthesia is a medical procedure performed by administering drugs that cause a loss of sensation. Local anesthesia occurs when sensation is lost to a limited part of the body without loss of consciousness. General anesthesia requires different classes of drugs that cause loss of sensation to the entire body, usually resulting in a loss of consciousness. This chapter will examine drugs used for both local and general anesthesia.

LOCAL ANESTHESIA

Local anesthesia is loss of sensation to a relatively small part of the body without loss of consciousness to the patient. This technique may be necessary when a relatively brief dental or medical procedure is performed.

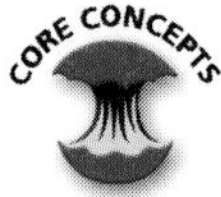

13.1 Local anesthesia causes a rapid loss of sensation to a limited part of the body.

Although local anesthesia often causes a loss of sensation to a small, limited area, it sometimes affects relatively large portions of the body, such as an entire limb. Because of this action, some local anesthetic treatments are more accurately called *surface anesthesia* or *regional anesthesia,* depending on how the drugs are administered and the results they produce.

The five major routes (Figure 13.1 ■) for applying local anesthetics include:

1. Topical
2. Infiltration
3. Nerve block
4. Spinal
5. Epidural

Fast Facts Anesthesia and Anesthetics

- Over 20 million people receive general anesthetics each year in the United States.
- About half of the general anesthetics are administered by a nurse anesthetist.
- The first medical applications of anesthetics were in 1842 with ether and in 1846 with nitrous oxide.
- Herbal products may interact with anesthetics; St. John's wort may intensify or prolong the effects of some opioids and anesthetics.

FIGURE 13.1

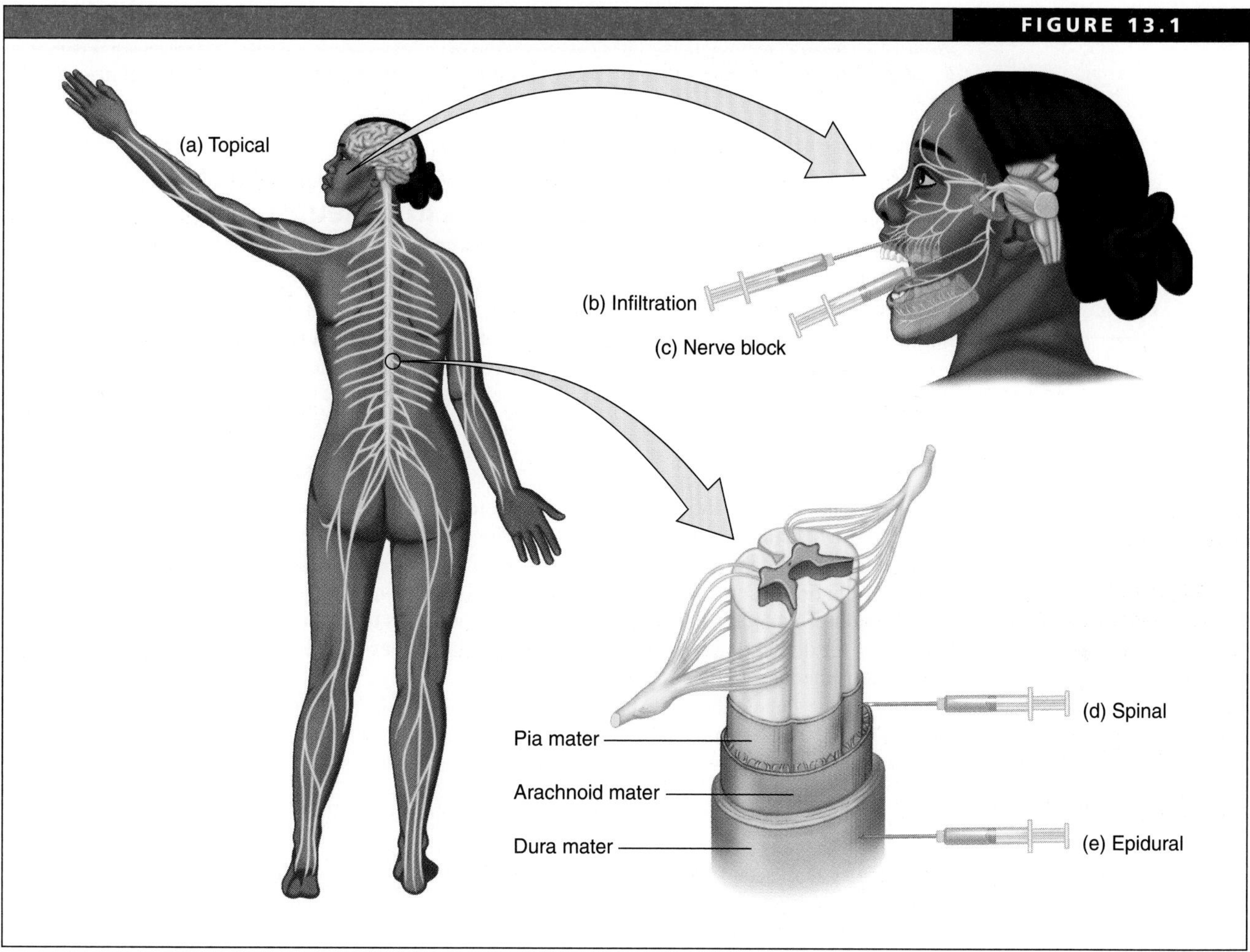

Routes for applying local anesthesia include (a) topical, (b) infiltration, (c) nerve block, (d) spinal, and (e) epidural.

The method used depends on the location and amount of anesthesia that is needed. For example, some local anesthetics are applied topically before a needle stick or minor skin surgery. Others are used to block sensations to large areas such as limb or the lower abdomen. The different methods of local and regional anesthesia are summarized in Table 13.1.

TABLE 13.1 Methods of Local and Regional Anesthesia

ROUTE	FORMULATION/METHOD	DESCRIPTION
Surface (topical) anesthesia	Creams, sprays, suppositories, drops, and lozenges	Applied to mucous membranes including the eyes, lips, gums, nasal membranes, and throat; very safe unless absorbed
Infiltration (field block) anesthesia	Direct injection into tissue immediate to the surgical site	Drug diffuses into tissue to block a specific group of nerves in a small area very close to the area to be operated upon
Nerve block anesthesia	Direct injection into tissue that may be distant from the operation site	Drug affects the bundle of nerves serving the area to be operated upon; used to block sensation in a limb or large area of the face
Spinal anesthesia	Injection into the cerebral spinal fluid (CSF)	Drug affects large, regional area such as the lower abdomen and legs
Epidural anesthesia	Injection into epidural space of spinal cord	Most commonly used in obstetrics during labor and delivery

Concept Review 13.1

- What is local anesthesia? Name the five general methods of local and regional anesthesia.

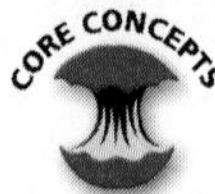
CORE CONCEPTS

13.2 Local anesthetics produce their therapeutic effect by blocking the entry of sodium ions into neurons.

The mechanism of action of local anesthetics is well known. Recall that the concentration of sodium ions is normally higher on the outside of neurons than on the inside. A rapid flood of sodium ions into cells is necessary for neurons to fire and conduct an action potential.

Local anesthetics act by blocking sodium channels, as illustrated in Figure 13.2 ■. The blocking of sodium channels by local anesthetics is nonselective; therefore, both sensory and motor impulses are affected. Sensation and muscle activity in the treated area will be decreased temporarily. Because of their mechanism of action, local anesthetics are sometimes called *sodium channel blockers.*

During a medical or surgical procedure, it is essential that the direction of action of the anesthetic lasts at least until the procedure is completed. Small amounts of epinephrine are sometimes added to the anesthetic solution to constrict blood vessels in the immediate area where the local anesthetic is applied. This keeps the anesthetic in the area longer and lengthens the duration of action of the drug. The addition of epinephrine to lidocaine (Xylocaine), for example, increases the duration of its local anesthetic effect from 20 minutes to as long as 60 minutes. This effect is important for dental or surgical procedures that take longer than 20 minutes; otherwise, a second injection of the anesthetic would be necessary.

Sometimes an alkaline substance, such as sodium hydroxide or sodium bicarbonate, is added to anesthetic solutions to increase the drug's effectiveness in areas with extensive local infection or abscesses. The reason for this is that bacteria tend to acidify an infected site, and local anes-

FIGURE 13.2

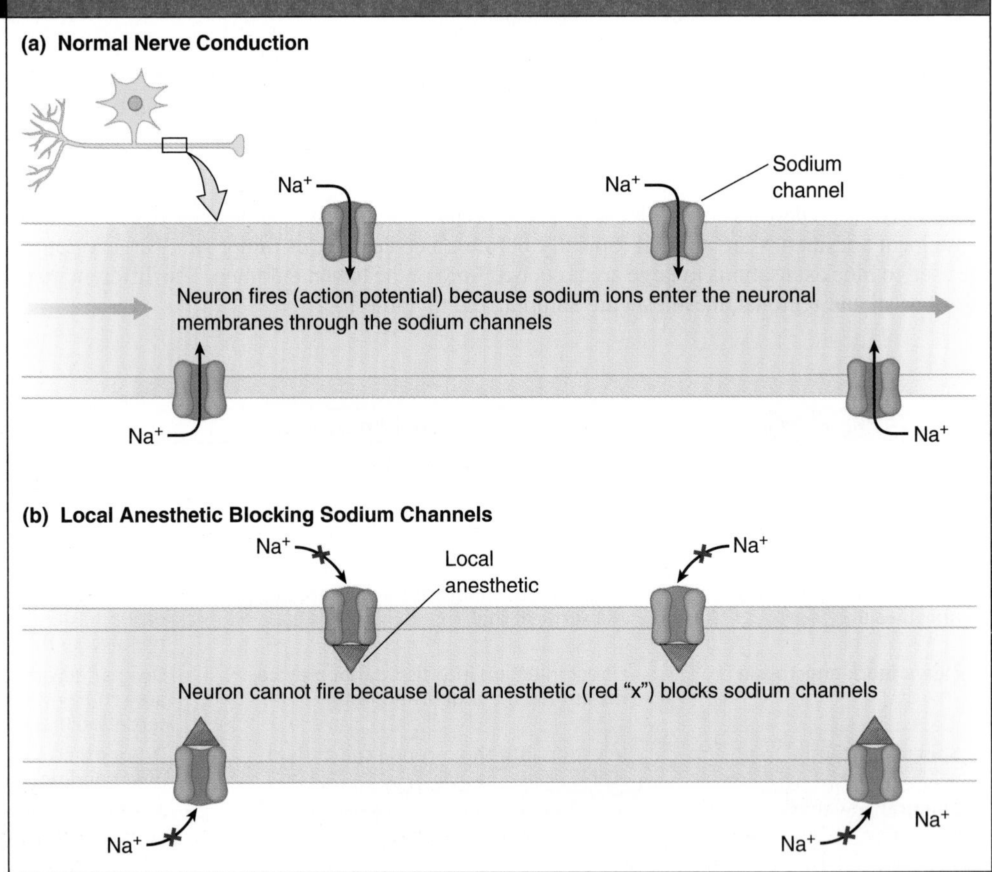
(a) Normal Nerve Conduction
Na+
Na+
Sodium channel
Neuron fires (action potential) because sodium ions enter the neuronal membranes through the sodium channels
Na+
Na+
(b) Local Anesthetic Blocking Sodium Channels
Na+
Local anesthetic
Na+
Neuron cannot fire because local anesthetic (red "x") blocks sodium channels
Na+
Na+
Na+

(a) In normal nerve conduction, sodium ions (Na^+) enter the sodium channels along a neuron and allow the neuron to fire (set off an action potential) and conduct an impulse. (b) Local anesthetics (shown by the red x) block the sodium channels. Sodium ions are not able to enter the neuronal membrane through the sodium channels. Therefore, no action potential can be conducted along the nerve.

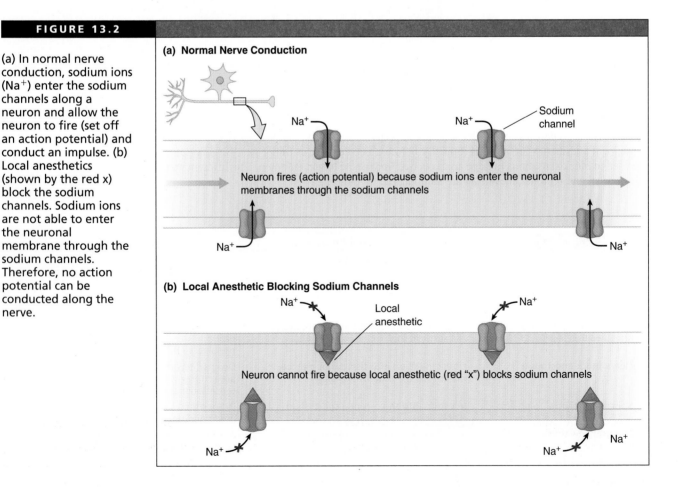

thetics are less effective in an acidic environment. Adding alkaline substances neutralizes the infected region and allows the anesthetic to work better.

13.3 Local anesthetics are classified by their chemical structures.

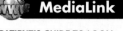

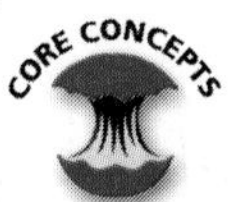

The two major classes of local anesthetics are esters and amides (Table 13.2). The terms **esters** and **amides** refer to types of chemical linkages found within the anesthetic molecules, as illustrated in Figure 13.3 ■. Although esters and amides have equal effectiveness, important differences exist. A small number of miscellaneous agents are neither esters nor amides.

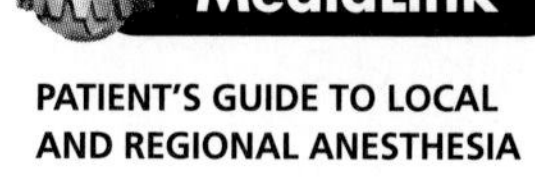

PATIENT'S GUIDE TO LOCAL AND REGIONAL ANESTHESIA

Cocaine was the first local anesthetic widely used for medical procedures, as far back as the 1880s. Cocaine is a natural ester, found in the leaves of the plant *Erythroxylon coca,* native to the Andes Mountains of Peru. As late as the 1980s, cocaine was routinely used for eye surgery, nerve blocks, and spinal anesthesia. Although still available for local anesthesia, cocaine is a Schedule II drug and rarely used therapeutically in the United States. The abuse potential of cocaine is discussed in Chapter 6.

TABLE 13.2 Selected Local Anesthetics

DRUG	USE	REMARKS
ESTERS		
benzocaine (Americaine, Solarcaine, others)	Topical anesthesia	For sunburn, sore throat, earache, hemorrhoids, and other minor skins conditions
chloroprocaine (Nesacaine)	Infiltration, nerve block, and epidural anesthesia	Short duration
cocaine	Topical anesthesia	For ear, nose, and throat procedures
procaine (Novocain)	Infiltration, nerve block, epidural, and spinal anesthesia	Short duration
tetracaine (Pontocaine)	Topical and spinal anesthesia	Long duration
AMIDES		
articaine (Septodont, Septanest)	Infiltration and nerve block anesthesia	Long duration
bupivicaine (Marcaine)	Infiltration and epidural anesthesia	Long duration
dibucaine (Nupercaine, Nupercainal)	Topical or spinal anesthesia	Long duration
etidocaine (Duranest)	Infiltration, nerve block, and epidural anesthesia	Long duration
Pr lidocaine (Xylocaine)	Topical, infiltration, nerve block, epidural, and spinal anesthesia	May be combined as a mixture of lidocaine and prilocaine (EMLA cream) for topical application
mepivacaine (Carbocaine)	Infiltration, nerve block, and epidural anesthesia	Intermediate duration
prilocaine (Citanest)	Infiltration, nerve block, and epidural anesthesia	Intermediate duration
ropivacaine (Naropine)	Infiltration, nerve block, and epidural anesthesia	Long duration
MISCELLANEOUS AGENTS		
dyclonine (Dyclone)	Topical anesthesia	For ear, nose, and throat procedures
pramoxine (Tronothane)	Topical anesthesia	For minor medical procedures

FIGURE 13.3

The amides contain a type of chemical linkage that includes carbon, nitrogen, and oxygen (-NH-CO-). The esters contain a type of chemical linkage that includes carbon and oxygen (-CO-O-).

Type	General formula	Example
Ester	R—C(=O)—O—R	H_2N—C_6H_4—C(=O)—O—C_2H_2—N(C_2H_5)$_2$ **Procaine**
Amide	R—NH—C(=O)—R	(CH_3)$_2C_6H_3$—NH—C(=O)—CH_2—N(C_2H_5)$_2$ **Lidocaine**

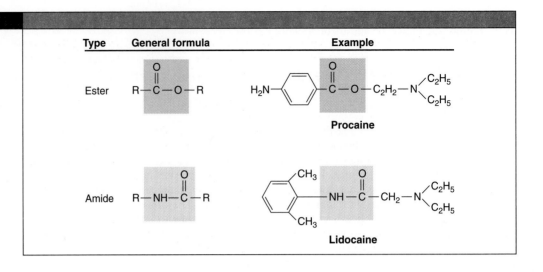

DRUG PROFILE: Local Anesthetic Amide: Pr *Lidocaine (Xylocaine)*

Actions and Uses:

Lidocaine is the most frequently used injectable local anesthetic. It is available in solutions ranging from 0.5% to 2% for infiltration, nerve block, spinal, or epidural anesthesia. A topical form is also available. When given for anesthesia, its onset of action is 5–15 minutes. Several hours may be needed for complete sensation to reappear. Lidocaine is also given IV, IM, or subcutaneously to treat dysrhythmias, as discussed in Chapter 17. Solutions of lidocaine containing preservatives or epinephrine are used for local anesthesia only and must never be given parenterally for dysrhythmias.

Adverse Effects and Interactions:

When used for anesthesia, side effects are uncommon. An early symptom of toxicity is excitement, leading to irritability and confusion. Serious adverse effects include convulsions, respiratory depression, and cardiac arrest. Until the effect of the anesthetic diminishes, patients may injure themselves by biting or chewing areas of the mouth that have no sensation following a dental procedure.

Barbiturates may decrease activity of lidocaine. Increased effects of lidocaine occur if taken with cimetidine, quinidine, and beta blockers. If lidocaine is used on a regular basis, its effectiveness may diminish when used with other medication.

Mechanism in Action: 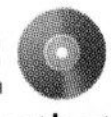

Lidocaine acts as a local anesthetic to block neuronal pain impulses and as an antidysrhythmic to correct ventricular fibrillation and tachycardia. These actions are achieved by blocking sodium channels located within the membranes of neurons and cardiac tissue.

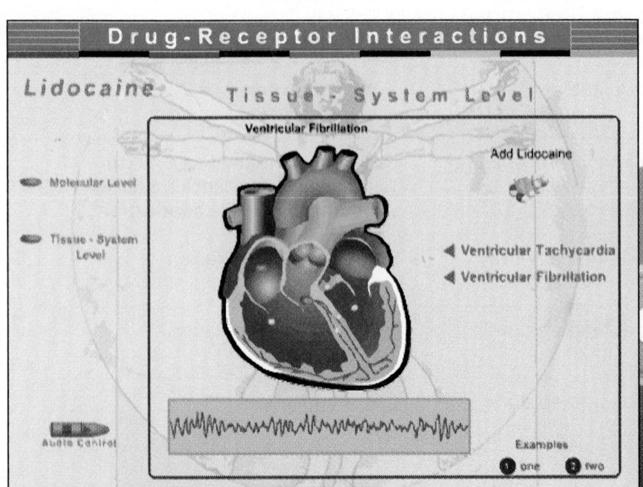

Use the student CD-ROM to see Mechanism in Action for Lidocaine.

See the Companion Website for a Nursing Process Focus specific to this drug.

Another ester, procaine (Novocain), was the drug of choice for dental procedures from the mid-1900s to the 1960s. About that time, amide anesthetics were developed and use of the ester anesthetics declined. One ester, benzocaine (Solarcaine and others) is used as a topical OTC agent for treating a large number of painful conditions, including sunburn, insect bites, hemorrhoids, sore throat, and minor wounds.

In most cases, amides have replaced the esters because they produce fewer side effects and generally have a longer duration of action. Lidocaine (Xylocaine) is the most widely used amide for short surgical procedures requiring local anesthesia.

Adverse effects to local anesthesia are uncommon. Allergy is rare. When it does occur, it is often due to sulfites, which are added as preservatives to prolong the shelf life of the anesthetic, or to methylparaben, which may be added to prevent bacterial growth in anesthetic solutions. Early signs of adverse effects of local anesthetics include symptoms of CNS stimulation such as restlessness or anxiety. Later, drowsiness and unresponsiveness may occur, which are due to CNS depression. Cardiovascular effects, including hypotension and dysrhythmias, are possible. Patients with a history of cardiovascular disease are often given forms of local anesthetics that contain no epinephrine to reduce the possible effects of this sympathomimetic on the heart and blood pressure. CNS and cardiovascular side effects are rare unless the local anesthetic is absorbed rapidly or is accidentally injected directly into a blood vessel.

NURSING PROCESS FOCUS

Patients Receiving Local Anesthesia

ASSESSMENT

Prior to administration:

- Assess for allergies to amide-type local anesthetics
- Check for the presence of broken skin, infection, burns, and wounds where medication is to be applied
- Assess for character, duration, location, and intensity of pain where medication is to be applied

POTENTIAL NURSING DIAGNOSES

- Risk for Aspiration
- Risk for Injury
- Deficient Knowledge, related to drug use

PLANNING: Patient Goals and Expected Outcomes

The patient will:

- Experience no pain during surgical procedure
- Experience no side effects or adverse reactions to anesthesia

IMPLEMENTATION

Interventions and (Rationales)	Patient Education/Discharge Planning
▪ Monitor for cardiovascular side effects. (These may occur if anesthetic is absorbed.)	▪ Instruct patient to report any unusual heart palpitations, lightheadedness, drowsiness, or confusion. If using medication on a regular basis, instruct patient to see the healthcare provider regularly.
▪ Monitor skin or mucous membranes for infection or inflammation. (Condition could be worsened by drug.)	▪ Instruct patient to report irritation or increase in discomfort in areas where medication was used.
▪ Monitor for length of effectiveness. (Local anesthetics are effective for 1–3 hours.)	▪ Instruct patient to report any discomfort during procedure.

continued...

(continued from page 221)

NURSING PROCESS FOCUS

Interventions and (Rationales)	Patient Education/Discharge Planning
■ Obtain information and monitor use of other medications.	■ Instruct patient to report use of any medication to healthcare provider.
■ Provide for patient safety. (There is a potential for injury related to area being treated having a lack of sensation.)	■ Inform patient about having no feeling in anesthetized area taking extra caution to avoid injury, including heat-related injury.
■ Monitor for gag reflex if used in the mouth or throat. (Xylocaine viscous may interfere with swallowing reflex.)	Instruct patient to: ■ Not eat within 1 hour of administration ■ Not chew gum while any portion of mouth or throat is anesthetized to prevent biting injuries

EVALUATION OF OUTCOME CRITERIA

Evaluate the effectiveness of drug therapy by confirming that patient goals and expected outcomes have been met (see "Planning").

See Table 13.2 for a list of drugs to which these nursing actions apply.

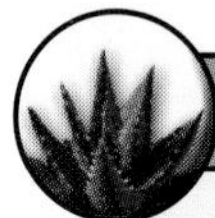

NATURAL ALTERNATIVES

Cloves and Anise as Natural Dental Remedies

You might not be aware that one natural remedy for tooth pain is oil of cloves. Extracted from the plant *Eugenia,* eugenol is the chemical extract found in cloves that is thought to produce its numbing effect. It works especially well for cavities. Soak a piece of cotton and pack it around the gums close to the painful area. Dentists sometimes recommend it for temporary relief of a toothache. Clove oil has an antiseptic effect that has been reported to kill bacteria, fungi, and helminths.

Another natural remedy is oil of anise, scientific name *Pimpinella,* for jaw pain caused by nerve pressure or gritting of teeth. Anise oil is an antispasmodic agent, which means it relaxes intense muscular pressure around the jaw angle, cheeks, and throat area. It has extra benefits in that it is also a natural expectorant, cough suppressant, and breath freshener. The pharmacological effects of anise are thought to be due to the chemical anethole, which is similar in structure to natural catecholamines. ■

Concept Review 13.2

- How does a local anesthetic work? How does the anesthetic action of lidocaine with epinephrine differ from that of lidocaine without epinephrine?

GENERAL ANESTHESIA

General anesthetics are used when it is necessary for patients to remain still and without pain for a longer period of time than could be achieved with local anesthetics.

TABLE 13.3	Stages of General Anesthesia
Stage 1	Loss of pain; the client loses general sensation but may be awake. This stage proceeds until the client loses consciousness.
Stage 2	Excitement and hyperactivity; the client may be delirious and try to resist treatment. Heartbeat and breathing may become irregular and blood pressure can increase. This is the stage when some IV agents are administered to calm the client.
Stage 3	Surgical anesthesia; skeletal muscles become relaxed and delirium stabilizes; cardiovascular and breathing activities stabilize. Eye movements slow down and the patient becomes very still. This is the stage when surgery begins and remains until the procedure ends.
Stage 4	Paralysis of the medulla region in the brain responsible for controlling respiratory and cardiovascular activity. If breathing or the heart stops, death could result. This stage is usually avoided during general anesthesia.

13.4 General anesthesia is a loss of sensation occurring throughout the entire body, accompanied by a loss of consciousness.

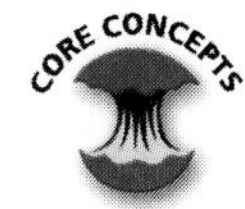

The goal of **general anesthesia** is to provide a rapid and complete loss of sensation. Signs of general anesthesia include total analgesia (no feeling of pain) and loss of consciousness, memory, and body movement. Although these signs are similar to those of sleeping, general anesthesia and sleep are not exactly the same. General anesthetics stop most nervous activity in the brain, whereas sleeping stops activity in only very specific areas. If fact, some brain activity actually increases during sleep, as described in Chapter 8.

General anesthesia usually requires more than one drug. Multiple medications are used to rapidly cause unconsciousness and muscle relaxation, and to maintain deep anesthesia. This approach, called *balanced anesthesia,* allows the dose of inhalation anesthetic to be lower so that the procedure is safer for the patient.

General anesthesia occurs in distinct steps, or stages. The most effective medications can quickly cause all four stages, whereas others are only able to cause stage 1 (light sedation). Most major surgery occurs in stage 3 when skeletal muscles are relaxed and the patient is sedated. Stage 3 anesthesia is called *surgical anesthesia.* When a patient is given surgical anesthesia, the anesthesiologist will try to move quickly through stage 2 because this stage produces symptoms such as hyperactivity and irregular breathing and heart rate. Often an IV agent will be given to calm the patient during this stage. The stages of anesthesia are shown in Table 13.3.

13.5 General anesthetics are usually administered by the IV or inhalation routes.

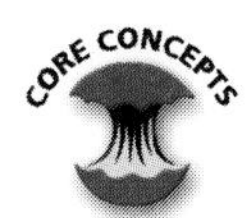

There are two primary methods of causing general anesthesia. Intravenous agents are usually administered first because they act within a few seconds. After the patient loses consciousness, inhaled agents are used to maintain the anesthesia. During short surgical procedures or those requiring lower stages of anesthesia, the IV agents may be used alone.

Inhaled general anesthetics, shown in Table 13.4, may be gasses or volatile liquids. These agents produce their effects by preventing the flow of sodium into neurons in the CNS, thus delaying nerve impulses and producing a dramatic reduction in neural activity. The exact mechanism for how this occurs is not exactly known, although it is likely that GABA receptors in the brain are activated. It is not the same mechanism as that of local anesthetics. There is some evidence suggesting that the mechanism may be related to how some antiseizure drugs work; however, this has not been proved. There is not a specific receptor that binds to general anesthetics, and they do not seem to affect neurotransmitter release.

The only gas used routinely for anesthesia is nitrous oxide, commonly called laughing gas. Nitrous oxide is used for dental procedures and for brief obstetrical and surgical procedures. It

TABLE 13.4	Inhaled General Anesthetics
DRUG	**USE**
VOLATILE LIQUID	
desflurane (Suprane)	Induction and maintenance of general anesthesia
enflurane (Ethrane)	Induction and maintenance of general anesthesia
Pr halothane (Fluothane)	Induction and maintenance of general anesthesia; use has declined because safer agents are available
isoflurane (Forane)	Induction and maintenance of general anesthesia; most widely used inhalation anesthetic
methoxyflurane (Penthrane)	Used during labor because it does not suppress uterine contractions as much as other agents
servoflurane (Ultane)	Induction and maintenance of general anesthesia
GAS	
Pr nitrous oxide	Used alone in dentistry, obstetrics, and short medical procedures; used in combination with more potent inhaled anesthetics

may also be used together with other general anesthetics, making it possible to decrease their dosages with greater effectiveness.

Nitrous oxide should be used cautiously in patients with myasthenia gravis because it may cause respiratory depression and prolonged hypnotic effects. Patients with cardiovascular disease, especially those with increased intracranial pressure, should be monitored carefully because the hypnotic effects of the drug may be prolonged or more powerful.

The volatile anesthetics are liquid at room temperature, but are converted into a vapor and inhaled to produce their anesthetic effects. Commonly administered volatile agents are halothane (Fluothane), enflurane (Ethrane), and isoflurane (Forane). The most potent of these is halothane (Fluothane). Some general anesthetics increase the sensitivity of the heart to drugs such as epinephrine, norepinephrine, dopamine, and serotonin. Most volatile liquids depress cardiovascular and respiratory function. Because it has less effect on the heart and does not damage the liver, isoflurane (Forane) has become the most widely used inhalation anesthetic. The volatile liquids are excreted almost entirely by the lungs, through exhalation.

DRUG PROFILE: General Anesthetic, Gas: Pr *Nitrous Oxide*

Actions and Uses:

The main action of nitrous oxide is analgesia caused by suppression of pain mechanisms in the CNS. This agent has a low potency and does not produce complete loss of consciousness or extreme relaxation of skeletal muscle. Because nitrous oxide does not cause surgical anesthesia (stage 3), it is commonly combined with other surgical anesthetic agents. Nitrous oxide is ideal for dental procedures because the patient remains conscious and can follow instruction while experiencing full analgesia.

Adverse Effects and Interactions:

When used in low to moderate doses, nitrous oxide produces few adverse effects. At higher doses, patients exhibit some adverse signs of stage 2 anesthesia such as anxiety, excitement, and combativeness. Lowering the inhaled dose will quickly reverse these adverse effects. As nitrous oxide is exhaled the patient may temporarily have some difficulty breathing at the end of a procedure. Nausea and vomiting following the procedure are more common with nitrous oxide than with other inhalation anesthetics. Nitorus oxide has the potential to be abused by users (sometimes medical personnel) who enjoy the relaxed, sedated state that the drug produces.

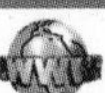
See the Companion Website for a Nursing Process Focus specific to this drug.

DRUG PROFILE: Volatile Anesthetic: Pr *Halothane (Fluothane)*

Actions and Uses:

Halothane produces a potent level of surgical anesthesia that is rapid in onset. Although potent, halothane does not produce as much muscle relaxation or analgesia as other volatile anesthetics. Therefore, halothane is primarily used with other anesthetic agents including muscle relaxants and analgesics. Nitrous oxide is sometimes combined with halothane. Patients recover from anesthesia rapidly after halothane is discontinued.

Adverse Effects and Interactions:

Halothane moderately sensitizes the heart muscle to epinephrine; therefore, dysrhythmias are a concern. This agent lowers blood pressure and the respiration rate. It also stops reflex mechanisms that normally keep the contents of the stomach from entering into the lungs. Because of potential liver toxicity, use of halothane has declined.

Malignant hyperthermia is rare, but can be a fatal adverse effect triggered by all inhalation anesthetics. It causes muscle rigidity and severe temperature elevation (up to 43°C). This risk is greatest when halothane is used with succinylcholine.

Levodopa taken at the same time increases the level of dopamine in the CNS, and should be stopped 6 to 8 hours before halothane administration.

Skeletal muscle weakness, respiratory depression, or apnea may occur if halothane is administered with polymyxins, lincomycin, or aminoglycosides.

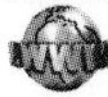
See the Companion Website for a Nursing Process Focus specific to this drug.

13.6 Intravenous anesthetics are important supplements to general anesthesia and include barbiturates, opioids, and benzodiazepines.

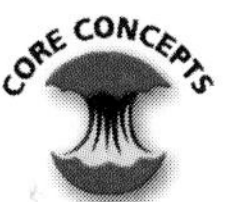

Although occasionally used alone, intravenous anesthetics are often administered with inhaled general anesthetics (Table 13.5). Administration of IV and inhaled anesthetics together allows the dose of the inhaled agent to be reduced, thereby lessening the possibility of serious side effects. Furthermore, when combined, they provide more analgesia and muscle relaxation than could be provided by the inhaled anesthetic alone. When IV anesthetics are administered without other anesthetics, they are generally used for medical procedures that take less than 15 minutes.

Drugs used as IV anesthetics include barbiturates, opioids, and benzodiazepines. Opioids offer the advantage of superior analgesia. For example, combining the opioid fentanyl (Sublimaze) with the antipsychotic agent droperidol (Inapsine) produces a state known as *neurolept analgesia.* In this state, patients are conscious but insensitive to pain and unaware of their surroundings. The premixed combination of these two agents is marketed as Innovar. A similar conscious, *dissociated* (that is, unaware) state is produced with ketamine (Ketalar).

Concept Review 13.3

- What is the role of IV anesthetics in surgical anesthesia? Why are these drugs not used by themselves for general anesthesia?

ADJUNCTS TO ANESTHESIA

A number of drugs are used either to complement the effects of general anesthetics or to treat anticipated side effects of the anesthesia. These agents, shown in Table 13.6, are called *adjuncts* to anesthesia. They may be given prior to, during, or after surgery.

TABLE 13.5 Intravenous Anesthetics

DRUG	REMARKS
BARBITURATE AND BARBITURATE-LIKE AGENTS	
etomidate (Amidate)	For induction of anesthesia; for short medical procedures
methohexital sodium (Brevital)	Ultrashort acting; for induction of anesthesia; used as a supplement to other anesthetic agents
propofol (Diprivan)	For induction and maintenance of general anesthesia; for short medical procedures
Pr thiopental sodium (Pentothal)	Ultrashort acting; for induction of anesthesia; used as a supplement to other anesthetic agents
BENZODIAZEPINES	
diazepam (Valium)	For induction of anesthesia; prototype drug for the benzodiazepines
lorazepam (Ativan)	For induction of anesthesia and to produce conscious sedation; for short medical procedures or surgery
midazolam hydrochloride (Versed)	For induction of anesthesia and to produce conscious sedation; for short diagnostic procedures
OPIOIDS	
alfentanil hydrochloride (Alfenta)	Rapid onset and short onset of action; for induction of anesthesia; used as a supplement to other anesthetic agents
fentanyl citrate (Sublimaze, others)	Short-acting analgesic used during the operative and perioperative period; used to supplement both general and regional anesthesia
remifentanil hydrochloride (Ultiva)	Short-acting analgesic; for induction and maintenance of general anesthesia
sufentanil citrate (Sufenta)	Approximately 7 times more potent than fentanyl; onset and duration of action more rapid than fentanyl; for induction and maintenance of anesthesia
OTHERS	
ketamine (Ketalar)	For sedation, amnesia, and analgesia; for short diagnostic, therapeutic, or surgical procedures; most often used in children

DRUG PROFILE: IV Anesthetic: Pr *Thiopental (Pentothal)*

Actions and Uses:

Thiopental is the oldest IV anesthetic. It is used for brief medical procedures or to rapidly cause unconsciousness prior to administering inhaled anesthetics. It is classified as an ultrashort-acting barbiturate, having an onset time of less than 30 seconds and a duration of only 10 to 30 minutes. Unlike some anesthetic agents, it has very low analgesic properties.

Adverse Effects and Interactions:

Like other barbiturates, thiopental can produce severe respiratory depression when used in high doses. It is used with caution in patients with cardiovascular disease because of its ability to depress the myocardium and cause dysrhythmias. Patients may experience emergence delirium postoperatively. This causes hallucinations, confusion, and excitability.

Thiopental interacts with many other drugs. For example, use of CNS depressants increases respiratory and CNS depression. Phenothiazines increase the risk of hypotension. Use with caution with herbal supplements, such as kava and valerian, which may increase sedation.

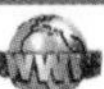

See the Companion Website for a Nursing Process Focus specific to this drug.

TABLE 13.6 Selected Adjuncts to Anesthesia

DRUG	REMARKS
BARBITURATE AND BARBITURATE-LIKE AGENTS	
amobarbital (Amytal)	Intermediate duration; for preoperative sedation.
butabarbital sodium (Butisol)	Intermediate duration; for preoperative sedation.
pentobarbital (Nembutal)	Short duration; for preoperative sedation; potent, causes respiratory depression.
secobarbital (Seconal)	Short duration; for preoperative sedation.
OPIOIDS	
alfentanil hydrochloride (Alfenta)	Short duration; for induction of anesthesia when endotracheal or mechanical ventilation is needed; provides analgesia.
fentanyl citrate (Duragesic, Actiq, others)	For analgesia during or after anesthesia; the combination of fentanyl and droperidol is called Innovar.
remifentanil hydrochloride (Ultiva)	For analgesia during or after anesthesia; shorter duration of action than fentanyl.
sufentanil citrate (Sufenta)	For primary anesthesia or to provide analgesia during or after anesthesia.
DOPAMINE BLOCKERS	
droperidol (Inapsine)	For nausea and vomiting caused by opioids; reduces anxiety and relaxes muscles.
promethazine (Pentazine, Phenazine, Phenergan, others)	For nausea and vomiting associated with obstetric sedation and opioids.
NEUROMUSCULAR BLOCKERS	
Pr succinylcholine chloride (Anectine, Quelicin, Sucostrin)	Short duration; depolarizing type.
tubocurarine	Long duration; prototype for the nondepolarizing type.
CHOLINERGIC AGENT	
bethanechol chloride (Duvoid, Urabeth, Urecholine)	For relief of constipation and urinary retention caused by opioids; stimulates GI motility. (See chapter 7 for the Drug Profile.)

13.7 Nonanesthetic drugs are used as adjuncts to anesthesia and include barbiturates, barbiturate-like drugs, opioids, neuromuscular blocking agents, and other miscellaneous drugs.

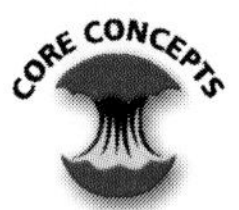

pre = *before*
operative = *surgery*

The preoperative drugs given to relieve anxiety and to provide mild sedation include barbiturates or benzodiazepines. Opioids such as morphine may be given to counteract pain that the patient will experience after surgery. Anticholinergics such as atropine may be administered to dry secretions and suppress the bradycardia caused by some anesthetics.

During surgery, the primary adjuncts are the *neuromuscular blockers.* These agents cause skeletal muscles to relax totally so that surgical procedures can be carried out safely. Administration of these drugs also allows the amount of anesthetic to be reduced. Neuromuscular blocking agents are classified as *depolarizing blockers* or *nondepolarizing blockers.* The only depolarizing blocker is succinylcholine (Anectine), which works by binding to acetylcholine receptors at neuromuscular junctions to cause total skeletal muscle relaxation. Succinylcholine is used in surgery for ease of tracheal intubation. Mivacurium (Mivacron) is the shortest acting of the nondepolarizing blockers, whereas tubocurarine is a longer-acting neuromuscular blocking agent. The nondepolarizing blockers cause muscle paralysis by competing with acetylcholine for cholinergic receptors at neuromuscular junctions. Once on the receptor, the nondepolarizing blockers prevent muscle contraction.

DRUG PROFILE: Neuromuscular Blocker: 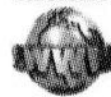 *Succinylcholine (Anectine)*

Actions and Uses:

Like the natural neurotransmitter acetylcholine, succinylcholine acts on cholinergic receptor sites at neuromuscular junctions. At first, depolarization occurs, and skeletal muscles contract. After repeated contractions, however, the membrane is unable to repolarize as long as the drug stays on the receptor. Effects are first noted as muscle weakness and muscle spasms. Eventually paralysis occurs. Succinylcholine is rapidly broken down by the enzyme pseudocholinesterase; when the IV infusion is stopped, the duration of action is only a few minutes. Use of succinylcholine reduces the amount of general anesthetic needed for procedures.

Adverse Effects and Interactions:

Succinylcholine can cause complete paralysis of the diaphragm and intercostal muscles; thus, mechanical ventilation is necessary during surgery. Bradycardia and respiratory depression and are expected adverse effects. If doses are high, tachycardia, hypotension, and urinary retention may occur. Patients with certain genetic defects may experience rapid onset of extremely high fever with muscle rigidity—a serious condition known as malignant hyperthermia.

Additive skeletal muscle blockade will occur if succinylcholine is given concurrently with clindamycin, aminoglycosides, furosemide, lithium, quinidine, or lidocaine.

Increased effect of succinylcholine may occur if given with phenothiazines oxytocin, promazine; acrine, or thiazide diuretics. Decreased effect of succinylcholine occurs if given with diazepam.

If this drug is given with halothane or nitrous oxide, an increased risk of bradycardia, dysrhythmias, sinus arrest, apnea, and malignant hyperthermia exists. If succinylcholine is given with cardiac glycosides, there is increased risk of cardiac dysrhythmias. If narcotics are given with succinylcholine, there is increased risk of bradycardia and sinus arrest.

See the Companion Website for a Nursing Process Focus specific to this drug.

post = *after*
operative = *surgery*

anti = *against*
emetic = *vomiting*

Postoperative drugs include analgesics for pain and antiemetics such as promethazine (Phenergan and others) for the nausea and vomiting that sometimes occur during recovery from the anesthesia. Occasionally, a parasympathomimetic such as bethanechol (Urecholine) is administered to stimulate the smooth muscle of the bowel and the urinary tract to begin working again following surgery.

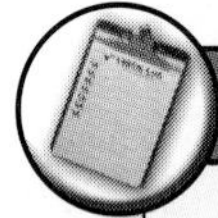

PATIENTS NEED TO KNOW

Patients treated with local anesthetic medications need to know the following:

1. When using topical anesthetics for skin conditions, avoid touching the eyes.
2. Never apply topical medications to large patches of skin or to areas where there is an open lesion or cut.
3. Notify your dentist or healthcare practitioners of any previous adverse reactions to local anesthesia before they give you additional anesthetic medications.
4. After receiving local anesthetic solutions for the mouth, do not consume food and drink until it is clear that the anesthetic has worn off.
5. Do not chew or pick at an area where a dental procedure has been performed while the area is still numb.
6. Be careful not to inhale anesthetic sprays used for topical application.
7. Get immediate assistance if drowsiness, confusion, or blurred vision has occurred after receiving a local anethetic. Other signs/symptoms to look for include lightheadedness, an irregular heartbeat, or feeling faint.
8. Report all medications and conditions to the healthcare provider before receiving anesthetics.
9. For outpatient dental or medical procedures involving anesthesia, someone should be available to assist with activities such as transportation.
10. Follow postprocedure instructions carefully after anesthesia.
11. Have sufficient pain medication readily available so that postprocedure pain can be managed after the effects of the anesthesia are no longer felt. ■

CHAPTER REVIEW

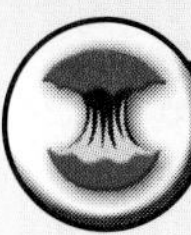

CORE CONCEPTS SUMMARY

13.1 Local anesthesia causes a rapid loss of sensation to a limited part of the body.

Local anesthesia is loss of sensation to a relatively small part of the body without causing loss of consciousness. Sometimes local anesthesia is applied to an entire limb. In these cases, it is more accurately called *surface anesthesia* or *regional anesthesia,* depending on how the drugs are administered and the results they produce.

13.2 Local anesthetics produce their therapeutic effect by blocking the entry of sodium ions into neurons.

Blocking sodium entry into neurons prevents transmission of the electrical impulse along the nerve. Epinephrine is sometimes added to anesthetic solutions to increase the duration of action of the anesthetic. A base such as sodium hydroxide is added to make an infected tissue environment more alkaline.

13.3 Local anesthetics are classified by their chemical structures.

The two major classes of local anesthetics are esters and amides. Benzocaine (Solarcaine, others) is the most commonly used ester, lidocaine (Xylocaine) is the most widely prescribed amide.

13.4 General anesthesia is a loss of sensation occurring throughout the entire body, accompanied by a loss of consciousness.

General anesthesia proceeds in stages from light sedation to total loss of consciousness. The less potent anesthetics cause stage 1 anesthesia, whereas more potent agents cause surgical anesthesia (stage 3).

13.5 General anesthetics are usually administered by the IV or inhalation routes.

Two primary methods for producing rapid unconsciousness and total analgesia are IV agents and inhaled general anesthetics. IV agents include barbiturates and barbiturate-like agents, opioids, and benzodiazepines. Inhalation agents include nitrous oxide, the only gaseous agent, and volatile liquids. Many agents may be used alone or in combination with other agents. The mechanism by which general anesthetics produce their effect is not completely known.

13.6 Intravenous anesthetics are important supplements to general anesthesia and include barbiturates, opioids, and benzodiazepines.

Intravenous agents may be used along with inhaled anesthetics to lower the potential for serious side effects. Barbiturates, opioids, and benzodiazepines are generally reserved for quick medical procedures and treatments requiring superior analgesia.

13.7 Nonanesthetic drugs are used as adjuncts to anesthesia and include barbiturates, barbiturate-like drugs, opioids, neuromuscular blocking agents, and other miscellaneous drugs.

A number of drugs are given prior to surgery to relieve anxiety, provide mild sedation, counteract pain, and dry secretions. Neuromuscular blockers, given during surgery, relax skeletal muscle and maintain a proper heart rate. Drugs after surgery include agents for pain and vomiting and to activate the bowel and urinary tract.

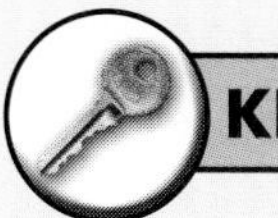

KEY TERMS

amides (AM-ides): type of chemical linkage found in some local anesthetics involving carbon, nitrogen, and oxygen (—NH—CO—) / ***page 219***

anesthesia (ANN-ess-THEE-zee-uh): medical procedure involving drugs that block the transmission of nerve impulses and cause loss of sensation and/or consciousness / ***page 216***

esters (ES-turs): type of chemical linkage found in some local anesthetics involving carbon and oxygen (—CO—O—) / ***page 219***

general anesthesia: medical procedure that produces loss of sensation throughout the entire body and unconsciousness / ***page 223***

local anesthesia: loss of sensation to a relatively small part of the body without loss of consciousness / ***page 216***

REVIEW QUESTIONS

The following questions are written in NCLEX-PN® style. Answer these questions to assess your knowledge of the chapter material, and go back and review any material that is not clear to you.

1. This herbal product may prolong or intensify the effects of anesthesia.

1. Kava kava
2. Cloves
3. Anise
4. St. John's wort

2. When toxic, this local anesthetic causes CNS excitement, irritability, and confusion.

1. Isoflurane (Forane)
2. Lidocaine (Xylocaine)
3. Nitrous oxide
4. Epinephrine

3. The patient in labor will most likely receive which type of anesthesia?

1. Nerve block
2. Epidural
3. Spinal
4. Surface

4. During anesthesia, the patient assessment reveals restlessness, blood pressure 196/110, pulse 128, and respirations 38. The patient is most likely in which of the following stages of anesthesia?

1. Stage 1
2. Stage 2
3. Stage 3
4. Stage 4

5. This is the stage of anesthesia when surgery begins.

1. Stage 1
2. Stage 2
3. Stage 3
4. Stage 4

6. The patient being prepared for surgery asks the nurse why he is receiving meperidine (Demerol) and atropine prior to surgery. The nurse's best response would be:

1. "You will need to speak with your physician."
2. "The meperidine (Demerol) will help to control pain before and after surgery, while the atropine will help to decrease secretions."
3. "The meperidine (Demerol) and atropine will help your anesthetic work more effectively."
4. "These medications are routinely used before we send a patient to surgery."

7. The patient with a history of cardiovascular disease should receive anesthetics without epinephrine because it can cause:

1. Tachycardia and hypertension
2. Bradycardia and hypotension
3. Tachycardia and hypotension
4. Bradycardia and hypertension

8. The patient receives nitrous oxide in addition to thiopental sodium (Pentothal):

1. To provide the additional anesthesia to put him in a sleep-like state
2. To increase the effectiveness of each drug at lower dosages
3. Because thiopental sodium (Pentothal) is not effective when used alone
4. Because nitrous oxide is not effective when used alone

9. The patient is having a cyst removed under local anesthesia. The physician requests lidocaine (Xylocaine) with epinephrine. The nurse understands the addition of epinephrine is to:

1. Prevent infection
2. Prevent an allergic reaction
3. Increase the duration of the anesthetic
4. Decrease pain after the procedure

10. The patient is experiencing nausea in the recovery room. The nurse anticipates which medication being ordered?

1. Meperidine (Demerol)
2. Bethanechol (Urecholine)
3. Phenergan
4. Succinylcholine

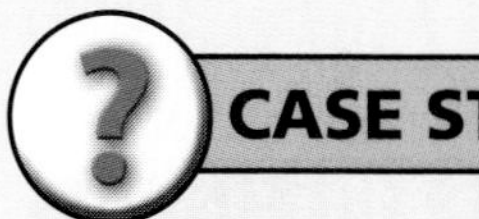

CASE STUDY QUESTIONS

For questions 1–5, please refer to the following case study, and choose the correct answer from choices 1–4.

Mr. Wand, age 77, has a history of cardiovascular disease. He has collapsed and sustained an injury to his scalp. The wound is substantial, and Mr. Wand is bleeding across his right forehead. The patient is rushed to the emergency room by his nephew. The nephew reports that his uncle is normally very fearful of doctors and nurses. It is unclear why Mr. Wand collapsed. The nurse decides to inject the tissue surrounding the wound with 1% lidocaine with epinephrine for local anesthesia prior to suturing the laceration.

1. The route of drug administration in this case is referred to as:

1. Topical (surface) anesthesia
2. Infiltration (field block) anesthesia
3. Nerve block anesthesia
4. Epidural anesthesia

2. Soon after administering this medication, the nurse should primarily be concerned with which of the following symptoms?

1. Constriction of airways
2. Anxiety
3. Tachycardia
4. Unresponsiveness

3. The medication administered to Mr. Wand is referred to as a(n):

1. Amide
2. Ester
3. Miscellaneous agent

4. Would it be advisable to give Mr. Wand a barbiturate to help him calm down due to his fear of doctors and nurses in this case?

1. No, a barbiturate might *increase toxicity symptoms* if Mr. Wand is allergic to lidocaine.
2. Yes, a barbiturate might *increase the effectiveness of lidocaine* in this situation and help the patient calm down.
3. No, a barbiturate might *decrease the effectiveness of lidocaine* in this situation and *make the patient more irritable.*
4. No, a barbiturate might *decrease the effectiveness of lidocaine* in this situation although the *medication would normally have a calming effect.*

5. Which serious side effect of lidocaine coincides with the possible cause of Mr. Wand's collapse and therefore is a reason why the nurse should be very cautious?

1. Convulsions
2. Cardiac arrest
3. Respiratory depression
4. All of the above

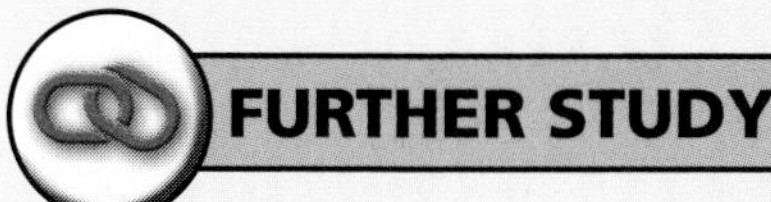

FURTHER STUDY

- The abuse potential of cocaine is discussed in Chapter 6.
- The use of barbiturates in treating insomnia is included in Chapter 8, and for seizures in Chapter 11.
- The use of benzodiazepines in treating anxiety is presented in Chapter 8, and for seizures in Chapter 11.
- The use of opiods in pain management is included in Chapter 12, and in treating GI disorders in Chapter 26.
- Bethanechol (Urecholine) is a profile cholinergic agent in Chapter 7.

EXPLORE MEDIALINK www.prenhall.com/holland

Additional resources for this chapter can be found on the CD-ROM accompanying this textbook, and on the Companion Website. Click on Chapter 13 to select activities for this chapter.

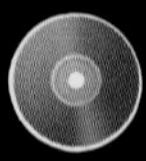

- **Mechanism in Action: Lidocaine**
- **Audio Glossary**
- **Concept Review**
- **NCLEX-PN® Review**
- **Nursing in Action**
- **Dosage Calculator**

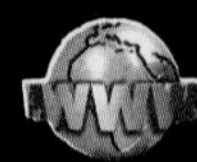

- **Virtual Anesthesia Textbook**
- **Patient's Guide to Local Regional Anesthesia**

UNIT

1 2 3 4 5 6 7

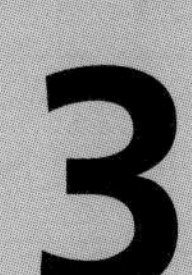

3 THE CARDIOVASCULAR SYSTEM

UNIT CONTENTS

CHAPTER

14 Drugs for Coagulation Disorders

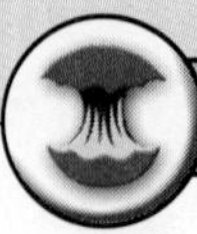

CORE CONCEPTS

14.1 Hemostasis is a complex process involving multiple steps and many clotting factors.

14.2 Removing a blood clot is essential to restoring normal circulation.

14.3 Drugs can modify the normal coagulation process.

14.4 Anticoagulants prevent the formation and enlargement of clots.

14.5 Antiplatelet agents prolong bleeding time by interfering with platelet aggregation.

14.6 Thrombolytics are used to dissolve existing clots.

14.7 Hemostatics are used to promote the formation of clots.

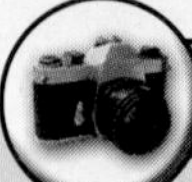

DRUG SNAPSHOT

The following drugs will be discussed in this chapter:

DRUG CLASSES	DRUG PROFILES
Anticoagulants	Pr heparin (Heplock)
	Pr warfarin (Coumadin)
Antiplatelet agents	Pr ticlopidine (Ticlid)
Thrombolytics	Pr alteplase (Activase)
Hemostatics	Pr aminocaproic acid (Amicar)

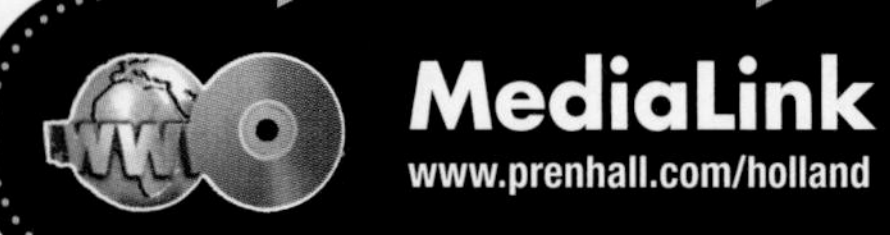

MediaLink
www.prenhall.com/holland

Interactive resources for this chapter can be found on the Companion Website. Click on Chapter 14 and "Begin" to select the activities for this chapter. For chapter-related animations, NCLEX-PN®-style questions, and an audio glossary, access the accompanying CD-ROM in this book.

OBJECTIVES

After reading this chapter, the student should be able to:

1. Explain the importance of hemostasis.
2. Construct a flow chart diagramming the important steps of hemostasis.
3. Identify the primary mechanisms by which coagulation-modifier drugs act.
4. For each of the following classes, identify representative medications and explain the mechanisms of drug action, primary actions, and important adverse effects:
   - **a.** Anticoagulants
   - **b.** Antiplatelet agents
   - **c.** Thrombolytics
   - **d.** Hemostatics
5. Categorize coagulation-modifying drugs based on their classifications and mechanisms of action.

The process of **hemostasis,** or the stopping of blood flow, is an essential mechanism protecting the body from both external and internal injury. Without efficient hemostasis, bleeding from wounds would lead to shock and perhaps death. Too much clotting, however, can be just as deadly as too little. Thus, hemostasis must maintain a delicate balance between fluidity and coagulation.

hemo = *blood*
stasis = *stopping*

A number of diseases and conditions can affect hemostasis. Some common disorders that may require pharmacological therapy with coagulation-modifying drugs are described in Table 14.1.

14.1 Hemostasis is a complex process involving multiple steps and many clotting factors.

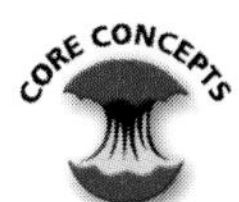

Hemostasis is complex and involves a number of substances called **clotting factors.** Hemostasis occurs in a series of sequential steps, sometimes referred to as a *cascade.* Drugs can be used to modify some of these steps.

When an injury occurs, cells lining the damaged blood vessel release chemicals that begin the clotting process. The vessel immediately spasms or constricts to limit blood flow to the injured area. Small blood components called platelets become sticky, adhere to the injured area, and aggregate or clump to plug the damaged vessel. Blood flow is further slowed, allowing **coagulation,** the formation of an insoluble clot. The three basic steps of hemostasis are shown in Figure 14.1 ■.

The **coagulation cascade** is a complex series of steps that begins when the injured cells release a chemical called *prothrombin activator* or *prothrombinase.* Prothrombin activator converts the clotting factor **prothrombin** to an enzyme called **thrombin.** Thrombin then converts **fibrinogen,** a plasma protein, to long strands of **fibrin.** Thus two of the factors essential to clotting, thrombin and

thrombo = *clot*
plastin = *to form*
pro = *before*
thrombin = *clot*

TABLE 14.1	Disorders Commonly Treated with Coagulation-modifying Drugs
DISORDER/CONDITION	**DESCRIPTION**
angina	narrowing of the coronary vessels
cerebrovascular accident (CVA)/stroke	clot within an artery serving the brain
deep vein thrombosis (DVT)	clot within a vein
indwelling devices	mechanical heart valves, stents
myocardial infarction	clot within a coronary artery
postoperative hemorrhage	bleeding following a surgical procedure
pulmonary embolus	clot within a pulmonary artery
valvular heart disease	disease of heart valves or replacement of a heart valve

Fast Facts Clotting Disorders

- Because the liver supplies many of the clotting factors, liver disease is one of the most common causes of coagulation disorders.
- More than 2 million patients each year develop a deep vein thrombosis (DVT).
- More than 60,000 patients each year die of pulmonary emboli.
- Von Willebrand's disease is the most common hereditary platelet disorder and is caused by a deficiency of a clotting protein.
- Hemophilia A is a hereditary lack of clotting factor VIII; it accounts for 80% of all hemophilia cases.
- Hemophilia B is a hereditary lack of clotting factor IX.
- More than 15,000 people in the United States have hemophilia A or B.

FIGURE 14.1

Basic steps in hemostasis

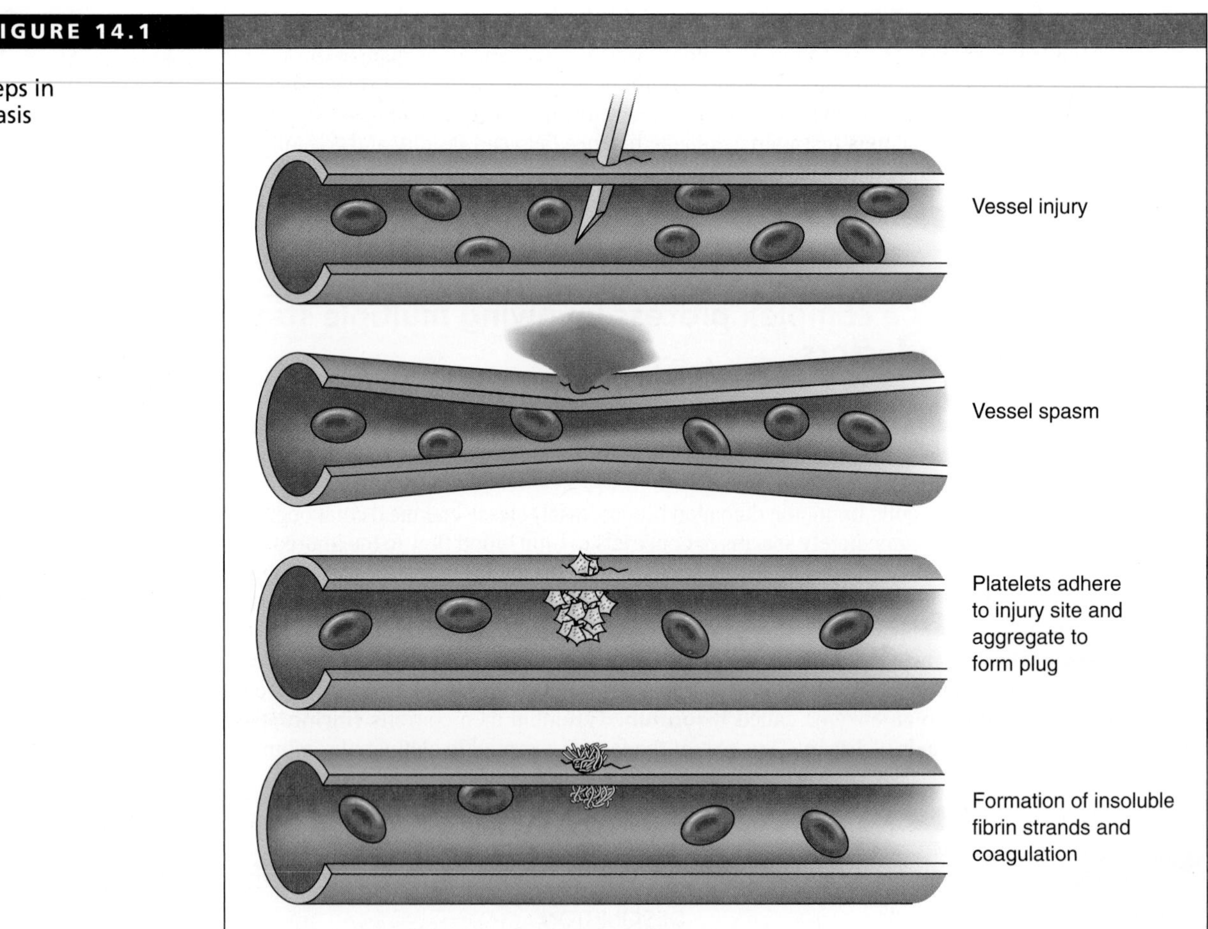

fibrin, are only formed *after* injury to the vessels. The fibrin strands form an insoluble web over the injured area to stop blood loss. Normal blood clotting occurs in about 6 minutes. The primary steps in the coagulation cascade are shown in Figure 14.2 ■.

It is important to note that several clotting factors, including thromboplastin and fibrinogen, are proteins made by the liver that are constantly circulating through the blood in an *inactive* form. Vitamin K is required for the liver to make four of the clotting factors. Because of the crucial importance of the liver in creating these clotting factors, patients with serious liver disorders often have abnormal coagulation.

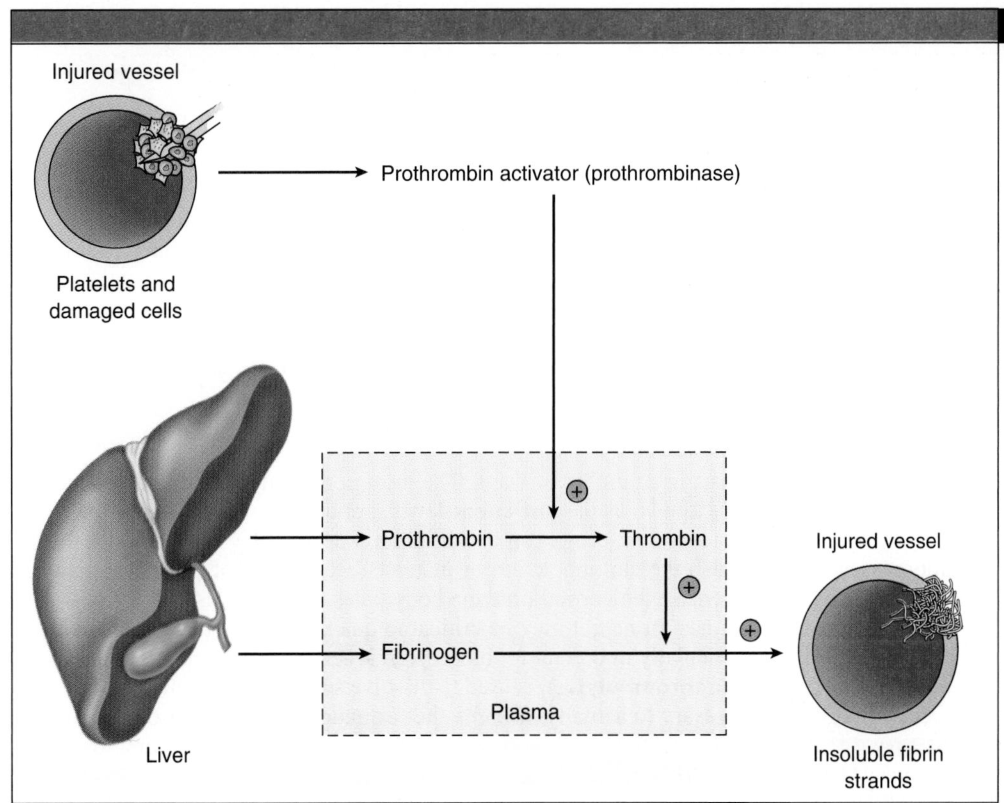

FIGURE 14.2

Major steps in the coagulation cascade

14.2 Removing a blood clot is essential to restoring normal circulation.

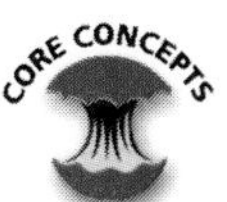

The goal of hemostasis has been achieved once a blood clot is formed and the body is protected from excessive hemorrhage. The clot, however, may prevent adequate blood flow to the affected area; circulation must eventually be restored so that the tissue can resume normal activities. The process of clot removal is called **fibrinolysis.**

fibrin = *fiber*
lysis = *break apart*

Fibrinolysis also involves several cascading steps. When the fibrin clot is formed, nearby blood vessel cells secrete **tissue plasminogen activator (tPA).** tPA converts the inactive protein **plasminogen,** which is present in the fibrin clot, to its active form called **plasmin.** Plasmin then digests the fibrin strands to remove the clot. The body normally regulates fibrinolysis such that *unwanted* fibrin clots are removed, whereas fibrin present in wounds is left to maintain hemostasis. The steps of fibrinolysis are shown in Figure 14.3 ■.

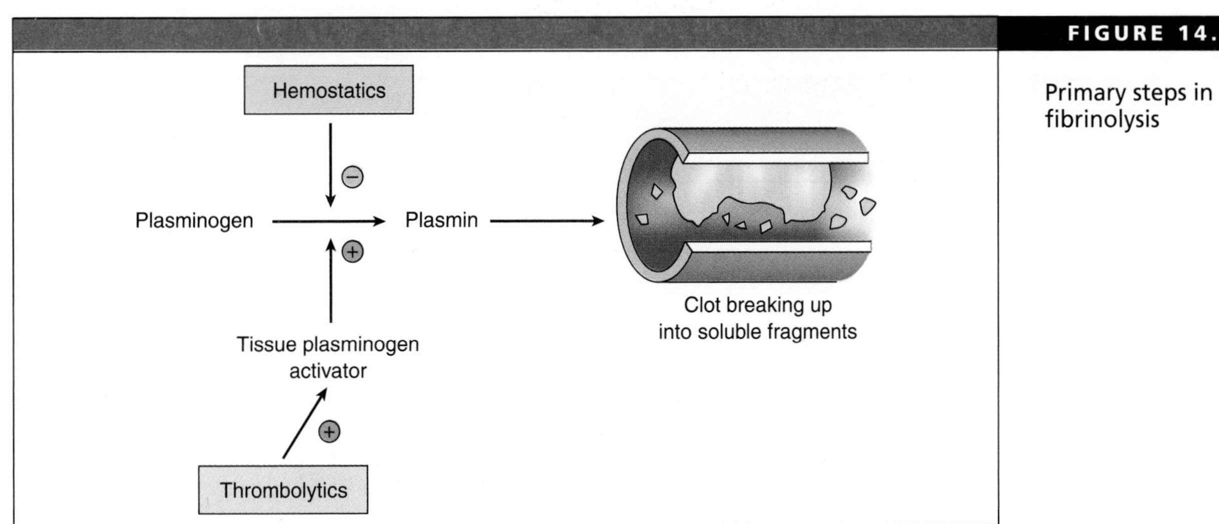

FIGURE 14.3

Primary steps in fibrinolysis

ABNORMAL COAGULATION

There are many types of disorders in which abnormal coagulation might occur. Examples are when the blood becomes gelatinous or semisolid, disrupting the normal flow of blood. Solid masses of blood or blood clots can place clients in extreme danger. Blood clots may become dislodged and move to another part of the body, such as the lungs or the brain. In some cases, the blood may not clot quickly enough, for example, following surgery. In this case, it is desirable to make the blood clot more quickly to prevent excessive bleeding.

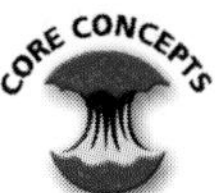

14.3 Drugs can be used to modify the normal coagulation process.

anti = *against*
coagulation = *clotting*

Drugs can modify hemostasis in a number of ways. The most commonly prescribed coagulation modifiers, the class of drugs known as the **anticoagulants,** are used to prevent the formation of clots. To accomplish clot prevention, drugs can either inhibit specific clotting factors in the coagulation cascade or diminish the clotting action of platelets. Regardless of the mechanism, all anticoagulant drugs will increase the normal time the body takes to form clots.

thrombo = *clot*
lytic = *remove/destroy*

Once an abnormal clot has formed, it may be critical to quickly remove it in order to restore normal function. This is particularly important for blood vessels serving the heart, lungs, and brain. A specific class of drugs, the **thrombolytics,** is used to dissolve such life-threatening clots.

Occasionally, it is necessary to actually *promote* the formation of clots. These drugs, called **hemostatics,** inhibit the normal removal of fibrin, thus keeping the clot in place for a longer period of time. Hemostatics are used to speed clot formation, or to limit bleeding from a surgical site. (See Figure 14.3 to view a graphic of these drugs.)

Concept Review 14.1

- Which clotting factors are always circulating in the blood? Which are only formed when coagulation is underway?

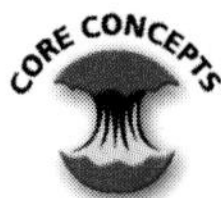

14.4 Anticoagulants prevent the formation and enlargement of clots.

Once a stationary clot, or **thrombus,** forms in a vessel, it often grows larger as more fibrin is added. Pieces of the thrombus may break off and travel in the bloodstream to affect other vessels. A traveling clot is called an **embolus.** The term **thromboembolic disease** refers to these types of clotting disorders.

NURSING PROCESS FOCUS

Patients Receiving Anticoagulant Therapy

ASSESSMENT	POTENTIAL NURSING DIAGNOSES
Prior to administration: ■ Obtain complete health history including recent surgeries or trauma, allergies, drug history, and possible drug interactions ■ Obtain vital signs; assess in context of patient's baseline values	■ Risk for Injury (bleeding), related to adverse effects of anticogulant therapy ■ Activity Intolerance (contact sports) ■ Ineffective Tissue Perfusion, related to hemorrhage ■ Impaired Tissue Integrity ■ Risk for Infection ■ Deficient Knowledge, related to drug therapy

continued...

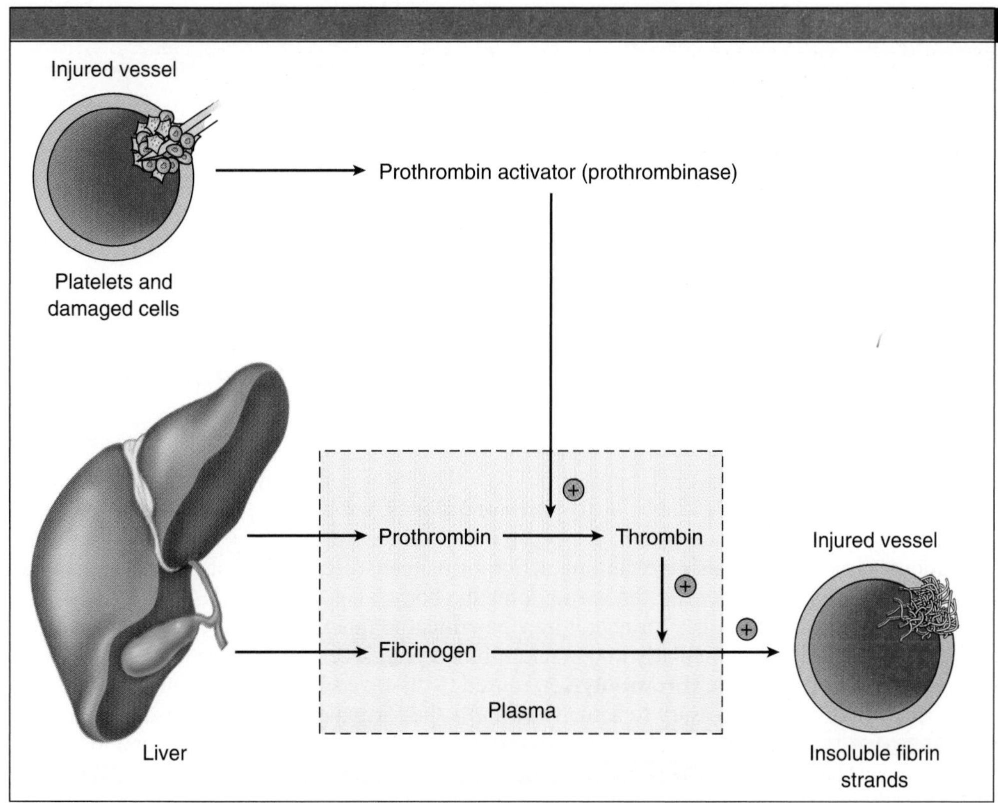

FIGURE 14.2

Major steps in the coagulation cascade

14.2 Removing a blood clot is essential to restoring normal circulation.

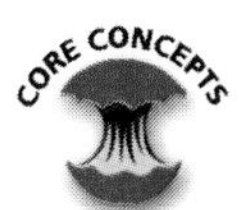

The goal of hemostasis has been achieved once a blood clot is formed and the body is protected from excessive hemorrhage. The clot, however, may prevent adequate blood flow to the affected area; circulation must eventually be restored so that the tissue can resume normal activities. The process of clot removal is called **fibrinolysis.**

fibrin = *fiber*
lysis = *break apart*

Fibrinolysis also involves several cascading steps. When the fibrin clot is formed, nearby blood vessel cells secrete **tissue plasminogen activator (tPA).** tPA converts the inactive protein **plasminogen,** which is present in the fibrin clot, to its active form called **plasmin.** Plasmin then digests the fibrin strands to remove the clot. The body normally regulates fibrinolysis such that *unwanted* fibrin clots are removed, whereas fibrin present in wounds is left to maintain hemostasis. The steps of fibrinolysis are shown in Figure 14.3 ■.

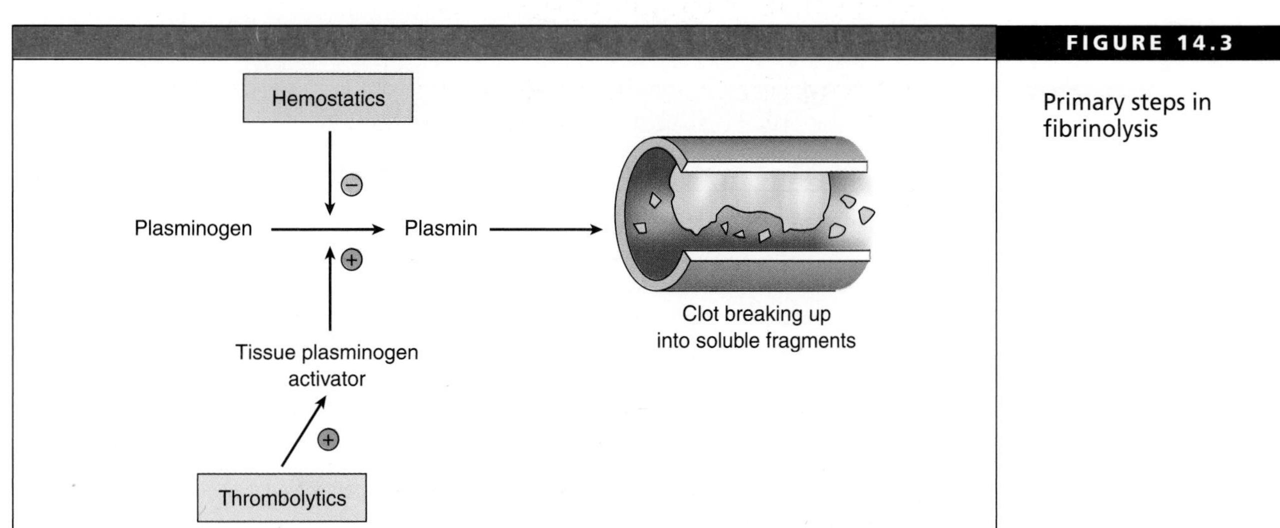

FIGURE 14.3

Primary steps in fibrinolysis

ABNORMAL COAGULATION

There are many types of disorders in which abnormal coagulation might occur. Examples are when the blood becomes gelatinous or semisolid, disrupting the normal flow of blood. Solid masses of blood or blood clots can place clients in extreme danger. Blood clots may become dislodged and move to another part of the body, such as the lungs or the brain. In some cases, the blood may not clot quickly enough, for example, following surgery. In this case, it is desirable to make the blood clot more quickly to prevent excessive bleeding.

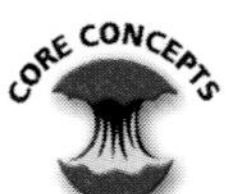

14.3 Drugs can be used to modify the normal coagulation process.

anti = *against*
coagulation = *clotting*

Drugs can modify hemostasis in a number of ways. The most commonly prescribed coagulation modifiers, the class of drugs known as the **anticoagulants,** are used to prevent the formation of clots. To accomplish clot prevention, drugs can either inhibit specific clotting factors in the coagulation cascade or diminish the clotting action of platelets. Regardless of the mechanism, all anticoagulant drugs will increase the normal time the body takes to form clots.

thrombo = *clot*
lytic = *remove/destroy*

Once an abnormal clot has formed, it may be critical to quickly remove it in order to restore normal function. This is particularly important for blood vessels serving the heart, lungs, and brain. A specific class of drugs, the **thrombolytics,** is used to dissolve such life-threatening clots.

Occasionally, it is necessary to actually *promote* the formation of clots. These drugs, called **hemostatics,** inhibit the normal removal of fibrin, thus keeping the clot in place for a longer period of time. Hemostatics are used to speed clot formation, or to limit bleeding from a surgical site. (See Figure 14.3 to view a graphic of these drugs.)

Concept Review 14.1

- Which clotting factors are always circulating in the blood? Which are only formed when coagulation is underway?

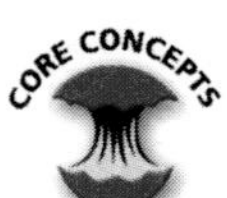

14.4 Anticoagulants prevent the formation and enlargement of clots.

Once a stationary clot, or **thrombus,** forms in a vessel, it often grows larger as more fibrin is added. Pieces of the thrombus may break off and travel in the bloodstream to affect other vessels. A traveling clot is called an **embolus.** The term **thromboembolic disease** refers to these types of clotting disorders.

NURSING PROCESS FOCUS

Patients Receiving Anticoagulant Therapy

ASSESSMENT	POTENTIAL NURSING DIAGNOSES
Prior to administration: ■ Obtain complete health history including recent surgeries or trauma, allergies, drug history, and possible drug interactions ■ Obtain vital signs; assess in context of patient's baseline values	■ Risk for Injury (bleeding), related to adverse effects of anticogulant therapy ■ Activity Intolerance (contact sports) ■ Ineffective Tissue Perfusion, related to hemorrhage ■ Impaired Tissue Integrity ■ Risk for Infection ■ Deficient Knowledge, related to drug therapy

continued...

TABLE 14.2 Anticoagulants

DRUG	ROUTE AND ADULT DOSE	REMARKS
anisindione (Miradon)	PO 25–250 mg/day	Therapy begins with a higher dose, which is gradually reduced; similar to warfarin
argatroban (Acova, Novastan)	IV 2–10 mcg/kg/min	Thrombin inhibitor; for prevention and treatment of thrombosis
bivalirudin (Angiomax)	IV 1 mg/kg bolus followed by 2.5 mg/kg/hr for 4h	Thrombin inhibitor; used with aspirin to prevent clots during angioplasty
foundaparinux (Arixtra)	Subcutaneously 2.5 mg/daily	For prevention of DVT and pulmonary emboli
Pr heparin (Heplock)	IV infusion 5000–40,000 units/day subcutaneously; 15,000–20,000 units/bid	For prevention and treatment of venous thrombosis and pulmonary edema; therapy begins with a higher dose, which is gradually reduced
lepirudin (Refludan)	IV 0.4 mg/kg bolus followed by 0.15–16.5 mg/kg/hr for 2–10 days	Thrombin inhibitor; for prevention of clots in clients with heparin-induced thrombocytopenia
pentoxifylline (Trental)	PO 400 mg tid	Reduces blood viscosity and increases the flexibility of red blood cells
Pr warfarin (Coumadin)	PO 2–15 mg/day	Same use as heparin but effect is more prolonged; IV form is available
LOW MOLECULAR WEIGHT (FRACTIONATED) HEPARINS (LMWHS)		
ardeparin (Normiflo)	Subcutaneously 50 units/kg q12h for 14 days	For prevention and treatment of DVT following knee or hip replacement or abdominal surgery, unstable angina, or acute coronary syndromes
dalteparin (Fragmin)	Subcutaneously 2500–5000 units/day	
danaparoid (Orgaran)	Subcutaneously 750 units q12h for 7–10 days	
enoxaparin (Lovenox)	Subcutaneously 1 mg/kg q12h for 7–10 days	
tinzaparin (Innohep)	Subcutaneously 175 units/kg daily for at least 6h	

The most common, and potentially serious, adverse effect of anticoagulant and antiplatelet agents is bleeding. The patient must be observed for signs of hemorrhage, such as bruising, bleeding gums, and blood in the urine or stools. Patients who have recently experienced a traumatic injury or surgery are especially at risk. Any symptoms of bleeding must be immediately reported to the healthcare provider. Specific blockers may be administered to reverse the anticoagulant effects: protamine sulfate is used for heparin, and vitamin K is administered for warfarin.

14.5 Antiplatelet agents prolong bleeding time by interfering with platelet aggregation.

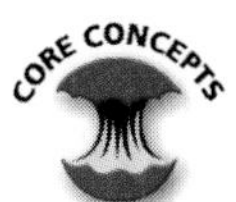

Antiplatelet medications exert an anticoagulant effect by interfering with various aspects of platelet function. Unlike the anticoagulants, which are used primarily to prevent thrombosis in *veins,* antiplatelet agents are used to prevent clot formation in *arteries.*

Platelets are a central component of the hemostasis process. Too few platelets or diminished platelet function can profoundly increase bleeding time. The three subclasses of antiplatelet agents are (1) aspirin, (2) adenosine diphosphate (ADP) receptor blockers, and (3) glycoprotein IIb/IIIa receptor blockers. Doses for antiplatelet agents are shown in Table 14.3.

Aspirin deserves special mention as an antiplatelet type of coagulation modifier. Because it is available over the counter, patients may not consider aspirin a strong medication. However, its anticoagulant activity is well documented. Aspirin acts by inhibiting thromboxane$_2$, which causes

DRUG PROFILE: Anticoagulant: 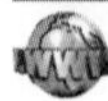 *Heparin (Heplock)*

Actions and Uses:

Heparin is a natural substance found in the lining of blood vessels. Its normal function is to prevent excessive clotting within blood vessels. When given as a drug, heparin provides immediate anticoagulant activity. The binding of heparin to a substance called *antithrombin II* results in an inactivation of some of the clotting factors and an inhibition of thrombin activity. Because heparin is not absorbed by the gastrointestinal mucosa, it must be given either subcutaneously or through IV infusion. The onset of action for IV heparin is immediate, whereas subcutaneous heparin may take up to an hour for maximum therapeutic effect.

In recent years, the heparin molecule has been shortened and modified to create a new class of drugs called **low molecular weight heparins (LMWHs).** LMWHs possess the same anticoagulant activity as heparin, but have several advantages. They produce a more stable response than heparin, thus fewer lab tests are needed, and family members or the patient can be trained to give the necessary subcutaneous injections at home. LMWHs have become the drugs of choice for many clotting disorders, including the prevention of deep vein thrombosis (DVT) following surgery.

Adverse Effects and Interactions:

Abnormal bleeding is common during heparin therapy. If aPTT becomes prolonged or toxicity is observed, stopping the heparin infusion will result in loss of anticoagulant activity within hours. If serious hemorrhage occurs, a specific blocker, protamine sulfate, may be administered to neutralize the anticoagulant activity of heparin. Protamine sulfate has an onset time of 5 minutes and is also a blocker of the LMWHs.

Oral anticoagulants, including warfarin, increase the action of heparin. Ibuprofen, ASA, and other drugs that inhibit platelet aggregation may induce bleeding. Nicotine, digoxin, tetracyclines, or antihistamines may inhibit anticoagulation.

Herbal supplements such as arnica, which contains a coumarin component, may increase the anticoagulant effect.

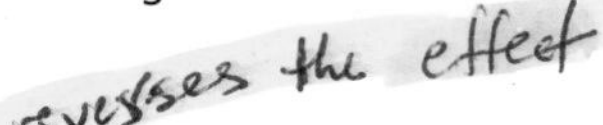

See the Companion Website for a Nursing Process Focus specific to this drug.

TABLE 14.3 Antiplatelet Agents

DRUG	ROUTE AND ADULT DOSE	REMARKS
aspirin (ASA, acetylsalicylic acid)	PO 80 mg daily–650 mg bid	Inhibits platelet aggregation; available without a prescription; higher doses are used to treat inflammation or pain; therapeutic serum level is 10–30 mcg/dl.
dipyridamole (Persantine)	PO 75–100 mg qid	Platelet inhibitor to prevent embolism in patients with prosthetic heart valves; often used with warfarin; IV form available
ADP RECEPTOR BLOCKERS		
clopidogrel bisulfate (Plavix)	PO 75 mg daily	Prolongs bleeding time
Pr ticlopidine (Ticlid)	PO 250 mg bid	Platelet aggregation inhibitor; prolongs bleeding time
GLYCOPROTEIN IIB/IIIA BLOCKERS		
abciximab (ReoPro)	IV 0.25 mg/kg initial bolus over 5 min; then 10 mcg/min for 12 hours	Used to prevent cardiac ischemia during coronary angioplasty; duration lasts up to 48 hr after infusion is stopped
eptifibatide (Integrilin)	IV 180 mcg/kg initial bolus over 1–2 min; then 2 mcg/kg/min for 24–72 hours	Also for unstable angina and other acute coronary syndromes; duration lasts up to 8 hr after infusion is stopped
tirofiban hydrochloride (Aggrastat)	IV 0.4 mcg/kg/min for 30 min; then 0.1 mcg/kg/min for 12–24 hours	Similar to eptifibatide; duration lasts up to 8 hr after infusion is stopped

DRUG PROFILE: Anticoagulant: Pr *Warfarin (Coumadin)*

Actions and Uses:

Unlike heparin, the anticoagulant activity of warfarin can take several days to reach its maximum effect. This explains why heparin and warfarin therapy are overlapped. Warfarin inhibits the action of vitamin K that is essential for the synthesis of several clotting factors. Because these clotting factors are normally circulating in the blood, it takes several days for them to clear the plasma and for the anticoagulant effect of warfarin to appear. Another reason for the slow onset is that 99% of warfarin binds to plasma proteins and is unavailable to produce its effect. This high level of protein binding is responsible for a significant number of drug-drug interactions that may occur during warfarin therapy.

Adverse Effects and Interactions:

Like all anticoagulants, the most serious adverse effect of warfarin is abnormal bleeding. On discontinuation of therapy, the activity of warfarin can take up to 10 days to diminish. If life-threatening bleeding occurs during therapy, the anticoagulant effects of warfarin can be reduced in 6 hours through the IM or subcutaneous administration of its blocker, vitamin K. The therapeutic range of serum warfarin levels varies from 1 to 10 mcg/ml, to achieve an INR value of 2–3.

Extensive protein binding is responsible for numerous drug interactions, some of which include NSAIDs, diuretics, SSRIs, and other antidepressants, steroids, antibiotics and vaccines, and vitamins (for example, vitamin K). Use with NSAIDs may increase bleeding risk.

Use of warfarin with herbal supplements, such as feverfew, garlic, and ginger, may increase the risk of bleeding; use with arnica may increase the anticoagulant effect.

Mechanism in Action: 

Many vitamin K–dependent clotting factors are essential for blood coagulation. The anticoagulant warfarin inhibits the amount of factors made available by the liver. Reducing vitamin K–dependent factors inhibits the formation of prothrombin, which is one of the final coagulation proteins in the clotting cascade. The result is slowed clot formation and increased bleeding time.

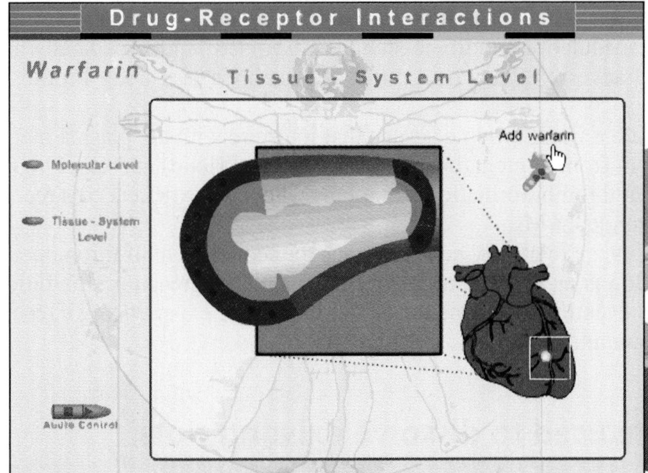

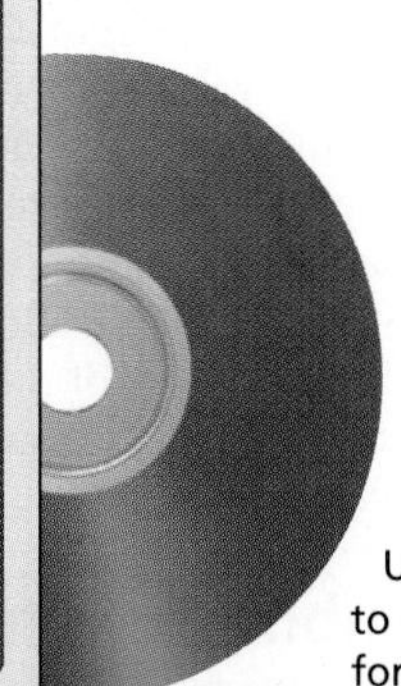

Use the student CD-ROM to see Mechanism in Action for Warfarin.

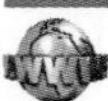 *See the Companion Website for a Nursing Process Focus specific to this drug.*

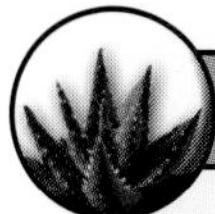

NATURAL ALTERNATIVES

Garlic for Cardiovascular Disease

Garlic (*Allium sativum*) is one of the best studied herbs. Indications for garlic are said to include arteriosclerosis, common cold, cough/bronchitis, high cholesterol, hypertension, tendency to infection, and many other conditions. It has been proven to be of value in only a few of these disorders.

A number of different substances, known as *alliaceous oils,* have been isolated from garlic and shown to have pharmacological activity. The supplement can be eaten as prepared garlic oil or fresh bulbs from the plant.

Garlic has been shown to decrease the aggregation or "stickiness" of platelets, thus producing an anticoagulant effect. Claims that garlic can reduce heart disease and the incidence of stroke may be related to this action. The healthcare provider may want to recommend that patients taking anticoagulant medications limit their intake of garlic to avoid bleeding complications. ■

DRUG PROFILE: Anticoagulant, Antiplatelet Agent: Pr *Ticlopidine (Ticlid)*

Actions and Uses:

Ticlopidine prolongs bleeding time by inhibiting platelet aggregation. It is given orally. Although its only approved use is to reduce the risk of stroke due to thrombi, is also given to prevent thrombi formations in patients with coronary artery stents, and to prevent postoperative deep vein thromboses (DVTs). Because it is expensive, it is usually only prescribed for patients unable to tolerate aspirin, which has similar anticoagulant activity. Clopidogrel (Plavix) acts by the same mechanism as ticlopidine, but generally causes fewer adverse effects.

Adverse Effects and Interactions:

The most serious adverse effects of ticlopidine are on blood cells. The drug can reduce the number of neutrophils. Although uncommon, ticlopidine can cause an acute blood disorder known as thrombotic thrombocytopenia purpura, which can be fatal in up to 30% of patients who develop the disorder. More common, though less serious, effects are nausea, diarrhea, abdominal pain, and rash.

Using ticlopidine with other anticoagulants increases the risk of bleeding. Cimetidine decreases the clearance of ticlopidine. Use of ticlopidine with cyclosporine can decrease the level of the latter. Theophylline and phenytoin blood levels may be increased when either is given with ticlopidine.

See the Companion Website for a Nursing Process Focus specific to this drug.

platelet aggregation. The anticoagulant effect of a single dose of aspirin may last for as long as a week. Use of aspirin with other coagulation modifiers should be avoided unless medically approved. The primary actions and adverse effects of aspirin are described in a Drug Profile in Chapter 12.

The ADP receptor blockers are a small group of drugs that interfere with the plasma membrane of platelets, preventing them from aggregating. Both ticlopidine (Ticlid) and clopidogrel (Plavix) are given orally to prevent thrombi formation in patients who have experienced a recent thromboembolic event such as a stroke or MI.

Glycoprotein IIb/IIIa inhibitors are relatively new additions to the treatment of thromboembolic disease. **Glycoprotein IIb/IIIa** is an enzyme necessary for platelet aggregation. Inhibition of this enzyme has the effect of preventing thrombus formation in patients experiencing a recent MI, stroke, or percutaneous transluminal coronary angioplasty (PTCA).

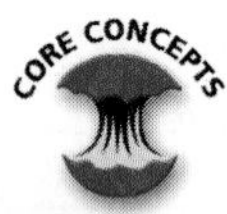

14.6 Thrombolytics are used to dissolve existing clots.

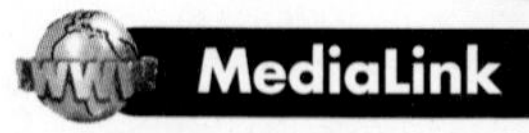

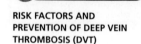

RISK FACTORS AND PREVENTION OF DEEP VEIN THROMBOSIS (DVT)

It is often mistakenly believed that the purpose of anticoagulants such as heparin and warfarin is to dissolve preexisting clots. This is not the case: A totally different type of drug is needed for this purpose. These drugs, called *thrombolytics,* are administered quite differently than the anticoagulants and produce their effects by different mechanisms. Thrombolytics are prescribed for a number of different disorders, including the following:

- Acute MI
- Pulmonary embolism
- Acute ischemic cerebrovascular accident (CVA)
- DVT
- Arterial thrombosis
- Coronary thrombosis
- To clear thrombi in arteriovenous cannulas and blocked IV catheters

Thrombolytics are nonspecific: They will dissolve whatever clots they encounter. Because clotting is a natural and desirable process to prevent excessive bleeding, thrombolytics

DRUG PROFILE: Thrombolytics: Pr *Alteplase (Activase)*

Actions and Uses:

Produced through recombinant DNA technology, alteplase is identical to the enzyme human tissue plasminogen activator (tPA). Like other thrombolytics, the primary action of alteplase is to convert plasminogen to plasmin, which then dissolves clots. Alteplase must be given within 6 hours of the onset of symptoms of MI and within 3 hours of thrombotic stroke to be effective. Peak effect occurs in 5–10 minutes. Alteplase does not cause allergic reactions, as does streptokinase. An unlabeled use is for restoration of patency (openness) of IV catheters.

Adverse Effects and Interactions:

Thrombolytics such as alteplase are contraindicated in patients with active bleeding or with a history of recent trauma. The client must be monitored carefully for signs of bleeding every 15 minutes for the first hour of therapy and every 30 minutes thereafter. Signs of bleeding such as bruising, hematomas, or nosebleeds should be reported to the physician immediately.

Alteplase should be used with caution with herbal supplements, such as ginkgo, which may cause an increased thrombolytic effect.

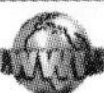
See the Companion Website for a Nursing Process Focus specific to this drug.

have a narrow margin of safety between dissolving normal and abnormal clots. Vital signs must be monitored continuously, and any signs of bleeding may call for discontinuation of therapy. Because these medications are rapidly destroyed in the bloodstream, discontinuation normally results in the immediate end of thrombolytic activity. After the clot is successfully dissolved with the thrombolytic, anticoagulant therapy is generally started prevent the reformation of clots.

Since the discovery of streptokinase, the first thrombolytic, there have been a number of generations of thrombolytics. The newer drugs such as tenecteplase (TNKase) have a more rapid onset and a longer duration and may produce fewer side effects than older drugs in this class. Table 14.4 lists the major thrombolytics.

Concept Review 14.2

- Both warfarin and heparin are effective anticoagulants. Why would a physician choose heparin over warfarin?

TABLE 14.4 Thrombolytics

DRUG	ROUTE AND ADULT DOSE	REMARKS
Pr alteplase recombinant (Activase)	IV begin with 60 mg and then infuse 20 mg/hour over next 2 hours	Naturally occurring tissue plasminogen activator; must be given within 6 hours of start of MI or 3 hours of thrombotic stroke
anistreplase (Eminase)	IV 30 units over 2–5 min	Usually given at the onset of an acute MI
reteplase recombinant (Retavase)	IV 10 units over 2 min; repeat dose in 30 min	Given during an acute MI to decrease chance of HF and death
streptokinase (Streptase, Kabikinase)	IV 250,000–1.5 million units over a short period of time	For acute DVT, pulmonary emboli, and MI
tenecteplase (TNKase)	IV 30–50 mg infused over 5 sec	Newer thrombolytic with fewer side effects than streptokinase
urokinase (Abbokinase)	IV 4400–6000 units administered over several minutes to 12 hours	For massive pulmonary emboli; restores patency in occluded IV catheters

NURSING PROCESS FOCUS

Patients Receiving Thrombolytic Therapy

ASSESSMENT

Prior to administration:

- Obtain complete health history including recent surgeries or trauma, allergies, drug history, and possible drug interations
- Obtain vital signs; assess in context of patient's baseline values
- Assess lab values: aPTT, PT, Hgb, Hct, platelet count

POTENTIAL NURSING DIAGNOSES

- Risk for Injury (bleeding), related to adverse effects of thrombolytic therapy
- Ineffective Tissue Perfusion, related to increase in size of thrombus due to ineffective thrombolytic therapy
- Deficient Knowledge, related to drug therapy

PLANNING: Patient Goals and Expected Outcomes

The patient will:

- Experience a dissolving of preexisting blood clot(s) as evidenced by laboratory values ordered by the healthcare provider
- Demonstrate an understanding of the drug's action by accurately describing drug side effects and precautions

IMPLEMENTATION

Interventions and (Rationales)	Patient Education/Discharge Planning
■ If necessary, have IV lines initiated or Foley catheter prior to beginning therapy. (This decreases the risk of bleeding from those sites).	■ Instruct patient about procedures and why they are necessary prior to beginning thrombolytic therapy.
■ Monitor vital signs every 15 minutes during first hour of infusion, then every 30 minutes during remainder of infusion. ■ Patient should be moved as little as possible during the infusion. (This is done to prevent internal injury.)	Advise patient: ■ Of the need for frequent vital signs ■ That activity will be limited during infusion and pressure dressing may be needed to prevent any active bleeding
■ If given for thrombotic CVA, monitor neurological status frequently. ■ Have cardiac rhythm monitored while medication is infusing. (Dysrhythmias may occur with reperfusion of myocardium.)	■ Advise patient about assessments and why they are necessary. ■ Advise patient that cardiac rhythm will be monitored during therapy.
■ Monitor blood tests (Hct, Hgb, platelet counts) during and after therapy for indications of blood loss due to internal bleeding. (Patient has increased risk of bleeding for 2–4 days postinfusion.)	■ Instruct patient of increased risk for bleeding and activity restriction and frequent monitoring during this time.

EVALUATION OF OUTCOME CRITERIA

Evaluate the effectiveness of drug therapy by confirming that patient goals and expected outcomes have been met (see "Planning").

See Table 14.4 for a list of drugs to which these nursing actions apply.

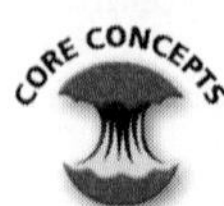

14.7 Hemostatics are used to promote the formation of clots.

Hemostatics, also called *antifibrinolytics,* have an action opposite to that of anticoagulants: to shorten bleeding time. The name *hemostatics* comes from their ability to slow blood flow. They are used to prevent excessive bleeding following surgery.

The final class of coagulation modifiers, the hemostatics, is a small group of drugs used to prevent and treat excessive bleeding from surgical sites. All of the hemostatics have specific indications for use, and none are commonly prescribed. Although their mechanisms differ, all drugs in this class prevent fibrin from dissolving, thus enhancing the stability of the clot. Desmopressin differs from the others in being a hormone similar to vasopressin, a hormone naturally present in the body that promotes the renal conservation of water. Unlike the other hemostatics, it has uses beyond hemostasis that include the control of excessive or nocturnal urination (enuresis). The hemostatics are listed in Table 14.5.

TABLE 14.5 Hemostatics

DRUG	ROUTE AND ADULT DOSE	REMARKS
Pr aminocaproic acid (Amicar)	IV 4–5 g for 1 hour, then 1–1.25 g/hour until bleeding is controlled	For control of excessive bleeding caused by a pathological condition known as *systemic hyperfibrinolysis;* oral form available
aprotinin (Trasylol)	IV 15,000 KIU as a test dose, then give 500,000 KIU during surgery	Used prior to coronary bypass surgery to reduce perioperative blood loss
desmopressin acetate (DDAVP)	IV 0.3 mcg/kg, repeated as needed	Unlabelled use is to help control bleeding in patients with hemophilia A; infusion occurs over 15–30 minutes, usually immediately prior to surgery; PO, subcutaneous, and intranasal forms available; also used for diabetes insipidus and nocturnal enuresis
tranexamic acid (Cyklokapron)	PO 25 mg/kg qid	Used just prior to and following dental surgery; IV form available

DRUG PROFILE: Hemostatics: Pr *Aminocaproic Acid (Amicar)*

Actions and Uses:

Aminocaproic acid acts by inactivating plasminogen, the precursor of the enzyme plasmin that dissolves the fibrin clot. Aminocaproic acid is prescribed in situations in which there is excessive bleeding as a result of clots being dissolved prematurely. During acute hemorrhages, it can be given IV to reduce bleeding in 1–2 hours. It is most commonly prescribed following surgery to reduce postoperative bleeding.

Adverse Effects and Interactions:

Because aminocaproic acid tends to stabilize clots, it should be used cautiously in patients with a history of thromboembolic disease. Side effects are generally mild. The therapeutic serum level is 100–400 mcg/ml.

Drug interactions include hypercoagulation when used with estrogens and oral contraceptives.

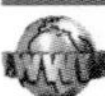

See the Companion Website for a Nursing Process Focus specific to this drug.

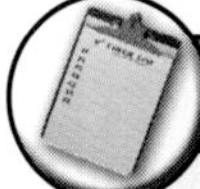

PATIENTS NEED TO KNOW

Patients treated for coagulation disorders need to know the following:

1. Keep all scheduled appointments for PT, aPTT, and INR laboratory tests. Test results are used in making decisions about drug dose adjustments.
2. Report unusual bruising or bleeding such as nose bleeds, bleeding gums, black or red stool, heavy menstrual periods, or spitting up blood to healthcare providers.
3. Inform dental hygienists and dentists about the use of anticoagulant medication.
4. Use caution when engaged in activities that can cause bleeding, such as shaving, brushing teeth, trimming nails, and using kitchen knives. A soft toothbrush and an electric razor are safe choices. Contact sports, with their high risk for injury, should be avoided.
5. Take medications on time and as directed. Do not skip a dose and do not double up on doses.
6. Speak with the practitioner before taking any other drugs, including OTC drugs or herbal supplements. Many drugs increase or decrease the action of anticoagulants. ■

CHAPTER REVIEW

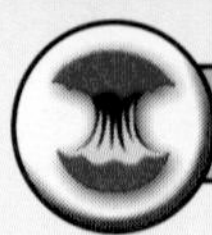

CORE CONCEPTS SUMMARY

14.1 Hemostasis is a complex process involving multiple steps and many clotting factors.

Hemostasis is an essential mechanism protecting the body from both external and internal injury that occurs in a sequential series of steps known as the coagulation cascade. The final result of coagulation is formation of the fibrin clot that protects the body from excessive blood loss.

14.2 Removing a blood clot is essential to restoring normal circulation.

Blood clots are removed by fibrinolysis. Plasmin digests the fibrin strands, thus restoring circulation to the injured area.

14.3 Drugs can be used to modify the normal coagulation process.

Articogaulants prevent the formation of clots, thrombolytics dissolve existing clots, and hemostatics promote the formation of clots. Coagulation is always carefully monitored through the use of PT or aPTT laboratory tests.

14.4 Anticoagulants prevent the formation and enlargement of blood clots.

Anticoagulants prolong coagulation time by inhibiting platelets or a specific clotting factor in the coagulation cascade. Heparin is given IV or subcutaneously to provide immediate anticoagulation activity, and warfarin is given orally to offer more prolonged action. Protamine sulfate can reverse the anticoagulant activity of heparin, and vitamin K can reverse the effects of warfarin.

14.5 Antiplatelet agents prolong bleeding time by interfering with platelet aggregation.

Aspirin, ADP receptor blockers, and glycoprotein IIb/IIIa receptor blockers prolong bleeding time by interfering with platelet function. They are used to prevent thrombus formation in arteries.

14.6 Thrombolytics are used to dissolve existing clots.

By dissolving existing clots, thrombolytics restore circulation to an injured area. For maximum effectiveness, they should be given as soon as possible after the thrombus is diagnosed.

14.7 Hemostatics are used to promote the formation of clots.

Hemostatics inhibit fibrin in a clot from dissolving and are used primarily to prevent excessive bleeding from surgical sites.

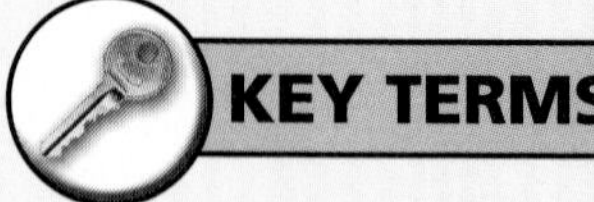

KEY TERMS

activated partial thromboplastin time (aPTT): (throm-bow-PLAS-tin): blood test used to determine how long it takes clots to form, to regulate heparin dosage / ***page 240***

anticoagulant (ANT-eye-co-AG-you-lent): an agent that inhibits the formation of blood clots / ***page 238***

clotting factors: substances contributing to the process of blood clotting / ***page 235***

coagulation (co-ag-you-LAY-shun): the process of blood clotting / ***page 235***

coagulation cascade (cass-KADE): complex series of steps by which blood flow stops / ***page 235***

embolus (EM-boh-luss): a blood clot carried in the blood stream / ***page 238***

fibrin (FEYE-brin): an insoluble protein formed from fibrinogen by the action of thrombin in the blood-clotting process / ***page 235***

fibrinogen (feye-BRIN-oh-jen): blood protein converted to fibrin by the action of thrombin in the blood-clotting process / ***page 235***

fibrinolysis (feye-brin-OL-oh-sis): removal of a blood clot / ***page 237***

glycoprotein IIb/IIIa (GLEYE-koh-proh-teen): enzyme responsible for platelet aggregation / ***page 244***

hemostasis (hee-moh-STAY-sis): the slowing or stopping of blood flow / ***page 235***

hemostatics (hee-moh-STAT-iks): drugs used to prevent and treat excessive bleeding from surgical sites / ***page 238***

international normalized ratio (INR): lab value used to monitor the degree of blood anticoagulation during warfarin therapy / ***page 240***

low molecular weight heparins (LMWHs): heparinlike drugs that inhibit blood clotting / ***page 242***

plasmin (PLAZ-min): enzyme formed from plasminogen that dissolves blood clots / *page 237*

plasminogen (plaz-MIN-oh-jen): protein that prevents fibrin clot formation / *page 237*

prothrombin (PRO-throm-bin): blood protein converted to thrombin in the blood-clotting process / *page 235*

prothrombin time (PT): blood test used to determine the time needed for plasma to clot to regulate warfarin dosage / *page 240*

thrombin (THROM-bin): enzyme formed in coagulating blood from prothrombin; it converts fibrinogen to fibrin, which forms the basis of a blood clot / *page 235*

thromboembolic disease (THROM-bow-EM-bow-lik): disorders in which patients have blood clots / *page 238*

thrombolytics (throm-bow-LIT-iks): drugs used to dissolve existing blood clots / *page 238*

thrombus (THROM-bus): blood clot / *page 238*

tissue plasminogen activator (tPA): natural enzyme and a drug that dissolves blood clots / *page 237*

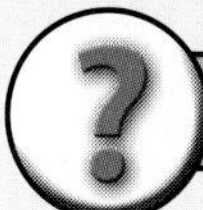

REVIEW QUESTIONS

The following questions are written in NCLEX-PN® style. Answer these questions to asses your knowledge of the chapter material, and go back and review any material that is not clear to you.

1. The patient's INR is 5.5. The nurse will:

1. Recheck the lab value
2. Notify the physician
3. Administer warfarin (Coumadin)
4. Hold the warfarin (Coumadin) and notify the physician

2. The patient has been started on warfarin (Coumadin) for DVT. The patient asks when the medication will break up the clots. The nurse's best response would be:

1. "It will 7 to 10 days for the clot to break down."
2. "This medication will not break down clots but will make it less likely that the clot will get larger."
3. "It will break down the clot within 8 to 12 hours of administration."
4. "You will need to be on this medication for a long time before it will break down the clot."

3. The patient on IV heparin is started on warfarin (Coumadin) because:

1. Additional medication is needed
2. Warfarin (Coumadin) is much more effective than heparin
3. Warfarin (Coumadin) is not effective until 12 to 24 hours after the first dose
4. Heparin has a low molecular weight and is effective for only a short time

4. The patient is receiving enoxaparin (Lovenox) subcutaneously every 12 hours following knee replacement surgery. The nurse should assess for:

1. Gingival hyperplasia
2. Signs and symptoms of bruising and bleeding
3. Clotting at the incision site
4. Increased pain

5. The patient has severe hepatic cirrhosis. The nurse understands the patient's abnormal coagulation times related to:

1. Inadequate tissue plasminogen activator
2. Inadequate prothrombin activator
3. Inadequate vitamin E
4. Inadequate vitamin K

6. The patient is receiving warfarin (Coumadin). Which of the following lab tests should be scheduled?

1. Prothrombin time (PT)
2. International normalized ratio (INR) and PT
3. Partial prothrombin time (PPT)
4. INR

7. The patient on anticoagulant therapy has had a minor surgical procedure. Which of the following would be appropriate for pain control?

1. Ibuprofen (Motrin)
2. Aspirin
3. Acetaminophen (Tylenol)
4. Naproxin sodium (Naprosyn)

8. The patient on intermittent heparin is found to have hematuria and bleeding from old IV sites. The nurse anticipates what being ordered?

1. Protamine sulfate
2. Vitamin K
3. Pentoxifylline (Trental)
4. Ardeparin (Normiflo)

9. Which drug would be appropriate for a patient experiencing an acute MI?

1. Dipyridamole (Persantine)
2. Aminocaproic acid (Amicar)
3. Desmopressin acetate (DDAVP)
4. Alteplase (Activase)

10. Hemophilia B is due to a lack of clotting factor:

1. VIII
2. X
3. IX
4. XI

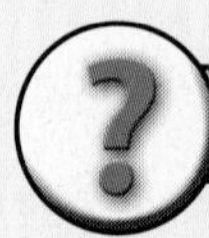

CASE STUDY QUESTIONS

For questions 1–5, please refer to the following case study, and choose the correct answer from choices 1–4.

Mr. Hawkins was recently admitted to the hospital with chest pain and suspected pulmonary embolus. He was immediately placed on heparin for 2 days and then switched to warfarin. He is now leaving the hospital with instructions to have laboratory testing every other day for the next 2 weeks.

1. What was the likely goal of placing Mr. Hawkins on heparin?

1. To dissolve pulmonary emboli
2. To prevent excessive bleeding
3. To reduce blood viscosity
4. To prevent additional thrombi from forming

2. Why did the physician first place Mr. Hawkins on heparin, instead of warfarin?

1. Heparin is more effective.
2. Heparin causes fewer side effects.
3. Heparin has a faster onset of action.
4. Heparin has a longer duration of action.

3. Which of the following is the most common and dangerous side effect of heparin therapy?

1. Nausea/vomiting
2. MI
3. Bleeding
4. Sedation

4. What was the likely reason why Mr. Hawkins was switched from heparin to warfarin before he was released from the hospital?

1. Warfarin is more effective.
2. Warfarin is given orally.
3. Warfarin causes less risk of hemorrhage.
4. Warfarin is less expensive.

5. What laboratory tests will likely be performed during the 2 weeks after his release?

1. PT/INR
2. Complete blood count (CBC)
3. aPTT
4. White blood cell count

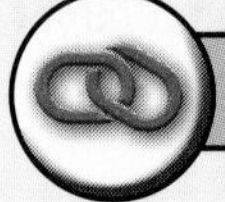

FURTHER STUDY

- The actions and adverse effects of aspirin are described in a Drug Profile in Chapter 12.
- The role of thrombolytics in the treatment of MI and cerebrovascular accident is presented in Chapter 18.

EXPLORE MEDIALINK www.prenhall.com/holland

Additional resources for this chapter can be found on the CD-ROM accompanying this texbook, and on the Companion Website. Click on Chapter 14 to select activities for this chapter.

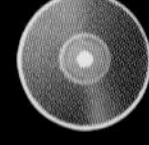

Mechanism in Action: Warfarin
Audio Glossary
Concept Review
NCLEX-PN® Review
Nursing in Action
Dosage Calculator

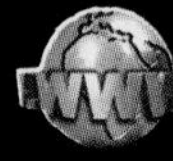

Immune Thrombocytopenic Purpura (ITP)
Risk Factors and Prevention of Deep Vein Thrombosis (DVT)

CHAPTER

15 Drugs for Hypertension

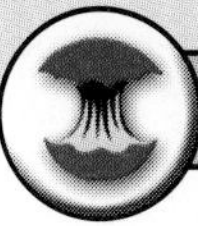

CORE CONCEPTS

15.1 Hypertension can lead to stroke, heart failure, or MI, if untreated.

15.2 Blood pressure is caused by the pumping action of the heart.

15.3 The primary factors responsible for blood pressure are cardiac output, the resistance of the small arteries, and blood volume.

15.4 Many nervous and hormonal factors help to keep blood pressure within normal limits.

15.5 The normal range of blood pressure varies throughout the lifespan.

15.6 Lifestyle changes can often reverse borderline hypertension.

15.7 Selection of specific antihypertension drugs depends on the severity of the disease.

15.8 Diuretics are often drugs of first choice for treating mild to moderate hypertension.

15.9 Calcium channel blockers have emerged as primary drugs in the treatment of hypertension.

15.10 Blocking the renin-angiotensin pathway leads to a decrease in blood pressure.

15.11 Alpha- and beta-adrenergic blockers are commonly used to treat hypertension.

15.12 Some vasodilators act directly on arteriolar smooth muscle to lower blood pressure.

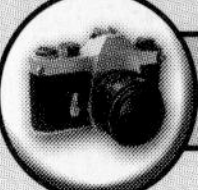

DRUG SNAPSHOT

The following drugs will be discussed in this chapter:

DRUG CLASSES	DRUG PROFILES
Diuretics (HydroDIURIL)	Pr hydrochlorothiazide
Calcium channel blockers	Pr nifedipine (Procardia)
Renin-angiotensin pathway modifiers	Pr enalapril (Vasotec)
Adrenergic blockers	Pr doxazosin (Cardura)
Direct-acting vasodilators	Pr hydralazine (Apresoline)

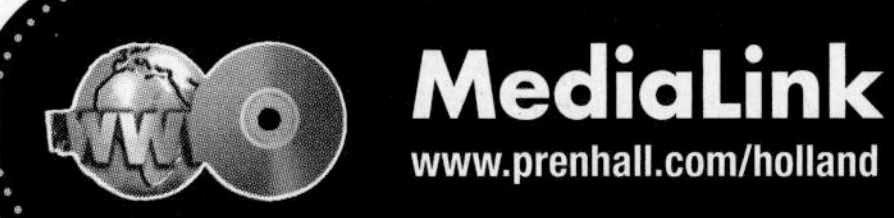

MediaLink
www.prenhall.com/holland

Interactive resources for this chapter can be found on the Companion Website. Click on Chapter 15 and "Begin" to select the activities for this chapter. For chapter-related animations, NCLEX-PN®-style questions, and an audio glossary, access the accompanying CD-ROM in this book.

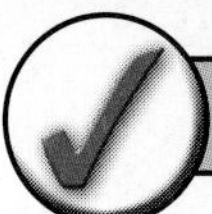

OBJECTIVES

After reading this chapter, the student should be able to:

1. Identify the major risk factors associated with hypertension.
2. Describe how the pumping action of the heart creates blood pressure.
3. Explain the effects of cardiac output, peripheral resistance, and blood volume on blood pressure.
4. Discuss how the vasomotor center, baroreceptors, emotions, and hormones influence blood pressure.
5. Describe how hypertension is classified.
6. Outline a method for controlling borderline hypertension without drugs.
7. Apply "stepped care" principles as they pertain to antihypertension drugs.
8. For each of the following classes, identify representative medications and explain the mechanism of drug action, primary actions, and important side effects.
   - **a.** Diuretics
   - **b.** Calcium channel blockers
   - **c.** Renin-angiotensin modifiers
   - **d.** Adrenergic blockers
   - **e.** Direct-acting vasodilators
9. Categorize antihypertensive drugs based on their classification and mechanism of action.

hyper = *high*
tension = *pressure*

Cardiovascular disease, which includes all conditions affecting the heart and blood vessels, is the most common cause of death in the United States. **Hypertension** or *high blood pressure* is the most common of the cardiovascular diseases. Because healthcare providers encounter numerous patients with this disease, a firm grasp of the underlying principles of antihypertensive therapy is critical.

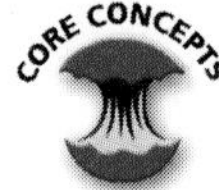

15.1 Hypertension can lead to stroke, heart failure, or MI if untreated.

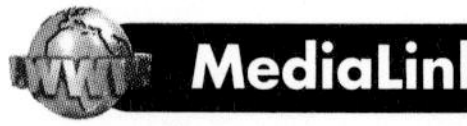

THE AMERICAN SOCIETY OF HYPERTENSION

The most common type of hypertension, accounting for 90% of all cases, is called *primary* or *essential.* Although the actual cause of primary hypertension is not known, many conditions or risk factors have been shown to be associated with the disease. Advancing age and weight gain, particularly around the hips and thighs, tends to be associated with hypertension. The disease is most prevalent in Blacks and least prevalent in Mexican Americans. Men in all ethnic groups experience more hypertension compared to women. The disease also has a hereditary component, with family members of hypertensive patients having greater risk of acquiring the disease than nonfamily members. Other factors, such as tobacco use and high-fat diets, contribute to the disease.

Fast Facts Hypertension

- Hypertension increases with age. It affects approximately:
  30% of those 50 years old and older; 64% of men older than age 65; 75% of women older than age 75
- Almost 19,250 people died of hypertension in the United States in 2001 (8.7 deaths per 100,000 population).
- Hypertension is responsible for more than 10 million ambulatory care visits.
- Hypertension affects one in three adult Americans, more than 60 million people per year.
- Blacks have the highest rate of hypertension.
- Fewer than 34% of Americans diagnosed with hypertension keep their blood pressure within recommended parameters.
- Hypertension is the most common complication of pregnancy.

Because chronic hypertension may produce no identifiable symptoms for as long as 10 to 20 years, many people are not aware of their condition. Convincing patients to control their diets, spend money on medication, and take drugs on a regular basis when they are feeling healthy is a difficult task for the healthcare practitioner. Failure to control hypertension, however, can result in serious consequences. Prolonged high blood pressure can lead to accelerated narrowing of the arteries resulting in strokes, kidney failure, and even cardiac arrest. One of the most serious consequences of chronic hypertension is that the heart must work harder to pump blood to organs and tissues. This excessive workload can cause the heart to fail and the lungs to fill with fluid, a condition known as **heart failure (HF).** Drug therapy of HF is covered in Chapter 16.

The death rate from cardiovascular-related diseases has dropped significantly over the past 20 years because, in large part, of the recognition and treatment of hypertension, as well as the acceptance of healthier lifestyle habits. Early treatment is essential; the long-term cardiovascular damage caused by hypertension may be irreversible if the disease is allowed to progress unchecked.

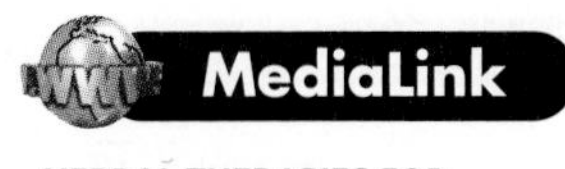

HERBAL THERAPIES FOR HYPERTENSION

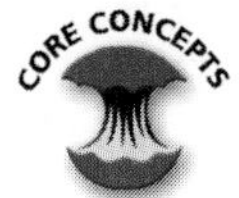

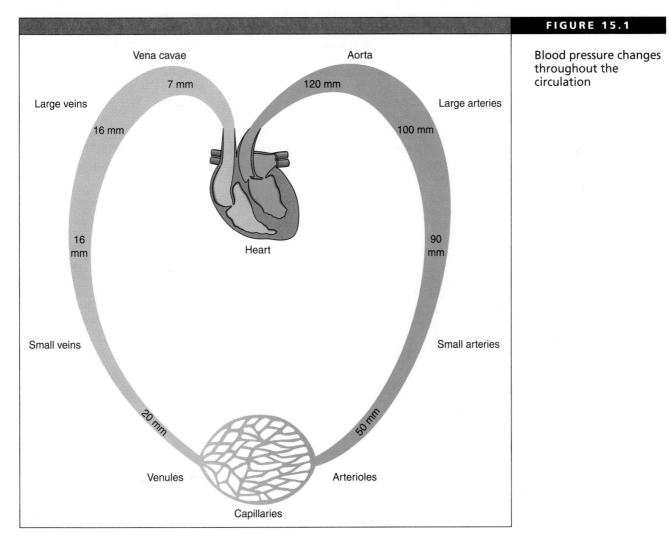

15.2 Blood pressure is caused by the pumping action of the heart.

Although pressure can be measured in nearly any vessel in the body, the term *blood pressure* commonly refers to pressure in the arteries. Because the pumping action of the heart is the source of blood pressure, those arteries closest to the heart, such as the aorta, have the highest pressure. Pressure decreases gradually as the blood travels farther from the heart, until it falls close to zero in the largest veins. This is illustrated in Figure 15.1 ■.

When the ventricles of the heart contract and eject blood, the pressure created in the arteries is called **systolic pressure.** When the ventricles relax and the heart temporarily stops ejecting blood,

FIGURE 15.1

Blood pressure changes throughout the circulation

FIGURE 15.2

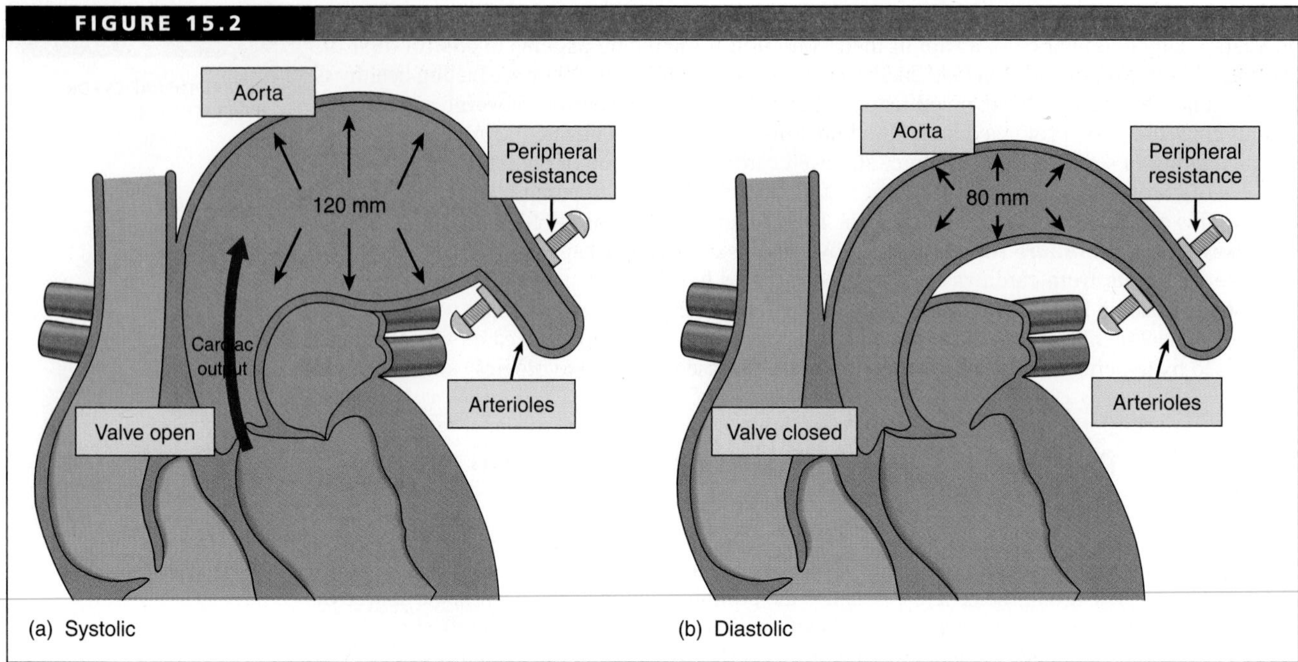

(a) Systolic pressure occurs when the heart ejects blood, creating high pressure in the arteries. (b) Diastolic pressure occurs when the heart relaxes, resulting in less pressure in the arteries.

pressure in the arteries will fall, and this results in **diastolic pressure.** Blood pressure is measured in units of millimeters mercury, abbreviated as mm Hg. (Hg is the chemical symbol for the element mercury.) The average normal systolic pressure in a healthy adult is considered to be less than 120 mm Hg, whereas the average normal diastolic pressure is less than 80 mm Hg. The systolic and diastolic pressures are usually measured and reported together, with the systolic given first. For example, average normal blood pressure is said to be less than 120/80 mm Hg. Figure 15.2 ■ illustrates how the pumping action of the heart determines sytolic and diastolic blood pressure.

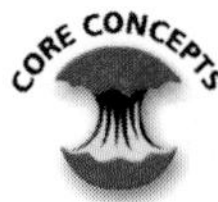

15.3 The primary factors responsible for blood pressure are cardiac output, the resistance of the small arteries, and blood volume.

While many factors can influence blood pressure, three factors are truly responsible for determining the pressure. The three primary factors—cardiac output, peripheral resistance, and blood volume—are shown in Figure 15.3 ■.

The volume of blood pumped per minute is called the **cardiac output.** Although resting cardiac output is approximately 5 liters per minute (L/min), strenuous exercise can increase this output to as much as 35 L/min. The higher the cardiac output, the higher the blood pressure. This is important to pharmacology because drugs that change the cardiac output have the potential to influence a patient's blood pressure.

As blood flows at high speeds through the vascular system, it bumps and drags across the walls of the vessels. Although the vessel walls are extremely smooth, this friction reduces the ve-

FIGURE 15.3

Primary factors affecting blood pressure

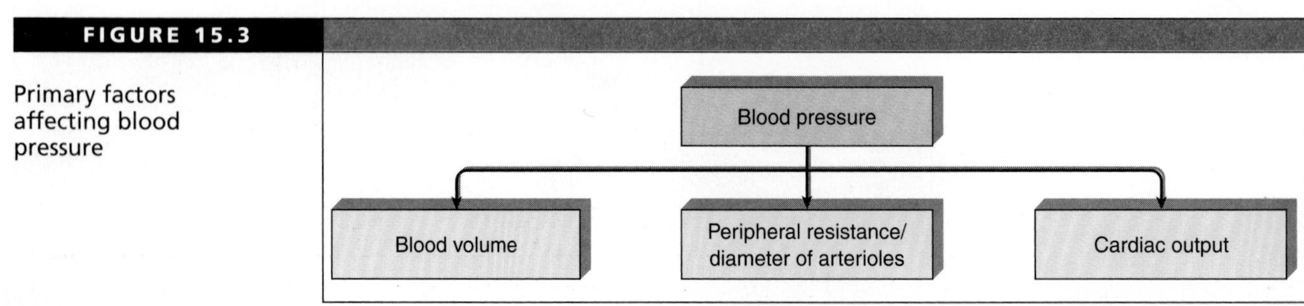

locity of the blood. This dragging or friction in the arteries is called **peripheral resistance.** Arteries have smooth muscle in their walls that, when constricted, will cause the inside diameter or **lumen** to become smaller, thus creating more resistance and higher pressure. This is how the body controls normal minute-by-minute changes in blood pressure. This is also important to pharmacology because a number of drugs affect vascular smooth muscle, causing vessels to constrict, thus raising blood pressure. Other drugs cause the smooth muscle to relax, thereby opening the lumen and lowering blood pressure. These drugs are among those used to treat hypertension. See Chapter 7 regarding the role of the autonomic nervous system in controlling peripheral resistance.

The third factor responsible for blood pressure is the total amount to blood in the vascular system, or *blood volume.* While the average person maintains a relatively constant blood volume of approximately 5 L, this can change as a result of certain regulatory factors and with certain disease states. More blood in the vascular system will exert additional pressure on the walls of the arteries and raise blood pressure. For example, high sodium diets cause water to be retained by the body, thus increasing blood volume and raising blood pressure. On the other hand, drugs called **diuretics** can cause fluid loss through urination, thus decreasing blood volume and lowering blood pressure. Diuretics are discussed later in this chapter and in Chapter 28.

15.4 Many nervous and hormonal factors help to keep blood pressure within normal limits.

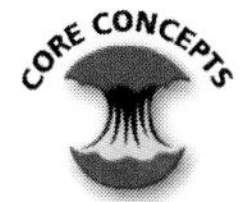

It is critical that the body maintains a normal range of blood pressure and that it has the ability to safely and rapidly change pressure as it proceeds through daily activities such as sleep and exercise. Too little blood pressure can cause dizziness and lack of urine formation, whereas too much pressure can cause vessels to rupture. A basic illustration of how the body maintains homeostasis during periods of blood pressure change is shown in Figure 15.4 ■.

Blood pressure is regulated on a minute-to-minute basis by a cluster of neurons in the medulla oblongata called the **vasomotor center.** Nerves travel from the vasomotor center to the arteries, where the smooth muscle is directed to either constrict (raise blood pressure) or relax (lower blood pressure).

Clusters of neurons in the aorta and the carotid artery act as sensors to provide the vasomotor center with vital information on current conditions in the vascular system. Some of these neurons, called **baroreceptors,** have the ability to sense blood pressure within these large vessels. The baroreceptors are important to the pharmacotherapy of hypertension. When a drug is given

baro = *pressure*
receptor = *sensor*

FIGURE 15.4

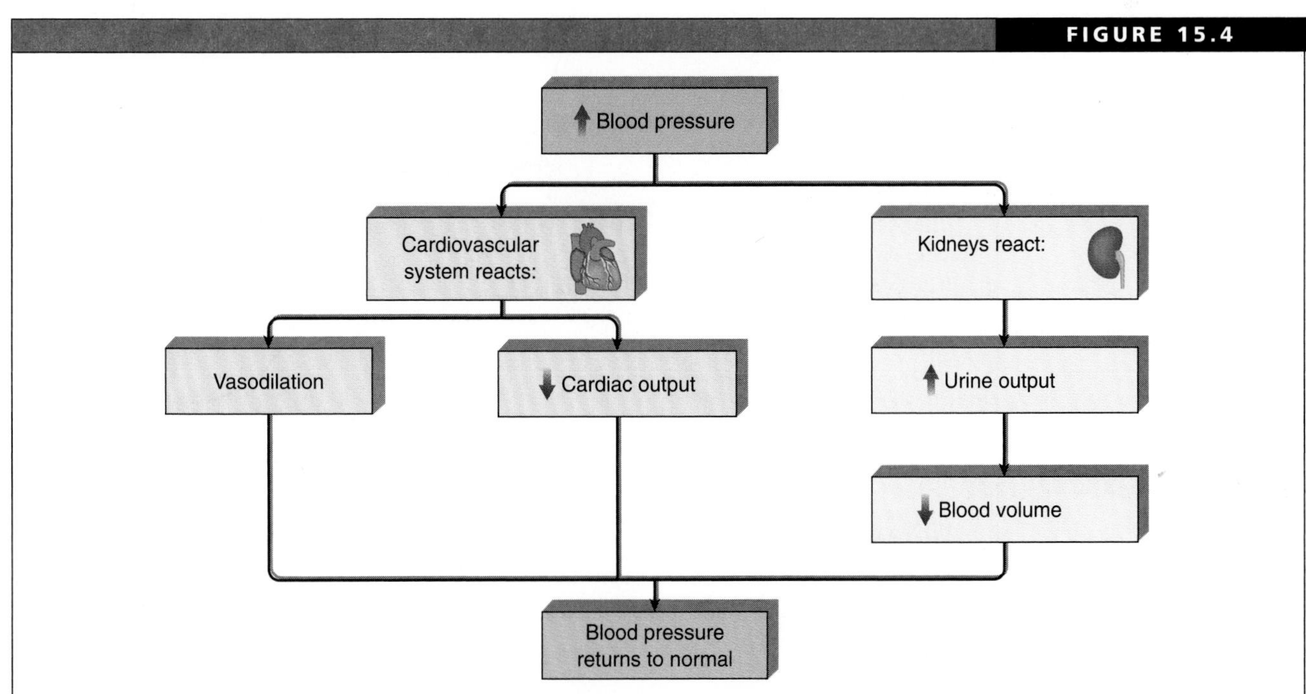

Blood pressure is controlled by the actions of the cardiovascular system and kidneys.

to lower blood pressure, the baroreceptors respond by trying to return pressure to its original (high) level. The baroreceptor response includes an immediate increase in heart rate, known as **reflex tachycardia.** In time, the body will recognize the lower blood pressure as normal, "reset" the baroreceptors, and reflex tachycardia will diminish. If reflex tachycardia does not decrease, a patient may be administered a beta-adrenergic blocker to prevent the heart rate increase.

Emotions can also have a profound effect on blood pressure. Anger and stress can cause blood pressure to rise, whereas mental depression and lethargy may cause it to fall. Strong emotions, if present for a long time, may be important contributors to chronic hypertension.

Certain hormones and other agents affect blood pressure on a daily basis. When given as drugs, some of these agents may have a profound effect on blood pressure. For example, injection of epinephrine or norepinephrine will immediately raise blood pressure. **Antidiuretic hormone (ADH)** is a strong vasoconstrictor that can increase blood pressure by raising blood volume. The **renin-angiotensin pathway** is particularly important in the drug therapy of hypertension and is discussed in Section 15.10. A summary of the various nervous and hormonal factors influencing blood pressure is shown in Figure 15.5 ■.

anti = *against*
diuretic = *urination*

Concept Review 15.1

- Because hypertension may cause no symptoms, how would you convince a patient to take his or her medication regularly?

FIGURE 15.5

Hormonal and nervous factors influencing blood pressure

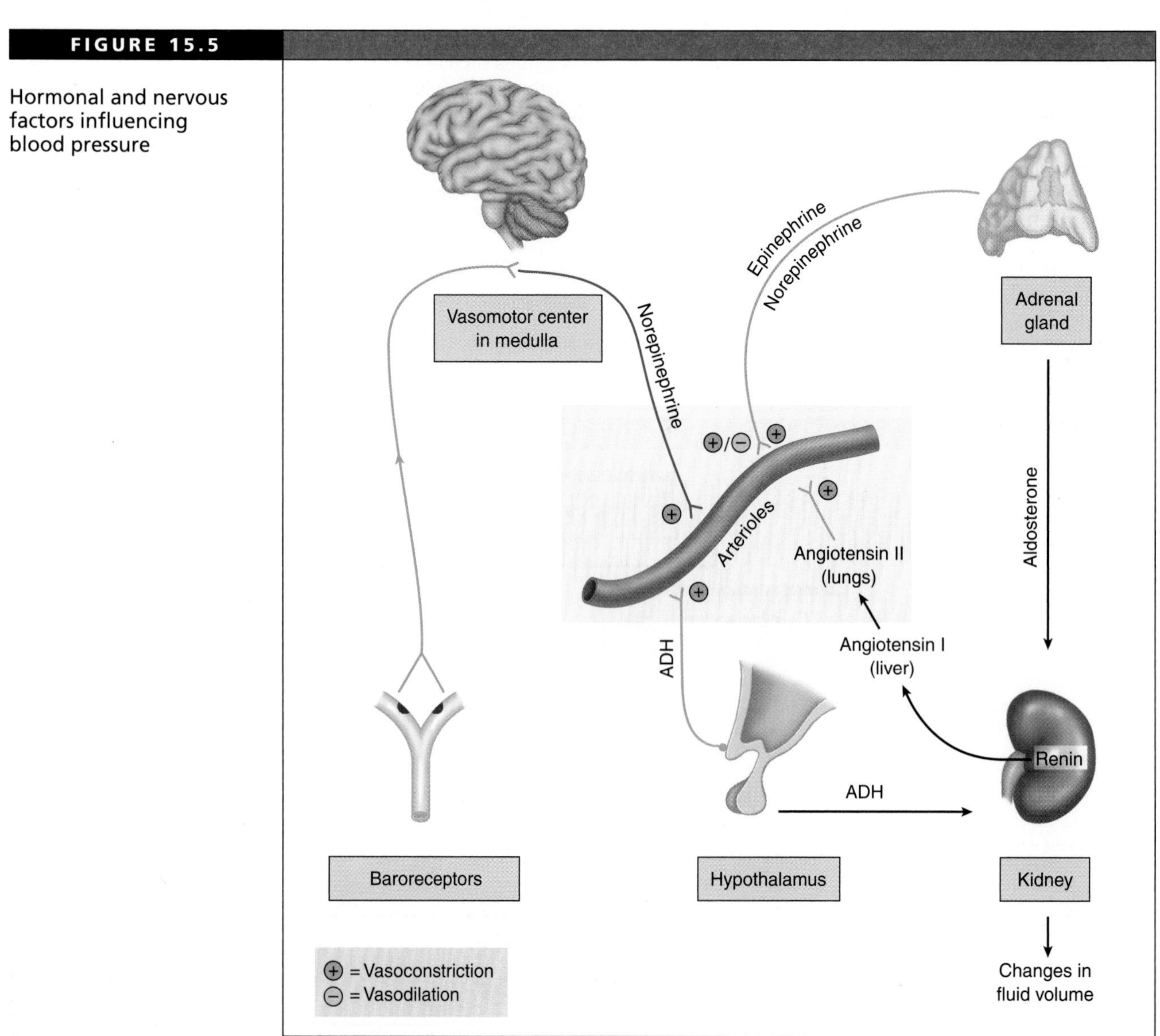

15.5 The normal range of blood pressure varies throughout the lifespan.

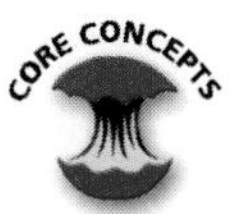

MediaLink

THE NATIONAL HEART, LUNG, AND BLOOD INSTITUTE

Although the average blood pressure of a healthy adult is defined as less than 120/80 mm Hg, many factors affect blood pressure, including normal aging. What is considered normal blood at one age may be considered abnormal in someone older or younger. Table 15.1 shows the normal variation in blood pressure that occurs throughout the lifespan.

The diagnosis of chronic hypertension is rarely made on a single blood pressure measurement. A patient having a sustained blood pressure of 140/90 mm Hg based on an average of three measurements made over several clinic visits is said to have hypertension. The disease is further subdivided according to the degree of pressure increase as shown in Table 15.2.

TABLE 15.1 Variation in Blood Pressure Throughout the Lifespan

AGE (YEARS)	MALE	FEMALE
1	96/66	95/65
5	92/62	92/62
10	103/69	103/70
20–24	123/76	116/72
30–34	126/79	120/75
40–44	129/81	127/80
50–54	135/83	137/84
60–64	142/85	144/85
70–74	145/82	159/85
80–84	145/82	157/83

TABLE 15.2 Classification and Management of Hypertension in Adults

				INITIAL DRUG THERAPY	
BP CLASSIFICATION	SBP* mm Hg	DBP* mm Hg	LIFESTYLE MODIFICATION	WITHOUT COMPELLING INDICATION	WITH COMPELLING INDICATION
Normal	<120	and <80	Encourage		
Prehypertension	120–139	or 80–89	Yes	No antihypertensive drug indicated.	Drug(s) for compelling indications‡
Stage 1 Hypertension	140–159	or 90–99	Yes	Thiazide-type diuretics for most. May consider ACEI, ARB, BB, CCB, or combination.	Drug(s) for the compelling indications:‡ Other antihypertensive drugs (diuretics, ACEI, ARB, BB, CCB) as needed.
Stage 2 Hypertension	≥160	or ≥100	Yes	Two-drug combination for most† (usually thiazide-type diuretic and ACEI or ARB or BB or CCB).	

DBP, diastolic blood pressure; SBP, systolic blood pressure.
Drug abbrevations: ACEI, angiotensin-converting enzyme inhibitor; ARB, angiotensin receptor blocker, BB, beta blocker; CCB, calcium channel blocker.

**Treatment determined by highest BP category.*
†Initial combined therapy should be used cautiously in those at risk for orthostatic hypotension.
‡Treat patients with chronic kidney disease or diabetes to BP goal of <130/80 mm Hg.

Compelling indications include HF, post-MI, high risk for coronary artery disease, diabetes, chronic kidney disease, and recurrent stroke prevention.

Source: JNC-7 Express. (2003) The Seventh Report of the Joint National Committee on Prevention, Detection, Evaluation and Treatment of High Blood Pressure by National High Blood Pressure Education Program, National Heart, Lung & Blood Institute. Retrieved June 14, 2005, from **www.nhlbi.nih.gov**

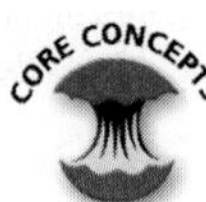

15.6 Lifestyle changes can often reverse borderline hypertension.

When a patient is first diagnosed with hypertension, the healthcare provider obtains a comprehensive medical history to determine if the disease can be controlled by nonpharmacological means. Changing certain personal habits may eliminate the need for drug therapy. Even if medications are needed to control the hypertension, it is important that the patient continue these lifestyle changes so that dosages can be minimized, thus lowering the potential for drug side effects. Nonpharmacological methods for controlling hypertension include the following:

- Implement a medically supervised, safe weight-reduction plan, if 20% or more over normal body weight.
- Stop using tobacco; smoking is a major contributor to hypertension.
- Watch mineral intake, limit salt (sodium) intake, and eat foods rich in potassium and magnesium.
- Limit alcohol consumption.
- Implement a medically supervised aerobic exercise plan.
- Reduce sources of stress and learn to implement coping strategies.

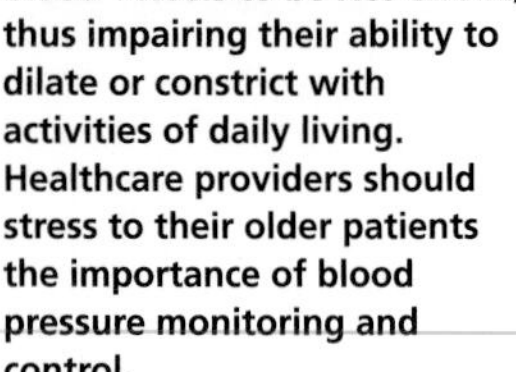

Control of blood pressure is particularly important in aging patients. Age often causes blood vessels to be less elastic, thus impairing their ability to dilate or constrict with activities of daily living. Healthcare providers should stress to their older patients the importance of blood pressure monitoring and control.

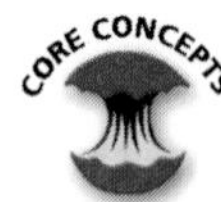

15.7 Selection of specific antihypertension drugs depends on the severity of the disease.

The goal of antihypertensive therapy is to reduce blood pressure to normal levels so that the long-term consequences of hypertension may be prevented. Keeping blood pressure within normal limits has been shown to reduce the risk of hypertension-related diseases such as stroke and heart failure. Several strategies are used to achieve this goal, as summarized in Figure 15.6 ■.

Management of hypertension depends on the degree of blood pressure increase, and whether a compelling indication such as MI, HF, or stroke has been experienced by the patient (see Table 15.2). Generally, pharmacological therapy of hypertension begins with low doses of a single medication having few side effects, usually a diuretic. If this does not control blood pressure in 2 to 4 weeks, the healthcare practitioner may increase the dose of the initial drug or substitute another antihypertensive drug from a different drug class.

A common strategy used in controlling hypertension is **stepped care.** This is the use of two drugs, from different classes, rather than one. The advantage of this approach is that it allows lower doses of each drug than would be needed if a single one were used. Lower doses usually produce fewer side effects and encourage patient compliance. Compliance decreases when patients need to take more than one drug or when they need to take them more often. In an effort to reduce noncompliance, drug manufacturers sometimes combine two drugs into a single pill or capsule. These combination drugs are quite common in the treatment of hypertension. One of the most widely used antihypertensive combinations is Dyazide, which contains two diuretics, hydrochlorothiazide (HydroDIURIL) and triamterene (Dyrenium). Another example is the drug Tarka that combines trandolapril (Mavik) and verapamil (Calan), two medications from different antihypertension classes.

The types of drugs used to treat chronic hypertension generally fall into five primary classes:

- Diuretics
- Calcium channel blockers (CCBs)
- Renin-angiotensin pathway modifiers
- Adrenergic blockers
- Direct-acting vasodilators

FIGURE 15.6

Mechanism of action of antihypertensive drugs

15.8 Diuretics are often drugs of first choice for treating mild to moderate hypertension.

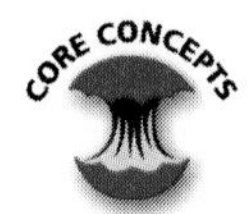

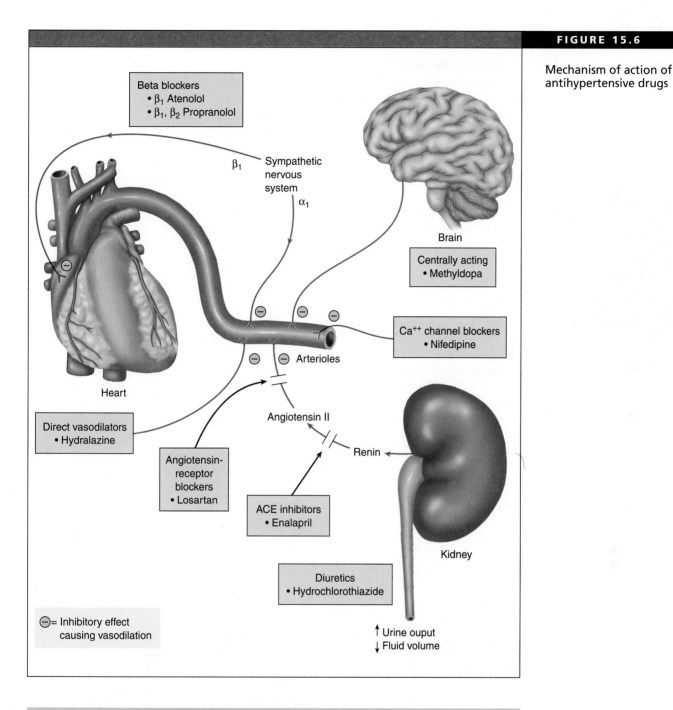

Diuretics act by increasing the amount of urine produced by the kidneys. They are widely used in the treatment of hypertension and heart failure. Table 15.3 lists diuretics commonly used to treat hypertension.

Diuretics were the first class of drugs used to treat hypertension in the 1950s. Despite many advances in drug therapy since then, diuretics are still considered drugs of first choice for this disease because they produce few adverse effects and are very effective at controlling mild to moderate hypertension. For more advanced disease, they are frequently prescribed with other antihypertensive medications. Diuretics are also used to treat heart failure (Chapter 16) and kidney disorders (Chapter 28).

TABLE 15.3 Diuretics Used for Hypertension

DRUG	ROUTE AND ADULT DOSE	REMARKS
amiloride (Midamor)	PO 5–20 mg in 1–2 divided doses (max: 20 mg/day)	Potassium sparing; acts by directly inhibiting sodium-potassium exchange in the distal tubule
chlorothiazide (Diuril)	PO/IV 250 mg–1 g in 1–2 divided doses (max: 2 g/day)	Thiazide type; acts by inhibiting sodium reabsorption in distal tubule; decreases blood potassium levels
chlorthalidone (Hygroton)	PO 12.5–25 mg daily (max: 100 mg/day)	Thiazide type; acts by inhibiting sodium reabsorption in distal tubule; decreases blood potassium levels
furosemide (Lasix)	PO 10–40 mg bid (max: 480 mg/day)	Loop diuretic; decreases blood potassium levels; acts by inhibiting sodium and chloride reabsorption in the loop of Henle; IV and IM forms available
Pr hydrochlorothiazide (Hydrodiuril, HCTZ)	PO 12.5–100 mg in 1–2 divided doses (max: 100 mg/day)	Thiazide type; acts by inhibiting sodium reabsorption in distal tubule; decreases blood potassium levels
indapamide (Lozol)	PO 2.5 mg daily; may increase to 5 mg daily if needed (max: 5 mg/day)	Similar to thiazide type; acts by inhibiting sodium reabsorption in distal tubule; decreases blood potassium levels
spironolactone (Aldactone)	PO 25–100 mg daily (max: 200 mg/day)	Potassium-sparing; acts by inhibiting aldosterone in the distal tubule
torsemide (Demedex)	PO/IV 5–10 mg daily	Loop diuretic;acts by inhibiting sodium and chloride reabsorption in the loop of Henle and distal tubule
triamterene (Dyrenium)	PO 100 mg bid (max: 300 mg/day).	Potassium sparing; acts by directly inhibiting sodium-potassium exchange in the distal tubule

Life Span Fact

Older adults are especially at risk for dyhydration and must be carefully monitored during the initial stages of diuretic therapy.

de = *high*
hydra = *water*
tion = *condition*

hyper = *high*
hypo = *low*
ka = *potassium*
emia = *blood*

Although many different diuretics are available for hypertension, all produce a similar result: the reduction of blood volume through the urinary excretion of water and electrolytes. **Electrolytes** are ions such as sodium (Na^+), calcium (Ca^{++}), chloride (Cl^-), and potassium (K^+). The mechanism by which diuretics reduce blood volume—specifically where and how the kidney is affected—differs among the various diuretics.

One of the most common adverse effects of diuretic therapy is *dehydration,* the excessive loss of water from the body. Early signs of dehydration include thirst, dry mouth, dizziness, lethargy, and a fall in blood pressure.

Electrolyte imbalances of potassium, sodium, and magnesium are additional adverse effects of diuretic therapy. Loss of potassium, or **hypokalemia,** is of particular concern because it can lead to serious abnormalities in cardiac rhythm. When taking thiazide or loop diuretics, patients should be encouraged to include a potassium supplement or to eat foods rich in potassium content, such as bananas, oranges, tomatoes, milk, salmon, and beef.

Certain diuretics such as triamterene (Dyrenium) have less tendency to cause K^+ depletion, and for this reason are called *potassium-sparing diuretics.* Taking potassium supplements with potassium-sparing diuretics may lead to dangerously high potassium levels in the blood, or **hyperkalemia,** that can cause cardiac conduction abnormalities.

Concept Review 15.2

- State the major reasons why patients should continue lifestyle changes even though their antihypertensive drugs appear to be effective.

DRUG PROFILE: Diuretic: Pr *Hydrochlorothiazide (HydroDIURIL)*

Actions and Uses:

Hydrochlorothiazide is the most widely prescribed diuretic for hypertension, belonging to a class of about 12 drugs known as the thiazides. Like many diuretics, it produces few adverse effects and is quite effective at producing a 10–20 mm Hg reduction in blood pressure. Patients with severe hypertension, however, may require the addition of a second drug from a different class to control the disease. Hydrochlorothiazide acts on the kidney tubule to decrease the reabsorption of Na^+. Normally, over 99% of the sodium entering the kidney is reabsorbed by the body so that very little leaves via the urine. When hydrochlorothiazide blocks this reabsorption, more Na^+ and water is sent into the urine, thus reducing blood volume and decreasing blood pressure. The volume of urine produced is directly proportional to the amount of sodium reabsorption blocked by the diuretic.

Adverse Effects and Interactions:

Hydrochlorothiazide has few serious adverse effects. The most common side effects involve potential electrolyte imbalances. In the case of hydrochlorothiazide, K^+ is lost along with the Na^+. Because potassium deficiency in the blood may cause conduction abnormalities in the heart, patients are usually asked to increase their intake of dietary potassium as a precaution.

Hydrochlorothiazide increases the action of other hypertensives and skeletal muscle relaxants. It may reduce the effectiveness of anticoagulants, antigout drugs, and antidiabetic drugs including insulin.

CNS depressants such as alcohol, barbiturates, and opioids may increase the orthostatic hypotension caused by hydrochlorothiazide. Steroids or amphotericin B increase potassium loss when given hydrochlorothiazide, leading to hypokalemia.

Hydrochlorothiazide increases the risk of serum toxicity of the following drugs: digitalis, lithium, allopurinol, diazoxide, anesthetics, and antineoplastics. It also alters vitamin D metabolism and calcium conservation; use of calcium supplements may cause hypercalcemia. Use with caution with herbal supplements, such as ginkgo biloba, which may actually cause an increase in blood pressure.

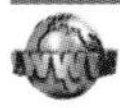
See the Companion Website for a Nursing Process Focus specific to this drug.

15.9 Calcium channel blockers have emerged as primary drugs in the treatment of hypertension.

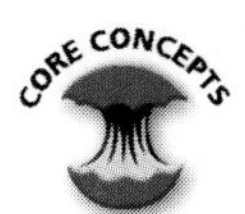

Calcium channel blockers (CCBs) comprise a group of about 10 drugs that are used to treat a number of cardiovascular diseases, including angina pectoris, cardiac dysrhythmias, and hypertension. When CCBs were first approved for the treatment of angina in the early 1980s, it was quickly noted that a side effect of the drugs was the lowering of blood pressure in hypertensive patients. CCBs have since become a widely prescribed class of drugs for hypertension. Table 15.4 lists CCBs, commonly used to treat hypertension.

Contraction of a muscle is regulated by the amount of calcium ion inside the muscle cell. When calcium enters the cell through channels in the plasma membrane, muscular contraction occurs. CCBs block these channels and prevent Ca^{++} from entering the cell, thus inhibiting muscular contraction. At low doses, CCBs cause vasodilation in arterioles, thus decreasing blood pressure. Some CCBs, such as nifedipine (Procardia), are selective for calcium channels in arterioles, while others, such as verapamil (Calan), affect channels in both arterioles and the myocardium. CCBs vary in their potency and the frequency and types of side effects produced. The use of CCBs in the treatment of dysrhythmias and angina are discussed in Chapters 17 and 18, respectively.

The high safety profile of CCBs has contributed to their popularity in treating hypertension. Common side effects related to their vasodilation action include headache, facial flushing, and dizziness. The CCBs that affect the heart should be used cautiously in patients with preexisting heart disease.

TABLE 15.4 Calcium Channel Blockers Used for Hypertension

DRUG	ROUTE AND ADULT DOSE	REMARKS
amlodipine (Norvasc)	PO 5–10 mg daily (max: 10 mg/day)	Works primarily on peripheral circulation; reduces systolic, diastolic, and mean blood pressure; also for angina
diltiazem (Cardizem)	PO 80–120 mg tid (max: 360 mg/day)	Dilates coronary arteries; affects calcium channels in both heart and blood vessels; sustained-release and IV forms available; also for angina and specific dysrhythmias
felodipine (Plendil)	PO 5–10 mg/day (max: 20 mg/day)	Selective for calcium channels in blood vessels; also for angina and heart failure
isradipine (DynaCirc)	PO 1.25–10 mg bid (max: 20 mg/day)	Affects calcium channels in both heart and blood vessels; also for angina
nicardipine (Cardene)	PO 20–40 mg tid (max: 120 mg/day)	Selective for calcium channels in blood vessels; also for angina; sustained-release and IV forms available
Pr nifedipine (Procardia, Aldalat)	PO 10–20 mg tid (max: 180 mg/day)	Selective for calcium channels in blood vessels; decreases peripheral vascular resistance and increases cardiac output; also for angina; sustained-release form available
nisoldipine (Nisocor, Sular)	PO 10–20 mg bid (max: 40 mg/day)	Structurally similar to nifedipine; affects calcium channels in both the heart and blood vessels; also for angina and heart failure
verapamil (Calan, Isoptin, Verelan)	PO 40–80 mg tid (max: 360 mg/day)	Affects calcium channels in both heart and blood vessels; sustained-release form available; IV form available for specific dysrhythmias

NURSING PROCESS FOCUS

Patients Receiving Calcium Channel Blocker Therapy

ASSESSMENT

Prior to administration:

- Obtain complete health history including data on recent cardiac events, allergies, drug history, and possible drug interactions
- Obtain ECG and vital signs; assess in context of patient's baseline values
- Assess neurological status and level of consciousness
- Auscultate chest sounds for rales or rhonchi that indicate pulmonary edema
- Assess lower limbs for edema; note character/level

POTENTIAL NURSING DIAGNOSES

- Ineffective Health Maintenance
- Deficient Knowledge, related to drug therapy
- Decreased Cardiac Output
- Altered Tissue Perfusion

PLANNING: Patient Goals and Expected Outcomes

The patient will:

- Exhibit a reduction in systolic/diastolic blood pressure
- Demonstrate an understanding of the drug's action by accurately describing drug side effects and precautions

continued...

NURSING PROCESS FOCUS

IMPLEMENTATION

Interventions and (Rationales)	Patient Education/Discharge Planning
■ Monitor vital signs. ■ Have ECG monitored during initial therapy. (Calcium channel blockers [CCBs] dilate the arteries, reducing blood pressure.)	Instruct patient to: ■ Monitor vital signs as specified by the nurse, particularly blood pressure, ensuring proper use of home equipment ■ Withhold medication for severe hypotensive readings as specified by the nurse (e.g., "hold for levels below 88/50 mm Hg") ■ Immediately report palpitations or rapid heartbeat
■ Observe for changes in level of consciousness, dizziness, fatigue, postural hypotension (caused by vasodilation). ■ Observe for paradoxical increase in chest pain, angina symptoms, or increase in heart rate (related to severe hypotension). ■ Obtain blood pressure readings in sitting, standing, and supine positions to monitor fluctuations in blood pressure.	Instruct patient to: ■ Report dizziness or lightheadedness ■ Report chest pain or other angina-like symptoms ■ Rise slowly from prolonged periods of sitting or lying down
■ Monitor for signs of HF. (CCBs can decrease myocardial contractility, increasing the risk of HF.)	■ Instruct patient to immediately report any severe shortness of breath, frothy sputum, profound fatigue, and swelling. These may be signs of HF or fluid accumulation in the lungs.
■ Monitor for fluid accumulation. ■ Measure intake and output, and daily weights. (Edema is a side effect of some CCBs.)	Instruct patient to: ■ Avoid excessive heat, which contributes to excessive sweating and fluid loss ■ Measure and monitor fluid intake and output, and weigh daily ■ Consume enough *plain* water to remain adequately, but not overly, hydrated
■ Observe for hypersensitivity reaction.	■ Instruct patient to immediately report difficulty breathing, throat tightness, hives or rash, muscle cramps, or tremors.
■ Monitor liver and kidney function. (CCBs are metabolized in the liver and excreted by the kidneys.)	Instruct patient to: ■ Report signs of liver toxicity: nausea, vomiting, anorexia, bleeding, severe upper abdominal pain, heartburn, jaundice, or a change in the color or character of stools ■ Report signs of renal toxicity: fever, flank pain, changes in urine output, color or character (cloudy, with sediment, etc.) ■ Adhere to laboratory testing regimens as ordered by the healthcare provider
■ Observe for constipation. May need to increase dietary fiber or administer laxatives.	Advise patient to: ■ Maintain adequate fluid and fiber intake to facilitate stool passage ■ Use a bulk laxative or stool softener, as recommended by the healthcare provider
■ Ensure patient safety. ■ Monitor ambulation until response to drug is known (because of postural hypotension caused by drug).	■ Instruct patient to avoid driving or other activities that require mental alertness or physical coordination until effects of the drug is known.

EVALUATION OF OUTCOME CRITERIA

Evaluate the effectiveness of drug therapy by confirming that patient goals and expected outcomes have been met (see "Planning").

See Table 15.4 for a list of drugs to which these nursing actions apply.

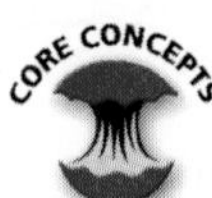

15.10 Blocking the renin-angiotensin pathway leads to a decrease in blood pressure.

Drugs that modify the renin-angiotensin pathway decrease blood pressure and increase urine volume. They are widely used in the treatment of hypertension, heart failure, and MI. Table 15.5 lists renin-angiotensin pathway modifiers commonly used to treat hypertension.

angio = *vessels*
tensin = *pressure*

The renin-angiotensin pathway is one of the primary homeostatic mechanisms controlling blood pressure and fluid balance in the body. Renin is an enzyme secreted by the kidneys when blood pressure falls or when there is a decrease in Na^+ flowing through the kidney tubules. In a series of enzymatic steps, **angiotensin II,** one of the most potent natural vasoconstrictors known, is formed. The enzyme reponsible for the final step of this pathway is called **angiotensin-converting enzyme (ACE).** The intense vasoconstriction of arterioles caused by angiotensin II raises blood pressure by increasing peripheral resistance.

A second, equally important effect of angiotensin II is stimulation of the secretion of **aldosterone,** a hormone from the adrenal gland that increases sodium reabsorption in the kidney. This increase in sodium reabsorption helps the body retain water, which raises blood volume and increases blood pressure. Drugs that inhibit the renin-angiotensin pathway block the effects of angiotensin II, thus decreasing blood pressure through *two* mechanisms: dilating arteries and decreasing blood volume.

TABLE 15.5 ACE Inhibitors and Angiotensin-Receptor Blockers Used for Hypertension

DRUG	ROUTE AND ADULT DOSE	REMARKS
ACE INHIBITORS		
benazepril (Lotensin)	PO 10–40 mg in 1–2 divided doses (max: 40 mg/day)	May be used in combination with thiazide diuretics
captopril (Capoten)	PO 6.25–25 mg tid (max: 450 mg/day)	Also for heart failure and MI
Pr enalapril (Vasotec) enalaprilat (Vasotec IV)	PO 5–40 mg in 1–2 divided doses (max: 40 mg/day)	Also for heart failure; IV form available
fosinopril (Monopril)	PO 5–40 mg daily (max: 80 mg/day)	Also for heart failure
lisinopril (Prinivil, Zestril)	PO 10 mg daily (max: 80 mg/day)	Also for heart failure and MI
moexipril (Univasc)	PO 7.5–30 mg daily (max: 30 mg/day)	Only approved for hypertension
perindopril (Aceon)	PO 4–8 mg daily (max: 16 mg/day)	Also for heart failure
quinapril (Accupril)	PO 10–20 mg daily (max: 80 mg/day)	Also for heart failure
ramipril (Altace)	PO 2.5–5 mg daily (max: 20 mg/day)	Also for heart failure
trandolapril (Mavik)	PO 1–4 mg daily (max: 8 mg/day)	Only approved for hypertension; discontinue diuretics 2–3 days before starting therapy
ANGIOTENSIN-RECEPTOR BLOCKERS		
candesartan (Atacand)	PO 8–32 mg daily (max: 800 mg/day)	Only approved for hypertension
eprosartan (Teveten)	PO 400–800 mg daily	Only approved for hypertension
irbesartan (Avapro)	PO 150–300 mg daily	Maximum effect may take 6–12 weeks
losartan potassium (Cozaar)	PO 25–50 mg in 1–2 divided doses (max: 100 mg/day)	Causes relaxation of smooth vascular muscle
olmesartan (Benicar)	PO 20–40 mg daily	Only approved for hypertension
telmisartan (Micardis)	PO 40–80 mg daily	Only approved for hypertension
valsartan (Diovan)	PO 80 mg daily (max: 320 mg/day)	Evidence of effectiveness of therapy in 2–4 weeks

DRUG PROFILE: Calcium Channel Blocker: *Nifedipine (Procardia)*

Actions and Uses:

Nifedipine is a CCB prescribed for angina as well as for hypertension. Nifedipine selectively blocks calcium channels in myocardial and vascular smooth muscle, including that in the coronary arteries. This results in reduced oxygen demands by the heart, an increase in cardiac output, and a fall in blood pressure. Nifedipine is as effective as diuretics and beta-adrenergic blockers at reducing blood pressure.

Adverse Effects and Interactions:

Side effects of nifedipine are generally minor and related to vasodilation such as headache, dizziness, and flushing. Fast-acting forms of nifedipine can cause significant reflex tachycardia. To avoid rebound hypotension, discontinuation of drug therapy should occur gradually.

Nifedipine may increase serum levels of digoxin, cimetidine, and ranitidine, and increase the effects of warfarin, resulting in increased PTT. It may also increase the effects of fentanyl anesthesia, resulting in severe hypotension and an increased need for fluids. Grapefruit juice may cause greater absorption of nifedipine.

Alcohol increases the vasodilating action of nifedipine and can lead to a severe drop in blood pressure. Nicotine causes vasoconstriction, countering the desired effect of nifedipine.

Use with caution with melatonin, which may increase blood pressure and heart rate.

Mechanism in Action: 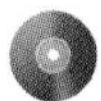

Blocking calcium influx into smooth muscle cells results in arteriolar vasodilation. When arterioles are dilated, peripheral resistance and cardiac workload are reduced, and the blood pressure returns to normal. ■

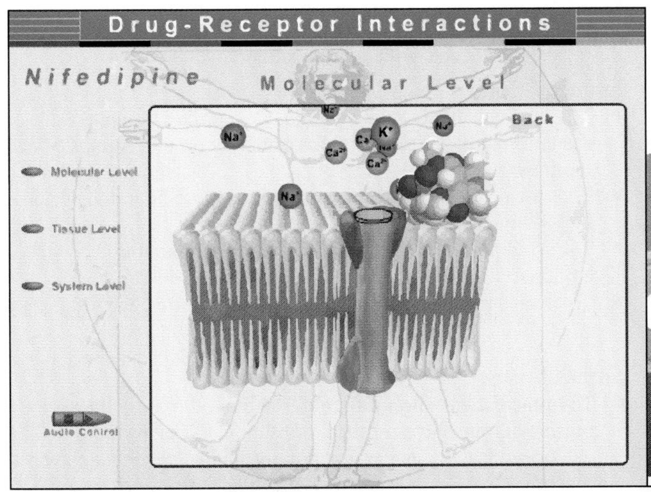

Use the student CD-ROM to see Mechanism in Action for Nifedipine.

 *See the Companion Website for a Nursing Process Focus specific to this drug.*

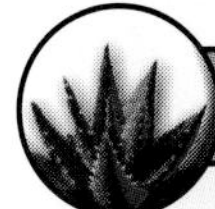

NATURAL ALTERNATIVES

Hawthorn for Hypertension

A number of botanicals have been claimed to have antihypertensive activity, including hawthorn, which is sometimes called *May bush.* Hawthorn (*Cretaegus*) is a thorny shrub or small tree that is widespread in North America, Europe, and Asia. Use of hawthorn dates back to ancient Greece. In some cultures, the shrub is used in magic and religious rites and is thought to ward off evil spirits. The ship *Mayflower* was named after this shrub.

Leaves, flowers, and berries of the plant are dried or extracted in liquid form. Active ingredients are flavonoids and procyanidins. Hawthorn has been purported to lower blood pressure after 4 weeks or longer of therapy, although the effect has been small. The mechanism of action may be inhibition of ACE or reduction of cardiac workload. Patients taking cardiac glycosides should avoid hawthorn, as it has the ability to decrease cardiac output. Patients should be advised not to rely on any botanical for the treatment of hypertension without consulting their healthcare practitioner, and frequent measurements of blood pressure must be taken to be certain that therapy is effective. ■

NURSING PROCESS FOCUS

Patients Receiving ACE Inhibitor Therapy

ASSESSMENT

Prior to administration:

- Obtain complete health history including data on recent cardiac events and any incidence of angioedema, allergies, drug history, and possible drug interactions
- Obtain ECG and vital signs; assess in context of patient's baseline values
- Assess neurological status and level of consciousness
- Obtain blood and urine specimens for laboratory analysis

POTENTIAL NURSING DIAGNOSES

- Risk for Injury, related to orthostatic hypotension
- Deficient Knowledge, related to drug therapy
- Ineffective Tissue Perfusion
- Risk for Imbalanced Nutrition: More than Body Requirements, related to hyperkalemia

PLANNING: Patient Goals and Expected Outcomes

The patient will:

- Exhibit a reduction in systolic/diastolic blood pressure
- Maintain normal serum electrolyte levels during drug therapy
- Demonstrate an understanding of the drug's action by accurately describing drug side effects and precautions

IMPLEMENTATION

Interventions and (Rationales)	Patient Education/Discharge Planning
■ Monitor for first-dose phenomenon of profound hypotension.	Warn the patient about the first-dose phenomenon; reassure that this effect diminishes with continued therapy. Instruct patient: ■ That changes in consciousness may occur due to rapid reduction in blood pressure; immediately report feelings of faintness ■ That the drug takes effect in approximately 1 hour and peaks in 3–4 hours ■ To rest in the supine position beginning 1 hour after administration and for 3 hours after the first dose ■ To always rise slowly, avoiding sudden posture changes
■ Observe for hypersensitivity reaction, particularly angioedema. (Angioedema may arise at any time during ACE inhibitor therapy, but is generally expected shortly after initiation of therapy.)	Instruct patient: ■ To immediately report difficult breathing, throat tightness, muscle cramps, hives or rash, or tremors (These symptoms can occur as early as the first dose or much later as a delayed reaction.) ■ That angioedema can be life threatening and to call emergency medical services if severe dyspnea or hoarseness is accompanied by swelling of the face or mouth
■ Monitor for the presence of blood dyscrasia. ■ Observe for signs of infection: fever, sore throat, malaise, joint pain, ecchymoses, profound fatigue, shortness of breath, or pallor. (Bruising is a sign of bleeding which can indicate the presence of a serious blood disorder.)	Instruct patient to: ■ Immediately report any flulike symptoms ■ Observe for bruising and signs of bleeding from the nose, mouth, GI tract ("coffee ground" vomit or tarry stools), menstrual flooding, or bright red rectal bleeding
■ Monitor for changes in level of consciousness, dizziness, drowsiness, or lightheadedness. (Signs of decreased blood flow to the brain are due to the drug's vasodilating hypotensive action. Sudden syncopal collapse is possible.)	Instruct patient to: ■ Report dizziness or fainting that persists beyond the first dose, as well as unusual sensations (e.g., numbness and tingling) or other changes in the face or limbs ■ Contact the healthcare provider, before the next scheduled dose of the drug, if fainting occurs

continued...

NURSING PROCESS FOCUS

Interventions and (Rationales)	Patient Education/Discharge Planning
■ Monitor for persistent dry cough (a possible side effect of the drug). ■ Monitor changes in cough pattern. (This may indicate another disease process.)	Instruct patient to: ■ Expect persistent dry cough ■ Report any change in the character or frequency of cough (Any cough accompanied by shortness of breath, fever, or chest pain should be reported *immediately* because it may indicate MI.) ■ Sleep with head elevated if cough becomes troublesome when in supine position ■ Use nonmedicated sugar-free lozenges or hard candies to relieve cough
■ Monitor for dehydration or fluid overload. (Dehydration causes low circulating blood volume and will exacerbate hypotension. Severe dehydration may trigger syncope and collapse. Pitting edema, a sign of fluid retention, can be a sign of HF and may indicate reduced drug effectiveness.)	Instruct patient to: ■ Observe for signs of dehydration such as oliguria, dry lips and mucous membranes, or poor skin turgor ■ Report any bodily swelling that leaves sunken marks on the skin when pressed ■ Measure and monitor fluid intake and output, and weigh daily ■ Monitor increased need for fluid caused by vomiting, diarrhea, or excessive sweating ■ Avoid excessive heat that contributes to sweating and fluid loss ■ Consume adequate amounts of *plain* water
■ Monitor for hyperkalemia. (May occur due to reduced aldosterone levels.)	Instruct patient to: ■ Immediately report signs of hyperkalemia: nausea, irregular heartbeat, profound fatigue/muscle weakness, and slow or faint pulse ■ Avoid consuming electrolyte-fortified snacks, or sports drinks that may contain potassium ■ Avoid using salt substitute (KCl) to flavor foods ■ Consult the healthcare provider before taking any nutritional supplements containing potassium
■ Monitor for liver and kidney function. (ACE inhibitors are metabolized by the liver and excreted by the kidneys.)	Instruct patient to: ■ Report signs of liver toxicity: nausea, vomiting, anorexia, diarrhea, rash, jaundice, abdominal pain, tenderness or distension, or change in the color or character of stools ■ Discontinue drug immediately, and contact the healthcare provider if jaundice occurs ■ Adhere to laboratory testing regimen as ordered by the healthcare provider
■ Ensure patient safety (due to postural hypotension caused by drug). ■ Monitor ambulation until response to the drug is known.	Instruct patient to: ■ Obtain help prior to getting out of bed or attempting to walk alone ■ Avoid driving or other activities that require mental alertness or physical coordination until effects of the drug are known

EVALUATION OF OUTCOME CRITERIA

Evaluate the effectiveness of drug therapy by confirming that patient goals and expected outcomes have been met (see "Planning").

See Table 15.5 for a list of drugs to which these nursing actions apply.

First detected in the venom of pit vipers in the 1960s, drugs that inhibit ACE have been approved for hypertension since the 1980s. Since then, the ACE inhibitors have become important drugs in the treatment of hypertension. ACE inhibitors are drugs of choice for diabetic patients with hypertension because they have been shown to reduce the progression to kidney failure that often occurs in diabetic patients. Because of cardiovascular changes associated with diabetes, these patients often require therapy with at least two antihypertensive drugs. Side effects are relatively minor and include persistent cough and hypotension following the first dose of the drug. Some ACE inhibitors have also been approved for the treatment of heart failure and myocardial infarction, and these are discussed in Chapters 16 and 18, respectively.

tachy = *rapid*
cardia = *heart*

A second method of altering the renin-angiotensin pathway is blocking the action of angiotensin II *after* it is formed. Several drugs, including irbesartan (Avapro), losartan (Cozaar), and valsartan (Diovan), block the receptors for angiotensin in arteriolar smooth muscle and in the adrenal gland, thus causing blood pressure to fall. Their actions of arteriolar dilation and increased renal sodium excretion are quite similar to those of the ACE inhibitors. Angiotensin-receptor blockers (ARBs) have relatively few side effects, such as headache, dizziness, and facial flushing, most of which are related to hypotension. Drugs in this class are often combined with drugs from other classes; for example, the drug Hyzaar combines losartan with the diuretic hydrochlorothiazide.

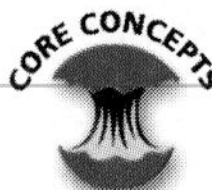

15.11 Alpha- and beta-adrenergic blockers are commonly used to treat hypertension.

Blockade of adrenergic receptors results in a number of beneficial effects on the heart and vessels. These autonomic drugs are used for a wide variety of cardiovascular disorders. Adrenergic blockers and centrally acting agents that are important in hypertension are listed in Table 15.6.

As discussed in Chapter 7, the autonomic nervous system controls involuntary functions of the body such as heart rate, pupil size, and smooth muscle contraction, including that in the arterial walls. Stimulation of the sympathetic division causes fight-or-flight responses such as faster heart rate, an increase in blood pressure, and bronchodilation. Most organs also receive signals from the parasympathetic division, which promote rest-and-digest actions that are generally

DRUG PROFILE: Renin-Angiotensin Pathway Modifier: Pr *Enalapril (Vasotec)*

Actions and Uses:

Enalapril is one of the most common ACE inhibitors prescribed for hypertension. Unlike captopril (Capoten), the first ACE inhibitor to be marketed, enalapril has a prolonged half-life, which permits administration once or twice daily. Enalapril acts by reducing angiotensin II and aldosterone levels to produce a significant reduction in blood pressure with few side effects. Enalapril has an effectiveness comparable to the thiazide diuretics and the beta-adrenergic blockers and may be used by itself or in combination with other antihypertensives to minimize side effects.

Adverse Effects and Interactions:

Unlike diuretics, ACE inhibitors such as enalapril have little effect on electrolyte balance, and unlike beta-adrenergic blockers, they cause few cardiac side effects. Like other antihypertensive drugs, enalapril may cause hypotension, especially when moving quickly from a supine to an upright position. This condition, known as postural or orthostatic hypotension, can cause lightheadedness and even fainting. Care must be taken because a rapid fall in blood pressure may occur following the first dose. Other side effects include headache, dizziness, and postural hypotension.

Thiazide diuretics increase potassium loss and potassium-sparing diuretics increase the risk of hyperkalemia when used with ACE inhibitors. Renin-releasing antihypertensives increase the action of enalapril and can cause profound hypotension.

Enalapril may induce lithium toxicity by reducing renal clearance of lithium. NSAIDs may reduce the effectiveness of ACE inhibitors.

See the Companion Website for a Nursing Process Focus specific to this drug.

TABLE 15.6 Adrenergic Blockers and Central-acting Agents Used for Hypertension

DRUG	ROUTE AND ADULT DOSE	REMARKS
atenolol (Tenormin)	PO 25–50 mg daily (max: 100 mg/day)	Selective $beta_1$ blocker; IV form available for MI; monitor apical pulse prior to administration
bisoprolol (Zebeta)	PO 2.5–5 mg daily (max: 20 mg/day)	Selective $beta_1$ blocker; also for angina; discontinue drug gradually to avoid rebound hypertension
carvedilol (Coreg)	PO 6.25 mg bid (max: 50 mg/day)	Blocks both alpha and beta receptors; also for heart failure
clonidine (Catapres)	PO 0.1 mg bid–tid (max: 0.8 mg/day)	Central acting $alpha_2$-adrenergic agent; transdermal patch available; epidural infusion form available for management of cancer pain
Pr doxazosin (Cardura)	PO 1 mg at bedtime; may increase to 16 mg/day in 1–2 divided doses (max: 16 mg/day)	Selective $alpha_1$ blocker; also for BPH
methyldopa (Aldomet)	PO 250 mg bid or tid (max: 3 g/day)	Central acting $alpha_2$-adrenergic agent; IV form available; lowers standing and supine blood pressure
metoprolol (Toprol, Lopressor)	PO 50–100 mg daily or bid. (max: 450 mg/day)	Selective $beta_1$ blocker; sustained-release and IV forms available; also for angina and MI
nadolol (Corgard)	PO 40–320 mg/day	Nonselective beta blocker; also for angina
prazosin (Minipress)	PO 1 mg at bedtime; increase to 1 mg bid–tid (max: 20 mg/day)	Selective $alpha_1$ blocker used in combination with other antihypertensives; also for BPH, Raynauds disease, and pheochromocytoma
propranolol (Inderal)	PO 40 mg bid but may be increased to 160–480 mg/day in divided doses (max: 480 mg/day)	Nonselective $beta_1$ and $beta_2$ blocker; also for angina, MI, dysrhythmias, and migraine prophylaxis; IV form available
terazosin (Hytrin)	PO 1 mg at bedtime; increase 1–5 mg/day (max: 20 mg/day)	Selective $alpha_1$ blocker; also for BPH

the opposite of the sympathetic division. An important exception is peripheral blood vessels, which receive only sympathetic nerves.

Antihypertensive drugs block the effects of the sympathetic division through a number of different mechanisms, although all have in common the effect of lowering blood pressure. These mechanisms include the following:

- Blockade of alpha receptors
- Selective blockade of $beta_1$ receptors
- Nonselective blockade of $beta_1$ and $beta_2$ receptors
- Stimulation of $alpha_2$ receptors in the brainstem (centrally acting)

Some drugs, such as epinephrine, affect both beta- and alpha-adrenergic receptors and can cause serious adverse effects. Drugs that affect only one receptor subtype produce fewer side effects. Prazosin (Minipress), for example, is specific to $alpha_1$ receptors and thus should have less effect on the heart, which contains $beta_1$ receptors. On the other hand, atenolol (Tenormin) and metoprolol (Toprol, Lopressor) are selective for $beta_1$ receptors and thus have little effect on the bronchi, which have $beta_2$ receptors.

The side effects of adrenergic blockers are generally quite predictable because they are extensions of the fight-or-flight response. The $alpha_1$ blockers tend to cause **orthostatic hypotension** in patients when they move quickly from a supine to an upright position. Dizziness, nausea, **bradycardia,** and dry mouth are also common. Less common, though sometimes a major cause for noncompliance, is their adverse effect on male sexual function (impotence). Nonselective beta blockers slow the heart rate and cause bronchoconstriction: Use with caution in patients with asthma or heart failure.

ortho = *straight*
static = *causing to stand*

brady = *slow*
cardia = *heart*

Some adrenergic blockers do not act directly on organs stimulated by peripheral autonomic nerves, but instead affect the production of neurotransmitters in the central nervous system. For example, methyldopa (Aldomet) is converted to a **false neurotransmitter** in the brainstem, thus causing a shortage of the "real" neurotransmitter and inhibition of the sympathetic nervous system. Clonidine (Catapres), an $alpha_2$ blocker, affects alpha-adrenergic receptors in the cardiovascular control centers in the brainstem. The central acting agents have a tendency to produce sedation and are rarely prescribed.

Concept Review 15.3

- Why is it important for the patient to weigh himself or herself on a regular basis when taking antihypertensive drugs?

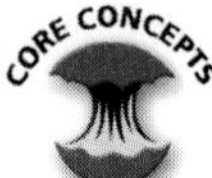

15.12 Some vasodilators act directly on arteriolar smooth muscle to lower blood pressure.

Drugs that directly affect arteriolar smooth muscle are effective at lowering blood pressure but produce too many side effects to be drugs of first choice. The direct-acting vasodilators used for hypertension are listed in Table 15.7.

Drugs discussed thus far lower blood pressure through indirect means—by affecting enzymes (ACE inhibitors), autonomic nerves (alpha and beta blockers), or fluid volume (diuretics). It would seem that a more efficient way to reduce blood pressure would be to cause a direct relaxation of arteriolar smooth muscle. Unfortunately, most drugs in this class of direct vasodilators produce reflex tachycardia that may be a serious concern for hypertensive patients.

DRUG PROFILE: Alpha-Adrenergic Blocker: Pr *Doxazosin (Cardura)*

Actions and Uses:

Doxazosin is a selective $alpha_1$-adrenergic blocker available only in oral form. Because it is selective for blocking $alpha_1$ receptors in vascular smooth muscle, it has few adverse effects on other autonomic organs and thus is preferred over nonselective beta blockers such as propranolol (Inderal). Doxazosin dilates both arteries and veins and is capable of causing a rapid, profound fall in blood pressure. Although prazosin (Minipress) was the first alpha-adrenergic blocker available for hypertension, other alpha blockers such as doxazosin and terazosin (Hytrin) are more widely used because they have prolonged half-lives that allow them to be taken once daily.

Doxazosin and several other alpha-adrenergic blockers also relax smooth muscle around the prostate gland. Patients who have dificulty urinating due to an enlarged prostate, a condition known as benign prostatic hyperplasia (BPH) sometimes receive these drugs to relieve symptoms of this disease, as discussed in Chapter 30.

Adverse Effects and Interactions:

When starting doxazosin therapy, some patients experience orthostatic hypotension, although tolerance normally develops to this side effect after a few doses. Dizziness and headache are also common side effects, although they are rarely severe enough to cause discontinuation of therapy. Oral cimetidine may cause a mild increase (10%) in the half-life of doxazosin. This is not considered to be clinically significant.

Mechanism in Action: 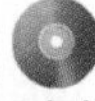

Doxazosin selectively blocks $alpha_1$-adrenergic receptors. By dilating vascular smooth muscle $alpha_1$ blockers reverse any frictional resistance to lower blood pressure. $Alpha_1$ blockers relax smooth muscle around the prostate gland.

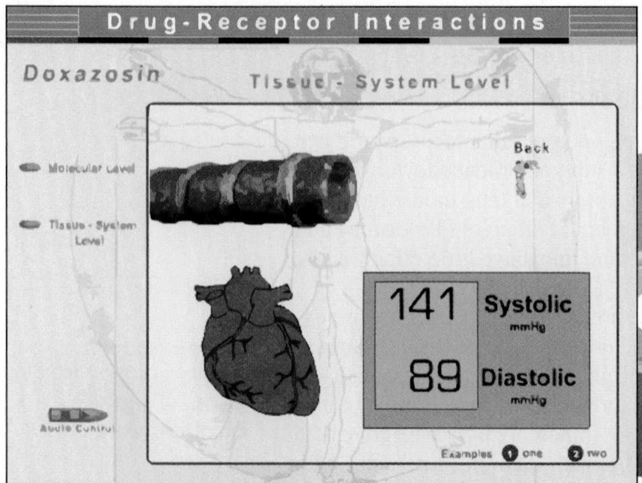

Use the student CD-ROM to see Mechanism in Action for Doxazosin.

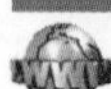
See the Companion Website for a Nursing Process Focus specific to this drug.

TABLE 15.7 Direct-acting Vasodilators Used for Hypertension

DRUG	ROUTE AND ADULT DOSE	REMARKS
diazoxide (Hyperstat IV)	IV 1–3 mg/kg by IV push (max: 150 mg)	Dose may be repeated every 15 min until blood pressure falls; may be given as infusion or by push for malignant hypertension
Pr hydralazine (Apresoline)	PO 10–50 mg qid (max: 300 mg/day)	Diastolic response usually greater than systolic; IV and IM forms available
minoxidil (Loniten)	PO 5–40 mg/day in single or divided doses (max: 100 mg/day)	Reserved for severe hypertension; topical form used to promote hair growth
nitroprusside (Nipride, Nitropress)	IV 0.5–10 mcg/kg/min	For hypertensive crisis; produces both arteriolar and venous dilation; infusion not to exceed 10 min

DRUG PROFILE: Direct-acting Vasodilator: Pr *Hydralazine (Apresoline)*

Actions and Uses:

Hydralazine was one of the first oral antihypertensive drugs marketed in the United States. Although it produces an effective reduction in blood pressure, drugs in other antihypertensive classes have largely replaced hydralazine because of its many side effects.

Adverse Effects and Interactions:

Hydralazine may produce many side effects, including severe reflex tachycardia. Patients taking hydralazine often receive a beta-adrenergic blocker that counteracts this effect on the heart. The drug may produce a lupus-like syndrome with extended use. Sodium and fluid retention is another potentially serious adverse effect. The use of hydralazine is mostly limited to patients whose hypertension cannot be controlled with other, safer medications.

MAO inhibitors may increase the hypotensive action of hydralazine. Other antihypertensive drugs taken with hydralazine can cause profound hypotension. NSAIDs may decrease the antihypertensive response.

See the Companion Website for a Nursing Process Focus specific to this drug.

One direct-acting vasodilator is specifically used for those patients who have an extremely high, life-threatening hypertension that must be quickly controlled. Nitroprusside (Nipride, Nitropress), with a half-life of only 2 minutes, has the capability of lowering blood pressure almost instantaneously on IV administration. Careful monitoring is critical to avoid serious effects of over treatment, such as hypotension.

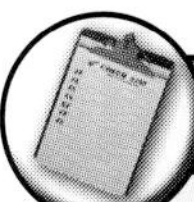

PATIENTS NEED TO KNOW

Patients treated for hypertension need to know the following:

1. Take medications as prescribed.
2. Never discontinue medication without approval from a healthcare provider.
3. To control hypertension, incorporate lifestyle changes such as diet and exercise, even if blood pressure is brought into normal limits by the medication.
4. Check blood pressure on a regular basis and report significant variations to the healthcare provider.
5. Get out of bed slowly to avoid dizziness.
6. Unless a potassium-sparing diuretic is prescribed, an increased intake of potassium-rich foods such as bananas, dried fruits, and orange juice may be necessary.
7. Take weight regularly and report abnormal weight gains or losses.
8. Do not take any OTC medications for colds, flu, or allergies without first checking with a healthcare provider. ■

NURSING PROCESS FOCUS

Patients Receiving Direct Vasodilator Therapy

ASSESSMENT

Prior to administration:

- Obtain complete health history including allergies, drug history, and possible drug interactions
- Obtain ECG and vital signs; assess in context of patient's baseline values
- Auscultate heart and chest sounds
- Assess neurological status and level of consciousness
- Obtain blood and urine specimens for laboratory analysis

POTENTIAL NURSING DIAGNOSES

- Ineffective Tissue Perfusion
- Excess Fluid Volume
- Risk for Injury, related to orthostatic hypotension
- Risk for Impaired Skin Integrity (e.g., IV vasodilators)
- Deficient Knowledge, related to drug therapy

PLANNING: Patient Goals and Expected Outcomes

The patient will:

- Exhibit a reduction in systolic/diastolic blood pressure
- Demonstrate an understanding of the drug's action by accurately describing drug side effects and precautions

IMPLEMENTATION

Interventions and (Rationales)	Patient Education/Discharge Planning
■ Observe for signs and symptoms of lupus.	■ Instruct patient to report classic "butterfly rash" over the nose and cheeks, muscle aches, and fatigue when taking hydralazine.
■ Monitor patient vital signs every 5–15 minutes and have infusion titrated based on prescribed parameters. (These drugs cause rapid hypotension.)	■ Instruct patient to report any burning or stinging pain, swelling, warmth, redness, or tenderness at the IV insertion site which may signal phlebitis or drug seepage into soft tissues.
■ Use with caution with impaired cardiac/cerebral circulation. (The hypotension produced by vasodilators may further compromise individuals who already suffer from ischemia.)	Instruct patient to: ■ Report angina-like symptoms: chest, arm, back and/or neck pain, palpitations ■ Report faintness, dizziness, drowsiness, any sensation of cold, numbness, tingling, pale or dusky look to the hands and feet ■ Report headache or signs of stroke: facial drooping, visual changes, limb weakness, or paralysis ■ Monitor vitals signs (especially blood pressure) daily or as often as advised by the nurse
■ Monitor for dizziness. (This is a sign of hypotension that occurs because the brain is not getting enough blood flow.)	Instruct patient to: ■ Avoid driving or other activities requiring mental alertness or physical coordination until effects of the drug are known ■ Always arise slowly, avoiding sudden posture changes
■ Evaluate for needed lifestyle modifications.	■ Instruct patient to comply with additional interventions for HTN such as weight reduction, modification of sodium intake, smoking cessation, exercise, and stress management.
■ Discontinue medication gradually. (Abrupt withdrawal of drug may cause rebound hypertension and anxiety.)	■ Instruct patient to not stop taking drug suddenly.

EVALUATION OF OUTCOME CRITERIA

Evaluate the effectiveness of drug therapy by confirming that patient goals and expected outcomes have been met (see "Planning").

See Table 15.7 for a list of drugs to which these nursing actions apply.

CHAPTER REVIEW

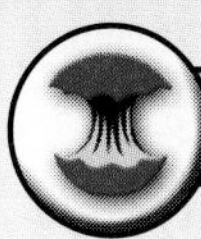

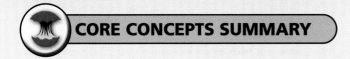

CORE CONCEPTS SUMMARY

15.1 Hypertension can lead to stroke, heart failure, or MI, if untreated.

Hypertension is one of the most common diseases. Uncontrolled hypertension can cause chronic and debilitating disorders such as stroke, heart attack, and heart failure.

15.2 Blood pressure is caused by the pumping action of the heart.

As the heart pumps, it creates pressure that is greatest in the arteries closest to the heart. The pressure created by the heart's contraction is called systolic pressure, and that present during the heart's relaxation is called diastolic pressure.

15.3 The primary factors responsible for blood pressure are cardiac output, the resistance of the small arteries, and blood volume.

As blood leaves the heart, its pressure depends on how much blood is present in the vessels (blood volume), how much is ejected per minute, and how much resistance it encounters from the small arteries (peripheral resistance). These are considered the primary factors controlling blood pressure.

15.4 Many nervous and hormonal factors help to keep blood pressure within normal limits.

Clusters of neurons in the medulla known as the vasomotor center regulate blood pressure. Feedback is provided to the vasomotor center by baroreceptors in the aorta and carotid arteries. Hormonal agents such as epinephrine or ADH may have profound effects on blood pressure.

15.5 The normal range of blood pressure varies throughout the lifespan.

A patient having a sustained blood pressure of 140/90 mm Hg after multiple measurements made over several clinic visits is said to have hypertension.

15.6 Lifestyle changes can often reverse borderline hypertension.

Because antihypertensive drugs may have uncomfortable side effects, lifestyle changes such as proper diet and exercise are often implemented prior to and during drug therapy to enable lower drug doses.

15.7 Selection of specific antihypertension drugs depends on the severity of the disease.

Drug therapy of hypertension often begins with low doses of a single drug. If ineffective, a second drug from a different class may be added to the regimen. Multidrug therapy is common.

15.8 Diuretics are often drugs of first choice for treating mild to moderate hypertension.

Diuretics are often drugs of first choice for hypertension because they have few side effects and can control minor to moderate hypertension. Electrolytes should be carefully monitored in patients taking diuretics.

15.9 Calcium channel blockers have emerged as primary drugs in the treatment of hypertension.

CCBs block calcium ions from entering smooth cells, muscle causing arterioles to relax, thus reducing blood pressure. Some CCBs are also used to treat angina, heart failure, and dysrhythmias.

15.10 Blocking the renin-angiotensin pathway leads to a decrease in blood pressure.

Blocking angiotensin-converting enzyme (ACE) or the angiotensin II receptor can prevent the intense vasoconstriction caused by angiotensin. These drugs also decrease blood volume, which aids in producing their antihypertensive effect.

15.11 Alpha- and beta-adrenergic blockers are commonly used to treat hypertension.

Autonomic drugs are available that block alpha$_1$ receptors, block beta$_1$ and/or beta$_2$ receptors, or stimulate alpha$_2$ receptors in the brain stem (centrally acting) to lower blood pressure. Although acting by different mechanisms, these drugs all lower blood pressure.

15.12 Some vasodilators act directly on arteriolar smooth muscle to lower blood pressure.

A few drugs lower blood pressure by acting directly to relax arteriolar smooth muscle. Other than their use in treating hypertensive crisis, drugs in this class are not widely used because of their numerous side effects.

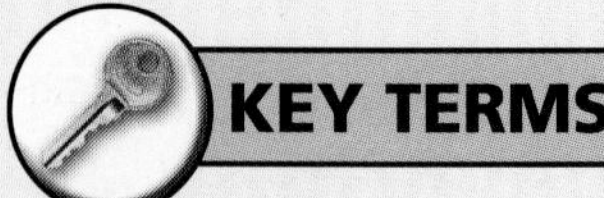

KEY TERMS

aldosterone (al-DOH-stair-own): hormone released by the adrenal cortex that regulates sodium reabsorption / *page 264*

angiotensin II (AN-geo-TEN-sin): chemical released in response to falling blood pressure that causes vasoconstriction and release of aldosterone / *page 264*

angiotensin-converting enzyme (ACE) (angeo-TEN-sin): enzyme responsible for converting angiotensin I to angiotensin II / *page 264*

antidiuretic hormone (ADH) (ANT-eye-deye-your-ET-ik): hormone produced by the hypothalamus that stimulates the kidneys to conserve water / *page 256*

baroreceptors (BARE-oh-ree-sep-tours): nerves located in the walls of the atria, aortic arch, vena cava, and carotid sinus that sense changes in blood pressure / *page 255*

bradycardia (bray-dee-KAR-DEE-ah): a condition of slow heartbeat / *page 269*

calcium channel blocker (CCB): drug that blocks the flow of calcium ions into myocardia cells / *page 260*

cardiac output: amount of blood pumped by each ventricle in 1 minute / *page 254*

diastolic pressure (DEYE-ah-stall-ik): blood pressure during the relaxation phase of heart activity / *page 254*

diuretic (deye-your-ET-ik): drug that increases urine flow / *page 255*

electrolytes (ee-LEK-troh-lites): charged substances in the blood such as sodium, potassium, calcium, chloride, and phosphate / *page 260*

false neurotransmittor (NYUR-oh-TRANS-mitt-ur): chemical that simulates a natural neurotransmitter but does not produce the same physiological effect / *page 270*

heart failure (HF): disease in which the heart muscle cannot contract with sufficient force to meet the body's metabolic needs / *page 253*

hyperkalemia (heye-purr-kah-LEE-mee-ah): high amounts of potassium in the blood / *page 260*

hypokalemia (heye-poh-kah-LEE-mee-ah): low amounts of potassium in the blood / *page 260*

hypertension (heye-purr-TEN-shun): high blood pressure / *page 252*

lumen (LOO-men): the inside diameter of a hollow tube such as a blood vessel / *page 255*

orthostatic hypotension (or-tho-STAT-ik): fall in blood pressure that occurs when someone changes position from recumbent to upright / *page 269*

peripheral resistance (per-IF-ur-ul): the amount of friction encountered by blood as it travels through the vessels / *page 255*

reflex tachycardia (ta-kee-CAR-dee-ah): temporary speeding up of heart rate that occurs when blood pressure falls / *page 256*

renin-angiotensin pathway (REN-in–an-geo-TEN-sin): series of enzymatic steps by which the body raises blood pressure / *page 256*

stepped care: a systematic approach to treatment of hypertension / *page 258*

systolic pressure (SIS-tol-ik): blood pressure during the contraction phase of heart activity / *page 253*

vasomotor center (VAZO-mo-tor): area of the medulla that controls baseline blood pressure / *page 255*

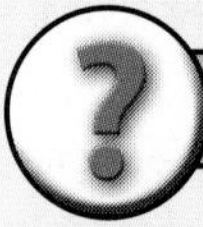

REVIEW QUESTIONS

The following questions are written in NCLEX-PN® style. Answer these questions to assess your knowledge of the chapter material, and go back and review any material that is not clear to you.

1. Which of the following is not a nonpharmacological method to control hypertension?

1. Weight loss
2. Smoking cessation
3. Moderate exercise
4. Decreased potassium and magnesium intake

2. An otherwise healthy man has been diagnosed with hypertension. You suspect the physician will order:

1. Hydrochlorothiazide (HydroDIURIL)
2. Captopril (Capoten)
3. Nifedipine (Procardia)
4. Enalapril (Vasotec)

3. The patient is on two antihypertensive drugs. The nurse recognizes that the advantage of multidrug treatment is:

1. Blood pressure decreases faster.
2. Side effects are fewer and patient compliance is greater.
3. There is less daily medication dosing.
4. Multidrug therapy treats the patient's other medical conditions.

4. The patient is taking furosemide (Lasix) 40 mg bid. The patient should be monitored for:

1. Hyperkalemia
2. Hypokalemia
3. Hypernatremia
4. Hypercalcemia

5. The patient has been taking losartan (Cozaar) for his hypertension. The physician has determined that the current medication regimen is not effective. Which of the following drugs may be added to the treatment plan?

1. Felodipine (Plendil)
2. Methyldopa (Aldomet)
3. Atenolol (Tenormin)
4. Hydrochlorothiazide (HCTZ)

6. The patient has been started on antihypertensives. The patient should be monitored for:

1. Nausea and vomiting
2. Diarrhea
3. Dizziness
4. Tetany

7. This antihypertensive medication is a potassium-sparing diuretic.

1. Furosemide (Lasix)
2. Spironolactone (Aldactone)
3. Chlorothiazide (Diuril)
4. Hydrochlorothiazide (HCTZ)

8. The type of antihypertensive that affects the renin-angiotensin pathway to increase urine is the:

1. Calcium channel blocker
2. Adrenergic blocker
3. ACE inhibitor
4. Direct-acting vasodilator

9. This class of antihypertensives that relax smooth muscles in the blood vessels to decrease peripheral resistance are the:

1. Calcium channel blockers
2. Adrenergic blockers
3. ACE inhibitors
4. Direct-acting vasodilators

10. The patient is on an ACE inhibitor. Which of the following may develop as a result of therapy?

1. Hypokalemia
2. Hyperkalemia
3. Hypernatremia
4. Hyperglycemia

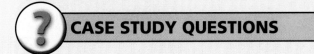

CASE STUDY QUESTIONS

For questions 1–5, please refer to the following case study, and choose the correct answer from choices 1–4.

Ms. Rodriguez was admitted to the emergency department unconscious with a possible stroke. Her blood pressure was measured as 210/120 mm Hg, and she was immediately placed on diazoxide (Hyperstat IV). She stayed in the hospital for 2 days and was discharged with a blood pressure of 135/88 mm Hg. She was given a prescription for Aldactazide, a combination drug that contains hydrochlorothiazide and spironolactone.

1. Why was diazoxide used in the emergency department, rather than Aldactazide?

1. Diazoxide is safer.
2. Diazoxide has a longer duration of action.
3. Diazoxide has a faster onset of action.
4. Ms. Rodriguez may have been allergic to Aldactazide.

2. At the time of her discharge, how would you describe Ms. Rodriguez's blood pressure?

1. Normal
2. Prehypertensive
3. Stage 1 hypertension
4. Stage 2 hypertension

3. What two drug classes are contained in Aldactazide?

1. Thiazide diuretic and beta blocker
2. Thiazide diuretic and potassium-sparing diuretic
3. ACE inhibitor and potassium-sparing diuretic
4. Alpha blocker and ACE inhibitor

4. What instructions should be given to the patient taking Aldactazide?

1. Weigh self regularly and report any abnormal weight gain or loss.
2. Take a daily potassium supplement.
3. Eat plenty of calcium-rich foods such as yogurt.
4. Do not exercise regularly because exercise may interfere with blood pressure regulation.

5. After 8 months on Aldactazide, the physician switched Ms. Rodriguez to nifedipine (Procardia). The patient stopped taking this drug because it made her dizzy, and she felt her heart was racing. This common side effect was probably due to:

1. Electrolyte imbalance
2. Overdose of nifedipine
3. Excessive vasodilation of arteries
4. Reflex tachycardia

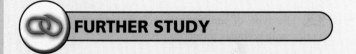

FURTHER STUDY

- Drugs for heart failure are discussed in Chapter 16.
- The role of the autonomic nervous system in controlling peripheral resistance is covered in Chapter 7.
- Diuretics used in the treatment of kidney disorders are discussed in Chapter 28; and Chapter 16 covers their use in the treatment of heart failure.
- The use of calcium channel blockers in treating dysrhythmia is discussed in Chapter 17; CCBs used to treat angina are covered in Chapter 18.
- ACE inhibitors approved for treating heart failure are covered in Chapter 16; Chapter 18 gives information on their use in myocardial infarction.
- More information on the autonomic nervous system and its functions is given in Chapter 7. Benign prostatic hyperplasia (BPH) is covered in Chapter 30.

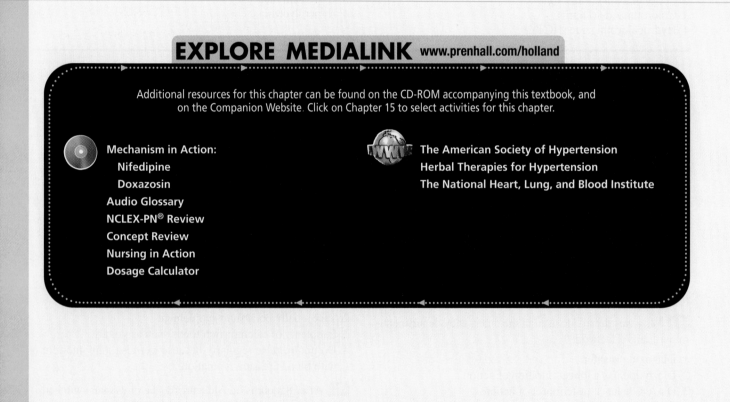

EXPLORE MEDIALINK www.prenhall.com/holland

Additional resources for this chapter can be found on the CD-ROM accompanying this textbook, and on the Companion Website. Click on Chapter 15 to select activities for this chapter.

Mechanism in Action:
- **Nifedipine**
- **Doxazosin**

Audio Glossary
NCLEX-PN® Review
Concept Review
Nursing in Action
Dosage Calculator

The American Society of Hypertension
Herbal Therapies for Hypertension
The National Heart, Lung, and Blood Institute

CHAPTER

16 Drugs for Heart Failure

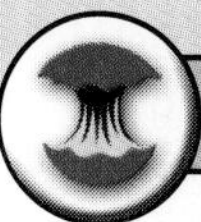

CORE CONCEPTS

16.1 Heart failure is closely associated with disorders such as chronic hypertension and diabetes.

16.2 The central cause of heart failure is weakened heart muscle.

16.3 The three primary characteristics of heart function are force of contraction, heart rate, and speed of impulse conduction.

16.4 The specific therapy for heart failure depends on the severity of the disease.

16.5 Cardiac glycosides increase the force of myocardial contraction and were once the traditional drugs of choice for heart failure.

16.6 Angiotensin-converting enzyme (ACE) inhibitors have become the preferred drugs for heart failure.

16.7 Diuretics relieve symptoms of heart failure by reducing blood volume.

16.8 Phosphodiesterase inhibitors are used for short-term therapy of advanced heart failure.

16.9 Vasodilators reduce symptoms of heart failure by decreasing cardiac oxygen demands.

16.10 Beta-adrenergic blockers are used in combination with other drugs to slow the progression of heart failure and to prolong patient survival.

16.11 Natriuretic peptides are the first new drugs to treat heart failure in more than 10 years.

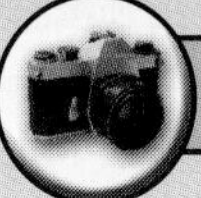

DRUG SNAPSHOT

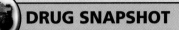

The following drugs will be discussed in this chapter:

DRUG CLASSES	DRUG PROFILES
Cardiac glycosides	Pr digoxin (Lanoxin)
Angiotensin-converting enzyme (ACE) inhibitors	Pr lisinopril (Prinivil)
Diuretics	Pr furosemide (Lasix)
Phosphodiesterase inhibitors	Pr milrinone (Primacor)
Vasodilators	Pr isosorbide dinitrate (Isordil)
Beta-adrenergic blockers	Pr carvedilol (Coreg)
Natriuretic peptides	

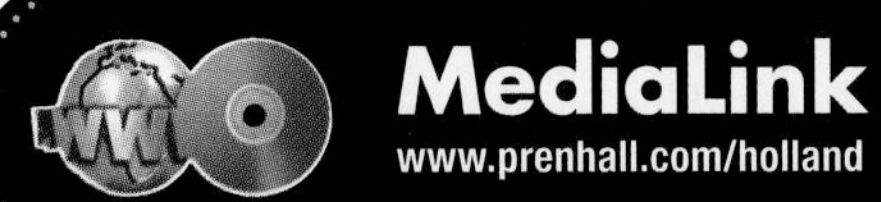

Interactive resources for this chapter can be found on the Companion Website. Click on Chapter 16 and "Begin" to select the activities for this chapter. For chapter-related animations, NCLEX-PN®-style questions, and an audio glossary, access the accompanying CD-ROM in this book.

OBJECTIVES

After reading this chapter, the student should be able to:

1. Identify the major risk factors associated with heart failure.
2. Relate how the classic symptoms associated with heart failure may be caused by weakened heart muscle.
3. Identify drug classes that are used for first- and second-choice pharmacotherapy of heart failure.
4. Explain several means by which patients may control their heart failure without drugs.
5. For each of the following classes, identify representative medications and explain the mechanism of drug action, primary actions, and important adverse effects.
   a. Cardiac glycosides
   b. ACE inhibitors
   c. Diuretics
   d. Phosphodiesterase inhibitors
   e. Vasodilators
   f. Beta-adrenergic blockers
   g. Natriuretic peptides
6. Categorize heart failure drugs based on their classification and mechanism of action.

Heart failure (HF) is one of the most common and fatal of the cardiovascular diseases, and its incidence is expected to increase as the population ages. Despite the dramatic decline in death rates for most cardiovascular diseases that has occurred over the past two decades, the death rate for HF has only recently begun to decrease. Although improved treatment of myocardial infarction (MI) and hypertension has led to declines in mortality due to HF, approximately one in five patients dies within 1 year of diagnosis of HF, and 50% die within 5 years.

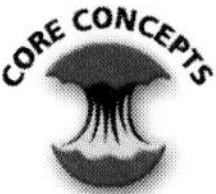

16.1 Heart failure is closely associated with disorders such as chronic hypertension and diabetes.

Heart failure (HF) is the inability of the ventricles to pump enough blood to meet the body's metabolic demands. It is not usually considered a distinct disease in itself, but is instead caused or worsened by certain underlying disorders. Indeed, while weakening of cardiac muscle is a natural consequence of aging, the process can be accelerated by a number of diseases associated with heart failure that are shown in Table 16.1. Because there is no cure for HF, the treatment goals are to prevent, treat, or remove the underlying causes, when possible, so that the patient's quality of life can be improved and life expectancy extended. Effective drug therapy can relieve many of the distressing symptoms of heart failure and may prolong patients' lives.

Fast Facts Heart Failure

- Heart failure increases with age. It affects:
  2% of those 40–50 years old
  5% of those 60–69 years old
  10% of those over age 70
- More than 40,000 people die of HF each year.
- Heart failure is responsible for more than 2.9 million office care visits and 875,000 hospitalizations.
- Blacks have 1.5 to 2 times the incidence of HF as whites.
- Heart failure occurs slightly more frequently in men than women.
- Heart failure is twice as frequent in hypertensive patients and 5 times as frequent in persons who have experienced an MI.

TABLE 16.1 Disorders Commonly Associated with Heart Failure

DISEASE	DESCRIPTION
Mitral stenosis	Inability of the mitral valve to open fully
Myocardial infarction	Clot within the coronary arteries
Chronic hypertension	High systemic blood pressure
Coronary artery disease	Atherosclerosis of the coronary arteries
Diabetes	Lack of insulin or inability to tolerate carbohydrates

16.2 The central cause of heart failure is weakened heart muscle.

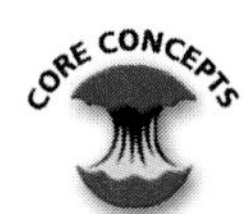

Although a number of diseases can lead to HF, the end result is the same: The heart is unable to pump out the volume of blood required to meet the body's metabolic needs. To understand how drugs act on the weakened heart muscle, it is essential to understand the underlying cardiac physiology.

The right side of the heart receives blood from the venous system and sends it to the lungs, where the blood receives oxygen and loses its carbon dioxide. The blood returns to the left side of the heart, which sends it out to the rest of the body through the aorta. The amount of blood received by the right side should exactly equal that sent out by the left side. If this does not happen, HF may occur. The amount of blood pumped by each ventricle per minute is the cardiac output. The relationship between cardiac output and blood pressure was explained in Chapter 15.

Although many variables affect cardiac output, the two most important factors are **preload** and **afterload.** Just before the chambers of the heart contract (*systole*), they are filled to their maximum capacity with blood. The degree to which the heart fibers are stretched just prior to contraction is preload. The more these fibers are stretched, the more forcefully they will contract. This is somewhat analogous to a rubber band: The more it is stretched, the more forcefully it will snap back. This strength of contraction of the heart is called **contractility.**

The second important factor affecting cardiac output is afterload. For the left ventricle to pump blood out of the heart, it must overcome a fairly substantial pressure in the aorta. The afterload is the pressure in the aorta that must be overcome for blood to be ejected from the left side of the heart.

In HF, the myocardium becomes weakened, and the heart cannot eject all the blood it receives. This weakening may occur on the left side, the right side, or both sides of the heart. If it occurs on the left side, excess blood accumulates in the left ventricle. The wall of the left ventricle may become thicker (*hypertrophy*) in an attempt to compensate for the extra blood. Because the left ventricle has limits to its ability to compensate, blood "backs up" into the lungs, resulting in the classic symptoms of cough and shortness of breath, particularly when the patient is lying down. Left heart failure is sometimes called *congestive heart failure.*

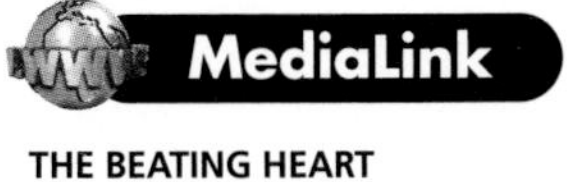

THE BEATING HEART

Although left heart failure is more common, the right side of the heart can also become weak, either simultaneously with the left side or independently from the left side. In right heart failure, the blood "backs up" into the peripheral veins. This results in swelling of the feet and ankles, a condition known as **peripheral edema,** and engorgement of organs such as the liver. Figure 16.1 ■ illustrates the underlying pathophysiology of HF. Figure 16.2 ■ illustrates the signs and symptoms of the patient in HF.

16.3 The three primary characteristics of heart function are force of contraction, heart rate, and speed of impulse conduction.

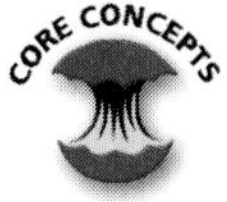

Cardiac physiology is quite complex, particularly when the heart is challenged with a chronic disease such as HF. A simplified method for understanding cardiac function, and one that is quite useful for understanding drug therapy, is to visualize the heart as having three fundamental characteristics:

1. It contracts with a specific force or strength (contractility).
2. It beats at a certain rate (beats per minute).
3. It conducts electrical impulses at a particular speed.

FIGURE 16.1

Pathophysiology of heart failure

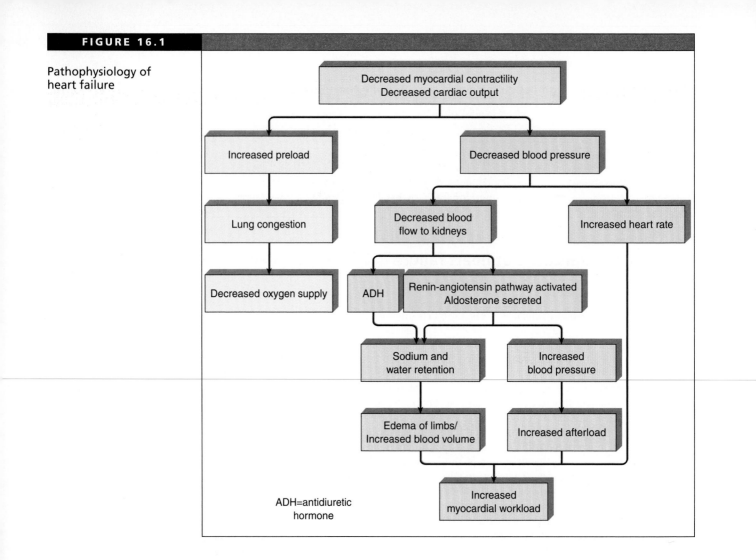

Decreased myocardial contractility
Decreased cardiac output

Increased preload

Decreased blood pressure

Lung congestion

Decreased blood flow to kidneys

Increased heart rate

Decreased oxygen supply

ADH

Renin-angiotensin pathway activated
Aldosterone secreted

Sodium and water retention

Increased blood pressure

Edema of limbs/
Increased blood volume

Increased afterload

Increased myocardial workload

ADH=antidiuretic hormone

FIGURE 16.2

Signs and symptoms of the patient with heart failure

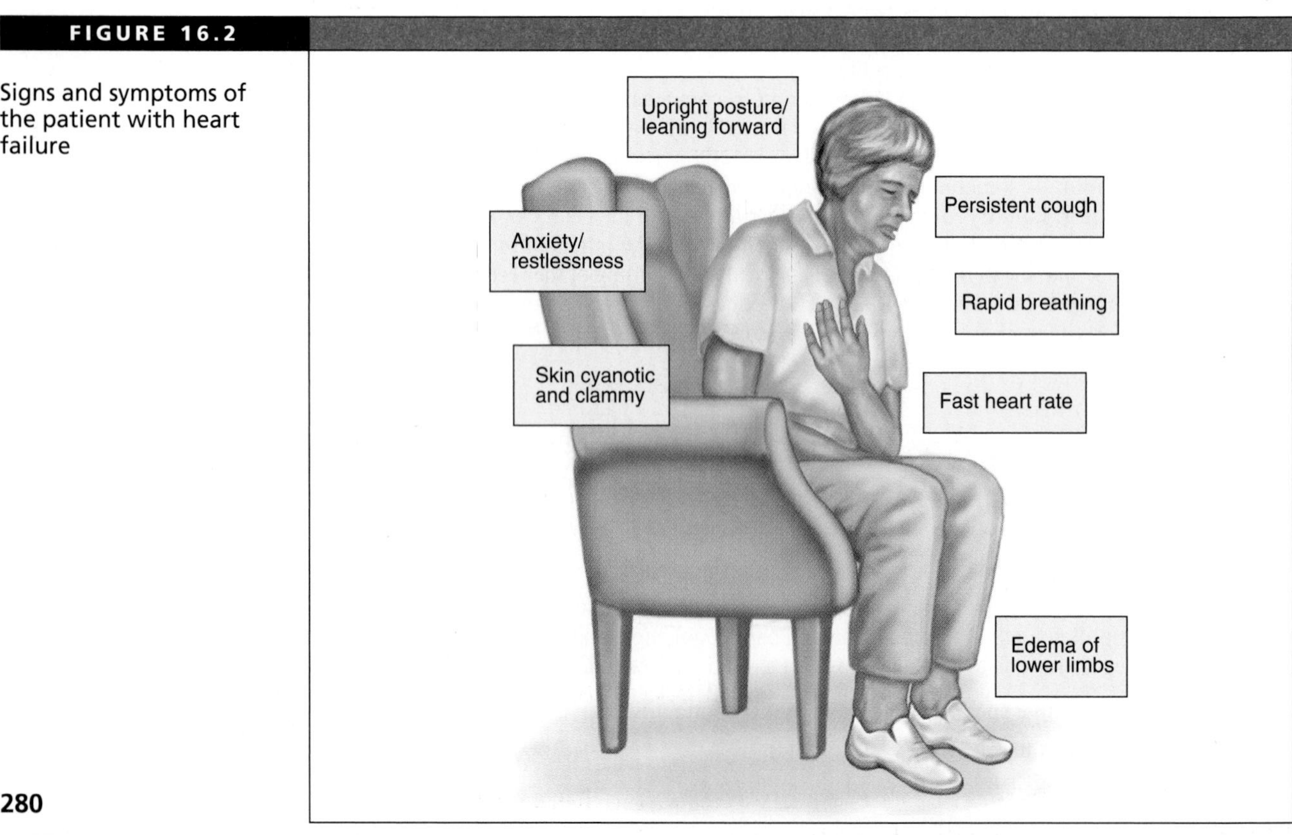

FIGURE 16.3

Mechanisms of action of drugs used for heart failure

Sympathetic neurons
Adrenergic blockers α_1, β_1, β_2 • Carvedilol
β_1
Heart rate
α_1
Cardiac output
Phosphodiesterase inhibitors • Milrinone
Cardiac glycosides • Digoxin
Heart
ACE inhibitors • Lisinopril
Arterioles
Direct vasodilators • Isosorbide dinitrate
⊕ = Stimulation
⊖ = Inhibition
Kidney
Diuretics • Furosemide
Increased urine output/ decreased blood volume

The ability to change the force of contraction is of particular interest to the pharmacotherapy of HF. Because the fundamental cause of HF is a weak myocardium, causing the muscle to beat more forcefully seems to be an ideal solution. The ability to increase the strength of contraction is called a positive **inotropic effect** and is a fundamental characteristic of the class of drugs known as the *cardiac glycosides.*

ino = *fiber*
tropic = *to influence*

The ability of the heart to speed up or slow down is a second characteristic important to pharmacology. A faster heart works harder but not necessarily more efficiently. A slower heart has a longer time to rest between beats.

A third fundamental characteristic of cardiac physiology is the electrical conduction through the heart. Some cardiovascular drugs influence the speed of this conduction. These drugs are covered in Chapter 17.

These primary characteristies of cardiac function can be modified through pharmacotherapy to assist the heart in meeting the body's metabolic demands. The mechanisms by which HF medications accomplish this are shown in Figure 16.3 ■.

16.4 The specific therapy for heart failure depends on the severity of the disease.

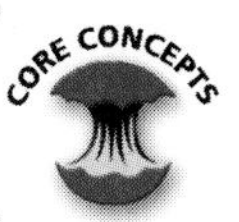

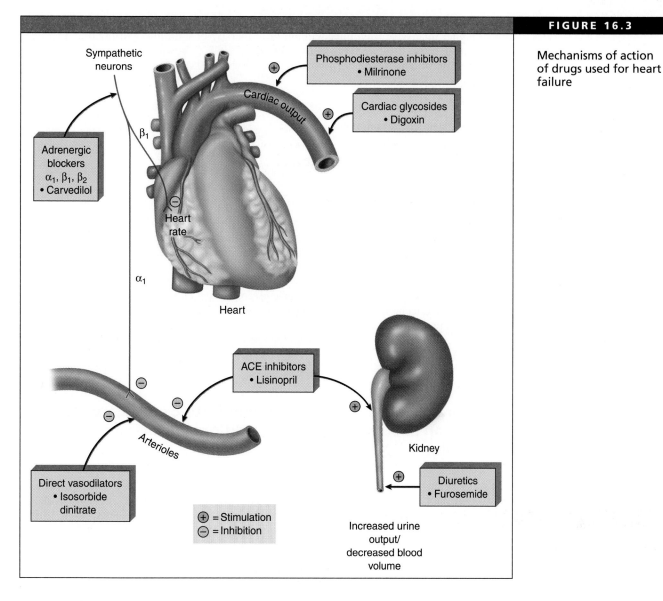

Although HF can be acute and require immediate treatment, it is often considered a progressive, chronic disorder. In its early stages, many of its symptoms can be alleviated through nonpharmacological intervention. Through certain lifestyle changes, the patient can experience a higher quality of life either without drug therapy or with lower drug doses that have less risk for adverse effects. Signs and symptoms of HF are shown in Figure 16.2. Following are nonpharmacological methods for controlling HF.

- Stop using tobacco.
- Limit salt (sodium) intake and be sure to eat foods rich in potassium and magnesium.
- Limit alcohol consumption.
- Implement a medically supervised exercise plan.
- Learn and use effective ways to deal with stress.
- Reduce weight to an optimum level.
- Limit caffeine consumption.

Once heart disease progresses such that it significantly affects activities of daily living, drug therapy is indicated. Drugs for HF may be classified as first- or second-choice drugs. If first-choice drugs do not work at all or completely, then second-choice drugs will be tried or added. The drugs of first choice are the ACE inhibitors and diuretics. These agents reduce most symptoms of mild to moderate HF, and produce the fewest number of significant side effects. Sometimes considered first-choice drugs, the cardiac glycosides are effective but have the potential for serious adverse effects. Drugs of second choice are those used in severe HF, or when the first-choice drugs prove ineffective. Second-choice drugs include the phosphodiesterase inhibitors, vasodilators, and beta-adrenergic blockers. The use of multiple drugs is common in the pharmacotherapy of HF.

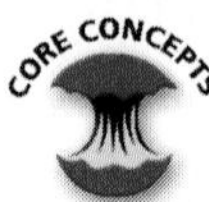

16.5 Cardiac glycosides increase the force of myocardial contraction and were once the traditional drugs of choice for heart failure.

The value of the cardiac glycosides in treating heart disorders has been known for over 2000 years. They have been used as arrow poisons by African tribes and as medicines by the ancient Egyptians and Romans. The route and doses of the cardiac glycosides are listed in Table 16.2.

Extracted from the common plants *Digitalis pupura* (purple foxglove) and *Digitalis lanata* (white foxglove), drugs from this class are sometimes called *digitalis glycosides.* Until the discovery of the ACE inhibitors, the cardiac glycosides were the mainstay of heart failure treatment. The two primary cardiac glycosides, digoxin and digitoxin, are quite similar in effectiveness. The primary difference is that digitoxin has a longer half-life than digoxin. Digitoxin is no longer available in the United States.

The primary action of the cardiac glycosides is an increase in the force of contraction. This action, a positive inotropic effect, allows the weakened heart to eject more blood per beat, thus increasing cardiac output. The increased cardiac output helps the heart to meet the metabolic demands of the tissues.

A second important action of the cardiac glycosides is their ability to slow electrical conduction through the heart. This results in fewer beats per minute. The reduced heart rate, combined with more forceful contractions, allows for much greater efficiency of the heart.

Unfortunately, the cardiac glycosides cause potentially serious adverse effects at high doses, and in certain patients. The margin of safety between a beneficial dose and a toxic dose is very small; thus, therapy should be closely monitored. Serum digoxin levels above 1.8 ng/ml are considered toxic. Initial side effects are GI related, and include loss of appetite, vomiting, and diarrhea. Headache, drowsiness, confusion, and blurred vision may occur. Excessive slowing of the heart rate and other cardiac abnormalities can be fatal if not corrected.

The antidote for digoxin toxicity is administration of digoxin immune fab (Ovine). This drug binds digoxin, preventing it from reaching the tissues. Onset of action is rapid: less than 1 minute after the IV infusion is begun.

Concept Review 16.1

- If cardiac glycosides are so effective at increasing myocardial contraction, why are they no longer drugs of first choice for heart failure?

TABLE 16.2 Drugs for Heart Failure

DRUG	ROUTE AND ADULT DOSE	REMARKS
CARDIAC GLYCOSIDE		
Pr digoxin (Lanoxin, Lanoxicaps)	PO 0.1–0.375 mg daily (max: 0.5 mg/day)	Increases cardiac output; larger dose is given to initiate therapy; IV form available; also used for dysrhythmias
ACE INHIBITORS		
captopril (Capoten)	PO 6.25–12.5 mg tid (max: 450 mg/day)	Decreases central venous and pulmonary wedge pressure; also for hypertension and acute MI
enalapril maleate (Vasotec) enalaprilat (Vasotec IV)	PO 2.5 mg daily or bid (max: 40 mg/day)	Increases cardiac output; IV form available; also for hypertension
Fosinopril (Monopril)	PO 5–40 mg daily (max: 40 mg/day)	Also for hypertension
Pr lisinopril (Prinivil, Zestril)	PO 10 mg daily (max: 80 mg/day)	Therapy should not begin until 2–3 days after diuretics are stopped; also for hypertension and acute MI
quinapril (Accupril)	PO 10–20 mg daily (max: 40 mg/day)	Observe for signs of hyperkalemia; also for hypertension
ramipril (Altace)	PO 2.5–5 mg bid (max: 10 mg/day)	Also for hypertension
DIRECT-ACTING VASODILATORS		
hydralazine (Apresoline)	PO 10–50 mg 4 times/day (max: 300 mg/day)	Increases heart rate and cardiac output; also for hypertension; IV and IM forms available
Pr isosorbide dinitrate (Isordil, Sorbitrate, Dilatrate SR)	PO 2.5–30 mg 4 times/day administer ac and at bedtime (max: 160 mg/day)	Decreases myocardial oxygen consumption; sustained-release form available; sublingual, chewable, and buccal forms available for angina
SELECTED DIURETICS		
bumetanide (Bumex)	PO 0.5–2 mg daily (max: 10 mg/day)	Affects loop of Henle; diuretic activity is 40 times greater and duration of action is shorter than furosemide; IM and IV forms available
chlorothiazide (Diuril)	PO 250 mg–1 g in 1–2 divided doses (max: 2 g/day)	Initially reduces cardiac output; also for hypertension; IV form available; thiazide diuretic
Pr furosemide (Lasix)	PO 20–80 mg in 1 or more divided doses (max: 600 mg/day)	Monitor for signs and symptoms of hypokalemia; also for hypertension; IV and IM forms available; loop diuretic
hydrochlorothiazide (HydroDIURIL, HCTZ)	PO 25–200 mg in 1–3 divided doses (max: 200 mg/day)	May bring on diabetes in the prediabetic patient; also for hypertension; thiazide diuretic
spironolactone (Aldactone)	PO 25–200 mg in divided doses (max: 200 mg/day)	Used for refractory edema with heart failure; also for hypertension; potassium-sparing diuretic
triamterene (Dyrenium)	PO 100 mg bid (max: 300 mg/day)	Used as adjunct therapy to manage edema with heart failure; also for hypertension; potassium-sparing diuretic
torsemide (Demadex)	PO 10–20 mg daily (max: 200 mg/day)	Affects loop of Henle; also for hypertension; IV form available
PHOSPHODIESTERASE INHIBITORS		
inamrinone (Inocor)	IV 0.75 mg/kg bolus given slowly over 2–3 min; then 5–10 mcg/kg/min (max: 10 mg/kg/day)	Larger dose is given to initiate therapy; peak effect reached in 10 min
Pr milrinone (Primacor)	IV 50 mcg/kg over 10 min; then 0.375–0.75 mcg/kg/min	Larger dose is given to initiate therapy; peak effect reached in 2 min

NURSING PROCESS FOCUS

Patients Receiving Cardiac Glycoside (Digoxin) Therapy

ASSESSMENT

Prior to administration:

- Obtain complete health history including allergies, drug history, and possible drug interactions
- Assess vital signs, urinary output, and cardiac output, initially and throughout therapy
- Determine the reason the medication is being administered

POTENTIAL NURSING DIAGNOSES

- Ineffective Tissue Perfusion, related to impaired cardiac status
- Decreased Cardiac Output
- Excess Fluid Volume
- Deficient Knowledge, related to drug therapy

PLANNING: Patient Goals and Expected Outcomes

The patient will:

- Report decreased symptoms of cardiac decompensation congestion related to fluid overload
- Exhibit evidence of improved organ perfusion, including kidney, heart, and brain
- Demonstrate an understanding of the drug's action by accurately describing drug side effects and precautions
- Immediately report side effects such as nausea, vomiting, diarrhea, heart rate less than 60 bpm, and vision changes

IMPLEMENTATION

Interventions and (Rationales)	Patient Education/Discharge Planning
■ Have ECG monitored for rate and rhythm changes during initial therapy. (Drug has a strong positive inotropic effect.) ■ Hold medication and report to healthcare provider/charge nurse if pulse is less than 60 bpm.	Instruct patient to: ■ Count pulse for 1 full minute, and record pulse with every dose ■ Contact healthcare provider if pulse rate is less than 60 bpm or greater than 100 bpm
■ Observe for side effects such as nausea, vomiting, diarrhea, anorexia, shortness of breath, vision changes, and leg muscle cramps. ■ Weigh patient daily.	■ Instruct patient to report side effects immediately to prevent toxicity. ■ Instruct patient to report weight gain of 2 lb or more per day.
■ Administer precise ordered dose at same time each day. (Overdose may cause serious toxicity.)	Instruct patient to: ■ Take as directed; do not double dose. ■ Not discontinue drug without advice of healthcare provider.
■ Monitor serum drug level (to determine therapeutic concentration and toxicity). Dosages may need to be adjusted. ■ Report serum drug levels greater than 1.8 ng/ml to healthcare provider.	■ Instruct patient to report to laboratory as scheduled by healthcare provider for ongoing drug level determinations.
■ Monitor levels of potassium, magnesium, calcium, BUN, and creatinine. (Hypokalemia predisposes the patient to digoxin toxicity.)	■ Instruct patient to consume foods high in potassium such as bananas, apricots, kidney beans, sweet potatoes, and peanut butter.
■ Monitor for signs and symptoms of digoxin toxicity.	■ Instruct patient to immediately report visual changes, mental depression, palpitations, weakness, loss of appetite, vomiting, and diarrhea.
■ Monitor for use of all other drugs.	■ Inform patient to consult with healthcare provider before taking any drugs including OTC and herbal supplements.

EVALUATION OF OUTCOME CRITERIA

Evaluate the effectiveness of drug therapy by confirming that patient goals and expected outcomes have been met (see "Planning").

16.6 Angiotensin-converting enzyme (ACE) inhibitors have become the preferred drugs for heart failure.

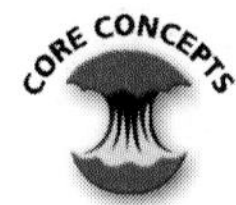

Drugs affecting the renin-angiotensin system reduce the afterload on the heart and lower blood pressure. They are drugs of choice in the treatment of HF. Table 16.2 lists the ACE inhibitors approved to treat HF.

The basic pharmacology of the ACE inhibitors and their effects on the renin-angiotensin pathway were discussed in Chapter 15. Approved for the treatment of hypertension since the 1980s, ACE inhibitors have since been shown to slow the progression of HF and to reduce deaths from this disease. They have largely replaced digoxin as the first-choice drug for the treatment of chronic HF.

The primary action of the ACE inhibitors is to lower blood pressure and reduce blood volume by enhancing the excretion of sodium and water. The resultant reduction of arterial blood pressure increases cardiac output. An additional effect of the ACE inhibitors is dilation of the veins returning blood to the heart. This action, which is probably not directly related to their inhibition of angiotensin, decreases preload and reduces peripheral edema. The combined actions of ACE inhibitors substantially decrease the workload on the heart and allow it to work more efficiently. Several ACE inhibitors have been shown to reduce mortality following acute MI when therapy is started soon after the onset of symptoms (Chapter 18).

dys = *difficult or bad*
rhythmia = *rhythm*

hypo = *below*
kal = *potassium*
emia = *blood*

DRUG PROFILE: Cardiac Glycoside: Pr *Digoxin (Lanoxin)*

Actions and Uses:

The primary benefit of digoxin is its ability to increase the contractility or strength of cardiac contraction. Digoxin accomplishes this by inhibiting Na^+–K^+ ATPase, an enzyme in myocardial cells.

By increasing myocardial contractility, digoxin directly increases cardiac output, thus alleviating symptoms of HF and improving exercise tolerance.

The increased cardiac output also results in increased urine production and a desirable reduction in blood volume, thus relieving the distressing symptoms of lung congestion and peripheral edema.

In addition to its positive inotropic effect, digoxin also affects impulse conduction in the heart. It has the ability to suppress the SA node (the pacemaker of the heart) and slow electrical conduction through the AV node. Because of these actions, digoxin is sometimes used to treat rhythm abnormalities known as **dysrhythmias,** as discussed in Chapter 7.

Adverse Effects and Interactions:

The most dangerous adverse effect of digoxin is its ability to create dysrhythmias, particularly in patients who have hypokalemia. Because diuretics can cause hypokalemia and are also often used to treat HF, use of digoxin and diuretics together must be carefully monitored. Other adverse effects of digoxin therapy include nausea, vomiting, and anorexia, and abnormalities of the nervous system such as blurred vision. Periodic serum levels are checked to determine if the digoxin level is within the therapeutic range, and the dosage may be adjusted based on the laboratory results. Digoxin also interacts with many other medications. Because small changes in digoxin levels can produce serious adverse effects, the healthcare provider must constantly be alert for drug/drug interactions.

Mechanism in Action: 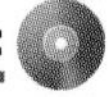

Digoxin's primary action is to inhibit the Na^+–K^+ ATPase enzyme. This enzyme is responsible for pumping sodium out of the myocardial cell in exchange for potassium. As Na^+ accumulates, calcium ions are released from their storage areas in the cell. The release of Ca^{++} produces a more forceful contraction of the muscle fibers.

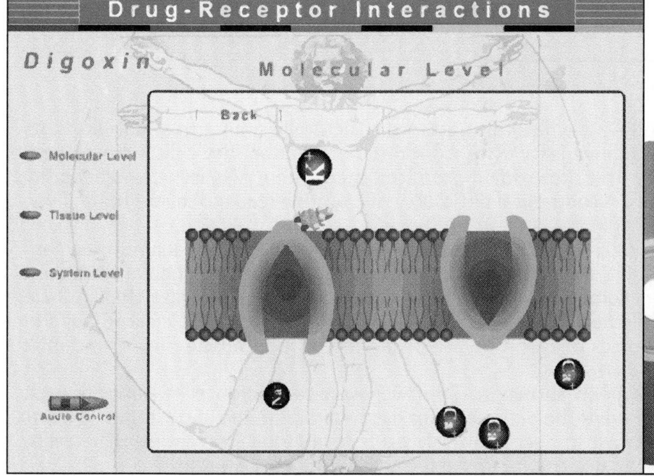

Use the student CD-ROM to see Mechanism in Action for Digoxin.

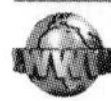 *See the Companion Website for a Nursing Process Focus specific to this drug.*

DRUG PROFILE: ACE Inhibitor: Pr *Lisinopril (Prinivil, Zestril)*

Actions and Uses:

Because of its value in the treatment of both HF and hypertension, lisinopril has become one of the most commonly prescribed drugs. Like other ACE inhibitors, doses of lisinopril may require 2–3 weeks of adjustment to reach maximum effectiveness and several months of therapy may be needed for a patient's functional status to return to normal. Because of their combined hypotensive action, concurrent therapy with lisinopril and diuretics should be carefully monitored.

Adverse Effects and Interactions:

Although lisinopril causes few side effects, high potassium levels may occur during therapy. Use of potassium supplements or potassium-sparing diuretics should be avoided during lisinopril therapy. Thus, electrolyte levels are usually monitored periodically. Other side effects include cough, taste disturbances, and hypotension.

Lisinopril interacts with indomethacin and other NSAIDs, causing decreased antihypertensive activity. When taken together with potassium-sparing diurectics, hyperkalemia may result. Lisinopril may increase lithium levels and toxicity.

Mechanism in Action:

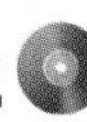

Angiotensin-converting enzyme (ACE) causes the conversion of angiotensin I to angiotensin II. Two major physiological actions result from this conversion: increased water/sodium retention and increased peripheral vascular resistance. Both actions contribute to hypertension. Lisinopril lowers blood pressure by blocking ACE.

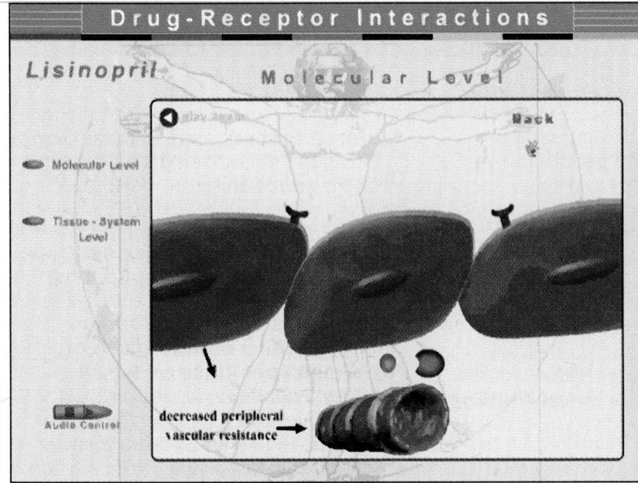

Use the student CD-ROM to see Mechanism in Action for Lisinopril.

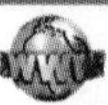

See the Companion Website for a Nursing Process Focus specific to this drug.

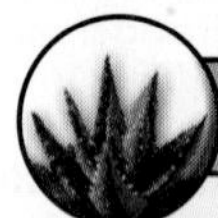

NATURAL ALTERNATIVES

Carnitine and Heart Disease

Once thought to be a vitamin, carnitine is a natural substance structurally similar to amino acids. Its primary function in metabolism is to move fatty acids from the bloodstream into cells, where carnitine assists in the breakdown of fats. This breakdown produces energy and increases the availability of oxygen, particularly in muscle cells. A congenital deficiency of carnitine leads to severe brain, liver, and heart damage.

Although a normal diet supplies 300 mg/day, certain patients may need additional amounts. Vegetarians are at risk for carnitine depletion, because plant protein supplies little or no carnitine. Endurance athletes and body builders sometimes use carnitine supplements to increase their muscle mass. Carnitine is available as a supplement in several forms, including L-carnitine, D, L-carnitine, and acetyl L-carnitine. The best food sources of carnitine are organ meat, fish, muscle meats, and milk products.

L-carnitine supplementation has been shown to improve exercise tolerance in patients with angina. The use of L-carnitine may prevent the occurrence of dysrhythmias in the early stages of heart disease. L-carnitine has also been shown to decrease triglyceride levels while increasing HDL levels, thus helping to minimize one of the major risk factors associated with heart disease.

Carnitine may have a number of additional effects including improvement of brain function in patients with Alzheimer's disease. Because of its role in fat metabolism, some claim it assists in treating obesity, although this has yet to be supported by research. ▪

16.7 Diuretics relieve symptoms of heart failure by reducing blood volume.

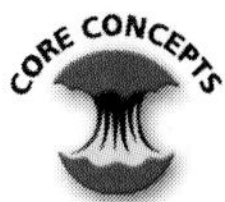

Diuretics increase urine flow, thus reducing blood volume and cardiac workload. They are widely used in the treatment of cardiovascular disease in patients with fluid overload (see Table 16.2).

Diuretics are commonly used for the treatment of HF. They produce few adverse effects and are effective at lowering blood volume, and reducing edema and congestion. As diuretics reduce fluid overload and lower blood pressure, the workload on the heart is reduced and cardiac output increases. Diuretics are rarely used alone, but instead are prescribed in combination with ACE inhibitors and other HF medications in patients who have adema.

The most common adverse effects from diuretic therapy are electrolyte imbalances. These can be especially important in patients taking cardiac glycosides; patients with potassium or magnesium deficiencies are at greater risk for toxicity from digoxin. Potassium or magnesium supplements may be prescribed to prevent this adverse effect. Even without digoxin, too little or too much potassium can greatly affect a failing heart. Frequent laboratory testing may be necessary to monitor electrolyte levels in patients with HF.

DRUG PROFILE: Diuretic: Pr *Furosemide (Lasix)*

Actions and Uses:

Furosemide is used in the treatment of acute HF because it has the ability to remove large amounts of edema fluid from the patient in a short time. Patients often receive quick relief from their distressing symptoms. Compared to other diuretics, furosemide is particularly beneficial when cardiac output and renal flow are severely diminished.

Adverse Effects Interactions:

Side effects of furosemide, like those of most diuretics, involve potential electrolyte imbalances, the most important of which is hypokalemia. Because hypokalemia may cause dysrhythmias in patients taking cardiac glycosides, combination therapy with furosemide and digoxin must be carefully monitored. When furosemide is given with corticosteroids and amphotericin B, it can increase hypokalemia. When given with lithium, elimination of lithium is decreased, causing higher risk of toxicity. When given with sulfonylureas and insulin, furosemide may diminish their hypoglycemic effects. Because furosemide is such a potent drug, fluid loss must be carefully monitored to avoid possible dehydration and hypotension.

Furosemide should be monitored carefully in patients receiving aminoglycoside antibiotics because additive ototoxicity may result. Patients allergic to sulfur or sulfonamide antibiotics should not receive furosemide because of potential allergic response.

Mechanism in Action:

Furosemide inhibits the combined transport of sodium, potassium, and chloride (called Na^+–K^+–$2Cl^-$ symport) across the loop of Henle. By blocking active NaCl reabsorption, furosemide interferes with water reabsorption. When water reabsorption is blocked, increased urination results. ■

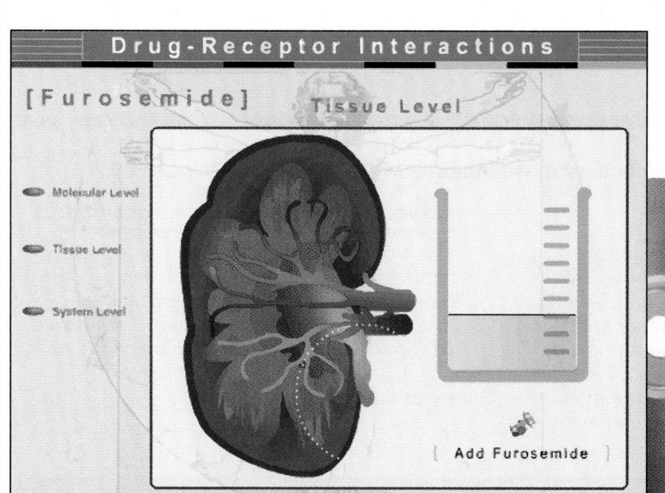

Use the student CD-ROM to see Mechanism in Action for Furosemide.

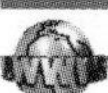

See the Companion Website for a Nursing Process Focus specific to this drug.

The mechanism by which diuretics reduce blood volume, specifically where and how the nephron of the kidney is affected, differs among the various drugs. Differences in mechanisms among the classes of diuretics are discussed in Chapter 28. The role of the thiazide diuretics in the treatment of hypertension is discussed in Chapter 15.

Concept Review 16.2

- Why are the ACE inhibitors preferred over both the nitrates and the diuretics in the treatment of HF?

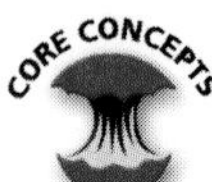

16.8 Phosphodiesterase inhibitors are used for short-term therapy of advanced heart failure.

Phosphodiesterase inhibitors have a brief half-life and are used for the short-term control of acute HF. The doses of phosphodiesterase inhibitors are given in Table 16.2.

In the 1980s, two drugs became available that block the enzyme **phosphodiesterase** in cardiac and smooth muscle. Blocking phosphodiesterase has the effect of increasing the amount of calcium available for myocardial contraction. The inhibition results in two main actions that benefit patients with HF: an increased force of contraction (positive inotropic response) and vasodilation. Because of their toxicity, phosphodiesterase inhibitors are normally reserved for patients who have not responded to ACE inhibitors or cardiac glycosides, and they are generally used only for 2 to 3 days.

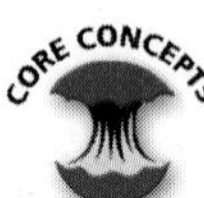

16.9 Vasodilators reduce symptoms of heart failure by decreasing cardiac oxygen demands.

Vasodilators play a minor role in the drug therapy of HF. They are also used for hypertension and angina pectoris (see Table 16.2).

The two drugs in this class act directly on vascular smooth muscle to relax blood vessels and lower blood pressure. Hydralazine (Apresoline) acts on arterioles, whereas isosorbide dinitrate (Isordil) acts on veins. Because the two drugs act synergistically, isosorbide dinitrate is usually combined with hydralazine in the treatment of HF. Because of the high incidence of side effects, they are generally reserved for patients with more severe disease, or those who cannot tolerate ACE inhibitors. The role of hydralazine in the treatment of hypertension is discussed in Chapter 15, and the use of isosorbide dinitrate for therapy of angina pectoris is presented in Chapter 18.

DRUG PROFILE: Phosphodiesterase Inhibitor: Pr *Milrinone (Primacor)*

Actions and Uses:

Of the two phosphodiesterase inhibitors available, milrinone is generally preferred because it has a shorter half-life and fewer side effects. It is only given intravenously and is primarily used for the short-term support of advanced HF. Peak effects occur in 2 minutes. Immediate effects of milrinone include an increased force of contraction and an increase in cardiac output.

Adverse Effects and Interactions:

The most serious side effect of milrinone is ventricular dysrhythmia, which can occur in more than 1 of every 10 patients taking the drug. The patient's ECG is usually monitored continuously during the infusion of the drug.

Use with disopyramide may cause excessive hypotension.

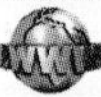

See the Companion Website for a Nursing Process Focus specific to this drug.

DRUG PROFILE: Vasodilator: Pr *Isosorbide dinitrate (Isordil)*

Actions and Uses:

Isosorbide dinitrate acts directly on veins to cause venodilation, thus reducing venous return (preload), decreasing cardiac workload, and increasing cardiac output. Isosorbide dinitrate also dilates the coronary arteries to bring more oxygen to the myocardium. Isosorbide dinitrate belongs to a class of drugs called *organic nitrates* that are widely used in the treatment of angina.

Adverse Effects and Interactions:

Side effects of isosorbide dinitrate include headache, hypotension, and reflex tachycardia. Use is contraindicated if the patient is also taking sildenafil (Viagra) because serious hypotension may result.

Use of alcohol, antihypertensive agents or phenothiazines may cause increased hypotensive effects.

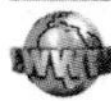

See the Companion Website for a Nursing Process Focus specific to this drug.

16.10 Beta-adrenergic blockers are used in combination with other drugs to slow the progression of heart failure and to prolong patient survival.

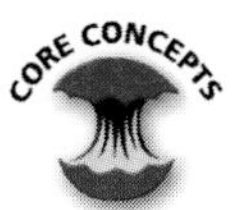

As has been seen with the cardiac glycosides and phosphodiesterase inhibitors, drugs that produce a positive inotropic effect play important roles in treating the diminished contractility that is the hallmark of HF. It may seem somewhat unusual, then, to find medications that exhibit a negative inotropic effect prescribed for this disease. Yet such is the case with the beta-adrenergic blockers. Beta blockers have been shown to dramatically reduce the number of hospitalizations and deaths associated with HF. Carvedilol and metoprolol are the two beta blockers used to treat HF. They are always used in combination with other agents. The basic pharmacology of the beta blockers is presented in Chapter 7. Other uses, routes, and dosages of the beta-adrenergic blockers are discussed elsewhere in this text: hypertension in Chapter 15, dysrhythmias in Chapter 17, and angina/myocardial infarction in Chapter 18.

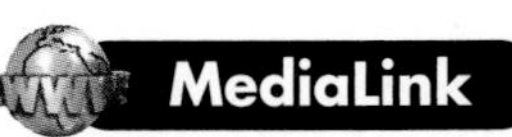

SUPPORT FOR HEART FAILURE PATIENTS AND HEALTH PROFESSIONALS

DRUG PROFILE: Beta-Adrenergic Blocker: Pr *Carvedilol (Coreg)*

Actions and Uses:

Carvedilol was the first beta-adrenergic blocker approved for the treatment of HF. It has been found to reduce symptoms, slow the progression of the disease, and increase exercise tolerance when combined with other HF drugs such as ACE inhibitors. Unlike many drugs in this class, carvedilol blocks $beta_1$ and $beta_2$ as well as $alpha_1$-adrenergic receptors. The primary therapeutic effects relevant to HF are a reduction in heart rate and a drop in blood pressure. The lower blood pressure decreases afterload and reduces the workload on the heart.

Adverse Effects and Interactions:

Carvedilol's ability to decrease the heart rate combined with its ability to reduce contractility has the potential to worsen HF, and dosage must be carefully monitored. Because of the potential for adverse cardiac effects, beta-adrenergic blockers such as carvedilol are not considered first-choice drugs in the treatment of HF.

Carvedilol interacts with many drugs. For example, levels of carvedilol are significantly increased when the drug is taken with rifampin. MAO inhibitors, clonidine, and reserpine can cause hypotension or bradycardia when given with carvedilol. When given with digoxin, carvedilol may increase digoxin levels. It may also enhance the hypoglycemic effects of insulin and oral hypoglycemic agents.

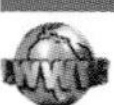

See the Companion Website for a Nursing Process Focus specific to this drug.

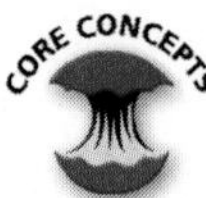

16.11 Natriuretic peptides are the first new drugs to treat heart failure in more than 10 years.

In 2001, the first new class of medications for HF in more than 10 years was approved. Nesiritide (Natrecor) is a small peptide hormone, produced through recombinant DNA technology, that is structurally identical to a hormone secreted by the heart.

natri = *sodium*
uretic = *urinary excretion*

When HF occurs, the ventricles begin to secrete a hormone known as beta-type **natriuretic peptide** (hBNP) in response to the increased stretch on the ventricular walls. hBNP acts on the kidney to increase the excretion of sodium and water, thus lowering blood pressure. hBNP also causes vasodilation, which contributes to reduced preload. Nesiritide, being the same molecule as hBNP, thus reduces both preload and afterload, improving cardiac efficiency in patients with HF.

Nesiritide has limited uses because of its ability to cause severe hypotension. The medication is only given by IV infusion, and patients require continuous monitoring. It is approved for patients with severe HF.

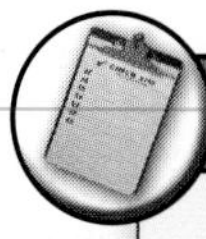

PATIENTS NEED TO KNOW

Patients treated for HF need to know the following:

In General

1. Take blood pressure regularly because many drugs for HF affect blood pressure. Report any persistent changes.
2. Take weight regularly and report abnormal weight gains or losses.
3. An increased intake of potassium-rich foods such as bananas, dried fruits, and orange juice, or a potassium supplement, may be necessary if certain diuretics are taken. Taking potassium supplements with food reduces stomach irritation. Salt intake should be limited.

Regarding ACE Inhibitors

4. Avoid sudden position changes because these can cause lightheadedness.

Regarding Cardiac Glycosides

5. Check pulse rate before taking digoxin. If the rate is less than 60 beats per minute, or the rate designated by a healthcare provider, the drug should not be taken.
6. Many drugs interact with digoxin to increase or decrease its effects on the heart. For this reason, it is important to consult with a healthcare provider before taking any other medication.
7. Report visual disturbances (seeing halos or a yellow-green tinge, blurring), nausea, headaches, or irregular heartbeat without delay because they are signs and symptoms of digoxin toxicity.

Regarding Diuretics

8. Limit salt intake.
9. Drink at least 6 to 8 glasses of water daily.
10. Report any of the following side/adverse effects: abdominal pain, jaundice, dark urine, flulike symptoms.
11. Avoid sudden position changes. ■

CHAPTER REVIEW

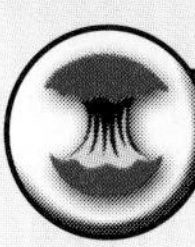

CORE CONCEPTS SUMMARY

16.1 Heart failure is closely associated with disorders such as chronic hypertension and diabetes.

Heart failure is not considered a distinct disease in itself. Instead, a number of diseases that affect the heart, such as chronic hypertension and diabetes, lead to the collection of symptoms known as HF.

16.2 The central cause of heart failure is weakened heart muscle.

Heart failure occurs when the heart cannot pump enough blood to meet the demands of the tissues. This usually occurs when the heart muscle cannot contract with sufficient force. Heart failure may occur on the right side, left side, or both sides of the heart, producing symptoms such as shortness of breath, coughing, and peripheral edema.

16.3 The three primary characteristics of heart function are force of contraction, heart rate, and speed of impulse conduction.

The ability of the heart to effectively pump blood depends on the strength of contraction of the myocardial fibers. Heart rate and the speed of the impulse conduction across the myocardium also directly affect the ability of the heart to pump blood.

16.4 The specific therapy for heart failure depends on the severity of the disease.

Mild HF can be improved through lifestyle changes such as tobacco cessation and maintaining optimum weight. As HF progresses, pharmacotherapy with drugs of first choice, such as ACE inhibitors or diuretics, is indicated. More advanced disease may require therapy with cardiac glycosides, phosphodiesterase inhibitors, beta blockers, or vasodilators.

16.5 Cardiac glycosides increase the force of myocardial contraction and were once the traditional drugs of choice for heart failure.

Cardiac glycosides, long the mainstay for pharmacotherapy of HF, increase myocardial contractility and are effective. The large number of drug-drug interactions and the potential for serious adverse effects such as dysrhythmias limit their use.

16.6 Angiotensin-converting enzyme (ACE) inhibitors have become the preferred drugs for heart failure.

ACE inhibitors improve HF by reducing peripheral edema and increasing cardiac output. Because of their effectiveness and their relatively low potential for serious adverse effects, they have become first-choice drugs in the treatment of HF.

16.7 Diuretics relieve symptoms of heart failure by reducing blood volume.

Diuretics produce few side effects and are often used in combination with other HF drugs to reduce patient symptoms. Potent diuretics such as furosemide are particularly valuable in treating acute HF.

16.8 Phosphodiesterase inhibitors are used for short-term therapy of advanced heart failure.

Phosphodiesterase inhibitors are a relatively new class of drugs used for the short-term treatment of HF. While effective, they are only given IV and can produce potentially serious adverse effects.

16.9 Vasodilators reduce symptoms of heart failure by decreasing cardiac oxygen demands.

Direct vasodilators are effective at relaxing blood vessels, thus reducing myocardial oxygen demand on the heart. Their use is limited by their high incidence of side effects.

16.10 Beta-adrenergic blockers are used in combination with other drugs to slow the progression of heart failure and to prolong patient survival.

Although beta blockers decrease myocardial contractility, they also lower heart rate and blood pressure, which are beneficial to reducing the symptoms of HF. When administered to treat patients with HF, they are nearly always used in combination with other drugs.

16.11 Natriuretic peptides are the first new drugs to treat heart failure in more than 10 years.

Nesiritide (Natrecor) is a small peptide hormone that is structurally identical to a hormone secreted by the heart, beta-type natriuretic peptide (hBNP). This new drug reduces blood pressure and causes vasodilation, thus helping a failing heart beat more efficiently. It is approved only for severe HF because of its potentially serious adverse effects.

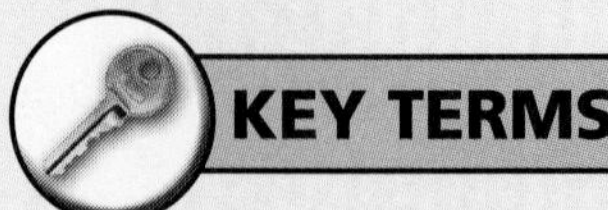

KEY TERMS

afterload: pressure that must be overcome for the ventricles to eject blood from the heart / *page 279*

contractility (kon-trak-TILL-eh-tee): the strength by which the myocardial fibers contract / *page 279*

dysrhythmia (diss-RITH-mee-uh): abnormal cardiac rhythm / *page 285*

heart failure (HF): disease in which the heart muscle cannot contract with sufficient force to meet the body's metabolic needs / *page 278*

inotropic effect (in-oh-TRO-pik): change in the strength or contractility of the heart / *page 281*

natriuretic peptide (na-tree-ur-ET-ik): hormone that increases the urinary excretion of sodium and dilates blood vessels / *page 290*

peripheral edema (purr-IF-ur-ul eh-DEE-mah): swelling in the limbs, particularly the feet and ankles due to an accumulation of interstitial fluid / *page 279*

phosphodiesterase (fos-fo-die-ES-tur-ase): enzyme in muscle cells that cleaves phosphodiester bonds; its inhibition increases myocardial contractility / *page 288*

preload: degree of stretch of the cardiac muscle fibers just before they contract / *page 279*

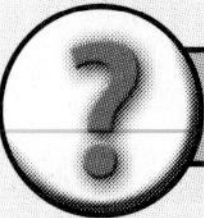

REVIEW QUESTIONS

The following questions are written in NCLEX-PN® style. Answer these questions to assess your knowledge of the chapter material, and go back and review any material that is not clear to you.

1. The patient has developed a cough and SOB when he lies down. The nurse suspects:

1. Right HF
2. Left HF
3. Liver engorgement
4. Peripheral edema

2. The patient has been started on digoxin (Lanoxin) therapy. Which of the following should be monitored?

1. BUN levels
2. Amylase levels
3. Sodium levels
4. Potassium levels

3. Which of the following should be expected with the use of digoxin (Lanoxin)?

1. Increased weight
2. Decreased edema
3. Increased blood volume
4. Increased heart rate

4. The patient with HF is also experiencing angina. Which of the following drugs would be appropriate for use?

1. Isosorbide dinitrate (Isordil)
2. Hydralazine (Apresoline)
3. Chlorothiazide (Diuril)
4. Milrinone (Primacor)

5. The patient is admitted with HF. The physician orders IV milrinone (Primacor). The most serious side effect of this drug is:

1. Headache
2. Dysrhythmias
3. Confusion
4. Drowsiness

6. Which of the following should not be included in the education provided to a patient on lisinopril (Prinivil)?

1. "It may take several months for your blood pressure to return to normal."
2. "You must have your potassium monitored from time to time."
3. "This medication may change your vision from time to time."
4. "You may notice a change in your sensation of taste."

7. In addition to decreasing cardiac contractility, beta blockers:

1. Lower heart rate and blood pressure
2. Increase heart rate and afterload
3. Produce systemic vasoconstriction
4. Increase the forces of the myocardial contraction

8. Which drug would the nurse expect to be ordered for a patient with digoxin toxicity?

1. Digoxin immune fab
2. Milrinone
3. Amrinone
4. Flecainide (Tambocor)

9. The patient on digoxin (Lanoxin) is complaining of blurred vision. The nurse suspects:

1. Retinal blindness
2. Digoxin (Lanoxin) toxicity
3. The need to increase the medication dosage
4. The patient has not had an eye exam in a long time

10. The patient with HF has noted a 5-pound weight gain over the last 3 days. The patient should:

1. Watch his diet
2. Take an additional dose of his medication
3. Notify his physician
4. Increase his exercise regimen

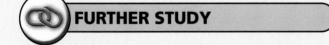

CASE STUDY QUESTIONS

For questions 1–5, please refer to the following case study, and choose the correct answer from choices 1–4.

Mr. Novi, age 45, has smoked since age 12. He recently has had trouble breathing when mowing the lawn, and he coughs when he lies down to sleep at night. The physician has diagnosed Mr. Novi with early HF.

1. Which of the following drugs would *most* likely be prescribed for Mr. Novi?

1. Isosorbide dinitrate (Isordil)
2. Enalapril (Vasotec)
3. Milrinone (Primacor)
4. Quinapril (Accupril)

2. Which of the following actions would be most desirable for a drug used to treat HF in Mr. Novi?

1. Speed up the heart rate
2. Increase the forcefulness of heart contractions
3. Increase arterial blood pressure
4. Increase blood volume by retaining water

3. After a year, Mr. Novi enters the emergency department with acute shortness of breath and severe congestion in both lungs. Which of the following medications would be a likely choice for this patient in the ER?

1. Inamrinone (Inocor)
2. Captopril (Capoten)
3. Carvedilol (Coreg)
4. Spironolactone (Aldactone)

4. Mr. Novi was also diagnosed with angina. Which of the following drugs is approved for both HF and angina?

1. Hydralazine (Apresoline)
2. Furosemide (Lasix)
3. Isosorbide dinitrate (Isordil)
4. Digoxin (Lanoxin)

5. Mr. Novi has been placed on digoxin and furosemide. Which of the following side effects of furosemide could lead to dysrhythmias and other cardiac disease in patients taking digoxin?

1. Hypotension
2. Bradycardia
3. Hypokalemia
4. Hyperkalemia

FURTHER STUDY

- The relationship between cardiac output and blood pressure is explained in Chapter 15.
- Chapter 15 describes the pharmacology of ACE inhibitors and how they affect the renin-angiotensin pathway.
- Dysrhythmia is discussed in Chapter 17.
- For further discussion of ACE inhibitor therapy in acute MI, see Chapter 18.
- More information on the role of hydralazine in the treatment of hypertension is found in Chapter 15.
- The use of isosorbide dinitrate in the treatment of angina pectoris is discussed in Chapter 18.
- Differences in mechanisms of action among diuretics is discussed in Chapter 27.
- Chapter 15 discusses how thiazide diuretics are used to treat hypertension.
- Chapter 7 explains the basic pharmacology of beta blockers.
- Uses, routes, and dosages of beta blockers are discussed in Chapter 15 (to treat hypertension); Chapter 17 (for dysrhythmias); and Chapter 18 (angina and MI).

EXPLORE MEDIALINK www.prenhall.com/holland

Additional resources for this chapter can be found on the CD-ROM accompanying this textbook, and on the Companion Website. Click on Chapter 16 to select activities for this chapter.

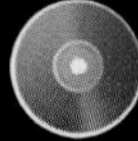

- Mechanism in Action:
  - Digoxin
  - Lisinopril
  - Furosemide
- Audio Glossary
- Concept Review
- NCLEX-PN® Review
- Nursing in Action
- Dosage Calculator

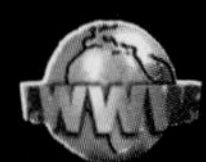

- The Beating Heart
- Support for Heart Failure Patients and Health Professionals

CHAPTER

17 Drugs for Dysrhythmias

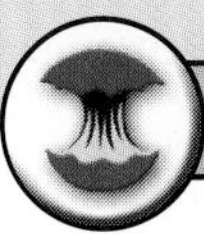

CORE CONCEPTS

17.1 Some types of dysrhythmias produce no patient symptoms, whereas others may be life threatening.

17.2 Dysrhythmias are classified by their location and type of rhythm abnormality produced.

17.3 The electrical conduction pathway in the myocardium keeps the heart beating in a synchronized manner.

17.4 Nonpharmacological therapy of certain dysrhythmias is often the treatment of choice.

17.5 Most antidysrhythmic drugs act by blocking ion channels in myocardial cells.

17.6 Antidysrhythmic drugs are classified by their mechanisms of action.

17.7 Sodium channel blockers slow the rate of impulse conduction through the heart.

17.8 Beta-adrenergic blockers reduce automaticity and slow conduction velocity in the heart.

17.9 Potassium channel blockers prolong the refractory period of the heart.

17.10 Two calcium channel blockers are available to treat supraventricular dysrhythmias.

17.11 Digoxin and adenosine are used for specific dysrhythmias, but do not act by blocking ion channels.

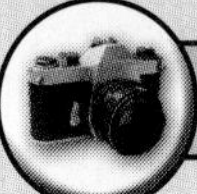

DRUG SNAPSHOT

The following drugs will be discussed in this chapter:

DRUG CLASSES	DRUG PROFILES
Sodium channel blockers	Pr quinidine (Quinidex)
Beta-adrenergic blockers	Pr propranolol (Inderal)
Potassium channel blockers	Pr amiodarone (Cordarone)
Calcium channel blockers	Pr verapamil (Calan)
Miscellaneous drugs	

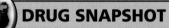

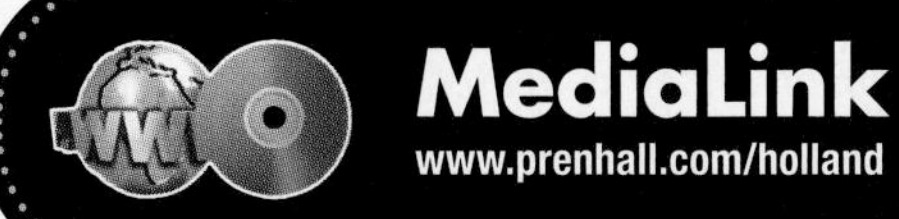

MediaLink
www.prenhall.com/holland

Interactive resources for this chapter can be found on the Companion Website. Click on Chapter 17 and "Begin" to select the activities for this chapter. For chapter-related animations, NCLEX-PN®-style questions, and an audio glossary, access the accompanying CD-ROM in this book.

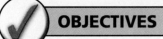

OBJECTIVES

After reading this chapter, the student should be able to:

1. Explain how rhythm abnormalities can affect cardiac function.
2. Illustrate the flow of electrical impulses through the normal heart.
3. Classify dysrhythmias based on their location and type of conduction abnormality.
4. Explain the importance of ion channels to myocardial function and the pharmacotherapy of dysrhythmias.
5. Identify the importance of nonpharmacological therapies in the treatment of dysrhythmias.
6. Identify basic mechanisms by which antidysrhythmic drugs act.
7. For each of the following classes, identify representative drugs, explain the mechanisms of drug action, primary actions, and important adverse effects:
   - **a.** Sodium channel blockers
   - **b.** Beta-adrenergic blockers
   - **c.** Potassium channel blockers
   - **d.** Calcium channel blockers
   - **e.** Miscellaneous antidysrhythmic drugs
8. Categorize antidysrhthmic drugs based on their classifications and mechanisms of action.

dys = *difficult or bad*
rhythm = *rhythm*
ia = *condition*

Dysrhythmias are abnormalities of electrical conduction or rhythm in the heart. Sometimes called arrhythmias, they encompass a number of different disorders that range from harmless to life threatening. Diagnosis is often difficult because patients usually must be connected to an electrocardiogram (ECG) and be experiencing symptoms to determine the exact type of rhythm disorder. Proper diagnosis and optimum pharmacological treatment can significantly affect the frequency of dysrhythmias and their consequences.

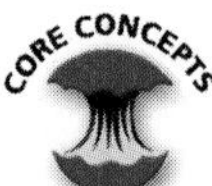

17.1 Some types of dysrhythmias produce no patient symptoms, whereas others may be life threatening.

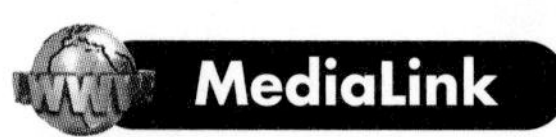

CHILDHOOD DYSRHYTHMIAS

a = *no or not*
symptomat = *symptoms*
ic = *pertaining to*

Whereas some dysrhythmias produce no symptoms and have negligible effects on heart function, others are life threatening and require immediate treatment. Typical symptoms include dizziness, weakness, decreased exercise tolerance, shortness of breath, and fainting. Many patients report palpitations or a sensation that their heart has skipped a beat. Persistent dysrhythmias are associated with increased risk of stroke and heart failure. Severe dysrhythmias may result in sudden death. Because asymptomatic patients may not seek medical attention, it is difficult to estimate the frequency of the disease, although it is likely that dysrhythmias are quite common in the population.

Fast Facts Dysrhythmias

- Dysrhythmias are responsible for more than 44,000 deaths each year.
- Atrial dysrhythmias occur more commonly in men than in women.
- The incidence of atrial dysrhythmias increases with age. They affect:
  Less than 0.5% of those aged 25–35
  1.5% of those up to age 60
  9% of those over age 75
- About 15% of strokes occur in patients with atrial dysrhythmias.
- A large majority of sudden cardiac deaths are thought to be caused by ventricular dysrhythmias.
- Sudden cardiac death occurs three to four times more frequently in Blacks.
- Atrial fibrillation affects 1.5 to 2.2 million people in the United States.

TABLE 17.1 Types of Dysrhythmias

NAME OF DYSRHYTHMIA	DESCRIPTION
Premature atrial or premature ventricular (PVC) contractions	An extra beat, often originating from a source other than the sinoatrial (SA) node; not normally serious unless it occurs in high frequency
Atrial or ventricular **tachycardia**	Rapid heart beat greater than 150 bpm; ventricular is more serious than atrial
Atrial or ventricular **flutter** and/or fibrillation	Very rapid, uncoordinated beats; atrial may require treatment but is not usually fatal; ventricular requires immediate treatment
Sinus **bradycardia**	Slow heartbeat, less than 50 bpm; may require a pacemaker
Heart block	Area of nonconduction in the myocardium; may be partial or complete; classified as first, second, or third degree

17.2 Dysrhythmias are classified by their location and type of rhythm abnormality produced.

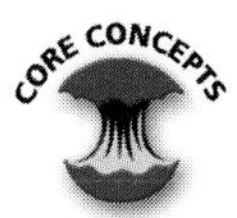

There are many types of dysrhythmias, and they may be classified by a number of different means. The simplest method is to name dysrhythmias according to the type of rhythm abnormality produced and its location. A summary of the different types of dysrhythmias along with a brief description of each abnormality is given in Table 17.1. Dysrhythmias that originate in the atria are sometimes referred to as **supraventricular.** Those that originate in the ventricles are generally more serious because they are more likely to interfere with the normal function of the heart. Although obtaining a correct diagnosis of the type of dysrhythmia is sometimes difficult, it is essential for effective treatment. Atrial **fibrillation,** a complete disorganization of rhythm, is thought to be the most common type of dysrhythmia.

supra = *above*
ventricular = *cardiac ventricle*

Dysrhythmias can occur in both healthy and diseased hearts. Although the actual cause of most dysrhythmias is elusive, dysrhythmias are often associated with certain conditions, primarily heart disease and myocardial infarction. Following are some of the diseases commonly associated with dysrhythmias:

- Hypertension
- Cardiac valve disease, such as mitral stenosis
- Coronary artery disease
- Medications such as digoxin
- Low potassium levels in the blood
- Myocardial infarction
- Adverse effect from antidysrhythmic medication
- Stroke
- Diabetes mellitus
- Congestive heart failure

17.3 The electrical conduction pathway in the myocardium keeps the heart beating in a synchronized manner.

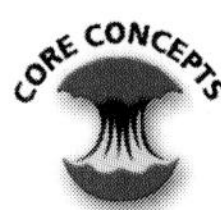

Although there are many different types of dysrhythmias, all have in common a defect in the formation or conduction of electrical impulses across the myocardium. These electrical impulses carry the signal for the cardiac muscle cells to contract and must be coordinated precisely for the chambers to beat in a synchronized manner. For the heart to function properly, the atria must contract simultaneously, sending their blood into the ventricles. Following atrial contraction, the right

FIGURE 17.1

Normal conduction pathway in the heart
SOURCE: Pearson Education/PH College

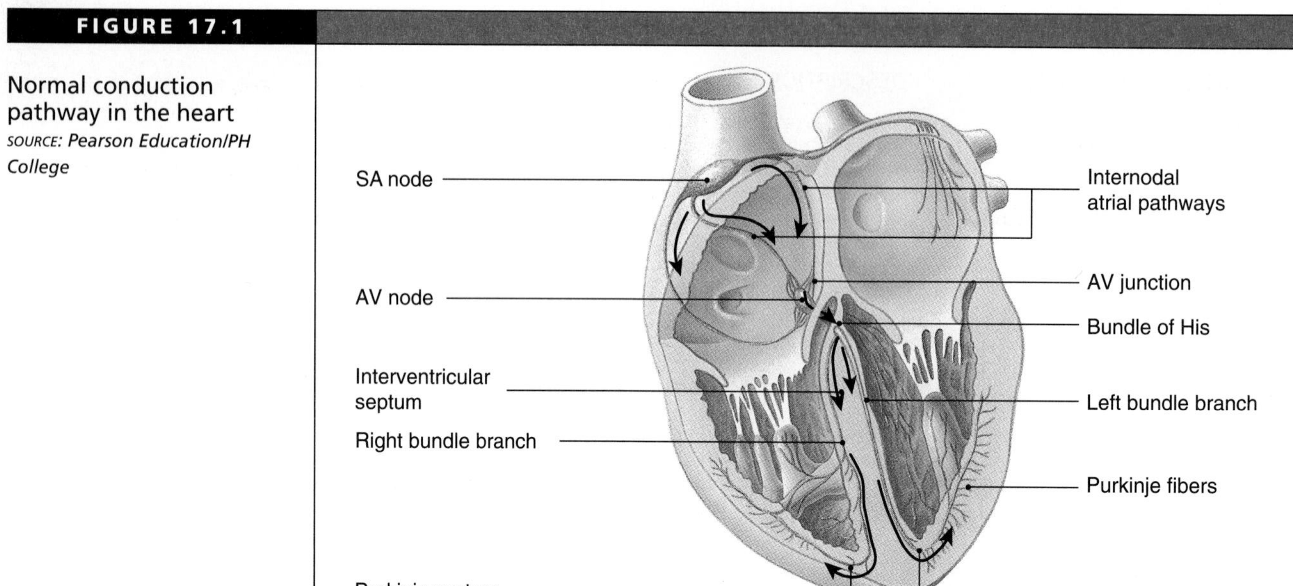

and left ventricles then must contract simultaneously. Lack of synchronization of the atria and ventricles or of the right and left sides of the heart may have serious consequences. The normal conduction pathway in the heart is illustrated in Figure 17.1 ■.

Normal control of this synchronization begins in a small area of tissue in the wall of the right atrium known as the **sinoatrial (SA) node.** The SA node or pacemaker of the heart has a property called **automaticity,** the ability of certain cells to spontaneously generate an electrical impulse known as an *action potential,* without instructions from the nervous system. The SA node generates a new action potential approximately 75 times every minute under resting conditions. This is referred to as the normal **sinus rhythm.**

On leaving the SA node, the action potential travels quickly across both atria to the **atrioventricular (AV) node.** The AV node also has the property of automaticity, although less so than the SA node. If the SA node malfunctions, the AV node has the ability to spontaneously generate action potentials and continue the heart's contraction.

As the action potential leaves the AV node, it travels rapidly to the **atrioventricular bundle** or bundle of His. The impulse is then conducted down the right and left **bundle branches** to the **Purkinje fibers,** which carry the impulse to all regions of the ventricles almost simultaneously.

The wave of electrical activity across the myocardium can be measured by the **electrocardiogram (ECG).** The total time for the electrical impulse to travel across the heart is about 0.22 second. A normal ECG and its relationship to impulse conduction in the heart are shown in Figure 17.2 ■.

ec = *outside*
top = *place*
ic = *pertaining to*

Although action potentials normally begin at the SA node and spread across the myocardium in a coordinated manner, other regions of the heart may begin to initiate beats. These areas, known as **ectopic foci** or **ectopic pacemakers,** may send impulses across the myocardium that compete with those from the normal conduction system. Although healthy hearts often experience an extra beat without incident, ectopic foci in diseased hearts have the potential to cause many of the types of dysrhythmias noted in Table 17.1.

It is important to understand that the underlying purpose of this conduction system is to keep the heart beating in a regular, synchronized manner so that cardiac output can be maintained. Some dysrhythmias occur sporadically, produce no symptoms, and cause little or no effect on cardiac output. These types of abnormalities may go unnoticed by the patient, and rarely require treatment. Some dysrhythmias, however, seriously affect cardiac output, producing patient symptoms and resulting in potentially serious, if not mortal, consequences. It is these types of dysrhythmias that require pharmacological treatment.

Concept Review 17.1

- Trace the flow of electrical conduction through the heart. What would happen if the impulse never reached the AV node?

FIGURE 17.2

Relationship of the ECG to electrical conduction in the heart

SOURCE: Pearson Education/PH College

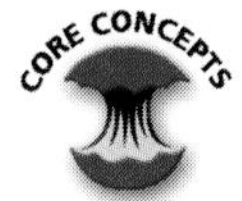

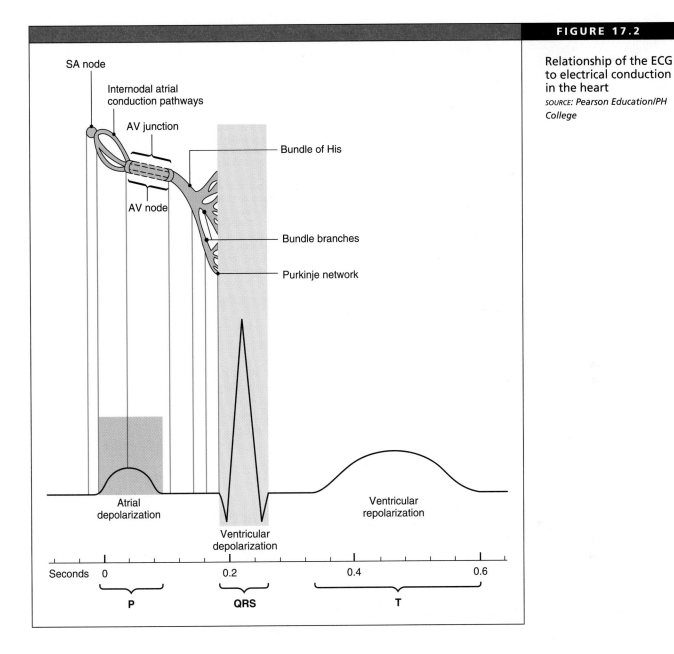

17.4 Nonpharmacological therapy of certain dysrhythmias is often the treatment of choice.

The goals of antidysrhythmic pharmacotherapy are to terminate dysrhythmias and to reduce the frequency of abnormal rhythms in order to decrease the possibility of sudden death, stroke, or other complications resulting from the disease. Because they can cause serious side effects, antidysrhythmic drugs are normally reserved for patients experiencing overt symptoms or for those whose condition cannot be controlled by other means. There is little or no benefit to the patient in treating asymptomatic dysrhythmias with drugs. There are several nonpharmacological strategies that physicians use to eliminate dysrhythmias.

The more serious types of dysrhythmias are corrected through electrical shock of the heart, a treatment called **cardioversion** or **defibrillation.** The electrical shock momentarily stops all electrical impulses in the heart, both normal and abnormal. Under ideal conditions, the temporary cessation of electrical activity allows the SA node to automatically return conduction to a normal sinus rhythm.

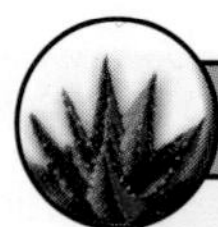

NATURAL ALTERNATIVES

Coenzyme Q10 and Cardiovascular Disease

Coenzyme Q10 is a vitaminlike substance found in most animal cells. It is an essential component in the cell's mitochondria for producing energy, or adenosine triphosphate (ATP). Because the heart requires high levels of ATP, a sufficient level of coenzyme Q10 is particularly important to that organ.

A normal dietary intake of coenzyme Q10 is 2–5 mg/day. Foods richest in this substance are pork, sardines, beef heart, salmon, broccoli, spinach, and nuts. Elderly adults appear to have an increased need for coenzyme Q10. Although coenzyme Q10 can be synthesized by the body, many amino acids and other substances are required; thus, patients having a number of different nutritional deficiencies may need supplementation.

In 1978, a Nobel Prize was awarded for research proving the importance of coenzyme Q10 in energy transfer, but it was not until the 1990s that the substance became the top-selling supplement in health food stores. Coenzyme Q10 is claimed to aid a wide range of conditions, including heart failure, hypertension, dysrhythmias, angina, diabetes, neurological disorders, cancer, and aging. A considerable body of research has begun to accumulate, particularly regarding the role of coenzyme Q10 in heart disease. Some data have found below-normal levels of coenzyme Q10 in patients with heart failure. Studies suggest that the frequency of preventricular contractions may be reduced in some patients by supplementation with coenzyme Q10. Although most studies have demonstrated positive results, coenzyme Q10 has not been widely accepted by the conventional medical community. ■

Other types of nonpharmacological treatment include identification and destruction of the myocardial cells responsible for the abnormal conduction through a surgical procedure called catheter ablation. Cardiac pacemakers are sometimes inserted to correct the types of dysrhythmias that cause the heart to beat too slowly. Implantable cardioverter defibrillators (ICDs) are placed in a patient to restore normal rhythm by either pacing the heart or giving it an electric shock when dysrhythmias occur. In addition, the ICD is capable of storing information regarding the heart rhythm for the physician to evaluate.

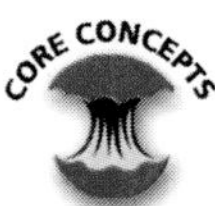

17.5 Most antidysrhythmic drugs act by blocking ion channels in myocardial cells.

Because most antidysrhythmic drugs act by interfering with the cardiac action potential, a firm grasp of this phenomenon is necessary for understanding drug mechanisms. Action potentials occur in both nervous and cardiac muscle cells because of changes in certain ions found inside and outside the cell. Under resting conditions, Na^+ and Ca^{++} are found in higher concentrations *outside* of myocardial cells, whereas K^+ is found in higher concentrations *inside* these cells. These imbalances are, in part, responsible for the inside of a myocardial cell membrane being slightly negatively charged, relative to the outside of the membrane. A cell having this negative membrane potential is said to be **polarized.**

An action potential begins when **sodium ion channels** located in the plasma membrane open and Na^+ rushes into the cell producing a rapid **depolarization,** or loss of membrane potential. During this period, Ca^{++} also enters the cell through **calcium ion channels.** It is this influx of Ca^{++} that is responsible for the contraction of cardiac muscle. The cell returns to its polarized state by the removal of K^+ through **potassium ion channels.** In cells located in the SA and AV nodes, it is the influx of Ca^{++}, rather than Na^+, that generates the rapid depolarization of the membrane. Although it may seem complicated to learn the different ions involved in an action potential, this is vital to cardiac pharmacology. Blocking potassium, sodium, or calcium ion channels is a pharmacological strategy used to terminate or prevent dysrhythmias. Figure 17.3 ■ illustrates the flow of ions during the action potential.

The pumping action of the heart requires alternating periods of contraction and relaxation. There is a brief period following depolarization that the cell cannot initiate another action potential. This time, known as the **refractory period,** ensures that the myocardial cell finishes contracting before a second action potential begins. The therapeutic effect of some antidysrhythmic agents is caused by their ability to prolong the refractory period.

FIGURE 17.3

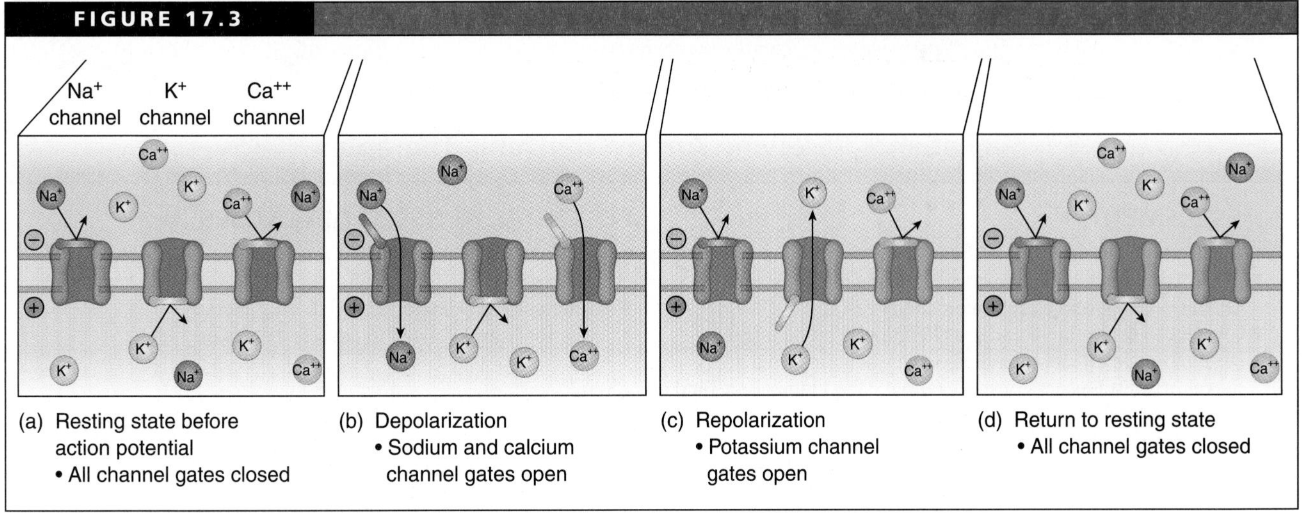

Ion channels in myocardial cells

17.6 Antidysrhythmic drugs are classified by their mechanisms of action.

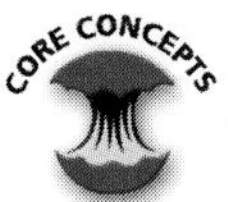

Antidysrhythmic drugs are classified by the stage at which they affect the action potential. These drugs fall into four primary classes and a miscellaneous group that does not act by one of the first four mechanisms. Categories of antidysrhythmics include the following.

- Sodium channel blockers (Class I)
- Beta-adrenergic blockers (Class II)
- Potassium channel blockers (Class III)
- Calcium channel blockers (Class IV)
- Miscellaneous antidysrhythmic drugs

All antidysrhythmic drugs have the potential to profoundly affect the heart's conduction system. The difference (called *safety margin*) between the optimal therapeutic dose and the toxic dose is narrow. As such, they not only have the ability to correct dysrhythmias; they also have the ability to worsen or even create new dysrhythmias. The healthcare provider must carefully monitor patients taking antidysrhythmic drugs. Often, the patient is hospitalized during the initial stages of therapy so that the optimum dose can be accurately determined.

17.7 Sodium channel blockers slow the rate of impulse conduction through the heart.

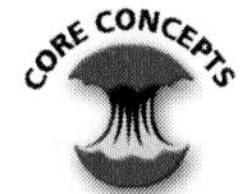

The first medical uses of the sodium channel blockers were recorded in the 18th century, and many are still widely prescribed. Sodium channel blockers used as antidysrhythmics are listed in Table 17.2.

Sodium channel blockers, the Class I drugs, are the largest group of antidysrhythmics. They are further divided into three subgroups, IA, IB, and IC, based on subtle differences in their mechanisms of action. Because progression of the action potential depends on the opening of sodium ion channels, a blockade of these channels will slow the spread of impulse conduction across the myocardium.

The sodium channel blockers are similar in structure and action to local anesthetics. In fact, lidocaine is a prototype local anesthetic in Chapter 13. This anesthetic action slows impulse conduction across the heart. Some, such as quinidine and procainamide, are effective against

NURSING PROCESS FOCUS

Patients Receiving Antidysrhythmic Therapies

ASSESSMENT

Prior to administration:

- Obtain complete health history including allergies, drug history, and possible drug interactions
- Assess to determine if cardiac alteration is producing a symptomatic effect on cardiac output including vital signs, level of consciousness, urinary output, skin temperature, and peripheral pulses
- Obtain baseline ECG to compare throughout therapy

POTENTIAL NURSING DIAGNOSES

- Ineffective Tissue Perfusion, related to cardiac conduction abnormality
- Deficient Knowledge, related to drug therapy
- Risk for Injury, related to adverse effects of drug

PLANNING: Patient Goals and Expected Outcomes

The patient will:

- Exhibit improved cardiac output as evidenced by stabilization of heart rate, heart rhythm, sensorium, urinary output, and vital signs
- State expected outcomes of drug therapy
- Demonstrate an understanding of the drug's action by accurately describing drug side effects and precautions

IMPLEMENTATION

Interventions and (Rationales)	Patient Education/Discharge Planning
■ Ensure cardiac rate and rhythm is monitored continuously if administering drug IV. (IV route is used when rapid therapeutic effects are needed. Constant monitoring is needed to detect any potential serious dysrhythmias.) ■ Monitor IV site. Administer all parenteral medication via infusion pump.	■ Explain the need for continuous ECG monitoring when administering the medication intravenously. ■ Instruct patient to report any burning or stinging pain, swelling, warmth, redness, or tenderness at the IV insertion site.
■ Investigate possible causes of the dysrhythmia such as electrolyte imbalances, hypoxia, pain, anxiety, caffeine ingestion, and tobacco use.	Instruct patient to: ■ Maintain a diet low in sodium and fat with sufficient potassium ■ Report illness such as flu, vomiting, diarrhea, and dehydration to healthcare provider to avoid adverse effects ■ Restrict use of caffeine and tobacco products
■ Observe for side effects specific to the antidysrhythmic used.	Instruct patient to: ■ Report adverse effects specific to prescribed antidysrhythmic ■ Report palpitations, chest pain, dyspnea, unusual fatigue, weakness, and visual disturbances
■ Monitor for proper use of medication.	Instruct patient to: ■ Never discontinue the drug abruptly ■ Take the drug exactly as prescribed, even if feeling well ■ Take pulse prior to taking the drug (Instruct patient regarding the normal range and rhythm of pulse; instruct to consult the healthcare provider regarding "reportable" pulse.)

EVALUATION OF OUTCOME CRITERIA

Evaluate the effectiveness of drug therapy by confirming that patient goals and expected outcomes have been met (see "Planning").

See Tables 17.2 through 17.6 for lists of drugs to which these nursing actions apply.

TABLE 17.2 Sodium Channel Blockers (Class I)

DRUG	RATE AND ADULT DOSE	REMARKS
disopyramide phosphate (Norpace, Nopamide)	PO 100–200 mg qid (max: 800 mg/day)	Class 1A; sustained-release form available; usually reserved for serious ventricular dysrhythmias
flecainide (Tambocor)	PO 100 mg bid; increase by 500 mg bid every 4 days (max: 400 mg/day)	Class 1C; usually reserved for serious ventricular dysrhythmias
lidocaine (Xylocaine)	IV 1–4 mg/min infusion; no more than 200–300 mg should be infused in a 1-hour period	Class 1B; usually reserved for rapid control of ventricular dysrhythmias; IM, subcutaneous, and topical forms available; also widely used as a local anesthetic
mexiletine (Mexitil)	PO 200–300 mg tid (max: 1200 mg/day)	Class 1B; usually reserved for serious ventricular dysrhythmias
moricizine (Ethmozine)	PO 200–300 mg tid (max: 900 mg/day)	Class 1B; usually reserved for serious ventricular dysrhythmias
phenytoin (Dilantin)	IV 50–100 mg every 10–15 min until dysrhythmia is terminated (max: 1 g/day)	Class 1B; unlabeled use for dysrhythmias induced by cardiac glycosides; oral form is used to treat convulsions
procainamide (Procan, Pronestyl, Procanbid)	PO 1-g loading dose followed by 250–500 mg every 3 hours	Class 1A; IM, IV, and sustained-release forms available; for both supraventricular and ventricular dysrhythmias
propafenone (Rythmol)	PO 150–300 mg tid (max: 900 mg/day)	Class 1C; usually reserved for serious ventricular dysrhythmias
quinidine gluconate (Duraquin, Quinaglute), Pr quinidine sulfate (Quinidex)	PO 200–600 mg tid or qid (max: 3–4 g/day)	Class 1A; gluconate salt is also available in IM and IV forms; sustained-release forms available for the sulfate and gluconate salts
tocainide (Tonocard)	PO 400–600 mg tid (max: 2.4 g/day)	Class 1B; usually reserved for serious ventricular dysrhythmias

many types of dysrhythmias. The remaining Class I drugs are more specific and indicated only for life-threatening ventricular dysrhythmias.

The side effects of the sodium blockers vary with each individual drug. All these agents can cause new dysrhythmias or worsen existing ones; thus, frequent ECGs should be obtained. The slowing of the heart can result in hypotension, dizziness, and fainting. Some Class I drugs have significant anticholinergic side effects such as dry mouth, constipation, and urinary retention.

Life Span Fact

Special attention should be given to older adults because anticholinergic side effects may worsen urinary hesitancy in patients with prostate enlargement.

Concept Review 17.2

- Why does slowing the speed of the electrical impulse across the myocardium sometimes correct a dysrhythmia?

17.8 Beta-adrenergic blockers reduce automaticity and slow conduction velocity in the heart.

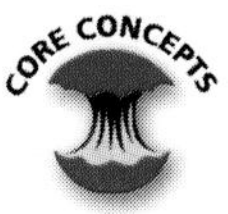

Beta blockers are widely used for cardiovascular disorders. Their ability to slow the heart rate and conduction velocity can suppress several types of dysrhythmias. Beta blockers of importance to dysrhythmias are listed in Table 17.3.

The basic pharmacology of beta-adrenergic blockers was explained in Chapter 7. Beta blockers are used to treat a large number of cardiovascular diseases, including hypertension, MI, heart failure, and dysrhythmias. Although the effects of beta blockers on the heart are complex,

DRUG PROFILE: Sodium Channel Blocker: *Quinidine sulfate (Quinidex)*

Actions and Uses:

Quinidine, the oldest antidysrhythmic drug, was originally obtained as a natural substance from the bark of the South American *Cinchona* tree. Like other drugs in this class, quinidine blocks sodium ion channels in myocardial cells, thus reducing automaticity and slowing conduction of the electrical impulse through the myocardium. This slight delay in conduction velocity can suppress dysrhythmias. Quinidine is referred to as a broad-spectrum drug because it has the ability to correct many different types of atrial and ventricular dysrhythmias.

Adverse Effects and Interactions:

The most common side effects of quinidine are gastrointestinal and include nausea, vomiting, and diarrhea. A potentially serious interaction can occur when quinidine is given concurrently with digoxin. Because quinidine has the potential to double digoxin levels in the blood, the dose of digoxin must be reduced accordingly and carefully monitored. Like all antidysrhythmic drugs, quinidine has the ability to produce new dysrhythmias or worsen existing ones; thus, patients should be frequently assessed for changes in cardiac status. Quinidine sulfate interacts with many other drugs. For example, it may increase digoxin levels by 50%. Amiodarone may increase quinidine levels, thus increasing the risk of heart block. Phenothiazines add to quinidine's cardiac depressant effects.

Use cautiously with herbal supplements. For example, because of their laxative effects, aloe and buckthorn may cause potassium deficiency and increase antidysrhythmic action.

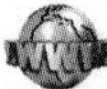

See the Companion Website for a Nursing Process Focus specific to this drug.

TABLE 17.3 Beta-adrenergic Blockers Used for Dysrhythmias (Class II)

DRUG	RATE AND ADULT DOSE	REMARKS
acebutolol (Sectral)	PO 200–600 mg bid (max: 1200 mg/day)	Cardioselective $beta_1$ blocker; usually reserved for ventricular dysrhythmias; also for hypertension and angina
esmolol (Brevibloc)	IV 50 mcg/kg/min maintenance dose (max: 200 mcg/kg/min)	Cardioselective $beta_1$ blocker; usually reserved for immediate control of severe atrial dysrhythmias; very short half-life of 9 min
propranolol (Inderal)	PO 10–30 mg tid or 4 times per day (max: 320 mg/day), IV 0.5–3 mg every 4 hours prn	Sustained-release forms available; also for hypertension, prevention of MI, angina, and migraines

their basic actions are to slow the heart rate and decrease conduction velocity through the AV node. Myocardial automaticity is reduced, and many types of dysrhythmias are stabilized. The main value of beta blockers as antidysrhythmic agents is to treat atrial dysrhythmias associated with heart failure.

Only three beta blockers are approved for dysrhythmias because of their potential side effects. Blockade of beta receptors in the heart may result in bradycardia. Hypotension may cause dizziness and possible fainting. Beta blockers that affect $beta_2$ receptors will also affect the lungs, causing bronchospasm. This is of particular concern in patients with asthma and in elderly patients with chronic obstructive pulmonary disease (COPD).

Concept Review 17.3

- Why are selective alpha-adrenergic blockers such as doxazosin (Cardura) of no value in treating dysrhythmias?

DRUG PROFILE: Beta-adrenergic Blocker: Propranolol (Inderal)

Actions and Uses:

Until 1978, propranolol was the only beta blocker approved to treat dysrhythmias. Propranolol is a nonselective beta-adrenergic blocker, affecting both $beta_1$ receptors in the heart and $beta_2$ receptors in the lungs. Propranolol reduces heart rate, slows conduction velocity, and lowers blood pressure. Propranolol is most effective against tachycardia and is often combined with other drugs such as digoxin (Lanoxin) or quinidine (Quinidex) in the treatment of cardiovascular disease. It is approved to treat a wide variety of disorders, including hypertension, angina, and migraine headaches. It is also used to help prevent MI.

Adverse Effects and Interactions:

Common side effects of propranolol include hypotension and bradycardia. Because of its ability to slow the heart rate, patients with other cardiac disorders such as heart failure must be carefully monitored. Side effects such as diminished sex drive and impotence may result in noncompliance.

Propranolol interacts with many other drugs, including phenothiazines, which have additive hypotensive effects. Propranolol should not be given within 2 weeks of an MAO inhibitor. Beta-adrenergic agents such as albuterol block the actions of propranolol.

Mechanism in Action: 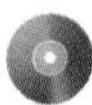

Propranolol is a nonspecific beta blocker that reduces automaticity and conduction velocity in the heart. These effects are achieved by interfering with the binding of natural adrenergic substances such as dopamine, epinephrine, and norepinephrine, all of which increase cardiac conduction, heart rate, force of contraction, and blood pressure.

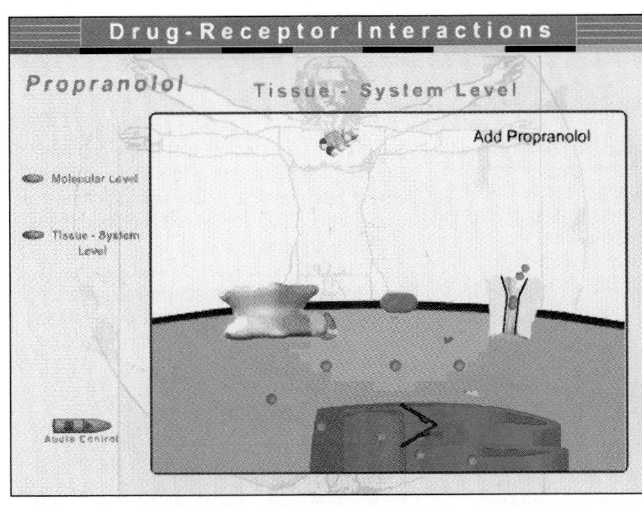

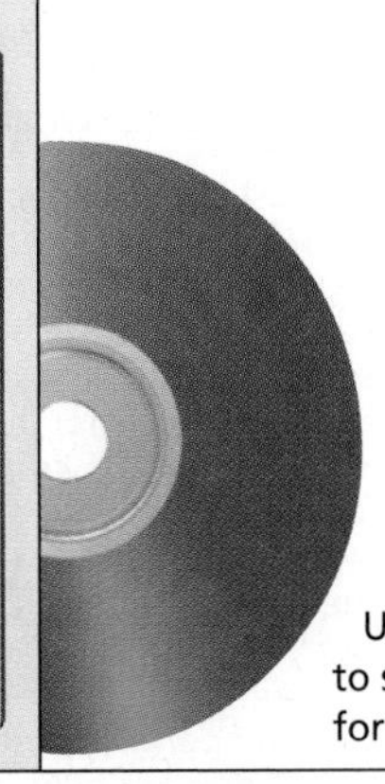

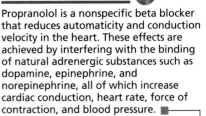

Use the student CD-ROM to see Mechanism in Action for Propranolol.

 *See the Companion Website for a Nursing Process Focus specific to this drug.*

17.9 Potassium channel blockers prolong the refractory period of the heart.

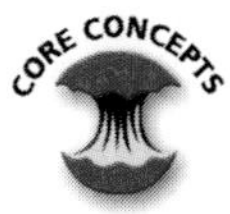

Although they comprise a small class of drugs, the potassium channel blockers (Class III) have important applications to the treatment of dysrhythmias. Potassium channel blockers used as antidysrhythmics are shown in Table 17.4.

The drugs in Class III exert their actions by blocking potassium ion channels in myocardial cells. After the action potential has passed and the myocardial cell is in a depolarized state, repolarization depends on removal of potassium from the cell. The Class III drugs prolong the duration of the action potential by lengthening the refractory period (resting stage), which tends to stabilize dysrhythmias.

Drugs in this class generally have restricted uses because of potentially serious side effects. Like other antidysrhythmics, potassium channel blockers slow the heart rate, resulting in bradycardia and possible hypotension. These side effects occur in a significant number of patients. These agents can worsen dysrhythmias, especially following the first few doses.

Life Span Fact

The health professional should carefully monitor older adults with preexisting heart failure because these patients are particularly at risk to the cardiac side effects of potassium channel blockers.

TABLE 17.4 Potassium Channel Blockers (Class III)

DRUG	RATE AND ADULT DOSE	REMARKS
Pr amiodarone (Cordarone, Pacerone)	PO 400–600 mg/day in 1–2 divided doses; maintenance dose (max: 1600 mg/day as loading dose)	IV form available; usually reserved for serious ventricular dysrhythmias
bretylium (Bretylol)	IV 1–2 mg/min continuous infusion (max: 30 mg/kg/day)	Approved for hypotension in 1959 but no longer used for that purpose; usually reserved for serious ventricular dysrhythmias; IM form available
dofetilide (Tikosyn)	PO 125–500 mcg bid based on creatinine clearance (no max dose available)	Usually for atrial dysrhythmias
ibutilide (Corvert)	IV 1 mg (10 ml) infused over 10 min	Usually reserved for atrial flutter or fibrillation
sotalol (Betapace)	PO 80 mg bid (max: 320 mg/day)	Usually reserved for serious ventricular dysrhythmias; also a nonselective beta-adrenergic blocker

DRUG PROFILE: Potassium Channel Blocker: Pr *Amiodarone (Cardarone)*

Actions and Uses:

Amiodarone is approved for the treatment of resistant ventricular tachycardia that may prove life threatening, and it has become a drug of choice for the treatment of atrial dysrhythmias in patients with heart failure. In addition to blocking potassium ion channels, some of amiodarone's actions on the heart relate to its blockade of sodium ion channels. Its onset of action may take several weeks when the drug is given orally. Its effects, however, can last 4–8 weeks after the drug is discontinued because it has an extended half-life that may exceed 100 days.

Adverse Effects and Interactions:

The most serious adverse effects from amiodarone occur in the lung, with the drug causing a pneumonia-like syndrome. The drug also causes blurred vision, rashes, photosensitivity, nausea, vomiting, anorexia, fatigue, dizziness, and hypotension. Amiodarone increases digoxin levels in the blood and enhances the actions of anticoagulants. As with other antidysrhythmics, patients must be closely monitored to avoid serious toxicity.

Amiodarone interacts with many other drugs. For example, it increases digoxin levels in the blood and enhances the actions of anticoagulants. If used together with beta-adrenergic blockers, sinus bradycardia may increase, and sinus arrest and atrioventricular block may occur. Amiodarone increases phenytoin levels two- to threefold.

Use cautiously with herbal supplements such as echinacea, which may cause increased liver toxicity. Aloe may increase the effect of amiodarone.

Mechanism in Action: 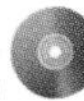

Amiodarone is effective in maintaining sinus rhythm in patients with atrial fibrillation, recurrent ventricular tachycardia, and fibrillations that are resistant to other drugs. Amiodarone blocks inactivated sodium and potassium channels and interferes with myocardial cell-to-cell coupling.

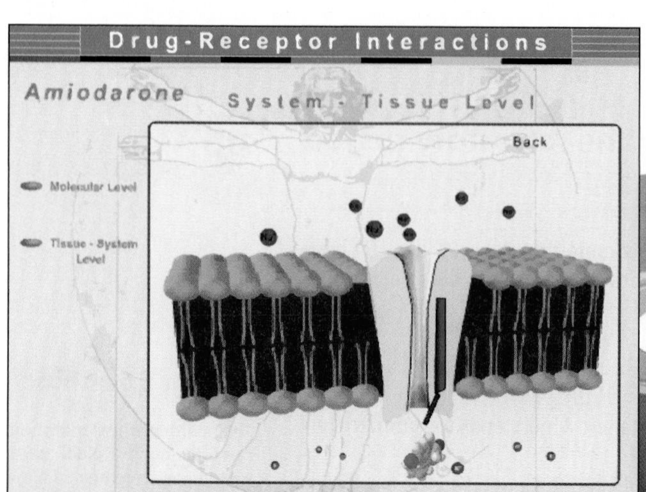

Use the student CD-ROM to see Mechanism in Action for Amiodarone.

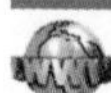 *See the Companion Website for a Nursing Process Focus specific to this drug.*

TABLE 17.5 Calcium Channel Blockers for Dysrhythmias (Class IV)

DRUG	RATE AND ADULT DOSE	REMARKS
diltiazem (Cardizem, Dilacor, Tiamate, Tiazac)	IV 5–15 mg/hr continuous infusion (max: 15 mg/hour) for a maximum of 24 hr	Oral and sustained-release forms available for hypertension and angina
Pr verapamil (Calan, Isoptin, Verelan)	PO 80–160 mg tid (max: 360 mg/day)	Sustained-release and IV forms available; also for hypertension, angina, and migraines

17.10 Two calcium channel blockers are available to treat supraventricular dysrhythmias.

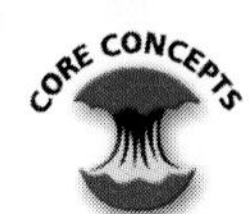

Like the beta blockers, the calcium channel blockers (Class IV) are widely prescribed for various cardiovascular disorders. By slowing conduction velocity, they are able to stabilize certain dysrhythmias. Two important calcium channel blockers used for treating dysrhythmias are listed in Table 17.5.

Although about 10 calcium channel blockers (CCBs) are available to treat cardiovascular diseases, only a limited number have been approved for dysrhythmias. The basic pharmacology of this drug class was presented in Chapter 15. (Diltiazem is a profile drug in Chapter 18 on page 323.)

Blockade of calcium ion channels has a number of effects on the heart, most of which are similar to those of beta-adrenergic blockers. Effects include reduced automaticity in the SA node and slowed impulse conduction through the AV node. This prolongs the refractory period and stabilizes many types of dysrhythmias. Calcium channel blockers are only effective against supraventricular dysrhythmias.

Calcium channel blockers are safe medications that are well tolerated by most patients. As with other antidysrhythmics, patients should be carefully monitored for bradycardia and hypotension. Because their cardiac effects are almost identical to those of beta-adrenergic blockers, patients concurrently taking drugs from both classes are especially at risk for bradycardia and possible heart failure. Because older patients often have multiple cardiovascular disorders, such as hypertension, heart failure, and dysrhythmias, it is not unusual to find elderly patients taking drugs from multiple classes.

DRUG PROFILE: Calcium Channel Blocker: Pr *Verapamil (Calan)*

Actions and Uses:

Verapamil was the first CCB approved by the FDA. It acts by inhibiting the flow of Ca^{++} into myocardial cells and in vascular smooth muscle. In the heart, this action slows conduction velocity and stabilizes dysrhythmias. In the vessels, calcium ion channel inhibition lowers blood pressure. Verapamil also dilates the coronary arteries, an action that is important when the drug is used to treat angina (Chapter 18).

Adverse Effects and Interactions:

Side effects are generally minor and may include headache, constipation, and hypotension. Because verapamil can cause bradycardia, patients with heart failure should be carefully monitored. Like many other antidysrhythmics, it has the ability to elevate blood levels of digoxin. Because both digoxin and verapamil have the effect of slowing conduction through the AV node, their concurrent use must be carefully monitored.

Like many other antidysrhythmics, verapamil has the ability to elevate blood levels of digoxin. Because both digoxin and verapamil have the effect of slowing conduction through the atrioventricular node, their use together must be carefully monitored.

Grapefruit juice may increase verapamil levels. Use cautiously with herbal supplements, such as hawthorn, which may have additive hypotensive effects.

See the Companion Website for a Nursing Process Focus specific to this drug.

Concept Review 17.4

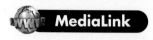

THE HEART RHYTHM SOCIETY

- Remembering the effects of digitalis on the heart from Chapter 16, explain why most antidysrhythmic drugs have the potential to cause serious side effects in patients taking cardiac glycosides.

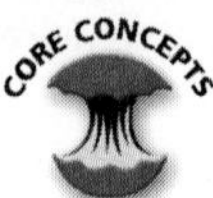

17.11 Digoxin and adenosine are used for specific dysrhythmias, but do not act by blocking ion channels.

Several other drugs are used to treat specific dysrhythmias, but do not act by the mechanisms described previously. These drugs are summarized in Table 17.6.

Although digoxin (Lanoxin) is primarily used to treat heart failure, it is also prescribed for certain types of atrial dysrhythmias because it decreases automaticity of the SA node and slows conduction through the AV node. Excessive levels of digoxin can produce serious dysrhythmias, and interactions with other medications are common; therefore, patients must be carefully monitored during therapy. The mechanism of action and adverse effects of digoxin are described in Chapter 16.

Adenosine (Adenocard) is given as a 1- to 2-second bolus IV injection to terminate serious atrial tachycardia by slowing conduction through the AV node and decreasing automaticity of the SA node. Its only indication is a specific dysrhythmia known as paroxysmal supraventricular tachycardia (PSVT), for which it is a drug of choice. Because of its 10-second half-life, side effects are generally self-limiting.

TABLE 17.6 Miscellaneous Drugs for Dysrhythmias

DRUG	RATE AND ADULT DOSE	REMARKS
adenosine (Adenocard, Adenoscan)	IV 6–12 mg given as a bolus injection	Usually reserved for atrial dysrhythmias; half-life is only 10 seconds
digoxin (Lanoxin)	PO 0.125–0.5 mg daily; dose is individualized for each patient	Usually reserved for atrial dysrhythmias; IV and IM forms available; also for heart failure

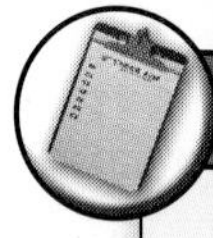

PATIENTS NEED TO KNOW

Patients treated for dysrhythmias need to know the following:

In General

1. Monitor heart rate and blood pressure regularly during treatment with adenosine (Adenocard, Adenoscan) or ibutilide (Corvert).
2. Monitor for a decreased rate and changes in rhythm while taking antidysrhythmic drugs. Report changes to a healthcare provider.

Regarding CCBs

3. Notify a healthcare provider if a very slow heart rate (less than 60 beats per minute), dizziness when standing up quickly, headache, or constipation is experienced.
4. Inform a healthcare practitioner if systolic blood pressure is less than 90 mm Hg, and do not take the next dose of CCB until instructed to do so.
5. Do not discontinue medication suddenly. It should be stopped gradually under the supervision of a healthcare provider.

Regarding Beta Blockers

6. Notify dentists, surgeons, and eye doctors if taking propranolol (Inderal). This drug lowers intraocular pressure.
7. For those with diabetes, check blood glucose regularly while taking beta blockers. These medications can change how the body uses sugars and starches. ■

CHAPTER REVIEW

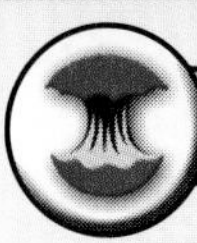

CORE CONCEPTS SUMMARY

17.1 Some types of dysrhythmias produce no patient symptoms, whereas others may be life threatening.

Some dysrhythmias produce no symptoms and are harmless, whereas others are life threatening. The frequency of dysrhythmias is difficult to ascertain, although it is thought to be quite common, particularly in the geriatric population.

17.2 Dysrhythmias are classified by their location and type of rhythm abnormality produced.

Dysrhythmias are classified by their site of origin, either atrial or ventricular, and by the type of rhythm abnormality produced, such as tachycardia, flutter, or fibrillation. Dysrhythmias are associated with diseases such as hypertension and heart failure.

17.3 The electrical conduction pathway in the myocardium keeps the heart beating in a synchronized manner.

The normal rhythm of the heart is established by the SA node, which ensures that the chambers beat in a synchronized manner. The central problem with dysrhythmias is their potential to affect the function of the heart, reduce cardiac output, and cause certain consequences such as stroke or heart failure.

17.4 Nonpharmacological therapy of certain dysrhythmias is often the treatment of choice.

All antidysrhythmic agents have the ability to cause rhythm abnormalities or worsen existing ones. Because of this, nonpharmacological treatment is sometimes preferred over drug therapy. Dysrhythmias may be corrected using cardioversion or catheter ablation.

17.5 Most antidysrhythmic drugs act by blocking ion channels in myocardial cells.

Antidysrhythmic drugs affect the action potential in myocardial cells. They act by blocking sodium, potassium, or calcium channels in the cell membrane.

17.6 Antidysrhythmic drugs are classified by their mechanisms of action.

Most antidysrhythmic medications are placed into one of five classes, based on their mechanisms of action. Class I agents are further subdivided into IA, IB, and IC. Agents within the same class have similar actions and adverse effects.

17.7 Sodium channel blockers slow the rate of impulse conduction through the heart.

Sodium channel blockers stabilize dysrhythmias by slowing the spread of impulse conduction across the myocardium. Quinidine, a Class IA agent, is the oldest antidysrhythmic drug.

17.8 Beta-adrenergic blockers reduce automaticity and slow conduction velocity in the heart.

Beta blockers such as propranolol stabilize dysrhythmias by slowing the heart rate and decreasing the conduction velocity through the AV node.

17.9 Potassium channel blockers prolong the refractory period of the heart.

Potassium channel blockers such as amiodarone stabilize dysrhythmias by prolonging the duration of the action potential and extending the refractory period.

17.10 Two calcium channel blockers are available to treat supraventricular dysrhythmias.

Calcium channel blockers such as verapamil have effects similar to those of beta-adrenergic blockers. These include reduced automaticity in the SA node, slowed impulse conduction through the AV node, and a prolonged refractory period.

17.11 Digoxin and adenosine are used for specific dysrhythmias, but do not act by blocking ion channels.

Digoxin and adenosine are used for specific dysrhythmias, but do not act by the mechanisms of Class I, II, III, or IV drugs. Adenosine is used for short-term, rapid termination of dysrhythmias.

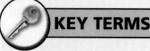

KEY TERMS

atrioventricular bundle (ay-tree-oh-ven-TRIK-you-lur BUN-dul): specialized cardiac tissue that receives electrical impulses from the AV node and sends them to the bundle branches, also known as the *bundle of His* / ***page 298***

atrioventricular (AV) node (ay-tree-oh-ven-TRIK-you-lur noad): mass of cardiac tissue that receives electrical impulses from the SA node and conveys them to the ventricles / ***page 298***

automaticity (aw-toh-muh-TISS-uh-tee): ability of certain myocardial cells to spontaneously generate an action potential / ***page 298***

bradycardia (bray-dee-KAR-DEE-uh): condition of slow heartbeat / ***page 297***

bundle branches (BUN-dul BRAN-chez): electrical conduction pathway in the heart leading from the AV bundle and through the wall between the ventricles / ***page 298***

calcium ion channel (KAL-see-um): pathway in a plasma membrane through which calcium ions enter and leave / ***page 300***

cardioversion/defibrillation (kar-dee-oh-VER-shun/dee-fib-ree-LAY-shun): conversion of fibrillation to a normal heart rhythm / ***page 299***

depolarization (dee-po-lur-eye-ZAY-shun): condition in which the plasma membrane charge is changed such that the inside is made less negative / ***page 300***

dysrhythmia (diss-RITH-mee-uh): abnormality in cardiac rhythm / ***page 296***

ectopic foci/pacemakers (ek-TOP-ik FO-si): cardiac tissue outside the normal cardiac conduction pathway that generates action potentials / ***page 298***

electrocardiogram (ECG) (e-lek-tro-KAR-dee-oh-gram): device that records the electrical activity of the heart / ***page 298***

fibrillation (fi-bruh-LAY-shun): type of dysrhythmia in which the chambers beat in a highly disorganized manner / ***page 297***

flutter (FLUH-tur): type of dysrhythmia in which the contractions become extremely rapid / ***page 297***

polarized (POLE-uh-rized): condition in which the inside of a cell is more negatively charged than the outside of the cell / ***page 300***

potassium ion channel (po-TASS-ee-um): pathway in a plasma membrane through which potassium ions enter and leave / ***page 300***

Purkinje fibers (purr-KEN-gee FI-burrs): electrical conduction pathway leading from the bundle branches to all portions of the ventricles / ***page 298***

refractory period (ree-FRAK-tor-ee): time during which the myocardial cells rest and are not able to contract / ***page 300***

sinoatrial (SA) node (si-no-AYE-tree-ul noad): pacemaker of the heart located in the wall of the right atrium / ***page 298***

sinus rhythm (SI-nuss): number of beats per minute normally generated by the SA node / ***page 298***

sodium ion channel (SO-dee-um): pathway in a plasma membrane through which sodium ions enter and leave / ***page 300***

supraventricular (sue-prah-ven-TRIK-you-lur): lying above the ventricles or in the atria / ***page 297***

tachycardia (tack-ee-KAR-dee-uh): condition of fast heartbeat / ***page 297***

REVIEW QUESTIONS

The following questions are written in NCLEX-PN® style. Answer these questions to assess your knowledge of the chapter material, and go back and review any material that is not clear to you.

1. This electrolyte produces depolarization.

1. Potassium
2. Magnesium
3. Sodium
4. Chloride

2. Sodium channel blockers:

1. Reduce automaticity
2. Slow the impulse conduction
3. Prolong the refractory period
4. Increase impulse conduction

3. This antiseizure medication is used off label to treat dysrhythmias.

1. Phenobarbital
2. Topiramate (Topamax)
3. Flecainide (Tambocor)
4. Phenytoin (Dilantin)

4. When the patient is on quinidine sulfate (Quinidex), the digoxin must be:

1. Discontinued
2. Increased
3. Decreased
4. Doubled

5. An expected outcome of a patient taking an antidysrhythmic drug would be:

1. Decreased cardiac output
2. Increased cardiac output
3. Increased renal insufficiency
4. Increased hepatic insufficiency

6. The patient taking an antidysrhythmic must be instructed to notify the physician if:

1. Constipation occurs
2. The heart rate is less than 60 beats/minute
3. The heart rate is greater than 90 beats/minute
4. The blood pressure does not decrease

7. Common side effects of antidysrhythmic medications include:

1. Dizziness, hypotension, and weakness
2. Headache, hypertension, and fatigue
3. Weakness, fatigue, and hypertension
4. Anorexia, diarrhea, and hypertension

8. Which of the following would be included in the teaching plan for a patient taking an antidysrhythmic medication?

1. "Take the drug only when you are feeling excessively tired."
2. "Take your blood pressure and pulse after you take your medication."
3. "Do not drink alcohol unless you have spoken with your physician."
4. "You will need to increase your sodium and potassium intake."

9. This antidysrhythmic also is used to treat angina.

1. Digoxin (Lanoxin)
2. Verapamil (Calan)
3. Adenosine (Adenocard)
4. Quinidine sulfate (Quinidex)

10. This antidysrhythmic is also used to treat hypertension and angina.

1. Diltiazem (Cardizem)
2. Digoxin (Lanoxin)
3. Adenosine (Adenocard)
4. Quinidine sulfate (Quinidex)

CASE STUDY QUESTIONS

For questions 1–5, please refer to the following case study, and choose the correct answer from choices 1–4.

Mr. Duncan, who has a history of hypertension, has arrived in the emergency room with a life-threatening ventricular dysrhythmia. He has been placed on a IV lidocaine infusion.

1. Lidocaine would be expected to terminate this dysrhythmia primarily by which of the following mechanisms?

1. Speeding up the heart rate
2. Lowering blood pressure
3. Increasing the strength of myocardial contractions
4. Slowing the speed of electrical conduction across the myocardium

2. When Mr. Duncan is discharged from the hospital, he is placed on propranolol. What effect would this drug have on his hypertension?

1. This drug will worsen the hypertension.
2. This drug will lower his hypertension.
3. This drug will have no effect on his hypertension.

3. Beta blockers such as propranolol have actions and side effects most similar to which other class of antidysrhythmics?

1. Calcium channel blockers
2. Cardiac glycosides
3. Potassium channel blockers
4. Sodium channel blockers

4. The physician lowers the dose of propranolol and adds amiodarone to the drug regimen. Mr. Duncan experiences dizziness, fainting spells, and fatigue. Which of the following would *most likely* explain these symptoms?

1. Mr. Duncan is not eating enough potassium-rich foods.
2. The drug combination is causing bradycardia or hypotension.
3. The drug combination is causing respiratory depression.
4. Mr. Duncan's hypertension is out of control.

5. When taking these medications, Mr. Duncan should be instructed to:

1. Check his pulse rate frequently
2. Keep a log of weight gain or loss
3. Eat plenty of foods containing potassium
4. Avoid taking aspirin, unless instructed to do so by the physician

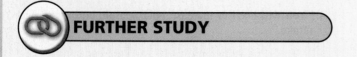

FURTHER STUDY

- The basic pharmacology of beta-adrenergic blockers is explained in Chapter 7.
- Calcium channel blockers are discussed in Chapter 15; diltiazem and verapamil are also discussed in Chapter 18.
- Chapter 16 covers the mechanism of action and adverse effects of digoxin.
- The actions of lidocaine, which are similar to those of the sodium channel blockers, are discussed in Chapter 13.

EXPLORE MEDIALINK www.prenhall.com/holland

Additional resources for this chapter can be found on the CD-ROM accompanying this textbook, and on the Companion Website. Click on Chapter 17 to select activities for this chapter.

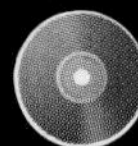

Mechanism in Action:
- **Propranolol**
- **Amiodarone**

Audio Glossary
Concept Review
NCLEX-PN® Review
Nursing in Action
Dosage Calculator

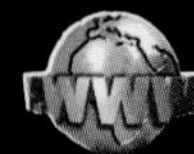

Childhood Dysrhythmias
The Heart Rhythm Society

CHAPTER

18 Drugs for Angina Pectoris, Myocardial Infarction, and Cerebrovascular Accident

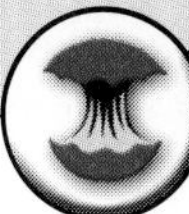

CORE CONCEPTS

18.1 Coronary heart disease is caused by a restriction in blood flow to the myocardium.

18.2 Angina pectoris is characterized by severe chest pain caused by lack of sufficient oxygen flow to heart muscle.

18.3 Anginal pain can often be controlled through lifestyle changes and surgical procedures.

18.4 The pharmacological goals for the treatment of angina are usually achieved by reducing cardiac workload.

18.5 The organic nitrates relieve anginal pain by dilating veins and the coronary arteries.

18.6 Beta-adrenergic blockers relieve anginal pain by decreasing the oxygen demands on the heart.

18.7 Calcium channel blockers relieve anginal pain by dilating the coronary vessels and reducing the workload on the heart.

18.8 Early diagnosis and treatment of myocardial infarction increases chances of survival.

18.9 Thrombolytics dissolve clots blocking the coronary arteries.

18.10 When given within 24 hours after the onset of MI, beta-adrenergic blockers can improve chances of survival.

18.11 A number of additional drugs are used to treat the symptoms and complications of acute MI.

18.12 Strokes are a major cause of death and disability.

18.13 Aggressive treatment of thrombotic stroke with anticoagulants, antihypertensives, and thrombolytics can increase survival.

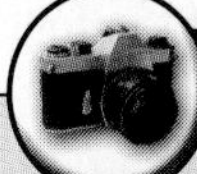

DRUG SNAPSHOT

The following drugs will be discussed in this chapter:

DRUG CLASSES	DRUG PROFILES
Organic nitrates	Pr nitroglycerin (Nitrostat)
Beta-adrenergic blockers	Pr atenolol (Tenormin)
	Pr metoprolol (Lopressor)
Calcium channel blockers	Pr diltiazem (Cardizem)
Thrombolytics	Pr reteplase (Retavase)

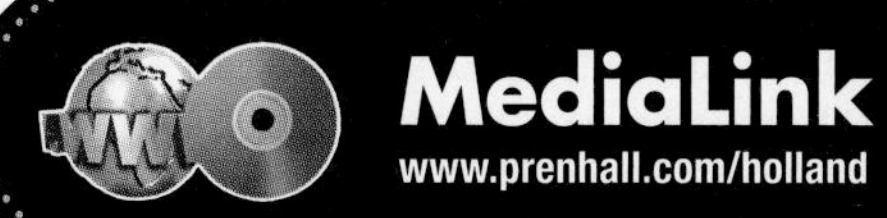

Interactive resources for this chapter can be found on the Companion Website. Click on Chapter 18 and "Begin" to select activities for this chapter. For chapter-related animations, NCLEX-PN®-style questions, and an audio glossary, access the accompanying CD-ROM in this book.

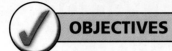

OBJECTIVES

After reading this chapter, the student should be able to:

1. Describe how the myocardium receives its oxygen and nutrient supply.
2. Explain the pathophysiology of angina pectoris.
3. Prescribe lifestyle changes by which a patient might control his or her angina.
4. For each of the following classes, identify representative drugs, explain the mechanisms of drug action, primary actions, and important adverse effects as they relate to the treatment of angina:
   - **a.** Organic nitrates
   - **b.** Beta-adrenergic blockers
   - **c.** Calcium channel blockers
5. Explain the pathophysiology of myocardial infarction.
6. For each of the following classes, identify representative drugs, explain the mechanisms of drug action, primary actions, and important adverse effects as they relate to the treatment of myocardial infarction:
   - **a.** Thrombolytics
   - **b.** Beta-adrenergic blockers
   - **c.** Anticoagulants and antiplatelet agents
   - **d.** Analgesics
7. Explain the pathophysiology of cerebrovascular accident (CVA).
8. Identify strategies used in the pharmacological treatment of CVA.
9. Categorize drugs used to treat angina, myocardial infarction, and CVA based on their classification and mechanisms of action.

All tissues in the body depend on an adequate supply of oxygen and other nutrients that are delivered via an extensive arterial system. When these vessels become clogged by fatty deposits or a clot, the tissues served by the affected arteries are starved for oxygen and their function is affected. This chapter covers the pharmacotherapy of three such diseases: angina pectoris, myocardial infarction, and cerebrovascular accident (CVA), also called stroke.

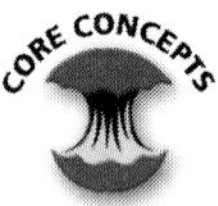

18.1 Coronary heart disease is caused by a restriction in blood flow to the myocardium.

The heart is the hardest working organ in the body. Whereas the activity of most organs slows considerably during rest and sleep, the heart must continue pumping so that the tissues can receive the nutrients they need and dispose of the wastes they have accumulated. Because it is such a vital organ, the heart muscle or myocardium must receive a continuous supply of oxygen and nutrients; disturbing this flow for even brief periods can have serious and even fatal consequences.

Because the heart chambers fill with blood more than 60 times per minute, one would think that the myocardium would have an ample supply of oxygen and nutrients. The myocardium, however, receives essentially no nutrients from the blood traveling through the heart's chambers. Instead, heart muscle receives its nutrients from the first two arteries branching off the aorta, the right and left **coronary arteries.** As these arteries branch, they circle the heart, bringing the myocardium its continuous supply of oxygen.

myo = *muscle*
cardium = *heart*

Coronary heart disease (CHD), also called coronary artery disease (CAD), is the term used to describe impaired blood flow in the coronary arteries. Moderate restriction of flow leads to angina pectoris. Severe impairment or complete loss of blood flow causes myocardial infarction and a high risk of sudden death. CHD can also cause dysrhythmias and lead to heart failure.

ANGINA PECTORIS

Angina pectoris is characterized by acute chest pain on physical exertion or emotional stress. Although it produces many of the same symptoms as a heart attack, its pharmacological treatment is quite different.

18.2 Angina pectoris is characterized by severe chest pain caused by lack of sufficient oxygen flow to heart muscle.

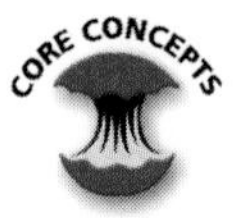

The most common cause of angina is **atherosclerosis:** a buildup of fatty, fibrous material called **plaque** in the walls of arteries. Although plaque may take as long as 40 to 50 years to accumulate to a level that would cause symptoms, plaque deposition actually begins very early in life. If plaque accumulates in a coronary artery, the myocardium downstream from the affected artery begins to receive less oxygen than it needs to perform its metabolic functions. This condition of having a reduced blood supply to cardiac muscle cells is called **myocardial ischemia.** Figure 18.1 ■ illustrates the progressive accumulation of plaque that is characteristic of atherosclerosis.

athero = *fatty*
sclera = *hard*
osis = *condition of*

The classic presentation of angina pectoris is sharp pain in the heart region, often moving to the left side of the neck and lower jaw and down the left arm. Most often this pain is preceded by physical exertion or emotional excitement. These events increase the oxygen demand of the heart, and the clogged artery is unable to supply the nutrients needed by the stressed myocardium. With rest, anginal pain usually diminishes in less than 15 minutes. Angina pectoris that is predictable in its frequency and duration is called **stable angina.** If angina episodes become more frequent or severe and occur during periods of rest, the condition is called **unstable angina.** Unstable angina requires more aggressive medical intervention. It is sometimes considered a medical emergency because it is associated with an increased risk of myocardial infarction (MI).

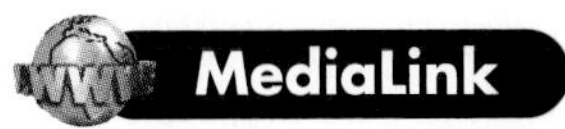

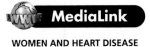

WOMEN AND HEART DISEASE

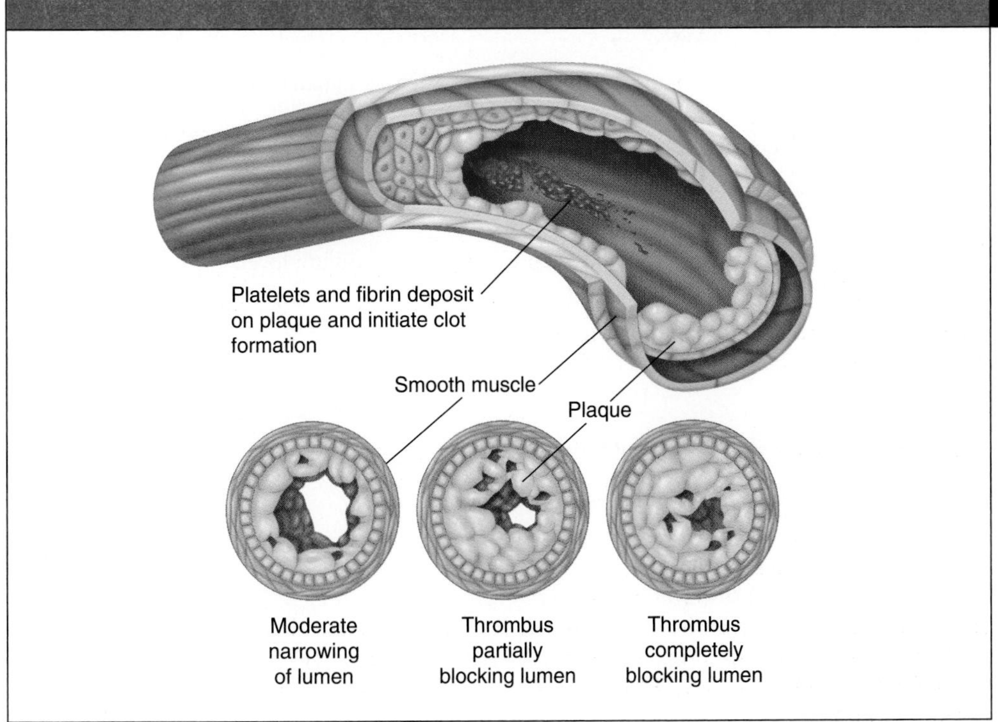

FIGURE 18.1

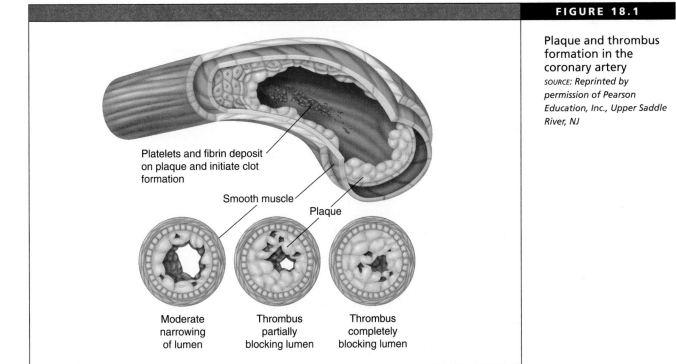

Plaque and thrombus formation in the coronary artery
SOURCE: Reprinted by permission of Pearson Education, Inc., Upper Saddle River, NJ

TABLE 18.1 Examples of Disorders That May Produce Chest Pain

NAME OF DISEASE	DESCRIPTION
Mitral stenosis	Inability of the mitral valve to fully open
Myocardial infarction	Clot within the coronary arteries
Hypertension	High systemic blood pressure
Coronary artery disease	Atherosclerosis of the coronary arteries
Diabetes	Lack of insulin or inability to tolerate carbohydrates
Peptic ulcer disease	Erosion of the mucosa of the stomach or small intestine
Gastric reflux	Backflow of stomach contents into the esophagus

Angina pain may closely mimic that of an MI. It is necessary for the healthcare provider to quickly distinguish between the two diseases because the pharmacologic treatment of angina is much different than that of MI. Whereas angina is rarely fatal, MI has a high mortality rate if treatment is delayed. Thus, drug therapy must begin immediately.

Chest pain is a common complaint of patients seeking care in physician offices and emergency rooms. It is also one of the most frightening symptoms for patients, who often equate their pain to having MI with a real risk of sudden death. The pain experienced by the patient, however, is only a symptom of an underlying disorder; a large number of diverse diseases can produce pain in the chest, and some of these are unrelated to the heart. A major goal of the healthcare provider is to quickly determine the cause of the pain so that the proper treatment can be administered. Table 18.1 lists some of the common diseases that can produce chest pain as a symptom.

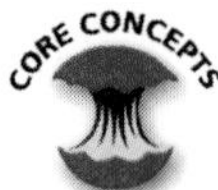

18.3 Anginal pain can often be controlled through lifestyle changes and surgical procedures.

A number of dietary and lifestyle factors are associated with an increased incidence of angina. The healthcare provider should help the patient control the frequency of anginal episodes by advising him or her to implement some or all of the following lifestyle changes:

- Stop using tobacco.
- Limit salt (sodium) intake.
- Eat foods rich in potassium and magnesium, such as bananas, beans, spinach, and tomatoes.
- Limit alcohol consumption.
- Implement a medically supervised exercise plan.
- Reduce stress levels as much as possible.
- Reduce dietary saturated fats and keep weight at an optimum level.
- If hyperlipidemia is present, have it treated.
- If hypertension is present, have it treated.

Fast Facts Angina Pectoris

- The incidence of angina peaks in the 75 to 84 age group:
  4% of those 65 to 74 years old
  6% of those 75 to 84 years old
  4% of those older than age 85
- About 6.2 million Americans have angina pectoris; 350,000 new cases occur each year.
- Among ethnic groups, the incidence of angina is highest among Blacks, intermediate in Mexican Americans, and lowest in non-Hispanic whites.
- Angina occurs more frequently in women than men; black women have twice the risk of black men.

When physicians discover that the coronary arteries are significantly blocked (or occluded), **coronary arterial bypass graft (CABG)** or **percutaneous transluminal coronary angioplasty (PTCA)** may be performed. CABG involves the use of a surgically implanted vein graft to bypass the area of obstruction in the coronary artery. PCTA is a procedure whereby the area of narrowing is opened using either a balloon catheter or a laser. The procedure carries some risk and is not 100% effective; however, it is less invasive than CABG and many patients benefit from the procedure.

angio = *vessel*
plasty = *shaped or molded by a surgical procedure*

per = *through*
cutaneous = *skin*

Concept Review 18.1

- How can a healthcare provider distinguish between stable angina and unstable angina?

18.4 The pharmacological goals for the treatment of angina are usually achieved by reducing cardiac workload.

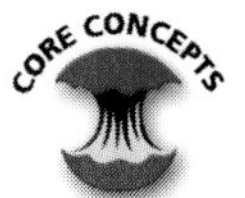

The treatment goals for a patient with angina are twofold: to *reduce the frequency* of anginal episodes and to *terminate* acute anginal pain in progress. The primary means by which antianginal drugs act is by reducing the myocardial demand for oxygen. This reduced demand can be accomplished by at least four mechanisms:

- Slowing the heart rate
- Causing the heart to receive less blood (reduced *preload*) by dilating veins
- Causing the heart to contract with less force (reduced *contractility*)
- Lowering blood pressure, thus giving the heart less resistance in pushing the blood out of its chambers (reduced *afterload*)

Three classes of drugs—organic nitrates, beta-adrenergic blockers, and calcium channel blockers—are used to treat angina. Drug therapy of stable angina is usually begun with the rapid-acting organic nitrates. If episodes become more frequent or severe, oral organic nitrates, beta-adrenergic blockers, or calcium channel blockers are added for prophylaxis. It is important to understand that the antianginal medications relieve symptoms but do not cure the underlying disorder. A summary of the means used to prevent and treat coronary artery disease is shown in Figure 18.2 ■.

18.5 The organic nitrates relieve anginal pain by dilating veins and the coronary arteries.

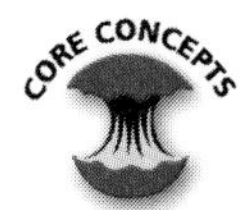

All drugs in this chemical class possess at least one nitrate (NO_2) group. The vasodilation effect of these agents is a result of the conversion of nitrate to its active form, nitric oxide (NO). Another nitrogen-containing drug, nitrous oxide (N_2O), is used in anesthesia (Chapter 13 ∞). Organic nitrates used to treat angina are listed in Table 18.2.

Since their medicinal properties were discovered in 1857, the organic nitrates have been the mainstay for the treatment of angina. The primary therapeutic action of these agents is their ability to relax both arterial and venous smooth muscle. When the organic nitrates cause venodilation, the amount of blood returning to the heart, or *preload,* is reduced and the chambers contain less blood. With less blood to eject, cardiac output (*afterload*) is reduced and the work required of the heart is decreased, thus lowering myocardial oxygen demand. This is the primary mechanism by which the organic nitrates reduce the frequency of acute anginal episodes and terminate chest pain in patients with stable angina.

Organic nitrates also have the ability to dilate coronary arteries, and this was once thought to be their primary mechanism of action. It seems logical that dilating a partially occluded coronary vessel would allow more oxygen to reach ischemic myocardial tissue. Although this effect does indeed occur, is not believed to be the primary mechanism of nitrate action in stable angina. This action, however, is important in treating a less common form of angina known as **variant angina,** in which the chest pain is caused by spasm of a coronary artery. The organic nitrates can relax these spasms and stop the pain.

FIGURE 18.2

Mechanisms of action of drugs used to treat angina pectoris

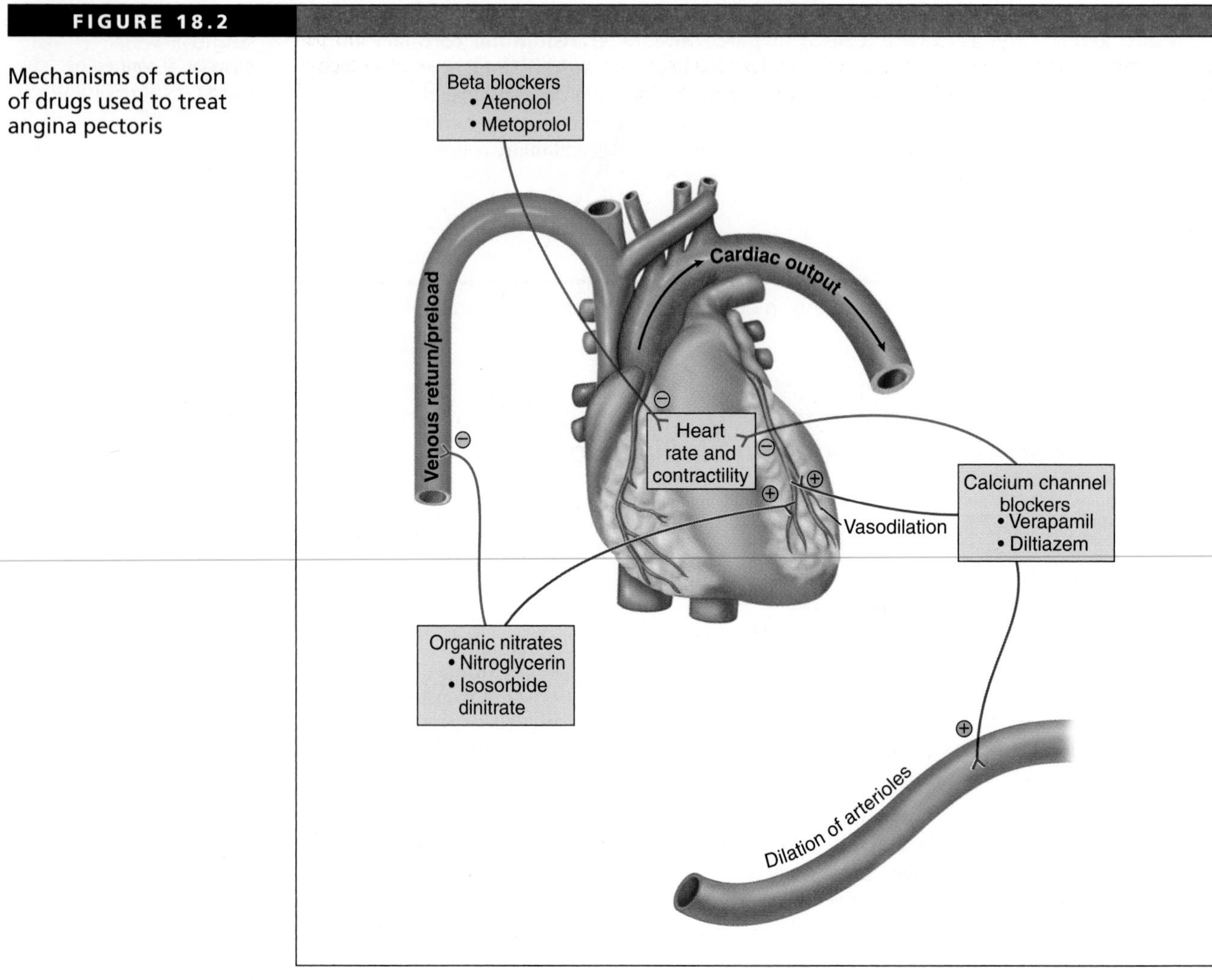

Organic nitrates are of two types: short acting and long acting. The short-acting agents, such as nitroglycerin, are taken sublingually to quickly stop an acute anginal attack in progress. Long-acting nitrates, such as isosorbide dinitrate, are taken orally or delivered through a transdermal patch to decrease the frequency and severity of anginal episodes.

trans = *across or through*
dermis = *skin*

TABLE 18.2 Organic Nitrates

DRUG	ROUTE AND ADULT DOSE	REMARKS
amyl nitrate (Vaporole)	Inhalation 1 ampule (0.18–0.3 ml) prn	Short acting; onset is 10–30 seconds; may be repeated in 3–5 minutes; also used as treatment for cyanide poisoning
isosorbide dinitrate (Dilatrate SR, Isordil, Sorbitrate)	PO 2.5–30 mg qid	For both acute attacks and long-term management; sublingual and chewable forms smaller dose is given to initiate therapy; extended-release form available
isosorbide mononitrate (Imdur, Ismo, Monoket)	PO 20 mg bid (max:240 mg/day with sustained release)	For the prevention of angina; a smaller dose is given to initiate therapy; extended-release form available
Pr nitroglycerin (Nitrostat, Nitrobid, Nitro-Dur, and others)	SL 1 tablet (0.3–0.6 mg) or 1 spray (0.4–0.8 mg) q 3–5 min (max: 3 doses in 15 min)	Dilates both arteries and veins; sublingual, oral, translingual, IV, transmucosal, transdermal, and topical forms available; extended-release form available
pentaerythrityl (Peritrate, Duotrate, Pentylan)	PO 10–20 mg tid or qid	Extended-release form available

Although the nitrates are safe drugs that have few serious adverse effects, some side effects may be troublesome to patients. Dilation of veins can reduce blood pressure and cause patients to become dizzy when moving to a standing position. This fall in blood pressure can result in reflex tachycardia, causing patients to feel as if their heart is having palpitations or skipping a beat. Dilation of cerebral vessels may cause headache, which can sometimes be severe. Flushing of the skin is common. Most of these effects are temporary and rarely cause discontinuation of drug therapy.

tachy = *rapid*
cardia = *heart*

Tolerance commonly occurs with the long-acting organic nitrates when they are taken for extended periods. The magnitude of the tolerance depends on the dosage and the frequency of drug administration. Patients are often instructed to remove the transdermal patch for 6 to 12 hours each day or withhold the evening dose of the oral organic nitrate to delay the development of tolerance.

Long-acting nitrates are also useful in reducing the symptoms of heart failure. Their role in the treatment of this disease was discussed in Chapter 16.

18.6 Beta-adrenergic blockers relieve anginal pain by decreasing the oxygen demands on the heart.

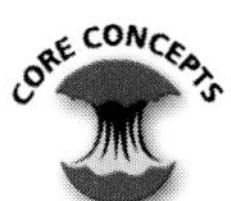

Beta-adrenergic blockers reduce the workload on the heart and are used for angina prophylaxis. Drugs for angina include cardioselective $beta_1$ blockers and mixed $beta_1$-$beta_2$ blockers. Selected beta-adrenergic blockers of importance in treating angina are listed in Table 18.3.

The pharmacology of the beta-adrenergic blockers was explained in Chapter 6 and in other chapters where the value of these drugs in the treatment of hypertension (Chapter 15), heart failure (Chapter 16), and dysrhythmias (Chapter 17) was presented. Because of their ability to reduce the workload on the heart by slowing heart rate and reducing contractility, several beta blockers are used to decrease the frequency and severity of anginal attacks caused by exertion. Patients should be advised against abruptly stopping beta-blocker therapy because this may result in a sudden increase in workload on the heart.

18.7 Calcium channel blockers relieve anginal pain by dilating the coronary vessels and reducing the workload on the heart.

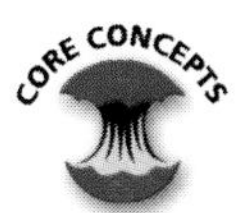

Several calcium channel blockers (CCBs) reduce myocardial oxygen demand by lowering blood pressure and slowing the heart rate. They are widely used in the treatment of cardiovascular disease. CCBs of importance to angina are listed in Table 18.4.

Like beta blockers, the CCBs have been discussed several times in this text for the treatment of hypertension (Chapter 15) and dysrhythmias (Chapter 17). The first approved use of CCBs

DRUG PROFILE: Organic Nitrate, Vasodilator: *Nitroglycerin (Nitrostat, Nitrobid, Nitro-Dur, and Others)*

Actions and Uses:

Nitroglycerin, the oldest and most widely used of the organic nitrates, can be delivered by a number of different routes, including sublingual, buccal, transdermal, topical, and IV. It is normally taken while an acute anginal episode is in progress or just prior to physical activity. When given sublingually, it reaches peak plasma levels in only 4 minutes and thus can stop anginal pain rapidly. Chest pain that does not respond quickly to sublingual nitroglycerin may indicate MI.

Adverse Effects and Interactions:

Side effects of nitroglycerin are usually cardiovascular, and rarely life threatening. Because nitroglycerin can dilate vessels in the head, headache is common and may be persistent and severe. Occasionally the venodilation created by nitroglycerin causes *reflex tachycardia.* A beta-adrenergic blocker may be prescribed to diminish this undesirable increase in heart rate. The side effects of nitroglycerin often diminish after a few doses.

Using with sildenafil (Viagra) may cause life-threatening hypotension and CV collapse. Nitrates should not be taken 24 hours before or after taking Viagra.

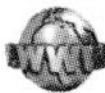

See the Companion Website for a Nursing Process Focus specific to this drug.

NURSING PROCESS FOCUS

Patients Receiving Nitroglycerin

ASSESSMENT

Prior to administration:

- Obtain complete health history including allergies, drug history, and possible drug interactions
- Assess vital signs, ECG, frequency and severity of angina, and alcohol use
- Obtain history of cardiac disorders and blood testing including cardiac enzymes, CBC, BUN, creatinine, and liver function tests
- Assess if patient has taken sildenafil (Viagra) within last 24 hours

POTENTIAL NURSING DIAGNOSES

- Risk for Ineffective Tissue Perfusion, related to hypotension from drug
- Risk for Injury (dizziness or fainting), related to hypotension from drug
- Acute Pain (headache), related to adverse effects of drug
- Deficient Knowledge, related to drug therapy

PLANNING: Patient Goals and Expected Outcomes

The patient will:

- Experience relief or prevention of chest pain
- Report immediately any chest pain unrelieved by nitroglycerin
- Demonstrate an understanding of the drug's action by accurately describing drug side effects and precautions

IMPLEMENTATION

Interventions and (Rationales)	Patient Education/Discharge Planning
■ Ask patient to describe and rate pain prior to drug administration for description/documentation of anginal episode. ■ Obtain a 12-lead ECG to differentiate between angina and infarction. (Pharmacotherapy depends on which disorder is presenting.)	Instruct patient to: ■ Take 1 tablet every 5 min until pain is relieved or for up to 3 doses during an acute anginal attack ■ Call EMS if chest pain is not relieved after 3 doses ■ Place SL tablet under tongue or spray under tongue; do not inhale spray
■ Monitor blood pressure and pulse. Do not administer drug if patient is hypotensive. (Drug will further reduce blood pressure.) ■ Monitor alcohol use. (Extremely low blood pressure may result, which could cause death.) ■ Monitor for headache in response to use of nitrates.	■ Instruct patient to sit or lie down before taking medication and to avoid abrupt changes in position. ■ Emphasize the importance of avoiding alcohol while taking nitroglycerin. Instruct patient that: ■ Headache is a common side effect, that usually decreases over time ■ OTC medicines usually relieve the headache
■ Monitor for use of sildenafil (Viagra) concurrently with nitrates, because cardiovascular disease is a major cause of erectile dysfunction in men. (Life-threatening hypotension may result with concurrent use of sildenafil.)	Instruct patient to: ■ Not take Viagra within 24 hours after taking nitrates ■ Wait at least 24 hours after taking Viagra to resume nitrate therapy
■ Monitor need for prophylactic nitrates.	■ Advise patient to take medication prior to a stressful event or physical activity to prevent angina.

EVALUATION OF OUTCOME CRITERIA

Evaluate the effectiveness of drug therapy by confirming that patient goals and expected outcomes have been met (see "Planning").

See Table 18.2 for a list of drugs to which these nursing actions apply.

TABLE 18.3 Beta-adrenergic Blockers Used for Angina

DRUG	ROUTE AND ADULT DOSE	REMARKS
Pr atenolol (Tenormin)	PO 25–50 mg daily (max: 100 mg/day)	Cardioselective $beta_1$ blocker; reduces rate and force of cardiac contractions; also for hypertension; IV form available for MI
bisoprolol (Zebeta)	PO 2.5–5 mg daily (max: 20 mg/day)	Cardioselective $beta_1$ blocker; improves exercise tolerance in angina; may take 2–4 weeks for therapeutic effect; also for hypertension
metoprolol (Lopressor, Toprol)	PO 100 mg bid (max: 400 mg/day)	Cardioselective $beta_1$ blocker; sustained-release form available; also for hypertension; IV form available for MI
nadolol (Corgard)	PO 40 mg daily (max: 240 mg/day)	Nonselective $beta_1$ and $beta_2$ blocker; indicated for long-term prevention of angina; also for hypertension
propranolol (Inderal)	PO 10–20 mg bid–tid (max: 320 mg/day)	Nonselective $beta_1$ and $beta_2$ blocker; IV form available; also for hypertension, dysrhythmias, MI, and migraine prophylaxis
timolol (Bliocadren)	PO 15–45 mg tid (max: 60 mg/day)	Nonselective $beta_1$ and $beta_2$ blocker; also for hypertension; topical form available for glaucoma

DRUG PROFILE: Beta-adrenergic Blocker: Pr *Atenolol (Tenormin)*

Actions and Uses:

Atenolol selectively blocks $beta_1$ receptors in the heart. Its effectiveness in angina is attributed to its ability to slow heart rate and reduce contractility (negative inotropic effect), both of which lower myocardial oxygen demand. It is also used in the treatment of hypertension and in the prevention of MI. Because of its 7- to 9-hour half-life, it may be taken once a day.

Adverse Effects and Interactions:

As a cardioselective $beta_1$ blocker, atenolol has few adverse effects on the lungs and is useful for patients experiencing bronchospasm. Like other beta blockers, therapy generally begins with low doses, which are gradually increased until the therapeutic effect is achieved. The most common side effects of atenolol include fatigue, weakness, and hypotension.

Using atenolol together with calcium channel blockers may cause excessive cardiac suppression. Using together with digoxin may cause slowed atrioventricular conduction leading to heart block. Patients should avoid using this drug with nicotine or caffeine because of their vasoconstricting effects.

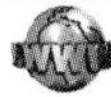
See the Companion Website for a Nursing Process Focus specific to this drug.

TABLE 18.4 Calcium Channel Blockers of Importance to Angina

DRUG	ROUTE AND ADULT DOSE	REMARKS
amlodipine (Norvasc)	PO 5–10 mg daily (max: 10 mg/day)	Also for hypertension; combined with the ACE inhibitor benazopril to form the drug Lotrel
bepridil (Vascor)	PO 200 mg daily (max: 400 mg/day)	Also blocks sodium channels; usually reserved for those patients unresponsive to safer antianginals
Pr diltiazem (Cardizem,Dilacor, Tiamate, Triazac)	PO 30 mg qid (max: 360 mg/day)	Dilates coronary arteries and decreases coronary artery spasm; sustained-release form available; also for hypertension; IV form available for dysrhythmias
nicardipine (Cardene)	PO 20–40 mg tid or 30–60 mg SR bid (max: 120 mg/day)	Also for hypertension; sustained-release and IV forms available
nifedipine (Procardia, Aldalat)	PO 10–20 mg tid (max: 180 mg/day)	Used in the treatment of vasospastic (Printzmetal's) angina; also for hypertension; sustained-release form available
verapamil (Calan, Isoptin, Verelan)	PO 80 mg tid–qid (max: 480 mg/day)	Dilates coronary arteries and inhibits coronary artery spasm; also for hypertension; sustained-release form available; IV form available for dysrhythmias

was for the treatment of angina. Blockade of calcium ion channels has a number of effects on the heart, most of which are similar to those of beta-adrenergic blockers.

CCBs cause arteriolar smooth muscle to relax, thus lowering peripheral resistance and reducing blood pressure. This reduction in afterload decreases the myocardial oxygen demand, thus reducing the frequency of anginal pain. Some CCBs are selective for arterioles. Others, such as verapamil and diltiazem, have an additional beneficial effect of slowing the heart rate (negative chronotropic effect). Because they relax arterial smooth muscle, the CCBs are useful in treating variant angina, in which the coronary vessels are constricted by acute spasm.

Concept Review 18.2

- How does decreasing the workload on the heart result in reduction in anginal pain?

MYOCARDIAL INFARCTION

A myocardial infarction (MI) is the result of a sudden occlusion of a coronary artery. Immediate pharmacological treatment may reduce patient mortality.

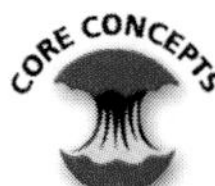

18.8 Early diagnosis and treatment of myocardial infarction increases chances of survival.

Myocardial infarctions are responsible for a substantial number of deaths each year. Some patients die before reaching a medical facility for treatment and many others die within 1 to 2 days after the initial MI. Clearly, MI is a serious and frightening disease and is responsible for a large percentage of sudden deaths.

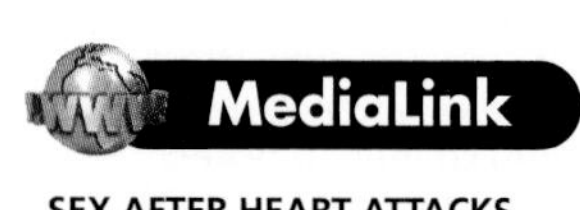

SEX AFTER HEART ATTACKS

The primary cause of MI is advanced coronary heart disease (CHD). Plaque buildup can narrow the coronary arteries that supply the myocardium with its essential nutrients. Pieces of plaque may break off and lodge in a small vessel that serves a portion of the myocardium. Deprived of its oxygen supply, this area becomes ischemic and cardiac cells can die unless the blood supply is quickly restored. Figure 18.3 ■ illustrates this blockage and the resulting reperfusion process.

The goals of the pharmacological treatment of acute MI include the following:

- To restore blood supply (perfusion) to the damaged myocardium as quickly as possible through the use of thrombolytics
- To reduce myocardial oxygen demand with organic nitrates or beta blockers to prevent another MI
- To control or prevent associated dysrhythmias with beta blockers or other antidysrhythmics
- To reduce post-MI mortality with aspirin and ACE inhibitors
- To control MI pain and associated anxiety with analgesics

Fast Facts Myocardial Infarction

- About 1.1 million Americans experience a new or recurrent MI each year.
- About one third of patients experiencing an MI will die.
- About 250,000 Americans each year die of an acute MI within 1 hour of the onset of the symptoms.
- About 60% of patients who died suddenly of MI had no previous symptoms of the disease.
- Mortality from MI is slightly higher in men than women.
- Because women have MIs, at older ages, they are more likely to die from them within a few weeks.
- More than 20% of men and 40% of women will die from an MI within 1 year after being diagnosed.

DRUG PROFILE: Calcium Channel Blocker: Pr *Diltiazem (Cardizem)*

Actions and Uses:

Diltiazem inhibits the transport of calcium ions into myocardial cells and has the ability to relax both coronary and peripheral blood vessels. It is useful in the treatment of atrial dysrhythmias and hypertension, as well as angina. When given as extended-release capsules, it may be administered once daily.

Adverse Effects and Interactions:

Side effects of diltiazem are generally not serious and are related to vasodilation: headache, dizziness, and edema of the ankles and feet. Although diltiazem produces few adverse effects on the heart or vessels, it should be used with caution in patients taking other cardiovascular medications, particularly digoxin or beta-adrenergic blockers; the combined effects of these drugs may cause heart failure or dysrhythmias.

Diltiazem increases the levels of digoxin or quinidine if taken together. Use cautiously with herbal supplements such as dong quai and ginger because these products interfere with blood clotting.

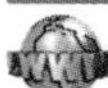
See the Companion Website for a Nursing Process Focus specific to this drug.

18.9 Thrombolytics dissolve clots blocking the coronary arteries.

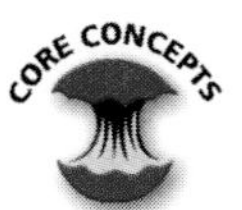

The basic pharmacology of the thrombolytics was presented in Chapter 14. In the treatment of MI, the goal of thrombolytic therapy is to dissolve clots that are obstructing the coronary arteries and restore circulation to the myocardium. Quick restoration of cardiac circulation has been found to reduce mortality from the disease. After the clot is successfully dissolved, anticoagulant or antiplatelet therapy is initiated to prevent the formation of additional thrombi. Dosages and descriptions of the various thrombolytics are given in Chapter 14.

Thrombolytics have a narrow margin of safety. The primary risk of thrombolytics is excessive bleeding from interference in the clotting process. Older patients have an increased risk of serious bleeding and intracranial hemorrhage. Patients with recent trauma or surgery should not receive these drugs. Vital signs must be monitored continuously and any signs of bleeding generally call for discontinuation of therapy. Because these medications are rapidly destroyed in the blood, stopping the infusion normally results in the rapid termination of any adverse effects.

18.10 When given within 24 hours after the onset of MI, beta-adrenergic blockers can improve chances of survival.

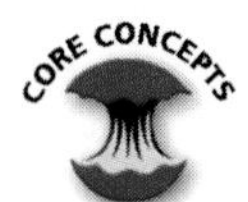

Beta blockers are used for MI, like they are for angina, to reduce the cardiac workload. Recent research suggests that their use may reduce mortality following an MI if given within 8 hours of the MI. Beta blockers of importance to MI are listed in Table 18.5.

The basic pharmacology and usefulness of the beta-adrenergic blockers in the treatment of cardiovascular disease has been discussed in a number of chapters in this text. This section will focus on their use in the treatment of MI.

Beta blockers have the ability to slow the heart rate, decrease contractility (negative inotropic effect), and reduce blood pressure. These three actions reduce myocardial oxygen demand, which is beneficial for those who experienced a recent MI. In addition, their ability to slow impulse conduction through the heart tends to suppress dysrhythmias, which can be serious and sometimes fatal complications following MI.

FIGURE 18.3

Blockade and reperfusion following myocardial infarction (MI): (a) blockage of left coronary artery with myocardial ischemia; (b) infusion of thrombolytics; (c) blood supply returning to myocardium; (d) thrombus dissolving and ischemia clearing *SOURCE: (a) and (c) Reprinted by permission of Pearson Education, Inc., Upper Saddle River, NJ*

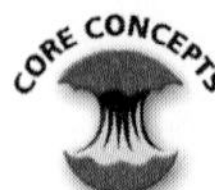

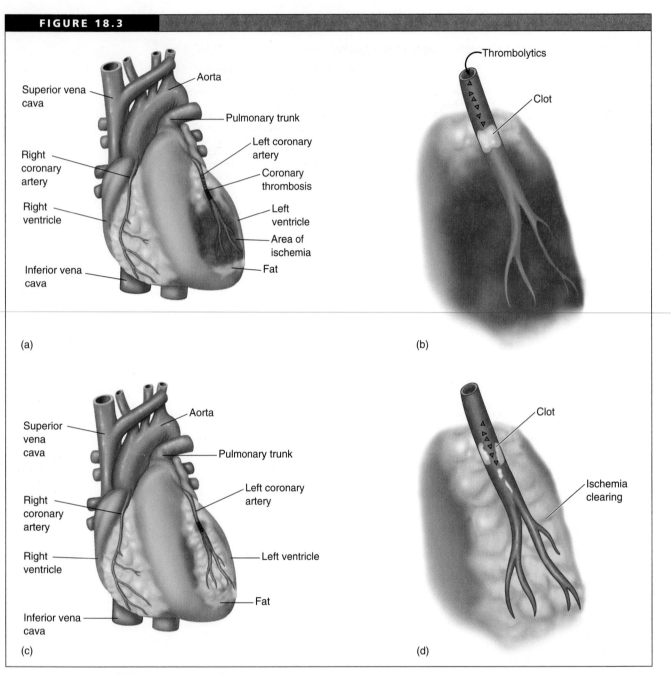

18.11 A number of additional drugs are used to treat the symptoms and complications of acute MI.

A number of additional drugs have proven useful in treating patients who experience an acute MI. Aspirin has been found to reduce mortality dramatically in the weeks following an acute MI. Unless contraindicated, 160 to 324 mg of aspirin is given as soon as possible following a suspected MI. The basic pharmacology of aspirin is covered in Chapter 21. Other coagulation modifiers, such as the glycoprotein IIb/IIIa blockers or the ADP receptor blockers, may be given to prevent further thrombi formation (Chapter 14).

TABLE 18.5 Beta-adrenergic Blockers Used for Myocardial Infarction

DRUG	ROUTE AND ADULT DOSE	REMARKS
acebutolol (Sectral)	PO 400–800 mg daily (max: 1200 mg/day)	Cardioselective $beta_1$ blocker; decreases cardiac output; also for hypertension, dysrhythmias, and angina
atenolol (Tenormin)	IV 5 mg q5 min for 2 doses then begin PO 50 mg daily (give 1st dose 10 min after 2nd IV dose) (max: 100 mg/day)	Cardioselective $beta_1$ blocker; also for hypertension
Pr metoprolol (Toprol, Lopressor)	IV 5 mg q2 min for 3 doses followed by PO doses	Cardioselective $beta_1$ blocker; also for hypertension and angina
propranolol (Inderal)	PO 60–80 mg tid (max: 240 mg/day)	Nonselective $beta_1$ and $beta_2$ blocker; IV form available; also for hypertension, dysrhythmias, angina, and migraine prophylaxis
timolol maleate (Blocadren)	PO 10 mg bid (max: 60 mg/day)	Nonselective $beta_1$ and $beta_2$ blocker; also for hypertension and angina; topical form available for glaucoma

DRUG PROFILE: Thrombolytic: Pr *Reteplase (Retavase)*

Actions and Uses:

Like other drugs in this class, reteplase is most effective if given within 30 minutes but not later than 12 hours after the onset of MI symptoms. It usually acts within 20 minutes. Restoration of circulation to the ischemic site may be faster with reteplase than with other thrombolytics. After the clot has been dissolved, heparin therapy is often started to prevent additional clots from forming.

Adverse Effects and Interactions:

Reteplase is contraindicated in patients with active bleeding. Healthcare providers must be vigilant in recognizing and reporting any abnormal bleeding that may occur during thrombolytic therapy.

Drug interactions with anticoagulants and platelet aggregation inhibitors will produce an additive effect and increase the risk of bleeding.

Mechanism in Action:

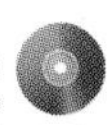

Reteplase dissolves blood clots by activating plasminogen, a protein found within many body tissues and the general circulation. On activation, plasminogen binds to fibrin, which is the meshlike substance forming the insoluble clot. Thrombolytics remove clots and restore circulation to injured or occluded blood vessels.

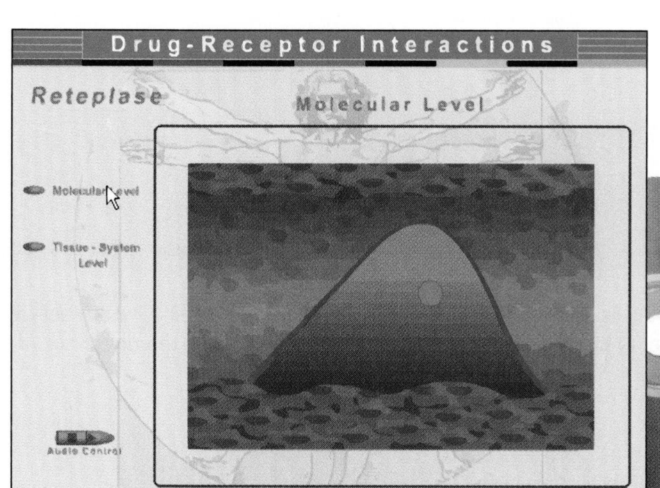

Use the student CD-ROM to see Mechanism in Action for Reteplase.

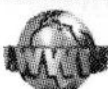

See the Companion Website for a Nursing Process Focus specific to this drug.

DRUG PROFILE: Beta-adrenergic Blocker: Pr *Metoprolol (Lopressor)*

Actions and Uses:

Metoprolol is a selective $beta_1$ blocker. When given intravenously, it quickly acts to reduce myocardial oxygen demand. Following an acute MI, metoprolol is infused slowly until a target heart rate is reached, usually 60–90 bpm. At hospital discharge, patients can be switched to oral forms of the drug. Metoprolol is also approved for angina, heart failure, hypertension, and MI.

Adverse Effects and Interactions:

Because it is selective for blocking $beta_1$ receptors in the heart, metoprolol has few adverse effects on other autonomic organs and thus is preferred over nonselective agents such as propranolol for patients with lung disorders. Side effects are generally minor and relate to its autonomic activity, such as bradycardia and hypotension. Because of its multiple effects on the heart, patients with disorders such as heart failure must be carefully monitored.

This drug is contraindicated in cardiogenic shock, sinus bradycardia, and heart block greater than first degree. If used together with digoxin, bradycardia may result. Oral contraceptives may cause increased effects of metoprolol.

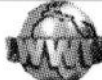
See the Companion Website for a Nursing Process Focus specific to this drug.

The ACE inhibitors, captopril (Capoten) and lisinopril (Prinivil, Zestril), have also been found to reduce mortality following MI. These drugs are most effective when therapy is started within 1 or 2 days after the onset of symptoms. Oral therapy with the ACE inhibitors normally begins after thrombolytic therapy has been completed and the patient's condition has stabilized. The pharmacology of the ACE inhibitors and the drug profile for lisinopril is presented in Chapter 16.

Pain control is essential following acute MI to ensure patient comfort and reduce stress. Narcotic analgesics such as morphine sulfate are sometimes given to ease the severe pain associated with acute MI and to sedate the anxious patient. Details on the pharmacology of the narcotic analgesics were presented in Chapter 12.

Concept Review 18.3

- Why is it important to treat an MI within the first 24 hours after symptoms have begun? What classes of drugs are used for this purpose?

CEREBROVASCULAR ACCIDENT (CVA)/STROKE

cerebro = *head or brain*
vascular = *vessels*

A cerebrovascular accident (CVA) is caused by a thrombus or bleeding within a vessel serving the brain. Although drug therapy is limited, immediate treatment may reduce the degree of permanent disability resulting from a CVA.

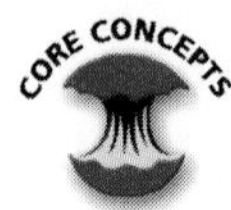

18.12 Strokes are a major cause of death and disability.

Cerebrovascular accident (CVA) or **stroke** is a major cause of permanent disability. The majority of strokes are caused by a thrombus in a vessel serving the brain (**thrombotic stroke**). Areas downstream from the clot lose their oxygen supply and neural tissue will begin to die unless circulation is quickly restored. A smaller percentage of strokes, about 20%, are caused by rupture

Fast Facts Cerebrovascular Accident

- CVA is the third leading cause of death, behind heart disease and cancer.
- The incidence of CVA increases with age (per 1000 population), although 25% of all CVAs occur in people younger than age 65:

  14% of those 65–74 years old
  25% of those 75–84 years old
  28% of those older than age 85
- About 4.4 million CVA survivors are alive in the United States; 600,000 new cases occur each year.
- The highest incidence of CVA is in black men—more than double that of white women.
- CVA occurs more frequently in men than women, although females account for about 60% of all deaths due to CVAs.
- Over 160,000 Americans die of CVAs each year.

of a cerebral vessel and its associated bleeding into neural tissue (**hemorrhagic stroke**). Symptoms are the same for the two types of strokes. Specific symptoms will vary widely depending on which area of the brain is affected and may include blindness, paralysis, speech problems, coma, and even dementia. Mortality from stroke is very high: As many as 40% of stroke victims will die within the first year following the stroke.

Many of the risk factors associated with CVA are the same as for other cardiovascular diseases such as hypertension and CHD. Lifestyle changes such as those in the following list may reduce the patients risk of experiencing a CVA:

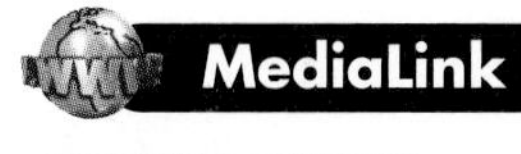

SUPPORT FOR STROKE VICTIMS

- Stop using tobacco.
- Limit salt (sodium) intake.
- Eat foods rich in potassium and magnesium, such as bananas, beans, spinach, and tomatoes.
- Limit alcohol consumption.
- Implement a medically supervised exercise plan.
- Reduce stress levels as much as possible.
- Reduce dietary saturated fats, and keep weight at an optimum level.
- If hyperlipidemia is present, have it treated.
- If hypertension is present, have it treated.

18.13 Aggressive treatment of thrombotic stroke with anticoagulants, antihypertensives, and thrombolytics can increase survival.

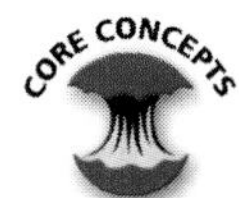

Drug therapy of thrombotic stroke focuses on two main goals: prevention of strokes through the use of anticoagulants and antihypertensive agents, and restoration of blood supply to the affected portion of the brain as quickly as possible after an acute stroke through the use of thrombolytics.

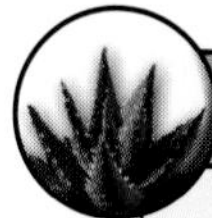

NATURAL ALTERNATIVES

Ginkgo Biloba for Cardiovascular Disease

Ginkgo biloba is a popular botanical that is often used for its effect on the brain. Ginkgo trees are native to China, Japan, and Korea and grow to be quite large. The trees are known for their extreme longevity, living to be more than 100 years old. They do not even flower for the first 20 years. The medicinal parts of the tree include the seeds and leaves. Ginkgo is available in liquid and solid forms and may be taken in drinks such as tea. The average daily dose is 120 mg of dried extract in 2–3 doses per day.

Many clinical studies have been conducted on ginkgo extracts. Active ingredients include flavenoids and terpenes. Effects include anticoagulant activity and an increase in blood flow to the brain and peripheral arteries. These effects are thought to be responsible for claims that ginkgo prevents CVAs and improves cerebral blood flow following CVAs. Controlled studies have not definitively proven these antistroke effects. ■

As discussed in Chapter 15, sustained, chronic hypertension is closely associated with stroke. Antihypertensive therapy with beta-adrenergic blockers, calcium channel blockers, diuretics, and/or ACE inhibitors can help control blood pressure and reduce the probability of stroke.

Aspirin, through its anticoagulant properties, has been found to reduce the incidence of stroke. When given in very low doses, aspirin discourages the formation of thrombi by inhibiting platelet aggregation. Patients are often placed on low-dose aspirin therapy on a continual basis following their first stroke. Ticlopidine (Ticlid) is an antiplatelet drug that may be used to provide anticoagulation in patients who cannot tolerate aspirin. Other anticoagulants such as warfarin may be given to prevent stroke in high-risk patients such as those with prosthetic heart valves. More detailed information on anticoagulant and antiplatelet agents is found in Chapter 14.

The single most important breakthrough in the treatment of stroke was development of the thrombolytic agents. Prior to the discovery of these drugs, the treatment of thrombotic stroke was largely a passive, wait-and-see strategy. Now, stroke is aggressively treated with thrombolytics as soon as the patient arrives at the hospital: These agents are most effective if administered within 3 hours of the attack. Use of aggressive thrombolytic therapy can completely restore brain function in a significant number of stroke patients. Because stroke is now viewed as a condition requiring immediate treatment, the disease has been renamed **brain attack.** Further information on the pharmacology of the thrombolytics can be found in Chapter 14.

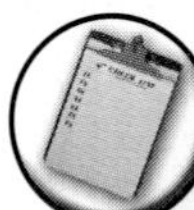

PATIENTS NEED TO KNOW

Patients treated for chest pain need to know the following:

Regarding Antianginals

1. Dissolve one nitroglycerin tablet under the tongue as soon as anginal pain is felt. If pain is not relieved in 5 minutes, use another. Many practitioners recommend a third nitroglycerin tablet for pain not relieved 5 minutes after the second dose. If chest pain/pressure is not relieved by 3 doses of nitroglycerin, call emergency medical services.
2. Rotate the application site of transdermal patches, and do not apply a new patch until after the old patch has been removed.
3. Change positions slowly. Postural hypotension may cause dizziness and even fainting.
4. Monitor blood pressure regularly, and report any consistent changes to a healthcare provider.

Regarding Anticoagulants

5. Do not eat large or inconsistent amounts of foods high in vitamin K while taking warfarin because this interferes with clotting time.
6. Do not take herbal supplements or OTC drugs before getting advice from a healthcare provider. Many drugs increase or decrease the effects of warfarin.
7. Report any symptoms of unusual bleeding or bruising to a healthcare provider. ▪

CHAPTER REVIEW

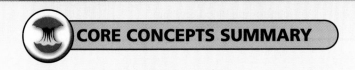

CORE CONCEPTS SUMMARY

18.1 Coronary heart disease is caused by a restriction in blood flow to the myocardium.

The high metabolic rate of the heart requires that a continuous supply of oxygen be maintained in the coronary arteries. Restriction of flow can lead to angina pectoris or myocardial infarction. Because both of these disorders can cause severe chest pain, the healthcare provider must quickly determine the cause of the pain, so that the appropriate treatment may be administered.

18.2 Angina pectoris is characterized by severe chest pain caused by lack of sufficient oxygen flow to heart muscle.

The coronary arteries can become partially occluded with plaque, resulting in ischemia. Lack of sufficient oxygen to the myocardium causes sharp chest pain on emotional or physical exertion, the characteristic symptom of angina.

18.3 Anginal pain can often be controlled through lifestyle changes and surgical procedures.

A number of lifestyle changes can reduce the deposition of plaque in the coronary arteries and help prevent coronary heart disease. These include stopping tobacco use, limiting alcohol consumption, and getting adequate exercise. Surgical procedures may be necessary to control severe angina.

18.4 The pharmacological goals for the treatment of angina are usually achieved by reducing cardiac workload.

Reducing the workload on the heart can relieve anginal pain. This can be accomplished by slowing the heart rate, dilating the vessels, reducing the force of myocardial contraction, or reducing blood pressure.

18.5 The organic nitrates relieve anginal pain by dilating veins and the coronary arteries.

Fast-acting organic nitrates can quickly terminate anginal pain by causing venodilation, which reduces the workload on the heart. They also dilate the coronary arteries, bringing more oxygen to the myocardium. Long-acting nitrates can prevent acute angina episodes, but the patient may become tolerant to their protective effect.

18.6 Beta-adrenergic blockers relieve anginal pain by decreasing the oxygen demands on the heart.

Beta blockers lower blood pressure, slow the heart rate and reduce the force of contraction, thus reducing the workload on the myocardium. They are prescribed to reduce the frequency of acute anginal episodes.

18.7 Calcium channel blockers relieve angina pain by dilating the coronary vessels and reducing the workload on the heart.

CCBs are effective at lowering blood pressure, thus reducing the workload on the heart. They are prescribed to reduce the frequency of acute anginal attacks.

18.8 Early diagnosis and treatment of myocardial infarction increases chances of survival.

Myocardial infarction is caused by a thrombus in a coronary artery and is responsible for a substantial number of sudden deaths. Fast, effective diagnosis and treatment can reduce mortality.

18.9 Thrombolytics dissolve clots blocking the coronary arteries.

When used within hours after the onset of MI, thrombolytics can dissolve clots and restore circulation to the myocardium.

18.10 When given within 24 hours after the onset of MI, beta-adrenergic blockers can improve chances of survival.

Beta blockers can slow the heart rate and reduce blood pressure, which have been shown to reduce mortality when given soon after MI symptoms appear.

18.11 A number of additional drugs are used to treat the symptoms and complications of acute MI.

Aspirin and ACE inhibitors have been shown to reduce mortality when given soon after the onset of MI. Narcotic analgesics are sometimes given to reduce the pain and anxiety associated with an MI.

18.12 Strokes are a major cause of death and disability.

Stroke, or brain attack, is caused by either a thrombus or bleeding in a cerebral vessel. It is a major cause of death and disability. Patients can lower their risk of stroke by adopting many of the same lifestyle changes required for coronary artery disease or hypertension.

18.13 Aggressive treatment of thrombotic stroke with anticoagulants, antihypertensives, and thrombolytics can increase survival.

Stroke, or brain attack, is now viewed as an emergency condition requiring immediate treatment to improve survival. Thrombolytics, when given quickly after the onset of stroke, can restore some or all brain function. Some degree of stroke prevention can be achieved by using anticoagulants and by controlling blood pressure.

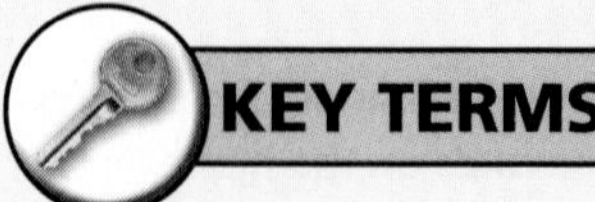

KEY TERMS

angina pectoris (an-JEYE-nuh PEK-tore-us): acute pain in the chest on physical or emotional exertion due to inadequate oxygen supply to the myocardium / ***page 315***

atherosclerosis (ath-ur-oh-skler-OH-sis): a buildup of fatty substances and loss of elasticity of the arterial walls / ***page 315***

cerebrovascular accident/stroke/brain attack (sir-ree-bro-VASK-u-lur): an acute condition of a blood clot or bleeding in a vessel in the brain / ***pages 326, 328***

coronary arteries (KOR-un-air-ee AR-tur-ees): vessels that bring oxygen and nutrients to the myocardium / ***page 314***

coronary arterial bypass graft (CABG): surgical procedure performed to restore blood flow to the myocardium by using a section of the saphenous vein or internal mammary artery to go around the obstructed coronary artery / ***page 317***

hemorrhagic stroke (hee-moh-RAJ-ik): type of stroke caused by bleeding from a blood vessel in the brain / ***page 327***

myocardial infarction (MI) (meye-oh-KAR-dee-ul in-FARK-shun): medical emergency of having a blood clot blocking a portion of a coronary artery / ***page 322***

myocardial ischemia (meye-oh-KAR-dee-ul ik-SKEE-mee-uh): condition in which there is a lack of blood supply to the myocardium due to a constriction or obstruction of a blood vessel / ***page 315***

percutaneous transluminal coronary angioplasty (PTCA) (per-cue-TAIN-ee-us trans-LOO-min-ul KOR-un-air-ee ANN-gee-oh-plas-tee): procedure by which a balloon-shaped catheter is used to compress fatty plaque against an arterial wall for the purpose of restoring normal blood flow / ***page 317***

plaque (plak): fatty material that builds up in the lining of blood vessels and may lead to hypertension, stroke, myocardial infarction, or angina / ***page 315***

stable angina: type of angina that occurs in a predictable pattern, usually relieved by rest / ***page 315***

thrombotic stroke (throm-BOT-ik): type of stroke caused by a blood clot blocking an artery in the brain / ***page 326***

unstable angina: type of angina that occurs frequently, with severe symptoms, and which is not relieved by rest / ***page 315***

variant angina: chest pain that is caused by acute spasm of the coronary arteries rather than by physical or emotional exertion / ***page 317***

REVIEW QUESTIONS

The following questions are written in NCLEX-PN® style. Answer these questions to assess your knowledge of the chapter material, and go back and review any material that is not clear to you.

1. The patient is being discharged with nitroglycerin (Nitrostat). Patient education would include:

1. "Swallow 3 tablets immediately for pain and call 911."
2. "Put 1 tablet under your tongue for chest pain."
3. "Call your physician when you have chest pain. The physician will tell you how many tablets to take."
4. "Place 3 tablets under your tongue and call 911."

2. The most common side effect of nitroglycerin is:

1. Headache
2. Hypertension
3. Diuresis
4. Bradycardia

3. This class of medications decreases heart rate, contractility, and blood pressure, and is used to increase survival rates in post MI.

1. Calcium channel blockers
2. Beta blockers
3. Vasodilators
4. Diuretics

4. The nurse assesses for the most common side effect of reteplase (Retavase), which is:

1. Dehydration
2. Bleeding
3. Confusion
4. Increased clotting times

5. The patient has a history of a CVA. Which of the following drugs would not be recommended for this patient?

1. Aspirin
2. Warfarin (Coumadin)
3. Protamine sulfate
4. Ticlopidine (Ticlid)

6. The patient should remove the transdermal nitroglycerin patch at night to:

1. Prevent overdose
2. Prevent adverse reactions
3. Ensure the dosage is appropriate
4. Delay development of tolerance

7. Warfarin (Coumadin) would be contraindicated in a patient with a history of:

1. Atrial fibrillation
2. Thrombolytic stroke
3. Hemorrhagic stroke
4. Mitral valve replacement

8. The patient on warfarin (Coumadin) should be advised to not consume a large amount of:

1. Red meats
2. Leafy green vegetables
3. Fiber-rich foods
4. Chicken

9. The patient taking calcium channel blockers should avoid which OTC medications?

1. Acetaminophen (Tylenol)
2. Ibuprofen (Motrin)
3. Calcium carbonate (Tums)
4. Ranitidine (Zantac)

10. The patient is complaining of a vicelike pain in his chest that subsides with rest. The patient is experiencing (a):

1. Stroke
2. Myocardial infarction
3. Angina
4. Cerebral vascular accident

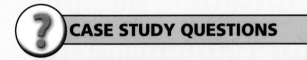

CASE STUDY QUESTIONS

For questions 1–5, please refer to the following case study, and choose the correct answer from choices 1–4.

Ms. Liu arrives in your office with a complaint of chest pain when she exercises. Subsequent tests show a 10% occlusion of two coronary arteries. Her blood pressure is 125/78 mm Hg. The physician prescribes one aspirin per day, sublingual nitroglycerin, and metoprolol.

1. The purpose of the nitroglycerin is to:

1. Prevent acute anginal attacks
2. End an angina attack in progress
3. Prevent MI or stroke
4. Relieve chest pain

2. What instructions should be given for the nitroglycerin?

1. Take before exercising.
2. Take on first indication of chest pain.
3. Take three or four times per day to prevent chest pain.
4. Take before bedtime and when rising.

3. The purpose of the metoprolol is to:

1. Prevent acute anginal attacks
2. End an angina attack in progress
3. Prevent MI or stroke
4. Lower blood pressure

Ms. Liu discontinues her drugs without notifying her physician. Three months later, she arrives in the ED with a possible stroke. Her blood pressure is 186/100 mm Hg. The physician orders a reteplase infusion.

4. The function of the reteplase is to:

1. Dissolve existing blood clots
2. Prevent possible formation of blood clots
3. Stabilize blood pressure
4. Reduce workload on the heart

5. The healthcare provider should be vigilant in observing for which of the following adverse effects during the reteplase infusion?

1. An increase in blood pressure
2. An increase in heart rate
3. Abnormal bleeding
4. Vomiting or diarrhea

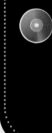

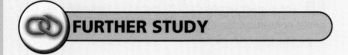

FURTHER STUDY

- The use of nitrous oxide as an anesthesia is discussed in Chapter 13.
- The role of long-acting nitrates for treating heart failure is covered in Chapter 16.
- Several chapters include information on beta-adrenergic blockers: Chapter 6 discusses their pharmacology; Chapter 15, their use in hypertension; Chapter 16, their use in heart failure; Chapter 17, their use for dysrhythmias.
- Information on chronic hypertension and the use of calcium channel blockers for treating it is found in Chapter 15.
- Chapter 17 considers the use of calcium channel blockers for dysrhythmias.
- Chapter 14 includes information on the basic pharmacology, dosages, and descriptions of thrombolytics, coagulation modifiers, and antiplatelet agents.
- For more information on aspirin, see Chapter 21.
- Chapter 16 presents the pharmacology of ACE inhibitors; and Chapter 12 provides more information on the narcotic analgesics.

EXPLORE MEDIALINK www.prenhall.com/holland

Additional resources for this chapter can be found on the CD-ROM accompanying this textbook, and on the Companion Website. Click on Chapter 18 to select activities for this chapter.

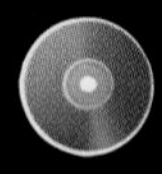

Mechanism in Action: Reteplase
Audio Glossary
Concept Review
NCLEX-PN® Review
Nursing in Action
Dosage Calculator

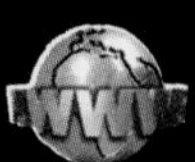

Women and Heart Disease
Sex after Heart Attacks
Support for Stroke Victims

CHAPTER

19 Drugs for Shock and Anaphylaxis

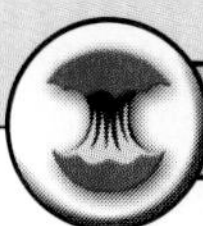

CORE CONCEPTS

19.1 Shock is a syndrome characterized by collapse of the circulatory system.

19.2 The initial treatment of shock includes basic life support and identification of the underlying cause.

19.3 Vasoconstrictors are administered during shock to maintain blood pressure.

19.4 Cardiotonic drugs are useful in reversing the decreased cardiac output resulting from shock.

19.5 Fluid replacement agents are infused to replace fluids lost during shock, which helps return blood pressure to normal.

19.6 Anaphylaxis is a special type of shock caused by a hyperresponse of body defense mechanisms.

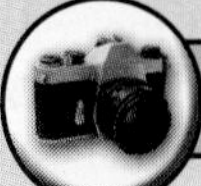

DRUG SNAPSHOT

The following drugs will be discussed in this chapter:

DRUG CLASSES	DRUG PROFILES
Vasoconstrictors	Pr norepinephrine (Levarterenol)
Cardiotonic agents	Pr dopamine (Dopastat, Intropin)
Fluid replacement agents	Pr normal serum albumin (Albuminar, Albutein)

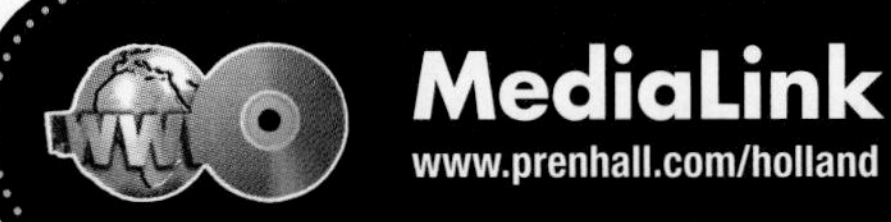

Interactive resources for this chapter can found on the Companion Website. Click on Chapter 19 and "Begin" to select the activities for this chapter. For chapter-related animations, NCLEX-PN®-style questions, and an audio glossary, access the accompanying CD-ROM in this book.

OBJECTIVES

After reading this chapter, the student should be able to:

1. Compare and contrast the different types of shock.
2. Relate the general symptoms of shock to their physiological causes.
3. Explain the initial treatment of a patient with shock.
4. For each of the following classes, identify representative drugs, explain the mechanisms of drug action, primary actions, and important adverse effects:
   - **a.** Sympathomimetics and other vasoconstrictors
   - **b.** Cardiotonic agents
   - **c.** Fluid replacement agents
   - **d.** Antihistamines
   - **e.** Corticosteroids
5. Categorize drugs used in the treatment of shock based on their classifications and mechanisms of action.

Shock is a condition in which vital tissues are not receiving enough blood to function properly. Without adequate oxygen and other nutrients, cells cannot carry on normal metabolism. Acute shock is considered a medical emergency; failure to reverse the causes and symptoms of shock may lead to irreversible organ damage and death. Most types of shock have a high mortality rate. This chapter will examine how drugs are used to aid in the treatment of different types of shock.

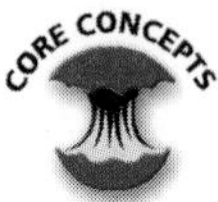

19.1 Shock is a syndrome characterized by collapse of the circulatory system.

There are several types of shock, each having different causes. The most useful method for classifying the different types is by naming the underlying pathological process or organ system causing the disease. Table 19.1 lists the different types of shock and their primary causes. This chapter focuses on the pharmacological therapy of two common types of shock: cardiogenic and anaphylactic.

Shock is a collection of signs and symptoms, many of which are nonspecific. Although symptoms vary somewhat among the different kinds of shock, there are some similarities. The patient may appear pale and claim to feel sick or weak without reporting any specific symptoms. Behavioral changes are often some of the earliest symptoms and may include restlessness, anxiety, confusion, depression, and lack of interest. Thirst is a common complaint; the skin may feel cold or clammy.

Assessing the patient's cardiovascular status may give some important signs for a diagnosis of acute shock. Blood pressure is often low with a diminished cardiac output. Heart rate may be rapid with a weak pulse. Breathing is usually rapid and shallow. Figure 19.1 ■ shows some of the common symptoms of a patient in shock.

Fast Facts Shock

- Cardiogenic shock occurs in 7%–10% of the patients suffering acute MI.
- Cardiogenic shock is the leading cause of death in patients hospitalized with acute MI, with a mortality rate of 70%–80%.
- The mortality rate for patients with sepsis who develop septic shock is 40%–70%.
- Incidence of anaphylaxis may be twice as high in women as in men.
- 0.4%–0.8% of the population experiences anaphylaxis from insect stings, resulting in approximately 250 deaths per year.

TABLE 19.1	Classification of Shock	
TYPE OF SHOCK	**DEFINITION**	**UNDERLYING PATHOLOGY**
Cardiogenic	Failure of the heart to pump sufficient blood to tissues	Left heart failure, myocardial ischemia, MI, dysrhythmias, pulmonary embolism, and myocardial or pericardial infection
Hypovolemic	Loss of blood volume	Hemorrhage, burns, profuse sweating, excessive urination, vomiting, or diarrhea
Neurogenic	Vasodilation due to overstimulation of the parasympathetic nervous system or understimulation of the sympathetic nervous system	Trauma to spinal cord or medulla, severe emotional stress or pain, drugs that depress the central nervous system
Septic	Multiple organ dysfunction as a result of pathogenic organisms in the blood	Widespread inflammatory response to bacterial, fungal, or parasitic infection
Anaphylactic	Acute allergic reaction	Severe reaction to allergens such as penicillin, nuts, shellfish, or animal proteins

FIGURE 19.1

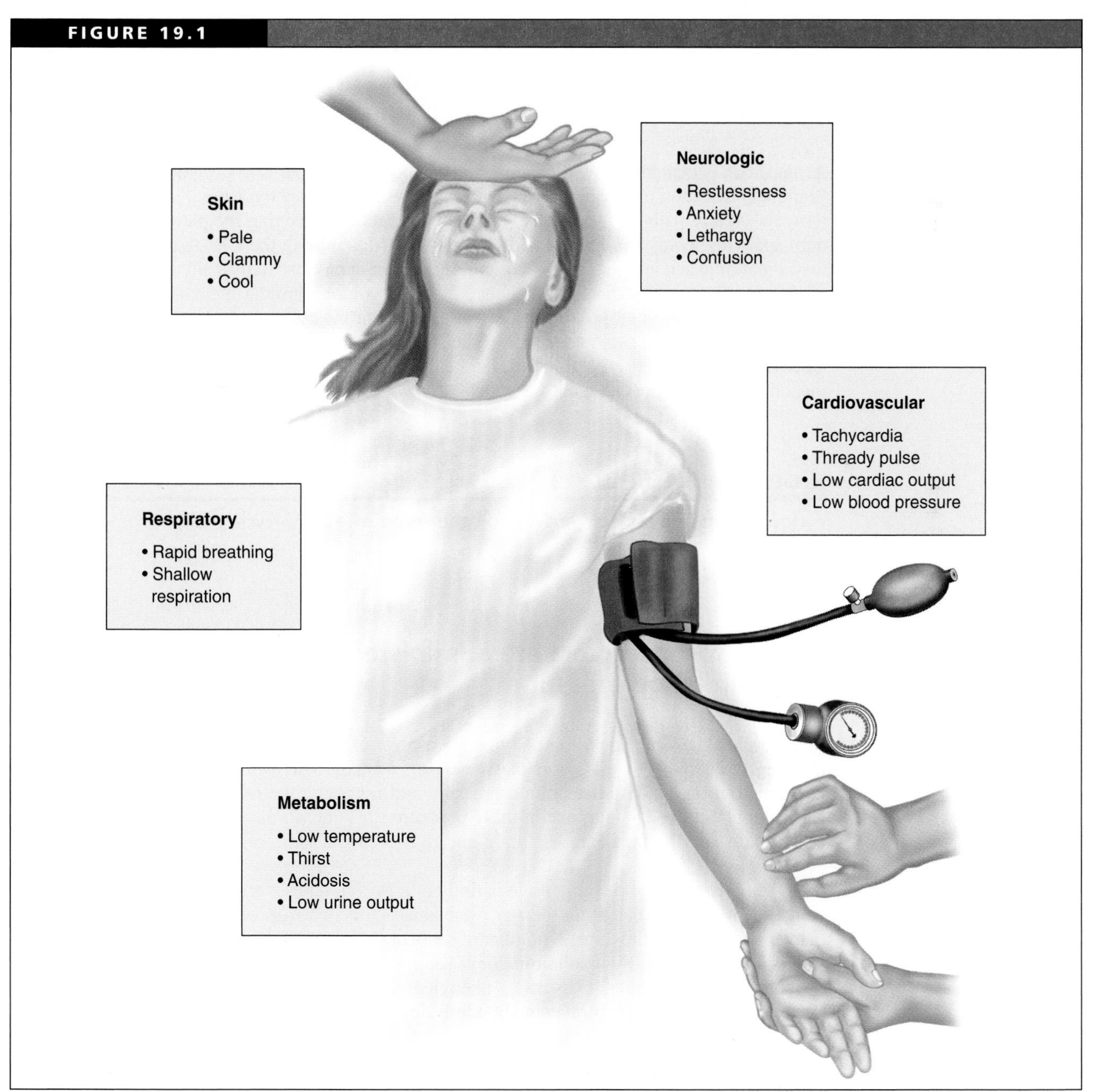

Symptoms of a patient in shock

hypo = *below*
vol = *volume*
emic = *pertaining to the blood*

neuro = *nervous system*
genic = *origin*

cardio = *heart*
genic = *origin*

Diagnosis of shock is rarely made on the basis of such nonspecific symptoms. A careful medical history, however, will give the healthcare provider valuable clues as to what type of shock may be present. For example, obvious trauma or bleeding combined with the symptoms mentioned previously would suggest **hypovolemic shock.** If trauma to the brain or spinal cord is evident, **neurogenic shock** may be suspected. A history of heart disease would suggest **cardiogenic shock,** whereas a recent infection may indicate **septic shock.** A history of allergy with a sudden onset of symptoms following food or drug intake may suggest **anaphylaxis.**

A hallmark of most types of shock is the inability of the cardiovascular system to send sufficient blood to the vital organs, with the heart and brain being affected early in the progression of the disease. Lack of blood to the brain may result in fainting, whereas disruption of blood supply to the myocardium may cause permanent damage to these vital cells. Without immediate treatment, other organ systems will be affected and respiratory failure or renal failure may result.

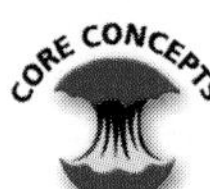

19.2 The initial treatment of shock includes basic life support and identification of the underlying cause.

Acute shock is treated as a medical emergency, and the first goal is to provide basic life support. Rapid identification of the underlying cause is essential because the patient's condition may deteriorate rapidly without specific and aggressive treatment. Keeping the patient quiet and warm until specific therapy can be initiated is important. Maintaining the ABCs of life support—airway, breathing, and circulation—is critical. If the patient has lost significant amounts of blood or other body fluids, immediate maintenance of blood volume through the administration of fluid and electrolytes or blood products is essential. Sodium bicarbonate may be administered to reverse the acidosis that may occur during shock. Unless contraindicated, oxygen is administered. Once basic life support is established, the healthcare practitioner can begin more specific treatment of the underlying causes of the shock.

Concept Review 19.1

- How would a paramedic arriving on the scene of a motorcycle accident determine the cause of the patient's shock?

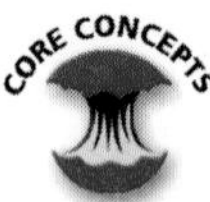

19.3 Vasoconstrictors are administered during shock to maintain blood pressure.

In the early stages of shock, the body compensates for the initial fall in blood pressure by increasing the activity of the sympathetic nervous system. This sympathetic activity results in vasoconstriction, which raises blood pressure and increases the heart rate and force of myocardial contraction. The purpose of these compensatory measures is to maintain blood flow to vital organs such as the heart and brain and to decrease flow to other organs such as the kidneys and liver.

The body's ability to compensate is limited, however, and severe hypotension may develop, which requires immediate drug therapy. Vasoconstrictors or vasopressors are medications useful in maintaining blood pressure. A number of vasoconstrictors may be used to stabilize blood pressure in shock patients. Sympathomimetics used for shock include norepinephrine (Levarterenol, Levophed), methoxamine (Vasoxyl), phenylephrine (Neo-Synephrine), and mephentermine (Wyamine). When given intravenously, these drugs can immediately raise blood pressure. Patients receiving these agents must be monitored continuously during the infusion to avoid hypertension due to overtreatment. The basic pharmacology of the adrenergic agents was discussed in Chapter 7. Table 19.2 gives the dosages for these agents.

TABLE 19.2 Vasoconstrictors for Shock

DRUG	RATE AND ADULT DOSE	REMARKS
Pr epinephrine	Subcutaneous 0.1–0.5 ml of 1:100 q10–15 min; IV 0.1–0.25 ml of 1:1000 q10–15 min	Nonselective adrenergic agent; also for cardiac arrest and asthma
mephentermine (Wyamine)	IV 20–60 mg as an infusion (1.2 mg/ml of D_5W)	Has alpha- and predominant beta-adrenergic activity; also for certain dysrhythmias
methoxamine hydrochloride (Vasoxyl)	IV 3–5 mg over 5–10 min	Selective to alpha receptors; used to maintain blood pressure during general anesthesia; also for certain dysrhythmias; IM form available
Pr norepinephrine (Levarterenol, Levophed)	IV 8–12 mcg/min until pressure stabilizes, then 2–4 mcg/min for maintenance	Has both alpha- and $beta_1$-adrenergic activity; also for cardiac arrest
phenylephrine (Neo-Synephrine and many others)	IV 0.1–0.18 mg/min until pressure stabilizes, then 0.04–0.06 mg/min for maintenance	Selective to alpha receptors; used to maintain blood pressure during general anesthesia; also for certain dysrhythmias, nasal congestion, and glaucoma, and to dilate the pupil during ophthalmic exams; subcutaneous, IM, ophthalmic, and nasal spray forms available

DRUG PROFILE: Vasoconstrictor/Sympathomimetic: Pr *Norepinephrine (Levarterenol, Levophed)*

Actions and Uses:

Norepinephrine is a sympathomimetic that acts directly on alpha-adrenergic receptors in the smooth muscle of blood vessels to rapidly raise blood pressure. Its stimulation of $beta_1$ receptors in the heart produces a positive inotropic response that increases cardiac output. Its primary uses are for acute shock and cardiac arrest. Because it is only administered by the IV route, its onset of action is immediate.

Adverse Effects and Interactions:

Norepinephrine is a powerful vasoconstrictor; thus, continuous monitoring of blood pressure is required to avoid hypertension. When first administered reflex bradycardia is sometimes experienced. It also has the ability to produce various types of dysrhythmias. Because of its potent effects on the cardiovascular system, it should be used with great caution in patients with heart disease.

Norepinephrine interacts with many drugs, including alpha and beta blockers, which may decrease the drug's pressor effects. Conversely, ergot alkaloids and tricyclic antidepressants may increase vasopressor effects. Halothane and cyclopropane may increase the risk of dysrhythmias.

See the Companion Website for a Nursing Process Focus specific to this drug.

19.4 Cardiotonic drugs are useful in reversing the decreased cardiac output resulting from shock.

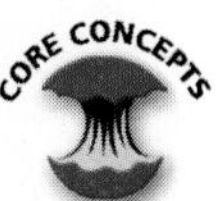

Cardiotonic drugs increase the force of contraction of the heart. In the treatment of shock, they are used to increase cardiac output. See Table 19.3.

As cardiogenic shock progresses, the heart begins to fail. Cardiac output decreases, lowering the amount of blood reaching vital tissues and worsening shock. Cardiotonic drugs, also known as **inotropic agents,** have the potential to reverse the cardiac symptoms of shock by increasing the force of myocardial contraction. In Chapter 16, the role of the cardiotonic drug digoxin

TABLE 19.3 Cardiotonic (Inotropic) Drugs of Importance to Shock

DRUG	RATE AND ADULT DOSE	REMARKS
digoxin (Lanoxin, Lanoxicaps)	IV digitalizing dose 2.5 mcg–5 mcg q6 hours × 24 hours; maintenance dose-0.125–0.5 mg daily	Doses are highly individualized for each patient; oral forms available; also for dysrhythmias and heart failure
dobutamine (Dobutrex)	IV infused at a rate of 2.5–40 mcg/kg/min for a max of 72 hours	Selective $beta_1$-adrenergic activity; for cardiac decompensation
Pr dopamine (Dopastat, Intropin)	IV 1.5 mcg/kg/min initial dose; may be increased to 30 mcg/kg/min	May stimulate dopaminergic, $beta_1$- or $alpha_1$-adrenergic receptors, depending on dose

(Lanoxin) in treating patients with heart failure was discussed. Digoxin increases myocardial contractility and cardiac output, thus rapidly bringing tissues their needed oxygen. Chapter 16 should be reviewed because drugs prescribed for heart failure are sometimes used for the treatment of shock.

Dobutamine (Dobutrex) is a $beta_1$-adrenergic agent that is often a drug of choice for the short-term treatment of certain types of shock because of its ability to cause the heart to beat more force-

DRUG PROFILE: Cardiotonic Agent: Pr *Dopamine (Dopastat, Intropin)*

Actions and Uses:

Dopamine is the immediate metabolic precursor to norepinephrine. Although classified as an sympathomimetic the mechanism of dopamine's action is dependent on the dose. At low doses, dopamine selectively stimulates receptors that cause an increased blood flow through the kidneys. This makes dopamine valuable in treating hypovolemic and cardiogenic shock. At higher doses, dopamine stimulates $beta_1$-adrenergic receptors, causing the heart to beat with more force and increasing cardiac output. Another beneficial effect of dopamine when given in higher doses is its ability to stimulate alpha-adrenergic receptors, thus causing vasoconstriction and raising blood pressure.

Adverse Effects and Interactions:

Because of its intense effects on the cardiovascular system, patients receiving dopamine are continuously monitored for signs of dysrhythmias and hypotension. Side effects are normally self-limiting because of the short half-life of the drug.

Dopamine interacts with many other drugs. For example, administering it with MAO inhibitors and ergot alkaloids increases alpha-adrenergic effects. Phenytoin may decrease dopamine action. Beta blockers may block dopamine's cardiac effects. Alpha blockers decrease peripheral vasoconstriction. Halothane increases the risk of hypertension and ventricular dysrhythmias.

Mechanism in Action: 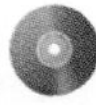

Dopamine is a naturally occurring neurotransmitter that relieves symptoms of heart failure or shock by increasing the force of cardiac contraction. This is accomplished through activation of $beta_1$-adrenergic receptors and an influx of calcium into myocardial cells.

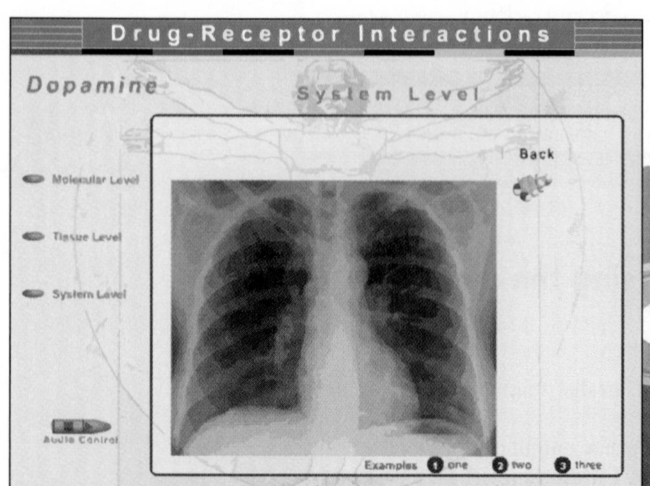

Use the student CD-ROM to see Mechanism in Action for Dopamine.

See the Companion Website for a Nursing Process Focus specific to this drug.

fully, without significantly increasing heart rate. The resulting increase in cardiac output assists in maintaining blood flow to vital organs. Although very effective, dobutamine has a half-life of only 2 minutes and therapy is limited to 72 hours.

19.5 Fluid replacement agents are infused to replace fluids lost during shock, which helps return blood pressure to normal.

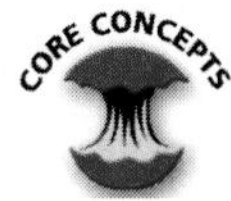

A number of agents are used to replace blood or other fluids lost during hypovolemic shock. Along with vasoconstrictors and cardiotonic agents, they help to reverse hypotension.

When a patient loses significant amounts of blood or other body fluids, immediate treatment with fluid replacement agents is essential. Fluid loss can occur due to hemorrhage, extensive burns, severe dehydration, persistent vomiting or diarrhea, or intensive diuretic therapy.

Fluid replacement agents are generally placed into the following three categories:

- Blood
- Colloids
- Crystalloids

Whole blood is indicated for the treatment of acute, massive blood loss when there is the need to replace plasma volume and supply red blood cells. The administration of whole blood has been largely replaced with the use of blood components. The supply of blood products depends on human donors and requires careful cross-matching to ensure compatibility between the donor and patient. Whole blood, although carefully screened, has the potential to transmit serious infections such as hepatitis or HIV.

Colloid and crystalloid infusions are often used when up to one third of an adult's blood volume is lost. **Colloids** are proteins or other large molecules that stay suspended in the blood for a long period and draw water molecules from the body's cells and tissues into the blood vessels. Colloids include normal human serum albumin, plasma protein fraction, dextran, and hetastarch.

Crystalloids are IV solutions that contain electrolytes in amounts resembling those of natural plasma. Unlike colloids, crystalloid solutions leave the blood and enter cells. They are used to replace fluids that have been lost and to increase urine output. Common crystalloids include normal saline, lactated Ringer's, hypertonic saline, and 5% dextrose in water (D_5W). Fluid replacement agents are presented in greater detail in Chapter 28.

DRUG PROFILE: Fluid Replacement Agent (Colloid): Pr *Normal Serum Albumin (Albuminar, Albutein, Buminate, Plasbumin)*

Actions and Uses:

Normal serum albumin is a protein extracted from whole blood or plasma. Albumin naturally comprises about 60% of all blood proteins. Its normal functions are to maintain plasma pressure and to shuttle certain substances through the blood, including a substantial number of drug molecules. After extraction from blood or plasma, it is sterilized to remove possible contamination by the hepatitis viruses or HIV.

Administered IV, albumin is used to restore plasma volume in hypovolemic shock, or to restore blood proteins in patients with hypoproteinemia. It has an immediate onset of action and is available in concentrations of 5% and 25%.

Adverse Effects and Interactions:

Because albumin is a natural blood product, allergic reactions are possible. Signs of allergy include fever, chills, rash, dyspnea, and possibly hypotension. Protein overload may occur if excessive albumin is infused.

No clinically significant drug interactions have been identified.

See the Nursing Process Focus in Chapter 28 for "Patients Receiving Fluid Replacement Agents," as well as the Companion Website for a Nursing Process Focus specific to this drug.

NURSING PROCESS FOCUS

Patients Receiving Fluid Replacement Therapy

ASSESSMENT

Prior to administration:

- Obtain complete health history, including allergies, drug history, and possible drug interactions.
- Assess lung sounds.
- Obtain vital signs.
- Assess level of consciousness.
- Assess renal function (BUN and creatinine).

POTENTIAL NURSING DIAGNOSES

- Risk for Injury, related to allergic reaction to drug
- Ineffective Tissue Perfusion, related to adverse effects of drug
- Excess Fluid Volume, related to increased intravascular volume
- Deficient Knowledge, related to drug therapy

PLANNING: Patient Goals and Expected Outcomes

The patient will:

- Immediately report difficulty breathing
- Report itching, flushing
- Maintain urinary output at least 50 ml/h
- Demonstrate an understanding of the drug's action by accurately describing drug side effects and precautions

IMPLEMENTATION

Interventions and (Rationales)	Patient Education/Discharge Planning
▪ Monitor respiratory status. (Effects of drugs and rapid infusion may result in fluid overload.)	Instruct patient to: ▪ Report any signs of respiratory distress ▪ Report changes in sensorium such as lightheadedness, drowsiness, or dizziness
▪ Monitor intake and output for changes in renal function.	▪ Instruct patient concerning rationale for Foley catheter insertion.
▪ Monitor electrolytes. (Crystalloid drugs may cause hypernatremia and resulting fluid retention.)	▪ Instruct patient to report any evidence of edema.
▪ Observe patient for signs of allergic reactions. (Administration of blood and blood products could cause allergic reactions.)	Instruct patient: ▪ To report itching, rash, chills, and difficulty breathing ▪ That frequent blood draws are necessary to monitor possible complications of drug administration
▪ Observe urine for changes in color. (Adverse reaction to blood could cause hematuria.)	▪ Instruct patient to notify the healthcare provider if changes in urine color occur.

EVALUATION OF OUTCOME CRITERIA

Evaluate the effectiveness of drug therapy by confirming that patient goals and expected outcomes have been met (see "Planning").

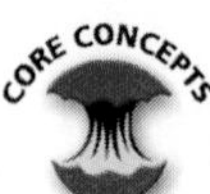

19.6 Anaphylaxis is a special type of shock caused by a hyperresponse of body defense mechanisms.

an = *without or against*
phylaxis = *protection*

Anaphylaxis is a condition in which the natural body defenses produce a hyperresponse to an **antigen.** An antigen may be defined as anything that is recognized as foreign by the body. Certain foods, industrial chemicals, drugs, pollen, animal proteins, and even latex gloves can be anti-

FIGURE 19.2

Symptoms of anaphylaxis

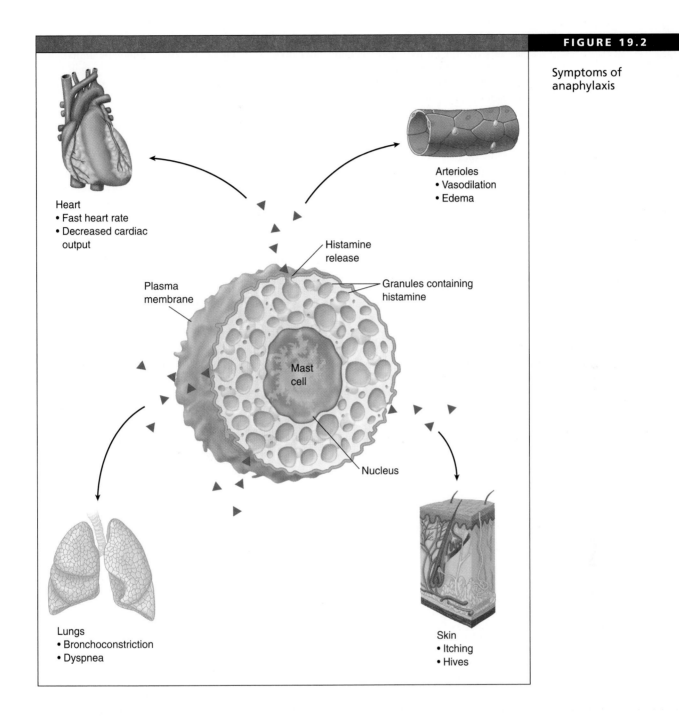

Heart
• Fast heart rate
• Decreased cardiac output

Arterioles
• Vasodilation
• Edema

Histamine release

Plasma membrane

Granules containing histamine

Mast cell

Nucleus

Lungs
• Bronchoconstriction
• Dyspnea

Skin
• Itching
• Hives

gens. A more detailed discussion of the immune system and the pharmacotherapy of immune disorders are included in Chapter 21.

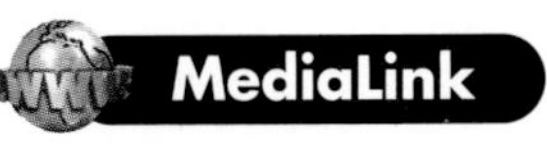

LATEX ALLERGIES

Normally the body responds to an antigen by processes such as inflammation, antibody production, and activation of lymphocytes that rid the body of the foreign agent. During anaphylaxis, the body responds quickly—usually within 20 minutes after exposure to the antigen—by releasing massive amounts of histamine and other defense mediators. Shortly after exposure to the antigen, the patient may experience itching, hives, and a tightness in the throat or chest. Swelling occurs around the larynx, causing the voice to become hoarse and a nonproductive cough. The patient may enter anaphylactic shock with acute symptoms such as a rapid fall in blood pressure and difficulty breathing due to bronchoconstriction. The fall in blood pressure causes *reflex tachycardia,* a rebound speeding up of the heart. Untreated anaphylactic shock is often fatal. Figure 19.2 ■ illustrates the symptoms of anaphylaxis.

Because anaphylaxis is potentially fatal, the patient and healthcare provider should take steps to prevent its occurrence. It is always easier to *prevent* anaphylaxis than it is to *treat* it. Patients should be strongly advised to avoid substances that trigger acute allergic reactions. This includes carefully reading all food and cosmetic labels to avoid exposure to known allergens. Individuals with known allergies to insect stings or food should carry injectable epinephrine, such as an EpiPen. The healthcare provider should always obtain a comprehensive drug allergy history before administering medications. Common allergies include the penicillin antibiotics and iodine-based contrast media used for radiological exams. The patient should be observed in the outpatient setting for 20 to 60 minutes after a drug injection because delayed anaphylactic reactions are possible.

Drug therapy of anaphylaxis is symptomatic and involves supporting the cardiovascular system and preventing further hyperreaction of body defenses. Several drugs are used to treat the symptoms of anaphylactic shock, depending on the severity of the condition. At the first suspicion of anaphylaxis, epinephrine and fluids are administered. Epinephrine is administered subcutaneously or IM to increase blood pressure and relieve bronchospasm. It may be necessary to use other vasoconstrictors, shown in Table 19.2, to overcome severe hypotension. Infusion of large amounts of fluids may be needed to overcome circulatory shock. These may include blood products, colloids, or crystalloids. The fluid infusions continue until systolic blood pressure reaches at least 90 mm Hg and is stable.

A number of other drugs are useful in treating anaphylaxis symptoms. Oxygen is usually administered immediately. Antihistamines such as diphenhydramine (Benadryl) may be administered IM or IV to prevent additional release of histamine. A bronchodilator such as albuterol (Ventolin, Proventil) is sometimes administered by inhalation to relieve the acute shortness of breath caused by histamine. Corticosteroids such as hydrocortisone may be administered to dampen the inflammatory response. Corticosteroids may be administered for 24 hours or longer to prevent the possibility of delayed anaphylactic reactions. The effects of antihistamines, bronchodilators, and corticosteroids are discussed in detail in Chapters 21, 24, and 28, respectively.

Concept Review 19.2

- How can cardiotonic drugs reduce the symptoms of shock without causing vasoconstriction?

DRUG PROFILE: Vasoconstrictor/Sympathomimetic: *Epinephrine (Adrenalin)*

Actions and Uses:

Subcutaneous or IV epinephrine is a drug of choice for acute anaphylactic shock because it can reverse many of the distressing symptoms within minutes. Epinephrine is a nonselective adrenergic activator, stimulating both alpha- and beta-adrenergic receptors. Almost immediately after injection, blood pressure rises due to stimulation of $alpha_1$ receptors. Activation of $beta_2$ receptors in the bronchi opens the airway and relieves the patient's shortness of breath. Cardiac output increases due to stimulation of $beta_1$ receptors in the heart.

Adverse Effects and Interactions:

When administered parenterally, epinephrine may cause serious adverse effects. Hypertension and dysrhythmias may occur rapidly; therefore, the patient is monitored continuously following IV or subcutaneous injections.

Epinephrine interacts with many drugs. For example, it may increase hypotension with phenothiazines and oxytocin. There may be additive toxicities with other sympathomimetics. MAO inhibitors, tricyclic antidepressants, and alpha- and beta-adrenergic agents inhibit the actions of epinephrine.

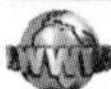
See the Companion Website for a Nursing Process Focus specific to this drug.

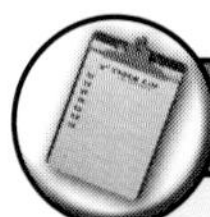

PATIENTS NEED TO KNOW

Patients treated for shock need to know the following:

1. Seek emergency medical assistance immediately if signs or symptoms of shock are being experienced.
2. While waiting for medical assistance, keep warm by using blankets.
3. If present, have caregiver monitor temperature, pulse, and blood pressure until emergency medical assistance arrives.
4. Do not move around. Lie down and elevate feet.
5. Report any changes in mental status, such as depression, confusion, or anxiety, to the healthcare provider immediately.
6. If allergies to bee or wasp stings are known, carry medications such as an EpiPen for all outside activities. Inform others of any allergies, where medications are kept, and how to administer them.
7. Take medications for shock (such as epinephrine) exactly as prescribed. ■

CHAPTER REVIEW

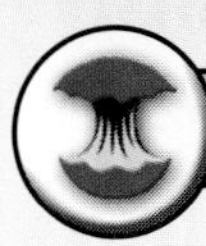

CORE CONCEPTS SUMMARY

19.1 Shock is a syndrome characterized by collapse of the circulatory system.

Basic types of shock include cardiogenic, hypovolemic, neurogenic, septic, and anaphylactic shock. Nonspecific symptoms of shock include hypotension, cold or clammy skin, reduced cardiac output, and behavioral changes such as confusion, apathy, or disorientation.

19.2 The initial treatment of shock includes basic life support and identification of the underlying cause.

Shock may be life threatening if allowed to proceed without medical intervention. Immediate therapy is targeted at restoring or maintaining vital processes such as respiratory function, blood pressure, and cardiac output. Immediate drug therapy includes vasoconstrictors, cardiotonic agents, and fluid replacement agents.

19.3 Vasoconstrictors are administered during shock to maintain blood pressure.

An immediate concern for the patient in shock is falling blood pressure. A variety of adrenergic agents, both selective and nonselective, are used to maintain blood pressure and cardiac function.

19.4 Cardiotonic drugs are useful in reversing the decreased cardiac output resulting from shock.

Circulatory failure can occur during shock if the cardiac output falls below a critical level. A number of cardiotonic drugs are used to strengthen myocardial function and improve cardiac output.

19.5 Fluid replacement agents are infused to replace fluids lost during shock, which helps return blood pressure to normal.

Fluid replacement agents include blood, colloids, and crystalloids. These agents help to maintain circulation and raise blood pressure.

19.6 Anaphylaxis is a special type of shock caused by a hyperresponse of body defense mechanisms.

When the body mounts a hyperresponse to an antigen, anaphylactic shock may result. Epinephrine is a drug of choice for immediately reversing the cardiovascular symptoms. Fluid replacement agents, antihistamines, and corticosteroids also serve roles in treating this form of shock.

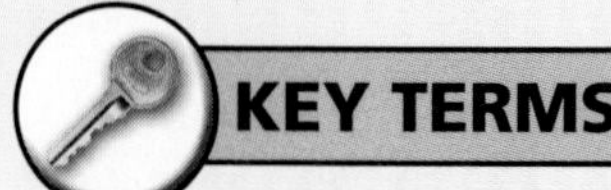

KEY TERMS

anaphylaxis (ann-uh-fuh-LAK-sis): potentially fatal condition caused by an acute allergic reaction to an antigen / *page 336*

antigen (ANN-tuh-jen): anything that is recognized as foreign by the immune system and produces an immune reaction / *page 340*

cardiogenic shock (kar-dee-oh-JEN-ik): type of shock caused when the heart is diseased such that it cannot maintain circulation to the tissues / *page 336*

colloids (KO-loyds): type of IV fluid replacement solution consisting of large protein molecules that are unable to cross membranes / *page 339*

crystalloids (KRIS-tuh-loyds): type of IV fluid replacement solution that resembles blood plasma and is capable of crossing membranes / *page 339*

hypovolemic snock (high-poh-voh-LEEM-ik): type of shock caused by loss of fluids such as occurs during hemorrhaging, extensive burns, or severe vomiting or diarrhea / *page 336*

inotropic agent (eye-noh-TROW-pik): drug or chemical that changes the force of contraction of the heart / *page 337*

neurogenic shock (nyoor-oh-JEN-ik): type of shock resulting from brain or spinal cord injury / *page 336*

septic shock (SEP-tik): type of shock caused by severe infection in the bloodstream / *page 336*

shock: condition in which there is inadequate blood flow to meet the body's needs / *page 334*

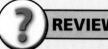

REVIEW QUESTIONS

The following questions are written in NCLEX-PN® style. Answer these questions to assess your knowledge of the chapter material, and go back and review any material that is not clear to you.

1. The patient with severe burns must be monitored for:

1. Cardiogenic shock
2. Hypovolemic shock
3. Septic shock
4. Anaphylactic shock

2. The most important intervention for a patient experiencing shock is assessing:

1. Temperature
2. Heart rate
3. Respirations
4. Blood pressure

3. Which IV solution would be most appropriate for a patient experiencing hypovolemic shock?

1. D5 0.45% NS
2. Normal serum albumin
3. 0.33% NS
4. Dextran

4. Which of the following is not correct regarding dopamine?

1. At low doses, dopamine causes increased blood flow to the kidneys.
2. At high doses, dopamine increases cardiac output.
3. Dopamine causes vasoconstriction and increases blood pressure.
4. At high doses, dopamine is used to treat anaphylaxis.

5. The patient is experiencing anaphylaxis. Which drug is used to increase blood pressure and treat bronchospasm related to anaphylaxis?

1. Epinephrine
2. Dobutamine (Dobutrex)
3. Digoxin (Lanoxin)
4. Dopamine

6. Which of the following medications is not used to treat anaphylaxis?

1. Antihistamines
2. Corticosteroids
3. Bronchodilators
4. Vasodilators

7. Use of cardiotonic agents in the treatment of shock:

1. Decreases cardiac output
2. Increases cardiac output
3. Slows the heart rate
4. Increases afterload

8. When using norepinephrine (Levophed):

1. Tachycardia may occur
2. Hypotension may occur
3. Hypertension may occur
4. Liver failure may occur

9. Dobutamine (Dobutrex) is used to treat shock because:

1. It increases myocardial contractility and heart rate
2. It increases myocardial contractility without increasing the heart rate
3. It decreases cardiac output
4. It is a powerful vasoconstrictor

10. When treating a shock patient, it is important to:

1. Keep the patient cool
2. Keep the patient warm
3. Elevate the patient's head
4. Monitor renal failure

CASE STUDY QUESTIONS

For questions 1–5, please refer to the following case study, and choose the correct answer from choices 1–4.

Mr. Hanks arrives in the emergency department having lost a considerable amount of blood in an automobile accident. His blood pressure is 60/30 mm Hg. His skin is clammy, and he is going in and out of consciousness. He is gasping for breath. The physician orders an infusion of D_5W, IV dobutamine, IM hydrocortisone, and subcutaneous epinephrine.

1. The healthcare provider notices that Mr. Hanks's breathing becomes less labored and he appears less anxious. Which drug most likely reduced Mr. Hanks's bronchospasm?

1. D_5W
2. Dobutamine
3. Hydrocortisone
4. Epinephrine

2. Which drug was given to replace the fluids lost during Mr. Hanks's accident?

1. D_5W
2. Dobutamine
3. Hydrocortisone
4. Epinephrine

3. Within 2 minutes, Mr. Hanks's blood pressure increases to 100/60 mm Hg. Which drug most likely caused this effect?

1. D_5W
2. Dobutamine
3. Hydrocortisone
4. Epinephrine

4. Why was dobutamine most likely given to Mr. Hanks?

1. To increase cardiac output
2. To replace lost fluids
3. To increase blood pressure
4. To reduce bronchospasm

5. After 4 hours, Mr. Hanks has stabilized, but he still has some difficulty breathing. Which of the following would most likely be prescribed for this symptom?

1. Diphenhydramine (Benadryl)
2. Hydrocortisone
3. Phenylephrine
4. Albuterol (Ventolin)

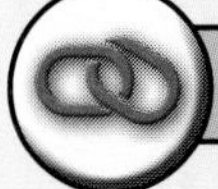

FURTHER STUDY

- Chapter 7 discusses the basic pharmacology of the adrenergic agents, or sympathomimetics.
- Chapter 16 discusses the role of the cardiotonic drug digoxin (Lanoxin) in treating patients with heart failure.
- Fluid replacement agents are presented in greater detail in Chapter 28.
- Chapter 21 provides a detailed discussion of the immune system and the pharmacology of immune disorders.
- See Chapter 21 for more information on antihistamines; Chapter 24, for bronchodilators; and Chapter 28 for corticosteroids.

EXPLORE MEDIALINK www.prenhall.com/holland

Additional resources for this chapter can be found on the CD-ROM accompanying this textbook, and on the Companion Website. Click on Chapter 19 to select activities for this chapter.

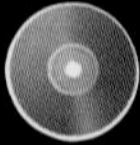

- Mechanism in Action: Dopamine
- Audio Glossary
- Concept Review
- NCLEX-PN® Review
- Nursing in Action
- Dosage Calculator

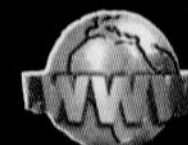

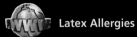

- Latex Allergies

CHAPTER

20 Drugs for Lipid Disorders

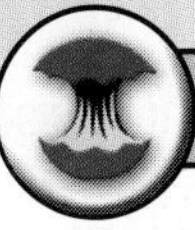

CORE CONCEPTS

20.1 High blood lipid levels can lead to cardiovascular disease.

20.2 The three classes of lipids are triglycerides, steroids, and phospholipids.

20.3 Lipoprotein levels are important predictors of cardiovascular disease.

20.4 Lipid levels can often be controlled through lifestyle changes.

20.5 Statins are drugs of first choice in reducing blood lipid levels.

20.6 Binding bile acids can increase cholesterol excretion and reduce LDL levels.

20.7 Nicotinic acid can reduce both triglyceride and LDL-cholesterol levels.

20.8 Fibric acid agents lower triglyceride levels but have little effect on LDLs.

20.9 Newer approaches to treating hyperlipidemia include ezetimibe and fixed-dose combination therapy.

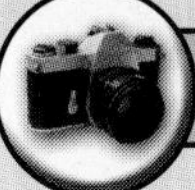

DRUG SNAPSHOT

The following drugs will be discussed in this chapter:

DRUG CLASSES	DRUG PROFILES
HMG-CoA reductase inhibitors (statins)	Pr atorvastatin (Lipitor)
Bile acid sequestrants	Pr cholestyramine (Questran)
Nicotinic acid	
Fibric acid agents (fibrates)	Pr gemfibrozil (Lopid)

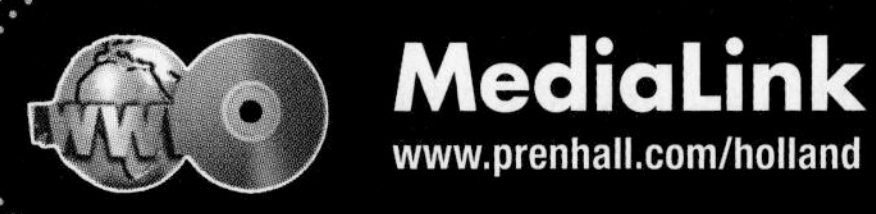

Interactive resources for this chapter can be found on the Companion Website. Click on Chapter 20 and "Begin" to select the activities for this chapter. For chapter-related animations, NCLEX-PN®-style questions, and an audio glossary, access the accompanying CD-ROM in this book.

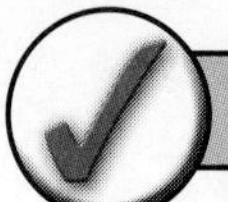

OBJECTIVES

After reading this chapter, the student should be able to:

1. Summarize the link between high blood cholesterol, LDL levels, and cardiovascular disease.
2. Compare and contrast the different types of lipids.
3. Illustrate how lipids are transported through the body.
4. Compare and contrast the different types of lipoproteins.
5. Give examples of how blood lipid levels can be controlled through nonpharmacological means.
6. For each of the following identify representative drugs, explain the mechanisms of drug action, primary actions, and important adverse effects:
   - **a.** HMG-CoA reductase inhibitors
   - **b.** Bile acid sequestrants
   - **c.** Nicotinic acid
   - **d.** Fibric acid agents
7. Categorize antilipidemic drugs based on their classifications and mechanisms of action.

Research during the 1960s and 1970s brought about a nutritional revolution as new knowledge about lipids and their relationship to obesity and cardiovascular disease allowed people to make more intelligent lifestyle choices. Since then, advances in the diagnosis of lipid disorders have helped to identify those patients at greatest risk for cardiovascular disease and those most likely to benefit from pharmacological intervention. Safe, effective drugs for lowering lipid levels are now available that decrease the risk of cardiovascular-related diseases. As a result of this knowledge and from advancements in pharmacology, the incidence of death due to most cardiovascular diseases has been declining. However, these disorders still remain the leading cause of death in the United States.

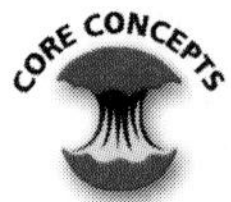

20.1 High blood lipid levels can lead to cardiovascular disease.

hyper = *above*
lipid = *fat*
emia = *blood*

Hyperlipidemia, the general term referring to high levels of lipids in the blood, is a major risk factor for cardiovascular disease. Elevated blood cholesterol, or **hypercholesterolemia,** is the type of hyperlipidemia that is most familiar to the general public. Cholesterol contributes to the fatty **plaque** that narrows arteries, thus contributing to angina, myocardial infarction (MI), and cerebrovascular accidents, as discussed in Chapter 18. Eating saturated fats plays a role in raising cholesterol levels in the blood. It is important that the healthcare provider have a firm grasp of lipid physiology to understand the pharmacology of the antilipidemics and, indeed, cardiovascular disease itself.

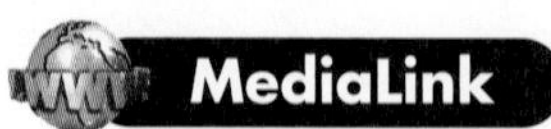

NATIONAL HEART, LUNG, AND BLOOD INSTITUTE

Fast Facts High Blood Cholesterol

- 30 million Americans (15% of all adults) are believed to have both hypertension and high blood cholesterol levels.
- The incidence of high blood cholesterol increases until age 65.
- Moderate alcohol intake does not reduce LDL cholesterol, but it does increase HDL cholesterol.
- Prior to menopause, high blood cholesterol occurs more frequently in men, but after age 50, the disease is more common in women.
- To lower blood cholesterol, both dietary cholesterol and saturated fats must be reduced.
- Familial hypercholesterolemia affects 1 in 500 people and is a genetic disease that predisposes people to high cholesterol levels.

20.2 The three classes of lipids are triglycerides, steroids, and phospholipids.

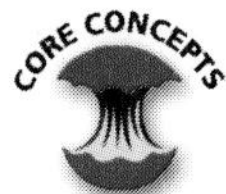

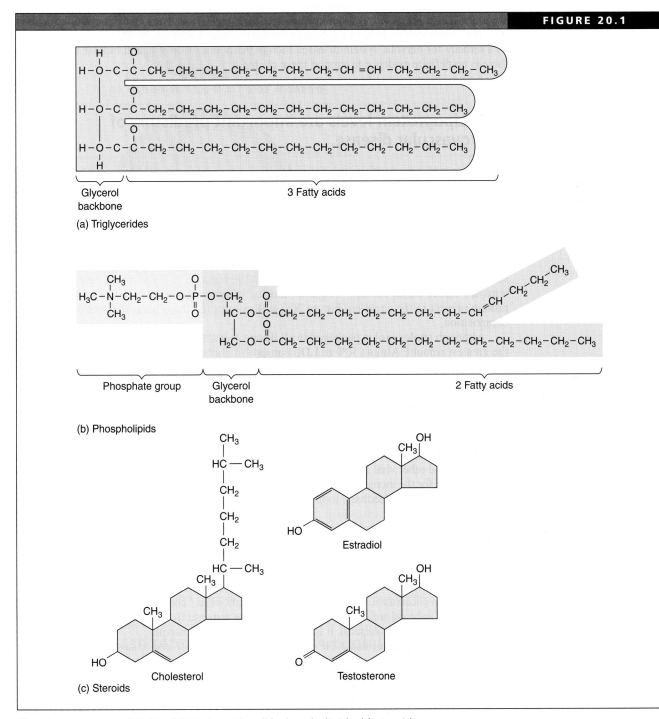

The three classes of lipids are illustrated in Figure 20.1■. The most common are the **triglycerides,** or neutral fats. Triglycerides form a large family of different lipids, all having three fatty acids attached to a chemical backbone of glycerol. Triglycerides are the major storage form of fat in the body and the only type of lipid that serves as an important energy source. They account for 90% of the total lipids in the body.

FIGURE 20.1

H–O–C–C–CH₂–CH₂–CH₂–CH₂–CH₂–CH₂–CH₂–CH =CH –CH₂–CH₂–CH₂–CH₃

H–O–C–C–CH₂–CH₂–CH₂–CH₂–CH₂–CH₂–CH₂–CH₂–CH₂–CH₂–CH₂–CH₃

H–O–C–C–CH₂–CH₂–CH₂–CH₂–CH₂–CH₂–CH₂–CH₂–CH₂–CH₂–CH₂–CH₃

Glycerol backbone

3 Fatty acids

(a) Triglycerides

$H_3C-N(CH_3)_2-CH_2-CH_2-O-P(=O)(O)-O-CH_2$

HC–O–C(=O)–CH₂–CH₂–CH₂–CH₂–CH₂–CH₂–CH₂–CH=CH–CH₂–CH₂–CH₃

H₂C–O–C(=O)–CH₂–CH₂–CH₂–CH₂–CH₂–CH₂–CH₂–CH₂–CH₂–CH₂–CH₂–CH₃

Phosphate group

Glycerol backbone

2 Fatty acids

(b) Phospholipids

Cholesterol

Estradiol

Testosterone

(c) Steroids

Chemical structure of lipids: (a) triglycerides, (b) phospholipids, (c) steroids

TABLE 20.1 Standard Laboratory Lipid Profiles

TYPE OF LIPID	LABORATORY VALUE (mg/dL)	STANDARD
Total cholesterol	<200	Desirable
	200–239	Borderline high
	>239	High
LDL cholesterol	<100	Optimal
	100–129	Near optimal/above optimal
	130–159	Borderline high
	160–189	High
	>189	Very high
HDL cholesterol	<40	Low
	>59	High
Triglycerides	<150	Normal
	150–199	Borderline high
	200–499	High
	>499	Very high

risk factors. The more risk factors present, the more aggressive is the therapy. Table 20.1 gives the desirable, borderline, and high laboratory values for each of the major lipids and lipoproteins.

Recommendations for the treatment of high blood cholesterol have been set by the National Cholesterol Education Program (NCEP) of the National Institute of Health. These recommendations, which are revised periodically, are the gold standard for treating this disorder. In some patients, high blood cholesterol levels can be controlled by initiating **therapeutic lifestyle changes,** without drug therapy. Even in high-risk patients for whom drug therapy is indicated, using these changes is important for reducing cholesterol levels. Following are the features of therapeutic lifestyle changes:

- Increase physical activity, which raises HDL levels and lowers triglycerides
- Maintain optimum weight because obesity is a major risk factor for coronary heart disease
- Maintain a healthy diet by observing a diet that:
  - Reduces saturated fat to 7% of total caloric intake
  - Reduces cholesterol intake to less than 200 mg/day
  - Increases intake of whole grains, vegetables, and fruits so that total dietary fiber is 10 to 25 g/day

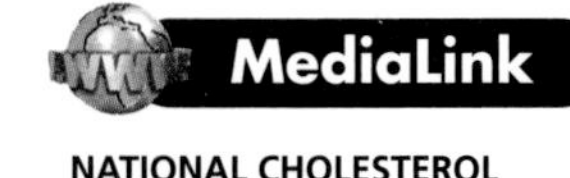

NATIONAL CHOLESTEROL EDUCATION PROGRAM

In addition to the recommendations of the NCEP, other lifestyle changes may contribute to keeping blood cholesterol levels within normal values and reducing the risk of CHD. These factors include stopping use of tobacco, maintaining blood pressure within normal limits, reducing stress, and limiting the intake of high-sugar foods. The particular type of fat ingested is also thought to play a role in blood cholesterol levels. Omega-3 fatty acids, which are found in high amounts in fatty fish (albacore tuna, salmon, sardines), tofu, and flaxseed oil, have been shown to reduce the risk of cardiovascular disease. Transfatty acids in the diet can raise blood cholesterol levels. Therefore, patients should be advised to avoid foods that are fried or contain vegetable shortening or partially hydrogenated oils.

Concept Review 20.1

- Why is the cholesterol in high-density lipoproteins considered to be "good" cholesterol?

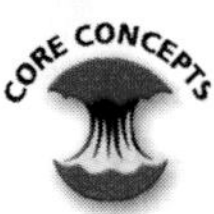

20.5 Statins are drugs of first choice in reducing blood lipid levels.

The statin class of antihyperlipidemics interferes with a critical enzyme in the synthesis of cholesterol. They are preferred drugs in the treatment of lipid disorders and involve some of the most widely prescribed drugs in the United States.

In the late 1970s, compounds were isolated from various species of fungi that were found to inhibit cholesterol production in human cells in the laboratory. This class of drugs, known as the *statins,* has since revolutionized the treatment of lipid disorders. Statins can produce a dramatic 20% to 40% reduction in LDL-cholesterol levels. In addition to decreasing LDL-cholesterol levels in the blood, statins can also lower triglyceride levels, lower VLDL levels, and raise "good" HDL-cholesterol levels.

Cholesterol is made in the liver by a series of more than 25 metabolic steps, beginning with acetyl CoA, a two-carbon unit that is produced from the breakdown of fatty acids. Of the many enzymes involved in this complex pathway, **HMG-CoA reductase** (hydroxymethylglutaryl-Coenzyme A reductase) serves as the primary regulatory site for cholesterol biosynthesis. Under normal conditions, this enzyme is controlled through negative feedback: High levels of LDL cholesterol in the blood will shut down production of HMG-CoA reductase, thus turning off the cholesterol pathway. Figure 20.3 ■ illustrates some of the steps in cholesterol biosynthesis and the importance of HMG-CoA reductase.

The statins act by inhibiting HMG-CoA reductase. As the liver makes less cholesterol, it responds by making more LDL receptors. These receptors remove more LDL from the blood; thus, blood levels of LDL cholesterol are reduced. The drop in lipid levels is not permanent, however, so patients need to remain on these drugs during the remainder of their lives or until their hyperlipidemia can be controlled through lifestyle changes. Statins have been shown to slow the progression of CHD and to reduce mortality from cardiovascular disease. Doses of the HMG-CoA reductase inhibitors are given in Table 20.2.

All the statins are given orally. Some may be administered in the evening because cholesterol biosynthesis in the body is higher at night.

FIGURE 20.3

Cholesterol biosynthesis and excretion

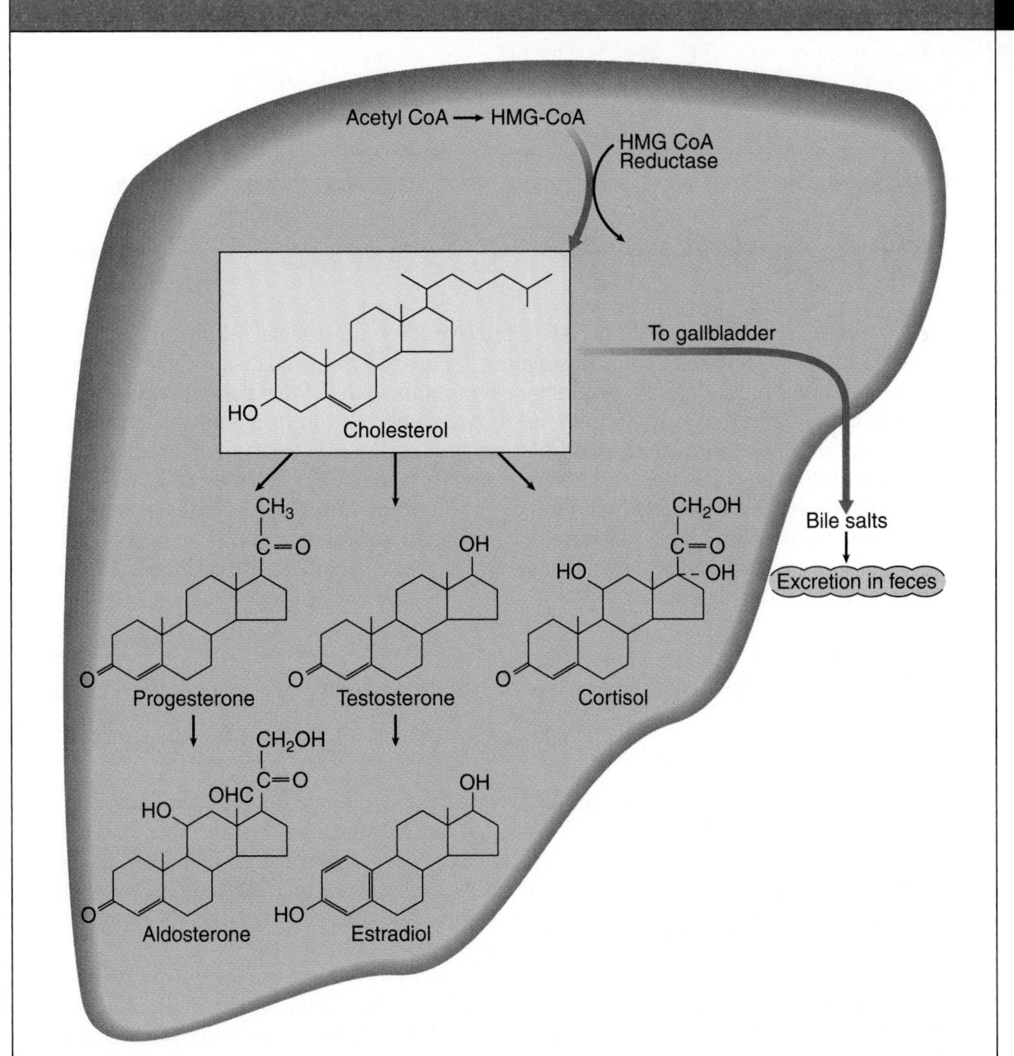

DRUG PROFILE: HMG-CoA Reductase Inhibitor (Statin): Pr *Atorvastatin (Lipitor)*

Actions and Uses:

Although lovastatin (Mevacor) was the first HMG-CoA reductase inhibitor approved for use in the United States, newer statins have been developed that offer certain advantages. For example, atorvastatin has a longer half-life and may be administered without regard to food or time of day. Maximum effects from atorvastatin are seen in 4–8 weeks, after which time a follow-up measurement of blood lipid levels is taken to determine whether the dosage is optimum.

Adverse Effects and Interactions:

Side effects of atorvastatin are rarely severe enough to cause discontinuation of therapy and include GI complaints such as intestinal cramping, diarrhea, and constipation. A small percentage of patients experience liver damage; thus, liver function is usually monitored periodically during therapy. Like other statins, atorvastatin is a pregnancy category X drug; birth defects have been noted in animal studies, and the risks to the fetus outweigh any potential benefits to the patient.

Atorvastatin interacts with many other drugs. For example, it may increase digoxin levels by 20%, as well as increase levels of oral contraceptives. Erythromycin may increase atorvastatin levels 40%.

Grapefruit juice inhibits the metabolism of statins, allowing them to reach toxic levels. Because HMG-CoA reductase inhibitors also decrease the synthesis of coenzyme Q10 (CoQ10), patients may benefit from CoQ10 supplements.

Mechanism in Action: 

Atorvastatin slows the biosynthesis of cholesterol by blocking the rate-limiting enzyme, HMG-CoA reductase. This enzyme is necessary for the availability of LDL and VLDL fragments to body cells including the liver. Atorvastatin also upregulates LDL receptors in the liver. The net effect is reduced cholesterol and trigylceride blood levels. ■

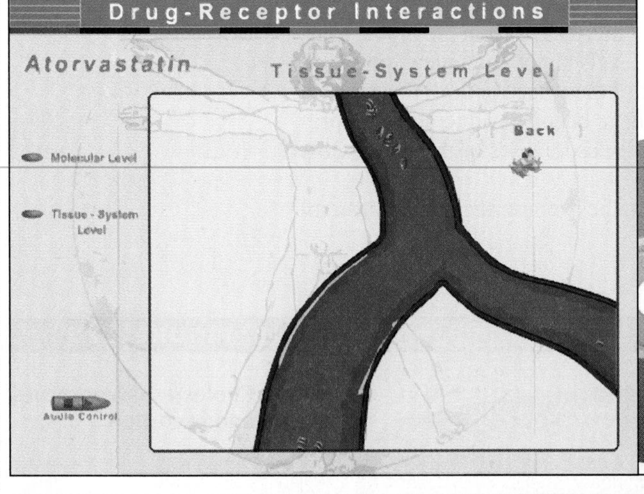

Use the student CD-ROM to see Mechanism in Action for Atorvastatin.

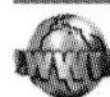 *See the Companion Website for a Nursing Process Focus specific to this drug.*

The statins are generally safe drugs, having few serious side effects. GI disturbances such as indigestion, flatulence, cramping, and constipation are usually mild and disappear with continued use. Statins can cause muscle injury, resulting in symptoms such as weakness, soreness, and pain. Muscle side effects are dose related and tend to occur more often in elderly patients. Patients should be carefully monitored for these symptoms because muscle injury may progress to more serious conditions. In 2001, cerivastatin was removed from the market because of 31 fatalities due to severe rhabdomyolysis associated with the use of the drug. *Rhabdomyolysis* is a medical condition in which muscle tissue becomes extremely inflamed, resulting in breakdown of muscle. Patients reporting muscular soreness or weakness may have their statin dosage reduced, or they may be switched to a different drug class.

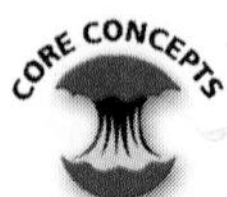

20.6 Binding bile acids can increase cholesterol excretion and reduce LDL levels.

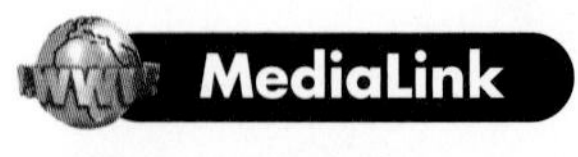

INTERNATIONAL FOOD INFORMATION COUNCIL

Bile acid sequestrants bind bile acids, thus increasing the excretion of cholesterol. They are sometimes used in combination with the statins. Doses of these drugs are given in Table 20.2.

Prior to the discovery of the statins, the primary means of lowering blood cholesterol was through use of bile acid sequestrants. **Bile acids** are substances that aid the digestion of fats, which contain a high concentration of cholesterol. Once bound in the intestine, the cholesterol in the bile acids becomes insoluble and is therefore eliminated in the feces.

Although effective at producing a 20% decrease in LDL-cholesterol levels, the bile acid sequestrants tend to cause more frequent side effects than do the statins. Taken orally, bile acid sequestrants are not absorbed into the circulation; therefore, their side effects are limited to the GI tract. Many patients, however, experience constipation, bloating, nausea, or indigestion. The

TABLE 20.2 Drugs for Dyslipidemias

DRUG	ROUTE AND ADULT DOSE	REMARKS
HMG-COA REDUCTASE INHIBITORS		
Pr atorvastatin (Lipitor)	PO 10–80 mg/day	May be taken with or without food any time of the day
fluvastatin (Lescol)	PO 20 mg/day (max: 80 mg/day)	May be taken with or without food in the evening
lovastatin (Mevacor)	PO 20–40 mg once or twice daily	Should be taken with meals in the evening
pravastatin (Pravachol)	PO 10–40 mg/day	May be taken with or without food in the evening
rosuvastatin (Crestor)	PO 5–40 mg/day	May be taken with or without food at any time of the day
simvastatin (Zocor)	PO 5–40 mg/day	May be taken with or without food in the evening
BILE ACID-BINDING AGENTS		
Pr cholestyramine (Questran)	PO 4–8 g bid–qid	Taken with large amounts of fluid; take other drugs 1 hour before or 4 hours after
colesevelam (Welchol)	PO 1350 mg/day	Taken with meals and with at least 8 oz of fluid
colestipol (Colestid)	PO 5–15 g bid–qid	Taken with large amounts of fluid; take other drugs 1 hour before or 4 hours after
FIBRIC ACID AGENTS		
fenofibrate (Tricor)	PO 54 mg/day (max: 160 mg/day)	Taken with meals. Assess periodically for symptoms of myopathy
Pr gemfibrozil (Lopid)	PO 600 mg bid (max: 1500 mg/day)	Take 30 min before morning and evening meals
OTHER AGENTS		
ezetimibe (Zetia)	PO 10 mg/day	One of the newest antihyperlipidemics Inhibits cholesterol absorption
niacin (Niac, Nicobid, others)	PO 1.5 to 3 g/day (max: 6 g/day)	Also used to treat niacin deficiency (10–20 mg/day) Give with meals

DRUG PROFILE: Bile Acid Sequestrant: Pr *Cholestyramine (Questran)*

Actions and Uses:

Cholestyramine is a powder that is mixed with fluid before being taken once or twice daily. It is not absorbed or metabolized once it enters the intestine; thus, it does not produce systemic effects. It may take 30 days or longer to produce its maximum effect.

Adverse Effects and Interactions:

Although cholestyramine rarely produces serious side effects, patients may experience constipation, bloating, gas, and nausea that may limit its use.

Because cholestyramine can bind to other drugs and interfere with their absorption, it should not be taken at the same time as other medications. Cholestyramine is sometimes combined with other cholesterol-lowering drugs such as the statins or nicotinic acid to produce additive effects.

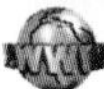

See the Companion Website for a Nursing Process Focus specific to this drug.

newest drug in this class, colesevelam (Welchol) is reported to have fewer side effects than the older drugs. Also of concern is that bile acid sequestrants can prevent the absorption of other medications and vitamins that may be taken at the same time. This can be avoided by teaching the patient to take these drugs 1 to 2 hours before, or 4 hours after, other medications.

NURSING PROCESS FOCUS

Patients Receiving HMG-CoA Reductase Inhibitor Therapy

ASSESSMENT

Prior to administration:

- Obtain a complete health history including allergies, drug history, and possible drug interactions
- Obtain baseline liver function tests, lipid studies, and a pregnancy test in women of childbearing age

POTENTIAL NURSING DIAGNOSES

- Deficient Knowledge, related to need for altered lifestyle
- Noncompliance, related to dietary and drug regimen
- Chronic Pain, related to drug-induced myopathy
- Impaired Health Maintenance, related to insufficient knowledge of actions and effects of prescribed drug therapy

PLANNING: Patient Goals and Expected Outcomes

The patient will:

- Immediately report skeletal muscle pain, unexplained muscle soreness, or weakness
- Demonstrate compliance with appropriate lifestyle changes
- Demonstrate an understanding of the drug's action by accurately describing drug side effects and precautions

IMPLEMENTATION

Interventions and (Rationales)	Patient Education/Discharge Planning
■ Monitor blood cholesterol and triglyceride levels at intervals during therapy (to determine effectiveness of therapy).	■ Advise patient of the importance of keeping appointments for laboratory testing.
■ Monitor patient compliance with dietary regimen. (Maintenance of controlled saturated fat diet is essential to effectiveness of medications.)	■ Provide patient with information needed to maintain low saturated fat, low cholesterol diet.
■ Monitor patient for alcohol abuse. (Excessive alcohol intake may result in liver damage and interfere with drug effectiveness.)	■ Instruct patient to avoid or limit alcohol use.
■ Monitor CPK level. (Elevated CPK may be indicative of impending myopathy.)	■ Instruct patient to report symptoms of leg or muscle pain to the healthcare provider.
■ Obtain patient's smoking history. (Smoking increases risk of cardiovascular disease and may decrease HDL levels.)	■ Encourage smoking cessation if appropriate.

EVALUATION OF OUTCOME CRITERIA

Evaluate the effectiveness of drug therapy by confirming that patient goals and expected outcomes have been met (see "Planning").

See Table 20.2 for a list of drugs to which these nursing actions apply.

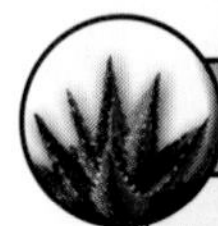

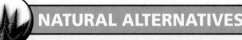

NATURAL ALTERNATIVES

Guggul Extracts for Lowering Blood Lipids

A number of herbal supplements are purported to lower blood cholesterol levels. One such botanical comes from the mukul tree (*Commiphora mukul*), a small, thorny shrub native to India. Extracts from the stems of this plant produce a thick resin called *guggul* or *guggul gum*. The resin contains a number of active agents that are classified as steroids called *guggulsterones*. In the Bible, this botanical is referred to as myrrh.

The benefits of mukul extracts were reported in ancient Indian literature. Guggulsterones have been reported to lower both cholesterol and triglyceride levels while raising HDL levels. They are also reported to have some antiplatelet activity.

The powdered mukul resin is available in capsule form. Dosage depends on the concentration of guggulsterones in the resin; however, a typical dosage is 25 mg of guggulsterones 3 times daily. ■

20.7 Nicotinic acid can reduce both triglyceride and LDL-cholesterol levels.

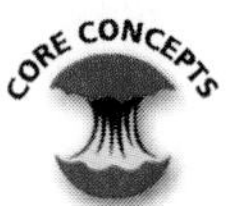

Nicotinic acid, or niacin, is a water-soluble B-complex vitamin that is occasionally used to lower lipid levels. It has a number of side effects that limit its use.

Its ability to lower lipid levels is unrelated to its role as a vitamin; very high doses are needed to achieve an antilipidemic effect. For lowering cholesterol, the usual dose is 2 to 3 g per day. When taken as a vitamin, the dose is only 25 mg per day.

The primary effect of nicotinic acid is to decrease VLDL levels. The patient experiences a reduction in LDL-cholesterol and triglyceride levels. It also has the desirable effects of reducing triglycerides and increasing HDL levels. Thus, niacin is unique in that it can improve all lipoprotein abnormalities. As with other lipid-lowering drugs, its maximum effects may take a month or longer to achieve.

Although effective at reducing LDL cholesterol by 20%, nicotinic acid produces more side effects than the statins. Flushing and hot flashes occur in almost every patient. In addition, a variety of uncomfortable intestinal effects such as nausea, excess gas, and diarrhea are commonly reported. More serious side effects such as liver toxicity and gout are possible. Because of these adverse effects, nicotinic acid is most often used in lower doses in combination with a statin or bile acid sequestrant because the beneficial effects of these drugs are additive. Extended-release niacin, which is taken once daily, causes less flushing and GI side effects.

As a vitamin, niacin is available without a prescription. However, patients should be instructed not to attempt self-medication with this drug. One form of niacin, available over the counter as a vitamin supplement called *nicotinamide,* has no lipid-lowering effects. Patients should be informed that if nicotinic acid is used to lower cholesterol, it should be done under medical supervision.

Concept Review 20.2

- How does the mechanism of the statins differ from that of nicotinic acid?

20.8 Fibric acid agents lower triglyceride levels but have little effect on LDLs.

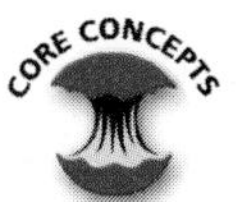

Once widely used to lower lipid levels, the fibric acid agents, or fibrates, have been largely replaced by the statins. They are sometimes used in combination with the statins. Doses of the fibrates are shown in Table 20.2.

The first fibric acid agent, clofibrate (Atromid-S), was widely prescribed until studies demonstrated it did not reduce mortality from cardiovascular disease. Although clofibrate is no longer available in the United States, another fibric acid agent, gemfibrozil, is sometimes used for patients who have excessive triglyceride (VLDL) levels. Fibrates are the most effective agents for reducing VLDLs and blood triglyceride levels. Elevation of "good" HDL cholesterol is another effect of fibrate therapy. Unfortunately, these drugs have little effect on LDL-cholesterol levels.

DRUG PROFILE: Fibric Acid Agent: Pr *Gemfibrozil (Lopid)*

Actions and Uses:

Gemfibrozil can cause up to a 50% reduction in VLDL with an increase in HDL. Because it is less effective than the statins, it is not a drug of first choice for reducing LDL-cholesterol levels. However, it is useful for patients with high triglyceride levels who have not responded favorably to diet modification and those at risk for pancreatitis.

Adverse Effects and Interactions:

Gemfibrozil produces few serious adverse effects, but it may increase the likelihood of gallstones and occasionally affect liver function. The most common side effects are GI related: diarrhea, nausea, and cramping.

Using with anticoagulants may increase the anticoagulant effects. Lovastatin increases the risk of myopathy and rhabdomyolysis if taken with gemfibrozil.

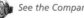

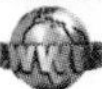
See the Companion Website for a Nursing Process Focus specific to this drug.

FIGURE 20.4

Mechanisms of action of lipid-lowering drugs

Fibrates cause few serious side effects. Rashes and GI complaints are the most common side effects. Patients have an increased risk of gallstones. Like the statins, some patients experience muscle pain or weakness; therefore, patients receiving combination therapy with both statins and fibrates should be monitored carefully. The mechanisms of action of the fibrates and other antihyperlipidemic drugs are shown in Figure 20.4 ■. Dosages of these drugs are listed in Table 20.2.

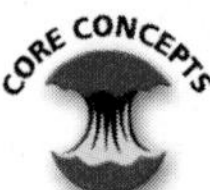

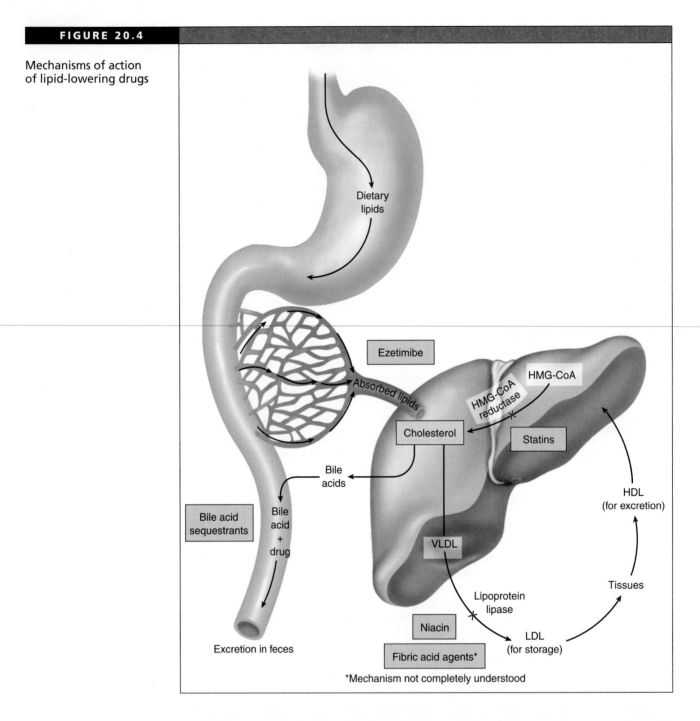

20.9 Newer approaches to treating hyperlipidemia include ezetimibe and fixed-dose combination therapy.

The newest drug for treating high blood cholesterol levels is ezetimibe (Zetia). Ezetimibe acts on the small intestine to block the absorption of dietary cholesterol. LDL-cholesterol and triglyceride levels are reduced, with a slight increase in HDL cholesterol. When used as monotherapy, it can decrease blood cholesterol levels by about 20%. It is well tolerated by patients. The dose for ezetimibe is listed in Table 20.2.

A recent trend in the treatment of hyperlipidemia is to combine drugs from two different classes in a single tablet. Vytorin combines 10 mg of ezetimibe with 10, 20, 40, or 80 mg of simvastatin. Advicor combines 20 mg of lovastatin with 500, 750, or 1000 mg of niacin. These fixed-dose combinations allow for lower doses of each individual agent, potentially resulting in fewer side effects. Taking a single tablet is easier for the patient to remember, thus increasing compliance. Because the combination agents attack cholesterol levels from two distinct mechanisms of action, it may be possible to get a synergistic, or additive, effect of the drugs on blood cholesterol levels.

A second trend in treating CHD is to combine an antihypertensive agent with an antihyperlipidemic drug. For example, Caduet combines the antihypertensive amlodipine with atorvastatin. Several fixed-dose combinations are available with 5 to 10 mg of amlodipine and 10 to 80 mg of atorvastatin. These combination agents are targeted for the estimated 30 million Americans who have both hypertension and elevated blood cholesterol levels.

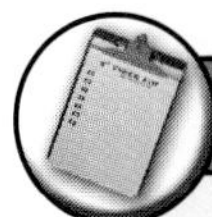

PATIENTS NEED TO KNOW

Patients treated for lipid disorders need to know the following:

In General

1. Because high cholesterol and triglyceride levels in the blood increase the risk for heart disease and stroke, follow the healthcare provider's instructions, even when feeling well.
2. Continuation of a low-fat, low-cholesterol diet while taking lipid-lowering drugs will provide the best results.

Regarding Statin Medications

3. Atorvastatin and rosuvastatin are effective regardless of the time of day they are taken. Taking other statin drugs in the evening makes them available to work on the higher amount of cholesterol that the body makes at night.
4. The healthcare provider may prescribe a fibric acid agent to lower triglycerides and another drug to lower cholesterol. One drug should not be stopped when the second drug is ordered, except on practitioner advice.

Regarding Acid-binding Agents

5. Self-medication with niacin can cause gout and liver damage from high doses. It will not lower cholesterol at low doses. Supervision by a healthcare practitioner supports safe and effective use of this drug.
6. If prescribed bile acid sequestrants, such as psyllium (Metamucil), cholestyramine (Questran), and colestipol (Colestid), take 1 hour after or 4 hours before other drugs to avoid counteracting drug effectiveness. Dissolving the bile acid sequestrant in water and keeping fluid intake high helps to avoid irritation of the mouth and constipation. ▪

CHAPTER REVIEW

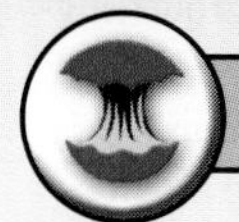

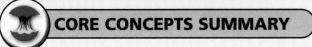

CORE CONCEPTS SUMMARY

20.1 High blood lipid levels can lead to cardiovascular disease.

Elevated levels of lipids in the blood can lead to plaque deposits on the walls of arteries. Narrowing of arteries may lead to angina pectoris, MI, stroke, or hypertension.

20.2 The three classes of lipids are triglycerides, steroids, and phospholipids.

Lipids can be classified into three types based on their chemical structures. Triglycerides contain three fatty acids connected to a backbone of glycerol. Phospholipids are similar to triglycerides, except a phosphate group and other components substitute for one of the fatty acids. Steroids, such as cholesterol, all contain a common ring structure called the steroid nucleus.

20.3 Lipoprotein levels are important predictors of cardiovascular disease.

Lipids are packaged for travel through the blood in lipoprotein complexes. High VLDL and LDL are associated with an increased incidence of cardiovascular disease, whereas HDL provides a protective effect.

20.4 Lipid levels can often be controlled through lifestyle changes.

Before starting pharmacotherapy for hyperlipidemia, patients are usually advised to control the condition through lifestyle changes such as restriction of dietary saturated fats and cholesterol, increased exercise, and smoking cessation.

20.5 Statins are drugs of first choice in reducing blood lipid levels.

Drugs in the statin class inhibit HMG-CoA reductase, a critical enzyme in the biosynthesis of cholesterol. They are safe and effective at lowering LDL cholesterol and are the most widely prescribed class of drugs for hyperlipidemias.

20.6 Binding bile acids can increase cholesterol excretion and reduce LDL levels.

The bile acid-binding drugs are effective at lowering LDL cholesterol although they produce more side effects than the statins. They should be taken separately from other medications because they can interfere with drug absorption.

20.7 Nicotinic acid can reduce both triglyceride and LDL-cholesterol levels.

Nicotinic acid, or niacin, can be effective at lowering LDL cholesterol and triglycerides when given in large amounts. It is not usually a first-choice drug but is sometimes combined in smaller doses with other lipid-lowering agents.

20.8 Fibric acid agents lower triglyceride levels but have little effect on LDLs.

Fibric acids such as gemfibrozil are effective at lowering triglycerides but less effective than the statins at lowering blood lipids. Their use is limited because of frequent side effects. However, they are sometimes combined with other agents to produce an additive effect.

20.9 Newer approaches to treating hyperlipidemia include ezetimibe and fixed-dose combination therapy.

Newer approaches to treating hyperlipidemia are emerging. These include ezetimibe, which blocks cholesterol absorption from the intestine, and combination drugs such as Advicor and Vytorin, which attack high blood cholesterol levels using two different mechanisms.

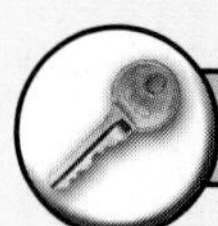

KEY TERMS

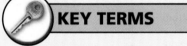

atherosclerosis (ath-ur-oh-sklur-OH-sis): condition characterized by a buildup of fatty plaque and loss of elasticity of the walls of the arteries / *page 350*

bile acid (BEYE-ul): chemicals secreted in bile that aid in the digestion of fats / *page 354*

high-density lipoprotein (HDL): lipid-carrying particle in the blood that contains high amounts of protein and lower amounts of cholesterol; considered to be "good" cholesterol / *page 350*

HMG-CoA reductase (ree-DUCK-tase): primary enzyme in the biochemical pathway for the synthesis of cholesterol / *page 353*

hypercholesterolemia (HEYE-purr-koh-LESS-tur-ol-EEM-ee-uh): high levels of cholesterol in the blood / *page 348*

hyperlipidemia (HEYE-purr-LIP-id-EEM-ee-uh): excess amounts of lipids in the blood / *page 348*

lecithin (LESS-ih-thin): phospholipid that is an important part of cell membranes / *page 350*

lipoprotein (LIP-oh-PROH-teen): substance carrying lipids in the bloodstream / *page 350*

low-density lipoprotein (LDL): lipid-carrying particle that contains lower amounts of protein and high amounts of cholesterol; considered to be "bad" cholesterol / *page 350*

phospholipid (FOS-foh-LIP-id): type of lipid that contains two fatty acids, a phosphate group, and a chemical backbone of glycerol / *page 350*

plaque (PLAK): fatty material that builds up in the lining of blood vessels and may lead to hypertension, stroke, myocardial infarction, or angina / *page 348*

steroid (STAIR-oyd): type of lipid that consists of four rings that comprises certain hormones and drugs / *page 350*

steroid nucleus (STAIR-ol NUK-lee-us): ring structure common to all steroids / *page 350*

therapeutic lifestyle changes: nondrug changes which, when implemented, can reduce blood cholesterol levels / *page 352*

triglyceride (tri-GLISS-ur-ide): type of lipid that contains three fatty acids and a chemical backbone of glycerol / *page 349*

very-low-density lipoprotein (VLDL): lipid-carrying particle that is converted to LDL in the liver / *page 350*

REVIEW QUESTIONS

The following questions are written in NCLEX-PN® style. Answer these questions to assess your knowledge of the chapter material, and go back and review any material that is not clear to you.

1. This lipoprotein is responsible for transporting cholesterol from the blood to the liver.

1. LDL
2. VLDL
3. HDL
4. Triglycerides

2. Which of the HMG-CoA reductase inhibitors should be taken with meals?

1. Atorvastatin (Lipitor)
2. Simvastatin (Zocor)
3. Simvastatin (Mevacor)
4. Digixon (Lanoxin)

3. Statin drugs are most effective when administered:

1. In the morning
2. In the evening
3. With other medications
4. On an empty stomach

4. When asked how an HMG-CoA reductase inhibitor lowers cholesterol, the nurse correctly answers that is by inhibiting the manufacture of cholesterol or by:

1. Increasing the secretion of bile acids
2. Decreasing triglyceride production
3. Removing cholesterol from the small intestine
4. Promoting the breakdown of cholesterol

5. Which of the following patient concerns would the nurse consider as an adverse reaction to a bile acid sequestrant?

1. Constipation
2. Headache
3. Anxiety
4. Double vision

6. When administering colestipol (Colestid), the nurse:

1. Administers the drug with meals to prevent GI upset
2. Administers the drug 30 minutes prior to meals
3. Administers the drug at least 1 hour before or 4 hours after meals
4. Administers the drug at bedtime

7. Which of the following antihyperlipidemic medications is most effective in reducing serum triglyceride levels?

1. Gemfibrozil (Lopid)
2. Niacin (Nicotinic acid)
3. Lovastatin (Mevacor)
4. Cholestyramine (Questran)

8. On assessment, the patient is found to have a cholesterol level of 326 mg/dL and an elevated blood pressure. The best treatment for this patient would be a low-fat diet and:

1. Exercise program
2. Cholesterol-lowering medication
3. Niacin
4. An antihypertensive

9. The patient has developed gallstones and elevated liver enzymes. Which of the following cholesterol-lowering medications could cause this?

1. Cholestyramine (Questran)
2. Niacin (Nicotinic acid)
3. Gemfibrozil (Lopid)
4. Lovastatin (Mevacor)

10. The preferred first-choice drugs to treat elevated cholesterol levels are?

1. Statins
2. Bile acids
3. Fibric acids
4. Nicotinic acids

CASE STUDY QUESTIONS

For questions 1–6, please refer to the following case study, and choose the correct answer from choices 1–4.

Mr. Long is a 50-year-old office worker who has gained 50 pounds over the past 5 years. His blood pressure has consistently been high, but he has declined to take medication for the condition. His LDL-cholesterol level has been above 210 mg/dL on his last three office visits. He claims to have no chronic diseases and is at the office seeking assistance for his weight gain.

1. Before starting therapy on antihyperlipidemics, the physician would likely try which of the following?

1. Therapeutic lifestyle changes
2. Therapy with an antihypertensive
3. A diet with strict limitations on carbohydrate intake
4. A diet with strict limitations on protein intake

2. The physician ordered cholestyramine for Mr. Long. This drug acts by:

1. Inhibiting enzymes that make cholesterol
2. Binding bile acids in the intestine, which increase cholesterol excretion
3. Increasing the breakdown of cholesterol in the liver
4. Making more bile acids, which bind cholesterol

3. You should teach Mr. Long that common side effects associated with cholestyramine include:

1. Decreased blood pressure
2. Drowsiness
3. Muscle weakness
4. Bloating, nausea, or constipation

4. After 2 months of therapy, the physician switched the prescription to lovastatin (Mevacor). This drug acts by:

1. Inhibiting enzymes that make cholesterol
2. Binding bile acids in the intestine, which increase cholesterol excretion
3. Increasing the breakdown of cholesterol in the liver
4. Making more bile acids, which bind cholesterol

5. After several weeks of lovastatin therapy, Mr. Long returns to the office for follow-up. What question should you ask to determine if he may be suffering from a very serious side effect of the statins?

1. Do you have bloody diarrhea more than once a week?
2. Have you felt confused, lethargic, or drowsy since starting the drug?
3. Have you experienced excessive muscle weakness or pain?
4. Have you experienced acid indigestion or nausea?

6. Which of the following is an expected, therapeutic effect of lovastatin?

1. Higher LDL level
2. Higher VLDL level
3. Lower HDL level
4. Higher HDL level

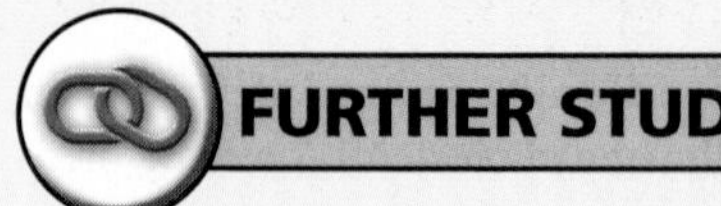

FURTHER STUDY

- Chapter 18 discusses fatty plaques that cause angina, myocardial infarction, and cerebrovascular accidents.
- The role of niacin as a vitamin is presented in Chapter 27.

EXPLORE MEDIALINK www.prenhall.com/holland

Additional resources for this chapter can be found on the CD-ROM accompanying this textbook, and on the Companion Website. Click on Chapter 20 to select activities for this chapter.

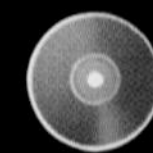

Mechanism in Action: Atorvastatin
Audio Glossary
Concept Review
NCLEX-PN® Review
Nursing in Action
Dosage Calculator

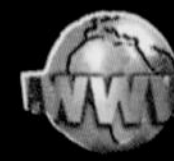

National Heart, Lung, and Blood Institute
National Cholesterol Education Program
International Food Information Council

UNIT

1 2 3 4 5 6 7

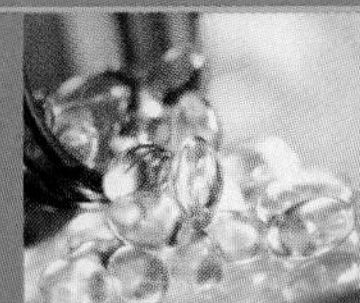

4 THE IMMUNE SYSTEM

UNIT CONTENTS

CHAPTER

21 Drugs for Inflammation, Allergies, and Immune Disorders

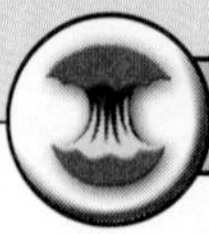

CORE CONCEPTS

21.1 Inflammation is a body defense that limits the spread of invading microorganisms and injury.

21.2 Histamine is a key chemical mediator in inflammation.

21.3 Histamine can produce its effects by interacting with two different receptors.

21.4 NSAIDs are the primary drugs for the treatment of mild inflammation.

21.5 Systemic glucocorticoids are effective in treating severe inflammation.

21.6 Allergic rhinitis is characterized by sneezing, watery eyes, and nasal congestion.

21.7 Antihistamines are useful for treating allergic rhinitis and several other disorders.

21.8 Intranasal glucocorticoids are drugs of choice in treating allergic rhinitis.

21.9 Sympathomimetics are used to alleviate nasal congestion due to allergic rhinitis and the common cold.

21.10 The immune response is obtained through activation of the humoral and cell-mediated immune systems.

21.11 Vaccines are biological drugs used to prevent illness.

21.12 Biologic response modifiers are used to boost the immune response.

21.13 Immunosuppressants are primarily used to avoid tissue rejection following organ transplant.

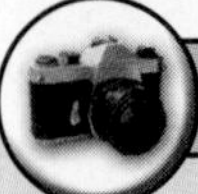

DRUG SNAPSHOT

The following drugs will be discussed in this chapter:

DRUG CLASSES	DRUG PROFILES
Nonsteroidal anti-inflammatory drugs (NSAIDs)	Pr naproxen (Naprosyn) and naproxen sodium (Aleve, Anaprox)
Systemic glucocorticoids	Pr prednisone (Meticorten, others)
H_1-receptor blockers (antihistamines)	Pr Sedating: diphenhydramine (Benadryl, others) Nonsedating: fexofenadine (Allegra)
Intranasal glucocorticoids	Pr fluticasone (Flonase)
Sympathomimetics (decongestants)	Pr oxymetazoline (Afrin, others)
Vaccines	Pr hepatitis B vaccine (Recombivax HB)
Immunosuppressants	Pr cyclosporine (Neoral, Sandimmune)

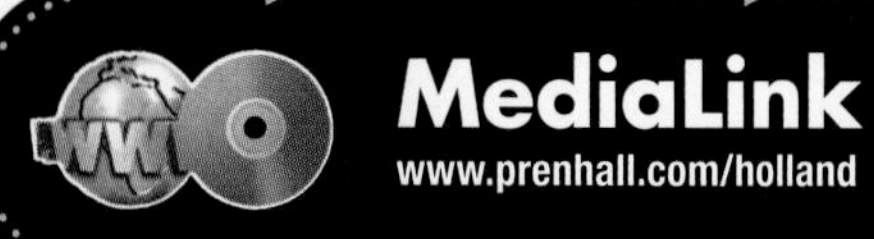

Interactive resources for this chapter can be found on the Companian Website. Click on Chapter 21 and "Begin" to select the activities for this chapter. For chapter-related animations, NCLEX-PN®-style questions, and an audio glossary, access the accompanying CD-ROM in this book.

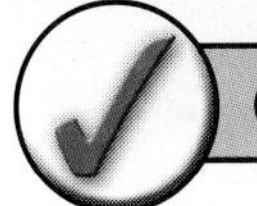

OBJECTIVES

After reading this chapter, the student should be able to:

1. Identify common signs and symptoms of inflammation.
2. Outline the basic steps in the acute inflammatory response.
3. Describe the central role of histamine in inflammation.
4. Compare and contrast the humoral and cell-mediated immune responses.
5. Differentiate between H_1- and H_2-histamine receptors.
6. Describe common causes and symptoms of allergic rhinitis.
7. For each of the following classes, identify representative drugs, explain the mechanisms of drug action, primary actions related to inflammation and/or the immune system, and important adverse effects:
   a. H_1-receptor blockers
   b. Nonsteroidal anti-inflammatory drugs
   c. Intranasal and systemic glucocorticoids
   d. Intranasal and oral sympathomimetics
   e. Immunosuppressants
   f. Vaccines
   g. Biologic response modifiers
8. Categorize drugs used in the treatment of inflammation, allergies, and immune disorders based on their classifications and mechanisms of action.
9. For each of the major vaccines, give the recommended dosage schedule.

The pain and redness of inflammation following minor abrasions and cuts is something everyone has experienced. Although there may be discomfort from such scrapes, inflammation is a normal and expected part of our body's defense against injury. For some diseases, however, inflammation can rage out of control, producing severe pain, fever, and other distressing symptoms. It is these sorts of conditions for which drug therapy may be needed.

Similarly, our bodies come under continuous attack from a host of foreign agents that include viruses, bacteria, fungi, and even single-celled animals. In defending the body, our immune system is capable of mounting a rapid and effective response against many of these pathogens. In some cases, vaccines or other drugs are given to stimulate body defenses so that disease can be prevented or controlled. On other occasions, it is desirable to decrease the immune response to allow a transplanted organ to survive. The purpose of this chapter is to examine the pharmacotherapy of diseases and conditions affecting our body defenses.

Fast Facts Inflammatory and Allergic Disorders

- Arthritis, the most common inflammatory disorder, is the leading cause of disability in the United States.
- Inflammatory bowel disease affects 300,000–500,000 Americans each year.
- More than 80 million prescriptions are written for NSAIDs each year, accounting for about 4.5% of all prescriptions written in the United States.
- More than 1% of the population uses NSAIDs on a daily basis.
- Worldwide, more than 30 million people consume NSAIDs daily, and, of these, 40% of the patients are older than 60 years.
- About 175 people die from food allergies each year in the United States.
- 85% of food allergies are related to milk, eggs, and nuts.
- About 3 million Americans (1.1%) are allergic to nuts.

INFLAMMATION

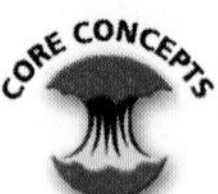

21.1 Inflammation is a body defense that limits the spread of invading microorganisms and injury.

The human body has developed complex ways to defend itself against injury and invasion by microorganisms. Inflammation is one of these defense mechanisms. **Inflammation** occurs in response to many different stimuli, including physical injury, exposure to toxic chemicals, extreme heat, invading microorganisms, or death of cells. The central purpose of inflammation is to contain the injury or destroy the microorganism. By removing cellular debris and dead cells, repair of the injured area can move at a faster pace. Inflammation proceeds in the same manner, regardless of its cause. Signs of inflammation include swelling, pain, warmth, and redness of the affected area.

Inflammation may be classified as *acute* or *chronic.* During acute inflammation, such as that caused by minor physical injury, 8 to 10 days are normally needed for the symptoms to resolve and for repair to begin. If the body cannot contain or neutralize the damaging agent, inflammation may continue for long periods and become chronic. In chronic diseases such as lupus and rheumatoid arthritis, inflammation may persist for years, with symptoms becoming progressively worse over time. Other disorders such as seasonal allergy arise at predictable times each year, and inflammation may produce only minor, annoying symptoms.

Treatment of inflammation may include drugs that decrease the natural inflammatory response. Most anti-inflammatory drugs are nonspecific: It does not matter whether the inflammation is caused from injury or allergy, the drug will exhibit the same actions. A few anti-inflammatory drugs are specific to certain diseases, such as those used to treat gout. Following are common diseases that have an inflammatory component:

- Allergic rhinitis
- Anaphylaxis
- Ankylosing spondylitis
- Contact dermatitis
- Crohn's disease
- Glomerulonephritis
- Hashimoto's thyroiditis
- Multiple sclerosis
- Peptic ulcers
- Rheumatoid arthritis
- Systemic lupus erythematosus
- Type 1 diabetes
- Ulcerative colitis

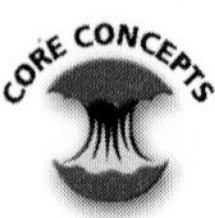

21.2 Histamine is a key chemical mediator in inflammation.

Whether the injury is due to pathogens, chemicals, or physical trauma, the damaged tissue releases a number of chemical mediators that act as "alarms" to notify the surrounding area of the injury. Chemical mediators of inflammation include histamine, leukotrienes, bradykinin, complement, and prostaglandins. Table 21.1 lists the sources and actions of these mediators.

Histamine is a key chemical mediator of inflammation. It is primarily stored within **mast cells** located in tissue spaces under epithelial membranes such as the skin, bronchial tree, and digestive tract, and along blood vessels. Mast cells detect foreign agents or injury and respond by releasing histamine, which initiates the inflammatory response within seconds. In addition, histamine directly stimulates pain receptors.

TABLE 21.1	Chemical Mediators of Inflammation
Bradykinin	Present in an inactive form in plasma and mast cells; vasodilator that causes pain; effects are similar to those of histamine
Complement	Series of at least 20 proteins that combine in a cascade fashion to neutralize or destroy an antigen
Histamine	Stored and released by mast cells; causes dilation of blood vessels, smooth muscle constriction, tissue swelling, and itching
Leukotrienes	Stored and released by mast cells; effects are similar to those of histamine
Prostaglandins	Present in most tissues; stored and released by mast cells; increase capillary permeability, attract white blood cells to site of inflammation, and cause pain

When released at an injury site, histamine dilates nearby blood vessels, causing the capillaries to become more permeable or leaky. Plasma and components such as complement proteins and phagocytes can then enter the area to neutralize foreign agents. The affected area may become congested with blood because of the permeable capillaries, which can lead to significant swelling and pain. Figure 21.1 ■ shows the basic steps in acute inflammation.

Rapid release of histamine on a larger scale throughout the body is responsible for **anaphylaxis,** a life-threatening allergic response that may result in shock and death. A number of chemicals, insect stings, foods, and some therapeutic drugs can cause this widespread release of histamine from mast cells. Drug therapy of anaphylactic shock is discussed in Chapter 19.

FIGURE 21.1

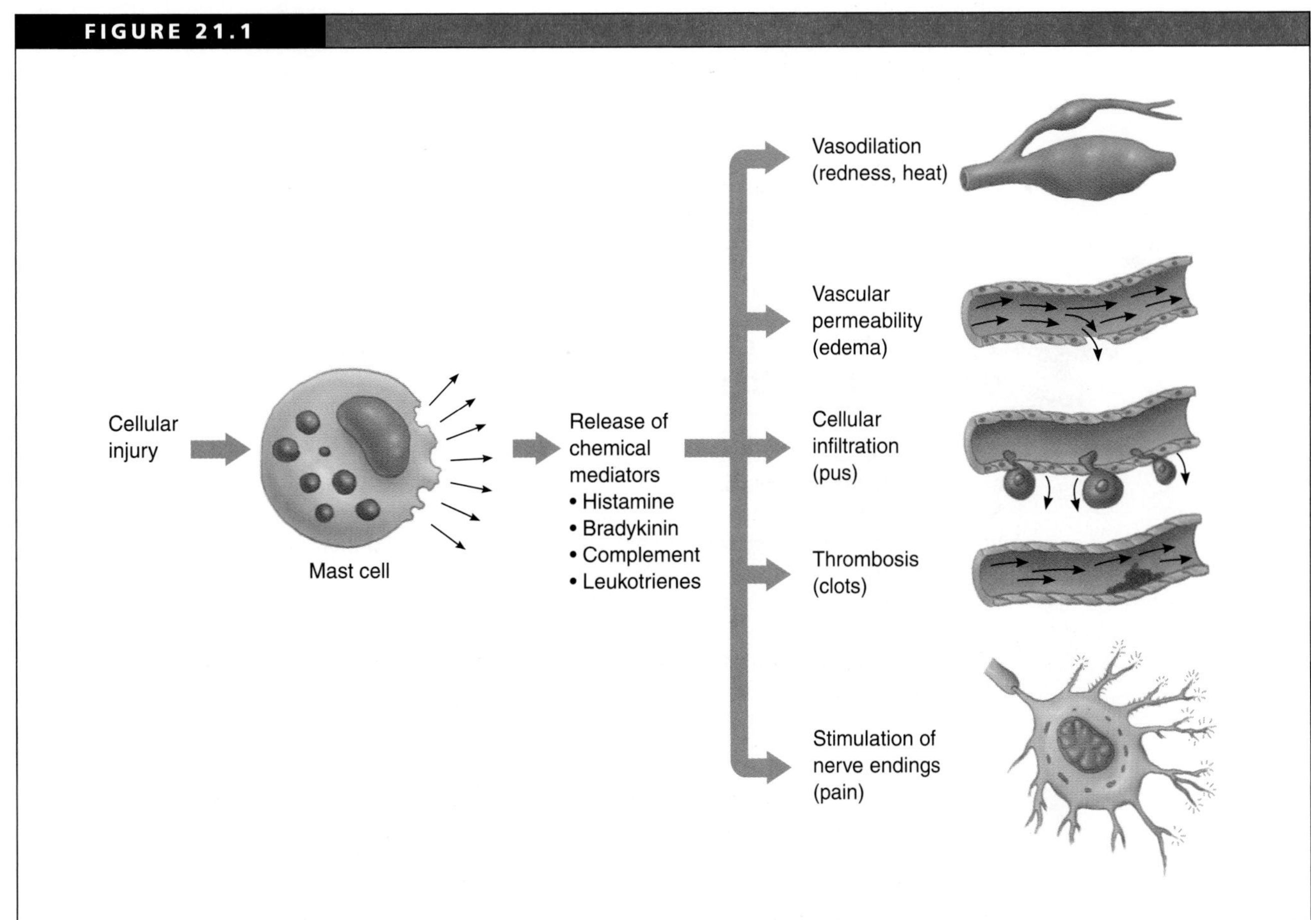

Steps in acute inflammation *Source: Pearson Education/PH College*

FIGURE 21.2

Mechanism of action of the antihistamines

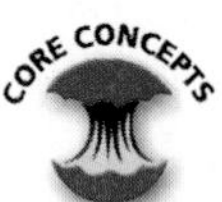

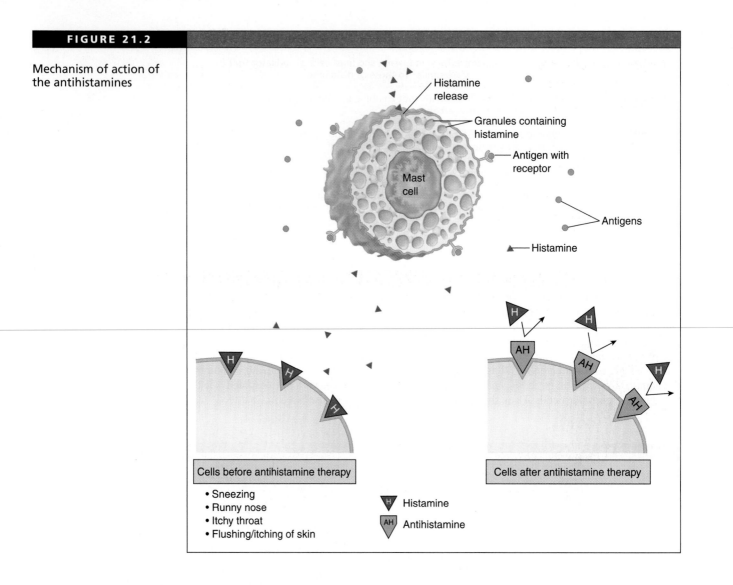

21.3 Histamine can produce its effects by interacting with two different receptors.

There are at least two different receptors by which histamine can cause a response. **H_1 receptors** are present in the smooth muscle of the vascular system, the bronchial tree, and the digestive tract. Stimulation of these receptors results in itching, pain, edema, vasodilation, and bronchoconstriction. In contrast, **H_2 receptors** are present in the stomach, and their stimulation results in the secretion of large amounts of hydrochloric acid.

Drugs that act as specific antagonists for H_1 and H_2 receptors are in widespread therapeutic use. H_1-receptor blockers, used to treat allergies and inflammation, are discussed in this chapter. H_2-receptor blockers are used to treat peptic ulcers and are discussed in Chapter 26. A simplified mechanism of action for the antihistamines is illustrated in Figure 21.2 ■.

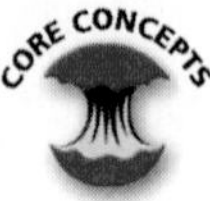

21.4 NSAIDs are the primary drugs for the treatment of mild inflammation.

Nonsteroidal anti-inflammatory drugs (NSAIDs) such as aspirin and ibuprofen have analgesic, antipyretic, and anti-inflammatory effects. They are drugs of choice in the treatment of mild to moderate inflammation. Some NSAIDs used for inflammation are listed in Table 21.2.

TABLE 21.2 Selected Nonsteroidal Anti-inflammatory Drugs

DRUG	ROUTE AND ADULT DOSE	REMARKS
aspirin (ASA and others)	PO 350–650 mg q4h (max: 4 g/day)	Inhibits the formation of prostaglandins; also for fever, pain, and prevention of stroke and MI
celecoxib (Celebrex)	PO 100–200 mg bid (max: 400 mg/day)	Selective COX-2 inhibitor
diclofenac (Voltaren, Cataflam)	PO 50 mg bid–qid (max: 200 mg/day)	Extended-release form available
diflunisal (Dolobid)	PO 250–500 mg bid (max: 1500 mg/day)	Similar to ibuprofen
etodolac (Lodine)	PO 200–400 mg tid–qid (max: 1200 mg/day)	Extended-release form available
fenoprofen (Nalfon)	PO 300–600 mg tid–qid (max: 3200 mg/day)	Similar to ibuprofen
flurbiprofen (Ansaid)	PO 50–100 tid–qid (max: 300 mg/day)	Similar to ibuprofen
ibuprofen (Motrin, Advil, others)	PO 400–800 mg tid–qid (max: 3200 mg/day)	Blocks prostaglandin synthesis as well as modulates T-cell function; also for dysmenorrhea
ketoprofen (Actron, Orudis, Oruvail)	PO 75 mg tid or 50 mg qid (max: 300 mg/day)	Extended-release form available; similar to ibuprofen; also for dysmenorrhea
nabumetone (Relafen)	PO 1000 mg daily (max: 2000 mg/day)	Inhibits COX-2 more than COX-1
Pr naproxen (Naprosyn)	PO 250–500 mg bid (max: 1000 mg/day)	Also for dysmenorrhea
naproxen sodium (Aleve, Anaprox, others)	PO 275 mg bid (max: 1100 mg/day)	Also for dysmenorrhea
oxaprozin (Daypro)	PO 600–1200 mg daily (max: 1800 mg/day)	Similar to naproxen; once-a-day dosage
piroxicam (Feldene)	PO 10–20 mg once or twice a day (max: 20 mg/day)	Has prolonged half-life
tolmetin (Tolectin)	PO 400 mg tid (max: 2 g/day)	Exact mode of anti-inflammatory action unknown

The analgesic action of (NSAIDs) was discussed in Chapter 12. This class includes some of the most widely used drugs, such as aspirin, ibuprofen, and the newer COX-2 inhibitors. Although acetaminophen shares the analgesic and antipyretic properties of these other drugs, it has no anti-inflammatory action and is thus not considered a NSAID.

Aspirin is useful in treating inflammation because it inhibits **cyclooxygenase (COX),** a key enzyme in the pathway of prostaglandin synthesis that is found in every tissue. Aspirin causes irreversible inhibition of both forms of cyclooxygenase, COX-1 and COX-2. Because it is readily available, inexpensive, and effective, aspirin is sometimes a drug of first choice for treating mild inflammation. The basic pharmacology and a drug profile of aspirin were presented in Chapter 12.

Unfortunately, large doses of aspirin are necessary to suppress severe inflammation, and these doses result in a greater incidence of side effects. The most common adverse effects observed during high-dose therapy relate to the digestive system. By increasing gastric acid secretion and irritating the stomach lining, aspirin may cause pain, heartburn, and even bleeding due to ulceration. Some aspirin formulations are buffered or given an enteric coating to minimize GI side effects. Because aspirin also has an anticoagulant effect (Chapter 14), the potential for bleeding must be carefully monitored by the healthcare provider. High doses may produce **salicylism,** a syndrome that includes symptoms such as ringing in the ears, dizziness, headache, and sweating. Patients with preexisting kidney disease should be monitored carefully because aspirin and other NSAIDs may affect kidney function.

DRUG PROFILE: Nonsteroidal Anti-inflammatory Drugs: Pr *Naproxen (Naprosyn) and Naproxen Sodium (Aleve, Anaprox)*

Actions and Uses:

Naproxen is a NSAID that inhibits prostaglandin synthesis through the nonselective inhibition of COX-1 and COX-2. Its efficacy at relieving pain and inflammation is similar to that of aspirin. Common indications include both rheumatoid arthritis and osteoarthritis, gout, and bursitis. In treating rheumatoid arthritis, the therapeutic effects may take 3 to 4 weeks to appear.

Adverse Effects and Interactions:

Side effects of naproxen are generally not serious and include GI upset, dizziness, and drowsiness. Administration with food will decrease the incidence of stomach upset, which is the most common side effect. Because naproxen may prolong bleeding time, the drug should be administered with caution to those with bleeding disorders. Patients taking naproxen should notify their dental hygienist before dental procedures are performed.

Using together with oral anticoagulants can prolong bleeding time. Lithium level may be increased. Bleeding potential increases when used with herbal agents such as feverfew, garlic, ginger, and ginkgo.

Mechanism in Action: 

Naproxen is a nonsteroidal anti-inflammatory drug (NSAID) that inhibits prostaglandin synthesis through the nonselective inhibition of cyclooxygenase type-1 (COX-1) and cyclooxygenase type-2 (COX-2) enzymes. It also inhibits platelet aggregation and prolongs bleeding time without affecting whole blood clotting, prothrombin time, or platelet count.

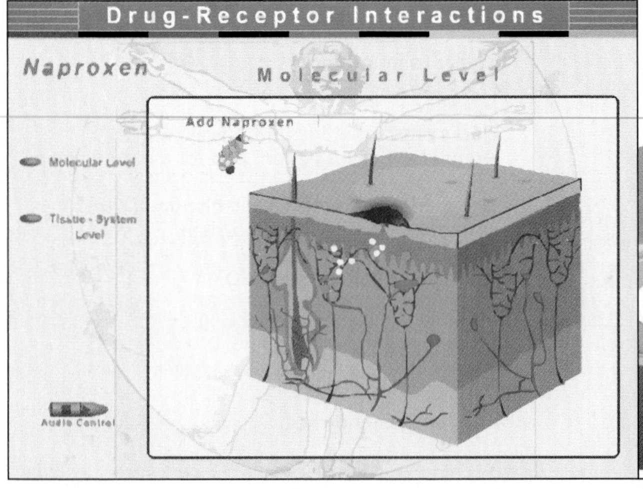

Use the student CD-ROM to see Mechanism in Action for Naproxen.

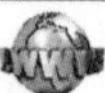 *See the Companion Website for a Nursing Process Focus specific to this drug.*

Many NSAIDs, such as ibuprofen, are available as alternatives to aspirin. Like aspirin, they exhibit their effects through inhibition of COX-1 and COX-2. Because of their similar mechanisms, they all have similar pharmacological properties and a low incidence of adverse effects. The most common side effects of these drugs are nausea and vomiting, although the incidence of gastric ulceration and bleeding is less than that of aspirin. Most have no significant effect on blood coagulation and are safe to use for patients who may be at risk for bleeding.

The newest, and most controversial, class of NSAIDs selectively inhibits COX-2. Inhibition of COX-2 produces the analgesic, anti-inflammatory, and antipyretic effects seen with the NSAIDs. Because they do not inhibit COX-1, these drugs—celecoxib (Celebrex), rofecoxib (Vioxx), and valdecoxib (Bextra)—do not produce adverse effects on the digestive system as does aspirin. Because they have no GI side effects and do not affect blood coagulation, these drugs quickly became the treatment of choice for moderate to severe inflammation.

However, in 2004, study data revealed that one of the drugs, rofecoxib, doubled the risk of heart attack and stroke in patients taking the drug for an extended time. More than 84 million people had used rofecoxib since its approval in 1999. Based on the data, the drug manufacturer voluntarily removed the drug from the market. In 2005, valdecoxib was also removed from the market. The FDA is examining the safety and future of the entire class of COX-2 inhibitors because studies suggest similar cardiovascular risk with long-term use of celecoxib. It is likely that these drugs will be withdrawn, or their use will be severely restricted.

NURSING PROCESS FOCUS

Patients Receiving NSAID Therapy

ASSESSMENT

Prior to administration:
- Obtain complete health history including allergies, drug history, and possible drug interactions
- Determine pain and analgesic usage patterns
- Identify infectious agents or other factors responsible for inflammation or pain

POTENTIAL NURSING DIAGNOSES

- Acute Pain, related to surgical procedure
- Chronic Pain, related to back injury
- Deficient Knowledge, related to drug therapy
- Ineffective Health Maintenance, related to chronic pain

PLANNING: Patient Goals and Expected Outcomes

The patient will:
- Report pain relief or a reduction in pain intensity
- Demonstrate an understanding of the drug's action by accurately describing drug side effects and precautions
- Report ability to manage activities of daily living
- Immediately report effects such as unresolved, untoward, or rebound pain; persistent fever; blurred vision; tinnitus; bleeding; changes in color of stool or urine

IMPLEMENTATION

Interventions and (Rationales)	Patient Education/Discharge Planning
■ NSAIDs may be administered PO or PR. When using suppositories, monitor integrity of rectum; observe for rectal bleeding.	Inform patient of the following: ■ Enteric-coated tablets must not be cut or crushed. Regular tablets may be broken or pulverized and mixed with food. ■ Administer liquid ASA immediately after mixing because it breaks down rapidly. ■ Different drugs and formulations, such as ibuprofen and naproxen, should not be taken concurrently. Consult the healthcare provider regarding appropriate OTC analgesics for specific types of pain. ■ ASA is an anticoagulant. The body needs time to manufacture new platelets to make clots that promote wound healing. Consult the nurse regarding ASA therapy following surgery. ■ Advise laboratory personnel of aspirin therapy when providing urine samples.
■ Monitor vital signs, especially temperature. (Increased pulse and blood pressure may indicate discomfort; accompanied by pallor and/or dizziness may indicate bleeding.)	Instruct patient to: ■ Report rapid heartbeat, palpitations, dizziness, or pallor ■ Monitor blood pressure and temperature ensuring proper use of home equipment
■ Monitor for signs of GI bleeding or hepatic toxicity. (NSAIDs can be a local irritant to the GI tract with anticoagulant action that is metabolized in the liver.) ■ Monitor gastrointestinal elimination; conduct guaiac stool testing for occult blood. ■ Monitor CBC for signs of anemia related to blood loss.	Instruct patient to: ■ Report any bleeding, abdominal pain, anorexia, heartburn, nausea, vomiting, jaundice, or a change in the color or character of stools. ■ Know the proper method of obtaining stool samples and home testing for occult blood. ■ Adhere to a regimen of laboratory testing as ordered by the healthcare provider. ■ Take NSAIDs with food to reduce stomach upset.
■ Assess for character, duration, location, and intensity of pain and the presence of inflammation.	■ Instruct patient to notify nurse if pain and/or inflammation remains unresolved. ■ Advise patient to take only the prescribed amount to decrease the potential for adverse effects.

continued...

(continued from page 371)

NURSING PROCESS FOCUS

Interventions and (Rationales)	Patient Education/Discharge Planning
■ Monitor for hypersensitivity reaction.	■ Advise the patient to immediately report shortness of breath, wheezing, throat tightness, itching, or hives. If these occur, stop taking ASA immediately and inform the healthcare provider.
■ Monitor urinary output and edema in feet/ankles. (Medication is excreted through the kidneys. Long-term use may lead to renal dysfunction.)	■ Report changes in urination, flank pain, or pitting edema. ■ Return to healthcare provider for prescribed follow-up appointments.
■ Monitor for sensory changes indicative of drug toxicity: tinnitus, blurred vision. ■ Evaluate blood salicylate levels.	■ Immediately report sensory changes in sight or hearing, especially blurred vision or ringing in the ears.

EVALUATION OF OUTCOME CRITERIA

Evaluate the effectiveness of drug therapy by confirming that patient goals and expected outcomes have been met (see "Planning").

See Table 21.2 for a list of drugs to which these nursing actions apply.

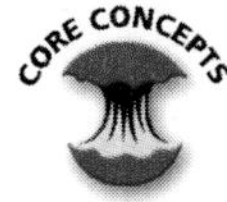

21.5 Systemic glucocorticoids are effective in treating severe inflammation.

Glucocorticoids have wide therapeutic application when given orally or parenterally. One of their most useful actions is their potent anti-inflammatory effect that can suppress severe cases of inflammation. Selected glucocorticoids used to treat severe inflammatory disease are listed in Table 21.3.

Glucocorticoids are natural hormones released by the cortex of the adrenal gland that have powerful effects on nearly every cell in the body. When used to treat inflammatory disorders, the drug doses are many times higher than those naturally present in the blood. The uses of glucocorticoids in treating hormonal imbalances are presented in detail in Chapter 29.

Glucocorticoids have the ability to suppress the actions of histamine and prostaglandins. In addition, they can inhibit the immune system by suppressing certain functions of phagocytes and lymphocytes. These multiple effects have the ability to markedly reduce inflammation, making glucocorticoids the most effective medications for the treatment of severe inflammatory disorders.

Unfortunately, the glucocorticoids have a number of serious adverse effects that limit their therapeutic use. These include suppression of the normal functions of the adrenal gland (adrenal insufficiency), elevated blood glucose, mood changes, cataracts, peptic ulcers, electrolyte imbalances, and osteoporosis. Because of their effectiveness at reducing the signs and symptoms of inflammation, glucocorticoids can mask infections that may be present in the patient. This combination of masking inflammation and suppressing the immune system creates a potential for existing infections to grow rapidly and undetected. An active infection is usually a contraindication for glucocorticoid therapy.

Because the appearance of these adverse effects is a function of the dose and duration of therapy, treatment is often limited to the short-term control of acute disease. When longer therapy is indicated, doses are kept as low as possible and **alternate-day therapy** is sometimes used; the medication is taken every other day to encourage the patient's adrenal glands to function on the days when no drug is taken. During long-term therapy, the healthcare provider must be alert for signs of overtreatment, a condition referred to as **Cushing's syndrome.** Signs in-

TABLE 21.3 Selected Glucocorticoids for Severe Inflammation

DRUG	ROUTE AND ADULT DOSE	REMARKS
betamethasone (Celestone, Betacort, others)	PO 0.6–7.2 mg/day	Topical, IM, and IV forms available
cortisone (Cortistan, Cortone)	PO 20–300 mg/day in divided doses	IM form available; also for adrenal insufficiency
dexamethasone (Decadron, others)	PO 0.25–4 mg bid–qid	IM and IV forms available; also for adrenal insufficiency and immunosuppression
hydrocortisone (Cetacort, Cortaid, others)	Topical 0.5% cream applied 1–4 times daily; PO 10–320 mg tid–qid	Used widely for skin inflammation; IM, PO, rectal, and IV forms available; may be injected intra-articular
methylprednisolone (Medrol)	PO 4–48 mg/day in divided doses	Available in IM, IV, and rectal forms; also for neoplasia and adrenal insufficiency
prednisolone (Delta-Cortef, Keypred, Prelone, others)	PO 5–60 mg 1–4 times daily	Available in IM and IV forms; also for neoplasia and adrenal insufficiency
Pr prednisone (Meticorten, others)	PO 5–60 mg 1–4 times daily	Only available in oral form; also for neoplasia
triamcinolone (Kenalog, Azmacort, others)	PO 4–48 mg 1–4 times daily	Available in IM, subcutaneous, intradermal, intra-articular, and aerosol forms

clude bruising and a characteristic pattern of fat deposits in the cheeks (moon face), shoulders (buffalo hump), and abdomen. The body becomes accustomed to the high doses of glucocorticoids and patients must discontinue the drug gradually because abrupt withdrawal can result in lack of adrenal function.

DRUG PROFILE: Glucocorticoid: Pr *Prednisone (Meticorten, Others)*

Actions and Uses:

Prednisone is a synthetic glucocorticoid. Its actions are the result of being metabolized to an active form, which is also available as a drug called *prednisolone* (Delta-Cortef, others). When used for inflammation, a 4- to 10-day duration for therapy is common. Alternate-day dosing is used for longer term therapy. Prednisone is occasionally used to terminate acute bronchospasm in patients with asthma (Chapter 25) and for patients with certain cancers such as Hodgkin's disease, acute leukemia, and lymphomas (Chapter 24).

Adverse Effects and Interactions:

When used for short-term therapy, prednisone has few adverse effects. Long-term therapy may result in Cushing's syndrome, a condition that includes elevated blood glucose, fat redistribution to the shoulders and face, muscle weakness, bruising, and bones that easily fracture. Glucocorticoids can raise blood glucose levels. Diabetic patients may require an adjustment in insulin dose. Gastric ulcers may occur with long-term therapy and an antiulcer medication may be prescribed prophylactically. Patients must report any potential infections immediately. This drug should be discontinued gradually.

Barbiturates, phenytoin, and rifampin increase the metabolism of prednisone: Increased doses of prednisone may be needed. Amphotericin B and diuretics together with prednisone can increase potassium loss. Prednisone may inhibit antibody response to vaccines and toxoids. In patients with myasthenia gravis, use of prednisone with ambenonium, neostigmine, or pyridostigmine can cause severe muscle weakness.

See the Companion Website for a Nursing Process Focus specific to this drug.

ALLERGY

Allergies are caused by a hyperresponse of body defenses. Many signs and symptoms are similar to those of inflammation because histamine is released during an allergic response. Allergies may also involve mediators of the immune system.

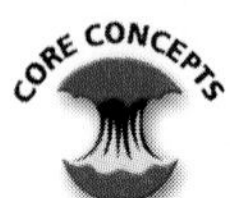

21.6 Allergic rhinitis is characterized by sneezing, watery eyes, and nasal congestion.

rhin = *nose*
itis = *inflammation*

Allergic rhinitis, or hay fever, is a common disorder affecting millions of people annually. Symptoms resemble those of the common cold: tearing eyes, sneezing, nasal congestion, postnasal drip, and itching of the throat. The exact cause of allergic rhinitis is often difficult to pinpoint; however, common causes include pollen from weeds, grasses, and trees; molds; dust mites; certain foods; and animal dander. Nonallergenic factors such as chemical fumes, tobacco smoke, or air pollutants such as ozone may contribute to the symptoms. Although some patients experience symptoms at specific times of the year, when pollen and mold are at high levels in the environment, others are bothered throughout the year.

The fundamental problem of allergic rhinitis is inflammation of the mucous membranes in the nose, throat, and airways. Chemical mediators such as histamine are released that initiate the distressing symptoms. The mechanism of allergic rhinitis is illustrated in Figure 21.3 ■.

Drugs used to treat allergic rhinitis may be grouped into two basic categories: preventers and relievers. Preventers are used for prophylaxis and include antihistamines, glucocorticoids, and mast cell stabilizers. Relievers are used to provide immediate, though temporary, relief for allergy symptoms once they have occurred. Relievers include the oral and intranasal sympathomimetics that are used as nasal decongestants.

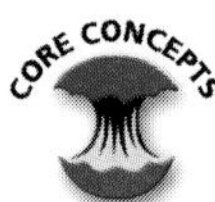

21.7 Antihistamines are useful for treating allergic rhinitis and several other disorders.

Antihistamines block the actions of histamine at the H_1 receptor; therefore, they are in a class known as **H_1-receptor blockers.** They are widely used OTC for relief of allergy symptoms, motion sickness, and insomnia. Common H_1-receptor blockers used to treat allergies and other disorders are shown in Table 21.4.

Because the term *antihistamine* is nonspecific and does not specify which of the two histamine receptors are affected, *H_1-receptor blocker* is the more accurate term. Although a large number of H_1-receptor blockers are available for use, their efficacies, therapeutic uses, and side effects are similar. A simple classification of these drugs is based on their ability to cause sedation. Older, first-generation H_1-receptor blockers have the potential to cause significant drowsiness, whereas the newer, second-generation agents lack this effect in most patients. Care must be taken to avoid alcohol and other CNS depressants when taking antihistamines, as their sedating effects may be additive.

The most common therapeutic use of H_1-receptor blockers is for the treatment of allergies. These drugs provide relief from the characteristic sneezing, runny nose, and itching of the eyes, nose, and throat of allergic rhinitis. Many H_1-receptor blockers are used in OTC cold and sinus medicines, often in combination with decongestants and antitussives. Some common OTC antihistamine combinations used to treat allergies are shown in Table 21.5.

Antihistamines are most effective when taken prophylactically to prevent allergic symptoms. Their effectiveness may diminish with long-term use. It should be noted that during severe allergic reactions such as anaphylaxis, histamine is just one of several chemical mediators released; thus, H_1-receptor blockers are not very efficacious in treating this disorder.

Although most antihistamines are given orally, azelastine (Astelin) was the first to be available by the intranasal route. Azelastine is as safe and effective as the oral antihistamines. Although a first-generation agent, it causes less drowsiness than others in its class because it is applied locally to the nasal mucosa, with little systemic absorption.

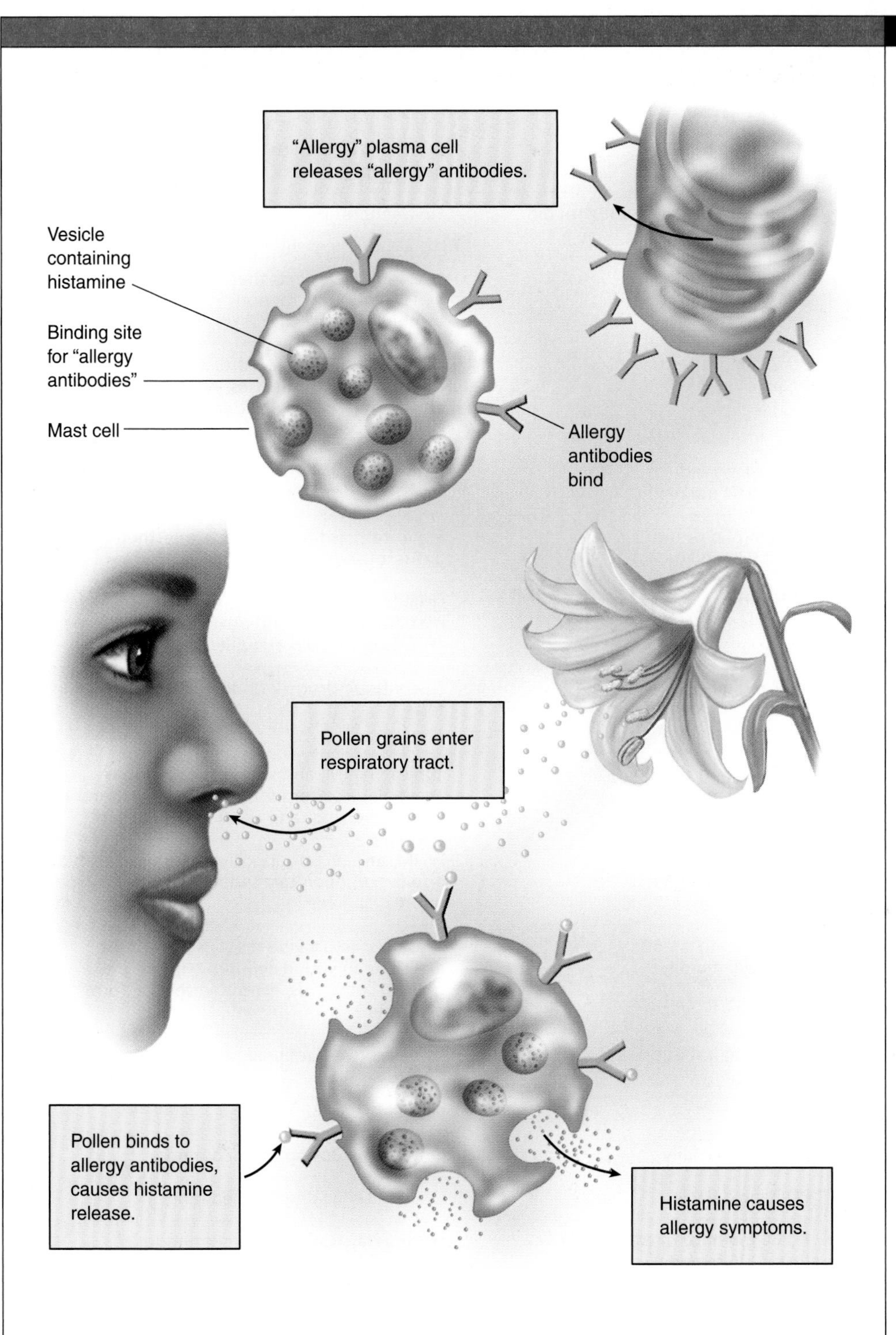
"Allergy" plasma cell releases "allergy" antibodies.
Vesicle containing histamine
Binding site for "allergy antibodies"
Mast cell
Allergy antibodies bind
Pollen grains enter respiratory tract.
Pollen binds to allergy antibodies, causes histamine release.
Histamine causes allergy symptoms.

FIGURE 21.3

Mechanism of action in allergic rhinitis

H_1-receptor blockers are effective in treating a number of other disorders. Motion sickness responds well to these medications. It is also one of the few classes of drugs available to treat *vertigo,* a form of dizziness that causes significant nausea. Some of the older antihistamines are marketed as OTC sleep aids, taking advantage of their ability to cause drowsiness.

Concept Review 21.1

- Why are the antihistamines most effective if given *before* inflammation occurs?

TABLE 21.4 H_1-Receptor Antagonists (Antihistamines)

DRUG	ROUTE AND ADULT DOSE	REMARKS
FIRST-GENERATION AGENTS		
azatadine (Optimine)	PO 1–2 mg bid	Trinalin is a combination of azatadine and pseudoephedrine
azelastine (Astelin)	Intranasal 2 sprays per nostril bid	First-generation antihistamine
brompheniramine (Codimal A, Dimetapp)	PO 4–8 mg tid–qid (max: 40 mg/day)	Less sedative effects than diphenhydramine; IV, IM, and subcutaneous forms available; combined with other drugs for OTC use
chlorpheniramine maleate (Chlor-Trimeton, others)	PO 2–4 mg tid–qid (max: 24 mg/day)	Also has antiemetic, antitussive, anticholinergic, and local anesthetic uses; IV, IM, subcutaneous, and extended-release forms available; combined with other drugs for OTC use
clemastine (Tavist)	PO 1.34 mg bid (max: 8.04 mg/day)	Central sedative effects are generally mild
cyproheptadine (Periactin)	PO 4 mg tid or qid (max: 0.5 mg/kg/day)	Significant antipruritic, local anesthetic, and antiserotonin effects
dexbrompheniramine (Drixoral)	PO 6 mg bid	Usually used in combination with pseudoephedrine and dextromethorphan as an OTC drug for cold and allergy
dexchlorpheniramine (Dexchlor, Poladex, Polargen, Polaramine)	PO 2 mg q4–6h (max: 12 mg/day)	Discontinue drug 72 hours before allergy skin tests
Pr diphenhydramine (Benadryl, others)	PO 25–50 mg tid–qid (max: 300 mg/day)	Topical, IV, IM, and subcutaneous forms available; also for motion sickness, Parkinson's disease, vertigo, and as an OTC sleep aid
promethazine (Phenazine, Phenergan, others)	PO 12.5 mg daily (max: 150 mg/day)	IV, IM, and rectal suppository forms available; also for preoperative sedation, motion sickness, nausea, and vertigo
tripelennamine (PBZ-SR, Pelamine)	PO 25–50 mg q4–6h (max: 600 mg/day)	Also used to provide mucous membrane analgesia in young children with herpetic gingivo stomatitis; extended-release form available
triprolidine (Actidil, Actifed)	PO 2.5 mg bid or tid	Long-acting; combined with other drugs for OTC use
SECOND-GENERATION AGENTS		
cetirizine (Zyrtec)	PO 5–10 mg daily	Once-a-day dosing; nonsedating
desloratadine (Clarinex)	PO 5 mg daily	Once-a-day dosing; nonsedating
Pr fexofenadine (Allegra)	PO 60 mg once or twice daily (max: 120 mg/day)	Once-a-day dosing; nonsedating
loratadine (Claritin)	PO 10 mg daily	Once-a-day dosing; nonsedating; take on an empty stomach

TABLE 21.5 Selected Antihistamine Combinations Available OTC for Allergic Rhinitis

BRAND NAME	ANTIHISTAMINE	DECONGESTANT	ANALGESIC
Actifed Cold and Allergy tablets	triprolidine	pseudoephedrine	
Actifed Cold and Sinus caplets	chlorpheniramine	pseudoephedrine	acetaminophen
Benadryl Allergy/Cold tablets	diphenhydramine	pseudoephedrine	acetaminophen
Chlor-trimeton Allergy-D tablets	chlorpheniramine	pseudoephedrine	
Dimetapp Cold and Allergy chewable tablets	brompheniramine	phenylpropanolamine	acetaminophen
Drixoral Allergy and Sinus extended release tablets	dexbrompheniramine	pseudoephedrine	acetaminophen
Sudafed Cold and Allergy tablets	chlorpheniramine	pseudoephedrine	
Tavist Allergy 12-hour tablets	clemastine		
Triaminic Cold/Allergy softchews	chlorpheniramine	pseudoephedrine	
Tylenol Allergy Sinus Nighttime caplets	diphenhydramine	pseudoephedrine	acetaminophen

DRUG PROFILE: Sedating Antihistamine: Pr *Diphenhydramine (Benadryl, Others)*

Actions and Uses:

Diphenhydramine is a first-generation H_1-receptor blocker that is a component of some OTC medications. Its primary use is to treat symptoms of allergy and the common cold such as sneezing, runny nose, and tearing of the eyes. Diphenhydramine is often combined with an analgesic, decongestant, or expectorant. Diphenhydramine is also used as a topical agent to treat rashes, and an IM form is available for severe allergic reactions. Other indications for diphenhydramine include Parkinson's disease, motion sickness, and insomnia.

Adverse Effects and Interactions:

As with most older H_1-receptor blockers, diphenhydramine causes significant drowsiness, although this usually diminishes with long-term use. Occasionally, a patient will exhibit CNS stimulation and excitability rather than drowsiness. Anticholinergic effects such as dry mouth, tachycardia, and mild hypotension are seen in some patients.

Use of diphenhydramine with alcohol, CNS depressants, or MAO inhibitors may cause additive CNS depression.

Mechanism in Action: 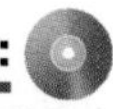

Diphenhydramine is an antihistamine used to treat disorders such as allergic rhinitis, Parkinson's disease, and insomnia. It reduces inflammation by blocking H_1-receptors found within smooth muscle cells of the respiratory tract and the endothelial cells lining blood vessels located in the skin.

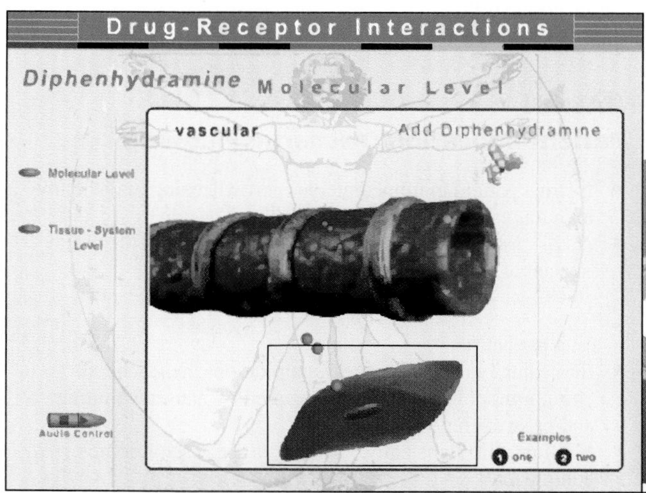

Use the student CD-ROM to see Mechanism in Action for Diphenhydramine.

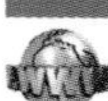 *See the Companion Website for a Nursing Process Focus specific to this drug.*

DRUG PROFILE: Nonsedating Antihistamine: 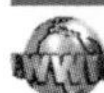 *Fexofenadine (Allegra)*

Actions and Uses:

Fexofenadine is a second-generation H_1-receptor blocker with effectiveness equal to that of diphenhydramine. Its primary action is to block the effects of histamine at H_1 receptors. When taken prophylactically, it reduces the severity of nasal congestion, sneezing, and tearing of the eyes. Its long half-life offers the advantage of once or twice daily administration. Fexofenadine is only available in oral form. Allegra-D combines fexofenadine with pseudoephedrine, a decongestant.

Adverse Effects and Interactions:

The major advantage of fexofenadine over first-generation antihistamines is that it causes less drowsiness. Although it is considered nonsedating, drowsiness can still occur in some patients. Other side effects are usually minor and include upset stomach.

No clinically significant interactions have been found.

See the Companion Website for a Nursing Process Focus specific to this drug.

NURSING PROCESS FOCUS

Patients Receiving Antihistamine Therapy

ASSESSMENT

Prior to administration:

- Obtain complete health history including data on anaphylaxis, asthma, or cardiac disease, plus allergies, drug history, and possible drug interactions
- Obtain EKG and vital signs; assess in context of patient's baseline values
- Assess respiratory status: breathing pattern
- Assess neurologic status and level of consciousness

POTENTIAL NURSING DIAGNOSES

- Ineffective Airway Clearance
- Ineffective Breathing Pattern
- Disturbed Sleep Pattern, related to somnolence or agitation

PLANNING: Patient Goals and Expected Outcomes

The patient will:

- Report relief from allergic symptoms such as congestion, itching, or postnasal drip
- Demonstrate an understanding of the drug's action by accurately describing drug side effects and precautions

IMPLEMENTATION

Interventions and (Rationales)	Patient Education/Discharge Planning
■ Auscultate breath sounds before administering. Use with extreme caution in patients with asthma or COPD. Keep resuscitative equipment accessible. (Anticholinergic effects of antihistamines may trigger bronchospasm.)	■ Instruct patient to immediately report wheezing or difficulty breathing. ■ Advise asthmatics to consult the nurse regarding the use of injectable epinephrine in emergency situations.
■ Monitor vital signs (including EKG) before administering. Use with extreme caution in patients with a history of cardiovascular disease. (Anticholinergic effects can increase heart rate and lower blood pressure. Fatal dysrhythmias and cardiovascular collapse have been reported in some patients receiving antihistamines.)	Instruct patient to: ■ Immediately report dizziness, palpitations, headache, or chest, arm, or back pain accompanied by nausea/vomiting and/or sweating ■ Monitor vital signs daily, ensuring proper use of home equipment
■ Monitor thyroid function. Use with caution in patients with a history of hyperthyroidism. (Antihistamines exacerbate CNS-stimulating effects of hyperthyroidism and may trigger thyroid storm.)	■ Instruct patient to immediately report nervousness or restlessness, insomnia, fever, profuse sweating, thirst, and mood changes.

continued...

NURSING PROCESS FOCUS

Interventions and (Rationales)	Patient Education/Discharge Planning
■ Monitor for vision changes. Use with caution in patients with narrow angle glaucoma. (Antihistamines can increase intraocular pressure and cause photosensitivity.)	Instruct patient to: ■ Immediately report head or eye pain and visual changes ■ Wear dark glasses, use sunscreen, and avoid excessive sun exposure
■ Monitor neurologic status, especially LOC. Use with caution in patients with a history of seizure disorder. (Antihistamines lower the seizure threshold. The elderly are at increased risk of serious sedation and other anticholinergic effects.)	Instruct patient to: ■ Immediately report seizure activity, including any changes in character and pattern of seizures ■ Avoid driving or performing hazardous activities until effects of the drug are known
■ Observe for signs of renal toxicity. Measure intake and output. Use with caution in patients with a history of kidney or urinary tract disease. (Antihistamines promote urinary retention.)	■ Instruct patient to immediately report flank pain, difficulty urinating, reduced urine output, and changes in the appearance of urine (cloudy, with sediment, odor, etc.).
■ Use with caution in patients with diabetes mellitus. Monitor serum glucose levels with increased frequency (e.g., from daily to tid, ac). (Antihistamines decrease serum glucose levels.)	Instruct patient to: ■ Immediately report symptoms of hypoglycemia ■ Consult the healthcare provider regarding timing of glucose monitoring and reportable results (e.g., "less than 70 mg/dL")
■ Monitor for GI side effects. Use with caution in patients with a history of GI disorders, especially peptic ulcers or liver disease. (Antihistamines block H_1 receptors, altering the mucosal lining of the stomach. These drugs are metabolized in the liver, increasing the risk of hepatotoxicity.)	Instruct patient to: ■ Immediately report nausea, vomiting, anorexia, bleeding, chest or abdominal pain, heartburn, jaundice, or a change in the color or character of stools ■ Avoid substances that irritate the stomach such as spicy foods, alcoholic beverages, and nicotine; take drug with food to avoid stomach upset
■ Monitor for side effects such as dry mouth; observe for signs of anticholinergic crisis.	Instruct patient to: ■ Immediately report fever or flushing accompanied by difficulty swallowing ("cotton mouth"), blurred vision, and confusion ■ Avoid mixing OTC antihistamines; always consult the healthcare provider before taking any OTC drugs or herbal supplements ■ Suck on hard candy to relieve dry mouth and maintain adequate fluid intake

EVALUATION OF OUTCOME CRITERIA

Evaluate the effectiveness of drug therapy by confirming that patient goals and expected outcomes have been met (see "Planning").

See Tables 21.4 and 21.5 for lists of drugs to which these nursing actions apply.

TABLE 21.6 Intranasal Glucocorticoids

DRUG	ROUTE AND ADULT DOSE	REMARKS
beclomethasone (Beconase, Vancenase)	Intranasal 1 spray bid–qid	Oral inhaler available (Beclovent) for asthma
budesonide (Rhinocort)	Intranasal 2 sprays bid	Oral inhaler available (Pulmicort) for asthma
flunisolide (Nasalide, Nasarel)	Intranasal 2 sprays bid, may increase to tid if needed	Oral inhaler available (AeroBid) for asthma
Pr fluticasone (Flonase)	Intranasal 1 spray once or twice daily (max: qid)	Oral inhaler available (Flovent) for asthma; topical form available (Cutivate) for dermatological use
mometasone (Nasonex)	Intranasal 2 sprays daily	Topical form available (Elocon) for dermatological use
triamcinolone (Nasacort AQ)	Intranasal 2–4 sprays qid	Oral inhaler available (Nasacort) for asthma; also available in IM, subcutaneous, intradermal, and intra-articular forms

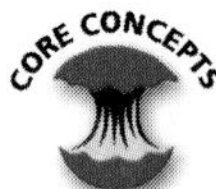

21.8 Intranasal glucocorticoids are drugs of choice in treating allergic rhinitis.

Glucocorticoids may be applied directly to the nasal mucosa to prevent symptoms of allergic rhinitis. They have begun to replace antihistamines in the treatment of chronic allergic rhinitis. The intranasal glucocorticoids and their doses are shown in Table 21.6. Some of these medications are also used to treat asthma.

Intranasal glucocorticoids are administered with a metered-spray device that delivers a consistent dose of drug per spray. Intranasal glucocorticoids produce none of the potentially serious adverse effects that are observed when these hormones are given orally. The most frequently reported side effects are an intense burning sensation in the nose immediately after spraying and drying of the nasal mucosa.

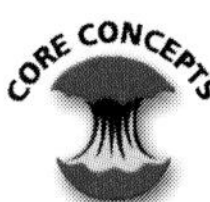

21.9 Sympathomimetics are used to alleviate nasal congestion due to allergic rhinitis and the common cold.

Sympathomimetics stimulate the sympathetic nervous system and relieve some of the symptoms associated with allergies and the common cold. Sympathomimetics used to treat allergic rhinitis are given in Table 21.7.

DRUG PROFILE: Intranasal Glucocorticoid: Pr *Fluticasone (Flonase)*

Actions and Uses:

Fluticasone is typical of the intranasal glucocorticoids used to treat allergic rhinitis. Therapy usually begins with 2 sprays in each nostril twice daily, and decreases to 1 dose per day. Fluticasone acts to decrease local inflammation in the nasal passages, thus reducing nasal stuffiness.

Adverse Effects and Interactions:

Side effects to fluticasone are rare. Small amounts of the intranasal glucocorticoids are sometimes swallowed, which increases their potential for causing systemic side effects. Nasal irritation and bleeding occur in a few patients.

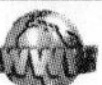

See the Companion Website for a Nursing Process Focus specific to this drug.

TABLE 21.7 Sympathomimetics for Allergic Rhinitis and Nasal Congestion

DRUG	ROUTE AND ADULT DOSE	REMARKS
ephedrine (Pretz-D)	Intranasal (0.5%) 2–4 drops no more than qid for 3–4 consecutive days	Oral, IV, IM, and subcutaneous forms available. Also for acute asthma, hypotension, myasthenia gravis, and urinary incontinence
epinephrine (Adrenalin)	Intranasal (0.1%) 1–2 drops bid	Subcutaneous, IV, and topical forms available; also for anaphylaxis, cardiac arrest, asthma, and glaucoma
naphazoline (Privine)	Intranasal 2 drops q3–6 hours	Also available as spray
Pr oxymetazoline (Afrin/12 hr, Neo-Synephrine/ 12 hr, others)	Intranasal (0.05%) 2–3 sprays bid for up to 3–5 days	Also available as drops
phenylephrine (Neo-Synephrine)	Intranasal (0.25–0.5%) 1–2 sprays q3–4h	Also available as drops, chewable tablets, and hemorrhoidal cream; also for hypotension and shock
pseudoephedrine (Sudafed)	PO 60 mg q4–6h (max: 120 mg/day)	Produces little congestive rebound or irritation; also available as drops and in extended-release form
xylometazoline (Otrivin)	Intranasal (0.1%) 1–2 sprays bid (max: 3 doses/day)	Also available as drops
tetrahydrozoline (Tyzine)	Intranasal (0.1%) 2–4 drops q3h	Ophthalmic solution is available for allergic reactions of the eye

Sympathomimetics are effective at relieving the nasal congestion associated with allergic rhinitis. Both oral and intranasal preparations are available. The intranasal drugs such as oxymetazoline (Afrin, others) are available over the counter as sprays or drops and produce an effective response within minutes. Because of their local action, intranasal sympathomimetics produce few systemic effects. The most serious, limiting side effect of the intranasal preparations is **rebound congestion;** prolonged use causes hypersecretion of mucus and worsened nasal congestion once the drug effects wear off. This rebound effect sometimes leads to a cycle of increased drug use as the condition worsens. Because of rebound congestion, intranasal sympathomimetics should be used for no longer than 3 to 5 days.

When administered orally, sympathomimetics do not produce rebound congestion. Their onset of action by this route, however, is much slower than the intranasal preparations, and they are less effective at relieving severe congestion. The possibility of systemic side effects is also greater with the oral drugs. Potential side effects include hypertension and CNS stimulation that may lead to insomnia or anxiety. Pseudoephedrine is the most common sympathomimetic found in OTC cold and allergy medicines. Because sympathomimetics only relieve nasal congestion, they are often combined with antihistamines to control the sneezing and tearing of allergic rhinitis. It is interesting to note that some OTC drugs having the same basic name (Neo-Synephrine, Afrin, Vicks) may contain different sympathomimetics. For example, Neo-Synephrine preparations with a 12-hour duration contain the drug oxymetazoline; preparations with the same name that last 4 to 6 hours contain phenylephrine. (See Table 21.5 for common combination drugs.)

Concept Review 21.2

- The sympathomimetics are the most effective drugs for relieving nasal congestion, but physicians often prefer to prescribe antihistamines or intranasal glucocorticoids. Why?

IMMUNE DISORDERS

Although inflammation is *nonspecific,* the body has also developed elaborate mechanisms of protection that target *specific* foreign agents. Drugs may be used to either *boost* the immune system (vaccines, biologic response modifiers) or *dampen* the immune system (immunosuppressants).

DRUG PROFILE: Sympathomimetics: Pr Oxymetazoline (Afrin, others)

Actions and Uses:

Oxymetazoline stimulates the alpha-adrenergic receptors of the sympathetic nervous system. This stimulation causes arterioles in the nasal passages to constrict, producing a drying of the mucous membranes. Relief from the symptoms of nasal congestion occurs within minutes and lasts for 10–12 hours. The drug is administered with a metered-spray device or by nose drops.

Adverse Effects and Interactions:

Rebound congestion is common when oxymetazoline is used for longer than 3–5 days. Minor stinging and dryness in the nasal mucosa may be experienced. Systemic side effects are unlikely, unless a considerable amount of the medicine is swallowed. Patients with thyroid disorders, hypertension, diabetes, or heart disease should use sympathomimetics only on the direction of their healthcare practitioner.

No clinically significant interactions have been found.

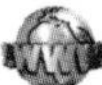
See the Companion Website for a Nursing Process Focus specific to this drug.

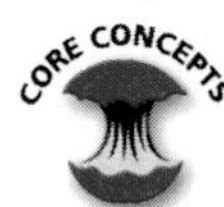

21.10 The immune response is obtained through activation of the humoral and cell-mediated immune systems.

anti = *against*
gen = *formation*

Foreign substances that cause a specific immune response are called **antigens.** Proteins such as those present on the surfaces of pollen grains, bacteria, and viruses are the strongest antigens. The primary cell of the immune system that interacts with antigens is the **lymphocyte.** Two basic types of lymphocytes are responsible for activating two very different branches of the immune system.

Humoral immunity is initiated when an antigen encounters a type of lymphocyte known as a **B cell.** The antigen activates the B cell, which then divides rapidly to form many copies, or clones, of itself. Most cells in this clone are called *plasma cells.* The primary function of the **plasma cells** is to secrete **antibodies,** sometimes called **immunoglobulins,** which are specific to the antigen that initiated the immune response. As they circulate through the body, antibodies physically interact with the antigen to neutralize it or target the foreign agent for destruction by other cells of the immune system. Peak production of antibodies occurs about 10 days after an immune response. Figure 21.4 ■ shows the basic steps in the humoral immune response.

Some B cells, called *memory B cells,* remember the initial antigen interaction. If the body is exposed to the same antigen in the future, the body will secrete higher levels of antibodies in a shorter time, approximately 2 to 3 days. For some antigens, memory is retained for an entire lifetime. Vaccines, discussed later in this chapter, are sometimes administered to produce these memory cells in advance of exposure to the antigen, so that when the body is exposed to the real organism it can mount a fast, strong response.

The second branch of the immune system involves lymphocytes called **T cells.** Two major types of T cells are **helper T cells** and **cytotoxic T cells.** These cells are often named after a protein receptor on their plasma membrane; the helper T cells have a CD4 receptor, and the cytotoxic T cells have a CD8 receptor. Helper T cells are particularly important because they are responsible for activating most other immune cells, including B cells.

cyto = *cell*
kine(sis) = *movement*

Like B cells, activated T cells rapidly form clones when they encounter their specific antigen. Unlike B cells, however, T cells do not produce antibodies. Instead, T cells produce huge amounts of chemicals called **cytokines.** Some cytokines kill foreign organisms directly, whereas others act as messengers to the immune system, stimulating T cells, B cells, and other white blood cells to rid the body of the foreign agent. Specific cytokines released by activated T cells include several interleukins, gamma interferon, and tumor necrosis factor (TNF). Some of these cytokines have been used to treat certain immune disorders and cancers. This class of medications, called *biologic response modifiers,* is discussed later in this chapter and in Chapter 24.

Cytotoxic T cells travel throughout the body searching for their specific antigen and can directly attack and kill certain bacteria, parasites, virus-infected cells, and cancer cells. As with B

FIGURE 21.4

IMMUNE RESPONSE
Activation of specific lymphocytes by an antigen
Humoral immunity
Cell-mediated immunity
Memory B cells
B cells activated
Antigen presentation
Helper T cells
T cells activated
Memory T cells
Regulatory activity
Regulatory activity
PLASMA CELLS
CYTOTOXIC T CELLS
Chemical attack by secreted antibodies
Boost nonspecific defenses
Direct physical attack on foreign or virus-infected cells

Steps in the humoral immune response *SOURCE: Pearson Education/PH College*

cells, some of the sensitized T cells become memory cells. If the body encounters the same antigen in the future, the memory T cells will assist in mounting a more rapid immune response.

21.11 Vaccines are biological drugs used to prevent illness.

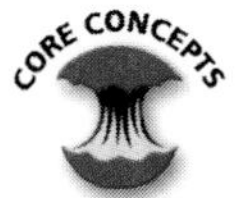

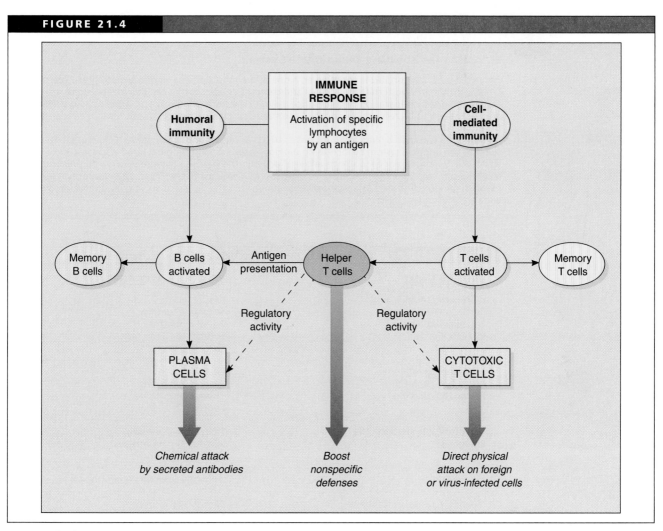

Lymphocytes attack antigens by recognizing certain foreign proteins on their surface. Sometimes they recognize a toxin or secretion produced by the microorganism. Pharmacologists have used this knowledge to create biological products, called **vaccines,** that prevent disease by stimulating body defenses. These vaccines consist of suspensions of one of the following:

- Microbes that have been killed
- Microbes that are alive but weakened (attenuated) so they are unable to produce disease
- Bacterial toxins—called **toxoids**—that have been modified to remove their hazardous properties

Table 21.8 gives some common vaccines and their recommended schedules.

Vaccination, or **immunization,** is performed to expose patients to the modified, harmless microorganism or its toxoid so that an immune response occurs in the following weeks or months. As a result of the vaccination, memory B cells form. When later exposed to the actual infectious organism, these cells react quickly by producing large quantities of antibodies. Although some immunizations are only needed once, most require follow-up vaccinations, called **boosters,** to provide continuous protection. The effectiveness of a vaccine can be assessed by measuring the amount of antibody produced by the body after the vaccine has been administered, a quantity called **titer.**

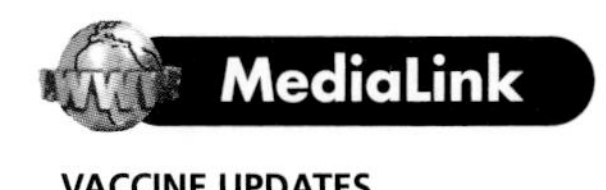

VACCINE UPDATES

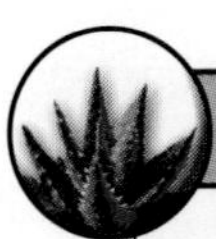

NATURAL ALTERNATIVES

Echinacea for Boosting the Immune System

Echinacea purpurea, or purple coneflower, is one of the most popular medicinal botanicals. This plant is native to the midwestern United States and central Canada; its flowers, leaves, and stems are harvested and dried. Preparations include dried powder, tincture, fluid extracts, and teas. No single ingredient seems to be responsible for the herb's activity; many active chemicals have been identified from the extracts.

Echinacea was used by Native Americans to treat various wounds and injuries. Echinacea is claimed to boost the immune system by increasing phagocytosis and inhibiting bacterial enzymes. Some substances in Echinacea appear to have antiviral activity; the herb is sometimes taken to prevent and treat the common cold and influenza, an indication for which it has received official approval in Germany. In general, it is used as a supportive treatment for any disease involving inflammation and to enhance the immune system. ■

TABLE 21.8 Common Childhood Vaccines and Their Schedules

VACCINE NAME	SCHEDULE AND AGE
diphtheria, tetanus, and pertussis (Tri-Immunol, Tripedia, Acel-Imune, Infanrix, Certiva)	First: 2 months Second: 4 months Third: 6 months Fourth: 15–18 months Fifth: 4–6 years
haemophilus influenza (HibTITER, OmniHIB, PedvaxHIB, ComVax)	First: 2 months Second: 4 months Third: 6 months Fourth: 12–15 months
hepatitis B (Recombivax HB, Energix-B)	First: birth–2 months Second: 1–4 months Third: 6–18 months
influenza	Annually from age 6 months–18 years
measles, mumps, and rubella (MMR II)	First: 12–15 months Second: 4–6 years
poliovirus, oral (Orimune)	First: 2 months Second: 4 months Third: 6–18 months Fourth: 4–6 years
varicella zoster/chickenpox (Varivax)	One dose: 12–18 months

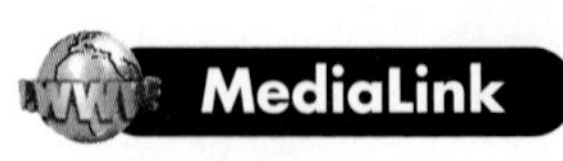

VACCINE UPDATES

Effective vaccines have been produced for a number of serious diseases. The widespread use of vaccines has prevented illness in millions of patients, particularly children. One disease—smallpox—has been virtually eliminated from the planet through immunization, and others such as polio have diminished to extremely low levels.

Vaccines may have adverse effects. Common side effects include redness and discomfort at the site of injection and fever. Although severe reactions are uncommon, anaphylaxis is possible. Vaccinations may be contraindicated for patient with a weakened immune system or who are currently experiencing symptoms such as diarrhea, vomiting, or fever.

The type of immunity achieved through the administration of a vaccine is called **active immunity.** In active immunity, the patient's immune system is stimulated by exposure to the vaccine to produce antibodies. **Passive immunity** may be obtained by administering antibodies to a patient. Examples of agents used to provide passive immunity include:

- Gamma globulin infused to counteract exposure to hepatitis
- Antivenoms administered to treat snake bites
- Sera used to treat botulism, tetanus, and rabies

Because these medications do not stimulate the patient's immune system, their protective effects last only until the antibodies disappear from the body, usually 2 to 3 weeks.

Fast Facts Vaccines and Organ Transplants

- Vaccines have erased smallpox from the world and the poliovirus from the Western hemisphere.
- Vaccines lowered the number of diphtheria cases in the United States from 175,000 in 1922 to 1 in 1998.
- Vaccines lowered the number of measles cases in the United States from more than 503,000 in 1962 to 89 in 1998.
- The most common transplanted organs are the kidney, liver, and heart.
- More than 79,000 patients are waiting for organ transplants, with 3000 added to the list every month.
- Because of the lack of available transplants, many patients die every year. This includes about:
    - 2000 kidney patients
    - 1300 liver patients
    - 450 heart patients
    - 361 lung patients

One particular vaccine that has received considerable attention in recent years is that for anthrax. Anthrax is caused by the bacterium *Bacillus anthracis,* which normally affects domestic and wild animals. In the fall of 2001, however, five people in the United States died as a result of exposure to anthrax, presumably due to purposeful, bioterrorist actions. Anthrax spores can remain viable in soil for hundreds, and perhaps thousands, of years. Anthrax spores are resistant to drying, heat, and some harsh chemicals, and can easily be applied to envelopes or other personal items to transmit disease.

Anthrax immunization (vaccination) has been licensed by the FDA for more than 30 years, but it has not been widely used because of the extremely low incidence of this disease in the United States before the fall of 2001. In addition, there is an ongoing controversy regarding the safety of the anthrax vaccine and whether it is effective at preventing the disease. At this time, the Centers for Disease Control and Prevention is recommending vaccination for only a few select populations:

- Laboratory personnel who work with anthrax
- Military personnel deployed to high-risk areas
- Those who deal with animal products imported from areas with a high incidence of the disease

21.12 Biologic response modifiers are used to boost the immune response.

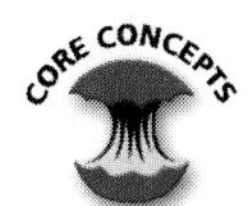

When challenged by antigens, certain cells in our body defenses secrete chemicals that help fight the invading organism. These natural chemicals, or cytokines, have been identified and, through recombinant DNA technology, have been made available to treat certain disorders. This class of drugs, the **biologic response modifiers** (sometimes called immunostimulants), has been approved to boost certain functions of the immune system. Only a few such medications have been approved.

Interferons are cytokines secreted by lymphocytes and macrophages that have been infected with a virus. Interferons slow the spread of viral infections and enhance the activity of leukocytes. The two major classes of interferons with clinical use are alpha and beta. The alpha class has the widest therapeutic application (when used as medications, the spelling is changed to *alfa*). Indications for interferon alpha therapy include cancers such as hairy cell leukemia, AIDS-related Kaposi's sarcoma, and chronic myelogenous leukemia (alfa-2a), and chronic hepatitis B or C (alfa- 2b). Interferon beta is primarily used for treatment of severe multiple sclerosis. Interferon alfa-2 (Roferon A, Intron A) is a profile drug in Chapter 24.

Interleukins are another class of cytokines secreted by lymphocytes, monocytes, and macrophages. At least 20 different interleukins have been identified, although only a few are available as medications. The interleukins have widespread effects on immune function, all of which boost the activity of natural defense mechanisms. Interleukin-2 is available as aldesleukin (Proleukin), which is approved for the treatment of metastatic renal carcinoma. Interleukin-11, derived from bone marrow cells, is a growth factor with multiple hematopoietic effects. It is marketed as

DRUG PROFILE: Vaccine: 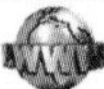 *Hepatitis B Vaccine (Recombinant)*

Actions and Uses:

Hepatitis B vaccine is administered IM to provide prophylaxis against exposure to the hepatitis B virus, which is of special interest because it is transmitted through infected blood and body fluids. Following injection, the body produces antibodies against the virus. The Centers for Disease Control and Prevention (CDC) strongly recommends that all healthcare professionals who have the potential for exposure to the virus receive the vaccine. The regimen involves 3 doses of the vaccine, usually followed by a titer to confirm that active immunity has been achieved.

Hepatitis B vaccine is sometimes given to patients *after* they have been exposed to the virus. In this case, it is often combined with hepatitis B immune globulin (HBIG), which will provide passive immunity while the body is building its own antibodies to the virus. Once a hepatitis B infection is acquired, it is difficult to eliminate; therefore, prevention is the best treatment.

Adverse Effects and Interactions:

The side effects of hepatitis B vaccine are similar to those of other vaccines. Pain and inflammation may appear at the injection site. A fever may develop, and the patient may feel tired and lethargic. Although anaphylaxis is rare, epinephrine should be kept available.

No clinically significant interactions have been found.

See the Companion Website for a Nursing Process Focus specific to this drug.

oprelvekin (Neumega) for its ability to stimulate platelet production in patients with weakened immune systems.

In addition to interferons and interleukins, a few additional biologic response modifiers are available to enhance the immune system. Levamisole (Ergamisole) is used to stimulate B cells, T cells, and macrophages in patients with colon cancer. Bacille Calmette-Guérin (BCG) vaccine (TICE, TheraCys) is an attenuated strain of *Mycobacterium tuberculosis,* used for the pharmacotherapy of certain types of bladder cancer.

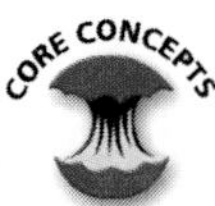

21.13 Immunosuppressants are primarily used to avoid tissue rejection following organ transplant.

The immune system is normally viewed as a life saver, protecting us from destructive pathogens in the environment. For those receiving organ or tissue transplants, however, the immune system is the enemy. Transplanted organs always contain some antigens that trigger the patient's immune response. This response, called **transplant rejection,** is sometimes acute, with antibodies rushing to destroy the transplanted tissue within a few days. The cell-mediated immune system reacts more slowly to the transplant, attacking it about 2 weeks following surgery. Even if the organ survives these attacks, chronic rejection of the transplant may occur months or even years after surgery.

Immunosuppressants are medications given to lessen the immune response. See Table 21.9. Transplantation would be impossible without the use of effective immunosuppressant drugs. In addition, these agents may be prescribed for severe cases of rheumatoid arthritis or other inflammatory diseases. The immunosuppressants are very toxic. Due to the suppressed immune system, infections are common and the patient must be protected from situations where exposure to infection is likely. Certain tumors such as lymphomas occur more frequently in transplant patients than in the general population. The mechanism of action of each of the immunosuppressant drugs differs, although most are toxic to bone marrow.

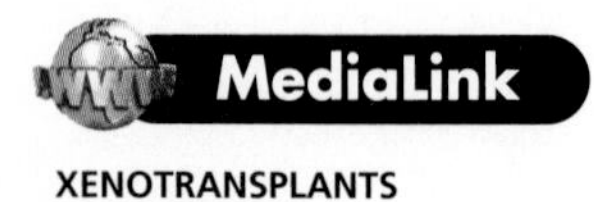

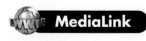

XENOTRANSPLANTS

Concept Review 21.3

- Why are oral glucocorticoids usually used concurrently with the immunosuppressant drugs following a transplant operation?

TABLE 21.9 Selected Immunosuppressants

DRUG	ROUTE AND ADULT DOSE	REMARKS
azathioprine (Imuran)	PO 3–5 mg/kg daily	IV form available; inhibits DNA, RNA, and protein synthesis; also for severe rheumatoid arthritis
Pr cyclosporine (Sandimmune, Neoral)	PO initial dose 14–18 mg/kg just prior to surgery; continue this dose for 1–2 weeks, then 5–10 mg/kg/day	IV form available; inhibits T cells; also for rheumatoid arthritis and severe psoriasis
lymphocyte immune globulin (antithymocyte globulin)	IV 10–30 mg/kg daily by slow infusion	Alters the formation of T cells and reduces their numbers
methotrexate (Amethopterin, Folex, Rheumatrex)	PO 2.5–5 mg bid 3 x week	IV, IM, and intrathecal forms available; blocks metabolism of folic acid; also for neoplasia, severe psoriasis, and severe rheumatoid arthritis
muromonab-CD3 (Orthoclone OKT 3)	IV 5 mg/day administered in less than 1 minute for 10–14 days	Antibodies specific for the CD3 receptor on T cells; for treatment of renal transplant rejection
mycophenolate mofetil (CellCept)	PO 1 g bid; begin within 24 hours of transplant	IV form available; inhibits B and T cells and antibody formation
sirolimus (Rapamune)	PO 6 mg loading dose, then 2 mg/day	Suppresses antibody production and acute transplant rejection
tacrolimus (FK-506) (Prograf)	PO 75–150 mcg/kg bid; begin 6 hours after transplant	IV form available; inhibits T cells; also for severe psoriasis

DRUG PROFILE: Immunosuppressants: Pr *Cyclosporine (Neoral, Sandimmune)*

Actions and Uses:

Cyclosporine is a complex chemical obtained from a soil fungus. Its primary mechanism of action is to inhibit helper T cells. Unlike some of the more cytotoxic immunosuppressants, it has little effect on bone marrow cells. When prescribed for transplant recipients, it is usually used in combination with high doses of glucocorticoids such as prednisone.

Adverse Effects and Interactions:

The primary adverse effect of cyclosporine occurs in the kidney, with up to 75% of patients experiencing reduction in urine flow. Frequent laboratory tests of kidney function are necessary. Other common side effects are tremor, hypertension, and elevated hepatic enzyme values. Although infections are common during cyclosporine therapy, they are fewer than with other immunosuppressants. Periodic blood counts are necessary to be certain that WBCs do not fall below 4000 or platelets below 75,000.

Because cyclosporine is extensively metabolized in the liver, many drug interactions are possible. The following drugs increase the metabolism of cyclosporine, making the drug *less effective:* phenytoin, carbamazepine, TMP-SMZ, and phenobarbitol. The following drugs decrease the metabolism of cyclosporine, causing the drug to build high concentrations and become *potentially toxic:* macrolide antibiotics, azole antifungals, and amphotericin B. Because cyclosporine can damage the kidneys, other nephrotoxic drugs such as amphotericin B, NSAIDs, or aminoglycosides should be administered with great caution.

See the Companion Website for a Nursing Process Focus specific to this drug.

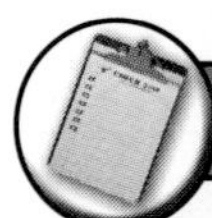

PATIENTS NEED TO KNOW

Patients treated for inflammatory or immune disorders need to know the following:

Regarding Antihistamines

1. If taking antihistamines for the first time, avoid operating machinery or performing other tasks requiring alertness because drowsiness may occur.
2. Use hard candies, chewing gum, or ice chips to reduce the dry mouth caused by antihistamines.
3. Stop taking antihistamines and notify a healthcare provider if excessive sedation, wheezing, chest tightness, or bleeding/bruising occur.
4. Do not take OTC cold or allergy medicines containing antihistamines at the same time as prescription antihistamines.

Regarding Anti-inflammatory Medications

5. Take NSAIDs with food to decrease stomach irritation.
6. Avoid drinking alcohol when taking high doses of NSAIDs or aspirin because it increases stomach irritation.
7. If signs of bleeding or bruising occur, discontinue aspirin use immediately and report the incident to a physician.
8. Take glucocorticoids exactly as prescribed because improper use may lead to serious adverse effects.

Regarding Vaccines

9. Maintain an accurate, written record of vaccinations, including the date of the vaccination, route and site of vaccination, type of vaccine (including manufacturer and lot number), and the address of the physician's office where the vaccination occurred.
10. Keep immunizations up to date to prevent illness. Because recommendations can change, seek current information from a healthcare provider periodically.
11. Vaccines may contain a number of additives, including antibiotics, formaldehyde, thimersol, and monosodium glutamate. If an allergy is known or suspected to any of these additives, notify a healthcare provider before getting a vaccination.
12. Never take cyclosporine with grapefruit juice; blood levels of the drug are increased by this combination. ■

CHAPTER REVIEW

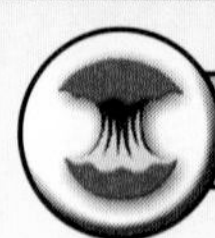

CORE CONCEPTS SUMMARY

21.1 Inflammation is a body defense that limits the spread of invading microorganisms and injury.

Inflammation is a nonspecific response designed to rid the body of invading pathogens or to contain the spread of injury. Acute inflammation occurs over a period of several days, whereas chronic inflammation may continue for months or years.

21.2 Histamine is a key chemical mediator in inflammation.

Inflammation is initiated by chemical mediators, the most important of which is histamine. Release of histamine causes vasodilation, allowing capillaries to become leaky, thus causing tissue swelling. Extremely rapid release of histamine throughout the body can trigger anaphylaxis.

21.3 Histamine can produce its effects by interacting with two different receptors.

Antihistamines used for allergies block H_1 receptors in vascular smooth muscle, in bronchi, and on sensory nerves. The H_2-receptor blockers are used to treat peptic ulcers.

21.4 NSAIDs are the primary drugs for the treatment of mild inflammation.

NSAIDs are drugs that inhibit the enzyme cyclooxygenase. Nonselective cyclooxygenase inhibitors, including aspirin, are effective at reducing inflammation and pain, but cause significant GI side effects in some patients.

21.5 Systemic glucocorticoids are effective in treating severe inflammation.

Glucocorticoids are hormones that are extremely effective at reducing inflammation. Because overtreatment with these drugs can cause Cushing's syndrome, glucocorticoid therapy for inflammation is generally short term.

21.6 Allergic rhinitis is characterized by sneezing, watery eyes, and nasal congestion.

Allergic rhinitis, also known as hay fever, is a chronic allergy triggered by a wide variety of antigens. The release of chemicals mediating the immune response can result in seasonal symptoms for some patients and chronic, continuous symptoms for others.

21.7 Antihistamines are useful for treating allergic rhinitis and several other disorders.

The H_1-receptor blockers, or antihistamines, are used to treat allergies, motion sickness, and insomnia. Newer drugs in this class are nonsedating and offer the advantage of once-a-day dosing.

21.8 Intranasal glucocorticoids are drugs of choice in treating allergic rhinitis.

Intranasal glucocorticoids are the treatment of choice for allergic rhinitis because of their high effectiveness and wide margin of safety. When used by this route, they do not produce the serious adverse effects observed when they are given orally or parenterally.

21.9 Sympathomimetics are used to alleviate nasal congestion due to allergic rhinitis and the common cold.

Oral and intranasal sympathomimetics are effective at relieving nasal congestion. The intranasal agents act more rapidly and are more effective. Use of the intranasal preparations, however, is usually limited to 3 to 5 days because of the potential for rebound congestion.

21.10 The immune response is obtained through activation of the humoral and cell-mediated immune systems.

B cells become plasma cells and secrete large quantities of antibodies. The antibodies are specific to the antigen and neutralize the foreign agent or destroy it. Some B cells remember the antigen for many years. T cells also recognize specific antigens, but instead of producing antibodies, they produce cytokines, which rid the body of the foreign agent. Memory B and T cells remember the antigen for many years and mount a faster immune response on subsequent exposures.

21.11 Vaccines are biological drugs used to prevent illness.

Vaccines are usually given to prevent a serious infectious disease. Vaccines may be live, attenuated, or toxoid. They are effective when taken according to schedule and rarely produce serious adverse effects.

21.12 Biologic response modifiers are used to boost the immune response.

Several drugs are available to boost a patient's immune function. Interleukins, interferons, and other agents enhance the body's natural defenses, primarily in the pharmacotherapy of cancer.

21.13 Immunosuppressants are primarily used to avoid tissue rejection following organ transplant.

For an organ or tissue transplant to be successful, the patient's immune system must be suppressed following surgery. Immunosuppressants are effective at lessening the immune system but must be monitored carefully because loss of immune function can lead to infections and cancer.

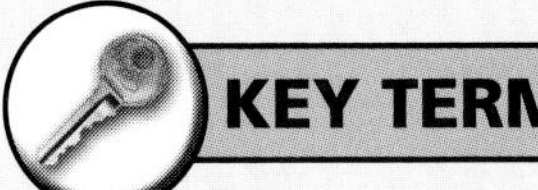

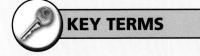

KEY TERMS

active immunity: stimulating the body to produce antibodies through the administration of a vaccine / *page 384*

allergic rhinitis (rye-NYE-tis): syndrome of sneezing, itchy throat, watery eyes, and nasal congestion resulting from exposure to antigens; also known as *hay fever* / *page 374*

alternate-day therapy: taking a drug every other day in order to minimize side effects / *page 372*

anaphylaxis (ANN-ah-fah-LAX-iss): acute allergic response to an antigen that results in severe hypotension and may cause death if untreated / *page 367*

antibody (ANN-tee-BOD-ee): protein produced by the body in response to an antigen; used interchangeably with the term *immunoglobulin* / *page 382*

antigen (ANN-tih-jen): a foreign organism or substance that induces the formation of antibodies / *page 382*

B cell: type of lymphocyte that is essential for the humoral immune response / *page 382*

biological response modifiers: agents that are able to enhance or stimulate the natural body defenses / *page 385*

booster: an additional dose of a vaccine given months or years after the initial dose to increase the effectiveness of the vaccine / ***page 383***

Cushing's syndrome (KUSH-ings): a condition of having too much corticosteroid in the blood / ***page 372***

cyclooxygenase (COX) (SEYE-kloh-OX-uh-jen-ase): key enzyme in the prostaglandin metabolic pathway that is blocked by aspirin and other NSAIDs / ***page 369***

cytokines (SYE-toh-kines): chemicals produced by white blood cells, such as interleukins, leukotrienes, interferon, and tumor necrosis factor, that guide the immune response / ***page 382***

cytotoxic T cell: type of lymphocyte that directly attacks and destroys antigens / ***page 382***

H_1 receptor: site located on smooth muscle cells in the bronchial tree that is stimulated by histamine / ***page 368***

H_2 receptor: site located on cells of the digestive system that is stimulated by histamine / ***page 368***

H_1-receptor blocker: drug that blocks the effects of histamine in smooth muscle in the bronchial tree / ***page 374***

helper T cell: type of lymphocyte that coordinates both the humoral and cell-mediated immune responses and that is the target of the human immunodeficiency virus / ***page 382***

histamine (HISS-tuh-meen): chemical released by mast cells in response to an antigen that causes dilation of blood vessels, smooth muscle constriction, tissue swelling, and itching / ***page 366***

humoral immunity (HYOU-mor-ul eh-MEWN-uh-tee): a specific body defense mechanism involving the production and release of antibodies / ***page 382***

immunoglobulin (ih-MEW-noh-GLOB-you-lin): proteins produced by the body in response to an antigen; used interchangeably with the term *antibody* / ***page 382***

immunosuppressant (ih-MEW-noh-suh-PRESS-ent): any drug, chemical, or physical agent that lowers the natural immune defense mechanisms of the body / ***page 386***

inflammation (IN-flah-MAY-shun): nonspecific body defense that occurs in response to an injury or antigen / ***page 366***

lymphocyte (LIM-foh-site): type of white blood cell formed in lymphoid tissue / ***page 382***

mast cell: connective tissue cell located in tissue spaces that releases histamine following injury / ***page 366***

passive immunity: administration of antibodies that provides short-term immunity / ***page 384***

plasma cell: type of cell derived from B cells that produces antibodies / ***page 382***

rebound congestion: a condition of hypersecretion of mucus following use of intranasal sympathomimetics / ***page 381***

salicylism (sal-IH-sill-izm): poisoning due to aspirin and aspirinlike drugs / ***page 368***

T cell: type of lymphocyte that is essential for the cell-mediated immune response / ***page 382***

titer (TIE-ter): measurement of the amount of a substance in the blood / ***page 383***

toxoid (TOX-oid): substance that has been chemically modified to remove its harmful nature but is still able to cause an immune response in the body / ***page 383***

transplant rejection: when the immune system recognizes a transplanted tissue as being foreign and attacks it / ***page 386***

vaccine (vaks-EEN): preparation of microorganism particles that is injected into a patient to stimulate the immune system, with the intention of preventing disease / ***page 383***

vaccination/immunization (VAK-sin-AYE-shun/IH-mewn-ize-AYE-shun): receiving a vaccine or toxoid to prevent disease / ***page 383***

REVIEW QUESTIONS

The following questions are written in NCLEX-PN® style. Answer these questions to assess your knowledge of the chapter material, and go back and review any material that is not clear to you.

1. Which of the following causes histamine release?

1. Prostaglandins
2. Leukotrienes
3. Bradykinin
4. Mast cells

2. H_1 receptors are located in the:

1. Brain, bronchioles, kidneys
2. Stomach
3. Smooth muscle, bronchial tree, and digestive tract
4. Kidneys, bladder, ureters

3. Patients on intranasal glucocorticoids may develop which adverse effect?

1. Rebound congestion
2. Nose bleeds
3. Drowsiness
4. Nervousness

4. Education for a patient using Afrin would include:

1. Not to use it for longer than 3–5 days to prevent rebound congestion from occurring
2. The importance of monitoring for hypertension
3. To notify the physician if nervousness occurs
4. Not to mix with any other medications

5. The most common side effect of NSAIDs is:

1. Edema
2. Rash
3. GI upset
4. Bleeding

6. The patient taking glucocorticoids is at risk for:

1. Bleeding
2. Respiratory distress
3. Dehydration
4. Infection

7. The diabetic patient taking prednisone states his blood sugar is higher than normal. The nurse's most appropriate response would be:

1. "You must not be following your diabetic diet."
2. "Prednisone can cause blood sugar levels to increase."
3. "You must be developing an illness."
4. "Your diabetes must be getting worse."

8. Which type of immunity occurs when the patient's immune system is stimulated to produce antibodies after exposure to a vaccine?

1. Passive
2. Attenuated
3. Live
4. Active

9. The patient on immunosuppressants must be assessed for:

1. Hyperglycemia
2. Infection
3. Hypoglycemia
4. Bleeding

10. Cytokines:

1. Produce antibodies
2. Are memory cells
3. Rid the body of foreign agents
4. Reduce inflammation

CASE STUDY QUESTIONS

For questions 1–5, please refer to the following case study, and choose the correct answer from choices 1–4.

Ms. Kuecken, age 38, has been suffering from rheumatoid arthritis for many years. In addition, it has been a terrible allergy season, and she has classic symptoms of severe allergic rhinitis. She has been self-treating herself with aspirin and Benadryl. She is at the physician's office, complaining that these drugs no longer work. The physician prescribed loratadine (Claritin) and Neo-Synephrine nasal spray.

1. Regarding Ms. Kuecken's aspirin use, what question should you ask to determine potential side effects?

1. Have you experienced excessive drowsiness?
2. Have you vomited any blood or passed any black stools?
3. Have you experienced excessive dryness or stinging sensations in your nose?
4. Have you experienced any rashes or dryness of the skin?

2. What instructions should you give Ms. Kuecken regarding the use of Neo-Synephrine?

1. Use only once per day.
2. Use as often as needed.
3. Use only for 3–5 days.
4. Use only at night.

3. What is the primary advantage of loratadine over Dramamine?

1. Less drowsiness
2. Less GI bleeding or pain
3. Less muscle stiffness or cramping
4. Less dryness of the nasal mucosa

4. If Ms. Kuecken's arthritis flares up and becomes acute, which of the following drug classes would likely be prescribed over a 10-day period?

1. Biologic response modifiers
2. Intranasal glucocorticoids
3. Systemic glucocorticoids
4. Sympathomimetics

5. Which of the following would likely be administered to Ms. Kuecken if she decided to go to school to become a nurse?

1. Biologic response modifiers
2. Hepatitis B vaccine
3. Systemic glucocorticoids
4. Immunosuppressants

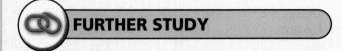

FURTHER STUDY

- Drug therapy for anaphylaxis is discussed in Chapter 19.
- Chapter 26 covers the use of H_2-receptor blockers for treating peptic ulcers.
- The analgesic action of NSAIDs and the basic pharmacology of aspirin are presented in Chapter 12.
- Chapter 29 presents details of glucocorticoids in treating hormonal imbalances.
- Chapter 25 discusses the use of prednisone to stop acute bronchospasm in asthma; Chapter 24 details its use in the treatment of certain cancers.
- Interferon alfa-2 is a profile drug in Chapter 24.

EXPLORE MEDIALINK www.prenhall.com/holland

Additional resources for this chapter can be found on the CD-ROM accompanying this textbook, and on the Companion Website. Click on Chapter 21 to select activities for this chapter.

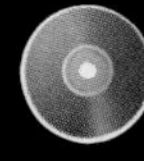

Mechanism in Action:
- **Naproxen**
- **Diphenhydramine**

Audio Glossary
Concept Review
NCLEX-PN® Review
Nursing in Action
Dosage Calculator

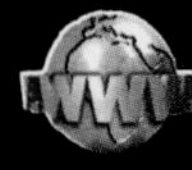

Pollen and Allergic Rhinitis
Vaccine Updates
Xenotransplants

CHAPTER

22 Drugs for Bacterial Infections

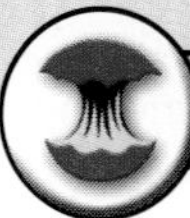

CORE CONCEPTS

22.1 Pathogens are organisms that cause disease because of their ability to divide rapidly or secrete toxins.

22.2 Anti-infective drugs are classified by their chemical structures or by their mechanisms of action.

22.3 Anti-infective drugs act by affecting the target organism's metabolism or life cycle.

22.4 Acquired resistance causes loss of antibiotic effectiveness and is worsened by the overprescribing of these agents.

22.5 Careful selection of the correct antibiotic is essential for effective pharmacotherapy and to limit adverse effects.

22.6 The penicillins are one of the oldest and safest groups of anti-infectives.

22.7 The cephalosporins are similar in structure and function to the penicillins and are one of the most widely prescribed anti-infective classes.

22.8 The tetracyclines have some of the broadest spectrums, but they are drugs of choice for few diseases.

22.9 The macrolides are safe alternatives to penicillin for many infections.

22.10 The aminoglycosides are narrow-spectrum drugs that have the potential to cause serious toxicity.

22.11 Fluoroquinolones have wide clinical applications because of their broad spectrum of activity and relative safety.

22.12 Widespread resistance has limited the clinical use of sulfonamides primarily to urinary tract infections.

22.13 A number of additional anti-infectives have distinct mechanisms of action and specific indications.

22.14 Pharmacotherapy of tuberculosis requires unique drugs because of the slow-growing, complex microbes.

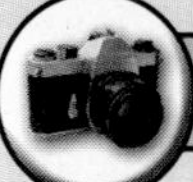

DRUG SNAPSHOT

The following drugs will be discussed in this chapter:

DRUG CLASSES	DRUG PROFILES
Penicillins	Pr penicillin G (Pentids)
Cephalosporins	Pr cefotaxime (Claforan)
Tetracyclines	Pr tetracycline (Achromycin, others)
Macrolides	Pr erythromycin (E-Mycin, Erythrocin)
Aminoglycosides	Pr gentamycin (Garamycin)
Fluoroquinolones	Pr ciprofloxacin (Cipro)
Sulfonamides	Pr trimethoprim-sulfamethoxazole (Bactrim, Septra)
Miscellaneous antibacterials	Pr vancomycin (Vancocin)
Antitubercular agents	Pr isoniazid (INH)

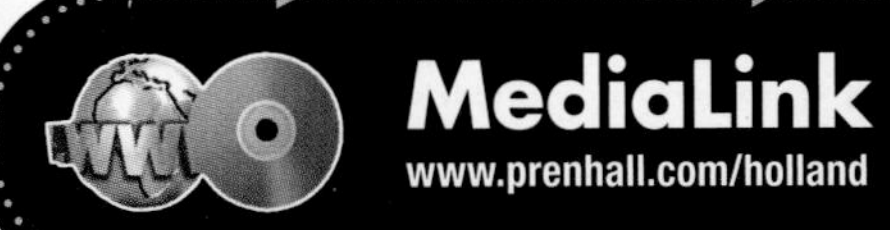

Interactive resources for this chapter can be found on the Companion Website. Click on Chapter 22 and "Begin" to select the activities for this chapter. For chapter-related animations, NCLEX-PN®-style questions, and an audio glossary, access the accompanying CD-ROM in this book.

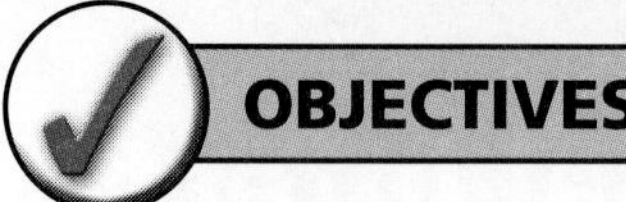

After reading this chapter, the student should be able to:

1. Compare and contrast the terms *pathogenicity* and *virulence.*
2. Explain how bacteria are described and classified.
3. Compare and contrast the terms *bacteriostatic* and *bacteriocidal.*
4. Using a specific example, explain how resistance can develop to an anti-infective drug.
5. Explain the importance of culture and sensitivity testing to anti-infective chemotherapy.
6. Identify the mechanism of development and symptoms of superinfections caused by anti-infective therapy.
7. For each of the following, identify representative drugs and explain the mechanisms of drug action, primary actions, and important adverse effects:
   a. Penicillins
   b. Cephalosporins
   c. Tetracyclines
   d. Macrolides
   e. Aminoglycosides
   f. Fluroquinolones
   g. Sulfonamides
   h. Miscellaneous antibiotics
8. Categorize antibacterial drugs based on their classification and mechanism of action.
9. Explain how the pharmacotherapy of tuberculosis differs from that of other infections.

The human body has adapted quite well to living in a world teeming with microorganisms. Present in the air, water, food, and soil, microbes are an essential component to life on the planet. In some cases, microorganisms such as those in the colon play a beneficial role in human health. When in an unnatural environment or when present in unusually high numbers, however, microorganisms can cause a variety of ailments ranging from mildly annoying to fatal. The development of the first anti-infective drugs in the mid-1900s was a milestone in the field of medicine. In the last 50 years, pharmacologists have attempted to keep pace with microbes that rapidly become resistant to therapeutic agents. This chapter examines two groups of anti-infectives: the antibacterial agents and the specialized drugs used to treat tuberculosis.

Fast Facts Bacterial Infections

- Infectious diseases are the third most common cause of death in the United States and the most common cause of death worldwide.
- Foodborne illness is responsible for 76 million illnesses, 300,000 hospitalizations, and 5000 deaths each year. About 500 people die of poisoning each year in the United States.
- Urinary tract infections (UTIs) are the most common infection acquired in hospitals. Nearly all are associated with the insertion of a urinary catheter. Hospital-acquired urinary infections add an average of 3.8 days to a hospital stay and can cost over $3,800 per infection.
- More than 2 million nosocomial infections are acquired each year. These infections add 1 day for UTI, 7 to 8 days for surgical site infections, and 6 to 30 days for pneumonia.
- Pneumococcal infections are the most common invasive bacterial infections in children, accounting for 1400 meningitis infections, 17,000 bloodstream infections, and 71,000 pneumonia infections in patients younger than age 5.
- Up to 30% of all *Streptococcus pneumoniae* found in some areas of the United States are resistant to penicillin.
- Nearly all strains of *Staphylococcus aureus* in the United States are resistant to penicillin.
- About 73,000 cases of *Escherichia coli* poisoning are reported annually in the United States, with the most common source being ground beef.

22.1 Pathogens are organisms that cause disease because of their ability to divide rapidly or secrete toxins.

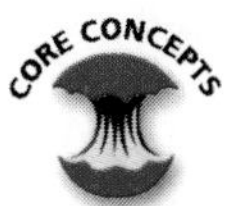

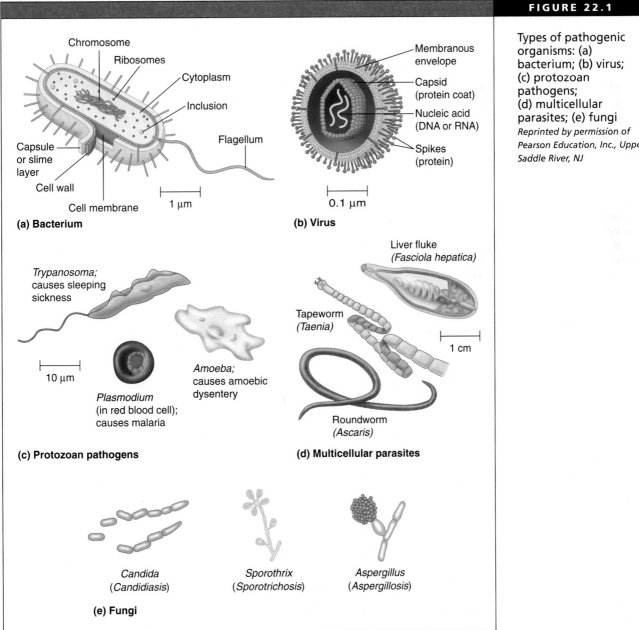

An organism that can cause disease in humans is called a **pathogen.** Human pathogens include viruses, bacteria, fungi, unicellular organisms, and multicellular animals. Examples of these pathogens are illustrated in Figure 22.1 ■. To infect humans, pathogens must bypass a number of elaborate body defenses, such as those described in Chapter 21. Pathogens may enter through broken skin, or by ingestion, inhalation, or contact with a mucous membrane such as the nasal, urinary, or vaginal mucosas.

path = *disease*
gen = *producing*

The ability of an organism to cause infection is called its **pathogenicity.** Pathogenicity depends on an organism's ability to bypass or overcome the body's immune system. Fortunately for us, only a few dozen pathogens commonly cause disease in humans. Some of these are listed in

FIGURE 22.1

Types of pathogenic organisms: (a) bacterium; (b) virus; (c) protozoan pathogens; (d) multicellular parasites; (e) fungi
Reprinted by permission of Pearson Education, Inc., Upper Saddle River, NJ

TABLE 22.1 Common Bacterial Pathogens

NAME OF ORGANISM	DISEASE(S)	REMARKS
Borrelia burgdorferi	Lyme disease	Acquired from ticks
Chlamydia trachomatis	Venereal disease, endometriosis	Most common cause of sexually transmitted diseases in the United States
Escherichia coli	Traveler's diarrhea, UTI, bacteremia, endometriosis	Part of normal flora of GI tract
Haemophilus	Pneumonia, meningitis in children, bacteremia, otitis media, sinusitis	Some *Haemophilus* species are normal flora in the upper respiratory tract
Klebsiella	Pneumonia, UTI	Usually infects immunosuppressed patients
Mycobacterium leprae	Leprosy	Most cases in the United States occur in immigrants from Africa or Asia
Mycobacterium tuberculosis	Tuberculosis	Incidence very high in HIV-infected patients
Mycoplasma pneumoniae	Pneumonia	Most common cause of pneumonia in patients age 5 to 35
Neisseria gonorrhoeae	Gonorrhea and other sexually transmitted diseases, endometriosis, neonatal eye infection	Some *Neisseria* species are normal host flora
Neisseria meningitidis	Meningitis in children	Some *Neisseria* species are normal host flora
Pneumococci	Pneumonia, otitis media, meningitis, bacteremia, endocarditis	Part of normal flora in upper respiratory tract
Proteus mirabilis	UTI, skin infections	Part of normal flora in GI tract
Pseudomonas aeroginosa	UTI, skin infections, septicemia	Usually infects immunosuppressed patients
Rickettsia rickettsii	Rocky Mountain spotted fever	Acquired from tick bites
Salmonella enteritidis	Food poisoning	From infected animal products, raw eggs, or undercooked meat or chicken
Salmonella typhi	Typhoid fever	From inadequately treated food or water supplies
Staphylococci aureus	Pneumonia, food poisoning, impetigo, abscesses, bacteremia, endocarditis, toxic shock syndrome	Some *Staphylococci* species are normal host flora
Streptococci	Pharyngitis, pneumonia, skin infections, septicemia, endocarditis	Some *Streptococci* species are normal host flora
Vibrio cholerae	Cholera	From inadequately treated food or water supplies

UTI = urinary tract infection

Table 22.1. Another common word used to describe a pathogen is **virulence.** A highly virulent organism is one that can produce disease when present in very small numbers.

After gaining entry, pathogens generally cause disease by one of two basic mechanisms. Some pathogens grow extremely rapidly and cause disease by their sheer numbers. This rapid growth can overcome the immune system and negatively impact cellular function. A second mechanism is the production of **toxins.** Even very small amounts of some bacterial toxins may disrupt normal cellular activity and, in extreme cases, result in death.

Several methods are used to describe and classify the millions of species of bacteria on the planet. The three most common methods are shown in Table 22.2. Healthcare providers must learn these organizational schemes because anti-infective drugs are often effective only for a specific type of bacteria, such as gram-positive bacilli or gram-negative anaerobes.

TABLE 22.2 Methods of Describing Bacteria

METHOD	DESCRIPTION
Staining	Gram positive and gram negative
Shape	Bacillus (rod), cocci (spherical), and spirilla (spirals)
Ability to use O_2	Aerobic (with O_2) or anaerobic (without O_2)

22.2 Anti-infective drugs are classified by their chemical structures or by their mechanisms of action.

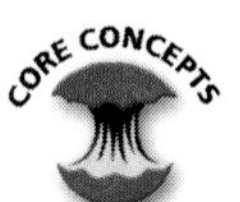

Anti-infective is a general term that applies to any drug that is effective against pathogens. Although **antibiotic** is a more frequently used word, it technically refers only to natural substances produced by microorganisms that can kill other microorganisms. In current practice, the terms *antibacterial, anti-infective, antimicrobial,* and *antibiotic* are often used interchangeably, as they are in this text.

anti = *against*
bio = *life*
ic = *pertaining to*

With more than 300 anti-infective drugs available, it is helpful to group these drugs into classes that have similar chemical or therapeutic properties. Chemical classes are widely used and the student will see names such as *aminoglycoside, fluoroquinolone,* and *sulfonamide* that refer to the fundamental chemical structure of a group of anti-infectives. Anti-infectives belonging to the same chemical class share similar mechanisms of action and side effects.

Another method of classifying anti-infectives is by mechanism of action. Examples include cell wall inhibitors, protein synthesis inhibitors, folic acid inhibitors, and reverse trancriptase inhibitors. These classifications are used in this text, where appropriate.

22.3 Anti-infective drugs act by affecting the target organism's metabolism or life cycle.

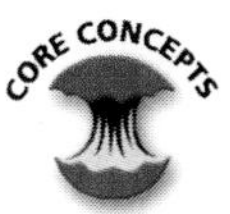

The primary goal of antimicrobial therapy is to rid the body of the infectious organism. Drugs that accomplish this goal by *killing* bacteria are called **bacteriocidal.** Some medications do not kill the bacteria, but instead slow their growth so that the body's natural defenses can dispose of the microorganisms. These *growth-slowing* drugs are called **bacteriostatic.**

bacteria = *bacteria*
cidal = *killing*
static = *staying the same*

Bacterial cells are quite different from human cells. Bacteria have cell walls and contain certain enzymes that human cells lack. Antibiotics exert selective toxicity on bacterial cells by targeting these unique differences. In that way, bacteria can be killed or their growth severely hampered without major effects on human cells. Of course there are limits to this selective toxicity, depending on the specific antibiotic and the dose used, and side effects can be expected from all the anti-infectives. The basic mechanisms of action of antimicrobial drugs are shown in Figure 22.2 ■.

22.4 Acquired resistance causes loss of antibiotic effectiveness and is worsened by the overprescribing of these agents.

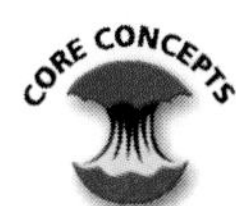

Microorganisms have the ability to replicate extremely rapidly. During cell division, bacteria make frequent errors duplicating their genetic codes. These errors, called **mutations,** occur spontaneously and randomly in the bacterial cell. Although most mutations are harmful to the organism, mutations occasionally result in a bacterial cell that has reproductive advantages over its neighbors. The mutated bacterium may be able to survive in harsher conditions or perhaps grow faster than other cells. One such mutation of particular importance to medicine is that which confers drug resistance on a microorganism.

Antibiotics promote the appearance of drug-resistant bacterial strains by killing the masses of bacteria that are sensitive to the drug. Consequently the only bacteria remaining are those microbes that possess mutations that make them *insensitive* to the effects of the antibiotic. These drug-resistant bacteria are then free to grow, unrestrained by their neighbors that were killed by the antibiotic. Soon the patient develops an infection that is resistant to conventional drug therapy. This

FIGURE 22.2

Mechanisms of action of antimicrobial drugs

Cell wall synthesis inhibitors:
• Carbapenums
• Cephalosporins
• Isoniazid
• Penicillins
• Vancomycin

RNA synthesis inhibitors:
• Rifampin

DNA

DNA synthesis inhibitors:
• Fluoroquinolones

Protein synthesis inhibitors:
• Aminoglycosides
• Chloramphenicol
• Clindamycin
• Linezolid
• Macrolides
• Streptogramins
• Tetracyclines

mRNA

Replication

Proteins

Enzymes or essential metabolites

Antimetabolites:
• Sulfonamides

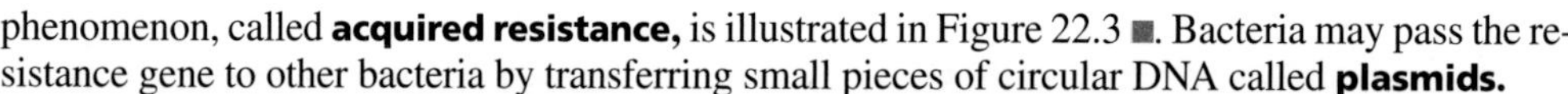

phenomenon, called **acquired resistance,** is illustrated in Figure 22.3 ■. Bacteria may pass the resistance gene to other bacteria by transferring small pieces of circular DNA called **plasmids.**

It is important to understand that the antibiotic did not *create* the mutation that caused the bacteria to become resistant. The mutation occurred randomly. The role of the antibiotic was to kill the surrounding cells that were susceptible to the drug, leaving the mutated ones plenty of room to divide and infect.

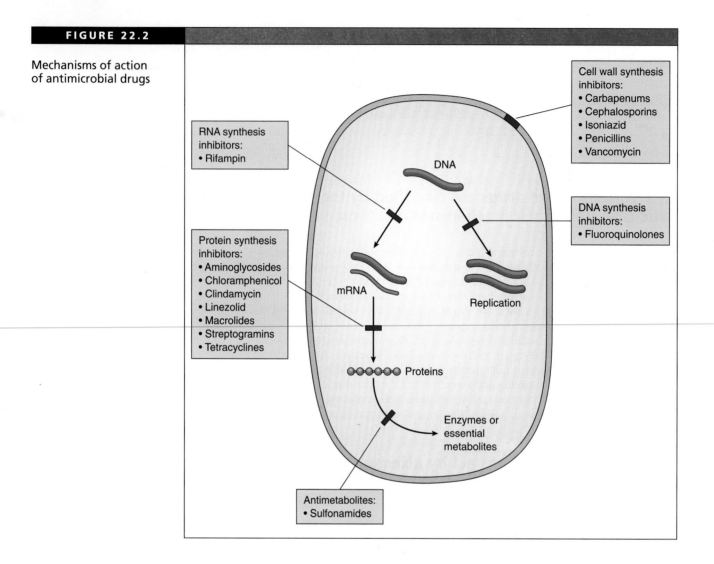

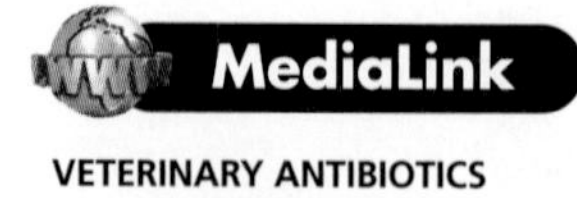

VETERINARY ANTIBIOTICS AND HUMAN HEALTH

The widespread and sometimes unwarranted use of antibiotics has led to many resistant strains. For example, 60% of all *Staphylococcus* bacteria are now resistant to penicillin. The longer an antibiotic is used in the population and the more often it is prescribed, the larger will be the percentage of resistant strains. Infections acquired in a hospital or other healthcare setting, called **nosocomial infections,** are often resistant to common antibiotics. Healthcare practitioners can play an important role in delaying the emergence of resistance by restricting the use of antibiotics to those conditions that are medically necessary.

Patients often discontinue taking their antibiotics when they begin feeling better. However, stopping antibiotic therapy early allows some microorganisms to survive, thus promoting the development of resistant strains. The patient should be instructed to take the medication for the entire treatment regimen—even if symptoms disappear before the prescription runs out.

In most cases, antibiotics are given when there is clear evidence of bacterial infection. Some patients, however, receive antibiotics to *prevent* an infection, a practice called *prophylactic use,* or **chemoprophylaxis.** Examples of patients who might receive prophylactic antibiotics include those who have suppressed immune systems, have experienced deep puncture wounds such as dog bites, and have prosthetic heart valves and are about to undergo medical or dental surgery.

Resistant organism

1. Infection

Antibiotic

2. Antibiotic kills all organisms except the resistant one.

Time

3. Resistant organism that remains rapidly divides to infect the patient. Antibiotic is no longer effective.

FIGURE 22.3

Acquired resistance

22.5 Careful selection of the correct antibiotic is essential for effective pharmacotherapy and to limit adverse effects.

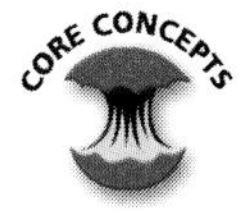

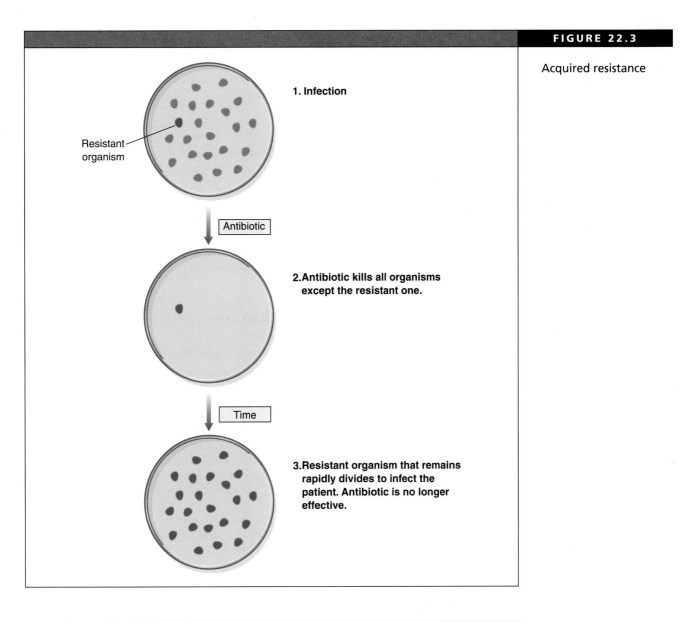

Some anti-infectives are effective against a wide variety of microorganisms. These are called **broad-spectrum antibiotics.** If the medication is effective against only one microorganism or a restricted group of microorganisms, it is referred to as a **narrow-spectrum antibiotic.**

Selection of an antibiotic that will be effective against a specific pathogen is an important task of the healthcare practitioner. Selecting an incorrect drug will not only delay proper treatment and give the microorganism more time to infect, but may cause unnecessary side effects in the patient as well.

Ideally, laboratory tests should be conducted to identify the organism prior to beginning anti-infective therapy. Lab tests may include examination of body specimens such as urine, sputum, blood, or pus for microorganisms. Organisms isolated from the specimens are grown in the laboratory so that they may be identified. After identification, the laboratory may test several different antibiotics to determine which is most effective against the identified pathogen. This process of growing the organism and identifying the effective antibiotic is called **culture and sensitivity testing.**

Proper testing and identification of bacteria may take several days and, in the case of viruses, several weeks. Some organisms cannot be cultured at all. If the infection is severe, then therapy will likely be started immediately with a broad-spectrum antibiotic. After the results of the culture and sensitivity tests are known, therapy may be changed to include the antibiotic found to be most effective against the identified microbe.

In most cases, anti-infective therapy uses a single drug, because combining two antibiotics may actually decrease each drug's effectiveness. This phenomenon is known as **antagonism.** Use of multiple antibiotics also has the potential to promote resistance. Multidrug therapy is warranted, however, if the patient's infection is caused by several different organisms or if therapy must be started before culture and sensitivity testing has been completed. Multidrug therapy is common in the treatment of tuberculosis and HIV infection.

One common side effect of anti-infective therapy is the appearance of secondary infections, called **superinfections,** that occur when microorganisms normally present in the body are killed by the drug. These normal microorganisms, or **host flora,** inhabit the skin and the upper respiratory, genitourinary, and intestinal tracts. Some of these organisms serve a useful purpose by producing antibacterial substances and by competing with pathogenic organisms for space and nutrients. Removal of host flora by an antibiotic gives pathogenic microorganisms space to grow, or allows for overgrowth of nonaffected normal flora. Appearance of a new infection while receiving anti-infective therapy is suspicious of a superinfection. Signs and symptoms of a superinfection may include diarrhea, bladder pain, painful urination, or abnormal vaginal discharges. Broad-spectrum antibiotics are more likely to cause superinfections because they kill so many different species of microorganisms. Figure 22.3 illustrates the production of a superinfection.

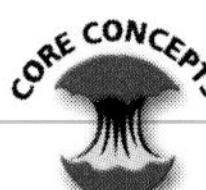

22.6 The penicillins are one of the oldest and safest groups of anti-infectives.

Although not the first anti-infective discovered, penicillin was the first *mass-produced* antibiotic. Isolated from the fungus *Penicillium* in 1941, penicillin quickly became a miracle drug by preventing thousands of deaths from what are now considered to be minor infections. Commonly prescribed penicillins are listed in Table 22.3.

Penicillins kill bacteria by disrupting their cell walls. The chemical structure of penicillin that is responsible for its antibacterial activity is called the **beta-lactam ring.** Some bacteria secrete an enzyme, called **beta-lactamase** or **penicillinase,** which splits the beta-lactam ring. This structural change allows these bacteria to become resistant to the effects of most penicillins. The action of penicillinase is illustrated in Figure 22.4 ■. Large numbers of resistant bacterial strains now limit the therapeutic usefulness of the penicillins.

Chemical modifications to the original penicillin molecule produced drugs offering several advantages. Oxacillin (Prostaphlin and others) and cloxacillin (Tegopen) are effective against penicillinase-producing bacteria and are thus called *penicillinase-resistant* penicillins. Although the original penicillin is effective against a narrow range of organisms, some in this class such as ampicillin (Polycillin and others) are effective against a wider range of microorganisms and are called broad-spectrum penicillins. The extended-spectrum penicillins, such as carbenicillin (Geocillin, Geopen) and piperacillin (Pipracil), are effective against even more species of microbes.

Several drugs are available that inhibit bacterial beta-lactamase. When combined with a penicillin, these agents protect the penicillin molecule from destruction, extending its spectrum of activity. The three beta-lactamase inhibitors—clavulanate, sulbactam and tazobactam—are only available in fixed-dose combinations with specific penicillins. These include Augmentin (amoxicillin plus clavulanate), Timentin (ticarcillin plus clavulanate), Unasyn (ampicillin plus sulbactam), and Zosyn (piperacillin plus tazobactam).

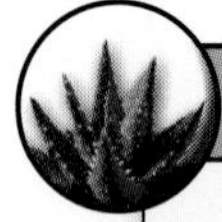

NATURAL ALTERNATIVES

The Antibacterial Properties of Goldenseal

Goldenseal (*Hydrastis canadensis*) was once a common plant found in woods in the eastern and midwestern United States. As word spread of its medicinal properties, the plant was harvested to near extinction. In particular, goldenseal was reported to mask the appearance of drugs in the urine of patients wanting to hide their drug abuse. This claim has been proven false.

The roots and leaves of goldenseal are dried and available as capsules, tablets, salves, and tinctures. One of the primary ingredients in goldenseal is hydrastine, which is reported to have antibacterial and antifungal properties. When used topically or locally, it is claimed to be of value in treating bacterial and fungal skin infections and oral conditions such as gingivitis and thrush. Other possible indications include hypertension, duodenal ulcers, and conjunctivitis. ■

TABLE 22.3 Penicillins

DRUG	ROUTE AND ADULT DOSE	REMARKS
ampicillin (Polycillin, Omnipen)	PO 250–500 mg qid	Broad spectrum; IM and IV forms available
amoxicillin (Amoxil, Trimox, Wymox)	PO 250–500 mg tid	Broad spectrum; IV form available; amoxicillin plus clavulanate is called Augmentin
bacampicillin (Spectrobid)	PO 400–800 mg bid	Broad spectrum
carbenicillin (Geocillin, Geopen)	PO 382–764 mg qid	Extended spectrum; IM and IV forms available
cloxacillin (Tegopen)	PO 250–500 mg qid	Penicillinase resistant
dicloxacillin (Dynapen)	PO 125–500 mg qid	Penicillinase resistant
mezlocillin (Mezlin)	IM 1.5–2 g qid (max: 24 g/day)	Extended spectrum; IV form available
nafcillin (Nafcin, Unipen)	PO 250 mg–1 g qid (max: 12 g/day)	Penicillinase resistant; IM and IV forms available
oxacillin (Prostaphlin, Bactocil)	PO 250 mg–1 g qid (max: 12 g/day)	Penicillinase resistant; IV and IM forms available
Pr penicillin G sodium/potassium (Pentids)	PO 400,000–800,000 units qid	IM and IV forms available; ineffective against most forms of *S. aureus*
penicillin G benzathine (Bicillin)	IM 1.2 million units as a single dose	Prolonged duration of action
penicillin G procaine (Crysticillin, Wycillin)	IM 600,000–1.2 million units daily	Prolonged duration of action
penicillin V (PenVee K, Veetids, Betapen VK)	PO 125–250 mg qid	Acid stable
piperacillin (Pipracil)	IM 2–4 g tid–qid (max: 24 g/day)	Extended spectrum
piperacillin/tazobactam (Zosyn)	IV 3.375 g qid over 30 min	Extended spectrum
ticarcillin (Ticar)	IM 1–2 g qid (max: 40 g/day)	Extended spectrum

FIGURE 22.4

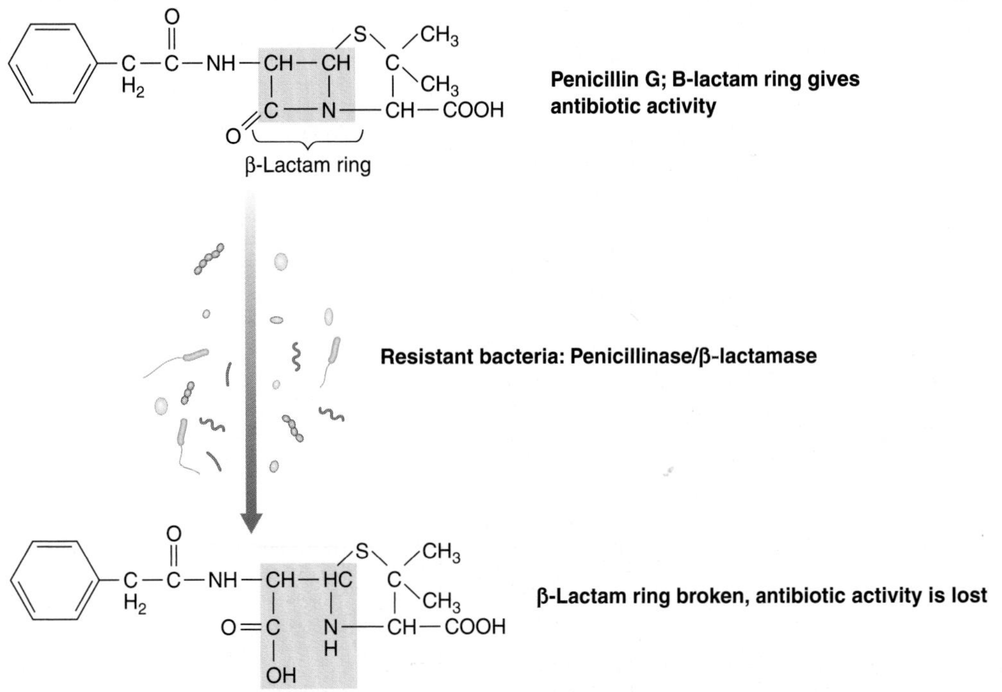

β-Lactam ring

Penicillin G; B-lactam ring gives antibiotic activity

Resistant bacteria: Penicillinase/β-lactamase

β-Lactam ring broken, antibiotic activity is lost

Action of penicillinase

In general, the adverse effects of penicillins are minor, and this has contributed to their widespread use for more than 60 years. Allergy is the most common adverse effect. Symptoms of penicillin allergy may include rash, fever, and anaphylaxis. The incidence of anaphylaxis is quite low, ranging from 0.04% to 2%. Allergy to one penicillin increases the risk of allergy to other drugs in the same class. Other less common side effects of the penicillins include skin rashes and lowered red blood cell, white blood cell, or platelet counts.

Concept Review 22.1

- Why does antibiotic resistance become more of a problem when antibiotics are prescribed too often?

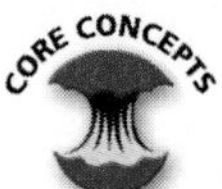

22.7 The cephalosporins are similar in structure and function to the penicillins and are one of the most widely prescribed anti-infective classes.

Isolated shortly after the penicillins, the four generations of cephalosporins comprise one of the largest antibiotic classes. Like the penicillins, the cephalosporins contain a beta-lactam ring that is primarily responsible for their antimicrobial activity. The cephalosporins are bacteriocidal and inhibit bacterial cell wall synthesis. Table 22.4 lists selected cephalosporins and their dosages.

TABLE 22.4 Selected Cephalosporins

DRUG	ROUTE AND ADULT DOSE	REMARKS
FIRST GENERATION		
cefadroxil (Duricef, Ultracef)	PO 500 mg–1 g once or twice daily (max: 2 g/day)	Binds to bacterial cell walls; bacteriocidal
cefazolin (Ancef, Kefzol)	IM 250 mg–2 g tid (max: 12 g/day)	IV form available
cephalexin (Keflex)	PO 250–500 mg qid	Binds to bacterial cell walls; bacteriocidal; broad spectrum
SECOND GENERATION		
cefaclor (Ceclor)	PO 250–500 mg tid	Binds to bacterial cell walls; extended/release form available; bacteriocidal
cefamandole (Mandol)	IM 500 mg–1g tid–qid (max: 12 g/day)	IV form available
cefonicid (Monocid)	IM 1 g daily (max: 2 g/day)	IV form available
cefprozil (Cefzil)	PO 250–500 mg once or twice daily	Binds to bacterial cell walls; bacteriocidal
cefuroxime (Ceftin, Kefurox, Zinacef)	PO 250–500 mg bid	Binds to bacterial cell walls; IM and IV forms available; bacteriocidal
THIRD AND FOURTH GENERATIONS		
cefdinir (Omnicef)	PO 300 mg bid	Third generation; broad spectrum
cefepime (Maxipime)	IM 0.5–1 g bid (max: 3 g/day)	Fourth generation; IV form available
cefixime (Suprax)	PO 400 mg daily or 200 mg bid	Third generation; binds to bacterial cell walls; bacteriocidal
Pr cefotaxime (Claforan)	IM 1–2 g bid–tid (max: 12 g/day)	Third generation; binds to bacterial cell walls; bacteriocidal; IV form available
ceftriaxone (Rocephin)	IM 1–2 g once or twice daily (max: 4 g/day)	Third generation; binds to bacterial cell walls; IV form also available; bacteriocida

DRUG PROFILE: Penicillins: Pr *Penicillin G Potassium (Pentids)*

Actions and Uses:

Similar to penicillin V, penicillin G is sometimes a drug of first choice against *streptococci, pneumococci,* and *staphylococci* organisms that do not produce penicillinase. It is also a drug of first choice for gonorrhea and syphilis caused by susceptible strains. Penicillin V is more acid stable; over 70% is absorbed after an oral dose compared to the 15% to 30% from penicillin G. Because of its low oral absorption, penicillin G is often given by the IV or IM routes. Penicillianase-producing organisms inactivate both penicillin G and penicillin V.

Adverse Effects and Interactions:

Penicillin G has few side effects. Although not serious, diarrhea, nausea, and vomiting are the most common adverse effects. Anaphylaxis is the most serious adverse effect, although its incidence is very low. Pain at the injection site may occur, and superinfections are possible.

Penicillin G may decrease the effectiveness of oral contraceptives. Colestipol decreases absorption of penicillin G. Potassium-sparing diurectics may cause hyperkalemia with penicillin G. Food increases the breakdown of penicillin in the stomach. Probenecid decreases renal excretion of penicillin G.

Mechanism in Action: 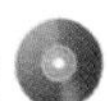

Penicillin G is a narrow-spectrum antibiotic that attaches to the penicillin-binding protein (PBP) at the active site of selected bacterial cell walls. Following attachment, penicillin G prevents the synthesis of new peptide bridges, causing fragmentation of the peptidoglycan cell wall matrix. Death of the bacterium soon follows. ■

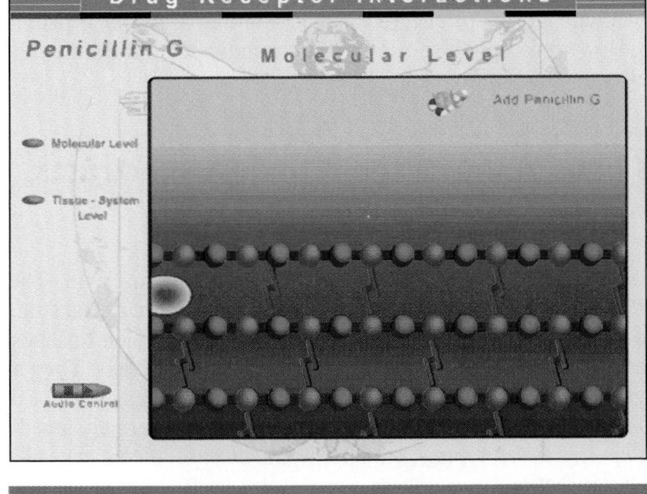

Use the student CD-ROM to see Mechanism in Action for Penicillin G.

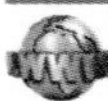
See the Companion Website for a Nursing Process Focus specific to this drug.

DRUG PROFILE: Cephalosporin: Pr *Cefotaxime (Claforan)*

Actions and Uses:

Cefotaxime is a third-generation cephalosporin with a broad spectrum of activity against gram-negative organisms. It is effective against many organisms that have developed resistance to earlier-generation cephalosporins and to other classes of anti-infectives. Cefotaxime exhibits bacteriocidal activity by inhibiting cell wall synthesis. It is prescribed for serious infections of the lower respiratory tract, CNS, genitourinary system, bones, and joints. It may also be used for blood infections such as bacteremia or septicemia. Like many of the cephalosporins, cefotaxime is not absorbed from the GI tract and must be given by the IM or IV routes.

Adverse Effects and Interactions:

For most patients, cefotaxime and the other cephalosporins are safe medications. Hypersensitivity is the most common adverse effect, although symptoms may include only a minor rash and itching. Anaphylaxis is possible; thus, the healthcare provider should be alert for this reaction. GI-related side effects such as diarrhea, vomiting, and nausea may occur. Some patients experience considerable pain at the injection site.

Probenecid decreases elimination by the kidneys. Alcohol produces a disulfiram reaction.

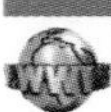
See the Companion Website for a Nursing Process Focus specific to this drug.

More than 20 cephalosporins are available, and they are classified by their "generation." The first-generation drugs contain a beta-lactam ring, and bacteria producing beta-lactamase will normally be resistant to these agents. The second-generation cephalosporins are more potent and more resistant to beta-lactamase, and exhibit a broader spectrum than the first-generation drugs. The third-generation cephalosporins generally have a longer duration of action, an even broader spectrum, and are resistant to beta-lactamases. Third-generation cephalosporins are sometimes the drugs of first choice against infections by *Pseudomonas, Klebsiella, Neisseria, Salmonella, Proteus,* and *Haemophilus influenza.* Newer, fourth-generation drugs are more effective against organisms that have developed resistance to earlier cephalosporins. There are not always clear distinctions among the generations.

The primary therapeutic use of the cephalosporins is for gram-negative infections and for patients who cannot tolerate the less-expensive penicillins. Like the penicillins, allergic reactions are the most common adverse effect. Skin rashes are a common sign of allergy and may appear several days following the initiation of therapy. Earlier generation cephalosporins exhibit kidney toxicity, but this is diminished with the newer drugs. The nurse must be aware that some patients (5% to 10%) who are allergic to penicillin will also be allergic to cephalosporins. Despite this small incidence of cross allergy, cephalosporins offer a reasonable alternative for *most* patients who are unable to take penicillins. However, cephalosporins are contraindicated if the patient has previously experienced a *severe* allergic reaction to a penicillin.

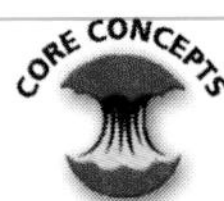

22.8 The tetracyclines have some of the broadest spectrums, but they are drugs of choice for few diseases.

The first tetracyclines were extracted from *Streptomyces* soil microorganisms in 1948. Their widespread use in the 1950s and 1960s has resulted in a large number of resistant bacterial strains that now limits their therapeutic usefulness. Table 22.5 lists the tetracyclines and their dosages.

Tetracyclines exert a bacteriostatic effect by inhibiting bacterial protein synthesis. They are effective against a wide range of gram-negative and gram-positive organisms and have one of the broadest spectrums of any class of antibiotics. They are drugs of first choice for relatively few diseases, including Rocky Mountain spotted fever, typhus, cholera, Lyme disease, ulcers caused by *Helicobacter pylori,* and *Chlamydial* infections.

The tetracyclines cause few *serious* adverse effects, but several side effects may limit therapy. Nausea, vomiting, and diarrhea are common. Patients should be urged *not* to drink milk with these medications because tetracyclines bind ions such as calcium and iron, thereby decreasing the drug's absorption by as much as 50%. Patients should be advised to avoid direct exposure to sunlight because tetracyclines can cause **photosensitivity** during therapy, making the skin particularly susceptible to sunburn. Unless suffering from a life-threatening infection, patients younger than 9 years are not given tetracyclines because these drugs may cause permanent yellow-brown teeth discoloration in young children. Because they are pregnancy category D agents, tetracyclines should not be used during pregnancy. Because of their broad spectrum, the risk for superinfection is relatively high, and nurses should always be observant for signs of a secondary infection.

TABLE 22.5 Tetracyclines

DRUG	ROUTE AND ADULT DOSE	REMARKS
demeclocycline (Declomycin)	PO 150–300 mg bid–qid (max: 2.4 g/day)	Intermediate duration of action; broad spectrum
doxycycline (Vibramycin, others)	PO 100 mg bid on day 1, then 100 mg daily (max: 200 mg/day)	Long duration of action; IV form available
minocycline (Minocin, others)	PO 200 mg as 1 dose followed by 100 mg bid	Long duration of action; IV form available; inhibits protein synthesis; bacteriostatic
oxytetracycline (Terramycin)	PO 250–500 mg bid–qid	Short acting; IM and IV forms available; broad spectrum
Pr tetracycline (Achromycin, Panmycin, Sumycin)	PO 250–500 mg bid–qid (max: 2 g/day)	Short acting; inhibits protein synthesis; bacteriostatic; IM and topical forms available

22.9 The macrolides are safe alternatives to penicillin for many infections.

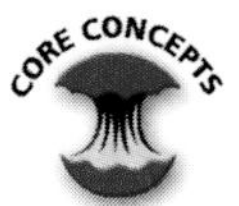

Erythromycin (E-Mycin, Erythrocin), the first macrolide antibiotic, was isolated from *Streptomcyes* in a soil sample in 1952. Macrolides are prescribed for infections that are resistant to penicillins. Commonly prescribed macrolides are shown in Table 22.6.

The macrolide antibiotics inhibit bacterial protein synthesis and may be either bacteriocidal or bacteriostatic, depending on the dose and the target organism. Macrolides are considered safe alternatives to penicillin, although they are drugs of first choice for relatively few infections. Common uses of macrolides include the treatment of whooping cough, Legionnaire's disease, and infections by *Streptococcus, Haemophilus influenza, Mycoplasma pneumoniae,* and *Chlamydia.*

The macrolides exhibit almost no serious side effects. Mild GI upset, diarrhea, and abdominal pain are the most common side effects. However, because macrolides are broad-spectrum agents, healthcare providers should observe patients for signs of superinfection. Other than prior allergic reactions to macrolides, there are no contraindications to therapy.

The newer macrolides have a longer half-life and cause less GI irritation than erythromycin. For example zithromycin (Zithromax) has such an extended half-life that it can be administered for only 3 or 4 days, rather the 10 days required for most antibiotics. The shorter duration of therapy could increase patient compliance.

Concept Review 22.2

- If penicillins are inexpensive, why might a physician prescribe a more expensive cephalosporin or macrolide antibiotic?

TABLE 22.6 Macrolides

DRUG	ROUTE AND ADULT DOSE	REMARKS
azithromycin (Zithromax)	PO 500 mg for 1 dose, then 250 mg daily for 4 days	Inhibits protein synthesis; bacteriostatic; IV form available
clarithromycin (Biaxin)	PO 250–500 mg bid	Inhibits protein synthesis; bacteriostatic
dirithromycin (Dynabac)	PO 500 mg daily	Should be taken with food to enhance its activity
Pr erythromycin (E-Mycin, Erythrocin)	PO 250–500 mg qid or 333 mg tid	Bacteriostatic or bacteriocidal, depending on nature of organism and drug concentration; IV form available

DRUG PROFILE: Tetracycline: Pr *Tetracycline (Achromycin, Others)*

Actions and Uses:

Tetracycline is effective against many different microorganisms, including some protozoans. It is given orally and has a short half-life. A topical preparation is available for treating acne. It should be administered 1–2 hours before or after meals to avoid drug interactions.

Adverse Effects and Interactions:

As a broad-spectrum antibiotic, tetracycline has a tendency to affect intestinal flora and cause superinfections. Diarrhea may be severe enough to cause discontinuation of therapy. Other common side effects include nausea, vomiting, and photosensitivity.

Tetracycline can decrease the effectiveness of oral contraceptives, thus alternative precautions should be taken during therapy to prevent pregnancy. Pregnant patients, and those breastfeeding, should not take tetracyclines, because they are pregnancy category D medications.

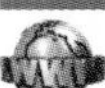

See the Companion Website for a Nursing Process Focus specific to this drug.

DRUG PROFILE: Macrolide: Pr Erythromycin (E-Mycin, Erythrocin)

Actions and Uses:

Erythromycin is inactivated by stomach acid and is thus administered as coated tablets or capsules that dissolve in the small intestine. The drug's main application is for patients who are allergic to penicillins or who may have a penicillin-resistant infection. It is a preferred drug for whooping cough and diphtheria.

Adverse Effects and Interactions:

The most common side effects from erythromycin are nausea, abdominal cramping, and vomiting, although these are rarely serious enough to cause discontinuation of therapy. Concurrent administration with food reduces this irritation. Its spectrum of activity is similar to that of the penicillins.

Anesthetic agents and anticonvulsant drugs may interact to cause serum drug levels to rise and result in toxicity. This drug interacts with cyclosporine, increasing the risk for kidney toxicity. It may increase the effects of warfarin. Erythromycin may interact with medications containing xanthine to cause an increase in theophylline levels.

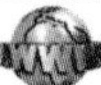
See the Companion Website for a Nursing Process Focus specific to this drug.

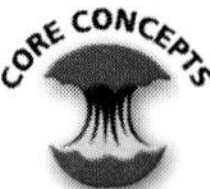

22.10 The aminoglycosides are narrow-spectrum drugs that have the potential to cause serious toxicity.

The aminoglycosides, first isolated from soil organisms in 1942, share a common chemical structure of an amino group (NH_2) and a sugar group. Although more toxic than most other antibiotic classes, they have important therapeutic applications for the treatment of a number of aerobic gram-negative bacteria, mycobacteria, and some protozoans. Table 22.7 lists selected aminoglycosides and their dosages.

The first aminoglycoside, streptomycin, was named after *Streptomyces griseus,* the soil organism from which it was isolated. Once widely used, streptomycin is now usually restricted to

TABLE 22.7 Aminoglycosides

DRUG	ROUTE AND ADULT DOSE	REMARKS
amikacin (Amikin)	IM 5–7.5 mg/kg as a loading dose, then 7.5 mg/kg bid	Broader spectrum than others in this class; usually bacteriocidal; IV form available
Pr gentamicin (Garamycin, G-mycin, Jenamicin)	IM 1.5–2 mg/kg as a loading dose, then 1–2 mg/kg bid–tid	IV, topical, and ophthalmic forms available
kanamycin (Kantrex)	IM 5–7.5 mg/kg bid–tid	Also used to sterilize the bowel prior to colon surgery; oral, inhalation, and IV forms available
neomycin (Mycifradin)	IM 1.3–2.6 mg/kg qid	Oral, topical, and IV forms available
netilmicin (Netromycin)	IM 1.3–2.2 mg/kg tid or 2–3.25 mg/kg bid	Also effective against gentimicin-resistant bacteria; IV form available
paromomycin (Humatin)	PO 7.5–12.5 mg/kg tid	For parasitic infections of the intestine; also used to treat hepatic coma
streptomycin	IM 15 mg/kg up to 1 g as a single dose	For tuberculosis, tularemia, and plague
tobramycin (Nebcin)	IM 1 mg/kg tid (max: 5 mg/kg/day)	Most effective against *Pseudomonas aeruginosa;* IV form available

DRUG PROFILE: Aminoglycoside: Pr Gentamicin (Garamycin)

Actions and Uses:

Gentamicin is a broad-spectrum, bacteriocidal antibiotic usually prescribed for serious urinary, respiratory, nervous, or GI infections when less toxic antibiotics are contraindicated. It is often used in combination with other antibiotics or when other antibiotics have proven ineffective. It is used parenterally, or as drops, in the case of eye infections.

Adverse Effects and Interactions:

As with other aminoglycosides, adverse effects from gentamicin may be severe. Ototoxicity is possible and may become permanent with continued use. Frequent hearing tests should be conducted so that gentamicin may be discontinued if early signs of ototoxicity are detected. The healthcare provider must also be alert for signs of nephrotoxicity, as this may limit drug therapy with gentamicin.

Using this drug together with amphotericin B, capreomycin, cisplatin, polymyxin B, or vancomycin increases the risk of nephrotoxicity. The risk of ototoxicity increases if the patient is currently taking amphotericin B, furosemide, aspirin, bumetanide, ethacrynic acid, cisplatin, or paromomycin.

See the Companion Website for a Nursing Process Focus specific to this drug.

the treatment of tuberculosis because of the development of a large number of resistant strains. A number of other aminoglycosides that share similar properties have since been discovered.

The aminoglycosides are capable of causing serious adverse effects in certain patients. Of greatest concern are their effects on the inner ear and the kidney. Damage to the inner ear, or **ototoxicity,** causes hearing impairment, dizziness, loss of balance, persistent headache, and ringing in the ears. Because ototoxicity may be irreversible, aminoglycosides are usually discontinued when these symptoms are first reported. Kidney damage, or **nephrotoxicity,** is recognized by abnormal urinary function tests, such as elevated serum creatinine or blood urea nitrogen (BUN). Nephrotoxicity caused by aminoglycosides is usually reversible.

oto = *ear*
toxicity = *poison*
nephron = *kidney*

Aminoglycosides are bacteriocidal and act by inhibiting bacterial protein synthesis. They are normally reserved for serious aerobic gram-negative infections, including those caused by *E. coli, Serratia, Proteus, Klebsiella,* and *Pseudomonas.* When used for systemic bacterial infections, they are given parenterally because they are poorly absorbed from the GI tract. Neomycin is available for topical infections of the skin, eyes, and ears. They are occasionally given orally to sterilize the bowel before intestinal surgery. Paromomycin (Humatin) is given orally for the treatment of parasitic infections. The student should note the differences in spelling of some of these drugs, from *-mycin* to *-micin,* which reflects the different organisms from which the drugs were originally isolated.

22.11 Fluoroquinolones have wide clinical applications because of their broad spectrum of activity and relative safety.

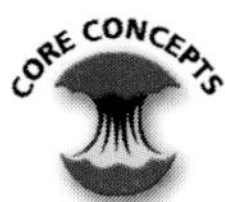

The class of drugs called fluoroquinolones was once reserved only for urinary tract infections because of their toxicity. However, the development of safer drugs in this class began in the late 1980s and has continued to present day. Newer fluoroquinolones have a broader spectrum of activity and are used for a variety of infections. The fluoroquinolones are shown in Table 22.8.

Although the first drug in this class, nalidixic acid (NegGram) was approved in 1962, it had a narrow spectrum of activity and its use was restricted to urinary tract infections (UTIs). Since then, four generations of fluoroquinolones have become available. All fluoroquinolones have activity against gram-negative pathogens; the newer ones are significantly more effective against gram-positive microbes.

The fluoroquinolones are bacteriocidal and act by inhibiting bacterial DNA synthesis. Agents in this class are extensively used as alternatives to other antibiotics. Clinical applications include

TABLE 22.8 Fluoroquinolones

DRUG	ROUTE AND ADULT DOSE	REMARKS
Cinoxacin (Cinobac)	PO 250–500 mg bid–qid	For UTI
Pr Ciprofloxacin (Cipro, Septra)	PO 250–750 mg bid	For lung, skin, bone and joint infections, and anthrax; broad spectrum
Enoxacin (Penetrex)	PO 200–400 mg bid	For UTI and gonorrhea
Gatifloxacin (Tequin)	PO 400 mg tid	For respiratory infections, UTI, and gonorrhea; IV form available
Gemifloxacin (Factive)	PO 320 mg daily	For respiratory infections
Levofloxacin (Levaquin)	PO 250–500 mg daily	For respiratory tract and skin infections; IV form available
Lomefloxacin (Maxaquin)	PO 400 mg daily	For UTI and respiratory infections
Moxifloxacin (Avelox)	PO 400 mg daily	For sinus and respiratory tract infections
Norfloxacin (Noroxin)	PO 400 mg bid	For UTI; ophthalmic form available
Ofloxacin (Floxin)	PO 200–400 mg bid	For UTI, respiratory tract infections, and gonorrhea
Sparfloxacin (Zagam)	PO 400 mg on day 1, then 200 mg daily	For respiratory tract infections
Trovafloxacin (Trovan)	PO 100–300 mg daily	For respiratory tract infections, gonorrhea, and sinusitis; IV form available

infections of the respiratory, gastrointestinal, and gynecologic tracts, and some skin and soft-tissue infections. Recent studies suggest that some fluoroquinolones may be effective against tuberculosis.

The most widely used drug in this class, ciprofloxacin (Cipro), is a drug of choice for exposure to anthrax (*Bacillus anthracis*), a potential bioterrorist threat. If exposure to anthrax is *suspected,* 500 mg of ciprofloxacin is administered by the oral route every 12 hours for 60 days. If exposure has been *confirmed,* ciprofloxacin is immediately administered IV, 400 mg every 12 hours. Other antibiotics are also effective against anthrax, including penicillin, vancomycin, ampicillin, erythromycin, tetracycline, and doxycycline.

A major advantage of the fluoroquinolones is that they are well absorbed orally and may be administered either once or twice a day. They should not be taken together with multivitamins or mineral supplements because these interact to reduce absorption of the antibiotic by as much as 90%.

Fluoroquinolones are safe for most patients, with nausea, vomiting, and diarrhea being the most common side effects. The most serious adverse effects are dysrhythmias (gatifloxacin and moxifloxacin) and liver failure (trovafloxacin). Use in children must be monitored carefully because of potential effects on cartilage development.

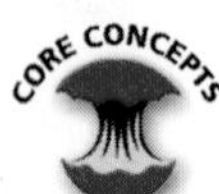

22.12 Widespread resistance has limited the clinical use of sulfonamides primarily to urinary tract infections.

Sulfonamides are older drugs that have been prescribed for a variety of infections over the past 70 years. Although their use has declined, sulfonamides are still useful in treating susceptible UTIs. The sulfonamides are shown in Table 22.9.

The discovery of the sulfonamides in the 1930s heralded a new era in the treatment of infectious disease. With their wide spectrum of activity, the sulfonamides significantly reduced deaths due to infections and earned its discoverer a Nobel Prize in medicine in 1938. Sulfonamides suppress bacterial growth by inhibiting folic acid, an essential substance in cellular metabolism.

DRUG PROFILE: Fluoroquinolone: Pr *Ciprofloxacin (Cipro)*

Actions and Uses:

Ciprofloxacin (Cipro), a second-generation fluoroquinolone, is the most widely used drug in this class. Ciprofloxacin inhibits bacterial replication and DNA repair, and is more effective against gram-negative than gram-positive organisms. It is prescribed for respiratory infections, bone and joint infections, GI infections, ophthalmic infections, sinusitis, and prostatitis. It is rapidly absorbed after oral administration. An IV form is available for severe infections.

Adverse Effects and Interactions:

Mild GI side effects may occur in as many as 20% of patients. Ciprofloxacin may be administered with food to lessen adverse GI effects; however, it should not be taken with antacids or mineral supplements because drug absorption will be diminished. Some patients report headache and dizziness.

Using this drug with warfarin may increase warfarin's anticoagulant effects. Ciprofloxacin can increase theophylline levels 15% to 30%. Antacids, ferrous sulfate, and sucralfate decrease the absorption of ciprofloxacin. Caffeine should be restricted to avoid excessive nervousness, anxiety, or tachycardia.

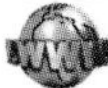
See the Companion Website for a Nursing Process Focus specific to this drug.

TABLE 22.9 Sulfonamides

DRUG	ROUTE AND ADULT DOSE	REMARKS
sulfacetamide (Cetamide, others)	Ophthalmic 1–3 drops of 10%, 15%, or 30% solution	10% ointment also available
sulfadiazine (Microsulfon)	PO 2–4 g daily in 4–6 divided doses	For malaria, toxoplasmosis, and prophylaxis of rheumatic fever
sulfamethizole (Thiosulfil Forte)	PO 2–4 g initially, followed by 1–2 g qid	For UTI
sulfisoxazole (Gantrisin)	PO 2–4 g initially, followed by 1–2 g qid	For UTI; short acting; vaginal form available
sulfamethoxazole (Gantanol)	PO 2 g initially, followed by 1 g bid–tid	For UTI; intermediate acting
Pr trimethoprim-sulfamethoxazole (TMP-SMZ) (Bactrim, Septra)	PO 160 mg TMP/800 mg SMZ bid	Combination drug; for UTI, pneumocystis, and ear infections

Several factors led to a significant decline in the use of sulfonamides. Their widespread use over many decades produced a substantial number of resistant strains. The development of the penicillins, cephalosporins, and macrolides gave physicians greater choices of safer agents. Despite their decline, approval of the combination antibiotic trimethoprim-sulfamethoxazole (Bactrim, Septra) marked a resurgence in the use of sulfonamides in treating urinary tract infections (UTIs).

Sulfonamides are classified by their route of administration: systemic or topical. Systemic agents, such as sulfisoxazole and sulfamethoxazole, are rapidly absorbed when given orally and excreted rapidly by the kidney. Other sulfonamides, including sulfadiazine, are used only for topical infections. The topical sulfonamides are not considered first-choice drugs because many patients are allergic to substances containing sulfur. One drug in this class, sulfadoxine, has an exceptionally long half-life and is occasionally prescribed for malarial prophylaxis.

In general, the sulfonamides are safe medications; however, some adverse effects may be serious. Adverse effects include the formation of crystals in the urine, allergic reactions, nausea, and vomiting. Although not common, sulfonamides can produce serious blood abnormalities, such as aplastic anemia and megaloblastic anemia.

DRUG PROFILE: Sulfonamide combination: Pr *Trimethoprim-sulfamethoxazole (Bactrim, Septra)*

Actions and Uses:

The combination of sulfamethoxazole (SMZ), a sulfonamide, with the anti-infective trimethoprim (TMP) is most commonly used in the pharmacotherapy of UTIs. It is also approved for the treatment of *Pneumocystis carinii* pneumonia, *Shigella* infections of the small bowel, and acute episodes of bronchitis.

Both SMZ and TMP are inhibitors of the bacterial metabolism of folic acid. Combining the two drugs produces a greater bacterial kill than would be achieved with either drug used separately. Another advantage of the combination is that development of resistance is lower than is observed when either of the agents is used alone.

Adverse Effects and Interactions:

The most common side effect of TMP-SMZ is skin rash, which is characteristic of other drugs in this class. Nausea and vomiting are common. This medication should be used cautiously in patients with preexisting kidney disease, because sulfonamides can adversely affect renal function. Periodic laboratory evaluations are usually performed to identify early signs of adverse blood effects.

TMP and SMZ may increase the effects of oral anticoagulants. These drugs may also increase methotrexate toxicity.

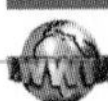
See the Companion Website for a Nursing Process Focus specific to this drug.

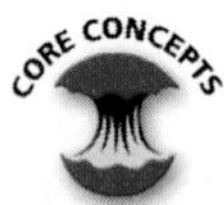

22.13 A number of additional anti-infectives have distinct mechanisms of action and specific indications.

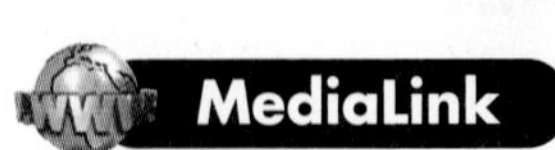

EMERGING INFECTIOUS DISEASES

Some anti-infectives cannot be grouped into classes, or the class is too small to require separate discussion. That is not to diminish their importance in medicine; some of these miscellaneous anti-infectives are critically important drugs in certain situations. For example, clindamycin (Cleocin) is sometimes the drug of choice for oral infections caused by *Bacteroides* species. It is considered to be appropriate treatment when less toxic alternatives are not effective. Vancomycin (Vancocin) is an antibiotic usually reserved for severe infections from gram-positive organisms such as *S. aureus* and *S. pneumoniae.* It is often used after bacteria have become resistant to other, safer antibiotics. Vancomycin is the most effective drug for treating methicillin-resistant *S. aureus* (MRSA) infections.

DRUG PROFILE: Miscellaneous Antibiotic: Pr *Vancomycin (Vancocin)*

Actions and Uses:

Vancomycin is usually reserved for severe infections from gram-positive organisms such as *Staphylococcus aureus* and *Streptococcus pneumoniae.* It is often used after bacteria have become resistant to other, safer antibiotics. It is bacteriocidal, inhibiting bacterial cell-wall synthesis. Because vancomycin was not used frequently during the first 30 years following its discovery, the incidence of vancomycin-resistant organisms is smaller than with other antibiotics. Vancomycin is the most effective drug for treating methicillin-resistant *S. aureus* infections, which have become a major problem in the United States. Vancomycin-resistant strains of *S. aureus,* however, have begun to appear in recent years. Vancomycin is normally given IV because it is not absorbed from the GI tract.

Adverse Effects and Interactions:

Frequent, minor side effects include flushing, hypotension, and rash on the upper body, sometimes called **red-man syndrome.** More serious adverse effects are possible with higher doses, including nephrotoxicity and ototoxicity. Some patients experience an acute allergic reaction and even anaphylaxis.

Vancomycin adds to toxicity of aminoglycosides, amphotericin B, cisplatin, cyclosporine, polymyxin B, and other ototoxic and nephrotoxic medications. Cholestyramine and colestipol can decrease the absorption of vancomycin.

See the Companion Website for a Nursing Process Focus specific to this drug.

NURSING PROCESS FOCUS

Patients Receiving Antibacterial Therapy

ASSESSMENT

Prior to administration:

- Obtain complete health history including allergies, drug history, and possible drug interactions
- Obtain specimens for culture and sensitivity before initiating therapy
- Perform infection-focused physical examination including vital signs, white blood cell count, and sedimentation rate

POTENTIAL NURSING DIAGNOSES

- Infection
- Risk for Injury, related to side effects of drug
- Deficient Knowledge, related to disease process, transmission, and drug therapy
- Noncompliance, related to therapeutic regimen

PLANNING: Patient Goals and Expected Outcomes

The patient will:

- Report reduction in symptoms related to the diagnosed infection, and have negative results for laboratory and diagnostic tests for the presenting infection
- Demonstrate an understanding of the drug's action by accurately describing drug side effects and precautions
- Immediately report significant side effects such as shortness of breath, swelling, fever, stomatitis, loose stools, vaginal discharge, or cough
- Complete full course of antibiotic therapy and comply with follow-up care

IMPLEMENTATION

Interventions and (Rationales)	Patient Education/Discharge Planning
■ Monitor vital signs and symptoms of infection to determine antibacterial effectiveness. (Another drug or different dosage may be required.)	■ Instruct patient to notify healthcare provider if symptoms persist or worsen.
■ Monitor for hypersensitivity reaction. (Immediate hypersensitivity reaction may occur within 2–30 minutes; accelerated occurs in 1–72 hours; and delayed after 72 hours.)	■ Instruct patient to discontinue the medication and inform healthcare provider if symptoms of hypersensitivity reaction develop such as wheezing; shortness of breath; swelling of face, tongue, or hands; and itching or rash.
■ Monitor for severe diarrhea. (The condition may occur due to superinfection or the possible adverse effect of antibiotic-associated pseudomembranous colitis, or AAPMC.)	Instruct patient to: ■ Consult healthcare provider before taking antidiarrheal drugs, which could cause retention of harmful bacteria ■ Consume cultured dairy products with live active cultures, such as kefir, yogurt, or buttermilk, to help maintain normal intestinal flora
■ Administer drug around the clock (to maintain effective blood levels).	Instruct patient to: ■ Take medication on schedule ■ Complete the entire prescription even if feeling better, to prevent development of resistant bacteria
■ Monitor for superinfection, especially in elderly, debilitated, or immunosuppressed patients. (Increased risk for superinfections is due to elimination of normal flora.) ■ Monitor intake of OTC products such as antacids, calcium supplements, iron products, and laxatives containing magnesium. (These products interfere with absorption of many antibiotics.)	■ Instruct patient to report signs and symptoms of superinfection such as fever; black hairy tongue; stomatitis; loose, foul-smelling stools; vaginal discharge; or cough. ■ Advise patient to consult with healthcare provider before using OTC medications or herbal products.

continued...

(continued from page 411)

NURSING PROCESS FOCUS

Interventions and (Rationales)	Patient Education/Discharge Planning
■ Monitor for photosensitivity. (Tetracyclines, fluoroquinolones, and sulfonamides can increase patient's sensitivity to ultraviolet light and increase risk of sunburn.) ■ Determine the interactions of the prescribed antibiotics with various foods and beverages.	Encourage patient to: ■ Avoid direct exposure to sunlight during and after therapy ■ Wear protective clothing, sunglasses, and sunscreen when in the sun Instruct patient regarding foods and beverages that should be avoided with specific antibiotic therapies: ■ No acidic fruit juices with penicillins ■ No alcohol intake with cephalosporins ■ No dairy product/calcium products with tetracyclines
■ Monitor IV site for signs and symptoms of tissue irritation, severe pain, and extravasation.	■ Instruct patient to immediately report pain or other symptoms of discomfort during intravenous infusion.
■ Monitor for side effects specific to various antibiotic therapies. (See "Nursing Considerations" for each antibiotic classification in this chapter.)	■ Instruct patient to report side effects specific to antibiotic therapy prescribed.
■ Monitor renal function such as intake and output ratios and urine color and consistency. Monitor lab work including serum creatinine and BUN. (Some antibiotics such as the aminoglycosides are nephrotoxic.)	■ Explain purpose of required laboratory tests and scheduled follow-up with healthcare provider. ■ Instruct patient to increase fluid intake to 2000–3000 ml/day.
■ Monitor for symptoms of ototoxicity. (Some antibiotics, such as the aminoglycosides and vancomycin, may cause vestibular or auditory nerve damage.)	Instruct patient to notify healthcare provider of: ■ Changes in hearing, ringing in ears, or full feeling in the ears ■ Nausea and vomiting with motion, ataxia, nystagmus, or dizziness
■ Monitor patient for compliance with antibiotic therapy.	Instruct patient in the importance of: ■ Completing the prescription as ordered ■ Follow-up care after antibiotic therapy is completed

EVALUATION OF OUTCOME CRITERIA

Evaluate the effectiveness of drug therapy by confirming that patient goals and expected outcomes have been met (see "Planning").

See Tables 22.3 through 22.10 for lists of drugs to which these nursing actions apply.

Two miscellaneous agents represent the first of several new classes of antibiotics. Linezolid (Zyvox) is the first drug in a new class called the oxazolidinones. This drug is effective against methicillin-resistant *S. aureus* infections. Quinupristin/dalfopristin (Synercid) is a combination drug that is the first in a new antibiotic class called streptogamins. This drug is primarily indicated for treatment of vancomycin-resistant *Enterococcus faecalis* infections. Table 22.10 lists some of these miscellaneous antibiotics and their dosages.

TUBERCULOSIS

Tuberculosis (TB) is a highly contagious infection caused by the organism *Mycobacterium tuberculosis.* Although the microorganisms typically invade the lung, they may also enter other body

TABLE 22.10 Miscellaneous Anti-infectives

DRUG	ROUTE AND ADULT DOSE	REMARKS
aztreonam (Azactam)	IM 0.5–2 g bid–qid (max: 8 g/day)	Monobactam class; for gram-negative aerobic bacteria; IV form available
chloramphenicol (Chloromycetin, others)	PO 12.5 mg/kg qid	Broad spectrum; for typhoid fever and meningitis; IV form available
clindamycin hydrochloride (Cleocin)	PO 150–450 mg qid	Bacteriostatic; effective against anaerobic organisms; topical, IM, and IV forms available
daptomycin (Cubicin)	IV 4 mg/kg once q24h for 7–14 days	Bacteriocidal; for serious skin infections
fosfomycin (Monurol)	PO 3 g sachet dissolved in 3–4 oz of water as a single dose	Bacteriocidal; for UTI
imipenem-cilastatin (Primaxin)	IV 250–500 mg tid–qid (max: 4 g/day)	Carbapenum class; combination drug; IM form available; one of the broadest spectrums of any anti-infective
lincomycin (Lincocin)	PO 500 mg tid–qid (max: 8 g/day)	Bacteriostatic; effective against anaerobic organisms; IM form available
linezolid (Zyvox)	PO 600 mg bid	For vancomycin-resistant *Enterococcus;* IV form available
meropenum (Merrem IV)	IV 1–2 g tid	Carbapenum class; for intra-abdominal infections, bacterial meningitis
methenamine (Mandelamine, Hiprex, Urex)	PO hippurate 1 g bid; mandelate 1 g qid	For chronic UTI; broad spectrum
metronidazole (Flagyl, others)	PO 7.5 mg/kg qid	For serious infections from anaerobic bacteria; also for protozoan infections; IV form available
nitrofurantoin (Furadantin, Marobid, Macrodantin)	PO 50–100 mg qid	For UTI; extended-release form available; interferes with bacterial enzymes; may be bacteriostatic or bacteriocidal
quinupristin-dalfopristin (Synercid)	IV 7.5 mg/kg infused over 50 min q8h	Streptogamins class; for serious infections resistant to vancomycin
spectinomycin (Trobicin)	IM 2 g as single dose	Bacteriostatic; for gonorrhea
teicoplanin (Targocid)	IV 6 mg/kg/day after 2 loading doses 12 hours apart	Glycopeptide class; for serious infections of the blood and heart
telithromycin (Ketek)	PO 800 mg daily	Ketolide class; for community-acquired respiratory tract infections
Pr vancomycin (Vancocin)	IV 500 mg qid–1 g bid	For *Staph*-resistant infections

systems, particularly bone. The slow-growing mycobacteria activate cells of the immune response, which attempt to isolate the pathogens by creating a wall around them. The mycobacteria usually become dormant, lying inside cavities called **tubercles.** They may remain dormant during an entire lifetime, or they may become reactivated if the immune system becomes suppressed. When active, tuberculosis can be quite infectious, being spread by contaminated sputum. With the immune suppression characteristic of AIDS, the incidence of TB has greatly increased: As many as 20% of all AIDS patients develop active tuberculosis. Two other types of mycobacteria infect humans. *Mycobacterium leprae* is responsible for leprosy, a rare disease in the United States and Canada. *M. leprae* is treated with multiple drugs, usually beginning with rifampin. *Mycobacterium avium* complex (MAC) causes an infection of the lungs, most commonly observed in AIDS patients. The most effective drugs against MAC are the macrolides azithromycin (Zithromax) and clarithromycin (Biaxin).

TABLE 22.11 First-choice Antitubercular Drugs

DRUG	ROUTE AND ADULT DOSE	REMARKS
ethambutol (Myambutol)	PO 15–25 mg/kg daily	Used in combination with other antituberculars
Pr isoniazid (INH, others)	PO 15 mg/kg daily	Used in combination with other antituberculars; IM form available
pyrazinamide	PO 5–15 mg/kg tid–qid (max: 2 g/day)	Rifater is a fixed-dose combination of pyrazinamide with isoniazid and rifampin
rifampin (Rifadin, Rimactane)	PO 600 mg daily	Used in combination with other antituberculars; IV form available; also for leprosy, *H. influenza*, and meningococcus infections
rifapentine (Priftin)	PO 600 mg twice a week for 2 months, then once a week for 4 months	Used in combination with other antituberculars
streptomycin	IM 15 mg/kg–1 g daily	Used in combination with other antituberculars; also for several other serious bacterial infections

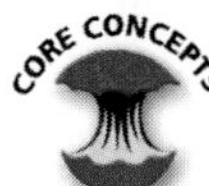

22.14 Pharmacotherapy of tuberculosis requires unique drugs because of the slow-growing, complex microbes.

Drug therapy of tuberculosis differs from that of most other infections. *Mycobacteria* have a cell wall that is resistant to penetration by anti-infective drugs. For medications to reach the isolated microorganisms in the tubercles, therapy must continue for 6 to 12 months. Although the patient may not be infectious this entire time and may have no symptoms, it is critical that therapy continue the entire period. Some patients develop multidrug-resistant infections and require therapy for as long as 24 months.

A second difference in the therapy of tuberculosis is that at least two—and sometimes four or more—antibiotics must be administered concurrently. During the 6- to 24-month treatment period, different combinations of drugs may be used. Multidrug therapy is necessary because the mycobacteria grow slowly, and resistance is common. Using multiple drugs and switching the combinations during the long treatment period lowers the potential for resistance and increases the success of therapy. Table 22.11 lists drugs used as first-choice therapy of tuberculosis. A second group of drugs are more toxic and less effective than the first-choice agents and are used when resistance develops.

DRUG PROFILE: Antitubercular: Pr *Isoniazid (INH)*

Actions and Uses:

Isoniazid has been a drug of choice for the treatment of *M. tuberculosis* for many years. It is bacteriocidal for actively growing organisms, but bacteriostatic for dormant mycobacteria. It is selective for *M. tuberculosis.* Isoniazid is used alone for chemoprophylaxis, or in combination with other antitubercular drugs for treating active disease.

Adverse Effects and Interactions:

The most common side effects of isoniazid are numbness of the hands and feet, rash, and fever. Although rare, liver toxicity is a serious adverse effect; thus, the healthcare provider should be alert for signs of jaundice, fatigue, elevated hepatic enzymes, or loss of appetite. Liver enzyme tests are usually performed monthly during therapy to identify early hepatotoxicity.

Aluminum-containing antacids decrease the absorption of isoniazid. When disulfiram is taken with INH, lack of coordination or psychotic reactions may result. Drinking alcohol with INH increases the risk of liver toxicity.

See the Companion Website for a Nursing Process Focus specific to this drug.

NURSING PROCESS FOCUS

Patients Receiving Antituberculosis Agents

ASSESSMENT

Prior to administration:

- Obtain complete health history including allergies, drug history, and possible drug interactions
- Perform complete physical examination including vital signs
- Assess for presence/history of the following:
  - Positive tuberculin skin test
  - Positive sputum culture or smear
  - Close contact with person recently infected with tuberculosis
  - HIV infection or AIDS
  - Immunosuppressant drug therapy
  - Alcohol abuse
  - Liver or kidney disease
  - Assess cognitive ability to comply with long-term therapy

POTENTIAL NURSING DIAGNOSES

- Risk for Infection
- Risk for Injury, related to side effects of medication
- Deficient Knowledge, related to drug therapy
- Noncompliance, related to therapeutic regimen

PLANNING: Patient Goals and Expected Outcomes

The patient will:

- Report reduction in tuberculosis symptoms and have negative results for laboratory and diagnostic tests indicating TB infection
- Demonstrate an understanding of the drug's action by accurately describing drug side effects and precautions
- Immediately report effects such as visual changes, difficulty voiding, changes in hearing, and symptoms of liver or kidney impairment
- Complete full course of antitubercular therapy and comply with follow-up care

IMPLEMENTATION

Interventions and (Rationales)	Patient Education/Discharge Planning
■ Monitor for hepatic side effects. (Antituberculosis agents, such as isoniazid and rifampin, cause hepatic impairment.)	■ Instruct patient to report yellow eyes and skin, loss of appetite, dark urine, and unusual tiredness.
■ Monitor for neurologic side effects such as numbness and tingling of the extremities. (Antituberculosis agents, such as isoniazid, cause peripheral neuropathy and depletion of vitamin B_6.)	Instruct patient to: ■ Report numbness and tingling of extremities ■ Take supplemental vitamin B_6 as ordered to reduce risk of side effects
■ Collect sputum specimens as directed by healthcare provider. (This will determine the effectiveness of the antituberculosis agent.)	■ Instruct patient in technique needed to collect a quality sputum specimen.
■ Monitor for dietary compliance when patient is taking isoniazid. (Foods high in tyramine can interact with the drug and cause palpitations, flushing, and hypertension.)	■ Advise patients taking isoniazid to avoid foods containing tyramine, such as aged cheese, smoked and pickled fish, beer and red wine, bananas, and chocolate.
■ Monitor for side effects specific to various antituberculosis drugs.	Instruct patient to report side effects specific to antituberculosis therapy prescribed: ■ Blurred vision or changes in color or vision field (ethambutol) ■ Difficulty in voiding (pyrazinamide) ■ Fever, yellowing of skin, weakness, dark urine (isoniazid, rifampin) ■ Gastrointestinal system disturbances (rifampin) ■ Changes in hearing (streptomycin) ■ Numbness and tingling of extremities (isoniazid) ■ Red discoloration of body fluids (rifampin) ■ Dark concentrated urine, weight gain, edema (streptomycin) ■ Establish infection control measures based on extent of disease condition, and established protocol

continued...

(continued from page 415)

NURSING PROCESS FOCUS

Interventions and (Rationales)	Patient Education/Discharge Planning
■ Establish therapeutic environment to ensure adequate rest, nutrition, hydration, and relaxation. (Symptoms of tuberculosis are manifested when the immune system is suppressed.)	■ Instruct patient in infectious control measures, such as frequent handwashing, covering the mouth when coughing or sneezing, and proper disposal of soiled tissues. ■ Teach patient to incorporate health-enhancing activities, such as adequate rest and sleep, intake of essential vitamins and nutrients, and intake of six to eight glasses of water/day.
■ Monitor patient's ability and motivation to comply with therapeutic regimen. (Treatment must continue for the full length of therapy to eliminate all *M. tuberculosis* organisms.)	Explain the importance of complying with the entire therapeutic plan, including: ■ Take all medications as directed by healthcare provider ■ Do not discontinue medication until instructed ■ Wear a medical alert bracelet ■ Keep all appointments for follow-up care

EVALUATION OF OUTCOME CRITERIA

Evaluate the effectiveness of drug therapy by confirming that patient goals and expected outcomes have been met (see "Planning").

 *See Table 22.11 for a list of drugs to which these nursing actions apply.*

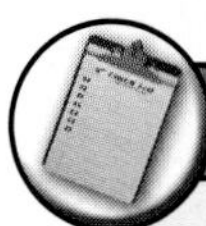

PATIENTS NEED TO KNOW

Patients treated for bacterial infections need to know the following:

In General

1. Take the entire prescription of anti-infective medication exactly as directed because partial doses, skipped doses, and shortened length of treatment encourage the development of resistant organisms.
2. Some antibiotics may cause GI upset. If this occurs, take the drug with food or milk as directed. Check prescription label for specific directions.
3. Eating active-culture yogurt or buttermilk may decrease the risks for diarrhea and vaginitis associated with antibiotic destruction of normal flora.
4. Antibiotics are most effective if taken around the clock, rather than just during normal waking hours.

Regarding Penicillins

5. It may be necessary to stay in the office for at least 30 minutes after receiving an injection of penicillin so the healthcare practitioners can monitor you for possible allergic reactions.
6. Avoid intake of caffeinated beverages, citrus fruits, and fruit juices for at least 1 hour before and 2 hours after taking oral penicillin to maximize the drug's absorption.

Regarding Sulfonamides and Tetracyclines

7. Take oral cephalosporins and oral lincomycin with food, and oral sulfonamides with food or milk to decrease GI upset. Drink a glass of water with each dose of sulfonamide, tetracycline, lincomycin, or fluoroquinolone, and drink a total of 2–3 L of fluid a day.
8. Avoid sun/tanning exposure while taking sulfonamides and tetracyclines because of photosensitivity the drug causes.
9. Antacids, dairy products, iron, baking soda, and kaolin-pectin bind and inactivate tetracycline. Separate intake by 2–3 hours for full antibiotic effectiveness.
10. Sulfonamides, tetracycline, and other antibiotics may interfere with the effectiveness of oral contraceptives. Ask a healthcare provider about the advisability of using an additional form of contraception. ■

A third difference is that antituberculosis drugs are used extensively for *preventing* the disease in addition to treating it. Chemoprophylaxis is common for close contacts or family members of recently infected tuberculosis patients. Therapy usually begins immediately after a patient receives a positive tuberculin test. Patients with immunosuppression, such as those with AIDS or those receiving immunosuppressant drugs, may receive preventative treatment with antituberculosis drugs. A short-term therapy of 2 months, consisting of a combination treatment with isoniazid (INH) and pyrazinamide, is approved for tuberculosis prophylaxis in HIV-positive patients.

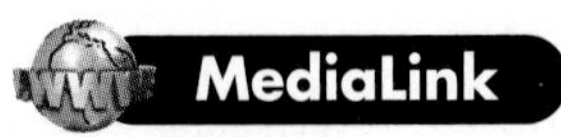

THE REEMERGENCE OF TUBERCULOSIS

Concept Review 22.3

- How does drug therapy of tuberculosis differ from that of conventional anti-infective chemotherapy? What are the rationales for these differences?

CHAPTER REVIEW

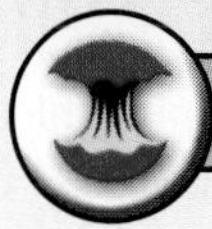

CORE CONCEPTS SUMMARY

22.1 **Pathogens are organisms that cause disease because of their ability to divide rapidly or secrete toxins.**

Pathogens can overwhelm natural immune defenses by growing extremely rapidly and invading normal tissues or by producing potent toxins. Bacteria are organized on the basis of their staining ability and structural and functional characteristics.

22.2 **Anti-infective drugs are classified by their chemical structures or by their mechanisms of action.**

Because of the large number of anti-infectives available, it is advantageous for the student to understand how to classify these drugs because medications in the same class exhibit similar pharmacological activity. Anti-infective drugs are classified based on similarities in their chemical structures or by their mechanisms of action.

22.3 **Anti-infective drugs act by affecting the target organism's metabolism or life cycle.**

Bacteria multiply rapidly, and drugs have been designed to take advantage of this characteristic. Anti-infectives may be bacteriocidal, bacteriostatic, or both, depending on the organism and dose.

22.4 **Acquired resistance causes loss of antibiotic effectiveness and is worsened by the overprescribing of these agents.**

Errors during replication result in random mutations of the bacterial DNA. Although rare, an occasional mutation may confer antibiotic resistance to a bacterium. Therapy with antibiotics kills the affected bacteria, leaving the resistant ones to multiply and infect the patient. To limit this problem, antibiotics should only be prescribed when medically necessary.

22.5 **Careful selection of the correct antibiotic is essential for effective pharmacotherapy and to limit adverse effects.**

Culture and sensitivity tests are used to identify the type of bacteria present and determine which antibiotics are most effective. Until test results are obtained, the patient may be started on a broad-spectrum antibiotic. Because broad-spectrum drugs are more likely to affect the patient's normal flora, a narrow-spectrum drug may be prescribed after the organism is identified.

22.6 **The penicillins are one of the oldest and safest groups of anti-infectives.**

Penicillins have been widely used because of their high margin of safety and effectiveness. Some patients are allergic to this class of drugs, and many bacterial species have become resistant to penicillins, thus limiting their use.

22.7 **The cephalosporins are similar in structure and function to the penicillins and are one of the most widely prescribed anti-infective classes.**

The cephalosporins consist of a large class of antibiotics, classified by generation, that are considered alternatives to penicillin. In general, they are used for serious gram-negative infections and for patients who are resistant to or cannot tolerate the penicillins.

22.8 The tetracyclines have some of the broadest spectrums, but they are drugs of choice for few diseases.

The tetracyclines have a broader spectrum of action and produce more side effects than the penicillins. Their use is limited to a small number of diseases such as Rocky Mountain spotted fever, typhus, cholera, Lyme disease, and Chlamydial infections.

22.9 The macrolides are safe alternatives to penicillin for many infections.

The macrolides are generally prescribed when a patient is allergic to penicillin or has a penicillin-resistant infection. They produce few side effects.

22.10 The aminoglycosides are narrow-spectrum drugs that have the potential to cause serious toxicity.

The aminoglycosides are usually reserved for severe gram-negative infections of the urinary tract, because they have the potential to cause serious side effects. Most of them are poorly absorbed from the GI tract and must be given parenterally.

22.11 Fluoroquinolones have wide clinical applications because of their broad spectrum of activity and relative safety.

Although fluoroquinolones are an older class of antibacterials, newer drugs in this class have been developed to greatly expand their use. They are effective oral alternatives to other antibiotics for both gram-negative and gram-positive organisms. Ciprofloxacin (Cipro) is one of the few agents approved for the treatment of anthrax.

22.12 Widespread resistance has limited the clinical use of sulfonamides primarily to urinary tract infections.

In the 1930s, the sulfonamides revolutionized the treatment of infectious disease. Present-day use of these agents is limited by bacterial resistance. The fixed combination of trimethoprim-sulfamethoxazole (Bactrim, Septra) is an important drug in the pharmacotherapy of UTIs.

22.13 A number of additional anti-infectives have distinct mechanisms of action and specific indications.

A number of important antibiotics do not belong to any of the previous classes. The streptogramins and oxazolidinones are small groups of drugs having specific applications. Vancomycin is known as the "last chance" antibiotic to be used when resistance has developed to most other anti-infectives.

22.14 Pharmacotherapy of tuberculosis requires unique drugs because of the slow-growing, complex microbes.

Drug therapy of tuberculosis involves taking multiple drugs for prolonged periods. Patients exhibiting a new, positive TB test are often given these drugs prophylactically, even if no signs of the disease are apparent.

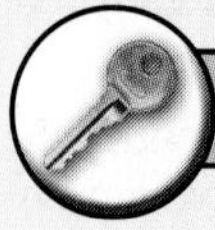

KEY TERMS

acquired resistance: when a microbe is no longer affected by a drug following treatment with anti-infectives / *page 398*

antagonism: type of drug interaction in which one drug inhibits the effectiveness of another / *page 400*

antibiotic (ann-tie-bye-OT-ik): substance produced by a microorganism that inhibits or kills other microorganisms / *page 397*

anti-infective (ann-tie-in-FEK-tive): general term for any medication effective against pathogens / *page 397*

bacteriocidal (bak-teer-ee-oh-SY-dall): substance that has ability to kill bacteria / *page 397*

bacteriostatic (bak-teer-ee-oh-STAT-ik): substance that can inhibit the growth of bacteria / *page 397*

beta-lactam ring (bay-tuh LAK-tam): chemical structure found in most penicillins and some cephalosporins / *page 400*

beta-lactamase/penicillinase (bay-tuh-LAK-tam-ace/pen-uh-SILL-in-ace): enzyme present in certain bacteria that is able to inactivate many penicillins and some cephalosporins / *page 400*

broad-spectrum antibiotic: anti-infective that is effective against many different gram-positive and gram-negative organisms / *page 399*

chemoprophylaxis (kee-moh-pro-fill-AX-is): use of a drug to prevent an infection / *page 398*

culture and sensitivity test: laboratory test used to identify bacteria and to determine which antibiotic is most effective / *page 399*

host flora (host FLOR-uh): normal microorganisms found in or on a patient / *page 400*

mutations (myou-TAY-shuns): permanent, inheritable changes to DNA / *page 397*

narrow-spectrum antibiotic: anti-infective that is effective against only one or a small number of organisms / *page 399*

nephrotoxicity (NEF-row-toks-ISS-ih-tee): an adverse effect on the kidneys / *page 407*

nosocomial infections (noh-soh-KOH-mee-ul): infections acquired in a healthcare setting such as a hospital, physician's office, or nursing home / *page 398*

ototoxicity (OH-toh-toks-ISS-ih-tee): an adverse effect on hearing / *page 407*

pathogen (PATH-oh-jen): organism that is capable of causing disease / *page 395*

pathogenicity (path-oh-jen-ISS-ih-tee): ability of an organism to cause disease in humans / ***page 395***

photosensitivity: condition that occurs when the skin is very sensitive to sunlight / ***page 404***

plasmid (PLAZ-mid): small piece of circular DNA found in some bacteria that is able to transfer resistance from one bacterium to another / ***page 398***

red-man syndrome: rash on the upper body caused by certain anti-infectives / ***page 410***

superinfection: condition caused when a microorganism grows rapidly as a result of having less competition in its environment / ***page 400***

toxin (TOX-in): chemical produced by a microorganism that is able to cause injury to its host / ***page 396***

tubercles (TOO-burr-kyouls): cavity-like lesions in the lung characteristic of infection by *Mycobacterium tuberculosis* / ***page 413***

virulence (VEER-you-lens): the severity of disease that an organism in able to cause / ***page 396***

REVIEW QUESTIONS

The following questions are written in NCLEX-PN® style. Answer these questions to assess your knowledge of the chapter material, and go back and review any material that is not clear to you.

1. The patient is taking amoxicillin (Amoxil). Which of the following statements by the patient demonstrates that he or she needs additional instruction?

1. "I will take this medication until it is gone."
2. "I will call my doctor if I develop a fever or a rash."
3. "Before I take my medication, I will avoid orange juice."
4. "I will take the medication until I feel better."

2. Children younger than 9 years should not be given tetracyclines because:

1. Photosensitivity may occur
2. Children's teeth may become discolored
3. Superinfections may occur
4. Children become dehydrated easily

3. The patient on tetracyclines should be instructed:

1. To take it with food or milk
2. That it is safe for pregnancy
3. To take it 1–2 hours before or after meals
4. That it has no adverse side effects

4. The patient on aminoglycosides should be monitored for:

1. Nephrotoxicity
2. Hepatic failure
3. Superinfection
4. Hypertension and rash

5. If ciprofloxin (Cipro) is administered with antacids, absorption is:

1. Increased
2. Decreased
3. Not affected
4. Delayed

6. The patient has a urinary tract infection. The nurse anticipates which of the following medications being ordered?

1. Sulfacetamide (Cetamide)
2. Sulfadiazine (Microsulfon)
3. Trimethoprim-sulfamethoxazole (Septra)
4. Vancomycin (Vancocin)

7. The patient with tuberculosis is now on isoniazid (INH). Which laboratory test should be monitored at least monthly?

1. PT and PTT
2. CBC
3. BUN
4. Liver enzymes

8. The patient asks why he must take two medications for his tuberculosis. The nurse's best response would be?

1. "You have TB throughout your body. It will take additional medications to cure you."
2. "You will need to speak with your physician."
3. "Taking multiple drugs increases the chances that therapy will be successful."
4. "With multiple drugs, we can decrease the time you need to take the medications."

9. Prophylactic treatment of TB in the HIV patient would include which of these drugs?

1. Streptomycin and isoniazid (INH)
2. Pyrazinamide and rifampin
3. Rifampin and streptomycin
4. Isoniazide (INH) and pyrazinamide

10. Patients on antibiotics should be instructed to:

1. Take the medication with food
2. Increase fluid intake to 2–3 L per day
3. Take all medication on an empty stomach
4. Take medication until symptoms subside

CASE STUDY QUESTIONS

For questions 1–5, please refer to the following case study, and choose the correct answer from choices 1–4.

Mr. Wu is a new patient at your clinic. Six months ago, he had a kidney transplant and is taking immunosuppressant drugs. Recently, he has been experiencing repeated bacterial infections due to resistant strains, and has been switched to different antibiotics throughout the last 6 months. The physician suspects a kidney infection.

1. Many factors promote the emergence of resistant bacterial strains. Which of the following is one of these factors?

1. Taking the medication for the full length of the prescription
2. Taking 2 or more antibiotics at the same time
3. Taking antibiotics that are not indicated for the infecting pathogen
4. Taking the drug with food that interferes with its absorption

2. Mr. Wu is admitted to the hospital and is administered gentamicin 300 mg daily by IV infusion. Which of the following tests should you monitor?

1. Input and output ratio
2. Serum transaminase levels
3. Visual acuity tests
4. Fasting blood glucose levels

3. Mr. Wu is showing signs of hearing loss due to gentamicin therapy and he is switched to ciprofloxacin (Cipro) 200 mg q12h. Which common side effect of ciprofloxacin therapy should you monitor?

1. Hearing loss
2. Diminished liver function
3. Nausea and vomiting
4. Nephrotoxicity

4. Mr. Wu is discharged from the hospital with a prescription for 4 g daily PO sulfamethoxazole. The primary use of this sulfonamide is for the pharmacotherapy of:

1. UTI
2. Resistant staph infections (MRSA)
3. Respiratory infections
4. Gonorrhea and other sexually transmitted bacterial infections

5. A year later, Mr. Wu returns for a follow-up and you note in the chart that he has been taking rifampin (Rifidin) and ethambutol (Myambutol) for the last 3 months. You can conclude that Mr. Wu:

1. is being treated for tuberculosis
2. has a severe respiratory infection
3. is being treated for a resistant staph infection (MRSA)
4. needs to have his medications reevaluated by the physician

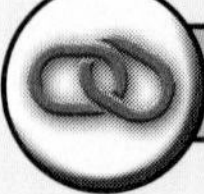

FURTHER STUDY

- Body defenses that pathogens must bypass to infect humans are discussed in detail in Chapter 21.
- Chapter 32 discusses some of the anti-infective agents for skin disorders.
- Chapter 23 discusses antiinfective drugs used to treat viral, fungal, and parasitic infections.

EXPLORE MEDIALINK www.prenhall.com/holland

Additional resources for this chapter can be found on the CD-ROM accompanying this textbook, and on the Companion Website. Click on Chapter 22 to select activities for this chapter.

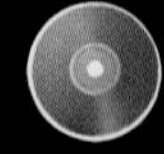

- Mechanism in Action: Penicillin G
- Audio Glossary
- Concept Review
- NCLEX -PN® Review
- Nursing in Action
- Dosage Calculator

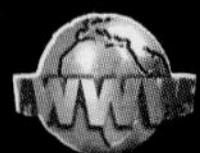

- Veterinary Antibiotics and Human Health
- Emerging Infectious Diseases
- The Reemergence of Tuberculosis

CHAPTER

23 Drugs for Fungal, Viral, and Parasitic Diseases

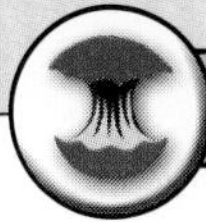

CORE CONCEPTS

23.1 Because fungi are more complex than bacteria, fungal infections require a different approach to pharmacotherapy.

23.2 Systemic antifungal drugs are used for serious infections of internal organs.

23.3 Superficial infections of the skin, nails, and mucous membranes are effectively treated with topical and oral antifungal drugs.

23.4 Viruses are nonliving parasites that require a host to replicate.

23.5 Antiretroviral drugs for HIV-AIDS do not cure the disease, but they do help many patients live longer.

23.6 A small number of antiviral drugs are available to treat herpes simplex and influenza infections.

23.7 Although not common in the United States, infections caused by helminths and protozoans cause significant disease worldwide.

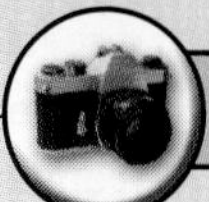

DRUG SNAPSHOT

The following drugs will be discussed in this chapter:

DRUG CLASSES	DRUG PROFILES
Antifungal drugs for systemic infections	Pr amphotericin B (Fungizone)
Antifungal drugs for superficial infections	Pr nystatin (Mycostatin)
Antiretroviral drugs for HIV-AIDS	Pr zidovudine (Retrovir, AZT)
Antiviral drugs for herpes simplex and influenza	Pr acyclovir (Zovirax)
Antiprotozoals and antihelmintics	Pr metronidazole (Flagyl)

MediaLink
www.prenhall.com/holland

Interactive resources for this chapter can be found on the Companion Website. Click on Chapter 23 and "Begin" to select the activities for this chapter. For chapter-related animations, NCLEX-PN®-style questions, and an audio glossary, access the accompanying CD-ROM in this book.

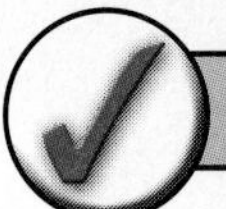

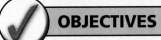

OBJECTIVES

After reading this chapter, the student should be able to:

1. Compare and contrast the pharmacotherapy of superficial and systemic fungal infections.
2. Identify the types of patients most likely to acquire serious fungal infections.
3. Describe the basic structure of a virus.
4. Identify viral diseases that may benefit from pharmacotherapy.
5. Explain the purpose and expected outcomes of HIV pharmacotherapy.
6. Define HAART, and explain why it is commonly used in the pharmacotherapy of HIV infection.
7. Identify protozoal and helminth infections that may benefit from pharmacotherapy.
8. For each of the following classes, identify representative drugs, explain the mechanisms of drug action, primary actions, and important adverse effects.
   - **a.** Systemic antifungal agents
   - **b.** Superficial antifungal agents
   - **c.** Antiretroviral and antiviral agents
   - **d.** Antiprotozoal agents
   - **e.** Antihelmintic agents
9. Categorize drugs used in the treatment of fungal, viral, protozoal, and helminth infections based on their classifications and mechanisms of action.

Fungi, protozoans, and multicellular parasites are exceedingly more complex than bacteria. Most antibacterial drugs are ineffective against these organisms because their structure and biochemistry are so different from that of bacteria. Although there are fewer medications to treat these diseases, the available medications are usually effective.

Viruses, on the other hand, are not living organisms. A virus infects by entering a host cell and using the host's internal machinery to replicate, or reproduce, itself. Antiviral drugs are the least effective of all the anti-infective classes. Although the number of antiviral medications has increased dramatically in recent years, they are relatively ineffective at preventing or treating viral infections.

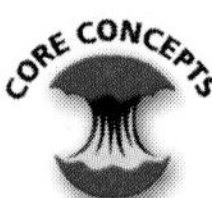

23.1 Because fungi are more complex than bacteria, fungal infections require a different approach to pharmacotherapy.

Fungi are single-celled or multicellular organisms that are much more complex than bacteria. Several species of fungi grow on skin and mucosal surfaces and are part of the normal host flora.

Fast Facts Fungal, Viral, and Parasitic Diseases

- About 45 million Americans are infected with genital herpes—1 of every 5 of the total adolescent and adult population.
- Genital herpes is more common in women than in men, and in Blacks than in other ethnic groups.
- More than 400,000 Americans are currently living with HIV infections; about 42,000 new infections occur each year.
- Approximately 70% of new HIV infections occur in men, with the largest risk category being men who have sex with other men.
- Of the new HIV infections in women, 75% are acquired through heterosexual contact.
- Since the beginning of the AIDS epidemic, more than 520,000 Americans have died of AIDS.
- Between 300 and 500 million cases of malaria occur worldwide each year, with an estimated 2.7 million deaths resulting from the disease.
- Of the more than 200,000 known species of fungi, fewer than 200 infect humans. About 90% of these infections are caused by just a few dozen species.

TABLE 23.1 Fungal Pathogens

NAME OF FUNGUS	DISEASE AND PRIMARY ORGAN SYSTEM
SYSTEMIC	
Aspergillus fumigatus and others	Aspergillosis: opportunistic; most commonly affects lung, but can spread to other organs
Blastomyces dermatitidis	Blastomycosis: begins in the lungs and spreads to other organs
Candida albicans and others	Candidiasis: most common opportunistic fungal infection; may occur in mucous membranes and nearly any organ
Coccidioides immitis	Coccidioidomycosis: begins in the lungs and spreads to the skin and other organs
Cryptococcus neoformans	Cryptococcosis: opportunistic; begins in lungs, but is the most common cause of meningitis in AIDS patients
Histoplasma capsulatum	Histoplasmosis: begins in the lungs and spreads to other organs
Mucorales (various species)	Mucormycosis: opportunistic; affects blood vessels; causes sinus infections, stomach ulcers, and others
Pneumocystis carinii	Pneumocystis pneumonia: opportunistic; primarily causes pneumonia of the lung, but can spread to other organs
SUPERFICIAL	
Candida albicans and others	Candidiasis: affects skin, nails, oral cavity (thrush), vagina
Epidermophyton floccosum	Athlete's foot (tinea pedis), jock itch (tinea cruris), and other skin disorders
Microsporum audouini and others	Ringworm of scalp (tinea capitus)
Sporothrix schenckii	Sporotrichosis: affects primarily skin and superficial lymph nodes
Trichophyton (various species)	Affects scalp, skin, and nails

The human body is remarkably resistant to infection by these organisms; patients with healthy immune systems experience few serious fungal diseases. Those with a suppressed immune system, however, such as patients infected with HIV, may acquire frequent fungal infections, some of which may require intensive drug therapy.

Fungal diseases are called **mycoses. Yeasts,** which include the common pathogen *Candida albicans,* are types of fungi. Molds are also classified as fungi. Table 23.1 lists the most common fungal pathogens.

myc = *fungus*
oses = *conditions*

A simple and useful method of classifying fungal infections is to consider them as either superficial or systemic. **Superficial mycoses** typically affect the scalp, skin, nails, and mucous membranes such as the oral cavity and vagina. Mycoses of this type are often treated with topical agents because the incidence of side effects is much lower by using this route of administration. Superficial fungal infections are sometimes called **dermatophytic.**

derma = *skin*
phyto = *something that grows*

Systemic mycoses are those affecting internal organs such as the lungs, brain, and digestive organs. Less common than superficial mycoses, systemic fungal infections may be serious and affect multiple body systems. In fact, systemic mycoses are sometimes fatal to patients with suppressed immune systems. Mycoses of this type often require aggressive oral or parenteral medications that produce more side effects than do the topical agents.

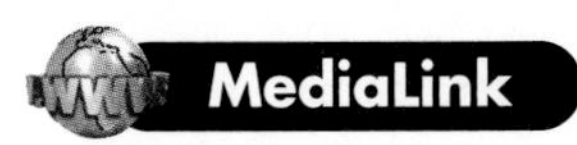

FUNGI IN THE WORLD

23.2 Systemic antifungal drugs are used for serious infections of internal organs.

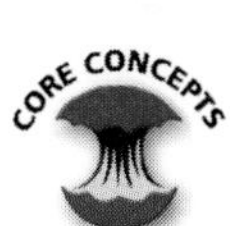

Systemic or invasive fungal disease may require intensive pharmacotherapy for extended periods. Amphotericin B and fluconazole are drugs of choice. Table 23.2 lists the primary antifungal drugs.

A number of drugs have become available for systemic fungal infections in the past 15 years, largely because of the development of medications for opportunistic fungal disease in

TABLE 23.2 Selected Antifungal Drugs

DRUG	ROUTE AND ADULT DOSE	REMARKS
Pr amphotericin B (Fungizone, others)	IV 0.25 mg/kg daily; may increase to 1 mg/kg daily or 1.5 mg/kg every other day (max: 1.5 mg/kg/day)	Cream, lotion, and PO suspension forms available for topical mycoses; must infuse a test dose first; has potential for severe adverse effects
butenafine (Mentax)	Topical apply daily × 4 weeks	For athlete's foot
butoconazole (Femstat)	Topical 1 applicator intravaginally at bedtime × 3 days	For vaginal mycoses
ciclopirox olamine (Loprox)	Topical apply bid × 4 weeks	For skin mycoses
clotrimazole (Gyne-Lotrimin, Mycelex, Femizole)	Topical for skin mycoses apply bid × 4 weeks; for vaginal mycoses, insert 1 applicatorful intravaginally at bedtime for 7 days	For vaginal and skin mycoses, athlete's foot, and candidiasis; vaginal tablet form also available
econazole (Spectazole)	Topical apply bid × 4 weeks	For skin mycoses
fluconazole (Diflucan)	PO 200–400 mg on day 1, then 100–200 mg daily × 2–4 weeks	For both systemic and superficial mycoses; 1% cream available for topical infections; IV form available
flucytosine (5-fluorocytosine, Ancobon)	PO 50–150 mg/kg in divided doses	For severe systemic infections such as candidiasis or cryptococcosis; IV form available
griseofulvin (Fulvicin)	PO 500 mg microsize or 330–375 mg ultramicrosize daily	For ringworm and other skin and nail infections
haloprogin (Halotex)	Topical apply bid × 2–3 weeks	For skin mycoses
itraconazole (Sporanox)	PO 200 mg daily; may increase to 200 mg bid (max: 400 mg/day)	For severe systemic lung mycoses and superficial nail mycoses
ketoconazole (Nizoral)	PO 200–400 mg daily	For severe systemic mycoses; topical form available for superficial mycoses
miconazole (Micatin, Monistat)	Topical apply bid × 2–4 weeks	For vaginal and skin mycoses; also available as vaginal suppositories and tampons
naftifine (Naftin)	Topical apply cream daily or gel bid × 4 weeks	For skin mycoses
Pr nystatin (Mycostatin, Nilstat, Nystex)	PO 500,000–1,000,000 units tid	For candidiasis; vaginal tablet form available
oxiconazole (Oxistat)	Topical apply daily in the evening × 2 months	For skin mycoses
sertaconazole (Ertaczo)	Topical 2% cream bid × 4 weeks	For tinea pedis
terbinafine (Lamisil)	Topical apply daily or bid × 7 weeks; PO 250 mg daily × 6–13 weeks	For skin and nail mycoses
terconazole (Terazol)	Topical insert one applicator intravaginally at bedtime × 3–7 days	For vulvovaginal candidiasis; vaginal suppository form available
tioconazole (Vagistat)	Topical insert one applicator intravaginally at bedtime × 1 day	For vulvovaginal candidiasis
tolnaftate (Aftate, Tinactin)	Topical apply bid × 4–6 weeks	For skin mycoses, ringworm, athlete's foot
undecylenic acid (Cruex, Desenex)	Topical apply once or twice daily	For athlete's foot, diaper rash
voriconazole (Vfend)	IV 6 mg/kg q l2h day 1, then 3–4 mg/kg q l2h	For systemic aspergillosis; oral form available

AIDS patients. Others who may experience systemic infections include patients receiving prolonged therapy with corticosteroids (Chapters 21 and 29), those with extensive burns, those receiving anticancer drugs (Chapter 24), and those who have recently received organ transplants (Chapter 21). Systemic antifungal medications have little or no antibacterial activity, and pharmacotherapy often lasts for several weeks or even months.

Amphotericin B (Fungizone) has been the drug of choice for systemic fungal infections for many years. However, the newer *azole* drugs such as fluconazole (Diflucan), itraconazole, (Sporanox), and ketoconazole (Nizoral) have come into widespread use. Ketoconazole has become a drug of choice for less severe systemic mycoses or for the prophylaxis of fungal infections. The *azole* drugs have a spectrum of activity similar to that of amphotericin B, are considerably less toxic, and have the major advantage that they can be administered orally. Several are available for both superficial and systemic mycoses.

Concept Review 23.1

- Why have the number of antifungal and antiviral drugs increased significantly over the past 15 years?

DRUG PROFILE: Systemic Antifungal: Pr *Amphotericin B (Fungizone)*

Actions and Uses:

Amphotericin B has a wide spectrum of activity that includes most of the fungi pathogenic to humans; thus, it is a drug of choice for severe systemic mycoses. It acts by binding to fungal cell membranes and causing them to become permeable or leaky. Because it is not absorbed from the GI tract, it is given by IV infusion. Treatment may continue for several months. Unlike antibiotics, resistance to amphotericin B is not common.

Adverse Effects and Interactions:

Amphotericin B can cause a number of serious side effects. Many patients develop fever and chills at the beginning of therapy, which subside as treatment continues. Phlebitis, or inflammation of the veins, is common during IV therapy. Some degree of nephrotoxicity is observed in most patients, and laboratory tests of kidney function are normally performed throughout the treatment period.

Amphotericin B interacts with many drugs. For example, therapy with aminoglycosides, vancomycin, carboplatin, and furosemide, which reduce renal function, is not recommended. Use with corticosteroids, skeletal muscle relaxants, and thiazole may cause hypokalemia. If hypokalemia is present, use with digoxin (Lanoxin) increases the risk of digoxin toxicity.

See the Companion Website for a Nursing Process Focus specific to this drug.

DRUG PROFILE: Topical Antifungal: Pr *Nystatin (Mycostatin, Nilstat, Nystex)*

Actions and Uses:

Although it belongs to the same chemical class as amphotericin B, nystatin is available in a wider variety of formulations, including cream, ointment, powder, tablets, and lozenges. It is used as a topical agent against *Candida* infections of the vagina, skin, and mouth. It may also be used orally to treat candidiasis of the intestine because it travels through the GI tract without being absorbed.

Adverse Effects and Interactions:

When given topically, nystatin produces few adverse effects other than minor skin irritation. When given orally, it may cause diarrhea, nausea, and vomiting.

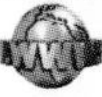

See the Companion Website for a Nursing Process Focus specific to this drug.

NURSING PROCESS FOCUS

Patients Receiving Superficial Antifungal Therapy

ASSESSMENT	POTENTIAL NURSING DIAGNOSES
Prior to administration: ■ Obtain complete health history including allergies, drug history, and possible drug interactions ■ Obtain a culture and sensitivity of suspected area of infection to determine need for therapy ■ Obtain baseline liver function tests	■ Risk for Injury (rash), related to side effect of drug ■ Deficient Knowledge, related to drug therapy ■ Risk for Impaired Skin Integrity

PLANNING: Patient Goals and Expected Outcomes

The patient will:

- Report healing of fungal infection
- Demonstrate an understanding of the drug's action by accurately describing drug side effects and precautions
- Immediately report effects such as hepatoxicity, GI distress, rash, or decreased urine output

IMPLEMENTATION

Interventions and (Rationales)	Patient Education/Discharge Planning
■ Monitor for possible side effects or hypersensitivity.	Instruct patient to report: ■ Burning, stinging, dryness, itching, erythema, urticaria, angioedema, and local irritation for superficial drugs ■ Symptoms of hepatic toxicity—jaundice, dark urine, light-colored stools, and pruritis ■ Nausea, vomiting, and diarrhea ■ Signs and symptoms of hypo- or hyperglycemia
■ Encourage compliance with instructions when taking oral antifungals (to increase medication effectiveness).	Instruct patient to: ■ Swish the oral suspension to coat all mucous membranes, then swallow medication ■ Spit out medication instead of swallowing if GI irritation occurs ■ Allow troche to dissolve completely, rather than chewing or swallowing; it may take 30 min for it to completely dissolve ■ Avoid food or drink for 30 min following administration ■ Remove dentures prior to using the oral suspension ■ Take ketoconazole with water, fruit juice, coffee, or tea to enhance dissolution and absorption
■ Monitor topical application. ■ Avoid occlusive dressings. (Dressings increase moisture in the infected areas and encourage development of additional yeast infections.)	■ Instruct patient to avoid wearing tight-fitting undergarments if using ointment in the vaginal or groin area.
■ Monitor for contact dermatitis with topical formulations. (This is related to the preservatives found in many of the formulations.)	■ Instruct patient to report any redness or skin rash.
■ Encourage infection control practices. Ensure that patient, family members, and other visitors also practice infection control techniques such as handwashing and avoiding affected area (to prevent the spread of infection).	Instruct patient to: ■ Clean affected area daily ■ Apply medication with a glove ■ Wash hands properly before and after application ■ Change socks daily if rash is on feet ■ Avoid sharing personal care items with family members/guests

EVALUATION OF OUTCOME CRITERIA

Evaluate the effectiveness of drug therapy by confirming that patient goals and expected outcomes have been met (see "Planning").

See Table 23.2 for a list of drugs to which these nursing actions apply.

23.3 Superficial infections of the skin, nails, and mucous membranes are effectively treated with topical and oral antifungal drugs.

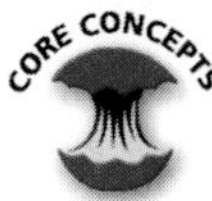

Superficial fungal infections of the hair, scalp, nails, and the mucous membranes of the mouth and vagina are rarely medical emergencies. Infections of the nails and skin, for example, may be ongoing for months or even years before a patient seeks treatment. Unlike systemic fungal infections, superficial infections may occur in any patient, not just those who have suppressed immune systems.

Topical antifungal medications are much safer than their systemic counterparts because only very small amounts are absorbed into the circulation. Many are available as OTC creams, gels, solutions, and ointments. Although a fungal infection may be diagnosed as superficial, oral antifungal drugs are occasionally prescribed along with the topical agents to be certain that the infection is completely eliminated from the deeper skin layers. The length of pharmacotherapy varies widely among the different types of superficial mycoses. Vaginal infections are sometimes treated successfully with a single vaginal tablet of clotrimazole, whereas nail mycoses may require several months of therapy with itraconazole or terbinafine.

Side effects from topical antifungal therapy are generally minor. If applied to the skin, irritation, redness, and itching may be experienced. Vaginal administration may result in burning, itching, or irritation. Antifungal drugs should not be applied to open sores or severely abraded skin because this may result in undesirable absorption of the drug and additional side effects.

23.4 Viruses are nonliving parasites that require a host to replicate.

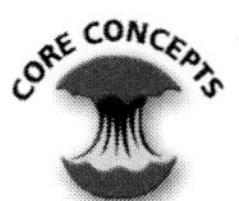

Viruses are nonliving particles that infect bacteria, plants, and animals. Viruses contain none of the cellular organelles necessary for self-survival that are present in living organisms. In fact, the structure of viruses is primitive compared to even the simplest living cell. Surrounded by a protein coat or **capsid,** a virus contains only a few dozen genes—either in the form of ribonucleic acid (RNA) or deoxyribonucleic acid (DNA)—that contain the necessary information needed for viral replication. Figure 23.1 ■ shows the basic structure of the human immunodeficiency virus (HIV).

FIGURE 23.1

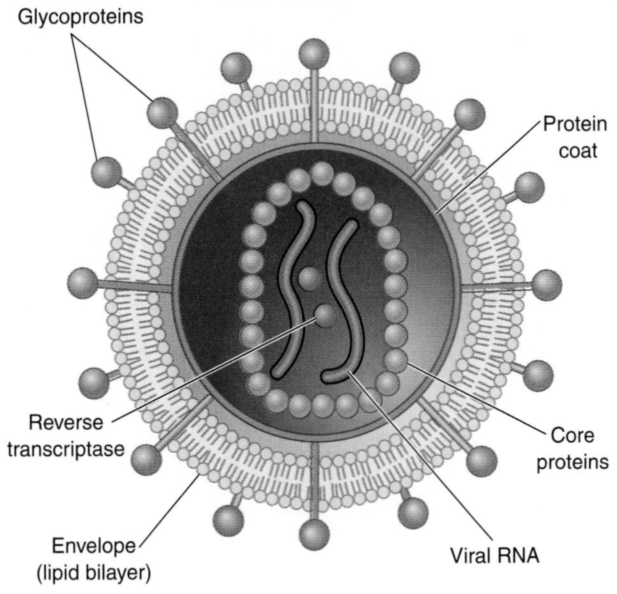

Glycoproteins
Protein coat
Reverse transcriptase
Core proteins
Envelope (lipid bilayer)
Viral RNA

Structure of the human immunodeficiency virus (HIV)

intra = *within*
cellular = *cell*

Although nonliving and structurally simple, viruses are capable of remarkable feats. They infect an organism, called the **host,** by entering a target cell and using the enzymes inside that cell to replicate. Thus viruses are called **intracellular parasites,** meaning that they must be inside a host cell to cause infection. The viral host is often very specific: It may be a single species of plant, bacteria, or animal, or even a single type of cell within that species. Most often, viruses that affect one species do not affect others, although cases have been documented where viruses can mutate and cross species, as is likely the case for HIV.

Many viral infections, such as the rhinoviruses that cause the common cold, are self-limiting and require no medical treatment. Although symptoms may be annoying, the virus disappears in 7 to 10 days and causes no permanent damage, if the patient is otherwise healthy. Other viruses, such as HIV, can cause serious and ultimately fatal disease and require aggressive drug therapy. Antiviral therapy is extremely challenging because of the rapid mutation rate of viruses, which can quickly render drugs ineffective. Also complicating therapy is the intracellular nature of the virus, which makes it difficult for medications to find their targets without giving excessively high doses that injure normal cells. Each of the antiviral drugs is specific to one particular virus. The antiviral medications are shown in Tables 23.3 and 23.4.

TABLE 23.3 Antiretroviral Drugs for HIV-AIDS

DRUG	ROUTE AND ADULT DOSE	REMARKS
NON-NUCLEOSIDE REVERSE TRANSCRIPTASE INHIBITORS (NNRTI)		
delavirdine (Rescriptor)	PO 400 mg tid	Used in combination with other antivirals
efavirenz (Sustiva)	PO 600 mg daily	Used in combination with other antivirals; a once-daily form is available
nevirapine (Viramune)	PO 200 mg daily × 14 days, then increase to bid	Used in combination with other antivirals
NUCLEOSIDE REVERSE TRANSCRIPTASE INHIBITORS (NRTI)		
abacavir (Ziagen)	PO 300 mg bid	
didanosine (Videx)	PO 125–300 mg bid	For use in patients who are intolerant to AZT
emtricitabine (Emtriva)	PO 200 mg daily	For use in combination with other antiretrovirals
lamivudine (Epivir, 3TC)	PO 150 mg bid	Usually given in combination with AZT
stavudine (Zerit, D4T)	PO 40 mg bid	For advanced HIV disease
zalcitabine (Hivid, ddC)	PO 0.75 mg tid	Given in combination with AZT
Pr zidovudine (Retrovir, AZT)	PO 200 mg q4h × 1 month then 100 mg q4h	For symptomatic or asymptomatic HIV; unlabeled use: postexposure chemoprophylaxis; IV form available
PROTEASE INHIBITORS		
amprenavir (Agenerase)	PO 1200 mg bid	The prodrug form is called fosamrenavir (Lexiva)
atazanavir (Reyataz)	PO 400 mg/day	Give with a light meal
idinavir (Crixivan)	PO 800 mg tid	Give 1 hour before or 2 hours after a meal
nelfinavir (Viracept)	PO 750 mg tid	Give with food
ritonavir (Norvir)	PO 600 mg bid	Give 1 hour before or 2 hours after a meal
saquinavir (Invirase, Fortovase)	PO 600 mg tid	
MISCELLANEOUS DRUGS		
enfuvirtide (Fuzeon)	Subcutaneous 90 mg bid	Fusion inhibitor
tenofovir (Viread)	PO 300 mg daily	Nucleotide reverse transcriptase inhibitor

23.5 Antiretroviral drugs for HIV-AIDS do not cure the disease, but they do help many patients live longer.

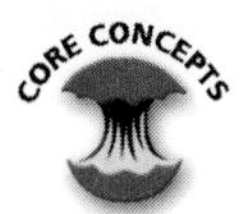

Drugs for viral infections are classified into those used to treat HIV-AIDS, and those used for other viral disorders such as herpes and influenza. Antiviral medications for HIV-AIDS have been developed that slow the growth of HIV by several different mechanisms.

The widespread appearance of HIV infection in 1981 created enormous challenges for public health and for the development of new antiviral drugs. HIV-AIDS is unlike any other infectious disease because it is uniformly fatal and demands a continuous supply of new drugs for patient survival. The challenges of HIV-AIDS have been met by the development of more than eight new antiviral drugs. Many others are in various states of clinical trials. Unfortunately, the initial hope of curing HIV-AIDS through antiviral therapy or vaccines has not been realized; none of these medications produces a cure for this disease. HIV mutates extremely rapidly and resistant strains develop so quickly that the creation of new, novel approaches to antiviral drug therapy is an ongoing process.

After initial exposure, HIV may remain dormant for several months to many years. During this *latent phase,* patients are asymptomatic and may not even realize they are infected. Once diagnosis is established, however, a decision must be made as to when to begin pharmacotherapy. The advantage of beginning during the latent stage is that early treatment may delay the onset of acute symptoms and the development of AIDS.

DRUG PROFILE: Antiretroviral: Pr *Zidovudine (Retrovir, AZT)*

Actions and Uses:

Zidovudine was first discovered in the 1960s, and its antiviral activity was demonstrated prior to the AIDS epidemic. As the HIV reverse transcriptase enzyme begins to synthesize viral DNA, it mistakenly uses zidovudine as one of the building blocks, thus creating a defective DNA strand. Because of its widespread use over the past 25 years, resistant HIV strains are common. It is usually used in combination with other antiretrovirals because this slows the development of resistance and allows HIV to be attacked by several different mechanisms.

Adverse Effects and Interactions:

Zidovudine can result in severe toxicity to blood cells at high doses. Reduced numbers of red blood cells (anemia) and white blood cells (leukopenia) are common and may limit therapy. Many patients report GI symptoms such as anorexia, nausea, and diarrhea. Patients may experience fatigue and report generalized weakness.

Zidovudine interacts with many drugs. Acetaminophen and ganciclovir may worsen bone marrow suppression. The following drugs may increase the risk of AZT toxicity: atovaquone, amphotericin B, aspirin, doxorubicin, fluconazole, methadone, and valproic acid. Other antiretroviral agents may cause lactic acidosis and severe hepatomegaly with steatosis.

Use with caution with herbal supplements, such as St. John's wort, which may cause a decrease in antiretroviral activity.

Mechanism in Action: 

Zidovudine resembles the chemical structure of thymidine, one of the building blocks of DNA. With the help of reverse transcriptase, the drug becomes incorporated into the infective strand of viral DNA. Once incorporated, zidovudine slows synthesis of HIV, thereby reducing symptoms associated with this disease. ■

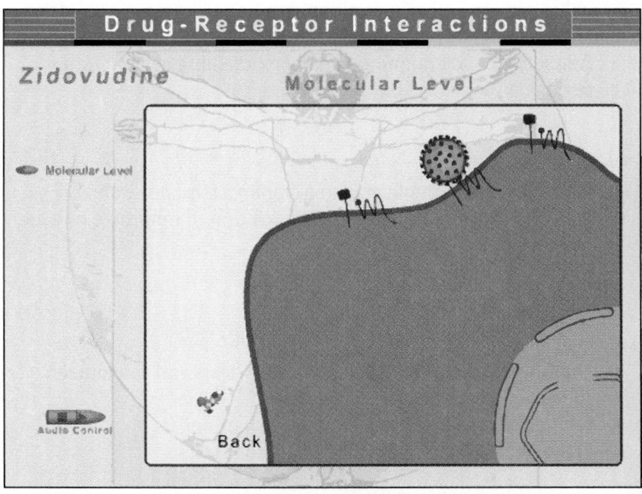

Use the student CD-ROM to see Mechanism in Action for Zidovudine.

See the Companion Website for a Nursing Process Focus specific to this drug.

NURSING PROCESS FOCUS

Patients Receiving Antiretroviral Agents

ASSESSMENT

Prior to administration:

- Obtain complete health history including allergies, drug history, and possible drug interactions
- Obtain complete physical examination
- Assess for the presence/history of HIV infection
- Obtain the following laboratory studies:
  - HIV RNA assay / CD4 count
  - Complete blood count (CBC)
  - Liver function
  - Renal function
  - Blood glucose

POTENTIAL NURSING DIAGNOSES

- Risk for Infection, related to compromised immune system
- Decisional Conflict, related to therapeutic regimen
- Fear, related to HIV diagnosis
- Risk for Injury, related to side effects of drugs
- Deficient Knowledge, related to disease process, transmission, and drug therapy

PLANNING: Patient Goals and Expected Outcomes

The patient will:

- Exhibit a decrease in viral load and an increase in CD4 counts
- Demonstrate knowledge of disease process, transmission, and treatment
- Identify side effects and report to healthcare provider
- Complete full course of therapy and comply with follow-up care

IMPLEMENTATION

Interventions and (Rationales)	Patient Education/Discharge Planning
■ Monitor for symptoms of hypersensitivity reactions. (Zalcitabine may cause anaphylactic reaction.)	■ Instruct patient to discontinue the medication and inform healthcare provider if symptoms of hypersensitivity reaction develop such as wheezing; shortness of breath; swelling of face, tongue, or hands; itching or rash.
■ Monitor vital signs, especially temperature, and for symptoms of infection. Monitor white blood cell count. (Antiretroviral drugs such as delavirdine may cause neutropenia.)	Instruct patient: ■ To report symptoms of infections such as fever, chills, sore throat, and cough ■ On methods to minimize exposure to infection such as frequent handwashing; avoiding crowds and people with colds, flu, and other infections; limiting exposure to children and animals; increasing fluid intake; emptying bladder frequently; and coughing and deep breathing several times per day
■ Monitor patient for signs of stomatitis. (Immunosuppression may result in the proliferation of oral bacteria.) ■ Monitor blood pressure. (Antiviral agents such as abacavir may cause significant decrease in blood pressure.)	Instruct patient to: ■ Be alert for mouth ulcers and to report their appearance. ■ Rise slowly from lying or sitting position to minimize effects of postural hypotension ■ Report changes in blood pressure
■ Monitor HIV RNA assay, CD4 counts, liver function, kidney function, complete blood count, blood glucose, and serum amylase and triglyceride levels. (These will determine effectiveness and toxicity of drug.)	Instruct patient: ■ On the purpose of required laboratory tests and scheduled follow-ups with healthcare provider ■ To monitor weight and presence of swelling ■ To keep all appointments for laboratory tests

continued...

NURSING PROCESS FOCUS

Interventions and (Rationales)	Patient Education/Discharge Planning
■ Determine potential drug-drug and drug-food interactions. (Antiretroviral medications have multiple drug-drug interactions and must be taken as prescribed.)	Instruct patient: ■ When to take the specific medication in relationship to food intake ■ About foods or beverages to avoid when taking medication some antiretrovirals should not be taken with acidic fruit juice ■ To take medication exactly as directed; do not skip any doses ■ To consult with healthcare provider before taking any OTC medications or herbal supplements
■ Monitor for symptoms of pancreatitis including severe abdominal pain, nausea, vomiting, and abdominal distention. (Antiretroviral agents such as didanosine may cause pancreatitis.)	■ Instruct patient to report the following immediately: fever, severe abdominal pain, nausea/vomiting, and abdominal distention
■ Monitor skin for rash; withhold medication and notify physician at first sign of rash. (Several antiretroviral drugs may cause Stevens-Johnson syndrome which may be fatal.)	■ Advise patient to check skin frequently and notify healthcare provider at first sign of any rash.
■ Establish therapeutic environment to ensure adequate rest, nutrition, hydration, and relaxation. (Support of the immune system is essential in HIV patients to minimize opportunistic infections.)	Teach patient to incorporate the following health-enhancing activities: ■ Adequate rest and sleep ■ Proper nutrition that provides essential vitamins and nutrients ■ Intake of six to eight glasses of water/day
■ Monitor blood glucose levels. (Antiretroviral drugs may cause hyperglycemia, especially in patients with type 1 diabetes.)	■ Instruct patient to report excessive thirst, hunger, and urination to healthcare provider. ■ Instruct diabetic patients to monitor blood glucose levels regularly.
■ Monitor for neurological side effects such as numbness and tingling of the extremities. (Many NRTI agents cause peripheral neuropathy.)	Instruct patient to: ■ Report numbness and tingling of extremities ■ Use caution when in contact with heat and cold due to possible peripheral neuropathy
■ Determine the effect of the prescribed antiretroviral agents on oral contraceptives. (Many agents reduce the effectiveness of oral contraceptives.)	■ Instruct patient to use an alternate form of birth control while taking antiretroviral medications.
■ Provide resources for medical and emotional support.	■ Advise patient on community resources and support groups.
■ Assess patient's knowledge level regarding use and effect of medication.	Advise patient: ■ That medication may decrease the level of HIV infection in the blood but will not prevent transmitting the disease ■ To use barrier protection during sexual activity ■ To avoid sharing needles ■ To not donate blood

EVALUATION OF OUTCOME CRITERIA

Evaluate the effectiveness of drug therapy by confirming that patient goals and expected outcomes have been met (see "Planning").

See Tables 23.3 and 23.4 for lists of drugs to which these nursing actions apply.

Unfortunately, the decision to begin treatment during the latent phase has negative consequences. Medications for HIV-AIDS are expensive; treatment with some of the newer agents may cost more than $20,000 per year. These drugs produce uncomfortable and potentially serious side effects. Therapy over many years promotes viral resistance; when the acute stage eventually develops, the medications may no longer be effective.

The decision to begin therapy during the acute phase is much easier because the severe symptoms of AIDS can rapidly lead to death. Thus, therapy is nearly always initiated during this phase.

The therapeutic goals for the pharmacotherapy of HIV-AIDS include the following:

- Evidence of reduction of HIV levels in the blood
- Increased lifespan
- Increased quality of life

Although drug therapy for HIV-AIDS has not produced a cure, it has resulted in a number of therapeutic successes. For example, many patients with HIV are able to live symptom-free with their disease for a much longer time because of antiviral therapy. Furthermore, the transmission of the virus from an HIV-infected mother to her newborn has been reduced dramatically because of drug therapy of the mother prior to delivery and of the baby immediately following birth. These two factors have resulted in a significant decline in the death rate due to HIV-AIDS in the United States.

Antiviral medications used for HIV-AIDS are called **antiretrovirals** because they block the replication cycle of HIV, which is classified as a retrovirus. The standard treatment for HIV-AIDS includes aggressive treatment with three to four drugs at a time, a regimen called **highly active antiretroviral therapy (HAART).** The goal of HAART is to reduce the amount of HIV in the plasma to its lowest possible level. It must be understood, however, that HIV is harbored in locations other than the blood, such as in lymph nodes; therefore, elimination of the virus from the blood is not a cure.

The replication of HIV is illustrated in Figure 23.2 ■. Antiretroviral drugs are classified into groups based on how they inhibit HIV replication.

- *Nucleoside reverse transcriptase inhibitors (NRTIs):* The oldest antiretroviral drug, zidovudine (see page 434) belongs to the NRTI class. Drugs in this class are structurally similar to nucleosides, the building blocks of DNA. NRTIs inhibit the action of the viral enzyme **reverse transcriptase,** which converts the viral RNA into viral DNA.
- *Nonnucleoside reverse transcriptase inhibitors (NNRTIs):* This class also inhibits the viral enzyme reverse transcriptase, but these drugs are not structurally similar to the building blocks of DNA. Instead, these agents bind directly to the reverse transcriptase molecule and inhibit its ability to build viral DNA.
- *Protease inhibitors:* These drugs block the final assembly of the HIV particle. They are quite effective at reducing plasma HIV to very low levels, although resistance develops quickly.
- Miscellaneous agents: Newer drugs are being developed as scientists discover more about the HIV replication cycle. Tenofovir (Viread) is a nucleoTide reverse transcriptase inhibitor that is incorporated into viral DNA in a manner like the NRTIs. Enfuvirtide (Fuzeon) blocks the fusion of HIV to the CD4 receptor on the lymphocyte.

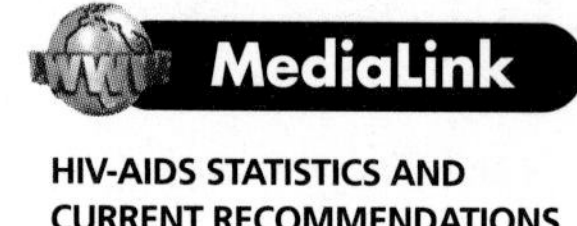

HIV-AIDS STATISTICS AND CURRENT RECOMMENDATIONS

Concept Review 23.2

■ Why are viral infections difficult to treat with current drugs?

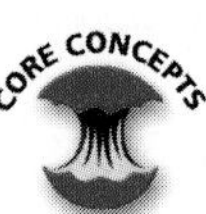

23.6 A small number of antiviral drugs are available to treat herpes simplex and influenza infections.

Other than the drugs used to treat HIV, only a few antivirals are available to treat other serious viral infections. These include drugs to treat infections from the herpesviruses and the influenza virus.

FIGURE 23.2

Coat
Envelope
Core
Viral RNA
Reverse transcriptase

1 Virus attaches to receptor on host's plasma membrane. Its core disintegrates, and viral RNA enters the cytoplasm.

2 Viral reverse transcriptase produces DNA, using viral RNA as template.

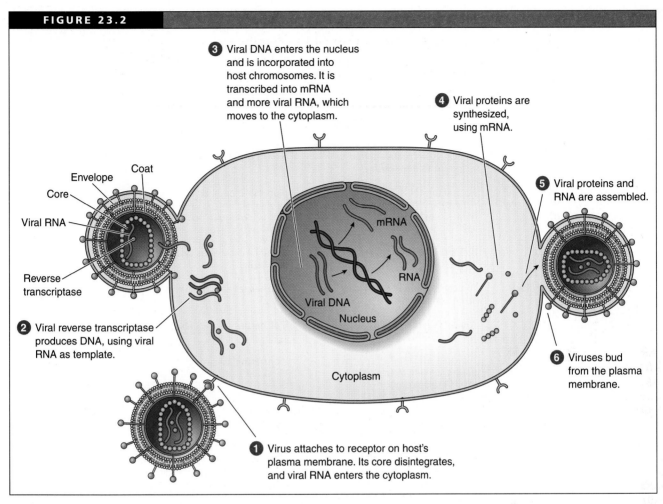

3 Viral DNA enters the nucleus and is incorporated into host chromosomes. It is transcribed into mRNA and more viral RNA, which moves to the cytoplasm.

4 Viral proteins are synthesized, using mRNA.

5 Viral proteins and RNA are assembled.

6 Viruses bud from the plasma membrane.

mRNA
RNA
Viral DNA
Nucleus
Cytoplasm

Replication of HIV

Herpes simplex viruses (HSV) are a family of viruses that cause repeated, blisterlike lesions on the skin, genitals, and other mucosal surfaces. Herpesviruses are acquired through sexual intercourse or other direct physical contact with an infected person. The herpesvirus family includes the following:

- HSV-type 1—nongenital infections of the eye, mouth, and lips (cold sores/fever blisters)
- HSV-type 2—genital infections
- Cytomegalovirus (CMV)—affects multiple body systems, usually in immunosuppressed patients

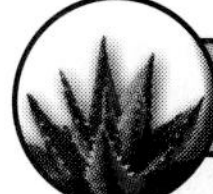

NATURAL ALTERNATIVES

The Antiviral Activity of Hyssop

Hyssop (*Hyssopus officianalis*) is a member of the mint family that originated from the Mediterranean region. The leaves of the plant are dried and available as capsules, tincture, or tea. Hyssop contains a number of substances claimed to have antiviral activity, including tannins and a polysaccharide called MR-10. It also contains a number of volatile oils, which give hyssop a strong, pleasant odor and are occasionally used as flavorings and scents.

Extracts of hyssop are sometimes used topically to treat skin lesions due to herpes virus. It can be used as a gargle for sore throats. It is claimed to have an expectorant action that may be of value in bronchitis and viral pneumonia. ■

TABLE 23.4 Antiviral Drugs for Herpes and Influenza Infections

DRUG	ROUTE AND ADULT DOSE	REMARKS
HERPES VIRUS DRUGS		
Pr acyclovir (Zovirax)	PO 400 mg tid	For HSV-1, HSV-2, and varicella-zoster; topical and IV forms available
cidofovir (Vistide)	IV 5 mg/kg q week × 2 weeks, then once q week	For cytomegalovirus retinitis in clients with AIDS; must give probenecid before and after infusion
docosanol (Abreva)	Topical 10% cream applied to lesion up to 5 times/day	For herpes simplex lesions on the face and lips
famciclovir (Famvir)	PO 500 mg tid × 7 days	For HSV-2 and zoster
foscarnet (Foscavir)	IV 40–60 mg/kg infused over 1–2 hours tid	For cytomegalovirus retinitis; for the treatment of acyclovir-resistant herpesvirus
ganciclovir (Cytovene)	IV 5 mg/kg infused over 1 hour bid	Drug of choice for cytomegalovirus; oral form available
idoxuridine (IDU) (Herplex)	Topical 1 drop in each eye q1h during the day and q2h at night	For herpes eye infections
penciclovir (Denavir)	Topical 0.5 inch of ointment to each eye q3h	For herpes simplex lesions on the face and lips
trifluridine (Viroptic)	Topical 1 drop in each eye q2h during waking hours (max: 9 drops/day)	For herpes eye infections
valacyclovir (Valtrex)	PO 1 g tid	For HSV-1, HSV-2, and zoster
vidarabine (Vira-A)	Topical 0.5 inch of ointment in each eye q3h, not to exceed 5 applications/day	For herpes eye infections
INFLUENZA DRUGS		
amantadine (Symmetrel)	PO 100 mg bid	For treatment and prevention of influenza A; also for Parkinson's disease
oseltamivir (Tamiflu)	PO 75 mg bid × 5 days	For treatment of influenza
rimantadine (Flumadine)	PO 100 mg bid	For treatment and prevention of influenza
zanamivir (Relenza)	Inhalation 2 inhalations × 5 days	For treatment of influenza

- Varicella-zoster virus—shingles (zoster) and chickenpox (varicella)
- Epstein-Barr virus—mononucleosis and Burkitt's lymphoma, a form of cancer

Following its initial entrance into the human host, HSV may remain in a latent, nonreplicating state in nerve cells for many years. Immunosuppression, physical challenge, or emotional stress can activate the virus, and cause the characteristic lesions to reappear. Although herpes lesions are often mild and require no drug therapy, patients who experience frequent recurrences may benefit from low doses of prophylactic antiviral therapy. Topical drugs are available for application on active lesions, but they are not as effective as oral medications. It should be noted that the antiviral drugs used to treat herpesviruses do not cure the patient; the virus remains in the patient for life. Drugs for treating herpesviruses are shown in Table 23.4.

Influenza is a viral infection characterized by acute symptoms that include sore throat, sneezing, coughing, fever, and chills. The virus is easily spread via airborne droplets. In immunosuppressed patients, an influenza infection may be fatal.

The best approach to influenza infection is prevention through annual vaccination. Those who benefit greatly from vaccinations include residents of long-term care facilities, those with chronic cardiopulmonary disease, women who will be in their second or third trimester during the peak flu season, and healthy adults older than age 50. Adequate immunity is achieved about 2 weeks after vaccination, and lasts for several months up to a year. Additional details on vaccines are presented in Chapter 21.

Antivirals may be used to prevent influenza or decrease the severity of influenza symptoms. The drug amantadine (Symmetrel) has been available to prevent and treat influenza for many years. Amantadine or rimantadine is indicated for unvaccinated high-risk patients, after a confirmed outbreak of influenza type A. Therapy with these antivirals is sometimes started at the same time as vaccination; the antiviral offers protection during the period before antibody titers are achieved from the vaccine. Antivirals for influenza are shown in Table 23.4.

A new class of drugs called the *neuroamidase inhibitors* was introduced in 1999 to treat active infections. If given within 48 hours of the onset of symptoms, oseltamivir (Tamiflu) and zanamivir (Relenza) are reported to shorten the normal 7-day duration of influenza symptoms to 5 days. Because the influenza antivirals produce only modest benefits for patients with an active infection, prevention through vaccination remains the best alternative.

23.7 Although not common in the United States, infections caused by helminths and protozoans cause significant disease worldwide.

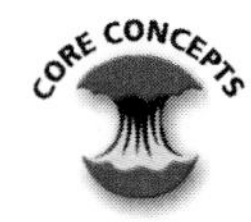

A number of pathogens other than bacteria and fungi may infect humans. These parasites include single-celled animals called **protozoans** and multicellular organisms such as mites, ticks, and worms. Although many of these diseases are rare in the United States and Canada, travelers to Africa, Asia, and South America may acquire them overseas and return home with the infection. Table 23.5 lists selected antiparasitics. Scabicides and pediculocides are covered in Chapter 31.

proto = *first*
zoans = *animals*

With a few exceptions, antibiotics, antifungal, and antiviral drugs are ineffective against these complex organisms. Drugs prescribed for parasitic diseases may be classified as antimalarials, antiprotozoas (other than antimalarial agents), antihelmintics, and scabicides/pediculicides.

Malaria is a disease caused by four species of the protozoan *Plasmodium.* Although rare in the United States and Canada, malaria is the second most common fatal infectious disease in the world, with 300 to 500 million cases occurring annually. The Centers for Disease Control and Prevention (CDC) recommends that travelers to infested areas receive prophylactic antimalarial drugs prior to and during their visit, and for 1 week after leaving. Proguanil (Paludrine) is an antimalarial commonly used for prophylaxis. Once a person is infected, the goal of drug therapy is

DRUG PROFILE: Antiviral: Pr *Acyclovir (Zovirax)*

Actions and Uses:

The antiviral activity of acyclovir is limited to the herpesviruses, for which it is the drug of choice. It is most effective against HSV-1 and HSV-2 and effective only at high doses against CMV and varicella-zoster. Acyclovir acts by inhibiting viral DNA synthesis. Resistance has developed to the drug, particularly in patients with HIV-AIDS. Acyclovir decreases the duration and severity of herpes episodes. When given for prophylaxis, it may decrease the frequency of active herpes episodes, but it does not cure the patient. It is available in topical form for placing directly on active lesions, in oral form for prophylaxis, and as an IV for particularly severe disease.

Adverse Effects and Interactions:

There are few adverse effects to acyclovir when administered topically or orally. When given IV, the drug may cause painful inflammation of vessels at the site of infusion. Because nephrotoxicity is possible, frequent laboratory tests may be performed to monitor kidney function.

Acyclovir interacts with several drugs. For example, probenecid decreases acyclovir elimination, and zidovudine may cause increased drowsiness and lethargy.

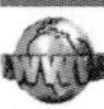
See the Companion Website for a Nursing Process Focus specific to this drug.

TABLE 23.5 Drugs for Helminth and Protozoal Infections

DRUG	ROUTE AND ADULT DOSE	REMARKS
AMEBICIDES		
doxycycline (Vibramycin)	PO 100 mg/day	For traveler's diarrhea; used also for malaria prophylaxis
iodoquinol (Yodoxin)	PO 630–650 mg tid × 20 days (max: 2 g/day)	For intestinal amebiasis
paromomycin (Humatin)	PO 25–35 mg/kg divided in 3 doses for 5–10 days	For acute and chronic amebiasis; can cause ototoxicity
ANTIHELMINTICS		
albendazole (Albenza)	PO 400 mg bid (max: 800 mg/day)	Only antihelmintic drug active against all stages of the helminth life cycle
ivermectin (Stromectol)	PO 150–200 mcg/kg × 1 dose	
mebendazole (Vermox)	PO 100 mg × 1 dose or 100 mg bid × 3 days	For the treatment of whipworm, roundworm, hookworm, and pinworm
praziquantel (Biltricide)	PO 5 mg/kg × 1 dose or 25 mg/kg tid	For all stages of schistosomiasis; bitter tablet
pyrantel (Antiminith)	PO 11 mg/kg × 1 dose (max: 1 g)	For the treatment of hookworm and roundworm
ANTIMALARIALS		
atovaquone (Mepron)	PO 750 mg bid × 21 days	Also for pneumocystis
chloroquine (Aralen)	PO 600 mg initial dose, then 300 mg weekly	A drug of choice for malaria; also for amebiasis and rheumatoid arthritis; IM form available; if administered IV, oral medication is ineffective
hydroxychloroquine (Plaquenil)	PO 620 mg initial dose, then 310 mg weekly	Also for rheumatoid arthritis and lupus erythematosus
mefloquine (Lariam)	PO prevention: begin with 250 mg once a week × 4 weeks, then 250 mg every other week; treatment: 1250 mg as a single dose	For prevention and treatment of malaria
primaquine (PRIM-ah-kwin)	PO 15 mg daily × 2 weeks	Removes *Plasmodium vivax* from the liver; used for malaria suppression
pyrimethamine (Daraprim)	PO 25 mg once per week × 10 weeks	Also antiprotozoan; drug of choice for toxoplasmosis
quinine (Quinamm)	PO 260–650 mg tid for 3 days	Largely replaced by other antimalarials; also for nocturnal leg cramps
ANTIPROTOZOALS (NONMALARIAL)		
melarsoprol (Arsobal)	IV 2–3.6 mg/kg for 3 days, then repeated on day 7 and days 10–21	Drug of choice for later stages of African trypanosomiasis
Pr metronidazole (Flagyl)	PO 250–750 mg tid	For many parasitic infections; IV form available
nifurtimox (Lampit)	PO 2–2.5 mg/kg q6h	Drug of choice for American trypanosomiasis
pentamidine (Pentam 300, Nebupent)	IV 4 mg/kg daily × 14–21 days; infuse over 60 min	For *Pneumocystis carinii* active infections and prophylaxis; IM and inhalation forms available
sodium stibogluconate (Pentostam)	IM 20 mg/kg/day	For leishmaniasis
suramin (Germanin)	IV 1 g on days 1, 3, 7, 14, and 21	Drug of choice for early stages of African trypanosomiasis
trimetrexate (Neutrexin)	IV 45 mg/m^2 daily	Alternate therapy for *Pneumocystis carinii* pneumonia

to interrupt the complex life cycle of the protozoan, which includes transmission by a bite from the female *Anopheles* mosquito. Once inside the body, *Plasmodium* grows in the liver and eventually infects red blood cells. Rupture of infected red blood cells causes severe fever and chills. Drug therapy is successful early in the course of the disease but becomes increasingly difficult because *Plasmodium* enters different stages of its life cycle in the body. Dormant parasites may remain in the liver for years and become resistant to medications. Chloroquine (Aralen) is the drug of choice for acute malaria; however, many other agents are also available because resistance to chloroquine is common. Primaquine is one of the few drugs available that can eliminate latent forms of *Plasmodium* residing in the liver.

Other species of protozoans that cause significant disease worldwide include *Entamoeba, Giardia, Leishmania, Pneumocystis, Toxoplasma,* and *Trypanosoma.* Amebiasis is a disease caused by *Entamoeba histolytica,* commonly found in Africa, Latin America, and Asia, where it frequently causes serious disease. Although primarily an intestinal disease, *E. histolytica* can invade the liver, where it causes abscesses. The primary symptom of amebiasis is a severe form of diarrhea known as amebic **dysentary.** Drugs used to treat amebiasis include those that act directly on amebas in the intestine and those that are administered for their systemic effects on the liver and other organs.

dys = *difficult or painful*
enter = *intestine*

Helminths consist of various species of parasitic worms, including hookworms, pinworms, roundworms, tapeworms, and flukes. Many of these worms attach to the mucosa of the human intestinal tract. Helminth diseases are quite common in areas of the world lacking high standards of sanitation. Helminth infections in the United States and Canada are generally neither common nor fatal, although drug therapy may be indicated. The most common helminth disease worldwide is caused by the roundworm *Ascaris;* however, infection by the pinworm *Enterobius* is more common in the United States.

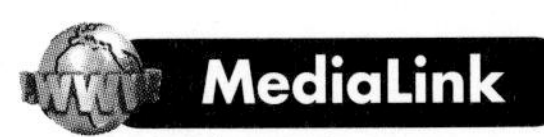

AVOIDING DISEASE WHILE TRAVELING ABROAD

Concept Review 23.3

- How do most patients in the United States and Canada acquire protozoan infections?

DRUG PROFILE: Antiprotozoal: Pr *Metronidazole (Flagyl)*

Actions and Uses:

Metronidazole is the drug of choice for most forms of amebiasis because it is effective against amebas in the intestine and in other organs. Metronidazole is also a drug of choice for two other protozoan infections: giardiasis from *Giardia lamblia* and trichonomiasis due to *Trichomonas vaginalis.* The drug is somewhat unique in that it also has antibiotic activity against anaerobic bacteria and thus is used to treat a number of respiratory, bone, skin, and CNS infections.

Adverse Effects and Interactions:

The most common side effects of metronidazole are anorexia, nausea, diarrhea, dizziness, and headache. Dryness of the mouth and an unpleasant metallic taste may be experienced. Although side effects are relatively common, most are not serious enough to cause discontinuation of therapy.

Metronidazole interacts with several drugs. For example, oral anticoagulants increase hypoprothombinemia. In combination with alcohol and medications that contain alcohol, metronidazole may cause a disulfiram reaction. It may also elevate lithium levels.

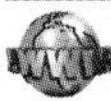
See the Companion Website for a Nursing Process Focus Specific to this drug.

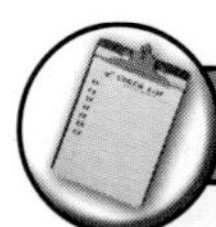

PATIENTS NEED TO KNOW

Patients treated for fungal, viral, or parasitic infections need to know the following:

Regarding Antifungals

1. Avoid alcohol and other drugs toxic to the liver while taking azole-type antifungals.
2. Griseofulvin, used to treat superficial mycoses, can decrease the effectiveness of oral contraceptives. An alternative method of contraception is advised.
3. Older children and adult patients should swish oral antifungal drugs around in their mouths and swallow them. Caregivers should swab the mouths of infants and toddlers. Wait at least 10 minutes after antifungal treatment to put anything else in the mouth.
4. Rinse the mouth after use of glucocorticoid inhalers to avoid a decrease in local immune defenses against oral candidiasis.
5. Refrain from sexual intercourse while taking antifungal drugs for a vaginal infection until the infection is resolved.

Regarding Antivirals

6. When taking antivirals, report bleeding and bruising as well as decreased resistance to infection. These are indications of possible bone marrow suppression that may require dosage adjustment or change of medication.
7. When taking antivirals, do not take any other medications or dietary supplements without consulting a healthcare practitioner because of the risk for interactions. ■

CHAPTER REVIEW

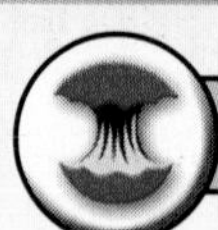

CORE CONCEPTS SUMMARY

23.1 Because fungi are more complex than bacteria, fungal infections require a different approach to pharmacotherapy.

Fungi are multicellular organisms. Because most are unaffected by antibiotics, they require different classes of medications. Fungal infections are usually only a serious problem in patients with compromised immune systems. Mycoses are classified as superficial or systemic.

23.2 Systemic antifungal drugs are used for serious infections of internal organs.

Systemic mycoses affect the internal organs and may require prolonged and aggressive drug therapy. Systemic antifungal agents may cause serious adverse effects.

23.3 Superficial infections of the skin, nails, and mucous membranes are effectively treated with topical and oral antifungal drugs.

Superficial mycoses of the hair, skin, nails, and mucous membranes are very common, though rarely serious. Antifungals given topically as powders, troches, and ointments produce few adverse effects.

23.4 Viruses are nonliving parasites that require a host to replicate.

Viruses take over the cellular machinery of their host and use it to replicate themselves. Although most viral infections require no pharmacotherapy, patients with infections by HIV, herpesviruses, and the influenza virus may benefit from drug treatment.

23.5 Antiretroviral drugs for HIV-AIDS do not cure the disease, but they do help many patients live longer.

Drugs used to treat HIV infections include the nucleoside and nonnucleoside reverse transcriptase inhibitors, protease inhibitors, and fusion inhibitors. These drugs may produce significant toxicity. Although none are able to cure the disease, they may extend the symptom-free period.

23.6 A small number of antiviral drugs are available to treat herpes simplex and influenza infections.

Drug therapy is used to extend the latent period of genital herpes and to speed the recovery from active lesions. A few antivirals are available to prevent influenza, and these are most useful when combined with vaccines. New drugs have been developed to shorten the discomfort period for influenza symptoms, although these have limited effectiveness.

23.7 Although not common in the United States, infections caused by helminths and protozoans cause significant disease worldwide.

Malaria is one of the most common infections in the world, and a significant number of drugs are available to disrupt the *Plasmodium* life cycle. Similarly, amebiasis is a common protozoal disease requiring intensive drug treatment. Diseases caused by helminths are common in areas of the world lacking adequate sanitation.

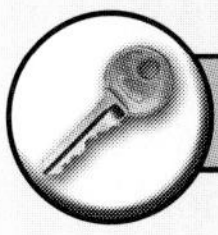

KEY TERMS

antiretroviral (an-tie-RET-roh-veye-ral): type of drug effective against retroviruses / *page 432*

capsid (CAP-sid): protein coat that surrounds a virus / *page 427*

dermatophytic (der-MAT-oh-FIT-ik): superficial fungal infection / *page 423*

dysentery (DISS-en-tare-ee): severe diarrhea that may include bleeding / *page 437*

fungi (FUN-jeye): kingdom of organisms that includes mushrooms, yeasts, and molds / *page 422*

highly active antiretroviral therapy (HAART): type of drug therapy for HIV infection that includes high doses of multiple medications that are given together / *page 432*

helminth (HELL-minth): type of flat, round, or segmented worm / *page 437*

host: an organism that is being infected by a microbe / *page 428*

influenza (in-flew-EN-zah): common viral infection of the respiratory system; often called *flu* / *page 434*

intracellular parasite: an infectious microbe that lives inside host cells / *page 428*

malaria (mah-LARE-ee-ah): tropical disease characterized by severe fever and chills caused by the protozoan *Plasmodium* / *page 435*

mycoses (my-KOH-sees): diseases caused by fungi/ *page 423*

protozoan (PRO-toh-ZOH-en): single-celled microorganism / *page 435*

reverse transcriptase (ree-VERS trans-CRIP-tace): viral enzyme that converts RNA to DNA / *page 432*

Superficial mycoses: fungal diseases of the hair, skin, nails, and mucous membranes / *page 423*

systemic mycoses: fungal diseases affecting internal organs / *page 423*

virus: nonliving particle containing RNA or DNA that is able to cause disease / *page 427*

yeast (YEEST): type of fungus that is unicellular and divides by budding / *page 423*

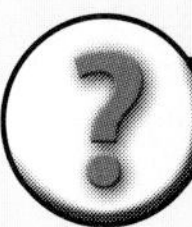

REVIEW QUESTIONS

The following questions are written in NCLEX-PN® style. Answer these questions to assess your knowledge of the chapter material, and go back and review any material that is not clear to you.

1. The patient on amphotericin B must be monitored for:

1. Ototoxicity
2. Hepatic toxicity
3. Nephrotoxicity
4. Anoxia

2. The patient has oral candidiasis. Which of the following medications does the nurse expect to be ordered?

1. Terbinafine (Lamisil)
2. Clotrimazole (Mycelex)
3. Ketoconazole (Nizoral)
4. Nystatin (Mycostatin)

3. The patient with a fungal infection of her toenails asks how long treatment must occur. The best response would be:

1. "Treatment is very quick, requiring only 1 tablet of clotrimazole."
2. "Treatment will occur daily for 3 days."
3. "Treatment will last for several months."
4. "You will need to speak to your physician."

4. Patient teaching for a patient on zidovudine (AZT) would include the:

1. Importance of taking the medication every 4 hours
2. Fact that medication is taken daily for 1 month only
3. Information that, if taken correctly, this medication will cure the disease
4. Fact that the medication is used to treat influenza

5. Which of the following drugs would be used to treat genital herpes?

1. Trifluridine (Viroptic)
2. Vidarabine (Vira-A)
3. Acyclovir (Zovirax)
4. Foscarnet (Foscavir)

6. The patient complains of flulike symptoms that started 24 hours ago. Which of the following class of medications would the nurse anticipate being ordered?

1. Protease inhibitors
2. Nonnucleoside reverse transcriptase inhibitors

3. Nucleoside reverse transcriptase inhibitors
4. Neuroamidase inhibitors

7. The drug of choice to treat *Trichomonas vaginalis* is:

1. Nifurtimox (Lampit)
2. Trimetrexate (Neutrexin)
3. Melarsoprol (Arsobal)
4. Metronidazole (Flagyl)

8. When applying topical antivirals, which of the following statements is true?

1. No other antivirals should be administered.
2. Gloves should be worn to prevent transmission.
3. Antivirals should not be applied to open areas.
4. Vitals signs should be assessed prior to administration.

9. The patient on oral glucocorticoid inhalers is at risk for developing:

1. Nephrotoxicity
2. Renal toxicity
3. Oral candidiasis
4. Nausea and diarrhea

10. The patient on antivirals has developed bruising. This could indicate which of the following?

1. The patient is most likely being abused.
2. The patient is experiencing minor adverse reactions.
3. The patient is not taking the medications as ordered.
4. The patient may be experiencing bone marrow suppression.

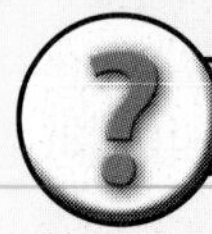

CASE STUDY QUESTIONS

1. Ms. Fasano is a 78-year-old retired auto worker who is frail and in ill health. What is her best option to avoid a potential life-threatening bout with the flu?

1. Begin taking oseltamivir (Tamiflu) 1 month before the flu season begins.
2. Take zanamavir (Relenza) within 48 hours on the onset of flu symptoms.
3. Receive a flu vaccination 30–60 days prior to the start of the flu season.
4. Take acyclovir (Zovirax) during the flu season.

2. During the flu season, Ms. Fasano reports vaginal itching and abnormal discharges, and the physician diagnoses vaginal candidiasis. Which of the following would be the most likely drug therapy?

1. Amphotericin B (Fungizone)
2. Clotrimazole (Gyne-Lotrimin)
3. Acyclovir (Zovirax)
4. Iodoquinol (Yodoxin)

3. While examining Mr. Walker's medical records, you note he is taking saquinavir (Invirase), abacavir (Ziagen), and efavirenz (Sustiva). Mr. Walker is most likely suffering from what type of infection?

1. HIV
2. Systemic fungal
3. Malaria
4. Herpes simplex

4. The type of drugs taken by Mr. Walker is called:

1. Antivirals
2. Antiretrovirals
3. Antifungals
4. Antiprotozoals

5. Mr. Gunter is planning a safari in the Congo and has been prescribed an 8-week therapy of chloroquine (Aralen), beginning 2 weeks before his flight. The purpose of this regimen is to prevent:

1. HIV infection
2. Amebiasis
3. Helminth infection
4. Malaria

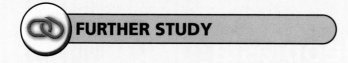

FURTHER STUDY

- Information on drugs that may cause patients to be more susceptible to systemic fungal infections is found in Chapters 21 and 29 (corticosteroids) and Chapter 24 (anticancer drugs). Chapter 21 also discusses organ transplants, which may also place patients at increased risk for system fungal infections.
- Information on vaccines is included in Chapter 21.
- Chapter 31 discusses scabicides and pediculicides.

EXPLORE MEDIALINK www.prenhall.com/holland

Additional resources for this chapter can be found on the CD-ROM accompanying this textbook, and on the Companion Website. Click on Chapter 23 to select activities for this chapter.

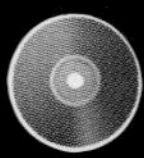

- Mechanism in Action: Zidovudine
- Audio Glossary
- Concept Review
- NCLEX-PN® Review
- Nursing in Action
- Dosage Calculator

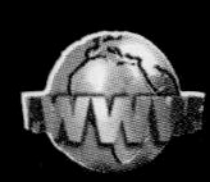

- Fungi in the World
- HIV-AIDS Statistics and Current Recommendations
- Avoiding Disease While Traveling Abroad

CHAPTER

24 Drugs for Neoplasia

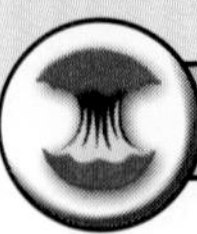

CORE CONCEPTS

24.1 Cancer is characterized by rapid, uncontrolled growth of cells.

24.2 The causes of cancer may be chemical, physical, or biological.

24.3 Personal risk of cancer may be lowered by a number of lifestyle factors.

24.4 Cancer may be treated using surgery, radiation therapy, and drugs.

24.5 To achieve a total cure, every malignant cell must be removed or killed.

24.6 Use of multiple drugs and special dosing schedules improve the success of chemotherapy.

24.7 Serious toxicity limits most of the antineoplastic agents.

24.8 Alkylating agents act by changing the structure of DNA in cancer cells.

24.9 Antimetabolites act by disrupting critical cell pathways in cancer cells.

24.10 Because of their cytotoxicity, a few antibiotics are used to treat cancer rather than infections.

24.11 Some plant extracts kill cancer cells by preventing cell division.

24.12 Some hormones and hormone antagonists are effective against prostate and breast cancer.

24.13 Biologic response modifiers and some additional antineoplastic drugs are effective against specific tumors.

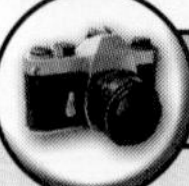

DRUG SNAPSHOT

The following drugs will be disscussed in this chapter:

DRUG CLASSES	DRUG PROFILES
Alkylating agents	Pr cyclophosphamide (Cytoxan)
Antimetabolites	Pr methotrexate (Mexate)
Antitumor antibiotics	Pr doxorubicin (Adriamycin)
Plant alkaloids/natural products	Pr vincristine (Oncovin)
Hormones and hormone antagonists	Pr tamoxifen (Nolvadex)
Biologic response modifiers and miscellaneous drugs for cancer patients	Pr interferon alfa-2 (Roferon-A, Intron A) Pr epoetin alfa (Epogen, Procrit)

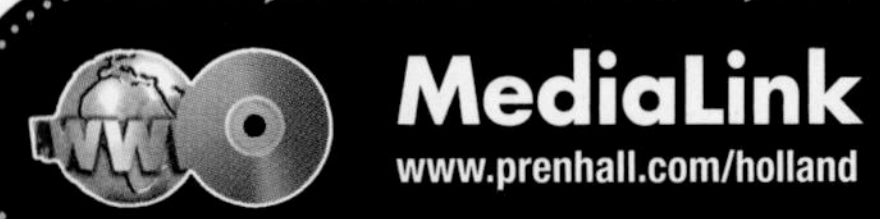

Interactive resources for this chapter can be found on the Companion Website. Click on Chapter 24 and "Begin" to select the activities for this chapter. For chapter-related animations, NCLEX-PN®-style questions, and an audio glossary, access the accompanying CD-ROM in this book.

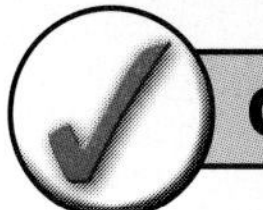

OBJECTIVES

After reading this chapter, the student should be able to:

1. Explain differences between normal cells and cancer cells.
2. Identify the primary causes of cancer.
3. Describe how the probability of acquiring cancer can be reduced by adopting certain lifestyle changes.
4. Differentiate among the terms *neoplasm, benign, malignant,* and *carcinoma.*
5. Identify the three primary treatments for cancer.
6. Explain why cancer is difficult to cure.
7. Explain why multiple drugs and special dosing schedules increase the effectiveness of chemotherapy.
8. Describe the general adverse effects of chemotherapeutic agents.
9. For each of the following, explain the mechanisms of drug action, primary actions, and important adverse effects.
   - **a.** alkylating agents
   - **b.** antimetabolites
   - **c.** antitumor antibiotics
   - **d.** hormones and hormone antagonists
   - **e.** plant extracts/natural products
   - **f.** biologic response modifiers and miscellaneous drugs for cancer patients
10. Categorize anticancer drugs based on their classifications and mechanisms of action.

Cancer is one of the most feared diseases for a number of valid reasons. It may be silent, producing no symptoms until it is too large to cure. It sometimes requires painful and disfiguring surgery. It may occur at an early age—even during childhood—depriving patients of a normal lifespan. Perhaps worst of all, the medical treatment of cancer often cannot offer a cure, and progression to death is sometimes slow, painful, and psychologically difficult for the patient and his or her loved ones.

Many advances have been made in the diagnosis, understanding, and treatment of cancer. Some types of cancer are now curable and therapy may provide the patient a longer, symptom-free life. This chapter examines the role of drugs in the treatment of cancer. Medications used to treat this disease are called anticancer drugs, antineoplastics, or cancer chemotherapeutic agents.

Fast Facts Cancer

- In 2004, 1,368,000 new cancer cases were estimated with 563,700 deaths (15,000 people every day).
- Cancer is the leading cause of death by disease in children younger than 15 years.
- Colorectal cancer is the third most common cancer in both men and women.
- Leukemia is the most common childhood cancer and is responsible for one quarter of all cancers occurring before age 20.
- Lung cancer accounts for 28% of all cancer deaths.
- Prostate cancer is the second leading cause of cancer death in men.
- The highest 5-year survival rates are for cancers of the prostate, testes, and thyroid. The lowest survival rates are for pancreatic and liver cancers.
- Among ethnic groups, Blacks have the highest incidence rates in many types of cancers, including lung, breast, and prostate. Since 1990, this gap has been narrowing.
- Although breast cancer is predominant in women (second in cancer deaths), about 1500 men are diagnosed with the disease each year.

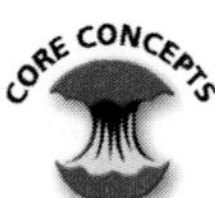

24.1 Cancer is characterized by rapid, uncontrolled growth of cells.

Cancer is a disease characterized by abnormal, uncontrolled cell division. Cell division is a normal process occurring extensively in most body tissues from conception to late childhood. At some point, however, cells suppress this rapid division by repressing the genes responsible for cell growth. This may result in a total lack of division in the case of muscle cells and, perhaps, brain cells. In other cells, the genes controlling division may be reactivated whenever it is necessary to replace worn-out cells, as in the case of blood cells and the lining of the digestive tract.

Cancer is thought to result from damage to the genes controlling cell growth. Once damaged, the cell is no longer responsive to normal chemical signals checking its growth. The cancer cells lose their normal functions, divide rapidly, and invade surrounding cells. The abnormal cells may travel to distant sites where they populate new tumors, a process called **metastasis.** Figure 24.1 ■ illustrates some characteristics of cancer cells.

neo = *new*
plasm = *thing formed*

The word **tumor** means swelling, abnormal enlargement, or mass. The word **neoplasm** is often used interchangeably with tumor. The suffix–*oma* signifies tumor. Tumors may be either benign or malignant.

Benign tumors grow slowly, do not metastasize, and rarely require drug treatment. Although they do not kill patients, their growth may cause pressure on nerves, blood vessels, or other tissues. When this occurs, they may be surgically removed; they do not normally grow back. Examples include **adenomas,** which are benign tumors of glandular tissue, and **lipomas,** which are tumors of adipose tissue.

adeno = *gland*
oma = *tumor*
lip = *fat*

Malignant tumors are called cancer. The word **malignant** refers to a disease that grows rapidly worse, becomes resistant to treatment, and normally results in death. The two major divisions of malignant neoplasms are carcinomas and sarcomas. Other types include cancer of the blood-forming cells in bone marrow (**leukemia**), lymphatic tissue (**lymphomas**), and the central nervous system (**gliomas**).

leuk = *white*
emia = *condition*

FIGURE 24.1

Invasion and metastasis by cancer cells

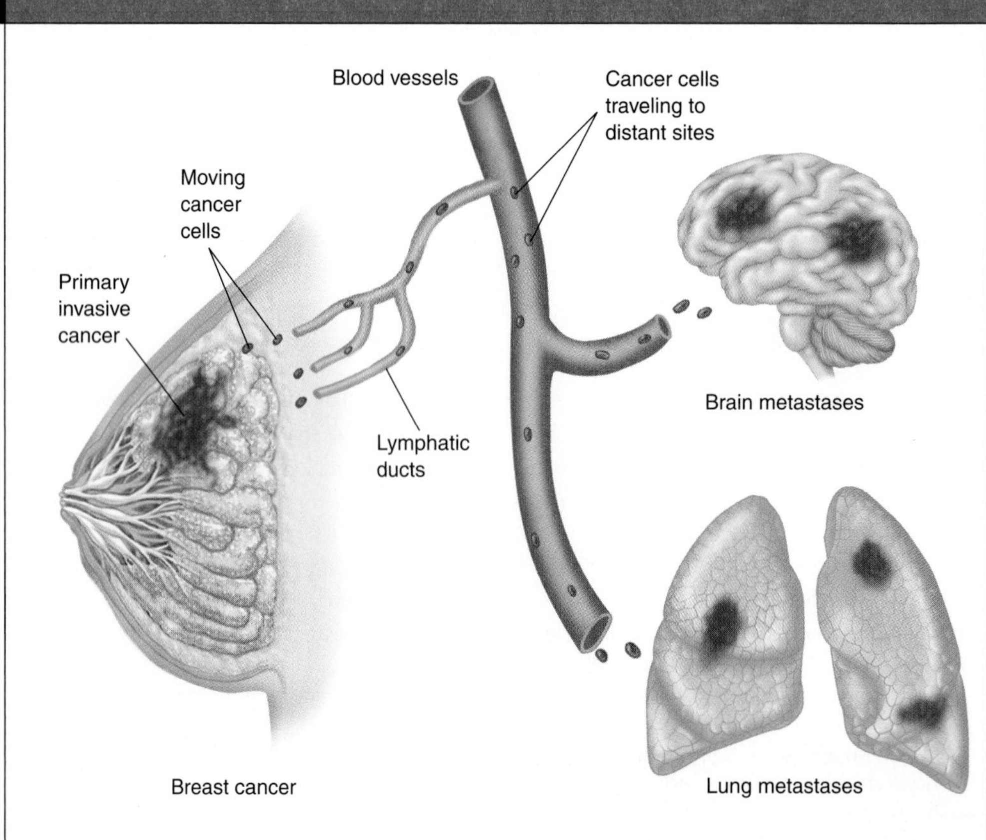

24.2 The causes of cancer may be chemical, physical, or biological.

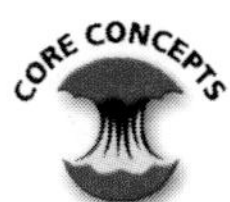

A large number of factors have been found to cause cancer or to be associated with a higher risk for acquiring the disease. These factors are known as **carcinogens.**

Many chemical carcinogens have been identified. Chemicals in tobacco smoke are thought to be responsible for about one third of all cancer in the United States. Some chemicals such as asbestos and benzene, have been associated with a higher incidence of cancer in the workplace. The actual site of the cancer may be distant from the entry location, as is the case of bladder cancer caused by the inhalation of certain industrial chemicals.

A number of physical factors are also associated with cancer. For example, exposure to large amounts of X-rays is associated with a higher risk of leukemia. Ultraviolet (UV) light from the sun is a known cause of skin cancer.

Viruses are associated with about 15% of all human cancers. Examples include herpes simplex viruses types I and II, Epstein-Barr virus, papillomavirus, cytomegalovirus, and human T-lymphotrophic viruses. Factors that suppress the immune system, such as HIV or drugs given after transplant surgery, may encourage the growth of cancer cells.

Some cancers have a strong genetic component. The fact that close relatives may acquire the same type of cancer suggests that the patient may have certain genes, called **oncogenes,** that predispose him or her to the condition. These abnormal genes interact with chemical, physical, and biological agents to promote cancer formation in the patient. Other genes, called **tumor suppressor genes,** may inhibit the formation of tumors. If these suppressor genes are damaged, cancer may result. Damage to the suppressor gene known as p53 is associated with cancers of the breast, lung, brain, colon, and bone.

Concept Review 24.1

- What is the fundamental feature that makes a cancer cell different from a normal cell?

24.3 Personal risk of cancer may be lowered by a number of lifestyle factors.

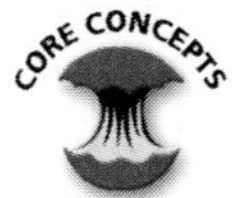

Fortunately, adopting healthy lifestyle habits such as those shown in the following list may reduce the risk of acquiring cancer. Eliminating tobacco use is the most important means of reducing cancer risk. Limiting exposure to exhaled, or secondhand, smoke is also thought to be important. Intake of alcoholic beverages and saturated fats should be limited and body weight kept within medically recommended ranges. The following list shows ways healthcare providers can teach their patients to reduce their risk of cancer:

- Eliminate tobacco use and exposure to secondhand tobacco smoke.
- Limit or eliminate alcoholic beverage use.
- Reduce fat in the diet, particularly that from animal sources.
- Choose most of the foods from plant sources; increase fiber in the diet.
- Exercise regularly and keep body weight within optimum guidelines.
- Self-examine your body monthly for abnormal lumps and skin lesions.
- When exposed to direct sun, use skin lotions with the highest SPF (Sun Protection Factor) value.
- Women should have periodic mammograms, as directed by their healthcare provider.
- Men should have a digital rectal prostate examination and a prostate-specific antigen (PSA) test annually after age 50.
- Have a fecal occult blood test (FOBT) and flexible sigmoidoscopy performed at age 50 with FOBT annually following age 50.
- Women who are sexually active or have reached age 18 should have an annual Pap test and pelvic examination.

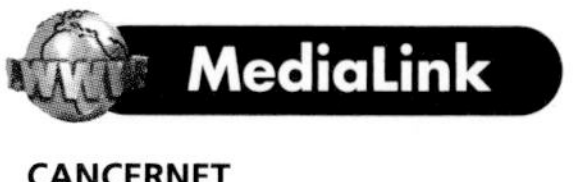

CANCERNET

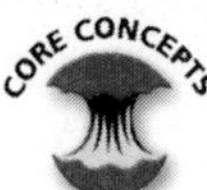

24.4 Cancer may be treated using surgery, radiation therapy, and drugs.

There is a much greater possibility for cure if the cancer is treated in its early stages, when the tumor is small and localized to a single area. Once the cancer has spread to distant sites, cure is much more difficult. Thus, it is important to diagnose the disease as early as possible. In an attempt to remove every cancer cell, three treatment approaches are used including surgery, radiation therapy, and drug therapy.

Surgery is performed to remove a tumor that is localized to one area or when the tumor is pressing on nerves, the airways, or other vital tissues. Surgery lowers the number of cancer cells in the body so that radiation and drug therapy can be more successful. Surgery is not an option for tumors of blood cells or when it would not be expected to extend a patient's lifespan or to improve the quality of his or her life.

Radiation therapy is an effective way to kill tumor cells through nonsurgical means. High doses of ionizing radiation are aimed directly at the tumor and confined to this area as much as possible. Radiation treatments may follow surgery to kill any cancer cells that were left behind following the operation. Radiation is sometimes given as **palliation** for inoperable cancers to shrink the size of a tumor that may be pressing on vital organs and to relieve pain or difficulty in breathing or swallowing.

Drug therapy of cancer is sometimes called **chemotherapy.** When these drugs are transported through the blood, they have the potential to reach cancer cells in any location. Some medications are even available to pass across the blood-brain barrier to treat brain tumors. Some are instilled directly into body cavities, such as the bladder to bring the highest dose possible to the cancer cells without producing systemic side effects. Anticancer drugs may be given to attempt cure, for palliation, or occasionally as prophylaxis to prevent cancer from occurring. Chemotherapy is often combined with surgery and radiation to increase the probability of a cure.

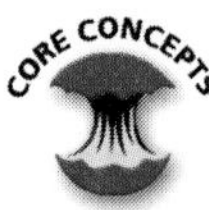

24.5 To achieve a total cure, every malignant cell must be removed or killed.

To cure a patient, it is believed that every single cancer cell must be destroyed or removed from the body. Even one malignant cell could potentially produce enough offspring to kill the patient. Unlike anti-infective therapy, in which the patient's immune system is an active partner in eliminating massive numbers of microorganisms, the immune system is able to eliminate only a small number of cancer cells.

Consider that a 1-cm breast tumor may contain 1 billion cancer cells before it is detected. A drug killing 99% of these cells would be considered a very effective drug. Yet even with this fantastic achievement, 10 million cancer cells would still remain, any one of which could cause the tumor to return and kill the patient. The relationship between cell kill and chemotherapy is shown in Figure 24.2 ■. This example illustrates the need to treat tumors at an early stage using several therapies such as chemotherapy, radiation, and surgery, when possible.

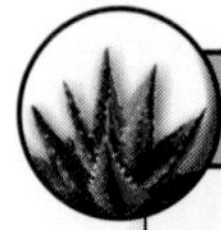

NATURAL ALTERNATIVES

Green Tea as an Antioxidant

Green tea is prepared from the dried leaves from plants grown in China, Ceylon, and India. Green tea—and to a lesser extent, black tea—have a number of chemicals shown to possess antioxidant activity. Antioxidants are thought to offer a protective effect against cancer because of their ability to eliminate free radicals—reactive substances that damage cells. Antioxidants in green tea include polyphenols, epigallocatechin gallate, and catechins.

Other than water, green tea is the world's most widely consumed liquid. The health effects of green tea have been reported since antiquity: the ancient Chinese believed the beverage increased longevity and protected against cancer. The caffeine in green tea also increases mental alertness and provides a mild diuretic effect. Green tea is reported to boost immune function and enhance cardiovascular health by inhibiting the production of low-density lipoproteins. ■

FIGURE 24.2

Cell kill and chemotherapy

Primary tumor
1 billion cells

First round of chemotherapy

Reduced tumor
99% kill
10 million cells

Second round of chemotherapy

Reduced tumor
99.9% kill
1 million cells

T cells removing
remaining cancer cells

24.6 Use of multiple drugs and special dosing schedules improve the success of chemotherapy.

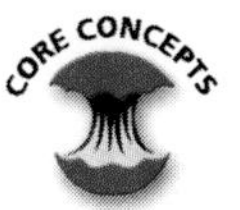

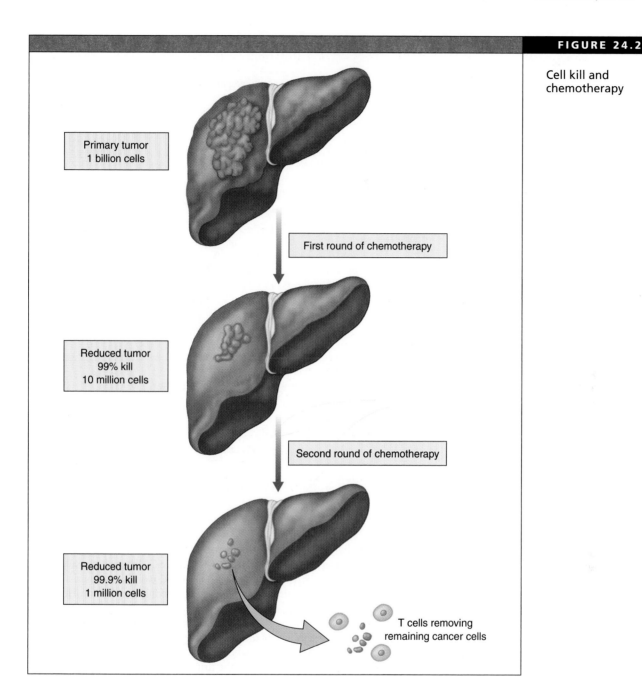

Many cancers are very difficult to treat using medications. Although cancer cells are clearly abnormal in many ways, much of their physiology is identical to that of normal cells. It is thus difficult to kill cancer cells selectively without seriously affecting normal cells. Complicating the chance for a pharmacological cure is the fact that cancer cells often develop resistance to antineoplastic drugs.

A number of treatment strategies have been found to increase the effectiveness of anticancer drugs. In most cases, multiple medications from different antineoplastic classes are given concurrently during a course of chemotherapy. Multiple classes will affect different stages of the cancer cell's life cycle, as illustrated in Figure 24.3 ■. This allows the tumor to be attacked from several mechanisms of action, thus increasing the percentage of cell kill. Using multiple drugs

FIGURE 24.3

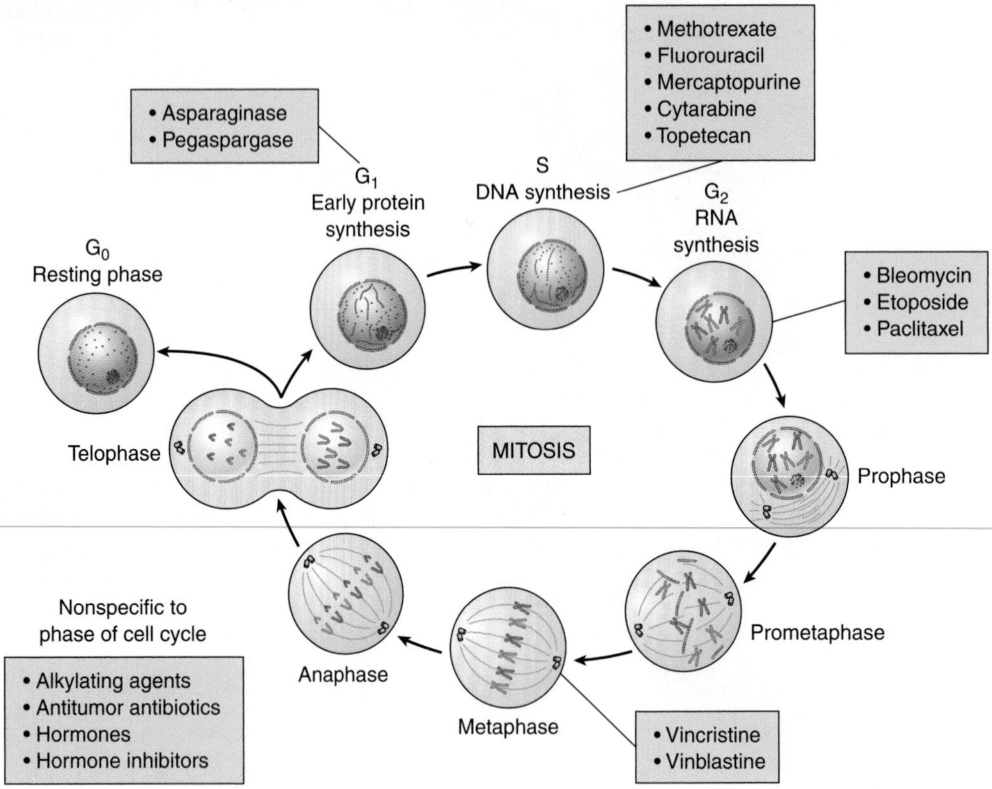

Antineoplastic agents and the cell cycle

also allows the dosages of each individual agent to be lowered, thereby reducing toxicity and slowing the development of resistance. Examples of common therapies include CMF (cyclophosphamide-methotrexate-fluorouracil) for breast cancer, CAV (cyclophosphamide-doxorubicin-vincristine) for lung cancer, and CHOP (cyclophosphamide-hydroxorubicin-oncovin-prednisone) for non-Hodgkins lymphoma.

Specific dosing schedules or cycles have been found to increase the effectiveness of the antineoplastic agents. For example, some anticancer drugs are given as single doses or perhaps a couple doses over a few days. Several weeks may pass before the next series of doses. This gives normal cells time to recover from the adverse effects of the drugs. It also allows tumor cells that may not have been replicating at the time of the first dose to begin dividing and become more sensitive to the next round of chemotherapy.

Concept Review 24.2

- Why is it important to kill or remove 100% of the cancer cells to cause a cure?

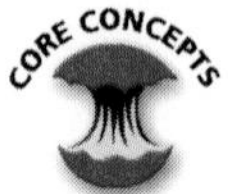

24.7 Serious toxicity limits most of the antineoplastic agents.

All anticancer drugs have the potential to cause serious toxicity. These drugs are often pushed to their maximum possible dosages so that the greatest tumor kill can be obtained. Such high dosages always result in adverse effects in the patient. A list of typical adverse effects of anticancer drugs is given in Table 24.1.

TABLE 24.1 Adverse Effects of Anticancer Drugs

CHANGES TO THE BLOOD	CHANGES TO THE GI TRACT	OTHER EFFECTS
anemia (low red blood cell count)	nausea	fatigue
thrombocytopenia	vomiting	opportunistic infections
(low platelet count)	diarrhea	ulceration and bleeding of the lips and gums
leukopenia (low white blood cell count)	anorexia (loss of appetite)	alopecia (loss of hair)

Because these drugs primarily affect rapidly growing cells, tissues that are still dividing in the adult are most susceptible to adverse effects. Hair follicles are damaged resulting in hair loss or **alopecia.** The lining of the digestive tract is affected, sometimes resulting in bleeding or severe diarrhea. The vomiting center in the medulla is triggered by many antineoplastics, resulting in severe nausea and vomiting. Vomiting is often so severe that patients may be treated with antiemetic drugs such as prochlorperazine (Compazine) or metoclopramide (Emex, Reglan) before beginning antineoplastic therapy. Blood cells in the bone marrow may be destroyed, causing a reduction in the number of red blood cells, white blood cells, and platelets. Severe effects on blood cells often cause discontinuation of chemotherapy. Efforts to minimize this toxicity may include therapy with growth factors such as filgrastim (Neupogen) or sargramostim (Leukine, Prokine). These drugs stimulate the production of white blood cells within the bone marrow.

MediaLink

CURRENT INDICATIONS FOR ANTINEOPLASTICS

Antineoplastic drugs act by many mechanisms, most of which involve cell killing or cytotoxicity. Classification is quite variable because some drugs kill cancer cells by several different mechanisms and have characteristics from more than one class. Furthermore, the mechanisms by which some of these medications act are not completely understood. A simple method of classifying this complex group of drugs includes six groups:

- Alkylating agents
- Antimetabolites
- Antitumor antibiotics
- Plant alkaloids/natural products
- Hormones and hormone blockers
- Miscellaneous drugs for cancer patients

24.8 Alkylating agents act by changing the structure of DNA in cancer cells.

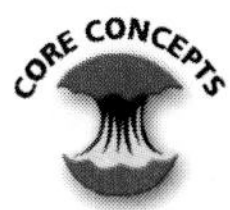

Alkylating agents act by chemically binding to nucleic acids and inhibiting cell division. They are some of the most widely used antineoplastic drugs. Table 24.2 lists the alkylating agents and their dosages.

The first alkylating agents, the **nitrogen mustards,** were developed in secrecy as chemical warfare agents during World War I. Although the drugs in this class have quite different chemical structures, all have the common characteristic of being able to form bonds or linkages with DNA. These agents physically attach to DNA, a process called **alkylation.** Alkylation changes the shape of DNA and prevents it from functioning normally. Although each alkylating agent attaches to DNA in a different manner, collectively they have the effect of killing—or at least slowing—the replication of tumor cells. The alkylation may occur in any cancer cell; however, the killing action does not occur until the affected cell divides. Figure 24.4 ■ illustrates the process of alkylation.

Blood cells are particularly sensitive to alkylating agents, and bone marrow suppression is the most important adverse effect of this class. Within days after administration, the numbers of red blood cells, white blood cells, and platelets begin to decline. Epithelial cells lining the GI tract are also damaged with this class of drugs, causing nausea, vomiting, and diarrhea.

TABLE 24.2 Alkylating Agents

DRUG	ROUTE AND ADULT DOSE	REMARKS
NITROGEN MUSTARDS		
chlorambucil (Leukeran)	PO initial dose 0.1–0.2 mg/kg daily; maintenance dose 4–10 mg daily	For chronic lymphocytic leukemia, non-Hodgkin's lymphoma, and cancer of the breast and ovary
Pr cyclophosphamide (Cytoxan, Neosar)	PO initial dose 1–5 mg/kg daily; maintenance dose 1–5 mg/kg q7–10 days	For Hodgkin's disease, non-Hodgkin's lymphoma, leukemias, multiple myeloma, cancer of the breast, ovary, and lung; IV form available
estramustine (Emcyt)	PO 5 mg/kg tid–qid	For palliative treatment of advanced prostate cancer
ifosfamide (Ifex)	IV 1.2 g/m^2 daily for 5 consecutive days	For testicular cancer
mechloroethamine (Mustargen)	IV 6 mg/m^2 on days 1 and 8 of a 28-day cycle	For Hodgkin's disease, non-Hodgkin's lymphoma, and lung cancer
melphalan (Alkeran)	PO 6 mg daily for 2–3 weeks	For multiple myeloma
thiotepa (Thioplex)	IV 0.3–0.4 mg/kg q1–4 weeks	For Hodgkin's disease and breast and ovarian cancer
NITROSOUREAS		
carmustine (BiCNU, Gliadel)	IV 200 mg/m^2 q6 weeks	For Hodgkin's disease, malignant melanoma, multiple myeloma, and brain cancer; topical form for mycosis fungoides
lomustine (CeeNU)	PO 130 mg/m^2 as a single dose	For Hodgkin's disease and brain cancer
streptozocin (Zanosar)	IV 500 mg/m^2 for 5 consecutive days	For pancreatic cancer
MISCELLANEOUS ALKYLATING AGENTS		
busulfan (Myleran)	PO 4–8 mg daily	For chronic myelogenous leukemia
carboplatin (Paraplatin)	IV 360 mg/m^2 q4 weeks	For cancer of the ovary
cisplatin (Platinol)	IV 20 mg/m^2 daily for 5 days	For testicular, bladder, ovarian, uterine, head, and neck carcinomas
dacarbazine (DTIC-Dome)	IV 2–4.5 mg/kg daily for 10 days	For Hodgkin's disease and malignant melanoma
oxaliplatin (Eloxatin)	IV 85 mg/m^2 infused over 120 min once q2 weeks	For metastatic colorectal cancer
temozolomide (Temodar)	PO 150 mg/m^2 daily for 5 consecutive days	For brain cancer

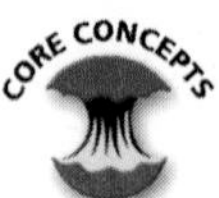

24.9 Antimetabolites act by disrupting critical cell pathways in cancer cells.

Antimetabolites interfere with aspects of the nutrient or nucleic acid metabolism of rapidly growing tumor cells. The antimetabolite drugs are shown in Table 24.3.

Rapidly growing cancer cells require large amounts of nutrients to build proteins and nucleic acids. Antimetabolites are drugs that chemically resemble essential building blocks of the cell. When cancer cells attempt to construct proteins or DNA, they use the antimetabolite drugs instead of the normal building blocks. By disrupting metabolic pathways in this manner, antimetabolites can kill cancer cells or slow their growth.

Several of these antimetabolites resemble **purines** and **pyrimidines,** chemicals that are the building blocks of DNA and RNA. These antimetabolites are called *purine* or *pyrimidine analogs.*

FIGURE 24.4

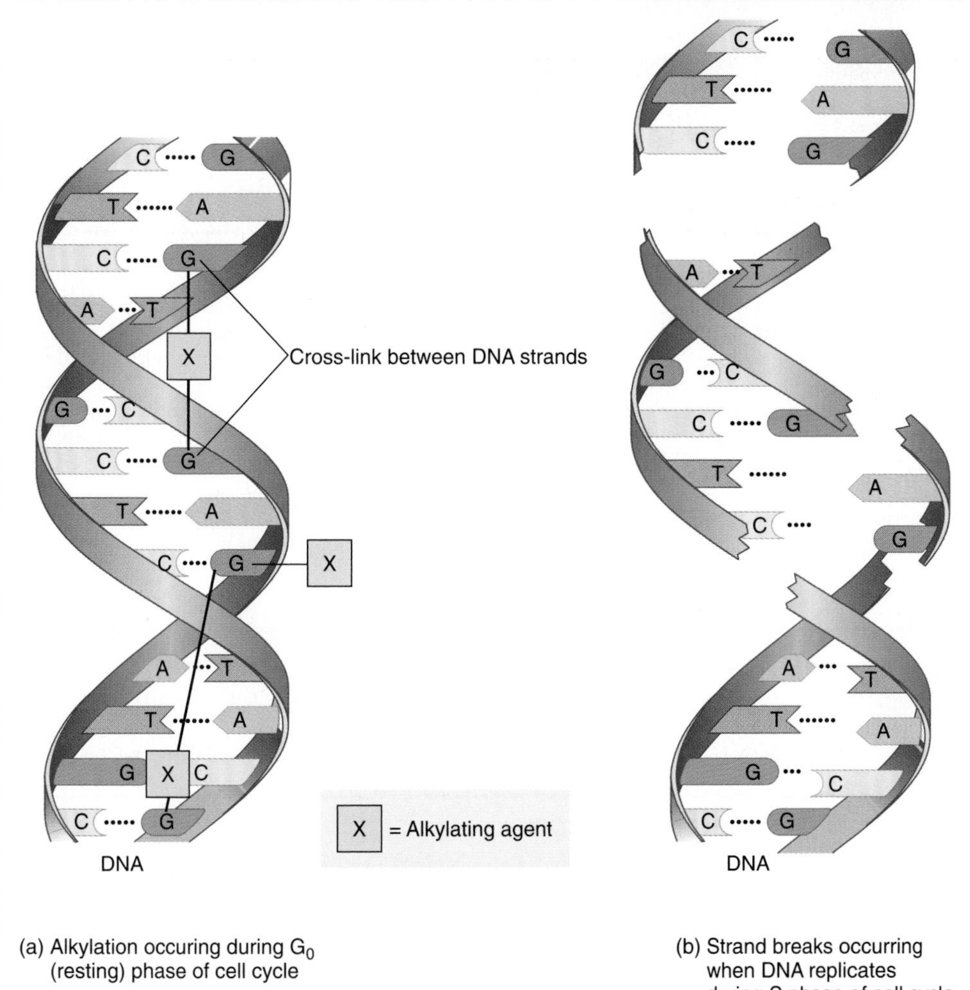

Mechanism of action of alkylating agents

DRUG PROFILE: Alkylating Agent: Pr *Cyclophosphamide (Cytoxan)*

Actions and Uses:

Cyclophosphamide is a commonly prescribed nitrogen mustard. It is used alone or in combination with other drugs against a wide variety of cancers, including Hodgkin's disease, lymphoma, multiple myeloma, breast cancer, and ovarian cancer. Cyclophosphamide acts by attaching to DNA and disrupting cell replication particularly in rapidly dividing cells. It is one of only a few anticancer drugs that are well absorbed when given orally.

Adverse Effects and Interactions:

Cyclophosphamide exerts a powerful immunosuppressant effect that peaks 1 to 2 days after administration. Thrombocytopenia is common, and thus bleeding and bruising may be observed. Nausea, vomiting, and diarrhea are frequently experienced. Cyclophosphamide damages hair follicles, causing alopecia, although this effect is usually reversible. Unlike other nitrogen mustards, cyclophosphamide causes little neurotoxicity.

Cyclophosphamide interacts with many drugs. For example, immunosuppressant agents may increase the risk of infections and further development of neoplasms. There is an increased chance of bone marrow toxicity if cyclophosphamide is used together with allopurinol. If anticoagulants are used together with cyclophosphamide, increased anticoagulant effects may occur, leading to hemorrhage.

If used with digoxin, decreased serum levels of digoxin occur. Using it with insulin may lead to increased hypoglycemia. Phenobarbital, phenytoin, or glucocorticoids may lead to an increased rate of cyclophosphamide metabolism by the liver. Thiazide diuretic use with cyclophosphamide may lead to leukopenia.

Herbal supplements, such as echinacea, which is an immune stimulator, may interfere with cyclophosphamide's immunosuppressant effects.

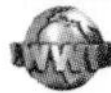
See the Companion Website for a Nursing Process Focus specific to this drug.

NURSING PROCESS FOCUS

Patients Receiving Antineoplastic Therapy

ASSESSMENT

Prior to administration:
- Obtain complete health history including lab values such as platelets, Hct, leukocyte count, liver and kidney function tests, and serum electrolytes
- Obtain drug history to determine possible drug interactions and allergies
- Assess neurological status including mood and/or sensory impairment
- Assess for history or presence of herpes zoster or chickenpox. (Immunosuppressive effects of cyclophosphamide and vincristine can cause life-threatening exacerbations.)

POTENTIAL NURSING DIAGNOSES

- Risk for Infection, related to compromised immune system
- Imbalanced Nutrition, Less than Body Requirements, related to nausea, vomiting, diarrhea, and anorexia as a result of drug side effects
- Impaired Skin Integrity, related to extravasation
- Risk for Disturbed Body Image, related to physical changes as a result of drug side effects
- Fatigue, related to side effects of drug

PLANNING: Patient Goals and Expected Outcomes

The patient will:
- Experience a reduction in tumor mass and/or progression of abnormal cell growth
- Demonstrate an understanding of the drug's action by accurately describing drug side effects, precautions, and therapeutic goals

IMPLEMENTATION

Interventions and (Rationales)	Patient Education/Discharge Planning
▪ Monitor hematological/immune status. ▪ Observe for signs and symptoms of myelosuppression. (This could be indicative of overdose.) ▪ Avoid consuming aspirin. ▪ Monitor complete blood count and temperature. ▪ Collect stool samples for guaiac testing of occult blood. (Antineoplastics may cause anemia.)	Instruct patient to: ▪ Immediately report profound fatigue, fever, sore throat, epigastric pain, coffee-grounds vomit, bruising, tarry stools, or frank bleeding ▪ Avoid persons with active infections ▪ Monitor vital signs (especially temperature) daily, ensuring proper use of home equipment ▪ Anticipate fatigue and balance daily activities to prevent exhaustion ▪ Avoid activities requiring mental alertness and physical strength until effects of the drug are known
▪ Monitor cardiorespiratory status. ▪ Monitor vital signs and chest/heart sounds. (Cyclophosphamide may cause myopericarditis and lung fibrosis. Doxorubicin may cause sinus tachycardia, cardiac depression, and delayed onset CHF.) ▪ Ensure that EKG are monitored for T-wave flattening, ST depression, or voltage reduction. ▪ Monitor for shortness of breath and pitting edema.	Instruct patient: ▪ To immediately report dyspnea; chest, arm, neck, or back pain; tachycardia; cough; frothy sputum; swelling; or activity intolerance ▪ To maintain a regular schedule of EKGs as advised by the healthcare provider ▪ That heart changes may be a sign of drug toxicity; HF may not appear for up to 6 months after completion of doxorubicin therapy
▪ Monitor renal status, urinary output, intake and output, and daily weights. (Cyclophosphamide may cause renal toxicity and/or hemorrhagic cystitis. Vincristine and methotrexate increase uric acid levels, contributing to renal calculi and gout. Vincristine may also cause water retention and highly concentrated urine.)	Instruct patient: ▪ To immediately report the following: changes in thirst; color, quantity, and character of urine (e.g., "cloudy," with odor or sediment); joint, abdominal, flank, or lower back pain; difficult urination; and weight gain ▪ That doxorubicin will turn urine red-brown for 1 to 2 days after administration; blood in the urine may occur several months after cyclophosphamide has been discontinued ▪ To consume 3 L of fluid on the day before treatment and daily for 72 hr after (when patient has no prescribed fluid restriction)

continued...

NURSING PROCESS FOCUS

Interventions and (Rationales)	Patient Education/Discharge Planning
■ Monitor GI status and nutrition. Administer antiemetics 30 to 45 minutes prior to antineoplastic administration or at the first sign of nausea. (Profound nausea, dry heaves, and/or vomiting are common with antineoplastic therapy. Dry mouth can also occur.)	Instruct patient to: ■ Report loss of appetite, nausea/vomiting, diarrhea, mouth redness, soreness, or ulcers ■ Consume frequent small meals, drink plenty of cold liquids; avoid strong odors and spicy foods to control nausea ■ Examine mouth daily for changes ■ Use a soft toothbrush; avoid toothpicks
■ Monitor for constipation. (Ileus or constipation and fecal impaction may occur with vincristine use, especially among the elderly.)	Instruct patient to: ■ Report changes in bowel habits ■ Increase activity, fiber, and fluids to reduce constipation
■ Monitor neurological/sensory status. (Antineoplastics may cause peripheral neuropathy and mental depression. Vincristine may cause ataxia and hand/foot drop. Tamoxifen may cause photophobia and decreased vision. Such neurological changes may be irreversible.)	Instruct patient to: ■ Report changes in skin color, vision, hearing, numbness or tingling, staggering gait, or depressed mood; obtain no self-harm contract ■ Limit sun exposure; wear sunscreen, sunglasses, and long sleeves when outdoors
■ Monitor genitourinary status. (Antineoplastic agents, including hormones, and especially tamoxifen, may alter menstrual cycles in women and may produce impotence in men. Tamoxifen increases the risk of endometrial cancer.)	Instruct patient to: ■ Report changes in menstruation, sexual functioning, and/or vaginal discharge ■ Recognize the risk of endometrial cancer before giving tamoxifen
■ Monitor for hypersensitivity or other adverse reactions.	■ Instruct patient to immediately report chest or throat tightness, difficulty swallowing, swelling (especially facial), abdominal pain, headache, or dizziness
■ Monitor hair and skin status. (Alopecia is associated with most chemotherapy and may be a sign of overdosage. Methotrexate can cause a variety of skin eruptions.)	Instruct patient to: ■ Immediately report desquamation of skin on hands and feet, rash, pruritus, acne, or boils ■ Wear a cold gel cap during chemotherapy to minimize hair loss
■ Monitor for conjunctivitis. (Doxorubicin may cause conjunctivitis.)	■ Instruct patient or caregiver to immediately report eye redness, stickiness, or pain or weeping
■ Monitor liver function tests. (Antineoplastics are metabolized by the liver, increasing the risk of hepatotoxicity.)	Instruct patient to: ■ Report jaundice, abdominal pain, tenderness or bloating, or change in stool color ■ Adhere to laboratory testing regimen for serum blood level tests of liver enzymes as directed
■ Administer with caution to patients with diabetes mellitus. (Hypoglycemia may occur secondary to combination of cyclophosphamide and insulin.)	Instruct patient to: ■ Report signs and symptoms of hypoglycemia (e.g., sudden weakness, tremors) ■ Monitor blood glucose daily; consult the healthcare provider regarding reportable results (e.g., less than 70 mg/dl)

EVALUATION OF OUTCOME CRITERIA

Evaluate the effectiveness of drug therapy by confirming that patient goals and expected outcomes have been met (see "Planning").

See Tables 24.2–24.7 for lists of drugs to which these nursing actions apply.

TABLE 24.3 Antimetabolites

DRUG	ROUTE AND ADULT DOSE	REMARKS
FOLIC ACID ANTAGONIST		
Pr methotrexate (Amethopterin, Folex, Mexate, Trexall, Rheumatrex)	IV 15–30 mg daily for 5 days	For acute lymphoblastic leukemia, choriocarcinoma, lymphoma, head and neck cancer, testicular cancer, bone cancer; oral and IM forms available
pemetrexed (Alimta)	IV 500 mg/m^2 on day 1 of each 21 day cycle	For malignant mesothelioma and non-small cell lung cancer
PYRIMIDINE ANALOGS		
capecitabine (Xeloda)	PO 2500 mg/m^2 daily for 2 weeks	For breast cancer
cytarabine (ARA-C, Cytosar-U, Tarabine, DepoCyt)	IV 200 mg/m^2 as a continuous infusion over 24 hours	For acute myelogenous leukemia; subcutaneous and intrathecal forms available
floxuridine (FUDR)	Intra-arterial; 0.1–0.6 mg/kg daily as a continuous infusion	For GI metastasis to the liver
fluorouracil (5-FU, Adrucil, Efudex, Fluorodex)	IV 12 mg/kg daily for 4 consecutive days	For cancer of the breast, colon, rectum, stomach, and pancreas; topical form available for basal cell carcinoma
gemcitabine (Gemzar)	IV 1000 mg/m^2 q week	For cancer of the pancreas and lung
PURINE ANALOGS		
cladribine (Leustatin)	IV 0.09 mg/m^2 daily as a continuous infusion	For hairy cell leukemia
clofarabine (Clolar)	IV 52 mg/m^2 over 2h for 5 consecutive days	For childhood acute lymphoblastic leukemia
fludarabine (Fludara)	IV 25 mg/m^2 daily for 5 consecutive days	For chronic lymphocytic leukemia
mercaptopurine (6-MP, Purinsthol)	PO 2.5 mg/kg daily	For childhood acute leukemia
pentostatin (Nipent)	IV 4 mg/m^2 q other week	For hairy cell leukemia
thioguanine (TG)	PO 2 mg/kg daily	For remission induction in adult acute leukemia

For example, floxuridine (FUDR) and fluorouracil (Adrucil) are able to block the formation of thymidylate, an essential chemical needed to make DNA. After becoming activated and incorporated into DNA, cytarabine (Cytosar) blocks DNA synthesis. Figure 24.5 ■ illustrates the similarities of some of these analogs to their natural counterparts.

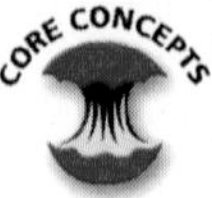

24.10 Because of their cytotoxicity, a few antibiotics are used to treat cancer rather than infections.

Antitumor antibiotics are antineoplastic drugs obtained from bacteria that have the ability to kill cancer cells. Although they are not widely prescribed, they are very effective against certain tumors. Table 24.4 lists the primary antitumor antibiotics.

A number of substances isolated from bacteria have been found to have antitumor properties. These chemicals are more toxic than the traditional antibiotics; thus, their use is restricted to treating specific cancers. All the antitumor antibiotics interact with DNA in a manner similar to the alkylating agents. Because of this, their general actions and side effects are similar to those of the alkylating agents. Unlike the alkylating agents, however, all the antitumor antibiotics must be administered intravenously or through direct instillation into a body cavity using a catheter.

FIGURE 24.5

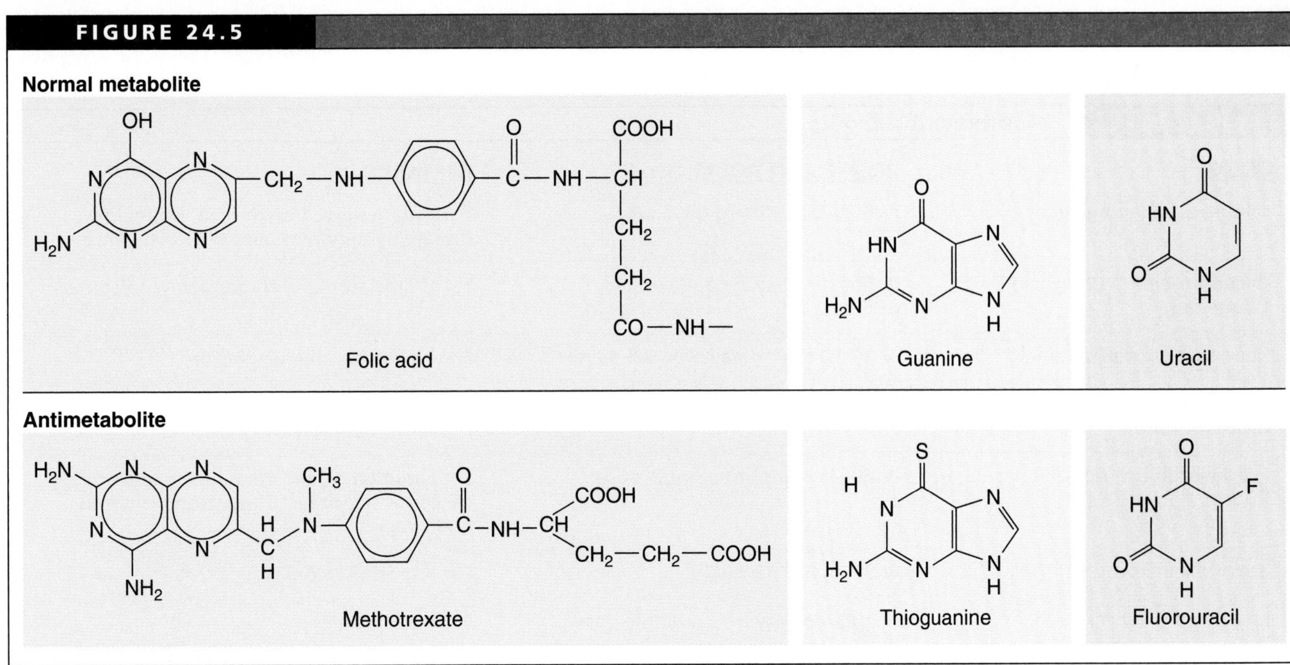

Structural similarities between antimetabolites and their natural counterparts

DRUG PROFILE: Antimetabolite: Pr *Methotrexate (Folex, Mexate, and others)*

Actions and Uses:

Methotrexate is classified as an antifolate because it inhibits folic acid metabolism. **Folic acid** is a water-soluble vitamin found in eggs, veal, liver, whole grains, and dark green vegetables. Folic acid is part of a coenzyme essential to the synthesis of nucleic acids.

Methotrexate is prescribed alone or in combination with other drugs for choriocarcinoma, bone cancers, leukemias, head and neck cancers, breast carcinoma, and lung carcinoma. It is occasionally used to treat non-neoplastic disorders such as severe psoriasis and rheumatoid arthritis that are unresponsive to other medications.

Adverse Effects and Interactions:

Like many antineoplastics, methotrexate is a potent immunosuppressant. Hemorrhage and bruising due to low platelet counts are often observed. Nausea, vomiting, and anorexia are common. Although rare, pulmonary toxicity may develop and be quite serious. Methotrexate is a pregnancy category X drug.

Methotrexate interacts with several drugs. Bone marrow suppressants such as other antineoplastic agents or radiation therapy may cause increased effects; the patient will require a lower dose of methotrexate. When used with NSAIDs, severe methotrexate toxicity may occur. Aspirin may interfere with excretion of methotrexate, leading to increased serum levels and toxicity. Administration with live oral vaccine may result in decreased antibody response and increased adverse reactions to the vaccine. Use with caution with herbal supplements, such as echinacea, which may interfere with the drug's immunosuppressant effects.

Mechanism in Action: 

Methotrexate interferes with the synthesis of folate. Folate is necessary for the synthesis of DNA, RNA, and protein in rapidly dividing cancer cells. By blocking the synthesis of folic acid, methotrexate is able to inhibit replication, particularly in rapidly dividing cells.

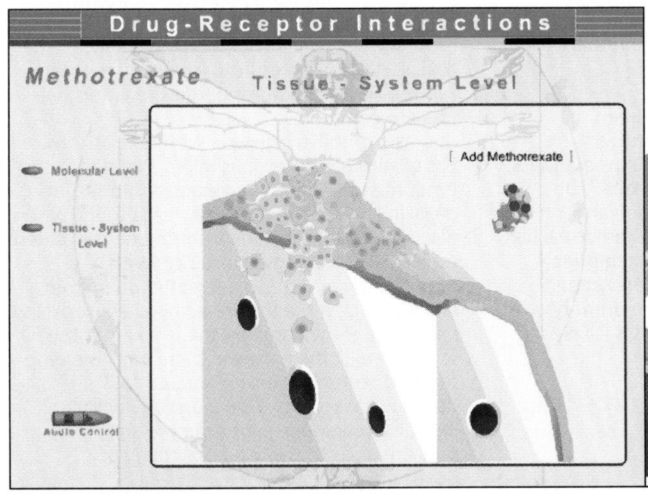

Use the student CD-ROM to see Mechanism in Action for Methotrexate.

See the Companion Website for a Nursing Process Focus specific to this drug.

TABLE 24.4 Antitumor Antibiotics

DRUG	ROUTE AND ADULT DOSE	REMARKS
bleomycin (Blenoxane)	IV 0.25–0.5 units/kg q4–7 days	For squamous cell carcinoma, Hodgkin's disease, lymphomas, and testicular cancer
dactinomycin (Actinomycin D, Cosmegan)	IV 500 mcg/day for a maximum of 5 days	For Wilms' tumor and rhabdomyosarcoma
daunorubicin (Cerubidine)	IV 30–60 mg/m^2 daily for 3–5 days	For leukemias and lymphomas
daunorubicin liposomal (DaunoXsome)	IV 40 mg/m^2 q2 weeks	For Kaposi's sarcoma
Pr doxorubicin (Adriamycin, Rubex)	IV 60–75 mg/m^2 as a single dose	For lymphomas, sarcomas, acute leukemia, cancer of the breast, lung, testes, thyroid, and ovary
doxorubicin liposomal (Doxil)	IV 20 mg/m^2 q3 weeks	For Kaposi's sarcoma
epirubicin (Ellence)	IV 100–120 mg/m^2 as a single dose	For breast cancer
idarubicin (Idamycin)	IV 8–12 mg/m^2 daily for 3 days	For acute myelogenous leukemia
mitomycin (Mutamycin)	IV 2 mg/m^2 as a single dose	For cancer of the colon, stomach, lung, head and neck, rectum, bladder, pancreas, and breast; also for malignant melanoma
mitoxantrone (Novantrone)	IV 12 mg/m^2 daily for 3 days	For acute nonlymphocytic leukemia
plicamycin (Mithramycin, Mithracin)	IV 25–30 mcg/kg daily for 8–10 days	For testicular cancer; also used to manage hypercalcemia
valrubicin (Valstar)	Intrabladder instillation; 800 mg q week for 6 weeks	For bladder cancer

DRUG PROFILE: Antitumor Antibiotic: Pr *Doxorubicin (Adriamycin)*

Actions and Uses:

Doxorubicin attaches to DNA, causing the double strands to be distorted, thus preventing cancer cell division. It is prescribed for solid tumors of the lung, breast, ovary, and bladder, and for various leukemias and lymphomas. It is structurally similar to daunorubicin (Cerubidine).

A novel delivery method has been developed for both doxorubicin and daunorubicin. The drug is enclosed in small sacs, or vesicles, of lipids called **liposomes.** The liposomal vesicle is designed to open and release the antitumor antibiotic when it reaches a cancer cell. The goal is to deliver a higher concentration of drug directly to the cancer cells, thus sparing normal cells. The primary indication for this delivery method is AIDS-related Kaposi's sarcoma.

Adverse Effects and Interactions:

Like many of the anticancer medications, doxorubicin may seriously lower blood cell counts. Leaking from an injection site can cause severe pain and tissue damage. The most serious concern is delayed cardiac toxicity that may result in irreversible heart failure. Nausea, vomiting, diarrhea, and hair loss are common.

Doxorubicin interacts with many drugs. For example, if digoxin is taken at the same time, the patient will have decreased serum digoxin levels. Phenobarbital leads to increased plasma clearance of doxorubicin and decreased effectiveness. Using doxorubicin with phenytoin may lead to decreased phenytoin levels and possible seizure activity. Liver toxicity may occur if mercaptopurine is taken at the same time. Using with verapamil may increase serum doxorubicin levels, leading to doxorubicin toxicity. Use cautiously with herbal supplements. For example, green tea may enhance the antitumor activity of doxorubicin.

See the Companion Website for a Nursing Process Focus specific to this drug.

TABLE 24.5	Plant Extracts/Natural Products	
DRUG	ROUTE AND ADULT DOSE	REMARKS
MITOTIC INHIBITORS		
vinblastine (Velban)	IV 3.7–18.5 mg/m^2 q week	For cancer of the breast and testicles; Hodgkin's disease
Pr vincristine (Oncovin)	IV 1.4 mg/m^2 q week (max: 2 mg/m^2)	For lymphomas, Hodgkin's disease, Wilms' tumor, and childhood acute leukemia
vinorelbine (Navelbine)	IV 30 mg/m^2 q week	For lung cancer
TAXOIDS		
docetaxel (Taxotere)	IV 60–100 mg/m^2 q3 weeks	For breast cancer
paclitaxel (Taxol)	IV 135–175 mg/m^2 q3 weeks	For ovarian and breast cancer
TOPOISOMERASE INHIBITORS		
topotecan (Hycamtin)	IV 1.5 mg/m^2 daily for 5 days	For ovarian cancer
etoposide (VePesid)	IV 50–100 mg/m^2 daily for 5 days	For testicular and lung cancer; choriocarcinomas; PO form available
teniposide (Vumon)	IV 165 mg/m^2 q 3–4 days for 4 weeks	For acute lymphocytic leukemia
irinotecan (Camptosar)	IV 125 mg/m^2 q week for 4 weeks	For colorectal cancer

24.11 Some plant extracts kill cancer cells by preventing cell division.

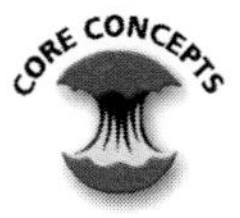

Plants have been a valuable source for antineoplastic agents. The primary plant extracts or alkaloids, used as antineoplastics, are shown in Table 24.5.

Chemicals with antineoplastic activity have been isolated from a number of plants, including the common periwinkle (*Vinca rosea*), the Pacific yew, the mandrake plant (May apple), and the shrub *Campothecus accuminata.* Although structurally very different, drugs in this class have the common ability to arrest cell division; thus they are sometimes called *mitotic inhibitors.*

The **vinca alkaloids,** vincristine (Oncovin) and vinblastine (Velban), are older medications derived from the periwinkle plant. Their biological properties were described in folklore for many years in various parts of the world prior to their use as anticancer drugs. Similarly, American Indians described uses of the May apple long before teniposide (Vumon) and etoposide (VePesid) were isolated from this plant and used for chemotherapy.

The **taxoids,** which include paclitaxel (Taxol) and docetaxel (Taxotere), were isolated from the Pacific yew, an evergreen found throughout the Western United States. Other recently isolated chemotherapeutic agents include topotecan (Hycamtin) and irinotecan (Camptosar). These agents are called **topoisomerase** inhibitors because they block the enzyme topoisomerase that helps repair DNA damage. Bone marrow suppression is a serious adverse effect of most natural product drugs.

24.12 Some hormones and hormone antagonists are effective against prostate and breast cancer.

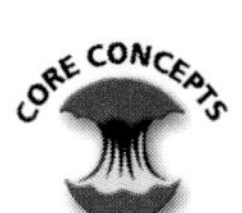

Use of natural or synthetic hormones or their antagonists as antineoplastic agents is a strategy used to slow the growth of hormone-dependent tumors. The major hormones and hormone blockers prescribed for cancer are given in Table 24.6.

The growth of certain tumors of reproductive tissues is greatly stimulated by natural hormones. Administering high doses of specific hormones or hormone antagonists can block these

TABLE 24.6 Hormones and Hormone Antagonists

DRUG	ROUTE AND ADULT DOSE	REMARKS
HORMONES		
diethylstilbestrol (DES, Stilbestrol)	PO for treatment of prostate cancer, 500 mg tid; for palliation, 1–15 mg daily	For cancer of the prostate and breast
ethinyl estradiol (Estinyl)	PO for treatment of breast cancer, 1 mg tid for 2–3 mos; for palliation of prostate cancer, 0.15–3 mg/day	For cancer of the prostate and breast
fluoxymesterone (Halotestin)	PO 10 mg tid	For breast cancer
medroxyprogesterone (Provera, Depo-Provera)	IM 400–1000 mg q week	For uterine and renal cancer
megestrol (Megace)	PO 40–160 mg bid–qid	For advanced cancer of the prostate and breast
prednisone (Deltasone, others)	PO 20–100 mg/m^2 daily	For acute leukemia, Hodgkin's disease, lymphomas
testolactone (Teslac)	PO 250 mg qid	For breast cancer
testosterone (Andro 100, Histerone, Testred, Delatest)	IM 200–400 mg q2–4 weeks	For breast cancer
HORMONE ANTAGONISTS		
abarelix (Plenaxis)	IM 100mg on day 1, 15, 29 and every 2 weeks thereafter	For palliative treatment of advanced prostate cancer
aminoglutethimide (Cytadren)	PO 250 mg bid–qid	For prostate, breast, adrenal cancer; must administer hydrocortisone in conjunction with this drug
anastrozole (Arimidex)	PO 1 mg daily	For advanced breast cancer
bicalutamide (Casodex)	PO 50 mg daily	For advanced prostate cancer
exemestane (Aromasin)	PO 25 mg daily after a meal	For advanced breast cancer
flutamide (Eulexin)	PO 250 mg tid	For prostate cancer
goserelin (Zoladex)	Subcutaneous 3.6 mg q28 days	For cancer of the prostate and breast
letrozole (Femara)	PO 2.5 mg daily	For advanced breast cancer
leuprolide (Lupron)	Subcutaneous 1 mg daily	For advanced prostate cancer
nilutamide (Nilandron)	PO 300 mg/daily for 30 days, then 150 mg daily	For metastatic prostate cancer
Pr tamoxifen (Nolvadex)	PO 10–20 mg bid	For breast cancer
toremifene (Fareston)	PO 60 mg daily	For metastatic breast cancer

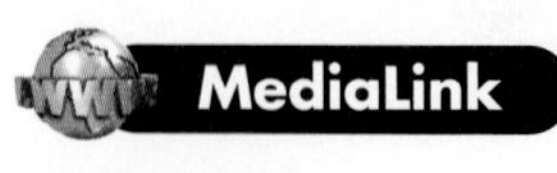

CLINICAL TRIALS

receptors and slow tumor growth. For example, administering the male hormone testosterone or the antiestrogen drug tamoxifen (Nolvadex) can slow specific types of breast cancer that depend on estrogen for growth. Tamoxifen is one of the most widely used drugs for this type of cancer. Administration of the female hormone estrogen slows the growth of prostate cancer. The other major class of hormones used for chemotherapy are the corticosteroids. When used for chemotherapy, the doses

DRUG PROFILE: Plant Extract: Pr *Vincristine (Oncovin)*

Actions and Uses:

Vincristine affects rapidly growing cells by inhibiting their ability to complete mitosis. Although it must be given IV, a major advantage of vincristine is that it causes minimal immunosuppression. It is usually prescribed in combination with other antineoplastics for the treatment of lymphoma, leukemias, Kaposi's sarcoma, Wilms' tumor, bladder carcinoma, and breast carcinoma.

Adverse Effects and Interactions:

The most serious limiting adverse effects of vincristine relate to nervous system toxicity. Symptoms include numbness and tingling in the limbs, muscular weakness, loss of neural reflexes, and pain. Severe constipation is common. Immunosuppression may occur, though it is less serious than with vinblastine, the other vinca alkaloid. Reversible alopecia occurs in most patients.

Vincristine interacts with many drugs. For example, asparaginase used together with or before vincristine may cause increased neurotoxicity secondary to decreased liver clearance of vincristine. Doxorubicin or prednisone may increase bone marrow depression. Calcium channel blockers may increase vincristine accumulation in cells. When used with digoxin, the patient may need an increased digoxin dose. When vincristine is given with methotrexate, the patient may need lower doses of methotrexate. Vincristine may decrease serum phenytoin levels, leading to increased seizure activity.

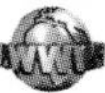
See the Companion Website for a Nursing Process Focus specific to this drug.

of these hormones are much higher than the levels normally found in the body. Additional indications for hormone pharmacotherapy are discussed in Chapters 29 and 30.

In general, hormones and hormone antagonists produce few of the cytotoxic side effects seen with other antineoplastics. They can, however, produce serious side effects when given at high doses for long periods. They are normally given for palliation because they rarely produce cancer cures when used singly.

DRUG PROFILE: Hormone Antagonist: Pr *Tamoxifen (Nolvadex)*

Actions and Uses:

Because it blocks estrogen receptors in cancer cells, tamoxifen is sometimes classified as an antiestrogenic agent. Tamoxifen is effective against breast tumors that require estrogen for their growth. These susceptible cancer cells are known as ER (estrogen receptor)-positive cells. The drug is unique among antineoplastics because it is not only given to patients with breast cancer, it is also given to high-risk patients to prevent the disease. Few if any other antineoplastics are given prophylactically because of their toxicity. Tamoxifen is given orally and is a drug of choice for treating breast cancer.

Adverse Effects and Interactions:

Other than nausea and vomiting, tamoxifen produces little of the serious toxicity observed with other antineoplastics. Of concern, however, is the association of tamoxifen therapy with an increased risk of uterine cancer. Hot flashes, fluid retention, venous blood clots, and abnormal vaginal bleeding are relatively common.

Tamoxifen interacts with several other drugs. For example, anticoagulants may increase the risk of bleeding. Using this drug with cytotoxic agents may increase the risk of thromboembolism.

See the Companion Website for a Nursing Process Focus specific to this drug.

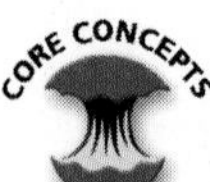

24.13 Biologic response modifiers and some additional antineoplastic drugs are effective against specific tumors.

A number of anticancer drugs act through mechanisms other than those previously described. For example, asparaginase deprives cancer cells of an essential amino acid. Mitotane (Lysodren) is similar to the insecticide DDT and poisons cancer cells by forming links to proteins. The uses of these miscellaneous antineoplastics are given in Table 24.7.

Biologic response modifiers are a relatively new class of drugs that do not kill tumor cells directly but instead stimulate the body's immune system to fight the cancer. These treatments are sometimes called immunotherapy. Some of the biologic response modifiers are given to minimize the toxic effects of other antineoplastics. For example, filgastrim (Neupogen) limits immunosuppressive effects.

Some miscellaneous drugs are given to limit or counteract the toxicity of antineoplastics. Oprelvekin (Neumega) stimulates platelet production and helps to prevent severe thrombocytopenia. Epoetin alfa (Epogen, Procrit) stimulates red blood cell production and is used to limit the anemia caused by certain antineoplastics. Further information about this drug follows.

Patients with neoplastic disorders have a high frequency of **hematopoietic** abnormalities. Anemia is one of the most common and important abnormalities, especially in patients undergoing chemotherapy. Hematopoietic abnormalities also occur in patients with AIDS, chronic renal failure, and older patients. The drug epoetin alfa (Epogen, Procrit) has significantly improved the quality of life for these patients. Although this drug does not cure the primary dis-

TABLE 24.7 Biologic Response Modifiers and Miscellaneous Anticancer Drugs

DRUG	ROUTE AND ADULT DOSE	REMARKS
altretamine (Hexalen)	PO 65 mg/m^2 four times a day	For ovarian cancer
asparaginase (Elspar)	IV 200 units/kg daily	For acute lymphocytic leukemia
bevacizumab (Avastin)	IV 5 mg/kg q14 days	For metastatic colorectal cancer
cetuximab (Erbitux)	IV 400 mg/m^2 over 2h, then 250 mg/m^2 over 1 hr weekly	For metastatic colorectal cancer
erlotinib (Tarceva)	PO 150 mg once daily	For metastatic non-small cell lung cancer
hydroxyurea (Hydrea)	PO 20–30 mg/kg daily	For palliative treatment of malignant melanoma and chronic granulocytic leukemia
imatinib (Gleevec)	PO 400–600 mg daily	For chronic myeloid leukemia after failure with interferon alfa therapy
Pr interferon alfa-2 (Roferon-A, Intron A)	Subcutaneous or IM 2–3 million units daily for leukemia; 36 million units daily for Kaposi's sarcoma	For hairy cell leukemia and Kaposi's sarcoma; also for hepatitis and other viral disorders
levamisole (Ergamisol)	PO 50 mg tid for 3 days	For colon cancer
mitotane (Lysodren)	PO 3–4 mg tid–qid	For adrenal cortex cancer
pegaspargase (Oncaspar, PEG-L-asparaginase)	IV 2500 IU/m^2 q14 days	For acute lymphocytic leukemia; IM form available
procarbazine (Matulane)	PO 2–4 mg/kg daily	For Hodgkin's disease
rituximab (Rituxan)	IV 375 mg/m^2 daily as a continuous infusion	For non-Hodgkin's lymphomas
trastuzumab (Herceptin)	IV 4 mg/kg as a single dose, then 2 mg/kg q week	For metastatic breast cancer

DRUG PROFILE: Biologic Response Modifier: Pr *Interferon alfa-2 (Roferon A, Intron A)*

Actions and Uses:

Interferon alfa-2 is a biologic response modifier that consists of two similar drugs; interferon alfa-2a (Roferon-A) and interferon alpha-2b (Intron A). Interferon alpha-2b is a natural protein that is produced by human lymphocytes 4 to 6 hours after viral stimulation. Large amounts of this drug are obtained through recombinant DNA technology in which the human gene for interferon alpha-2b has been spliced into the bacterium *Escherichia coli*. Interferon alpha-2b affects cancer cells by two mechanisms. First, it enhances or stimulates the immune system to remove more antigens. Second, the drug suppresses the growth of cancer cells. As expected from its origin, interferon alfa-2 also has antiviral activity.

Adverse Effects and Interactions:

Like most biologic response modifiers, the most common side effect is a flu-like syndrome of fever, chills, dizziness, and fatigue that usually diminishes as therapy progresses. Nausea, vomiting, diarrhea, and anorexia are relatively common. With prolonged therapy, more serious toxicity such as immunosuppression, hepatotoxicity, and neurotoxicity may be observed.

This drug may increase theophylline levels. Use with other antineoplastics may increase myelosuppression. Zidovudine can increase hematologic toxicity. Interferon alfa-2 can increase doxorubicin toxicity. Neurotoxicity is increased if this drug is used with vinblastine.

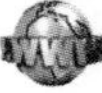

See the Companion Website for a Nursing Process Focus specific to this drug.

ease condition, it helps reduce the anemia that dramatically affects the patient's ability to perform daily activities.

Concept Review 24.3

- Why are the biologic response modifiers less toxic to normal body cells than other antineoplastics?

DRUG PROFILE: Hematopoietic Growth Factor: Pr Epoetin Alfa (Epogen, Procrit)

Actions and Uses:

Epoetin alfa is made through recombinant DNA technology and functions like human erythropoietin. Because of its ability to stimulate red blood cell formation, epoetin alfa is effective in treating specific disorders caused by a deficiency in the number of red blood cells: Patients with chronic renal failure often cannot secrete enough erythropoietin, and thus will benefit from epoetin administration. Epoetin is sometimes given to patients undergoing cancer chemotherapy, to counteract the anemia caused by antineoplastic agents. It is occasionally prescribed for patients prior to blood transfusions or surgery and to treat anemia in HIV-infected patients. Epoetin alfa is usually administered three times per week until a therapeutic response is achieved.

Adverse Effects and Interactions:

The most common adverse effect of epoetin alfa is hypertension, which may occur in as many as 30% of patients receiving the drug. Blood pressure should be monitored during therapy, and an anti-hypertensive drug may be indicated. The risk of thromboembolic events is increased.

Patients who are on dialysis may require increased doses of heparin. Transient ischemic attacks (TIAs), heart attacks, and strokes have occurred in chronic renal failure patients on dialysis who are also being treated with epoetin alfa.

The effectiveness of epoetin alfa will be greatly reduced in patients with iron deficiency or other vitamin depleted states, because erythropoiesis cannot be enhanced without these vital nutrients.

There are no clinically significant drug interactions with epoetin alfa.

See the Companion Website for a Nursing Process Focus specific to this drug.

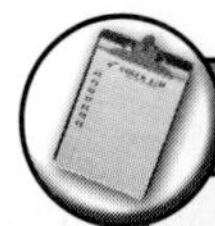

PATIENTS NEED TO KNOW

Patients treated for cancer need to know the following:

1. If hair loss is expected, cut long hair and be fitted for a wig or hairpiece before starting treatment. Select hats, scarves, or turbans. Use mild shampoo and conditioner.
2. Limit sun exposure; wear sunscreen, sunglasses, and long sleeves when outdoors. When hair is lost, protect the scalp from sunburn with sunscreen or a hat.
3. Eat foods that appeal in small amounts at frequent intervals if appetite is decreased. A healthcare provider may provide an appetite stimulant such as megestrol acetate (Megace).
4. Discuss drugs to control nausea with a practitioner if nausea is a problem. Drink liquids between meals rather than with food.
5. As the mouth may become irritated or ulcerated, avoid alcohol-based mouthwash, and use plain water or mild salt solution instead. Use a soft toothbrush. Avoid spicy foods and very hot or very cold food and drink. Ask about a mouth rinse to coat, soothe, and numb, such as BMX (Benadryl, Maalox, and xylocaine).
6. Because chemotherapy may decrease sperm production or increase the risk of genetic damage to sperm, consider sperm banking prior to receiving chemotherapy.
7. Increase fluid intake to decrease the risk of kidney damage and uric acid crystal formation.
8. Avoid exposure to crowds and individuals with infections or recent vaccinations because the immune system may be less able to protect you. Report temperatures of 101°F or higher.
9. Follow a neutropenic diet if white blood cell count is significantly reduced. Avoid raw fruits and vegetables, peppercorns, and raw fish and meat.
10. Report easy bruising, blood in the stool or urine, vomiting, severe fatigue, epigastric pain, and difficulty clotting. Many chemotherapeutic agents reduce platelet production needed for clot formation. ■

CHAPTER REVIEW

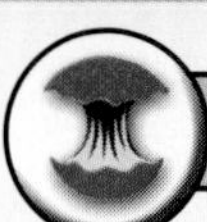

CORE CONCEPTS SUMMARY

24.1 Cancer is characterized by rapid, uncontrolled growth of cells.

Cancer cells grow rapidly, seemingly unaffected by their host surroundings. Cancer cells continue dividing until they invade normal tissues and eventually metastasize. Benign neoplasms grow slowly and rarely result in death. Malignant neoplasms, also known as cancer, are fast-growing and often fatal.

24.2 The causes of cancer may be chemical, physical, or biological.

Many factors have been found to cause or promote cancer. These include industrial chemicals, X-rays, UV light, and viruses. The genetic make-up of the patient plays an important role in whether or not cancer will develop after exposure to carcinogens.

24.3 Personal risk of cancer may be lowered by a number of lifestyle factors.

Eliminating tobacco use and limiting the intake of saturated fats and alcohol are important factors in reducing the risk of contracting cancer. Periodic self-examinations and physician check-ups are important in catching cancer at an early, more treatable stage.

24.4 Cancer may be treated using surgery, radiation therapy, and drugs.

Drugs are only one means of treating cancer. If the tumor is solid and located in a single area, surgical removal is sometimes needed. Radiation therapy may be used to kill microscopic cancer cells left behind following surgery or to shrink the size of inoperable tumors.

24.5 To achieve a total cure, every malignant cell must be removed or killed.

A single cancer cell may be able to divide rapidly enough to kill its host. Therefore, to achieve a complete cure, every single cancer cell must be eliminated through surgery, radiation, drugs, or by the patient's immune system.

24.6 Use of multiple drugs and special dosing schedules improve the success of chemotherapy.

Combinations of antineoplastic drugs are often used to attack cancer cells through several different mechanisms and to allow lower doses than if a single agent were used. The schedule of drug administration is critical to the success of the chemotherapy.

24.7 Serious toxicity limits most of the antineoplastic agents.

Antineoplastic drugs are among the most toxic medications available. Adverse effects are expected and may be severe. Whereas each agent has somewhat different toxicity, common adverse effects include thrombocytopenia, anemia, leukopenia, alopecia, severe nausea, vomiting, and diarrhea.

24.8 Alkylating agents act by changing the structure of DNA in cancer cells.

Alkylating agents are some of the oldest and most reliable of the antineoplastic drugs. By attaching to DNA, they prevent the cancer cell from replicating.

24.9 Antimetabolites act by disrupting critical cell pathways in cancer cells.

Antimetabolites block a specific step in cancer cell metabolism. By blocking the synthesis of critical cellular molecules, the drugs can slow the growth of cancer cells.

24.10 Because of their cytotoxicity, a few antibiotics are used to treat cancer rather than infections.

Antitumor antibiotics attach to the DNA of cancer cells, thereby inhibiting their growth. Their properties and side effects resemble those of the alkylating agents.

24.11 Some plant extracts kill cancer cells by preventing cell division.

Natural products of the periwinkle plant and the Pacific yew have provided several important antineoplastic agents. Drugs in this class also include the topoisomerase inhibitors.

24.12 Some hormones and hormone antagonists are effective against prostate and breast cancer.

A number of estrogens, androgens, corticosteroids, and hormone inhibitors have antitumor activity. They have very specific uses, usually for tumors of reproductive-related organs such as the breast, prostate, or uterus.

24.13 Biologic response modifiers and some additional antineoplastic drugs are effective against specific tumors.

Biologic response modifiers are a small group of drugs used to stimulate the immune system. Although much research has focused on this approach to chemotherapy, these drugs have only limited success.

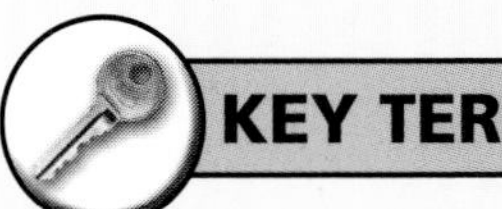

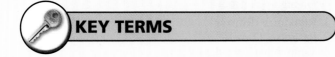

KEY TERMS

adenoma (AH-den-OH-mah): benign tumor of glandular tissue / *page 444*

alkylation (AL-kill-AYE-shun): process by which certain chemicals attach to DNA and change its structure and function / *page 449*

alopecia (AL-oh-PEESH-ee-uh): hair loss / *page 449*

anemia (ah-NEE-mee-ah): shortage of functional red blood cells / *page 449*

benign (bee-NINE): neither life-threatening nor fatal / *page 444*

biologic response modifiers: natural substances that are able to enhance or stimulate the immune system / *page 460*

cancer (KAN-sir): malignant disease characterized by rapidly growing, invasive cells that spread to other regions of the body and eventually kill the host / *page 444*

carcinogen (kar-SIN-oh-jen): any physical, chemical, or biological factor that causes or promotes cancer / *page 445*

chemotherapy: drug treatment of cancer / *page 446*

folic acid (FOH-lik): water-soluble vitamin that is part of a coenzyme essential to the synthesis of nucleic acids / *page 455*

glioma (glee-OH-muh): malignant tumor of the brain / *page 444*

hematopoietic (HEE-mah-toe-poy-ETIK): related to the number of blood cells / *page 460*

leukemia (lew-KEE-mee-ah): cancer of the blood characterized by overproduction of white blood cells / *page 444*

lipoma (lip-OH-mah): benign tumor of fat tissue / *page 444*

liposomes (LIP-oh-sohms): small sacs of lipids designed to carry drugs inside them / *page 456*

lymphoma (lim-FOH-mah): cancer of lymphatic tissue / *page 444*

malignant (mah-LIG-nent): life-threatening or fatal / *page 444*

metastasis (mah-TAS-tah-sis): travel of cancer cells from their original site to a distant tissue / *page 444*

nitrogen mustards: class of chemicals that are alkylating agents / *page 449*

neoplasm (NEE-oh-PLAZ-um): same as *tumor;* an abnormal swelling or mass / *page 444*

oncogenes (ON-koh-jeans): genes responsible for the conversion of normal cells into cancer cells / *page 445*

palliation (PAL-ee-AYE-shun): form of chemotherapy intended to alleviate symptoms rather than cure the disease / *page 446*

purine (PYUR-een): building block of DNA and RNA, either adenine or guanine / *page 450*

pyrimidine (peer-IM-uh-deen): building block of DNA and RNA, either thymine or cytosine in DNA, and cytosine and uracil in RNA / *page 450*

radiation therapy: the delivery of high-dose radiation with the intent of killing tumor cells / ***page 446***

taxoids (TAKS-oids): antineoplastic drugs obtained from the Pacific yew tree / ***page 457***

topoisomerase (TOH-poh-eye-SOM-er-ase): enzyme that assists in the repair of DNA damage / ***page 457***

tumor (TOO-more): abnormal swelling or mass / ***page 444***

tumor suppressor genes: genes that inhibit the transformation of normal cells into cancer cells / ***page 445***

vinca alkaloids (VIN-ka AL-kah-loids): chemicals obtained from the periwinkle plant / ***page 457***

REVIEW QUESTIONS

The following questions are written in NCLEX-PN® style. Answer these questions to assess your knowledge of the chapter material, and go back and review any material that is not clear to you.

1. When should the nurse administer antiemetic drugs to a patient receiving chemotherapy?

1. When vomiting occurs
2. Once the treatment is completed
3. Prior to treatment
4. Only if the patient requests to be medicated

2. The patient with testicular cancer is receiving cisplatin (Platinol) IV. The healthcare provider understands that she must assess for:

1. Irreversible heart failure
2. Bone marrow suppression
3. Cardiac toxicity
4. Peripheral neuropathy

3. Which classification of antineoplastic drugs functions to disrupt metabolic pathways to kill or slow cancer growth?

1. Biologic response modifiers
2. Plant alkaloids
3. Antitumor antibiotics
4. Antimetabolites

4. The patient with breast cancer has been receiving IV doxorubicin (Adriamycin). The patient is now complaining of severe pain at the injection site. The nurse understands that the following most likely occurred:

1. An allergic reaction
2. Leaking at the injection site
3. Loss of neural reflexes
4. Development of a blood clot

5. The prostate cancer patient is receiving leuprolide (Lupron). This is what type of antineoplastic drug?

1. Hormone/hormone antagonist
2. Antitumor antibiotic
3. Alkylating agent
4. Antimetabolite

6. The patient on cyclosphosphamide (Cytoxan) should be taught:

1. That alopecia is irreversible
2. About signs and symptoms of neurotoxicity
3. About signs and symptoms of renal toxicity
4. That nausea, vomiting, and diarrhea may occur 1 or 2 days after treatment

7. Rheumatoid arthritis may be treated with which of the following antineoplastic agents?

1. Fluorouracil (5-FU)
2. Methotrexate (Mexate)
3. Tamoxifen (Nolvadex)
4. Leuprolide (Lupron)

8. This antineoplastic drug is given to prevent breast cancer in high-risk patients.

1. Rituximab (Rituxan)
2. Paclitaxel (Taxol)
3. Tamoxifen (Nolvadex)
4. Vincristine (Oncovin)

9. The patient with a decreased white blood cell count should be instructed to:

1. Use alcohol-based mouthwash for mouth sores
2. Increase liquid intake with meals
3. Avoid raw foods
4. Ask his physician about ordering megestrol acetate (Megace)

10. The patient on tamoxifen (Nolvadex) must be assessed for:

1. Flu-like symptoms
2. Uterine cancer
3. Alopecia
4. Thrombocytopenia

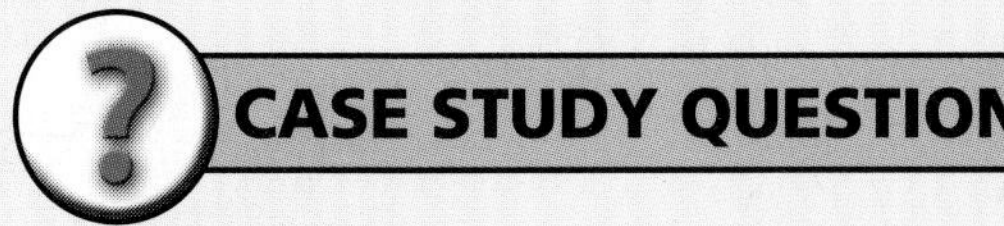

CASE STUDY QUESTIONS

For questions 1–5, please refer to the following case study, and choose the correct answer from choices 1–4.

Ms. Novak is being treated for invasive cancer, and is receiving the following drugs:

vincristine (Oncovin)
interferon alfa-2 (Roferon-A, Intron A)
tamoxifen (Nolvadex)
epoetin alfa (Epogen)

1. Which drug acts by boosting the patient's immune system?

1. Vincristine (Oncovin)
2. Epoetin alfa (Epogen)
3. Interferon alfa 2 (Roferon-A, Intron A)
4. Tamoxifen (Nolvadex)

2. Epoetin alfa (Epogen) is likely being administered to:

1. Boost the patient's immune system
2. Boost the number of red blood cells
3. Reduce possible neurotoxicity
4. Kill cancer cells

3. During vincristine (Oncovin) therapy, the nurse must regularly assess:

1. Blood glucose levels
2. For signs of peripheral neuropathy
3. For ototoxicity
4. For confusion and hallucinations

4. With interferon alfa-2 (Roferon-A, Intron A), the nurse should monitor for which common side effect?

1. Flu-like syndrome
2. Decreases in platelets and white blood cells
3. Anemia
4. Weakness or loss of sensation in the extremities

5. After 6 weeks of therapy, the physician discontinued vincristine due to possible liver damage. He added methotrexate to Ms. Novak's chemotherapy regimen. This drug acts by:

1. Blocking mitosis
2. Blocking RNA synthesis
3. Inhibiting folate metabolism
4. Blocking hormone synthesis

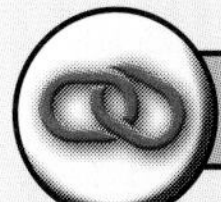

FURTHER STUDY

- Additional indications for hormone pharmacotherapy are discussed in Chapters 29 and 30.
- Drugs for nausea and vomiting (antiemetics) are presented in Chapter 26.
- The use of glucocorticoids in the pharmacotherapy of pulmonary disorders is covered in Chapter 25.

EXPLORE MEDIALINK www.prenhall.com/holland

Additional resources for this chapter can be found on the CD-ROM accompanying this textbook, and on the Companion Website. Click on Chapter 24 to select activities for this chapter.

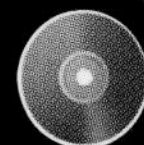

- Mechanism in Action: Methotrexate
- Audio Glossary
- Concept Review
- NCLEX-PN® Review
- Nursing in Action
- Dosage Calculator

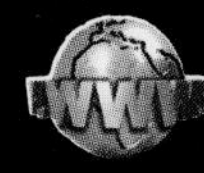

- Cancernet
- Current Indications for Antineoplastics
- Clinical Trials

UNIT

1 2 3 4 5 6 7

5 THE RESPIRATORY, DIGESTIVE, AND RENAL SYSTEMS

UNIT CONTENTS

CHAPTER

25 Drugs for Pulmonary Disorders

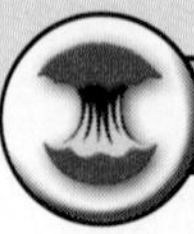

CORE CONCEPTS

25.1 The physiology of the respiratory system involves two main processes: ventilation and respiration.

25.2 Bronchioles are lined with smooth muscle that controls the amount of air entering the lungs.

25.3 The inhalation route of drug administration quickly delivers medications directly to their sites of action.

25.4 Asthma is a chronic inflammatory disease characterized by bronchospasm.

25.5 Beta-adrenergic agents are first-choice drugs for relieving acute bronchospasm.

25.6 Glucocorticoids are the most effective drugs for the long-term prophylaxis of asthma.

25.7 Mast cell stabilizers and leukotriene modifiers are alternative anti-inflammatory drugs for the prophylaxis of asthma.

25.8 Several drugs are effective at loosening bronchial secretions and relieving cough.

25.9 Chronic obstructive pulmonary disease is a progressive disorder treated with multiple drugs.

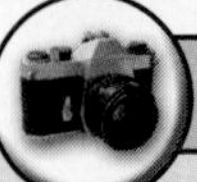

DRUG SNAPSHOT

The following drugs will be discussed in this chapter:

DRUG CLASSES	DRUG PROFILES
Beta-adrenergic agents	Pr salmeterol (Serevent)
Xanthines	
Anticholinergics	
Glucocorticoids	Pr beclomethasone (Beclovent, Beconase, Vancenase, Vanceril)
Mast cell stabilizers	
Leukotriene modifiers	
Antitussives, Expectorants, and Mucolytics	

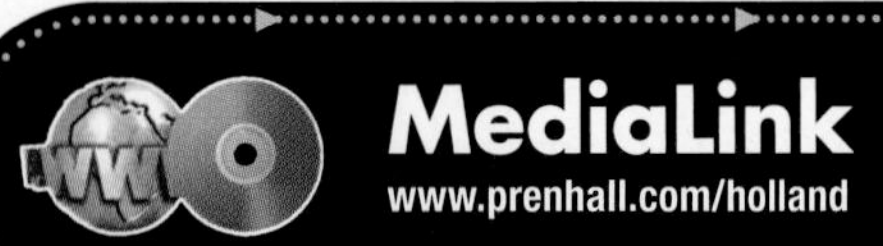

Interactive resources for this chapter can be found on the Companion Website. Click on Chapter 25 and "Begin" to select the activities for this chapter. For chapter-related animations, NCLEX-PN®-style questions, and an audio glossary, access the accompanying CD-ROM in this book.

OBJECTIVES

After reading this chapter, the student should be able to:

1. Identify basic anatomical structures associated with the respiratory system.
2. Explain how the autonomic nervous system controls airflow in the bronchial tree.
3. Explain why inhalation is an effective route of drug administration for pulmonary medicines.
4. Describe the types of devices used to deliver medications via the inhalation route.
5. Describe some common causes and symptoms of asthma, chronic bronchitis, and emphysema.
6. For each of the following classes, identify representative drugs, explain the mechanisms of drug action, primary actions on the respiratory system, and important adverse effects:
   a. beta-adrenergic agents/sympathomimetics
   b. glucocorticoids
   c. anticholinergics
   d. mast-cell stabilizers
   e. leukotriene modifiers
   f. expectorants
   g. antitussives
   h. mucolytics
7. Categorize drugs used in the treatment of pulmonary disorders based on their classifications and mechanisms of action.

The respiratory system is one of the most important organ systems; a mere 5 to 6 minutes without breathing may result in death. When functioning properly, the respiratory system provides the body with the oxygen critical for all cells to function. Measuring respiration rate and depth and listening to chest sounds with a stethoscope give the healthcare provider valuable clues as to what may be happening internally. The respiratory system also provides a means by which the body can rid itself of excess acids and bases, a topic that is covered in Chapter 28.

This chapter examines medications used in the therapy of asthma, a disease characterized by inflammation and acute constriction of the airway. Drugs used for seasonal allergies are covered in Chapter 21. Anti-infectives used in the treatment of lung infections such as pneumonia and tuberculosis are covered in Chapters 22 and 23.

25.1 The physiology of the respiratory system involves two main processes: Ventilation and respiration.

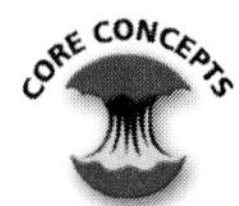

The primary function of the respiratory system is to bring oxygen into the body and to remove carbon dioxide. The process by which gasses are exchanged is called **respiration**. The basic structures of the respiratory system are shown in Figure 25.1 ■.

Ventilation is the process of moving air into and out of the lungs. As the muscular diaphragm contracts and lowers in position, it creates a negative pressure that draws air into the lungs. This process, known as inspiration, requires energy to produce the contraction. During expiration, the diaphragm relaxes and air leaves the lung passively, with no energy expenditure required. Ventilation is a purely mechanical process that occurs approximately 12–18 times per minute in adults, a rate determined by neurons in the brainstem. This rate may be modified by a number of factors, including emotions, fever, stress, and the pH of the blood.

Air entering the respiratory system travels through the nose, the pharynx, and the trachea and into the **bronchi,** which divide into smaller and smaller passages called **bronchioles.** The bronchial tree ends in dilated sacs called **alveoli.** Although they have no smooth muscle, the alveoli are abundantly rich in capillaries. An extremely thin membrane in the alveoli separates the airway from the pulmonary capillaries, allowing gasses to readily move between the internal environment of the blood and the inspired air. As oxygen crosses this membrane, it is exchanged for carbon dioxide, a cellular waste product that travels from the blood to the air. The lung is richly supplied with blood. Blood flow through the lung is called **perfusion.** The process of gas exchange is shown in Figure 25.1.

FIGURE 25.1

Pharynx
Vocal cord
Esophagus
Right lung
Right bronchus
Alveoli
Diaphragm
Nasal cavity
Tongue
Larynx
Trachea
Left lung
Left bronchus
Expired air
Alveolus
O_2
CO_2
Oxygenated blood circulated back to the heart
Deoxygenated blood from the heart

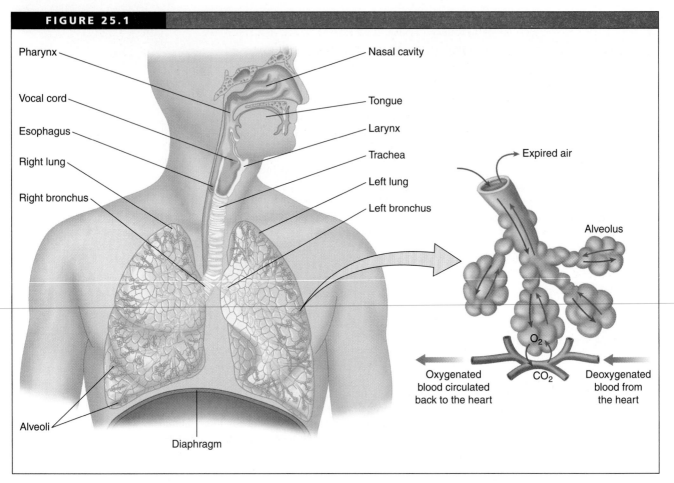

The respiratory system and the process of gas exchange

Concept Review 25.1

- What is the difference between ventilation and perfusion?

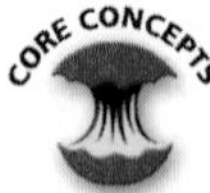

25.2 Bronchioles are lined with smooth muscle that controls the amount of air entering the lungs.

Bronchioles are elastic structures that are able to vary the size of their diameter, or *lumen,* with the specific needs of the body. Changes in the diameter of the bronchiolar lumen are made possible by smooth muscle lining the bronchial tree. This smooth muscle is controlled by the autonomic nervous system. During the fight-or-flight response, beta$_2$-adrenergic receptors of the sympathetic nervous system are stimulated, the bronchiolar smooth muscle relaxes, and **bronchodilation** results. This allows more air to enter the alveoli, thus increasing the oxygen supply to the body during periods of stress or exercise. Drugs that cause bronchodilation are some of the most common medications for treating pulmonary disorders.

When nerves from the parasympathetic nervous system are activated, bronchiolar smooth muscle contracts and the airway lumen narrows, resulting in **bronchoconstriction.** When this occurs quickly, it is called **bronchospasm.** Bronchospasm can cause great distress, leaving the patient gasping for breath. Parasympathetic stimulation also has the effect of slowing respiration rate; sympathetic stimulation has the opposite effect. Autonomic nerves serving bronchiolar smooth muscle are frequent targets for medications.

25.3 The inhalation route of drug administration quickly delivers medications directly to their sites of action.

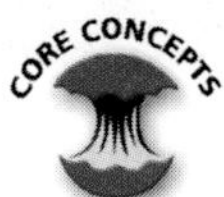

The respiratory system offers a rapid and efficient mechanism for delivering drugs. The enormous surface area of the bronchioles and alveoli, and the rich blood supply to these areas, results in an almost instantaneous onset of action for inhaled substances.

Medications are delivered to the respiratory system by aerosol therapy. An **aerosol** is a suspension of very small liquid droplets or fine solid particles suspended in a gas. Aerosol therapy can give immediate relief for bronchospasm. Drugs may also be given to loosen thick mucus in the bronchial tree. The major advantage of aerosal therapy is that it delivers the medications to their immediate site of action, thus reducing systemic side effects. To produce the same therapeutic action, an oral medication would have to be given at higher doses and would be distributed to all body tissues.

It should be clearly understood that agents delivered by inhalation can produce systemic effects due to absorption. For example, anesthetics such as nitrous oxide and halothane (Fluothane) are delivered via the inhalation route and are rapidly distributed to cause CNS depression, as presented in Chapter 13. Solvents such as paint thinners and glues are sometimes intentionally inhaled and can cause serious adverse effects on the nervous system, and even death.

Several devices are used to deliver medications via the inhalation route. **Nebulizers** are small machines that vaporize a liquid drug into a fine mist that can be inhaled, often using a facemask. If the drug is a solid, it may be administered using a **dry powder inhaler (DPI).** A DPI is a small device that is activated by the process of inhalation to deliver a fine powder directly to the bronchial tree. Turbohalers and rotahalers are types of DPIs. **Metered-dose inhalers (MDIs)** are a third type of device commonly used to deliver respiratory medicines. MDIs use a propellant to deliver a measured dose of drugs to the lungs during each breath. The patient times the inhalation to the puffs of drug emitted from the MDI. Patients must be carefully instructed on the correct use of these devices because drug dose depends on their correct use. In addition, swallowing medication that has been deposited in the oral cavity may cause the drug to be absorbed in the GI tract, causing potential side effects. Two devices used to deliver respiratory agents are shown in Figure 25.2 ■.

The primary goal of drug therapy for pulmonary disorders is keeping the airways open. Drugs include bronchodilators, which directly open the airways, and anti-inflammatory drugs, which

FIGURE 25.2

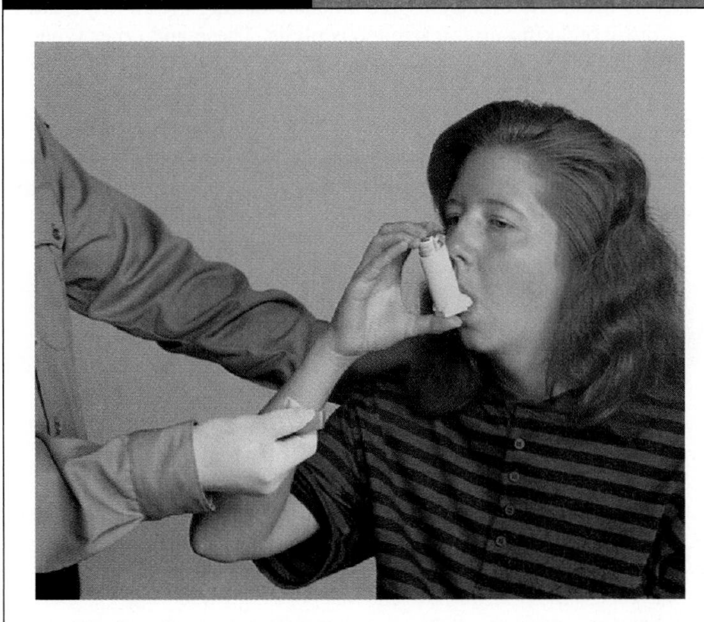

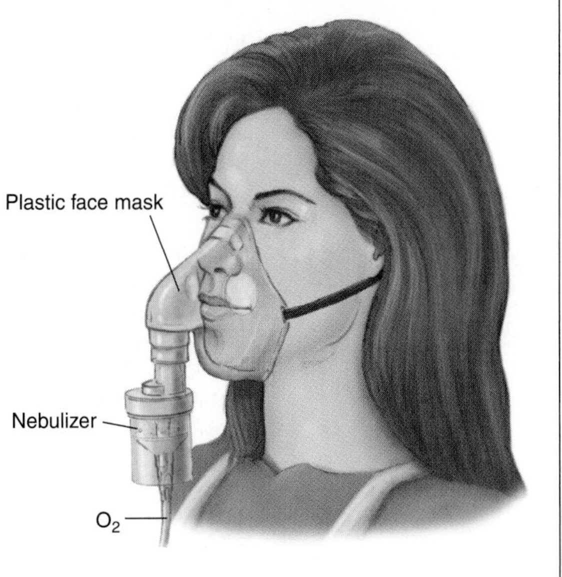

Devices used to deliver respiratory drugs *SOURCE: Pearson Education/PH College*

FIGURE 25.3

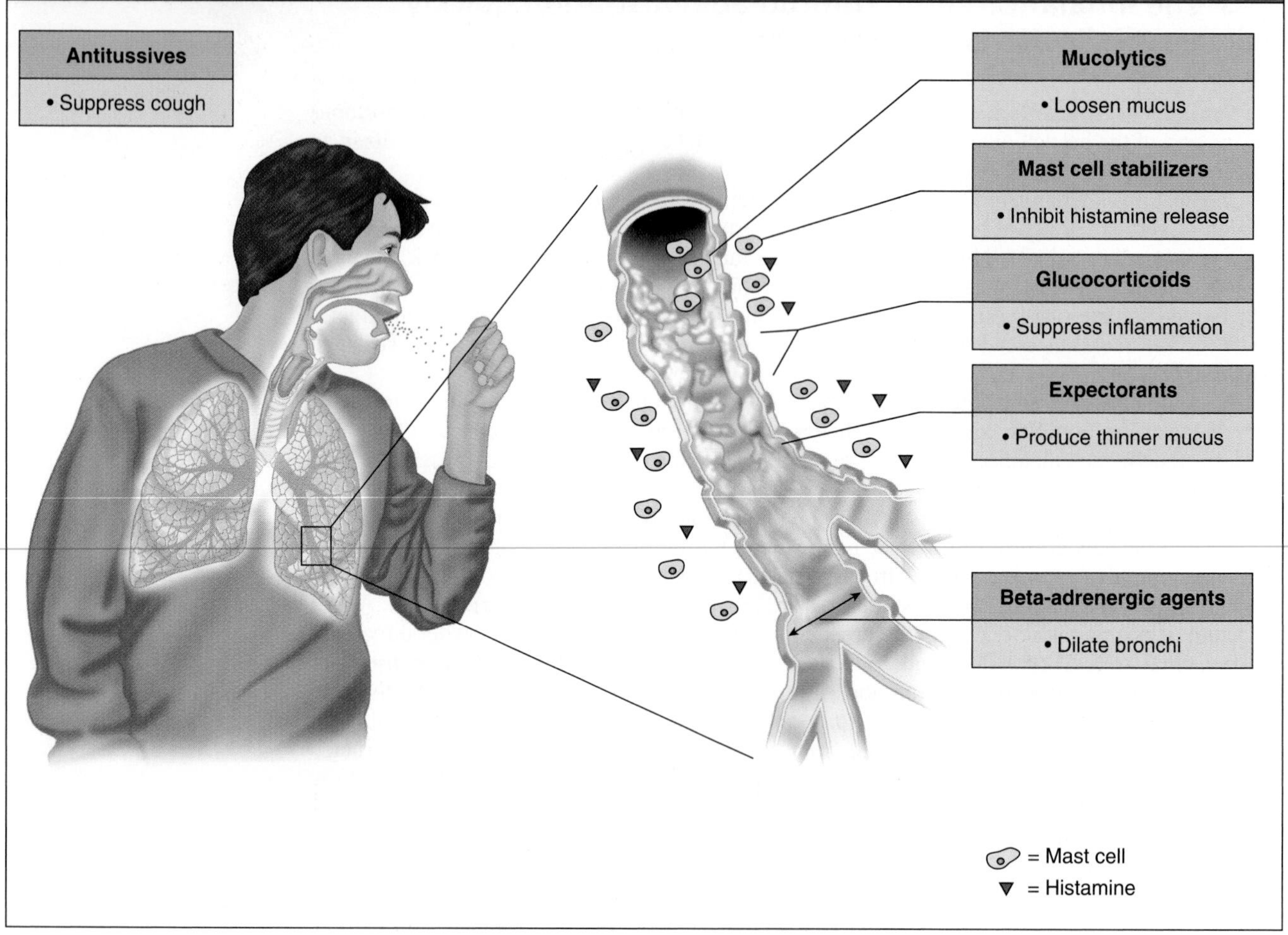

Antitussives
• Suppress cough

Mucolytics
• Loosen mucus

Mast cell stabilizers
• Inhibit histamine release

Glucocorticoids
• Suppress inflammation

Expectorants
• Produce thinner mucus

Beta-adrenergic agents
• Dilate bronchi

= Mast cell
▼ = Histamine

Drugs used to treat respiratory disorders

prevent their closure. Drugs may be used to act on excessive mucus blocking the airways, either by causing it to become thinner or by breaking up thick mucous plugs. These and other types of drugs used to treat pulmonary disorders are illustrated in Figure 25.3 ■.

Concept Review 25.2

- Name the three types of devices used to deliver drugs by the inhalation route. What are the differences among them?

ASTHMA

Asthma is a chronic disease with both inflammatory and bronchospasm components. Drugs are given to either decrease the frequency of asthmatic attacks or to terminate attacks in progress.

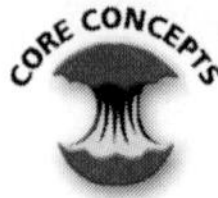

25.4 Asthma is a chronic inflammatory disease characterized by bronchospasm.

dys = *painful or difficult*
pnea = *breathing*

Asthma is one of the most common chronic conditions in the United States, affecting almost 15 million Americans. The disease is characterized by acute bronchospasm, which causes intense breathlessness, or **dyspnea,** coughing, and gasping for air. Along with bronchoconstriction, the

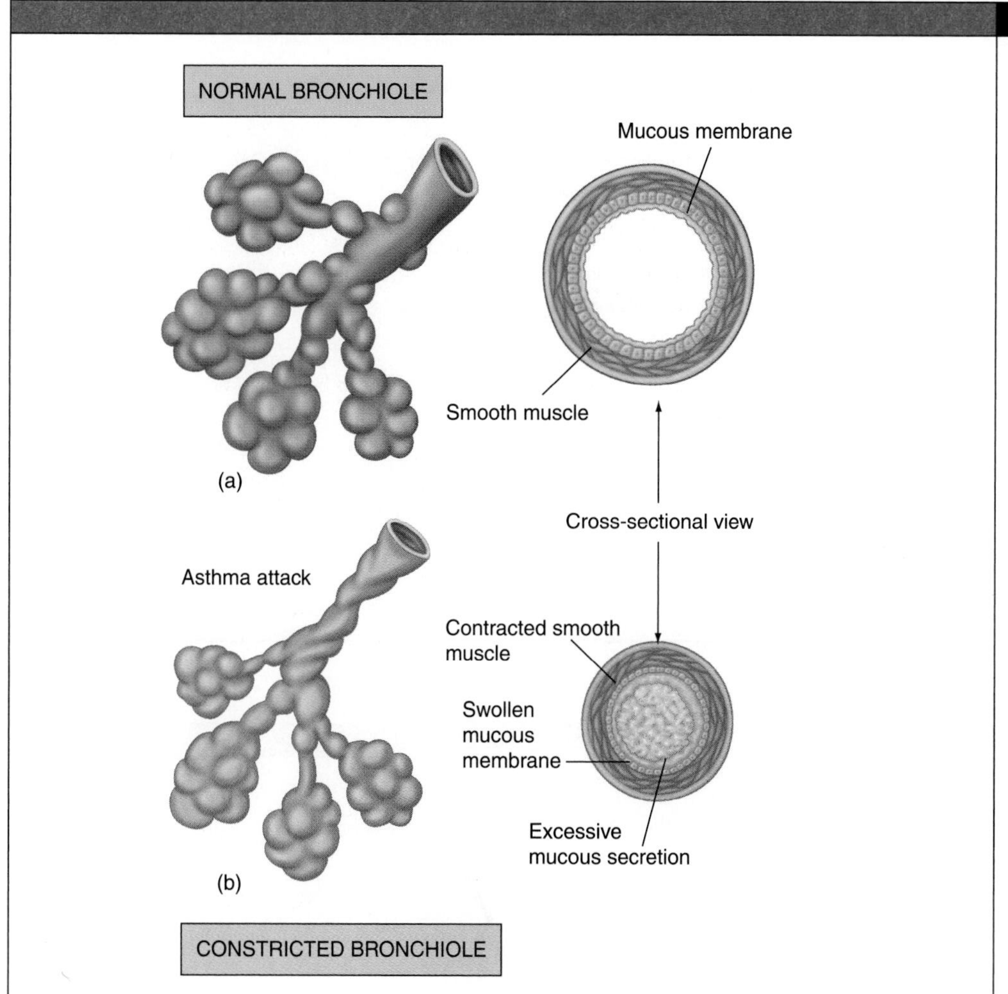

FIGURE 25.4

Changes in bronchioles during an asthma attack: (a) normal bronchiole, and (b) constricted bronchiole in asthma attack

Reprinted by permission of Pearson Education, Inc., Upper Saddle River, NJ

acute inflammatory response is initiated, stimulating mucous secretion and edema of the airway. These conditions are illustrated in Figure. 25.4 ■. **Status asthmaticus** is a severe, prolonged form of asthma that is unresponsive to drug treatment and may lead to respiratory failure. Typical causes of asthmatic attacks are shown in Table 25.1.

Although the exact cause of asthma is sometimes unknown, it is believed to be the result of chronic airway inflammation. Because asthma has both a bronchoconstriction component and an inflammatory component, drug therapy of the disease focuses on one or both of these mechanisms. The goals of drug therapy are twofold: to terminate acute bronchospasms in progress and to reduce the frequency of acute asthma attacks. Different drugs are usually needed to achieve each of these goals. The various classes of drugs used for asthma are shown in Figure 25.5 ■.

25.5 Beta-adrenergic agents are first-choice drugs for relieving acute bronchospasm.

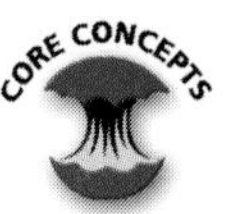

Bronchodilators are drugs used to rapidly relieve the acute bronchospasm characteristic of an asthmatic attack. Although the beta-adrenergic agents are the most commonly prescribed bronchodilators, theophylline and ipratropium may also be used. Bronchodilators used for asthma are listed in Table 25.2.

Beta-adrenergic agents, or sympathomimetics, are drugs of choice in the treatment of acute bronchoconstriction. In most cases, the agents used for pulmonary disease are selective for $beta_2$ receptors in the lung; thus, they produce fewer cardiac side effects than the nonselective beta agents. When inhaled, they produce rapid bronchodilation by relaxing bronchiolar smooth muscle. Inhaled beta-adrenergic agents produce little systemic toxicity because only small amounts

TABLE 25.1	Common Causes of Asthma
air pollutants	tobacco smoke ozone nitrous and sulfur oxides fumes from cleaning fluids or solvents burning leaves
allergens	pollen from trees, grasses, and weeds animal dander household dust mold
chemicals and food	drugs such as aspirin, ibuprofen, and beta blockers sulfite preservatives food such as nuts, monosodium glutamate (MSG), shellfish, and dairy products
respiratory infections	bacterial, fungal, and viral
stress	emotional stress or anxiety exercise in dry, cold climates

FIGURE 25.5

Drug classes used in the pharmacotherapy of asthma

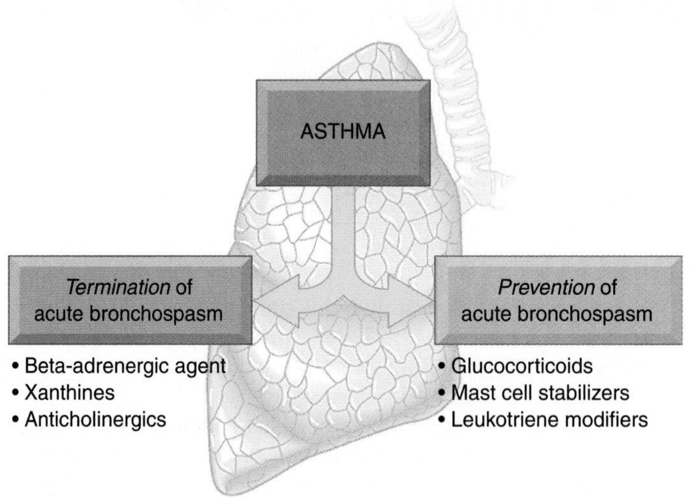

Fast Facts Asthma

- More than 15 million people have asthma.
- Asthma is responsible for more than 1.5 million emergency room visits and more than 500,000 hospitalizations each year.
- More than 5500 patients die of asthma each year.
- The incidence of asthma has been dramatically increasing each year since 1980 in all age, gender, and ethnic groups. The highest rate of increase has been among Blacks.
- The highest incidence of asthma is in those younger than age 18. From 7–10% of children have the disease.
- In adults, asthma is slightly more common in women than in men. In children, however, the disease affects twice as many boys as girls.

TABLE 25.2 Bronchodilators for Asthma

DRUG	ROUTE AND ADULT DOSE	REMARKS
BETA-ADRENERGIC AGENTS		
albuterol (Proventil, others)	PO 2–4 mg tid–qid	Relaxes smooth muscle of the bronchial tree; nebulizer form available
bitolterol (Tornalate)	MDI 2 inhalations tid–qid	Short acting; nebulizer form available
epinephrine (Adrenalin, Bronkaid, Primatene)	Subcutaneous 0.1–0.5 ml of 1:1000 q 20 min–4 hours	Subcutaneous and IV forms are given for emergency situations; available via inhalation to terminate asthmatic attacks
formoterol (Foradil)	DPI 12 mcg capsule q12hr	Long acting
isoetharine (Bronkosol, Bronkometer)	MDI 1–2 inhalations q4h up to 5 days	Increases vital capacity and decreases airway resistance; nebulizer form available
isoproteronol (Isuprel, Medihaler-Iso)	MDI 1–2 inhalations q4 hours–qid	IV and subcutaneous forms available
levalbuterol (Xopenex)	Nebulizer 0.63 mg tid–qid	Short acting; facilitates mucous drainage; increases vital capacity
metaproterenol (Alupent, Metaprel)	MDI 2–3 inhalations q3–4h (max: 12 inhalations/day)	Short acting; relaxes smooth muscle of bronchi; nebulizer form available
pirbuterol (Maxair)	MDI 2 inhalations four times a day (max: 12 inhalations/day)	Short acting
Pr salmeterol (Serevent)	MDI 2 inhalations bid	Long acting; facilitates mucous drainage and decreases reaction to allergens; DPI form available
terbutaline (Brethaire, Brethine)	PO 2.5–5 mg tid	Extended-release form available
XANTHINES		
aminophylline (Truphylline)	PO 0.25–0.75 mg/kg/hr divided four times a day	IV form available
theophylline (Theo-dur)	PO 0.4–0.6 mg/kg/hr divided tid–qid	IV and extended-release form available
ANTICHOLINERGICS		
ipratropium (Atrovent, Combivent)	MDI 2 inhalations four times a day (max: 12 inhalations/day)	Combivent is a combination of ipratropium plus albuterol
tiotropium (Spiriva)	Inhalation: Inhale contents of one capsule daily	Handihaler device is used to puncture capsule

of the drugs are absorbed. When given orally, a longer duration of action is achieved, but systemic side effects such as tachycardia and tremor are more frequently experienced. Tolerance may develop to the therapeutic effects of the beta-adrenergic agents; therefore, the patient must be instructed to seek medical attention if the drugs prove to be less effective with continued use.

As discussed in Chapter 7, blocking the parasympathetic nervous system produces similar effects to stimulation of the sympathetic nervous system. It is predictable, then, that anticholinergic drugs would cause bronchodilation and have potential use in the pharmacotherapy of asthma and other pulmonary diseases. The most widely used drug in this class, ipratropium (Atrovent, Combivent), is taken via inhalation to rapidly relieve bronchospasm. Because it is not readily absorbed from the lungs, it produces few systemic side effects, although it is considered less effective than beta-adrenergic agents. Inhaled anticholinergics are more effective when used with other bronchodilators; Combivent is a combination of ipratropium and albuterol in a single MDI canister. In 2005, a new anticholinergic tiotropium (Spiriva) was approved which has a long duration of action that allows for once daily dosing.

The third class of bronchodilators is the xanthines. Chemically related to caffeine, theophylline (Theo-dur, others) and aminophylline (Truphylline) were drugs of choice for bronchoconstriction

DRUG PROFILE: Bronchodilator/Beta-adrenergic agent: Pr *Salmeterol (Serevent)*

Actions and Uses:

Salmeterol is approved for prevention of bronchospasm in asthma patients and for the prevention of exercise-induced bronchospasm. Its 12-hour duration of action is longer than that of many other bronchodilators. Because salmeterol takes 10–25 minutes to act, it should not be used for the termination of acute bronchospasm.

Adverse Effects and Interactions:

Serious adverse effects from salmeterol are uncommon. Some patients may experience headaches, nervousness, and restlessness. Because of its potential to cause tachycardia, patients with heart disease, or dysrhythmias should be monitored regularly.

Use of beta blockers with salmeterol will block the effects of the drug.

Mechanism in Action:

Salmeterol relieves bronchospasm by binding selectively with $beta_2$ receptors located on the cellular membranes of bronchiolar smooth muscle. Because salmeterol is a selective $beta_2$ stimulator, there is less potential for activating $beta_1$-cardiac receptors, especially if it is administered as an aerosol. It is primarily used to treat asthma.

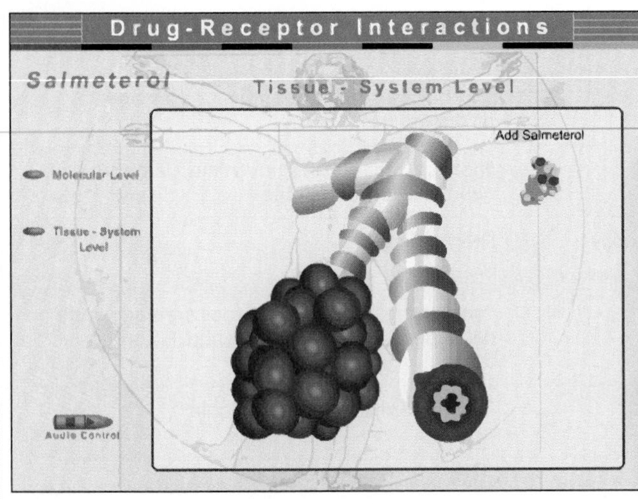

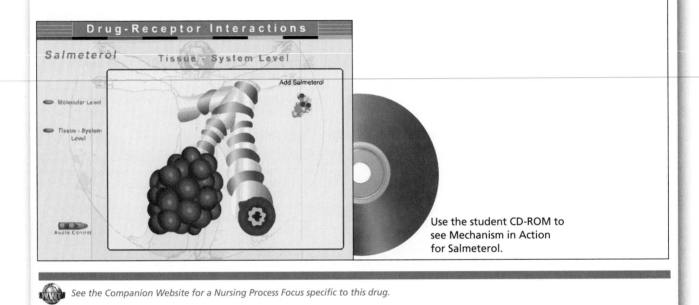

Use the student CD-ROM to see Mechanism in Action for Salmeterol.

See the Companion Website for a Nursing Process Focus specific to this drug.

NURSING PROCESS FOCUS

Patients Receiving Bronchodilators

ASSESSMENT

Prior to administration:

- Obtain complete health history including allergies, drug history, and possible drug reactions
- Assess for symptoms related to respiratory deficiency such as dyspnea, orthopnea, cyanosis, nasal flaring, wheezing, and weakness
- Obtain vital signs
- Auscultate bilateral breath sounds for air movement and adventitious sounds (crackles, rhonchi, wheezes)
- Assess pulmonary function with pulse oximeter, peak expiratory flow meter, and/or arterial blood gasses to establish baseline

POTENTIAL NURSING DIAGNOSES

- Impaired Gas Exchange, related to bronchial constriction
- Activity Intolerance, related to ineffective drug therapy
- Deficient Knowledge, related to drug therapy
- Anxiety, related to difficulty in breathing
- Disturbed Sleep Pattern, related to side effects of drugs
- Ineffective Tissue Perfusion, related to adverse effects of drugs

continued...

NURSING PROCESS FOCUS

PLANNING: Patient Goals and Expected Outcomes

The patient will:

- Exhibit adequate oxygenation as evidenced by improved lung sounds and pulmonary function values
- Report a reduction in subjective symptoms of respiratory deficiency
- Demonstrate an understanding of the drug's action by accurately describing drug side effects and precautions
- Report at least 6 hours of uninterrupted sleep

IMPLEMENTATION

Interventions and (Rationales)	Patient Education/Discharge Planning
■ Monitor vital signs including pulse, blood pressure, and respiratory rate.	Instruct patient to: ■ Use medication as directed even if asymptomatic ■ Report difficulty with breathing
■ Ensure pulmonary function is monitored using pulse oximeter, peak expiratory flow meter, and/or arterial blood gasses. (Monitoring is necessary to assess drug effectiveness.)	■ Instruct patient to report symptoms of deteriorating respiratory status such as increased dyspnea, breathlessness with speech, and/or orthopnea.
■ Monitor the patient's ability to use inhaler. (Proper use ensures correct dosage.)	Instruct patient: ■ In proper use of metered-dose inhaler ■ To strictly use the medication as prescribed; do not "double up" on doses ■ To rinse mouth thoroughly following use
■ Observe for side effects specific to the medication used.	■ Instruct patient regarding side effects and to report specific drug side effects.
■ Maintain environment free of respiratory contaminants such as dust, dry air, flowers, and smoke. (These substances may exacerbate bronchial constriction.)	Instruct patient to: ■ Avoid respiratory irritants ■ Maintain "clean air environment" ■ Stop smoking and avoid secondhand smoke, if applicable
■ Maintain dietary intake adequate in essential nutrients and vitamins. (Dyspnea interferes with proper nutrition.) ■ Ensure patient maintains adequate hydration of 3 to 4 L/day (to liquefy pulmonary secretions).	Instruct patient to: ■ Maintain nutrition with foods high in essential nutrients ■ Consume small frequent meals to prevent fatigue ■ Consume 3 to 4 L of fluid/day if not contraindicated ■ Avoid caffeine (increases CNS irritability)
■ Provide emotional and psychosocial support during periods of shortness of breath. ■ Monitor patient compliance. (Maintaining therapeutic drug levels is essential to effective therapy.)	■ Instruct patient in relaxation techniques and controlled breathing techniques. ■ Inform the patient of the importance of ongoing medication compliance and follow-up.

EVALUATION OF OUTCOME CRITERIA

Evaluate the effectiveness of drug therapy by confirming that patient goals and expected outcomes have been met (see "Planning").

See Table 25.2 for a list of drugs to which these nursing actions apply.

20 years ago. Theophylline, however, has a narrow margin of safety and interacts with a large number of other drugs. Side effects such as nausea, vomiting, and CNS stimulation are relatively common, and dysrthymias may occur at high doses. Having been largely replaced by safer and more effective drugs, theophylline is now primarily used for the long-term oral prophylaxis of persistent asthma.

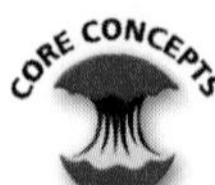

25.6 Glucocorticoids are the most effective drugs for the long-term prophylaxis of asthma.

Several classes of anti-inflammatory drugs are used to decrease the incidence of asthma attacks. The inhaled glucocorticoids are most commonly used for this purpose, although mast cell stabilizers and leukotriene inhibitors are also effective. Doses of the anti-inflammatory drugs used for asthma are given in Table 25.3.

Glucocorticoids are the most effective drugs available for the *prevention* of acute asthmatic episodes. When inhaled on a daily schedule, glucocorticoids suppress inflammation without producing major side effects. Patients should be informed that inhaled glucocorticoids must be taken daily to produce their therapeutic effect and that these medications are not effective at terminating episodes in progress. For some patients, a beta-adrenergic agent may be prescribed along with an inhaled glucocorticoid because this permits the dose of the glucocorticoid to be reduced as much as 50%.

TABLE 25.3 Anti-inflammatory Drugs

DRUG	ROUTE AND ADULT DOSE	REMARKS
GLUCOCORTICOIDS		
Pr beclomethasone (Beclovent, Vanceril, others)	MDI 1–2 inhalations tid or qid (max: 20 inhalations/day)	Intranasal form available for allergic rhinitis
budesonide (Pulmicort Turbuhaler)	DPI 1–2 inhalations (200 mcg/inhalation) daily (max: 800 mcg/day)	Intranasal form available for allergic rhinitis
flunisolide (AeroBid)	MDI 2–3 inhalations bid or tid (max: 12 inhalations/day)	Intranasal form available for allergic rhinitis
fluticasone (Flovent)	MDI (44 mcg); 2 inhalations bid (max: 10 inhalations/day)	Intranasal form available for allergic rhinitis; also available in 110 and 120 mcg inhalers
methylprednisolone (Depo-Medrol, others)	PO 4–48 mg daily	Available in IM, IV forms; also for neoplasia and adrenal insufficiency
prednisone (Deltasone, Meticorten, others)	PO 5–60 mg daily	Only available in oral form; also for neoplasia
triamcinolone (Azmacort) topical, and	MDI 2 inhalations tid or qid (max: 16 inhalations/day)	Also available in IM, subcutaneous, intradermal, oral forms
MAST CELL STABILIZERS		
cromolyn (Intal)	MDI 1 inhalation qid	Topical form available for ophthalmic use
nedocromil sodium (Tilade)	MDI 2 inhalations qid	Topical form available for ophthalmic use
LEUKOTRIENE MODIFIERS		
montelukast (Singulair)	PO 10 mg/day in evening	Also for allergic rhinitis
zafirlukast (Accolate)	PO 20 mg bid 1 h before or 2 h after meals	Not for acute bronchospasm
Zileuton (Zyflo)	PO 600 mg qid	Not for acute bronchospasm

DRUG PROFILE: Glucocorticoid: Pr *Beclomethasone (Beclovent, Beconase, Vancenase, Vanceril)*

Actions and Uses:

Beclomethasone is a glucocorticoid available through aerosol inhalation for asthma or as a nasal spray for allergic rhinitis. For asthma, two inhalations 2–3 times per day usually provide adequate prophylaxis. Beclomethasone acts by reducing inflammation, thus decreasing the frequency of asthma attacks. It is not a bronchodilator and should not be used to terminate asthma attacks in progress.

Adverse Effects:

Inhaled beclomethasone produces few systemic side effects. Because small amounts may be swallowed with each dose, the patient should be observed for signs of glucocorticoid toxicity when taking the drug for long periods. Local effects may include hoarseness in the voice. Like all glucocorticoids, the anti-inflammatory properties of beclomethasone can mask infections. A large percentage of patients taking beclomethasone on a long-term basis will develop candidiasis, a fungal infection in the throat, due to the constant deposits of drug in the oral cavity.

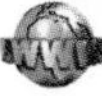

See the Companion Website for a Nursing Process Focus specific to this drug.

For severe, persistent asthma that is unresponsive to other treatments, oral glucocorticoids may be prescribed. Treatment time is limited to the shortest length possible, usually 5 to 7 days. If taken for longer than 10 days, oral glucocorticoids may produce significant adverse effects such as adrenal gland suppression, peptic ulcers, and hyperglycemia. Other uses and adverse effects of glucocorticoids are presented in Chapters 21 and 29.

25.7 Mast cell stabilizers and leukotriene modifiers are alternative anti-inflammatory drugs for the prophylaxis of asthma.

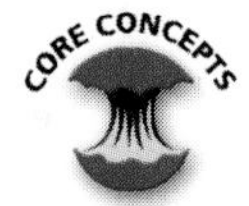

Two mast cell inhibitors play a limited though important role in the prophylaxis of asthma. These drugs act by inhibiting the release of histamine from mast cells.

Cromolyn (Intal) is an anti-inflammatory drug that is useful in preventing asthma attacks. When administered via an MDI or a nebulizer, cromolyn is a safe alternative to the glucocorticoids. Maximum therapeutic benefit may take several weeks. Patients must be informed that cromolyn should be taken on a daily basis and should not be used to terminate acute attacks. An intranasal form of cromolyn (Nasalcrom) is used in the treatment of seasonal allergies.

Nedocromil (Tilade) is an anti-inflammatory drug that has actions and uses similar to cromolyn. The drug has few adverse effects when administered with an MDI, although some patients experience an unpleasant taste.

The leukotriene modifiers are newer drugs, approved in the 1990s, that are used to reduce inflammation and ease bronchoconstriction. They modify the action of leukotrienes, which are mediators of the inflammatory response in asthmatic patients.

The leukotriene modifiers are approved for the prophylaxis of chronic asthma; they are ineffective in relieving bronchospasm. They are all given orally. Zileuton has a more rapid onset of action (2 hours), whereas the other two leukotriene modifiers take as long as a week to provide therapeutic benefit. Few serious adverse effects are associated with the leukotriene modifiers. Headache, cough, nasal congestion, or GI upset may occur.

Concept Review 25.3

- Distinguish the classes of drugs that *prevent* asthma attacks from those that can *terminate* an attack in progress. Name at least one drug in each class.

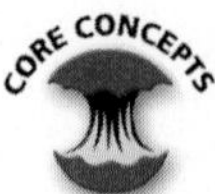

25.8 Several drugs are effective at loosening bronchial secretions and relieving cough.

A small number of drugs are available to suppress cough and control excess mucous production. Antitussives reduce the cough reflex, and expectorants and mucolytics help the client to remove thick bronchial secretions.

Cough is a common symptom that brings patients to seek medical attention. There are many possible causes of cough, ranging from the acute cough of an upper respiratory infection to the chronic cough of tobacco smoking. Some drugs, such as the ACE inhibitors and beta-adrenergic blockers, can trigger cough. Because cough is merely a symptom, the ultimate goal is to identify and treat the underlying disorder. Dry, hacking, nonproductive cough, however, can be quite irritating to the membranes of the throat and can deprive a patient of much needed rest. It is these types of conditions in which therapy with drugs that control cough, known as **antitussives,** may be needed.

anti = *against*
tussive = *pertaining to a cough*

Cough is a reflex mechanism controlled by neurons in the cough center, which is located in the medulla of the brain. The most popular antitussives, codeine and dextromethorphan, act by raising the cough threshold in the cough center, thereby decreasing both the frequency and intensity of cough.

Opioids are the most effective class of antitussives. Hydrocodone and codeine are the most frequently used opioid antitussives. Doses needed to suppress the cough reflex are low, and there is minimal potential for dependence. Most codeine cough mixtures are classified as Schedule III, IV, or V drugs, and are reserved for more serious cough conditions. The amount of codeine in cough mixtures is low and rarely causes serious side effects. However, care must be taken not to give these mixtures to patients allergic to codeine or other opioids. In addition, the drug must be kept secure from children because accidental overdose of opioids in infants can cause severe respiratory depression and even death.

The most frequently used OTC antitussive is dextromethorphan. This medication is included in most severe cold and flu preparations. Side effects are rare. Although not as effective as codeine, dextromethorphan has no risk for dependence.

Benzonatate (Tessalon) is a third antitussive in popular use. This drug does not act on the cough center. Instead, benzonatate has an anesthetic-like effect on stretch receptors in the lung, which essentially interrupts the cough message. The patient must be instructed not to chew the soft capsules, as they will cause numbness of the throat and tongue.

During acute respiratory infections, mucus becomes thick and requires forceful and painful coughing to remove. **Expectorants** are drugs that stimulate the flow of bronchial secretions. The increased bronchial secretions thin the mucus, allowing it to be removed with less forceful coughing.

The most effective OTC expectorant is guaifenesin. Like dextromethorphan, guaifenesin produces few adverse effects and is a common ingredient in many OTC cold and flu preparations. Higher doses of guaifenesin are available by prescription.

muco = *mucus*
lytic = *destruction or disintegration*

Acetylcysteine (Mucomyst) is one of the few drugs available to directly loosen thick, viscous bronchial secretions by breaking down mucous molecules. Drugs of this type are called **mucolytics.** Acetylcysteine is delivered by the inhalation route and is not available OTC. It is used in patients who have cystic fibrosis or other diseases that produce large amounts of thick bronchial secretions. Acetylcysteine is also given as a 5% oral solution for acetaminophen overdose. When given within 24 hours of the overdose, acetylcysteine prevents acute liver damage by blocking the formation of toxic metabolites of acetaminophen.

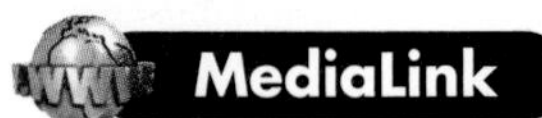

CANADIAN LUNG ASSOCIATION

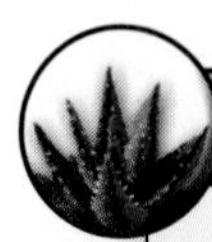

NATURAL ALTERNATIVES

Horehound for Respiratory Disorders

Horehound has been used as an herbal remedy since the ancient Egyptians and was popular with American Indians. In folklore, it was reported to aid in a number of respiratory disorders including asthma, bronchitis, whooping cough, and infections such as tuberculosis. Nonrespiratory uses include bowel disorders, jaundice, and wound healing.

Active ingredients of horehound are found throughout the flowering plant. The chief constituent is a bitter substance called *marrubium* that stimulates secretions. Formulations include tea, dried or fresh leaves, and liquid extracts. Horehound has an expectorant action when treating colds and is also available as cough drops. It is claimed to restore normal secretions to the lung and other organs. ■

CHRONIC OBSTRUCTIVE PULMONARY DISEASE (COPD)

Chronic obstructive pulmonary disease (COPD) includes progressive lung disorders primarily caused by tobacco smoking. COPD is a major cause of death and disability. Drugs may bring symptomatic relief but do not cure the disorders.

25.9 Chronic obstructive pulmonary disease is a progressive disorder treated with multiple drugs.

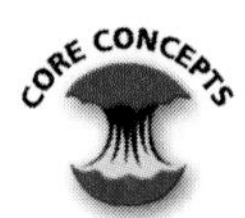

The two primary disorders classified as COPD are chronic bronchitis and emphysema. Both are strongly associated with smoking tobacco products and, secondarily, air pollutants. In **chronic bronchitis,** excess mucus is produced in the respiratory tree due to inflammation and irritation from smoke or pollutants. The airway becomes partially obstructed with mucus, resulting in the classic signs of dyspnea and coughing. Because microbes enjoy the mucus-rich environment, pulmonary infections are common. Gas exchange may be impaired.

bronch = *bronchus*
itis = *inflammation*

COPD is a progressive disease, with the terminal stage being **emphysema.** After years of chronic inflammation, the bronchioles lose their elasticity and the alveoli dilate to maximum size to get more air into the lungs. The patient suffers from extreme dyspnea from even the slightest physical activity.

Patients with COPD may receive a number of pulmonary drugs for symptomatic relief of their disorder. The goals of pharmacotherapy are to treat infections and to control cough and bronchospasm. Most patients receive bronchodilators such as ipratropium, $beta_2$-agents, or inhaled glucocorticoids. Mucolytics and expectorants are sometimes indicated to reduce the thickness of the bronchial mucus and to aid in its removal. Oxygen therapy may also be used in patients with emphysema. Patients should be taught to avoid taking any drugs that have beta-blocking activity or that otherwise cause bronchoconstriction. Respiratory depressants should be avoided. It is important to note that none of the pharmacotherapies offer a cure for COPD; they only treat the symptoms of a progressively worsening disease.

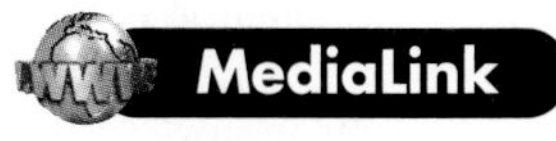

AMERICAN LUNG ASSOCIATION

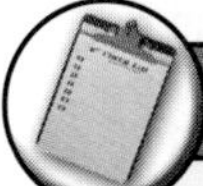

PATIENTS NEED TO KNOW

Patients treated for pulmonary disorders need to know the following:

In General

1. Since tolerance to some medications may occur, if medication is no longer effective, report this tolerance to a healthcare provider. Do not take extra medication without notifying a healthcare provider.

Regarding Inhaled Medications

2. When using MDIs or DPIs, allow an interval of at least 1 minute to pass between puffs.
3. When taking more than one respiratory medicine, take the bronchodilator first. This opens the airways and increases the effectiveness of the second medication.
4. Rinse the mouth thoroughly following inhaler use, to reduce the oral absorption of inhaled medicines.
5. Take inhaled glucocorticoids on a regular basis—not as needed. These medications are not used to stop acute asthma attacks.
6. Do not use decongestant nasal sprays for more than 2 or 3 days, unless instructed to do so by a healthcare provider.

Regarding Bronchodilators

7. Avoid caffeine-containing foods and beverages, if taking theophylline.
8. Immediately report any abnormalities in pulse rate, changes in blood pressure, or sensations of palpitations, when taking beta-adrenergic stimulators.

Regarding Antihistamines and Decongestants

9. Avoid operating machinery or performing other tasks requiring alertness, if taking antihistamines for the first time because drowsiness may occur.
10. Use hard candies, chewing gum, or ice chips to reduce the dry mouth caused by some decongestants and antihistamines. ▪

CHAPTER REVIEW

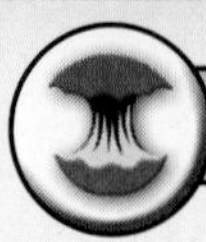

CORE CONCEPTS SUMMARY

25.1 The physiology of the respiratory system involves two main processes: ventilation and respiration.

The respiratory system brings needed oxygen into the body through inspiration and removes carbon dioxide through expiration. The process of moving air into and out of the lungs, or ventilation, is distinct from the process of gas exchange across the alveoli, a process known as respiration.

25.2 Bronchioles are lined with smooth muscle that controls the amount of air entering the lungs.

The autonomic nervous system affects the amount of air entering the bronchial tree by constricting or relaxing bronchial smooth muscle. Bronchoconstriction can produce severe shortness of breath.

25.3 The inhalation route of drug administration quickly delivers medications directly to their sites of action.

Inhalation is frequently used as a route of drug administration for those medications targeted for the respiratory system. Nebulizers, DPIs, and MDIs are used to deliver drugs via the inhalation route.

25.4 Asthma is a chronic inflammatory disease characterized by bronchospasm.

Asthma is a common disease characterized by bronchospasm and chronic airway inflammation. Exposure to a number of factors, including allergens, can cause an acute episode.

25.5 Beta-adrenergic agents are first-choice drugs for relieving acute bronchospasm.

Inhaled $beta_2$-adrenergic agents are drugs of choice for relieving bronchospasm. Anticholinergics are sometimes used for bronchodilation, but fewer are available because of their incidence of side effects. Xanthines, once widely used in pulmonary medicine, are now second-choice drugs in relieving bronchospasm because of their higher potential for side effects.

25.6 Glucocorticoids are the most effective drugs for the long-term prophylaxis of asthma.

Inhaled glucocorticoids are the drugs of choice for asthma prophylaxis. The inhaled glucocorticoids, even when used on a long-term basis, produce few side effects compared to oral glucocorticoids.

25.7 Mast cell stabilizers and leukotriene modifiers are alternative anti-inflammatory drugs for the prophylaxis of asthma.

Mast cell stabilizers such as cromolyn are sometimes used for asthma prophylaxis, although they are not as effective as the glucocorticoids. The leukotriene modifiers offer another option for the prophylaxis of chronic asthma.

25.8 Several drugs are effective at loosening bronchial secretions and relieving cough.

Antitussives are effective at inhibiting the cough reflex. Although opioids are the most effective, there is some risk of physical dependence. Guaifenesin is an OTC drug used to increase bronchial secretions so that cough may be more productive. Mucolytics loosen mucus so that it may be more easily removed from the bronchial tree.

25.9 Chronic obstructive pulmonary disease is a progressive disorder treated with multiple drugs.

Chronic bronchitis and emphysema are two types of COPD that often require multiple drug therapy. Bronchodilators, expectorants, mucolytics, antibiotics, and oxygen may offer symptomatic relief.

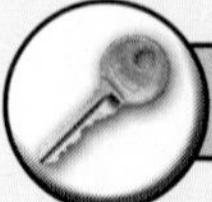

KEY TERMS

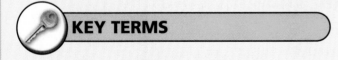

aerosol (AIR-oh-sol): suspension of small liquid droplets of drug, usually to cause bronchodilation / ***page 471***

alveoli (al-VEE-oh-lie): dilated sacs at the end of the bronchial tree where gas exchange occurs / ***page 469***

antitussive (anti-TUSS-ive): drug used to suppress cough / ***page 480***

asthma (AZ-muh): chronic inflammatory disease of the airways / ***page 472***

bronchi (BRON-ky): primary passageway of the bronchial tree that contains smooth muscle / ***page 469***

bronchioles (BRON-key-oles): very small bronchi / ***page 469***

bronchoconstriction (BRON-koh-kun-STRIK-shun): decrease in diameter of the airway due to contraction of bronchial smooth muscle / *page 470*

bronchodilation (BRON-koh-dye-LAY-shun): increase in diameter of the airway due to relaxation of bronchial smooth muscle / *page 470*

bronchospasm (bron-koh-SPAZ-um): rapid constriction of the airways / *page 470*

chronic bronchitis (KRON-ik bron-KEYE-tis): chronic disease of the lungs characterized by excess mucous production and inflammation / *page 481*

dry powder inhaler (DPI): device used to convert a solid drug to a fine powder for the purpose of inhalation / *page 471*

dyspnea (DISP-nee-uh): shortness of breath / *page 472*

emphysema (em-fuss-EE-muh): terminal lung disease characterized by dilation of the alveoli / *page 481*

expectorant (eks-PEK-tor-ent): drug used to increase bronchial secretions / *page 480*

metered-dose inhaler (MDIs): device used to deliver a precise amount of drug to the respiratory system / *page 471*

mucolytic: drug used to loosen thick mucus / *page 480*

nebulizer (NEB-you-lyes-ur): device used to convert liquid drugs into a fine mist for the purpose of inhalation / *page 471*

perfusion (purr-FEW-shun): blood flow through a tissue or organ / *page 469*

respiration (res-purr-AY-shun): exchange of oxygen and carbon dioxide / *page 469*

status asthmaticus (STAT-us az-MAT-ik-us): acute form of asthma requiring immediate medical attention / *page 473*

ventilation (ven-tah-LAY-shun): process by which air is moved into and out of the lungs / *page 469*

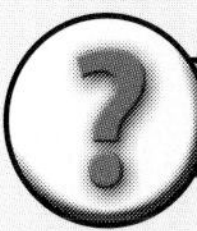

REVIEW QUESTIONS

The following questions are written in NCLEX-PN® style. Answer these questions to assess your knowledge of the chapter material, and go back and review any material that is not clear to you.

1. When assessing the asthmatic patient, which of the following would not be a potential cause of asthma?

1. Ibuprofen
2. Tobacco smoke
3. Exercise
4. Dairy products

2. The patient is having an acute asthma attack. Which of the following drugs would be most appropriate?

1. Pirbuterol (Maxair)
2. Budesonide (Pulmicort)
3. Fluticasone (Flovent)
4. Zafirlukast (Accolate)

3. Theophylline (Theo-Dur) has been added to your patient's treatment regimen. Which of the following would be highest-priority patient teaching?

1. Nausea and vomiting may be a side effect.
2. It is important to monitor for tachycardia.
3. The drug causes nervousness.
4. Avoid caffeine-containing foods and beverages.

4. When teaching a patient on multiple inhalers how to properly use this medication, which of the following would be correct?

1. Take inhaled glucocorticoids only for acute attacks.
2. Do not use for more than 3 days unless instructed by physician.
3. Space inhalers throughout the day to prevent side effects.
4. Use bronchodilators first.

5. Instructions to a patient taking zafirlukast (Accolate) would include:

1. "Take medication with food or milk."
2. "Take medication only in the morning."
3. "Take medication 1 hour before or 2 hours after meals."
4. "Take medication only at bedtime."

6. The physician has ordered montelukast (Singular). The patient wants to know how soon the medication will begin working. The best response would be:

1. "The medication has a rapid onset—within 2 hours."
2. "It will take about a week to become effective."
3. "This medication is used to treat acute bronchospasms only."
4. "Therapeutic benefits may take several weeks."

7. The patient asks what the difference is between antitussives and mucolytics. The nurse's best reply would be:

1. "Antitussives loosen bronchial secretions, and mucolytics stimulate removal of bronchial secretions."
2. "Antitussives suppress cough, whereas mucolytics loosen bronchial secretions."
3. "The terms are interchangeable."
4. "Both types of drugs work to loosen and remove secretions."

8. The most commonly used antitussive is:

1. Guaifenesin
2. Benzonatate (Tessalon)
3. Acetylcysteine (Mucomyst)
4. Dextromethorphan

9. The patient complains of numbness of the throat and tongue after taking benzonatate (Tessalon). The nurse should instruct the patient:

1. To swallow, not chew, medication.
2. To decrease the dosage of medication.
3. To stop taking medication immediately.
4. This is a common side effect and that will subside over time.

10. A patient taking inhaled glucocorticoids states he does not feel his medication is working. The best action this patient can take is to:

1. Increase frequency of medication administration
2. Take only as needed because he is building tolerance
3. Stop using it for a few days so it will become effective
4. Notify his physician

CASE STUDY QUESTIONS

For questions 1–5, please refer to the following case study, and choose the correct answer from choices 1–4.

Mr. Thomas arrives at your office with what appears to be an acute upper respiratory tract infection. He is complaining of nonproductive cough, low-grade fever, and shortness of breath when walking. He is 60 years old and smokes a pack of cigarettes daily. The physician prescribes Hycotuss, a combination drug containing hydrocodone and guaifenesin, acetaminophen, and an ipratropium (Atrovent) inhaler.

1. Which of the prescribed drugs will directly benefit Mr. Thomas' shortness of breath?

1. Hydrocodone
2. Acetaminophen
3. Guaifenesin
4. Ipratropium

2. Which of the prescribed drugs would increase bronchial secretions?

1. Hydrocodone
2. Acetaminophen
3. Guaifenesin
4. Ipratropium

3. Which of the prescribed drugs is classified as an opioid?

1. Hydrocodone
2. Acetaminophen
3. Guaifenesin
4. Ipratropium

4. Mr. Thomas calls the office the next day, complaining that he is unable to drive his car because of excessive drowsiness. Which drug most likely is causing this drowsiness?

1. Hydrocodone
2. Acetaminophen
3. Guaifenesin
4. Ipratropium

5. Mr. Thomas also has asthma, which has become worse over the past few months. He stated that when an acute asthma attack occurs, budesonide (Pulmicort Turbuhaler) does not stop the episode. The nurse should advise Mr. Thomas:

1. To use 4 inhalations of budesonide instead of 2
2. That budesonide must be taken on a regular schedule, not just during acute episodes
3. To request a tablet form of glucocorticoid, rather than an inhaler
4. To always gently clear his nose just prior to using budesonide

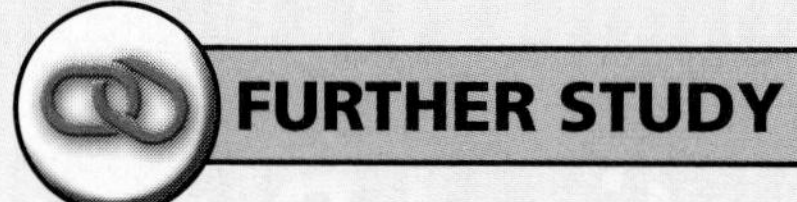

FURTHER STUDY

- Drugs for maintaining acid and base balance are covered in Chapter 28.
- Chapter 21 discusses drugs used for seasonal allergies.
- Anti-infectives, used in the treatment of lung infections, are discussed in Chapters 22 and 23.
- Chapter 13 presents information on anesthetics such as nitrous oxide and halothane (Fluothane), which are delivered via the inhalation route.
- Chapter 7 discusses in further detail the autonomic nervous system and its effects on the respiratory system.
- Uses and adverse effects of the glucocorticoids are detailed in Chapters 21 and 29.

EXPLORE MEDIALINK www.prenhall.com/holland

Additional resources for this chapter can be found on the CD-ROM accompanying this textbook, and on the Companion Website. Click on Chapter 25 to select activities for this chapter.

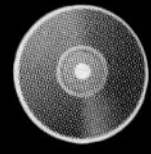

Mechanism in Action: Salmeterol
Audio Glossary
Concept Review
NCLEX-PN® Review
Nursing in Action
Dosage Calculator

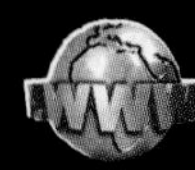

Canadian Lung Association
American Lung Association

FIGURE 26.3

Mechanism of peptic ulcer formation
Reprinted by permission of Pearson Education, Inc., Upper Saddle River, NJ

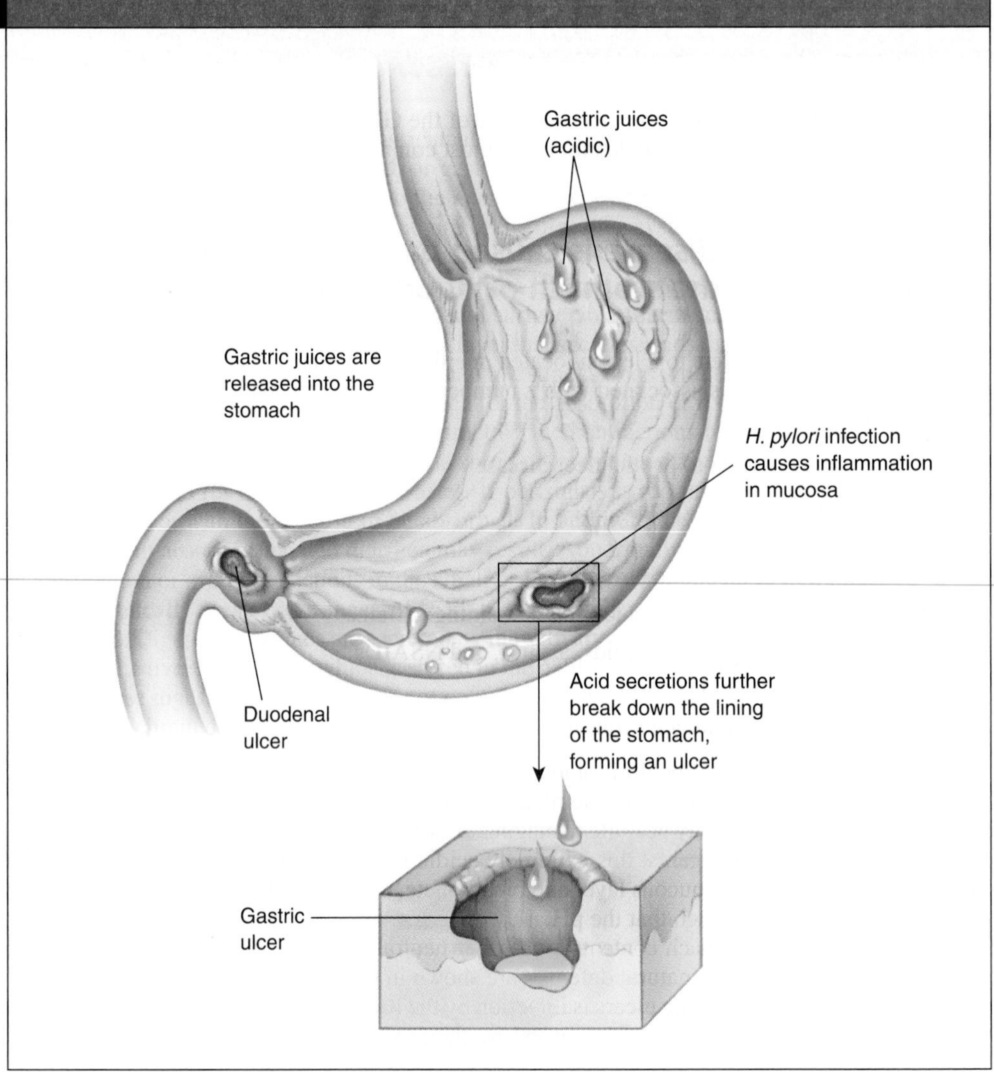

drugs (NSAIDs). Secondary factors that contribute to the ulcer and its subsequent inflammation include secretion of excess stomach acid and hyposecretion of adequate mucous protection. Figure 26.3 ■ illustrates the mechanism of peptic ulcer formation.

The characteristic symptom of duodenal ulcer is a gnawing or burning upper abdominal pain that occurs 1 to 3 hours after a meal. The pain is worse when the stomach is empty and often disappears following ingestion of food. Nighttime pain, nausea, and vomiting are uncommon. If the erosion progresses deeper into the mucosa, bleeding will occur and this may be evident as bright red blood in vomit or black, tarry stools. Many duodenal ulcers heal spontaneously, although they often reoccur after months of remission.

an = *not or without*
orexia = *appetite*

Gastric ulcers are less common than the duodenal type and have different symptoms. Although relieved by food, pain may continue even after a meal. Loss of appetite, known as **anorexia,** weight loss, and vomiting are more common. Remissions may be infrequent or absent. Medical follow-up of gastric ulcers sometimes proceeds for many years because a small percentage of the erosions become cancerous. The most severe ulcers may penetrate through the wall of the stomach and cause death. Whereas duodenal ulcers occur most frequently in the 30- to 50-year-old age group, gastric ulcers are more common in those older than age 60.

Ulceration in the lower small intestine is known as **Crohn's disease,** and erosions in the large intestine are called **ulcerative colitis.** These diseases are categorized as inflammatory bowel disease, and are treated with the anti-inflammatory medications discussed in Chapter 21. Particularly severe cases may require immunosuppressant drugs such as cyclosporine (Neoral, Sandimmune) or methotrexate (Folex, Mexate, others).

Gastroesophageal reflux disease (GERD) is a condition in which the acidic contents of the stomach move upwards into the esophagus. This causes an intense burning known as *heartburn,* and may lead to ulcers in the esophagus. The cause of GERD is usually a loosening of the sphincter located between the esophagus and the stomach. Many of the drugs prescribed for peptic ulcers are also used to treat GERD.

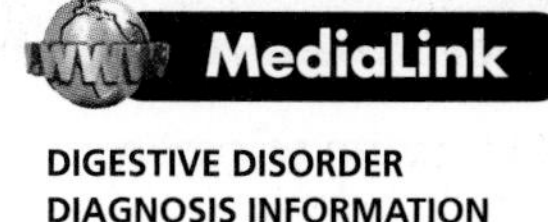

DIGESTIVE DISORDER DIAGNOSIS INFORMATION

Concept Review 26.1

- What are the similarities and differences between duodenal ulcers and gastric ulcers?

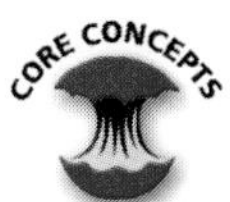

26.3 Peptic ulcer disease is treated by a combination of lifestyle changes and pharmacotherapy.

Before starting drug therapy, patients are usually advised to change lifestyle factors that contribute to peptic ulcer disease. For example, eliminating tobacco and alcohol use and reducing stress often cause an ulcer to go into remission.

For patients requiring drug therapy, a wide variety of both prescription and OTC medications are available. These agents fall into four primary classes, plus one miscellaneous group:

- H_2-receptor blockers
- Antibiotics
- Proton-pump inhibitors
- Antacids
- Miscellaneous agents

The goals of pharmacotherapy are to provide immediate relief from symptoms, promote healing of the ulcer, and prevent recurrence of the disease. The choice of medication depends on the source of the disease (infectious versus inflammatory), the severity of symptoms, and the convenience of OTC versus prescription drugs. The mechanisms of action of the four major classes of drugs used to treat peptic ulcer disease are shown in Figure 26.4 ■.

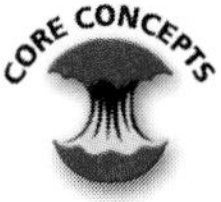

26.4 H_2-receptor blockers are often drugs of first choice in treating peptic ulcers.

The discovery of the H_2-receptor blockers in the 1970s marked a major breakthrough in the treatment of peptic ulcer disease. Since then, they have become available OTC and are drugs of choice in the treatment of peptic ulcer disease. Doses of the H_2-receptor blockers are given in Table 26.1.

As discussed in Chapter 21, histamine has two types of receptors: H_1 and H_2. Activation of H_1 receptors produces the classic symptoms of allergy, whereas the H_2 receptors are responsible for increasing acid secretion in the stomach. Cimetidine (Tagamet), the first **H_2-receptor blocker,** and other drugs in this class are quite effective at suppressing the volume and acidity of stomach acid. These drugs are also used to treat the symptoms of GERD. Several of these agents are available OTC for the treatment of heartburn.

Side effects of the H_2-receptor blockers are minor and rarely cause discontinuation of therapy. Patients taking high doses, or those with renal or hepatic disease, may experience confusion, restlessness, hallucinations, or depression. Patients should be advised not to take antacids at the same time as H_2-receptor blockers because the absorption of these drugs will be lessened.

Concept Review 26.2

- Explain the following statement: All H_2-receptor blockers are antihistamines, but not all antihistamines are H_2-receptor blockers.

FIGURE 26.4

Mechanism of action of antiulcer drugs: (a) proton-pump inhibitors act by blocking acid secretion by the HCl pump; (b) H_2-receptor blockers act by decreasing acid secretion; (c) antibiotics act by removing *H. pylori;* (d) antacids act by neutralizing acids.

Proton-pump inhibitor
Proton pump
(a) Proton-pump inhibitors
H_2-receptor blocker
H_2 receptor
(b) H_2-receptor blocker
HCl
K^+
Parietal cell with proton pump
Parietal cell with H_2-receptor
Ulcer with H.pylori
Antibiotic
(c) Antibiotic
Antacid
+ HCl ⟶ water + salt
(d) Antacid

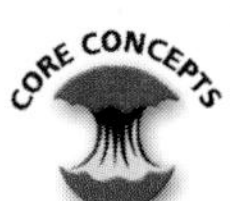

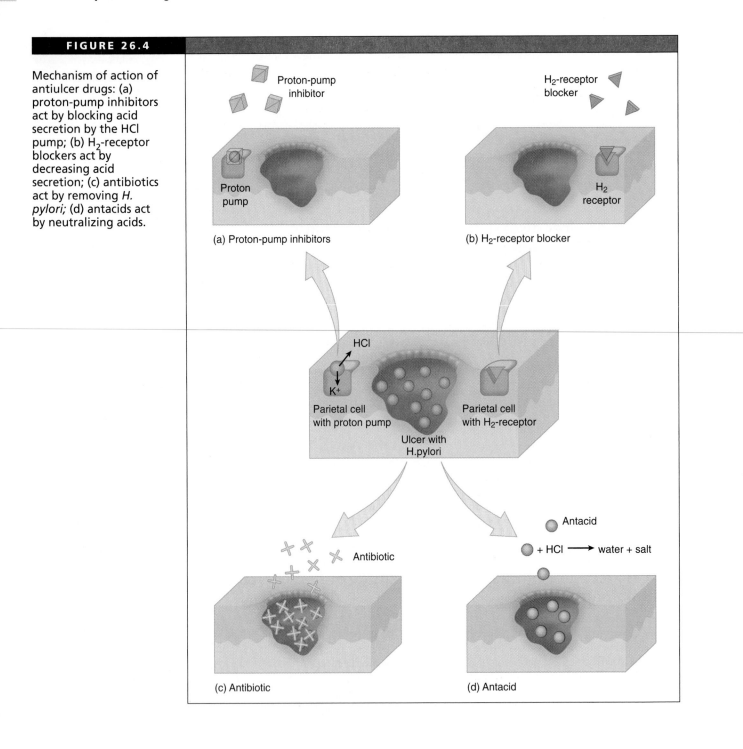

26.5 Proton-pump inhibitors are effective at reducing gastric acid secretion.

Proton-pump inhibitors act by blocking the enzyme responsible for secreting hydrochloric acid in the stomach. The proton-pump inhibitors are shown in Table 26.1.

Proton-pump inhibitors are relatively new drugs that have become widely used in the treatment of peptic ulcer disease and GERD. Drugs in this class reduce acid secretion in the stomach by binding irreversibly to the enzyme **H^+, K^+-ATPase.** In the mucosal cells of the stomach, this enzyme acts as a pump to release acid (also called H^+, or protons) onto the surface of the GI mu-

TABLE 26.1 Drugs for Peptic Ulcer Disease

DRUG	ROUTE AND ADULT DOSE	REMARKS
H_2-RECEPTOR BLOCKERS		
cimetidine (Tagamet)	PO 300–400 mg bid–qid or 800 mg at bedtime for active ulcers; 300 mg bid or 400 mg at bedtime for ulcer prophylaxis	For short-term treatment; decreases the metabolism of many medications; IM and IV forms available
famotidine (Pepcid)	PO 20 mg bid or 40 mg at bedtime for active ulcers; 20 mg at bedtime for ulcer prophylaxis	No identified drug interactions; IV form available
nizatidine (Axid)	PO 300 mg at bedtime for active ulcers; 150 mg at bedtime for ulcer prophylaxis	Newest drug in this class; rapid onset with few side effects
Pr ranitidine (Zantac)	PO 100–150 mg bid or 300 mg at bedtime for active ulcers; 150 mg at bedtime for ulcer prophylaxis	IM and IV forms available; ranitidine with bismuth citrate is given together with clarithromycin for *Helicobacter* infections
PROTON-PUMP INHIBITORS		
esomeprazole (Nexium)	PO 20–40 mg/day	Also for GERD
lansoprazole (Prevacid)	PO 15–60 mg/day	Often used in combination with antibiotics for *Helicobacter* infections; Prevac combines lansoprazole, amoxacillin, and clarithromycin
Pr omeprazole (Prilosec)	PO 20–60 mg once or twice daily	Often used in combination with antibiotics for *Helicobacter* infections; also for GERD
pantoprazole (Protonix)	PO 40 mg/day	Primarily for GERD; IV form available
rabeprazole sodium (AcipHex)	PO 20 mg/day for 4–8 weeks	Also for GERD
ANTACIDS		
aluminum hydroxide (Amphojel)	PO 600 mg tid–qid	Not absorbed; may cause constipation
calcium carbonate (Titralac, Tums)	PO 1–2 g bid–tid	Also for calcium replacement therapy; may cause constipation
calcium carbonate with magnesium hydroxide (Mylanta Gel-caps, Rolaids)	PO 2–4 capsules or tablets prn (max: 12 tablets/day)	Common OTC therapy
magaldrate (Riopan)	PO 480–1080 mg (5–10 ml suspension or 1–2 tablets) four times a day (max: 20 tablets or 100 ml/day)	Less incidence of bowel side effects than magnesium or aluminum antacids
magnesium hydroxide (Milk of Magnesia)	PO 2.4–4.8 g (30–60 ml) daily in 1 or more divided doses	Also used as a laxative; may cause diarrhea
magnesium hydroxide and aluminum hydroxide with simethicone (Mylanta, Maalox Plus)	PO 10–20 ml prn (max: 120 ml/day) or 2–4 tablets prn (max: 24 tablets/day)	Common OTC therapy
sodium bicarbonate (Alka-Seltzer, baking soda)	PO 0.3–2 g 1–4 times/day or 1/2 tsp of powder in glass of water	IV form available to treat metabolic acidosis and cardiac arrest

cosa. The proton-pump inhibitors reduce acid secretion to a greater extent than do the H_2-receptor blockers and have a longer duration of action.

Patients should be advised that it may take several days of therapy before they gain relief from ulcer pain. Beneficial effects last 3 to 5 days after therapy is stopped. These drugs are used only for the *short-term* control of peptic ulcers and GERD: typical length of therapy is 4 weeks.

Side effects from proton-pump inhibitors are uncommon. Headache, abdominal pain, diarrhea, nausea, and vomiting are the most commonly reported side effects.

DRUG PROFILE: H_2-Receptor Blocker: Pr *Ranitidine (Zantac)*

Actions and Uses:

Ranitidine has become a drug of choice for peptic ulcer disease. It has a higher potency than cimetidine that allows it to be administered once daily, usually at bedtime. Adequate healing of the ulcer takes 4 to 8 weeks. Patients with persistent disease may continue on drug maintenance for long periods to prevent recurrence. Gastric ulcers heal more slowly than duodenal ulcers, and require longer drug therapy. IV and IM forms are available for the treatment of acute stress-induced bleeding ulcers.

Adverse Effects and Interactions:

Ranitidine does not cross the blood-brain barrier to any appreciable extent, so the confusion and CNS depression observed with cimetidine is not expected with ranitidine. Ranitidine has fewer drug-drug interactions than cimetidine. Although rare, severe reductions in the number of red and white blood cells and platelets are possible; thus, periodic laboratory blood counts may be performed. High doses may result in impotence or a loss of libido in men.

Although ranitidine has fewer drug-drug interactions than cimetidine, it interacts with several drugs. For example, ranitidine may reduce the absorption of cefpodoxime, ketoconazole, and itraconazole.

Mechanism in Action: 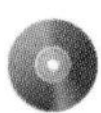

Ranitidine blocks the H_2 receptor and provides relief of pain due to gastric acid secretion in patients with peptic ulcer disease or GERD. ■

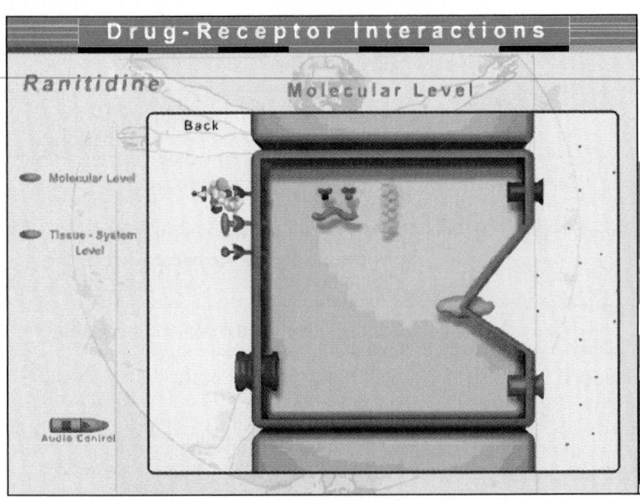

Use the student CD-ROM to see Mechanism in Action for Ranitidine.

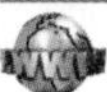 *See the Companion Website for a Nursing Process Focus specific to this drug.*

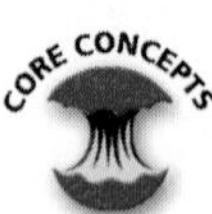

26.6 Antacids rapidly neutralize stomach acid and reduce the symptoms of peptic ulcer disease and GERD.

Antacids are alkaline substances that have been used to neutralize stomach acid for hundreds of years. Doses of the antacids are shown in Table 26.1.

Prior to the development of H_2-receptor blockers and proton-pump inhibitors, **antacids** were the mainstay of peptic ulcer and GERD pharmacotherapy. Indeed, many patients still use these inexpensive and readily available OTC medications. Antacids, however, are no longer recommended as the sole medication for peptic ulcer disease.

Antacids are alkaline, inorganic compounds of aluminum, magnesium, or calcium. Combinations of aluminum hydroxide and magnesium hydroxide are the most common type. Both aluminum hydroxide and magnesium hydroxide are bases, capable of rapidly neutralizing stomach acid. A few products combine antacids and H_2-receptor blockers into a single tablet; for example, Pepcid Complete contains calcium carbonate, magnesium hydroxide, and famotidine.

Simethicone is sometimes added to antacid preparations because it reduces gas bubbles that cause bloating and discomfort. For example, Mylanta contains simethicone, aluminum hydroxide, and magnesium hydroxide. Simethicone is classified as an **antiflatulent** because it reduces gas. It also is available by itself in OTC products such as Gas-X and Mylanta Gas.

anti = *against*
flatus = *gas in the GI tract*

NURSING PROCESS FOCUS

Patients Receiving H_2-Receptor Blocker Therapy

ASSESSMENT

Prior to administration:

- Obtain a complete health history including allergies, drug history, and possible drug interactions
- Assess patient for signs of GI bleeding
- Obtain vital signs
- Assess level of consciousness
- Obtain results of CBC, liver, and renal function tests

POTENTIAL NURSING DIAGNOSES

- Risk for Falls, related to adverse effect of drug
- Deficient Knowledge, related to drug therapy
- Acute Pain, related to gastric irritation from ineffective drug therapy
- Imbalanced Nutrition: Less than Body Requirements, related to adverse effects of drug

PLANNING: Patient Goals and Expected Outcomes

The patient will:

- Report episodes of drowsiness, dizziness
- Demonstrate an understanding of drug therapy
- Report reoccurrence of abdominal pain or discomfort during drug therapy
- Maintain body weight throughout course of treatment

IMPLEMENTATION

Interventions and (Rationales)	Patient Education/Discharge Planning
■ Monitor use of OTC drugs to avoid drug interactions especially with cimetidine therapy.	■ Instruct patient to consult with healthcare provider before taking other medications or herbal products.
■ Monitor level of abdominal pain or discomfort to assess effectiveness of drug therapy.	■ Advise patient that pain relief may not occur for several days after beginning therapy.
■ Monitor patient use of alcohol. (Alcohol can increase gastric irritation.)	■ Instruct patient to avoid alcohol use.
■ Discuss possible drug interactions. (Antacids can decrease the effectiveness of other drugs taken concurrently.)	■ Instruct patient to take H_2-receptor antagonists and other medications at least 1 hour before antacids.
■ Institute effective safety measures regarding falls. (Drugs may cause drowsiness or dizziness.)	■ Instruct patient to avoid driving or performing hazardous activities until drug effects are known.
■ Explain need for lifestyle changes. (Smoking and certain foods increase gastric acid secretion.)	Encourage patient to: ■ Stop smoking; provide information on smoke cessation programs ■ Avoid foods that cause stomach discomfort
■ Observe patient for signs of GI bleeding.	■ Instruct patient to immediately report episodes of blood in stool or vomitus or increase in abdominal discomfort.

EVALUATION OF OUTCOME CRITERIA

Evaluate the effectiveness of drug therapy by confirming that patient goals and expected outcomes have been met (see "Planning").

See Table 26.1 for a list of drugs to which these nursing actions apply.

DRUG PROFILE: Proton-Pump Inhibitor: 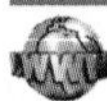 *Omeprazole (Prilosec)*

Actions and Uses:

Omeprazole was the first proton-pump inhibitor approved for peptic ulcer disease. Although this agent may take 2 hours to reach therapeutic levels, its effects last up to 72 hours. It is used for the short-term, 4- to 8-week therapy of peptic ulcers and GERD. Most patients are symptom-free after 2 weeks of therapy. It is used for longer periods in patients who have chronic hypersecretion of gastric acid, a condition known as **Zollinger-Ellison syndrome.** It is the most effective drug for this syndrome. Omeprazole is only available in oral form.

Adverse Effects and Interactions:

Adverse effects are generally minor and include headache, nausea, diarrhea, and abdominal pain. The main concern with proton-pump inhibitors is that long-term use has been associated with an increased risk of gastric cancer in laboratory animals. Because of this potential effect, therapy is generally limited to 2 months.

Omeprazole interacts with several drugs. For example, using it together with diazepam, phenytoin, and CNS depressants will cause increased blood levels of these drugs. Using it with warfarin may increase the likelihood of bleeding.

See the Companion Website for a Nursing Process Focus specific to this drug.

Unless taken in extremely large amounts, antacids are very safe. Although they act within 10 to 15 minutes, their duration of action lasts only 2 hours. Therefore, they must be taken often during the day. Products containing sodium, calcium, or magnesium can result in absorption of these minerals to the general circulation. When given in high doses, aluminum compounds may interfere with phosphate metabolism and cause constipation. Magnesium compounds may cause diarrhea. Patients should follow the label instructions very carefully and not take more than the recommended dosages.

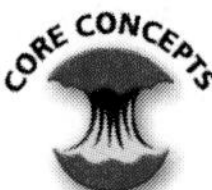

26.7 Antibiotics are administered to eliminate *Helicobacter pylori,* the cause of many peptic ulcers.

The bacterium *Helicobacter pylori* is associated with 90% of all duodenal ulcers and 70% of all gastric ulcers. This organism has adapted well as a human pathogen by devising ways to neutralize the high acidity surrounding it and by making chemicals called *adhesins* that allow it to stick tightly to the GI mucosa. *H. pylori* infections can remain active for life if not treated appropriately. Elimination of this organism causes ulcers to heal more rapidly and to remain in remission longer. The following antibiotics are commonly used for this purpose:

- Amoxacillin (Amoxil, others)
- Clarithromycin (Biaxin)
- Metronidazole (Flagyl)
- Tetracycline (Achromycin, others)

Two or more antibiotics are given together to increase the effectiveness of therapy and to lower the potential for bacterial resistance. Antibiotic therapy generally continues for 7 to 14 days. Bismuth compounds (Pepto-Bismol, Tritec) are sometimes added to the antibiotic regimen. While not antibiotics, bismuth compounds do inhibit bacterial growth and prevent *H. pylori* from adhering to the surface of the gastric mucosa. Dosages and additional information for these anti-infectives can be found in Chapters 22 and 23.

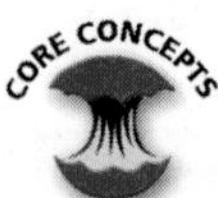

26.8 Several miscellaneous drugs are also beneficial in treating peptic ulcer disease.

Three additional drugs are beneficial in treating peptic ulcer disease. Sucralfate (Carafate) consists of sucrose (a sugar) plus aluminum hydroxide (an antacid). The drug produces a thick, gel-like substance that coats the ulcer, protecting it against further erosion and promoting healing.

Very little of the drug is absorbed from the GI tract. Other than constipation, side effects are minimal. A major disadvantage of sucralfate is that it must be taken four times a day.

Misoprostol (Cytotec) is a prostaglandin-like substance that inhibits gastric acid secretion and stimulates the production of protective mucus. Its primary use is for the prevention of peptic ulcers in patients taking high doses of NSAIDs or glucocorticoids. Diarrhea and abdominal cramping are relatively common. Classified as a pregnancy category X drug, misoprostol is contraindicated during pregnancy. In fact, misoprostol is sometimes used to terminate pregnancies, as discussed in Chapter 30.

Pirenzepine (Gastozepine) is a cholinergic-blocker (available in Canada) that inhibits gastric acid secretion. Although the action of pirenzepine is somewhat selective to the stomach, other anticholinergic effects such as dry mouth and constipation are possible. Anticholinergics were once widely used to treat peptic ulcer disease, but they are now rarely used for this purpose because of the availability of safer, more effective drugs.

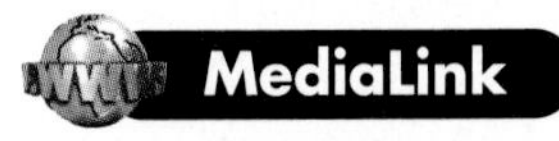

JOHNS HOPKINS' PEPTIC ULCER DISEASE SITE

Concept Review 26.3

- Is peptic ulcer disease considered an infection, an inflammation, or both?

CONSTIPATION

A major function of the large intestine is to reabsorb water from stools. If the waste material remains in the colon for an extended period, however, too much water will be reabsorbed, leading to small, hard stools. Difficult or infrequent bowel movements, known as **constipation,** is a common problem with a large number of different causes that include lack of exercise, insufficient food or fluid intake, lack of sufficient insoluble **dietary fiber,** and certain medications such as opioids. Positive dietary changes and increased physical activity should be considered before drugs are used. The normal frequency of bowel movements varies widely among individuals, from two to three per day to as few as one per week.

Occasional constipation is common and does not require drug therapy. However, chronic, infrequent, and painful bowel movements, accompanied by severe straining, may justify pharmacotherapy. Also, pharmacotherapy may be indicated following surgical procedures to prevent the patient from straining or bearing down when attempting a bowel movement. Drugs are given to cleanse the bowel prior to surgery or for diagnostic procedures of the colon, such as a colonoscopy or barium enema.

Life Span Fact

Constipation occurs more frequently in older adults because fecal transit time through the colon slows with aging; this population also exercises less and has more chronic disorders that cause constipation.

26.9 Laxatives are used to promote defecation.

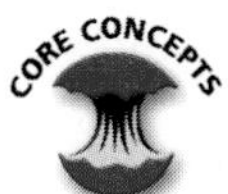

Laxatives are drugs that promote emptying of the bowel, or **defecation. Cathartic** is a related term that implies a stronger and more complete bowel emptying. When taken in prescribed amounts, laxatives have few side effects. Selected medications used to treat constipation are listed in Table 26.2. These drugs are often classified into four primary groups and a miscellaneous category.

laxat = *to loosen*
ive = *nature of, quality of*

- Bulk-forming: absorb water, thus adding size to the fecal mass; often taken prophylactically to prevent constipation
- Stimulant: irritate the bowel to increase peristalsis; may cause cramping
- Saline/osmotic: cause water to be retained in the fecal mass, causing a more watery stool
- Stool softeners/surfactant: cause more water and fat to be absorbed into the stools; often prescribed postoperatively to relieve straining
- Miscellaneous: act by mechanisms other than the above

Although laxatives are safe drugs, there are several conditions and side effects that must be monitored carefully. Laxatives are contraindicated in any patient with a suspected bowel obstruction because their use could cause the bowel to perforate. If acute abdominal cramping or diarrhea

TABLE 26.2 Laxatives

DRUG	ROUTE AND ADULT DOSE	REMARKS
bisacodyl (Dulcolax)	PO 5–15 mg daily prn	Stimulant type; also available as a rectal suppository
calcium polycarbophil (FiberCon, Fiberall, Mitrolan)	PO 1 g four times a day	Bulk-forming type
castor oil (Emulsoil, Neoloid, Purge)	PO 15–60 ml daily	Stimulant type; the only laxative to act on the small intestine
docusate (Surfak, Dialose, Colace)	PO 50–500 mg daily	Stool softener/surfactant type
magnesium citrate	PO 240 ml once	Saline/osmotic type
magnesium hydroxide (Milk of Magnesia)	PO 20–60 ml daily	Saline type
methylcellulose (Citrucel)	PO 5–20 ml tid in 8–10 oz water	Bulk-forming type
mineral oil	PO 45 ml bid	Miscellaneous type; lubricates the stools
phenolphthalein (Ex-Lax, Feen-A-Mint, Correctol)	PO 60–240 mg daily	Stimulant type
Pr psyllium muciloid (Metamucil, Naturcil)	PO 1–2 tsp in 8 oz water daily	Bulk-forming type; also used for diarrhea and as an aid in lowering blood cholesterol
sodium biphosphate (Fleet Phospho-Soda)	PO 15–30 ml mixed in water daily	Saline type; available as enema

Life Span Fact

Because of their reduced food intake and diminished physical activity, elderly patients are most prone to laxative misuse. Health professionals should advise these patients to increase their fluid intake, fiber consumption, and level of exercise.

occurs, the drug should be discontinued. Patients should be advised not to overuse laxatives because the smooth muscle in the bowel can lose its tone. Chronic constipation is the result.

Concept Review 26.4

- Bismuth compounds are used to treat several digestive disorders. Describe these agents and their uses.

DIARRHEA

dia = *through/between*
rrhea = *flow/discharge*

Occasionally, the colon does not reabsorb enough water from the fecal mass and stools become watery. **Diarrhea** is an increase in the frequency and fluidity of bowel movements. Like constipation, occasional diarrhea is a common, self-limiting disorder that does not require drug therapy. When prolonged or severe, especially in children, diarrhea can result in significant loss of body fluids and medications may be indicated. Prolonged diarrhea may lead to acid-base or electrolyte disorders, as discussed in Chapter 28.

Diarrhea is not a disease; it is a symptom of an underlying disorder. Diarrhea may be caused by certain medications, infections of the bowel, inflammatory bowel disorders such as Crohn's disease or ulcerative colitis, and chemicals such as lactate. Superinfections occurring during anti-infective therapy are common causes of diarrhea because they disrupt the normal microbial flora in the colon.

Drug therapy of diarrhea depends on the severity of the condition and whether or not a specific cause can be identified. If the cause is an infectious disease, an antibiotic or antiparasitic drug such as metronidazole (Flagyl) is indicated. If the cause is inflammatory in nature, anti-inflammatory drugs are needed. If the cause appears to be drug-induced the medication should be discontinued and another substituted.

NURSING PROCESS FOCUS

Patients Receiving Laxative Therapy

ASSESSMENT	POTENTIAL NURSING DIAGNOSES
Prior to administration: ■ Obtain complete health history including allergies, drug history, and possible drug interactions ■ Assess bowel elimination pattern ■ Assess bowel sounds	■ Risk for Injury (intestinal obstruction), related to adverse effects from drug therapy ■ Constipation

PLANNING: Patient Goals and Expected Outcomes

The patient will:

- Report relief from constipation
- Demonstrate an understanding of the drug's action by accurately describing drug side effects and precautions
- Immediately report effects such as nausea, vomiting, diarrhea, abdominal pain, and lack of bowel movement

IMPLEMENTATION

Interventions and (Rationales)	Patient Education/Discharge Planning
■ Monitor frequency volume and consistency of bowel movements. (Changes in bowel habits can indicate a serious condition.)	Advise patient to: ■ Discontinue laxative use if diarrhea occurs ■ Notify healthcare provider if constipation continues ■ Take medication as prescribed ■ Increase fluids and dietary fiber, such as whole grains, fibrous fruits, and vegetables ■ Expect results from medication within 2 to 3 days after initial dose
■ Monitor patient's ability to swallow. (Bulk laxatives can swell and cause obstruction in the esophagus.)	■ Instruct patient to discontinue medication and notify healthcare provider if having difficulty swallowing.
■ Monitor patient's fluid intake. (Esophageal or intestinal obstruction may result if the patient does not take in adequate amounts of fluid with the medication.)	Instruct patient to: ■ Drink six 8-oz glasses of fluid per day ■ Mix medication in 8 full oz of liquid ■ Drink at least 8 oz of additional fluid

EVALUATION OF OUTCOME CRITERIA

Evaluate the effectiveness of drug therapy by confirming that patient goals and expected outcomes have been met (see "Planning").

See Table 26.2 for a list of drugs to which these nursing actions apply.

Antidiarrheals act by relaxing the colon's smooth muscle, thus relieving cramping. Slower transit through the large intestine allows for better-formed stools. The selection of a particular agent depends on the severity of the diarrhea. Some antidiarrheals are shown in Table 26.3.

26.10 Opioids are the most effective drugs for controlling severe diarrhea.

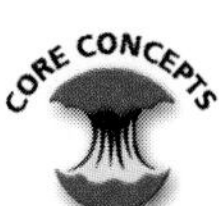

Acute or long-lasting diarrhea can lead to serious and even life-threatening conditions. The opioids are drugs of choice for this type of diarrhea because of their rapid onset and effectiveness.

DRUG PROFILE: Laxative: Pr *Psyllium Mucilloid (Metamucil, others)*

Actions and Uses:

Like other bulk-forming laxatives, psyllium is an insoluble fiber that is indigestible and not absorbed from the GI tract. When taken with plenty of water, psyllium swells and increases the size of the fecal mass by drawing water into the intestine. The larger the size of the fecal mass, the more the defecation reflex will be stimulated to promote bowel movements. Several doses of psyllium may be needed to produce a therapeutic effect. More frequent doses of psyllium may cause a small reduction in blood cholesterol level.

Adverse Effects and Interactions:

Psyllium rarely produces side effects. It generally causes less cramping than the stimulant-type laxatives and produces a more natural bowel movement. If taken with insufficient water, it may cause obstructions in the esophagus or intestine.

Psyllium may decrease absorption and clinical effects of antibiotics, warfarin, digoxin, nitrofurantoin, and salicylates.

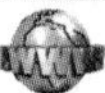

See the Companion Website for a Nursing Process Focus specific to this drug.

TABLE 26.3 Antidiarrheals

DRUG	ROUTE AND ADULT DOSE	REMARKS
bismuth salts (Pepto-Bismol)	PO 2 tabs or 30 ml prn	OTC adsorbent
difenoxin with atropine (Motofen)	PO 1–2 mg after each diarrhea episode (max: 8 mg/day)	Opioid; Schedule IV drug
Pr diphenoxylate with atropine (Lomotil)	PO 1–2 tabs or 5–10 ml tid–qid	Opioid; Schedule V drug
furazolidone (Furoxone)	PO 100 mg four times a day	For bacterial or protozoal GI infections
kaolin-pectin (Kao-Span, Kaolain	PO 60–120 ml after each diarrhea episode	OTC adsorbent
loperamide (Imodium, Kaopectate-III, others)	PO 4 mg as a single dose, then 2 mg after each diarrhea episode (max: 16 mg/day)	Opioid with no physical dependence; abuse is so low, it is not classified as a controlled substance
paregoric (Camphorated opium tincture)	PO 5–10 ml q2h to qid prn	Opioid; Schedule III drug

At doses used for diarrhea, opioids do not produce dependence or serious side effects. The most common opioid antidiarrheal is diphenoxylate (Lomotil), which is a Schedule V controlled substance. Loperamide (Imodium) is an opioid that carries no risk for dependence and is available OTC.

Nonopioid antidiarrheals include bismuth subsalicylate (Pepto-Bismol), which acts by binding and absorbing toxins. The psyllium and pectin preparations slow diarrhea by absorbing large amounts of fluid to form bulkier stools. Intestinal flora modifiers are supplements that help to correct the altered GI flora; a good source of healthy bacteria is yogurt with active cultures.

NAUSEA AND VOMITING

Nausea is an uncomfortable, subjective sensation that is sometimes accompanied by dizziness and an urge to vomit. Vomiting, or **emesis,** is a reflex primarily controlled by a portion of the medulla of the brain, known as the vomiting center. Nausea and vomiting are common symptoms associ-

TABLE 26.4 Antiemetics

DRUG	ROUTE AND ADULT DOSE	REMARKS
cyclizine (Marezine)	PO 50 mg q4h–qid	Antihistamine; for prevention of motion sickness and postop nausea and vomiting; IM form available
dexamethasone (Decadron)	IV 10–20 mg before chemotherapy	Glucocorticoid; IM, inhalation, and IV forms available; also for inflammatory disorders, severe allergies, acute asthma, and neoplasia
dimenhydrinate (Dramamine, others)	PO 50–100 mg q4h–qid (max: 400 mg/day)	Antihistamine; also used for allergies and cold/flu symptoms; IM and IV forms available
diphenhydramine (Benadryl)	PO 25–50 mg tid–qid (max: 300 mg/day)	Antihistamine; IM, IV, and topical forms available; also for allergies, Parkinson's disease, and anaphylaxis
dolasetron (Anzemet)	PO 100 mg 1 h before chemotherapy	Serotonin-receptor blocker; IV form available
granisetron (Kytril)	IV 10 mcg/kg 30 minutes before chemotherapy	Serotonin-receptor blocker; oral form available
hydroxyzine (Atarax, Vistaril)	PO 25–100 mg tid or qid	Antihistamine; IM form available; also for anxiety and as a pre-op medication
lorazepam (Ativan)	IV 1.0–1.5 mg before chemotherapy	Benzodiazepine; IM and IV forms available; also for anxiety, insomnia, and as a pre-op medication
meclizine (Antivert, Bonine)	PO 25–50 mg/day, 1 h before travel	Antihistamine; for motion sickness and nausea associated with vertigo
methylprednisolone (Medrol, Solu-medrol)	IV 2 doses of 125–500 mg 6 hours apart before chemotherapy	Glucocorticoid; IM and IV forms available; also for inflammatory disorders, severe allergies, acute asthma, and neoplasia
metoclopramide (Reglan)	PO 2 mg/kg 1 h before chemotherapy	Phenothiazine-like; IV and IM forms available; also for GERD, facilitation of small-bowel intubation, and gastric stasis
ondansetron (Zofran)	IV 4 mg tid prn	Serotonin-receptor blocker; IM and PO forms available
perphenazine (Phenazine, Trilafon)	PO 8–16 mg bid–qid	Phenothiazine; IM and IV forms available; also for psychoses
Pr prochlorperazine (Compazine)	PO 5–10 mg tid or qid	Phenothiazine; IM, IV, and suppository forms available; also for treatment of psychoses
promethazine (Phenergan)	PO 12.5–25 mg q4h–qid	Both a phenothiazine and an antihistamine; IM, IV, and suppository forms available; also for allergic disorders and as an adjunct to anesthesia and surgery
scopolamine (Hyoscine, Transderm Scop)	Transdermal; 0.5 mg q72h	Anticholinergic; oral, IV, IM, and subcutaneous forms available
thiethylperazine (Torecan)	PO 10 mg once to three times daily	Phenothiazine; IM form available

ated with a wide variety of conditions such as food poisoning, early pregnancy, extreme pain, migraines, trauma to the head or abdominal organs, inner ear disorders, and emotional disturbances. In treating nausea or vomiting, an important therapeutic goal is to remove the cause, whenever feasible.

Drugs from several different pharmacologic classes are prescribed to prevent nausea and vomiting. Patients receiving antineoplastic medications may receive three or more antiemetics to reduce the nausea and vomiting from the anticancer drugs. The individual antiemetic drugs are shown in Table 26.4.

DRUG PROFILE: Antidiarrheal:  *Diphenoxylate with Atropine (Lomotil)*

Actions and Uses:

The primary antidiarrheal ingredient in Lomotil is diphenoxylate. Like other opioids, diphenoxylate slows peristalsis, resulting in additional water being reabsorbed from the colon and formation of more solid stools. It is effective for moderate to severe diarrhea. The atropine in Lomotil is not added for its anticholinergic effect; it is added to discourage patients from taking too much of the drug.

Adverse Effects and Interactions:

Unlike most opioids, diphenoxylate has no analgesic properties and has an extremely low potential for abuse. Some patients experience dizziness or drowsiness and care should be taken not to operate machinery until the effects of the drug are known. At higher doses, the anticholinergic effects of atropine may be observed, which include drowsiness, dry mouth, and tachycardia.

MAO inhibitors may cause hypertensive crisis. Alcohol and other CNS depressants may enhance CNS effects.

See the Companion Website for a Nursing Process Focus specific to this drug.

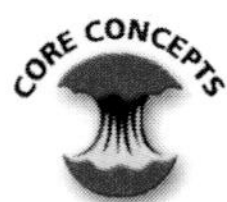

26.11 Antiemetics are prescribed to treat nausea, vomiting, and motion sickness.

anti = *against*
emetic = *vomit*

Many drugs *cause* nausea or vomiting as a side effect. The most extreme example of this is the antineoplastic agents, almost all of which cause some degree of nausea or vomiting. In fact, therapy with antineoplastic drugs is one of the most common reasons why **antiemetic** medications are prescribed. When cancer chemotherapy is initiated, it is common for a patient to receive three or more antiemetics. Antiemetic drugs belong to a number of different classes, including the following:

- Phenothiazines
- Antihistamines
- Serotonin-receptor blockers
- Glucocorticoids
- Benzodiazepines

To avoid losing antiemetic medication because of vomiting, many of these agents are available through the IM, IV, and/or suppository routes. The most effective antiemetics are serotonin-receptor blockers.

Motion sickness is a disorder affecting a portion of the inner ear known as the **vestibular apparatus** that is associated with significant nausea. The most common drug used for motion sickness is scopolamine, which is administered as a transdermal patch placed behind the ear. Antihistamines such as dimenhydrinate (Dramamine) and meclizine (Antivert) are also effective, but may cause significant drowsiness in some patients. Drugs used to treat motion sickness are most effective when taken 20 to 60 minutes before travel is expected.

On some occasions, it is desirable to *stimulate* the vomiting reflex with drugs called **emetics.** Indications for emetics include ingestion of poisons and overdoses of oral drugs. Ipecac syrup, given orally, or apomorphine, given subcutaneously, will induce vomiting in about 15 minutes. Drugs used to stimulate emesis should only be used in emergency situations under the direction of a healthcare provider.

WEIGHT LOSS

Hunger occurs when the hypothalamus in the brain recognizes the levels of certain chemicals (glucose) or hormones (insulin) in the blood. Hunger is a normal physiological response that drives people to seek nourishment. Appetite is somewhat different than hunger. Appetite is a psy-

DRUG PROFILE: Antiemetic: 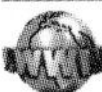 *Prochlorperazine (Compazine)*

Actions and Uses:

Prochlorperazine is a phenothiazine, a class of drugs usually prescribed for psychotic disorders as discussed in Chapter 10. The phenothiazines are actually the largest class of medications prescribed for severe nausea and vomiting and prochlorperazine is the most frequently prescribed antiemetic drug in its class. Prochlorperazine depresses the vomiting center in the medulla. It is frequently given by the rectal route, where absorption is rapid.

Adverse Effects and Interactions:

Prochlorperazine produces dose-related anticholinergic side effects such as dry mouth, constipation, and tachycardia. When used for prolonged periods at higher doses, extrapyramidal symptoms resembling those of Parkinson's disease are a serious concern (Chapters 10 and 11).

Prochlorperazine interacts with alcohol to increase CNS depression. Antacids and antidiarrheals inhibit absorption of prochlorperazine. When taken with phenobarbital, metabolism of prochlorperazine is increased.

See the Companion Website for a Nursing Process Focus specific to this drug.

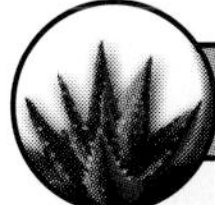

NATURAL ALTERNATIVES

Ginger for Nausea

Ginger is obtained from the roots of the herb *Zingiber officinale* that grows in a wide variety of places across the world. Active ingredients include aromatic oils that give the herb its characteristic scent and antiemetic activity. Because of its widespread use as a spice in Asian cooking, ginger is widely available in a number of forms, including tincture, tea, dried and fresh root, and capsules. Commercial products that use ginger as a flavoring include ginger cookies, gingerbread, and ginger ale. Consumers should check the product ingredients to be certain that the item truly contains ginger extract, rather than artificial ginger flavoring.

Ginger has been used in Chinese medicine for thousands of years. Indications relating to the digestive system include nausea, vomiting, morning sickness, and motion sickness. Studies have shown its effectiveness to be comparable to OTC medications.

Ginger is purported to have other significant benefits. The herb is said to have anti-inflammatory properties that are of benefit to patients with arthritis. It is sometimes given to patients with flu symptoms to help coughs and lower fever. Because of a possible effect on blood clotting, patients taking anticoagulants should avoid ginger unless otherwise directed by their healthcare provider. ■

chological response that drives food intake based on associations and memory. For example, people often eat not because they are experiencing hunger, but because it is a particular time of day or they find the act of eating pleasurable or social.

26.12 Anorexiants are drugs used for the short-term management of obesity.

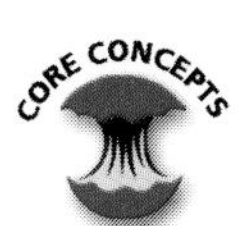

Despite the public's desire for effective agents to promote weight loss, there are few such drugs available. The approved drugs are used for the treatment of obesity, although they produce only modest weight loss.

Obesity may be defined as being more than 20% above the ideal body weight. Because of the prevalence of obesity in society and the difficulty most patients experience when following weight-reduction plans for extended periods of time, drug manufacturers have long sought to develop safe drugs that cause weight loss. In the 1970s, amphetamine and dextroamphetamine (Dexedrine) were widely prescribed as **anorexiants** to reduce appetite. These drugs, however, are addictive and amphetamines are rarely prescribed for this purpose today. In the 1990s, the combination of fenfluramine and phenteramine, known as fen-phen, was widely prescribed until fenfluramine was removed from the market for causing heart valve defects.

DRUG PROFILE: Anorexiant: 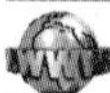 *Sibutramine (Meridia)*

Actions and Uses:

Sibutramine, a serotonin reuptake inhibitor, is the most widely prescribed appetite suppressant for the short-term control of obesity. When combined with a reduced calorie diet, sibutramine may produce a gradual weight loss of at least 10% of initial body weight over a period of a year. Sibutramine therapy is not recommended for longer than 1 year.

Adverse Effects and Interactions:

Headache is the most common complaint reported during sibutramine therapy, although insomnia and dry mouth are also possible. The drug should be used with great care in patients with cardiac disorders because it may cause tachycardia and raise blood pressure. It is a schedule IV drug with low potential for dependence.

Sibutramine interacts with several other drugs. For example, decongestants, cough, and allergy medications may cause elevated blood pressure. Ketoconazole and erythromycin may inhibit the metabolism of sibutramine. Using it together with an MAOI or SSRI may cause serotonin syndrome.

See the Companion Website for a Nursing Process Focus specific to this drug.

The two anorexiants currently on the market are sibutramine (Meridia) and orlistat (Xenical). Sibutramine is the most widely prescribed appetite suppressant for the short-term control of obesity. It suppresses appetite, probably by affecting the hunger center in the brain. Orlistat acts by a totally different mechanism—blocking fat absorption in the GI tract. Unfortunately, orlistat may also decrease absorption of other substances, including fat-soluble vitamins and coumadin. The effectiveness of sibutramine and orlistat is very limited, producing only a small increase in weight reduction compared to placebos.

PANCREATIC DISORDERS

The pancreas is responsible for the secretion of essential digestive enzymes. Lack of secretion, or **pancreatic insufficiency,** will result in malabsorption disorders. Replacement therapy with pancreatic enzymes is sometimes necessary.

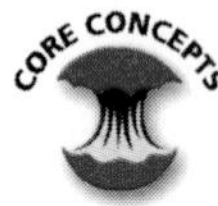

26.13 Pancreatic enzymes are administered as replacement therapy for patients with pancreatitis or malabsorption syndromes.

The pancreas secretes more than 1 L of pancreatic juice daily, which contains enzymes that split proteins, fats, and carbohydrates. Because these nutrients must be broken down into simpler molecules before they can be absorbed, lack of sufficient pancreatic juice can cause malabsorption syndromes. Lipase, the enzyme that digests fats, is most affected. The most common cause of pancreatic insufficiency is chronic pancreatitis. This disorder also occurs in most patients with cystic fibrosis.

Symptoms of pancreatic insufficiency include upper abdominal pain, loss of appetite, nausea, vomiting, and weight loss. *Steatorrhea,* the passing of bulky, foul-smelling fatty stools, occurs because dietary fats are passing through the GI tract without being broken down.

Pancreatic enzyme supplements include pancrelipase (Cotazym, Pancrease, others) and pancreatin (Entozyme, Viokase, others). These drugs are obtained from either pork or beef pancreas and contain the necessary enzymes to digest fats, carbohydrates, and proteins. Pancrelipase is generally preferred because it has significantly more enzyme activity. To avoid destruction by

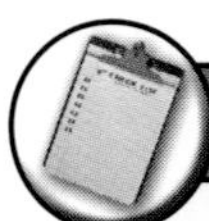

PATIENTS NEED TO KNOW

Patients treated for digestive disorders need to know the following:

Regarding Antiulcer Medications

1. Do not smoke tobacco when taking H_2-receptor blockers because this interferes with the drug action.
2. As drowsiness may occur when starting therapy with H_2-receptor blockers or proton-pump inhibitors; monitor operating equipment or using alcohol or other CNS drugs carefully.
3. When taking medications for peptic ulcer, avoid drugs that may cause stomach irritation such as aspirin or NSAIDs.
4. Shake liquid antacids well before pouring. Chewable tablets should be thoroughly chewed before swallowing.

Regarding Laxatives

5. As bulk-forming laxatives and stool softeners may take several days for results, be patient and do not take more than prescribed.
6. Take bulk-forming laxatives with at least two full glasses of water because this aids in forming larger stools.
7. If constipation is a frequent problem, try drinking more fluids and adding fiber to the diet rather than taking laxatives on a continual basis. Foods rich in fiber include all fruits and vegetables, bran cereals, and whole grain breads.

Regarding Antiemetics

8. Before taking antiemetic medications, try other methods of relieving nausea, such as drinking flat carbonated beverages or weak tea or eating small amounts of crackers or dry toast.
9. When taking phenothiazines or antihistamines as antiemetics, use sugarless candy, gum, or ice chips to minimize dry mouth.
10. Recall that medications taken to suppress hunger produce only modest weight loss and are not effective without a reduced-calorie diet. True, sustained weight loss can only be achieved by modification of dietary habits. ▪

stomach acid, capsules are made with an enteric coating. Dosing is individualized to the degree of pancreatic insufficiency in each patient. Administration of the drug is timed to coincide with meals so that the enzymes are available when food reaches the duodenum. Overtreatment can cause nausea, vomiting, and diarrhea.

CHAPTER REVIEW

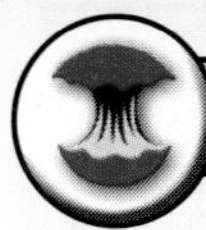

CORE CONCEPTS SUMMARY

26.1 The digestive system breaks down food, absorbs nutrients, and eliminates wastes.

The alimentary canal provides a large surface area for the absorption of nutrients and drugs. Substances are propelled through the GI tract by peristalsis. Abnormally fast or slow peristalsis can affect nutrient, drug, and water absorption.

26.2 Peptic ulcer disease is caused by an erosion of the mucosal layer of the stomach or duodenum.

Infection with *H. pylori* and therapy with NSAIDs are the most common causes of peptic ulcers. A gnawing pain in the upper abdomen that is relieved by eating is the most common symptom of duodenal ulcer. Though less common, gastric ulcers may be more serious and require longer treatment and follow-up. GERD gives similar symptoms to peptic ulcers and is treated with some of the same medications.

26.3 Peptic ulcer disease is treated by a combination of lifestyle changes and pharmacotherapy.

Before beginning drug therapy, the patient should eliminate tobacco and alcohol use and reduce stress levels, as these changes will favor remission of peptic ulcer disease. Goals of drug therapy include relief of symptoms, promotion of ulcer healing, and prevention of recurrences.

26.4 H_2-receptor blockers are often drugs of first choice in treating peptic ulcers.

H_2-receptor blockers reduce the volume and acidity of stomach acid. Healing of duodenal ulcers occurs in 4 to 8 weeks, and side effects are uncommon.

26.5 Proton-pump inhibitors are effective at reducing gastric acid secretion.

Proton-pump inhibitors diminish gastric acid secretion by interfering with the enzyme H^+, K^+-ATPase, which is present in the mucosal cells in the stomach. Although very effective, use is usually limited to 2 months because of the possibility of long-term adverse effects.

26.6 Antacids rapidly neutralize stomach acid and reduce the symptoms of peptic ulcer disease and GERD.

Once drugs of choice for treating peptic ulcer disease, antacids are now primarily used to give immediate relief for the heartburn associated with GERD or peptic ulcers.

26.7 Antibiotics are administered to eliminate *Helicobacter pylori*, the cause of many peptic ulcers.

Elimination of *H. pylori* using combination therapy with several different antibiotics has been found to promote more rapid ulcer healing and longer remissions.

26.8 Several miscellaneous drugs are also beneficial in treating peptic ulcer disease.

Sucralfate produces a gel-like substance that provides a protective coating for ulcers. Misoprostol inhibits gastric acid secretion and promotes the secretion of protective mucus. Pirenzepine inhibits acid secretion by blocking cholinergic receptors.

26.9 Laxatives are used to promote defecation.

Laxatives are given to promote emptying of the colon. Laxatives act by stimulating peristalsis or by adding more bulk or water to the fecal mass.

26.10 Opioids are the most effective drugs for controlling severe diarrhea.

Diarrhea is treated by addressing its cause, which may include anti-inflammatory drugs or anti-infectives. Opioids are the most effective drugs for relieving severe diarrhea, but they have some abuse potential. OTC bismuth compounds can help with simple diarrhea.

26.11 Antiemetics are prescribed to treat nausea, vomiting, and motion sickness.

Symptomatic treatment of nausea and vomiting includes drugs from many different classes, including phenothiazines, antihistamines, corticosteroids, benzodiazepines, and serotonin-receptor blockers. Motion sickness can be controlled through medications such as transdermal scopolamine or dimenhydrinate (Dramamine).

26.12 Anorexiants are drugs used for the short-term management of obesity.

Only a few drugs are available for the short-term management of obesity and these drugs produce only modest weight loss. The anorexiant sibutramine and the lipid-absorption blocker orlistat are used to help obese clients lose weight.

26.13 Pancreatic enzymes are administered as replacement therapy for patients with pancreatitis or malabsorption syndromes.

Pancreatic insufficiency leads to lack of breakdown and absorption of sufficient quantities of fats, carbohydrates, and proteins. This can lead to malabsorption syndromes. Pancrelipase and pancreatin are used to restore the deficient enzymes.

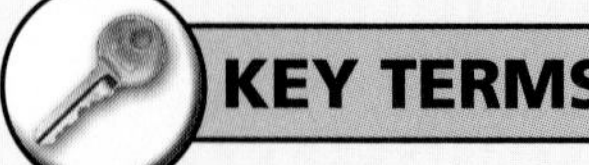

KEY TERMS

alimentary canal (AL-uh-MEN-tare-ee): the hollow tube in the digestive system that starts in the mouth and includes the esophagus, stomach, small intestine, and large intestine / ***page 488***

anorexia (AN-oh-REX-ee-uh): loss of appetite / ***page 490***

anorexiant (AN-oh-REX-ee-ant): drug used to suppress appetite / ***page 503***

antacid (an-TASS-id): drug that neutralizes stomach acid / ***page 494***

antiemetic (AN-tie-ee-MET-ik): drug that prevents vomiting / ***page 502***

antiflatulent (an-tie-FLAT-u-lent): drug that reduces gas formation in the GI tract / ***page 494***

cathartic (kah-THAR-tik): drug that causes complete evacuation of the bowel / ***page 497***

constipation (kon-stah-PAY-shun): Infrequent passage of abnormally hard and dry stools / ***page 497***

Crohn's disease (KROHNS): chronic inflammatory bowel disease affecting the ileum and sometimes the colon / ***page 490***

defecation (def-ah-KAY-shun): evacuation of the colon; bowel movement / ***page 497***

diarrhea: abnormal frequency and liquidity of bowel movements / ***page 498***

dietary fiber: substance neither digested nor absorbed that contributes to the fecal mass / ***page 497***

digestion (dye-JES-chun): process by which the body breaks down ingested food into small molecules that can be absorbed / ***page 488***

emesis (EM-eh-sis): vomiting / ***page 500***

emetic (ee-MET-ik): drug used to induce vomiting / ***page 502***

gastroesophageal reflux disease (GERD) (GAS-troh-ee-SOF-ah-JEEL REE-flux): the regurgitation of stomach contents into the esophagus / ***page 491***

H^+, K^+-ATPase: enzyme responsible for pumping acid onto the mucosal surface of the stomach / ***page 492***

H_2-receptor blocker: drug that inhibits the effects of histamine at its receptors in the GI tract / ***page 491***

Helicobacter pylori **(hee-lick-oh-BAK-tur py-LOR-eye):** bacterium associated with a large percentage of peptic ulcer disease / ***page 489***

pancreatic insufficiency: condition in which the pancreas is not secreting sufficient amounts of digestive enzymes, resulting in malabsorption syndromes / ***page 504***

peptic ulcer: erosion of the mucosa in the alimentary canal, most commonly in the stomach and duodenum / ***page 489***

peristalsis (pair-ih-STAL-sis): involuntary wave-like contraction that occurs in the alimentary canal / ***page 488***

proton-pump inhibitor: drugs that inhibit the enzyme H^+, K^+-ATPase / ***page 492***

ulcerative colitis (UL-sir-ah-tiv koh-LIE-tuss): inflammatory bowel disease of the colon / ***page 490***

vestibular apparatus (vest-IB-you-lar): portion of the inner ear responsible for the sense of position / ***page 502***

Zollinger-Ellison syndrome (ZOLL-in-jer ELL-ih-sun): disorder of having excess acid secretion in the stomach / ***page 496***

REVIEW QUESTIONS

The following questions are written in NCLEX-PN® style. Answer these questions to assess your knowledge of the chapter material, and go back and review any material that is not clear to you.

1. The primary cause of peptic ulcers is:

1. Stress
2. Smoking
3. *H. pylori* bacteria
4. Family history

2. The patient with a gastric ulcer has been started on ranitidine (Zantac). Instructions should include:

1. Drug therapy will extend over several weeks or months.
2. Information about the signs and symptoms of CNS depression.
3. Drug therapy will extend over a few days.
4. Information about the signs and symptoms of hepatic disease.

3. Your patient is taking nizatidine (Axid) and magaldrate (Riopan). The patient should:

1. Not take the medications at the same time
2. Take the medications at the same time
3. Switch to another antacid that is safer with this drug
4. Not be taking magaldrate because it is not effective

4. Important teaching to be included for a patient on omeprazole (Prilosec) should include which of the following?

1. This drug is safe for long-term use.
2. This drug should not be taken for more than 2 months.
3. Therapeutic effects may take weeks.
4. This drug must be used with antacids to be effective.

5. When the patient is receiving a magnesium hydroxide (Mylanta), the nurse must assess for:

1. Diarrhea
2. Peripheral disease
3. Neuropathy
4. Respiratory disorders

6. The nurse instructs patients on laxatives to:

1. Use daily for best results
2. Not overuse them because it can cause chronic constipation
3. Decrease fluid intake
4. Decrease food intake

7. After administering an antiemetic, the patient should be placed in what position?

1. Face up
2. Side-lying
3. Upright
4. Face down

8. Which of the following medications should be avoided when the patient has a peptic ulcer?

1. Aspirin
2. Raw foods
3. Anorexiants
4. Antiemetics

9. The patient on sibutramine (Meridia) must be assessed for:

1. Hepatic toxicity
2. Renal disease
3. Hypertension and tachycardia
4. Severe diarrhea

10. The patient demonstrates an understanding of pancrelipase (Cotazym) when she states:

1. "I will take this medication with meals."
2. "I will take this medication on an empty stomach."
3. "I will only take this medication when I am eating carbohydrates."
4. "If I develop nausea, vomiting, or diarrhea, I will increase my dosage."

CASE STUDY QUESTIONS

For questions 1–3 please refer to the following case study, and choose the correct answer from choices 1–4.

Ms. Han is a 32-year-old stock broker with a very stressful job. She has just been diagnosed with a duodenal ulcer. Initially, the physician prescribed ranitidine (Zantac), clarithromycin, and amoxicillin, with OTC antacids as needed.

1. Which drug was prescribed primarily to reduce the inflammation caused by the ulcer?

1. Ranitidine
2. Antacid
3. Clarithromycin
4. Amoxicillin

2. Which drug was prescribed to eradicate *H. pylori?*

1. Ranitidine
2. Clarithromycin
3. Amoxicillin
4. Both b and c

3. Ms. Han has been taking aluminum-based antacids for her ulcer and is experiencing constipation. Which of the following would you recommend that she obtain OTC to promote bowel movements?

1. Methylcellulose (Citrucel)
2. Famotidine (Pepcid)
3. Omeprazole (Prilosec)
4. Bismuth salts (Pepto-Bismol)

4. Mr. Tanner is 320 pounds and has tried numerous weight-loss plans. Which of the following drugs might assist Mr. Tanner in losing weight?

1. Pancreatin (Entozyme, Viokase, others)
2. Prochlorperazine (Compazine)
3. Lorazepam (Ativan)
4. Orlistat (Xenical)

5. Mr. Griffith is looking forward with anticipation to an Alaskan cruise but fears motion sickness. Which of the following might be beneficial for Mr. Griffith?

1. Sibutramine (Meridia)
2. Meclizine (Antivert)
3. Omeprazole (Prilosec)
4. Loperamide (Imodium)

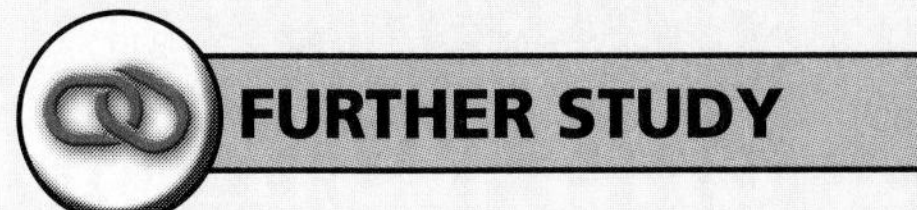

FURTHER STUDY

- Chapter 21 discusses anti-inflammatory medications that can be used in treating inflammatory bowel disease.
- Histamine is discussed in Chapter 21.
- Chapters 22 and 23 contain dosages and additional information for anti-infectives.
- Chapter 30 discusses the use of misoprostol to end pregnancies.
- Acid-base and electrolyte disorders are discussed in Chapter 28.
- Phenothiazines, used for psychotic disorders, are discussed in Chapter 10. Extrapyramidal symptoms, resembling those of Parkinson's disease, are discussed in Chapters 10 and 11.
- Antineoplastic drugs that cause significant nausea and vomiting are presented in Chapter 24.
- Additional applications for opioids are presented in Chapter 12.

EXPLORE MEDIALINK www.prenhall.com/holland

Additional resources for this chapter can be found on the CD-ROM accompanying this textbook, and on the Companion Website. Click on Chapter 26 to select activities for this chapter.

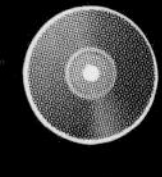

Mechanism in Action: Ranitidine
Audio Glossary
Concept Review
NCLEX-PN®
Nursing in Action
Dosage Calculator

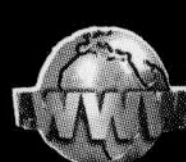

Digestive Disorder Diagnosis Information
Johns Hopkins' Peptic Ulcer Disease Site

CHAPTER

27 Vitamins, Minerals, and Nutritional Supplements

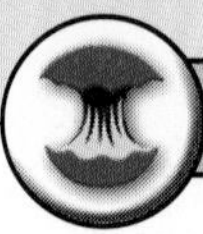

CORE CONCEPTS

27.1 Vitamins are organic substances that are needed in small amounts to promote growth and maintain health.

27.2 Vitamins are classified as fat soluble or water soluble.

27.3 Recommended dietary allowances (RDAs) for vitamins have been established for the average, healthy adult.

27.4 Vitamin therapy is indicated for specific conditions.

27.5 Minerals are inorganic substances needed in very small amounts to maintain normal body metabolism.

27.6 Enteral and total parenteral nutrition are therapies that deliver essential nutrients to patients with deficiencies.

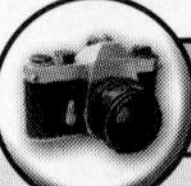

DRUG SNAPSHOT

The following drugs will be discussed in this chapter:

DRUG CLASSES	DRUG PROFILES
Vitamins	Pr cyanocobalamin (Cyanabin, others)
Minerals	Pr ferrous sulfate (Ferralyn, others)
NUTRITIONAL SUPPLEMENTS	
Enteral nutrition	
Total parenteral nutrition	

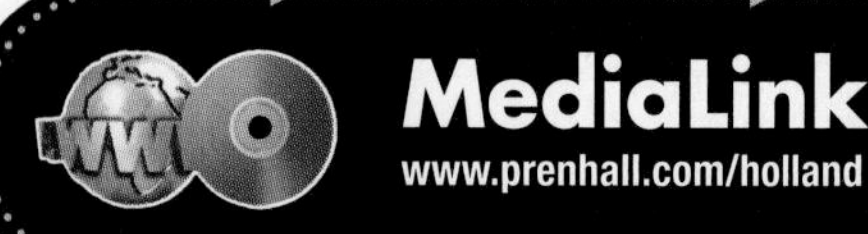

Interactive resources for this chapter can be found on the Companion Website. Click on Chapter 27 and "Begin" to select the activities for this chapter. For chapter-related animations, NCLEX-PN®-style questions, and an audio glossary, access the accompanying CD-ROM in this book.

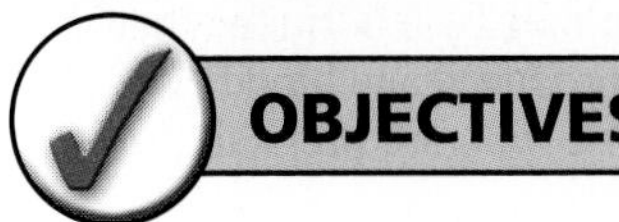

OBJECTIVES

After reading this chapter, the student should be able to:

1. Identify characteristics that differentiate vitamins from other nutrients.
2. Describe the functions of common vitamins and minerals.
3. Explain the rationale behind recommended dietary allowances (RDAs).
4. Describe the role of vitamin and mineral therapies in the treatment of deficiency disorders.
5. Identify several drug-vitamin and drug-mineral interactions.
6. Compare and contrast the functions of major minerals and trace minerals.
7. Compare and contrast enteral and parenteral methods of providing nutrition.

The vitamin, mineral, and nutritional supplement business is a multibillion dollar industry. Although aggresive marketing often leads patients to believe that dietary supplements are essential to maintain health, most people obtain all necessary nutrients through their normal diet. Once the body has obtained the amount of vitamin or mineral it needs to carry on metabolism, the excess is simply excreted or stored. There are some conditions, however, where dietary supplementation is necessary and will benefit the patient's health. This chapter will focus on these conditions and explore the role of vitamins, minerals, and nutritional supplements in pharmacology.

27.1 Vitamins are organic substances that are needed in small amounts to promote growth and maintain health.

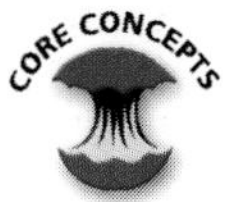

Vitamins are organic compounds required by the body in very small amounts for growth and for the maintenance of normal metabolic processes. Since the discovery of thiamine in 1911, over a dozen substances have been identified as vitamins. Because scientists did not know the chemical structures of the vitamins when they were discovered, they were assigned letters and numbers such as A, B_{12}, and C. These names are still widely used today.

An important characteristic of vitamins is that, with the exception of vitamin D, human cells cannot synthesize them. They or their precursors—known as **provitamins**—must be supplied in the diet. A second important characteristic is that if the vitamin is not present in adequate amounts, the body's metabolism will be disrupted and disease will result. Furthermore, the symptoms of the deficiency can be reversed by the administration of the missing vitamin.

pro = *before*
vitamin = *essential substance*

Vitamins serve diverse and important roles in human physiology. For example, the B complex vitamins are coenzymes essential to many metabolic pathways. Vitamin A is a precursor of

Fast Facts Vitamins, Minerals, and Dietary Supplements

- About 40% of Americans take vitamin supplements daily.
- There is no difference between the chemical structure of a natural vitamin and a synthetic vitamin, yet consumers pay much more for the natural type.
- Vitamin B_{12} is only present in animal products. Vegetarians may find adequate amounts in fortified cereals, nutritional supplements, or yeast.
- Administration of folic acid during pregnancy has been found to reduce birth defects in the nervous system of the baby.
- Patients who never go outside or never receive sun exposure may need vitamin D supplements.
- Heavy menstrual periods may result in considerable iron loss.
- Technically, vitamins and minerals cannot increase a patient's energy levels. Energy can only be provided by adding calories in carbohydrates, proteins, and fats.
- "Organic" foods do not necessarily contain a higher concentration of vitamins or minerals than non-organic foods.

retinal, a pigment needed for normal vision. Calcium metabolism is regulated by a hormone that is derived from vitamin D. Without vitamin K, abnormal prothrombin is produced and blood clotting is affected. Patients having a low or unbalanced dietary intake, those who are pregnant, or those experiencing a chronic disease may benefit from vitamin therapy.

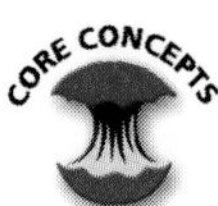

27.2 Vitamins are classified as fat soluble or water soluble.

A simple way to classify vitamins is by their ability to mix with water. Those that dissolve easily in water are called water-soluble vitamins. Examples include vitamin C and the B vitamins. Those that dissolve in lipids are called fat soluble and include vitamins A, D, E, and K.

The difference in solubility affects the way the vitamins are absorbed by the GI tract and stored in the body. The water-soluble vitamins are absorbed along with water in the digestive tract and readily dissolve in blood and body fluids. When excess water-soluble vitamins are ingested, they cannot be stored for later use and are simply excreted in the urine. Because they are not stored to any significant degree, they must be ingested daily; otherwise deficiencies will quickly develop.

Fat-soluble vitamins, however, cannot be absorbed in sufficient quantity in the small intestine unless they are ingested with other fats. These vitamins can be stored in large quantities in the liver and fat. Should the patient not ingest sufficient quantities, fat-soluble vitamins are removed from storage depots in the body as needed. Unfortunately, this storage can lead to dangerously high levels of the fat-soluble vitamins if they are taken in excessive amounts.

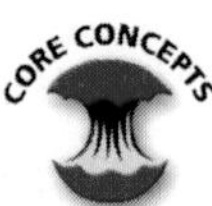

27.3 Recommended dietary allowances (RDAs) for vitamins have been established for the average, healthy adult.

Based on scientific research on humans and animals, the Food and Drug Administration has established levels for the intake of vitamins and minerals called **recommended dietary allowances (RDAs).** Canada publishes similar data called the recommended nutrient intake (RNI). The RDA values represent the minimum amount of vitamin or mineral needed to prevent a deficiency in a healthy adult. The RDAs are revised periodically to reflect the latest scientific research. Current RDAs for vitamins are shown in Table 27.1.

The need for certain vitamins and minerals may vary widely. Patients who are pregnant, have chronic disease, or who exercise vigorously have different nutritional needs than the average adult. One of the best known examples is the increased need for folic acid during pregnancy. Taking 400 mcg of **folic acid,** a B vitamin, daily prior to conception and during pregnancy can help prevent serious birth defects known as neural tube defects. Recognizing and adjusting for these nutritional differences are essential to maintaining good health.

Vitamin, mineral, or nutritional supplements should never substitute for a balanced diet. Sufficient intake of proteins, carbohydrates, and fats is needed for proper health. Furthermore, although the label on a vitamin supplement may indicate that it contains 100% of the RDA for a particular vitamin, the body may absorb as little as 10–15% of the amount ingested. With the exception of vitamins A and D, it is not harmful for most patients to consume 2 to 3 times the recommended levels of vitamins.

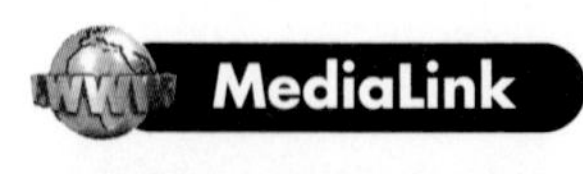

NATIONAL COUNCIL AGAINST HEALTH FRAUD

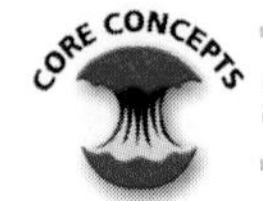

27.4 Vitamin therapy is indicated for specific conditions.

hyper = *above*
vitamin = *vitamin*
osis = *condition*

Life Span Fact

Infancy and childhood are times of potential vitamin deficiency due to the high growth demands placed on the body.

Most people who eat a normal, balanced diet obtain all the necessary nutrients without vitamin supplementation. Indeed, megavitamin therapy is not only expensive but may be harmful to health if taken for long periods. **Hypervitaminosis,** or toxic levels of vitamins, has been reported for vitamins A, C, D, E, B_6, niacin, and folic acid. In the United States, it is actually more common to observe syndromes of vitamin *excess* than those of vitamin *deficiency*.

Vitamin deficiencies may have a number of causes. In the United States deficiencies are most often the result of poverty, fad diets, chronic alcoholism, or prolonged parenteral feeding. In addition, requirements for all nutrients are increased during pregnancy and lactation. Vitamin deficiencies in patients with chronic liver and kidney disease are well documented. Patients with

TABLE 27.1 Vitamins

VITAMIN	FUNCTION(S)	RDA MEN	RDA WOMEN	COMMON CAUSE(S) OF DEFICIENCY
A	Visual pigments, epithelial cells	1000 RE*	800 RE	Prolonged dietary deprivation, particularly where rice is the main food source; pancreatic disease; cirrhosis
B complex:				
biotin	Coenzyme in metabolic reactions	30 mcg	30 mcg	Deficiencies are rare
Pr cyanocobalamin B_{12}	Coenzyme in nucleic acid metabolism	2.4 mcg	2.4 mcg	Lack of intrinsic factor, inadequate intake of foods from animal origin
folate	Coenzyme in amino acid and nucleic acid metabolism	400 mcg	400 mcg	Pregnancy, alcoholism, cancer, oral contraceptive use
niacin B_3	Coenzyme in metabolic reactions	16 mg	14 mg	Prolonged dietary deprivation, particularly where Indian corn (maize) or millet is the main food source; chronic diarrhea; liver disease; alcoholism
pantothenic acid	Coenzyme in metabolic reactions	5 mg	5 mg	Deficiencies are rare
pyridoxine B_6	Coenzyme in amino acid metabolism	1.3 mg	1.3 mg	Alcoholism; oral contraceptive use; malabsorption diseases
riboflavin B_2	Coenzyme in metabolic reactions	1.3 mg	1.1 mg	Inadequate consumption of milk or animal products; chronic diarrhea; liver disease; alcoholism
thiamine B_1	Coenzyme in metabolic reactions	1.2 mg	1.1 mg	Prolonged dietary deprivation, particularly where rice is the main food source; hyperthyroidism, pregnancy, liver disease; alcoholism
C	Coenzyme and antioxidant	60 mg	60 mg	Inadequate intake of fruits and vegetables; pregnancy; chronic inflammatory disease; burns; diarrhea, alcoholism
D	Calcium and phosphate metabolism	5 mcg	5 mcg	Low dietary intake; inadequate exposure to sunlight
E	Antioxidant	10 TE**	8 TE	Premature infants; malabsorption diseases
K	Cofactor in blood clotting	70 mcg	65 mcg	Newborns; liver disease; long-term parenteral nutrition; certain drugs such as cephalosporins and salicylates

**RE = retinoid equivalents*

***TE = alpha-tocopherol equivalents*

DRUG PROFILE: Vitamin: Pr *Cyanocobalamin (Cyanabin and Others)*

Actions and Uses:

Cyanocobalamin is a purified form of vitamin B_{12} that is administered in deficiency states. Vitamin B_{12} is not synthesized by either plants or animals; only bacteria perform this function. Because only miniscule amounts of vitamin B_{12} are required (3 mcg/day), deficiency of this vitamin is not usually caused by insufficient dietary intake. The most common cause of vitamin B_{12} deficiency is lack of a chemical called **intrinsic factor,** which is secreted by stomach cells. Intrinsic factor is required for vitamin B_{12} to be absorbed from the intestine. Figure 27.1 ■ illustrates the metabolism of vitamin B_{12}/cyanocobalamin. Inflammatory diseases of the stomach or surgical removal of the stomach (gastrectomy) may result in deficiency of intrinsic factor. Inflammatory diseases of the small intestine that affect food and nutrient absorption may also cause vitamin B_{12} deficiency.

Adverse Effects and Interactions:

Side effects from cyanocobalamin are uncommon. Hypokalemia is possible and serum potassium levels are monitored periodically.

Alcohol, aminosalicylic acid, neomycin, and colchicines may decrease absorption of oral cyanocobalamin. Chloramphenicol may interfere with therapeutic response to cyanocobalamin.

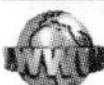

See the Companion Website for a Nursing Process Focus specific to this drug.

FIGURE 27.1

Metabolism of vitamin B_{12}

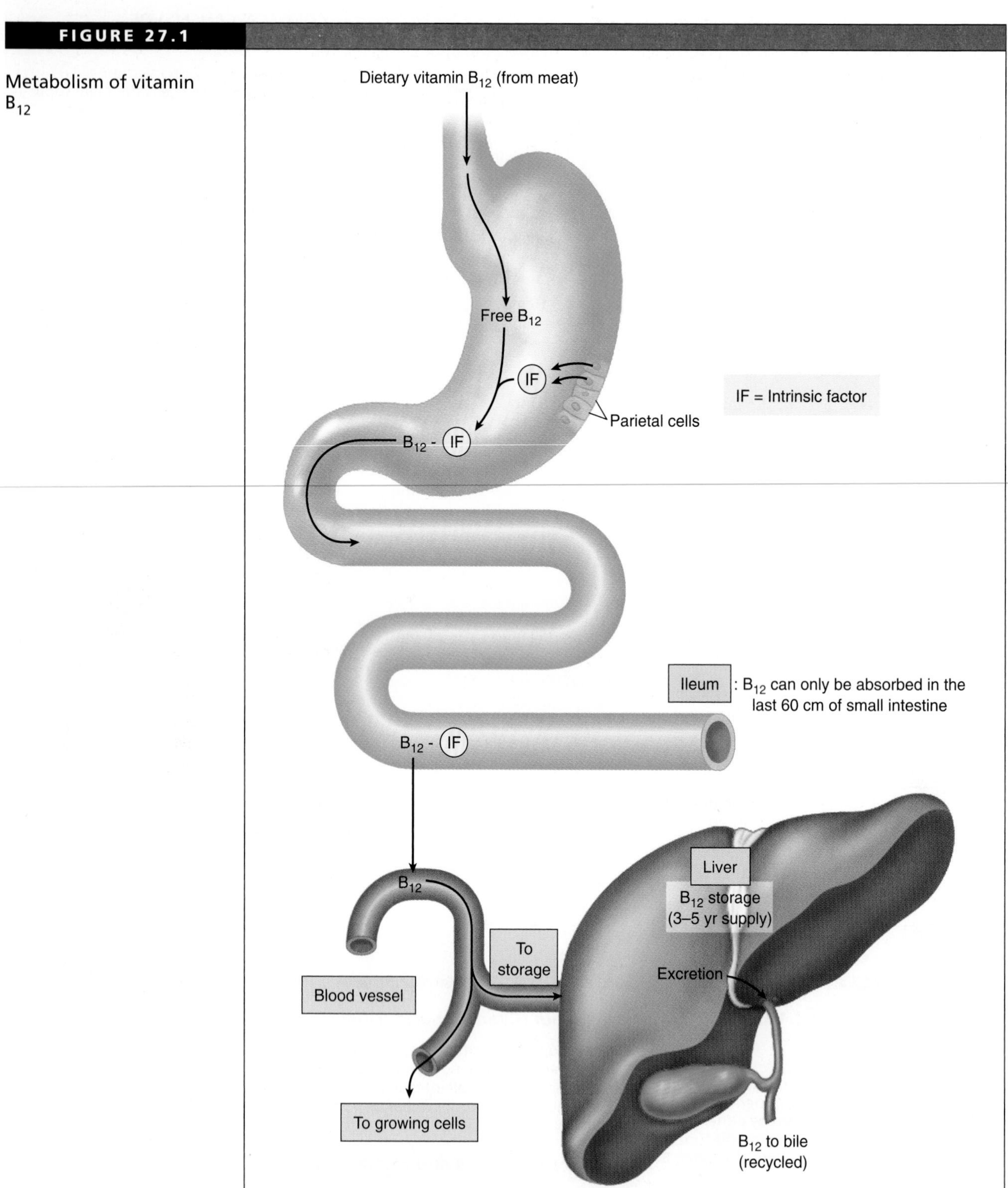

Life Span Fact

The absorption of food diminishes with age and often the quantity of ingested food is reduced, leading to vitamin deficiencies in elderly patients.

alcohol or serious drug dependency are often deficient in the quality and quantity of their nutritional intake. Table 27.1 shows the functions of the vitamins and some common causes of deficiencies.

Certain drugs affect vitamin metabolism. Alcohol is well known for its ability to inhibit the absorption of thiamine and folic acid; alcohol abuse is the most common cause of thiamine deficiency in the United States. Folic acid levels may be reduced in patients taking phenothiazines, oral contraceptives, phenytoin (Dilantin), or barbiturates. Vitamin D deficiency can be caused by therapy with certain anticonvulsants. Inhibition of vitamin B_{12} absorption has been reported with a number of drugs including trifluoperazine (Stelazine), alcohol, and oral contraceptives.

One of the most common and clinically important vitamin syndromes is deficiency of vitamin B_{12}. The most obvious consequence of B_{12} deficiency is a type of anemia called **pernicious** or **megaloblastic anemia.** Insufficient vitamin B_{12} creates a lack of activated folic acid, which is essential for DNA synthesis and cell division. Lack of vitamin B_{12} will also affect the nervous system, causing tingling or numbness in the limbs, mood disturbances, and even hallucinations in severe deficiencies.

megalo = *large*
blastic = *embryonic state*

an = *lack of*
emia = *blood condition*

Treatment of vitamin B_{12} deficiency is most often accomplished by weekly or biweekly IM or subcutaneous injections. Although oral supplements are available, they are only effective in patients who have sufficient intrinsic factor and normal absorption in the small intestine (see Drug Profile for cyanocobalamin). Parenteral administration rapidly reverses most signs and symptoms of B_{12} deficiency. If the disease has been prolonged, symptoms may take longer to resolve, and some neurological damage may be permanent. Treatment may need to continue for the remainder of the patient's life.

Vitamins are indicated for several additional conditions. Vitamin K is administered to patients with certain clotting disorders and as an antidote to warfarin (Coumadin) overdose. B complex vitamins such as folic acid, thiamine, and riboflavin are commonly administered to patients with chronic alcoholism. The role of vitamin D therapy in the pharmacotherapy of bone disorders is discussed in Chapter 31.

Life Span Fact

Elderly patients who have less direct exposure to sunlight may need vitamin D supplements.

Life Span Fact

Infants fed only breast milk receive insufficient amounts of vitamin D, which can result in rickets.

Concept Review 27.1

- What are some conditions in which the RDA for a vitamin may not be sufficient?

27.5 Minerals are inorganic substances needed in very small amounts to maintain normal body metabolism.

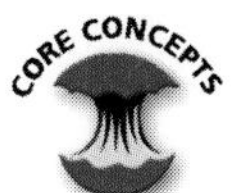

Minerals are inorganic substances that constitute about 4% of body weight. The most common minerals are the bone salts, calcium and phosphorous, which make up about 75% of the total mineral content in the body. Minerals are classified as **major minerals (macrominerals) or trace minerals,** depending on how much is needed in the diet. The seven major minerals must be obtained daily from dietary sources in amounts of 100 mg or higher. Required daily amounts of the nine trace minerals are 20 mg or less. These minerals are listed in Table 27.2.

TABLE 27.2 Minerals

MAJOR MINERALS	RECOMMENDED DAILY INTAKE	TRACE MINERALS	RECOMMENDED DAILY INTAKE
calcium	800–1200 mg	chromium	0.05–20 mg
chloride	750 mg	copper	0.1 mcg
magnesium	Men: 420 mg Women: 320 mg	fluoride	1.5–4 mg
phosphorous	700 mg	iodide	150 mcg
potassium	2.0 g	iron	Men: 10 mg Women: 15 mg
sodium	500 mg	manganese	2–5 mg
sulfur	not established	molybdenum	75–250 mg
		selenium	Men: 70 mcg Women: 55 mcg
		zinc	12–15 mg

Minerals serve many important and diverse functions in the body. Some minerals, such as sodium and magnesium, appear primarily as ions in body fluids. Others, such as iron and cobalt, are usually bound to organic molecules. The functions of many of the minerals in human physiology, such as calcium, sodium, and potassium, are well known. The functions of some of the trace minerals, such as aluminum, silicon, arsenic, and nickel, are less understood.

Most minerals are needed in very small amounts for human metabolism; a normal, balanced diet will supply the necessary quantities. Indeed, like vitamins, excess amounts of some minerals can lead to toxicity. For example, arsenic, chromium, and nickel have been implicated as human carcinogens and excess sodium intake can lead to water retention and hypertension.

Mineral therapy is indicated for certain disorders. Iron-deficiency anemia is the most common nutritional deficiency in the world, and is a primary indication for iron supplements.

osteo = *bone*
por = *passage*
osis = *condition*

Women at high risk for osteoporosis are advised to consume extra calcium, either in their diet or as a supplement (Chapter 31). Magnesium deficiencies are promptly treated with oral or IV magnesium salts because lack of sufficient amounts of this electrolyte can lead to weakness, dysrhythmias, and hypertension. Iodine-based drugs serve a number of functions including use as topical antiseptics, contrast agents in radiologic procedures of the urinary and cardiovascular systems, and the treatment of thyroid abnormalities (Chapter 29). Selected minerals used in pharmacotherapy are shown in Table 27.3.

Certain drugs affect mineral metabolism. For example, patients taking loop or thiazide diuretics are usually advised to add potassium to their diets. Corticosteroids, oral contraceptives, and a number of other drugs can cause sodium retention. The uptake of iodine by the thyroid gland can be impaired by certain oral hypoglycemics and lithium carbonate (Eskalith). Oral contraceptives have been reported to lower the plasma levels of zinc and increase those of copper.

Life Span Fact

For each decade after age 40, bone mass decreases approximately 3–5%. To avoid bone fractures, older adults must ensure a substantial dietary intake of calcium or take calcium supplements.

Concept Review 27.2

- What is the difference between a vitamin and a mineral?

DRUG PROFILE: Mineral: *Ferrous Sulfate (Ferralyn and Others)*

Actions and Uses:

Ferrous sulfate is an iron supplement. Iron is a mineral essential to the function of several biological molecules, the most significant of which is **hemoglobin.** Each molecule of hemoglobin in a red blood cell contains four iron atoms, each of which can bind reversibly to an oxygen atom. Sixty to eighty percent of all iron in the body is associated with hemoglobin.

Because free iron is toxic, the body binds the mineral to protein complexes called ferritin, hemosiderin, and transferrin. After red blood cells die, nearly all of the iron in their hemoglobin is recycled for later use. Because of this recycling, very little iron is excreted; thus, dietary iron requirements in most clients are small.

Iron deficiency is a common cause of anemia. The usual cause of iron-deficiency anemia is blood loss, such as may occur during menstruation or from peptic ulcers. Certain patients have an increased demand for iron, including those who are pregnant and those undergoing intensive athletic training. Ferrous sulfate is available in a wide variety of dosage forms to prevent or rapidly reverse symptoms of iron-deficiency anemia.

Adverse Effects and Interactions:

The most common side effect of iron sulfate is GI upset. Although taking iron with meals will lessen GI upset, food can decrease the absorption of iron by as much as 70%. It is recommended that iron preparations be administered 1 hour before or 2 hours after a meal. However if major gastric irritation is experienced the iron may be taken with meals. Patients should be advised that iron preparations may darken stools and that this is a harmless side effect. Excessive doses of iron are very toxic and patients should be advised to take their medication exactly as directed.

Antacids and food decrease the absorption of iron. Vitamin C increases the absorption of iron, whereas calcium (including dairy products) and bran block its absorption. Ferrous sulfate may decrease the absorption of penicillamine. Vitamin C may increase the absorption of ferrous sulfate.

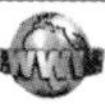
See the Companion Website for a Nursing Process Focus specific to this drug.

TABLE 27.3 Selected Minerals Used for Pharmacotherapy

DRUG	ROUTE AND ADULT DOSE	REMARKS
potassium chloride (K-Dur, Micro-K, Klor-Con, others)	PO 10–100 mEq/h divided doses IV 10–40 mEq/h diluted to at least 10–20 mEq/100 ml of solution (max: 200–400 mEq/day)	Electrolyte levels should be frequently assessed and the drug discontinued immediately if hyperkalemia is suspected
sodium bicarbonate	PO 0.3–2.0 g once or twice daily or 1 tsp of powder in glass of water	For treatment of metabolic acidosis, to enhance renal excretion of certain drugs and as an antacid
CALCIUM		
calcium carbonate (BioCal, Titralac, others)	PO 1–2 g bid–tid	For calcium supplementation and as an antacid
calcium citrate (Citracal)	PO 1–2 g bid–tid	For calcium supplementation
calcium gluceptate (Glucalcium, Calcitrans)	IV 1.1–4.4 g/day IM 0.5–1.1 g/day	For emergency treatment of hypocalcemia
calcium gluconate (Kalcinate)	PO 1–2 g bid–qid	For calcium supplementation and to reverse cardiac signs of hyperkalemia
calcium lactate (Cal-Lac, Calcimax, others)	PO 325 mg–1.3 g tid with meals	To correct mild hypocalemia
IRON		
ferrous fumarate (Feco-T, Femiron, Feostate, others)	200 mg tid–qid	For iron supplementation
ferrous gluconate (Fergon, Simron)	325–600 mg qid; may be gradually increased to 650 mg qid as needed and tolerated	For iron supplementation
Pr ferrous sulfate (Feosol, Fer-Iron, others)	750–1500 mg/day in 1–3 divided doses	For iron supplementation
iron dextran (Dexferrum, Imfed, Imferon)	IM/IV dose is individualized and determined from a table of correlations between patient's weight and hemoglobin, per package insert (max: 100 mg [2 ml] of iron dextran within 24 hours)	For iron supplementation when oral administration is not indicated
MAGNESIUM		
magnesium chloride (Chloromag, Slo-Mag)	PO 270–400 mg/day	For magnesium supplementation
magnesium oxide (Mag-Ox, Maox, others)	PO 400–1200 mg/day in divided doses	For constipation, hyperacidity or magnesium supplementation
magnesium sulfate (Epson salt)	IV/IM 0.5–3.0 g/day	For constipation, to control seizures or magnesium supplementation
PHOSPHOROUS		
monobasic potassium phosphate (K-Phos original)	PO 1 g qid	For correction of phosphate deficiency and to lower urinary calcium concentration
potassium phosphate (Neutra-Phos-K)	PO 1.45 g qid IV 10 mmol phosphorous/day	For correction of phosphate deficiency and to lower urinary calcium concentration
ZINC		
zinc gluconate	PO 20–100 mg (20-mg lozenges may be taken to a max of 6/day)	For correction of zinc deficiency
zinc sulfate (Orazinc, Zincate, others)	PO 15–220 mg/day	For correction of zinc deficiency

TPN is able to provide all the patient's nutritional needs with solutions containing amino acids, fats, carbohydrate (as dextrose), electrolytes, vitamins, and minerals. The particular formulation may be specific to the disease state, such as products for renal failure or hepatic failure. TPN is administered through an infusion pump so that nutrition can be precisely monitored. Patients in various settings such as acute care, long-term care, and home health care often benefit from TPN therapy.

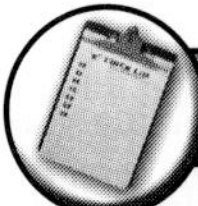

PATIENTS NEED TO KNOW

Patients treated with vitamins, minerals, or herbs need to know the following:

In General

1. If receiving regular monthly injections of vitamin B_{12}, do not take additional oral supplements of vitamin B_{12} or folic acid without the advice of a healthcare provider.
2. Do not take more than the recommended doses of any vitamin or mineral without first checking with a healthcare provider. Although small amounts of these substances are beneficial, large amounts may be dangerous.
3. Ensure that diet is nutritionally adequate, adding foods that naturally supply the needed vitamins and minerals before taking supplements. See a dietician for advice, particularly for special needs such as pregnancy or diabetes.
4. Avoid foods with high zinc or oxalate content if a calcium supplement is being taken because these may interfere with absorption. These foods include nuts, peas, beans, spinach, and soy products.
5. Know that niacin, or vitamin B_3, is also effective at lowering lipid levels. The dose for lowering cholesterol, however, is 2 to 3 grams per day whereas the vitamin dose is only 25 mg per day.
6. When providing a medical or drug history to the physician or dentist, always report vitamins, minerals, herbs, or dietary supplements being taken. If allergies to any dietary supplements are known, be sure to report these also.

Regarding Iron Preparations

7. Since liquid iron preparations can stain teeth, dilute these solutions with juice or water and rinse the mouth after taking the medication to reduce staining.
8. Take oral forms of ferrous sulfate (iron) 1 hour before or 2 hours after meals for better absoption. Take with a full glass of water or juice. ■

CHAPTER REVIEW

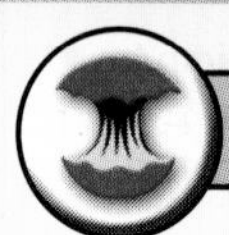

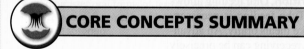

CORE CONCEPTS SUMMARY

27.1 Vitamins are organic substances that are needed in small amounts to promote growth and maintain health.

With the exception of vitamin D, vitamins cannot be synthesized by the body and must be provided in the diet. Although only very small amounts of vitamins are needed, lack of sufficient quantity will result in disease.

27.2 Vitamins are classified as fat soluble or water soluble.

Water-soluble vitamins include vitamins C and B. Fat-soluble vitamins include vitamins A, D, E, and K. Water-soluble vitamins cannot be stored and must be ingested daily, whereas excess fat-soluble vitamins can be stored for later use.

27.3 Recommended dietary allowances (RDAs) for vitamins have been established for the average, healthy adult.

RDA values represent the minimum amount of vitamin or mineral needed to prevent a deficiency in a healthy adult. These values must be adjusted for changes in health status, such as athletic training, pregnancy, or chronic disease.

27.4 Vitamin therapy is indicated for specific conditions.

Most people do not need vitamin supplementation, and excess intake may lead to hypervitaminosis. Indications for vitamin therapy include alcoholism, pregnancy or breast-feeding, chronic kidney or liver disease, therapy with certain drugs that affect vitamin metabolism, and reduced food intake in elderly patients.

27.5 Minerals are inorganic substances needed in very small amounts to maintain normal body metabolism.

Like vitamins, most people receive all the minerals they need through a balanced diet. Certain conditions, such as osteoporosis or iron-deficiency anemia, do warrant mineral therapy.

27.6 Enteral and total parenteral nutrition are therapies that deliver essential nutrients to patients with deficiencies.

Enteral nutrition supplies patients all the essential nutrients through the oral route or by a feeding tube. For patients who cannot take oral supplements, nutrients are supplied parenterally by way of total parenteral nutrition.

KEY TERMS

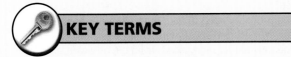

enteral nutrition: treatment of undernutrition by the oral route, or through a feeding tube / ***page 519***

folic acid (foh-lik): B vitamin that is a coenzyme in protein and nucleic acid metabolism; also known as *folate* / ***page 512***

hemoglobin (HEE-moh-glow-bin): substance in a red blood cell that contains iron and transports oxygen and CO_2 / ***page 516***

hypervitaminosis: excess intake of vitamins / ***page 512***

intrinsic factor: chemical secreted by the stomach that is required for absorption of vitamin B_{12} / ***page 513***

major mineral (macromineral): inorganic compound needed by the body in amounts of 100 mg or more daily / ***page 515***

perniclious (megaloblastic) anemia (pur-NISH-us ah-NEE-mee-ah): type of anemia usually caused by lack of secretion of intrinsic factor / ***page 515***

provitamin: an inactive chemical that is converted to a vitamin in the body / ***page 511***

recommended dietary allowance (RDA): amount of vitamin or mineral needed daily to avoid a deficiency in a healthy adult / ***page 512***

total parenteral nutrition (TPN): treatment of undernutrition through the parenteral infusion of dextrose, amino acids, emulsified fats, vitamins, and minerals / ***page 519***

trace mineral: inorganic compound needed by the body in amounts of 20 mg or less daily / ***page 515***

undernutrition: taking in or absorbing fewer nutrients than required for normal body growth and maintenance / ***page 519***

vitamins: organic compounds required by the body in small amounts / ***page 511***

REVIEW QUESTIONS

The following questions are written in NCLEX-PN® style. Answer these questions to assess your knowledge of the chapter material, and go back and review any material that is not clear to you.

1. Vitamin B_{12} is indicated for which of the following conditions?

1. Liver disease
2. Chronic inflammatory disease
3. Pernicious anemia
4. Inadequate exposure to sunlight

2. This vitamin is indicated for the patient who is experiencing warfarin (Coumadin) overdose.

1. Vitamin A
2. Vitamin D
3. Vitamin E
4. Vitamin K

3. If the patient is taking ferrous sulfate, what instructions should be given?

1. Do not take antacids with this medication.
2. This medication can cause severe diarrhea.
3. This medication should never be taken on an empty stomach.
4. Blood pressure must be monitored closely.

4. Patients with a history of alcohol abuse should be monitored for a ___________ deficiency.

1. Biotin
2. Thiamine
3. Niacin
4. Riboflavin

5. The patient on bumetamide (Bumex) should have which electrolyte monitored?

1. Sodium
2. Calcium
3. Potassium
4. Magnesium

6. The patient taking liquid iron should be instructed to:

1. Swish medication in his mouth for 1 minute
2. Take medication with food
3. Avoid foods with high iron content
4. Rinse his mouth with water afterwards

7. Your patient is exhibiting weakness, hypertension, and dysrhythmias. Which of the following should be checked?

1. Sodium
2. Magnesium
3. Aluminum
4. Chromium

8. Vitamins A, D, E, and K are:

1. Trace minerals
2. Minerals
3. Water-soluble vitamins
4. Fat-soluble vitamins

9. Your patient's GI tract is not functioning. Which type of feeding is the patient receiving?

1. Oral
2. Enteral
3. TPN
4. GI

10. The patient asks the nurse if it would be okay to increase her vitamin intake. The nurse's best response would be:

1. "While you can safely take additional vitamins, there is no need."
2. "You probably need to take more vitamins every day."
3. "You will need to speak with your physician."
4. "You may safely increase your intake of water-soluble vitamins only."

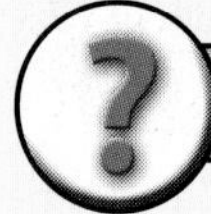

CASE STUDY QUESTIONS

For questions 1–3, please refer to the following case study, and choose the correct answer from choices 1–4.

Ms. Davis has been taking a multivitamin for several years. Lately, she has been taking 4 times the label dose because she heard that this can prevent colds.

1. In Ms. Davis' multivitamin, which of the following is a water-soluble vitamin?

1. A
2. B complex
3. D
4. E

2. Ms. Davis asks you the meaning of RDA. What would be the best response?

1. "It is the amount of nutrient required by all people."
2. "It is the maximum amount of nutrient required by all people."
3. "It is the amount of nutrient needed by an average person."
4. "It is the minimum amount of nutrient required by all people."

3. What would be your advice to Ms. Davis?

1. Stop taking multivitamins.
2. Continue taking 4 times the label dose because this is considered safe.
3. Take only the dose stated on the label.
4. Continue taking 4 times the label dose until she develops abnormal symptoms.

4. Mr. Yung is comatose and in the terminal stages of throat cancer. What type of nutrition is Mr. Yung likely receiving?

1. Total parenteral
2. Enteral
3. Tube
4. Hypervitamin

5. Which of the following are common indications for vitamin or mineral pharmacotherapy?

1. Chronic alcoholism
2. Liver failure
3. Iron-deficiency anemia
4. All of the above

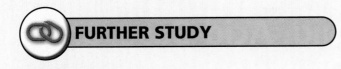

FURTHER STUDY

- The role of vitamin D and calcium therapy in the pharmacotherapy of bone disorders is discussed in Chapter 31.
- Iodine-based drugs serve a number of functions including the treatment of thyroid abnormalities, which is discussed in Chapter 29.

EXPLORE MEDIALINK www.prenhall.com/holland

Additional resources for this chapter can be found on the CD-ROM accompanying this textbook, and on the Companion Website. Click on Chapter 27 to select activities for this chapter.

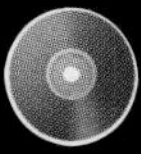

Audio Glossary
Concept Review
NCLEX-PN® Review
Nursing in Action
Dosage Calculator

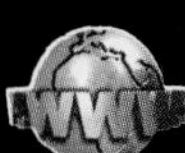

National Council Against Health Fraud

CHAPTER

28 Drugs for Fluid, Acid-Base, and Electrolyte Disorders

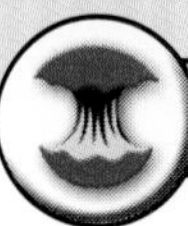

CORE CONCEPTS

28.1 The kidneys regulate fluid volume, electrolytes, acids, and bases.

28.2 The composition of filtrate changes dramatically as a result of the processes of reabsorption and secretion.

28.3 Renal failure significantly impacts pharmacotherapy.

28.4 Most diuretics act by blocking sodium reabsorption in the nephron.

28.5 The most effective diuretics are those that affect the loop of Henle.

28.6 The thiazides are the most widely prescribed class of diuretics.

28.7 Although less effective than the loop diuretics, potassium-sparing diuretics may help prevent hypokalemia.

28.8 Several less commonly prescribed diuretics have specific indications.

28.9 Intravenous fluid therapy with crystalloids and colloids is used to replace lost fluids.

28.10 Acidic and basic drugs can be administered to maintain normal body pH.

28.11 Electrolytes are charged substances that play important roles in body chemistry.

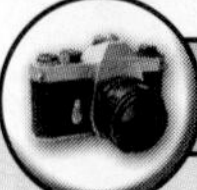

DRUG SNAPSHOT

The following drugs will be discussed in this chapter:

DRUG CLASSES	DRUG PROFILES
Loop (high-ceiling) diuretics	
Thiazide and thiazide-like diuretics	Pr chlorothiazide (Diuril)
Potassium-sparing diuretics	Pr spironolactone (Aldactone)
Carbonic anhydrase inhibitor diuretics	
Osmotic diuretics	
Fluid-replacement agents	Pr dextran 40 (Gentran 40, others)
Acid-base agents	Pr sodium bicarbonate
Electrolytes	Pr potassium chloride

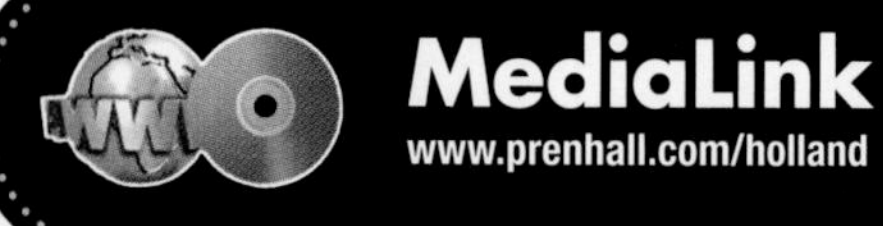

Interactive resources for this chapter can be found on the Companion Website. Click on Chapter 28 and "Begin" to select the activities for this chapter. For chapter-related animations, NCLEX-PN®-style questions, and an audio glossary, access the accompanying CD-ROM in this book.

OBJECTIVES

After reading this chapter, the student should be able to:

1. Explain the role of the urinary system in maintaining fluid, electrolyte, and acid-base balance.
2. Compare and contrast the three major classes of diuretics.
3. Identify common causes of alkalosis and acidosis and the drugs used to treat these disorders.
4. Describe conditions in which therapy with IV fluids may be indicated.
5. Explain the pharmacotherapy of sodium and potassium imbalances.
6. Compare and contrast colloids and crystalloids used in IV therapy.
7. For each of the following classes, identify representative drugs, and explain the mechanisms of drug action, primary actions, and important adverse effects:
   a. loop diuretics
   b. thiazide diuretics
   c. potassium-sparing diuretics
   d. acidic agents
   e. basic agents
   f. electrolytes
   g. colloids
   h. crystalloids
8. Categorize drugs used in the treatment of urinary system, acid-base, fluid, and electrolyte disorders based on their classifications and mechanisms of action.

The volume and composition of fluids in the body must be maintained within narrow limits. Excess fluid volume can lead to hypertension or congestive heart failure whereas depletion results in dehydration. Body fluids must also contain specific amounts of essential ions or electrolytes and be maintained at particular pH values. Imbalances in electrolytes may have fatal consequences. In addition, accumulation of excess acids or bases can change the pH of body fluids and rapidly result in death if left untreated. The kidneys serve a remarkable role in keeping the volume and composition of body fluids within normal limits. This chapter will examine drugs used to reverse symptoms of fluid volume, electrolyte, or acid-base imbalance.

28.1 The kidneys regulate fluid volume, electrolytes, acids, and bases.

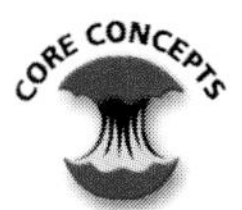

When most people think of the kidneys, they think of excretion. Although this is certainly one of their roles, the kidneys have many other essential functions. The kidneys are the primary organs for regulating fluid balance, electrolyte composition, and the acid-base balance of body fluids.

Fast Facts Renal Disorders

- More than 12,000 kidney transplants were performed in 1999.
- More than 47,000 people are currently on a waiting list for kidney transplants.
- One out of every 750 people is born with a single kidney. A single kidney is larger and more vulnerable to injury from heavy contact sports.
- About 260,000 Americans suffer from chronic kidney failure, and 50,000 die annually from causes related to the disease.
- Type 2 diabetes is the leading cause of chronic kidney failure, accounting for 30–40% of all new cases each year.
- Hypertension is the second leading cause of chronic kidney failure, accounting for about 25% of all new cases each year.

FIGURE 28.1

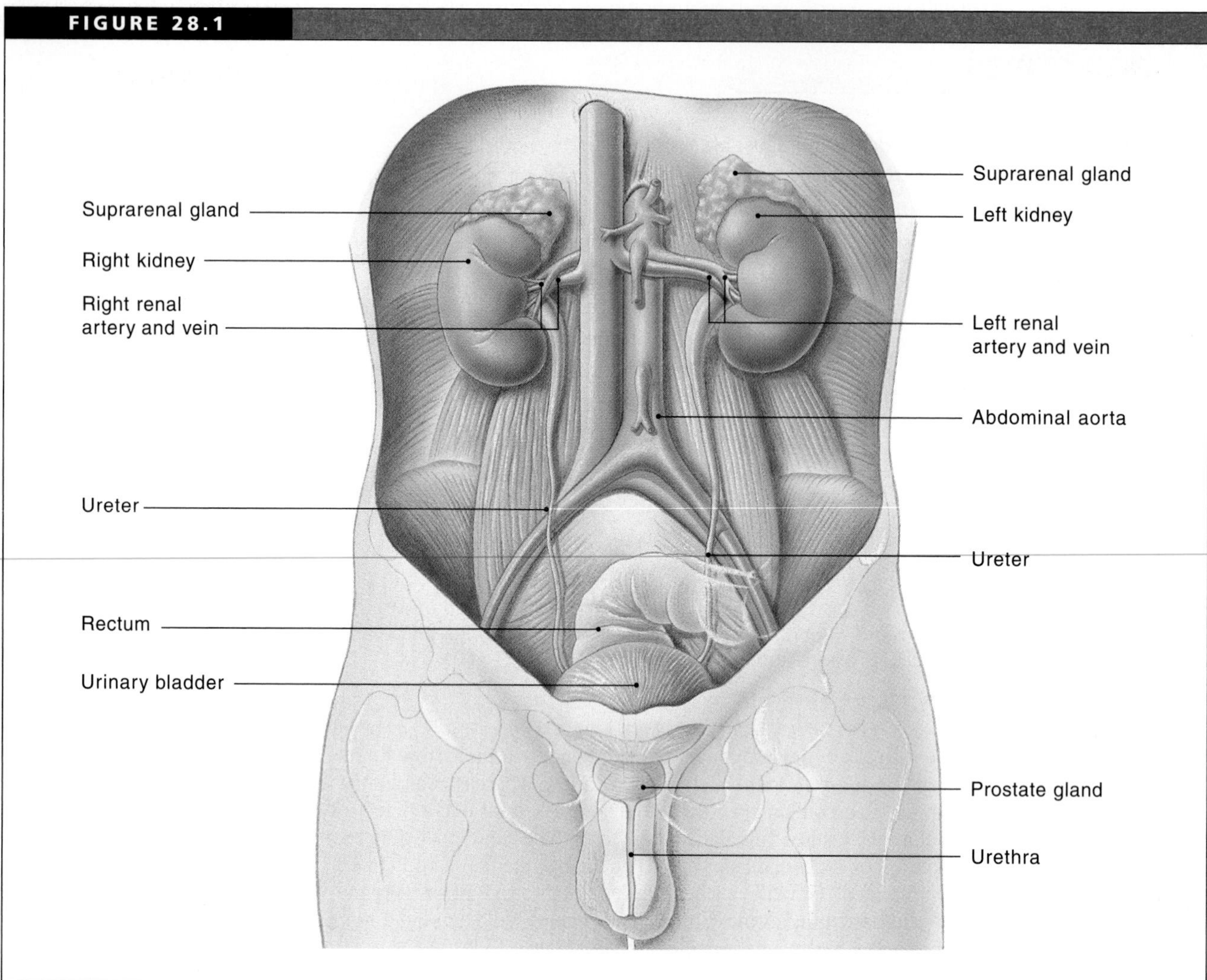

The urinary system *SOURCE: Pearson Education/PH College*

They also secrete the enzyme renin, which helps to regulate blood pressure (Chapter 15), and erythropoietin, a hormone that stimulates red blood cell production. In addition, the kidneys are responsible for the production of calcitriol, the active form of vitamin D, that helps maintain bone homeostasis (Chapter 31). It is not surprising that the overall health of the patient is strongly dependent on proper functioning of the kidneys.

The urinary system consists of two kidneys, two ureters, a urinary bladder, and a urethra. These structures are shown in Figure 28.1 ■. Each kidney contains more than 2 million **nephrons,** the functional units of the kidney. As blood enters a nephron, it is filtered through a semipermeable membrane known as *Bowman's capsule*. Water and other small molecules readily pass through Bowman's capsule and enter the first section of the nephron called the *proximal tubule*. Once in the nephron, the fluid is called **filtrate.** After leaving the proximal tubule, the filtrate travels through the *loop of Henle* and, subsequently, the *distal tubule*. Nephrons empty their filtrate into tubes called *common collecting ducts*, and then into larger and larger collecting structures inside the kidney. Fluid leaving the collecting ducts and entering subsequent portions of the kidney is called *urine*. The parts of the nephron are illustrated in Figure 28.2 ■.

Concept Review 28.1

- How does the composition of filtrate differ from that of blood?

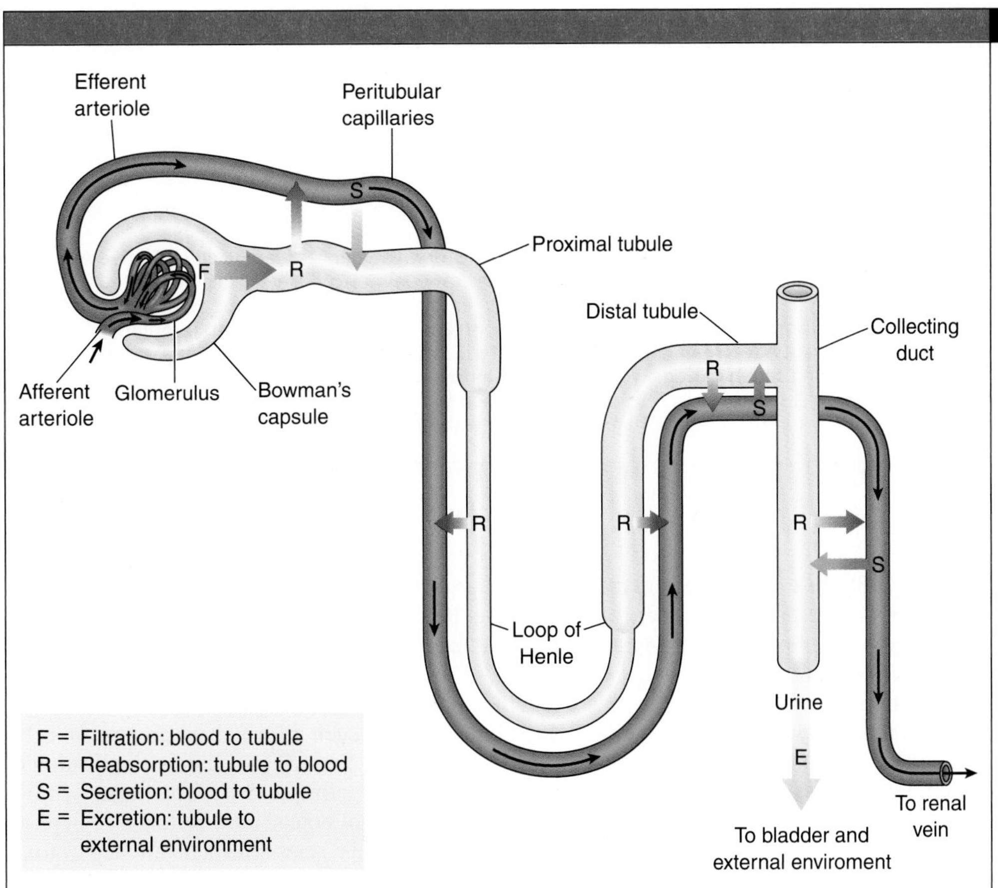

FIGURE 28.2

The nephron

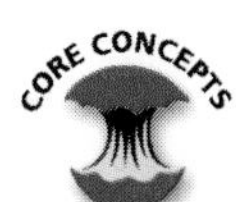

28.2 The composition of filtrate changes dramatically as a result of the processes of reabsorption and secretion.

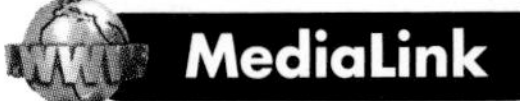

THE NEPHROLOGY CHANNEL

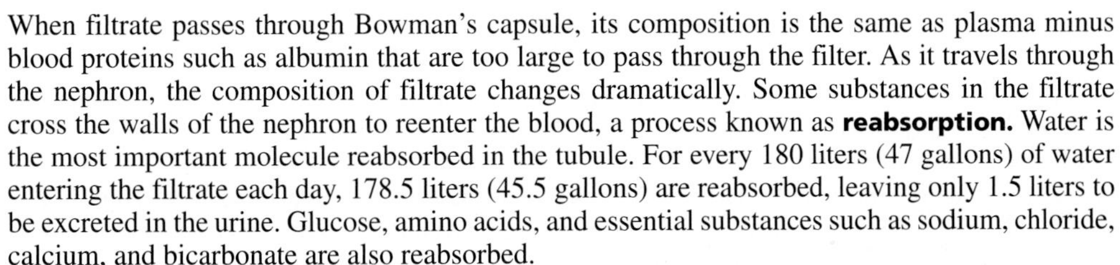

When filtrate passes through Bowman's capsule, its composition is the same as plasma minus blood proteins such as albumin that are too large to pass through the filter. As it travels through the nephron, the composition of filtrate changes dramatically. Some substances in the filtrate cross the walls of the nephron to reenter the blood, a process known as **reabsorption.** Water is the most important molecule reabsorbed in the tubule. For every 180 liters (47 gallons) of water entering the filtrate each day, 178.5 liters (45.5 gallons) are reabsorbed, leaving only 1.5 liters to be excreted in the urine. Glucose, amino acids, and essential substances such as sodium, chloride, calcium, and bicarbonate are also reabsorbed.

Certain ions and molecules too large to pass through Bowman's capsule can still enter the urine by crossing from the blood to the filtrate using a process known as **secretion.** Potassium, phosphate, hydrogen, and ammonium ions and many organic acids enter the filtrate through, secretion.

Reabsorption and secretion are critical to the pharmacokinetics of many drugs. Some drugs are reabsorbed, whereas others are secreted into the filtrate. For example, approximately 90% of a dose of penicillin G enters the urine through secretion. The processes of reabsorption and secretion are shown in Figure 28.2.

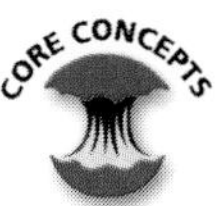

28.3 Renal failure significantly impacts pharmacotherapy.

As has been discussed previously in this chapter, the kidneys are truly essential organs for homeostasis. When the kidneys become impaired, doses of almost all drugs must be adjusted. If excretion is limited, drugs will accumulate to high concentrations in the blood and tissues, resulting

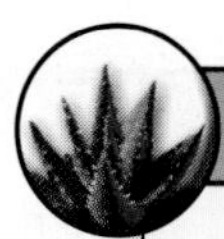

NATURAL ALTERNATIVES

Saw Palmetto for Urinary and Prostate Disorders

Saw palmetto is obtained from the sable palm *Serenoa repens*, which grows in the southeastern United States. The active ingredients come from the *ripe berries* that contain a number of sterols and alcoholic compounds. Some of these compounds are antiestrogenic, blocking estrogen receptors. Preparations include dried berries, capsules, and tinctures. A tea is available but not common because the taste and smell of saw palmetto is unpleasant.

Saw palmetto has an interesting pharmacological history. The berries were used by Native Americans as food, not medicines. During the 19th century, saw palmetto berry extract was listed in the National Formulary as an official treatment but was removed in 1950. As the population began to age and prostate disorders became more widely recognized, saw palmetto gained popularity.

Perhaps the most widespread use of saw palmetto is in the treatment of benign prostatic hypertrophy (BPH). When used in eatings with BPH, saw palmetto stimulates urinary flow, reduces painful urination, and decreases nocturia. The extract is claimed to reduce swelling of the prostate. Other indications include cold, flu, cough, inflammation, and asthma. ■

in toxicity. Because the kidneys excrete most drugs, the majority of medications will require a significant dosage reduction in patients with moderate to severe renal failure. *The importance of this cannot be overemphasized: administering the "average" dose to a patient in severe renal failure can kill a patient.*

The nurse has a critical role in preventing the potentially serious adverse drug effects resulting from renal impairment. Monitoring kidney function tests such as urinalysis and serum creatinine helps to identify impending renal failure. Notifying the prescriber at the first indication of renal failure allows drug dosages to be lowered, thereby preventing toxicity. The nurse will frequently encounter patients with renal failure; therefore, special note should be taken of nephrotoxic drugs when learning pharmacology. Once a diagnosis is established, all nephrotoxic medications should be either discontinued or used with extreme caution.

Renal failure can be acute or chronic. Acute renal failure requires immediate treatment because accumulation of waste products such as urea and creatinine can result in death if untreated. The most common cause of acute renal failure is lack of sufficient blood flow through the kidneys. The cause of acute renal failure must be quickly identified and corrected. Potential causes include heart failure, dysrhythmias, hemorrhage, and dehydration.

Chronic renal failure occurs over months or years. More than half of the cases of chronic renal failure occur in patients with longstanding hypertension or diabetes mellitus. Because of its long development and nonspecific symptoms, chronic renal failure may go undiagnosed for many years until the impairment becomes irreversible.

Pharmacotherapy of renal impairment includes administering diuretics, which can increase urine output. Cardiovascular agents are commonly administered to treat underlying hypertension or heart failure.

Patients with chronic renal failure often cannot secrete enough **erythropoietin,** a hormone secreted by the kidney, which serves as a primary signal to increase red blood cell production in the bone marrow. A synthetic form of erythropoietin, epoetin alfa (Epogen, Procrit) is effective in treating several disorders caused by a deficiency in red blood cells. Epoetin is sometimes given to patients undergoing cancer chemotherapy to counteract the anemia caused by antineoplastic agents (Chapter 24). It is occasionally prescribed for patients prior to blood transfusions or surgery and to treat anemia in HIV-infected patients. Epoetin alfa is usually administered three times per week until an increase in the number of red blood cells is achieved.

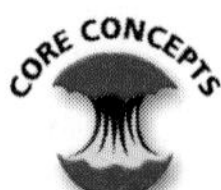

28.4 Most diuretics act by blocking sodium reabsorption in the nephron.

dia = *thoroughly*
uretic = *to urinate*

A **diuretic** is a drug that increases urine output. Excretion of excess fluid in the body is particularly desirable in the following conditions:

- Hypertension (Chapter 15)
- Heart failure (Chapter 16)

FIGURE 28.3

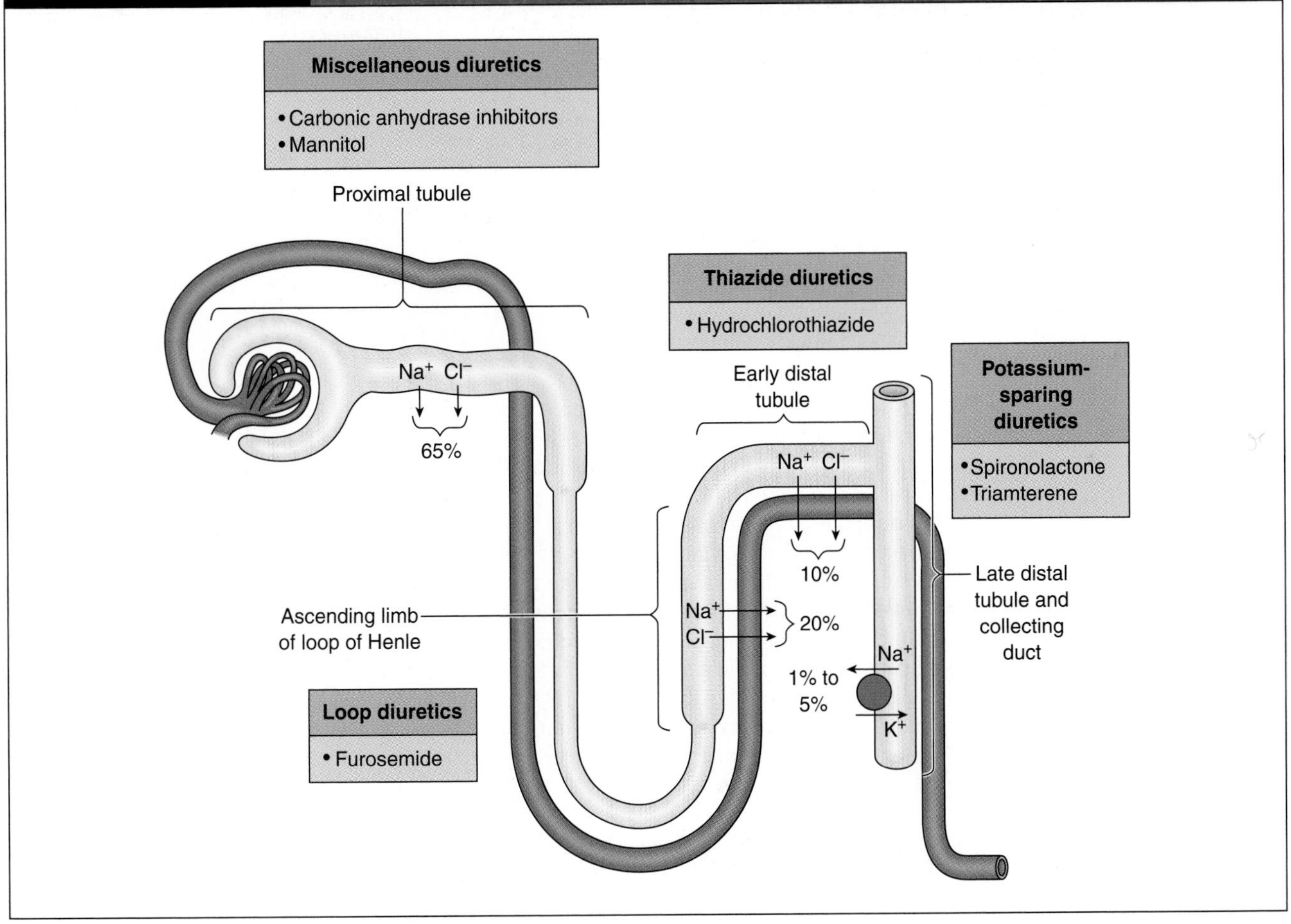

Miscellaneous diuretics
- Carbonic anhydrase inhibitors
- Mannitol

Proximal tubule

Na^+ Cl^-

65%

Thiazide diuretics
- Hydrochlorothiazide

Early distal tubule

Na^+ Cl^-

10%

Potassium-sparing diuretics
- Spironolactone
- Triamterene

Late distal tubule and collecting duct

Ascending limb of loop of Henle

Na^+ Cl^- 20%

Na^+ 1% to 5% K^+

Loop diuretics
- Furosemide

Sites of action of the diuretics

- Kidney failure
- Pulmonary edema
- Liver failure or cirrhosis

The most common way in which diureties act is by blocking sodium reabsorption in the nephron, thus sending more of this into the urine. Chloride ion (Cl^-) follows sodium. Because water molecules also tend to stay with sodium ions, blocking the reabsorption of sodium will keep more water in the filtrate. The more water retained in the filtrate, the greater the volume of urination, or diuresis. Some drugs, like furosemide (Lasix), act by preventing the reabsorption of sodium in the loop of Henle. Because of the abundance of sodium in the loop of Henle, furosemide is capable of producing large increases in urine output. Other drugs, such as the thiazides, act on the distal tubule. Because most sodium has already been reabsorbed from the filtrate by the time it reaches this point in the nephron, the thiazides produce less diuresis than does furosemide. The sites at which the various diuretics act are shown in Figure 28.3 ■.

28.5 The most effective diuretics are those that affect the loop of Henle.

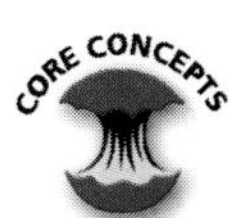

The most effective diuretics are called *loop* or *high-ceiling diuretics*. Drugs in this class act by blocking the reabsorption of sodium and chloride in the loop of Henle. When given IV, they have the ability to rapidly move large amounts of fluid through the kidney. Loop diuretics are used to reduce the edema associated with heart failure, hepatic cirrhosis, or chronic renal failure. Furosemide (Lasix) and torsemide (Demadex) are also approved for hypertension.

TABLE 28.1 Loop Diuretics

DRUG	ROUTE AND ADULT DOSE	REMARKS
bumetanide (Bumex)	PO 0.5–2 mg daily (max: 10 mg/day)	IV form available
ethacrynic acid (Edecrin)	PO 50–100 mg once or twice per day (max: 400 mg/day)	IV form available
furosemide (Lasix)	PO 20–80 mg daily (max: 600 mg/day)	IV and IM forms available
torsemide (Demadex)	PO 4–20 mg daily	Also for liver cirrhosis; IV form available

Furosemide is the most frequently prescribed loop diuretic. A drug profile for furosemide is found in Chapter 16. Unlike the thiazide diuretics, furosemide is able to increase urine output even when blood flow to the kidneys is diminished. Torsemide (Demadex) has a longer half-life than furosemide, which offers the advantage of once-a-day dosing. Bumetanide (Bumex) is 40 times more potent than furosemide, but has a shorter duration of action.

de = *not/without*
hydration = *water*

hypo = *low or below normal*
kal = *potassium*
emia = *blood condition*

The rapid excretion of large amounts of water caused by loop diuretics may produce adverse effects such as dehydration and electrolyte imbalances. Signs of dehydration include thirst, dry mouth, weight loss, and headache. Hypotension, dizziness, and even fainting can result from the rapid fluid loss. Potassium loss, or **hypokalemia,** may result in dysrhythmias, and potassium supplements may be indicated. Potassium loss is of particular concern to patients who are also taking digoxin (Lanoxin). Although rare, ototoxicity is possible. Because of the potential for serious side effects, the loop diuretics are normally reserved for patients with moderate to severe fluid retention, or when other diuretics have failed to produce a therapeutic effect. Information on the loop diuretics is given in Table 28.1.

Concept Review 28.2

- Why are drugs that block sodium reabsorption at the loop of Henle more effective than those that act on the distal tubule?

DRUG PROFILE: Thiazide Diuretic: *Chlorothiazide (Diuril)*

Actions and Uses:

Chlorothiazide is commonly prescribed for mild to moderate hypertension and may be combined with other antihypertensives in the treatment of severe hypertension. It is also used to treat edema due to heart failure, liver disease, and corticosteroid or estrogen therapy. When given orally, it may take as long as 4 weeks to obtain the optimum therapeutic effect. When given IV, results are seen in 15 to 30 minutes.

Adverse Effects and Interactions:

Excess loss of water and electrolytes can occur. Symptoms may include thirst, weakness, lethargy, muscle cramping, hypotension, or tachycardia. Due to the potentially serious consequences of hypokalemia, patients taking digoxin should be carefully monitored. The intake of potassium-rich foods should be increased and potassium supplements may be indicated.

Chlorothiazide interacts with several drugs. For example, when administered with amphotericin B or corticosteroids, hypokalemic effects are increased. Antidiabetic medications such as sulfonylureas and insulin may be less effective when taken with chlorothiazide. Cholestyramine and colestipol decrease the absorption of chlorothiazide. Alcohol increases the hypotensive action of some thiazide diuretics, and caffeine may increase diuresis.

Use cautiously with herbal supplements, such as licorice, which, in large amounts, will create an additive effect of hypokalemia. Aloe may also increase potassium loss.

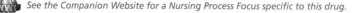

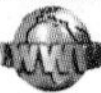
See the Companion Website for a Nursing Process Focus specific to this drug.

TABLE 28.2 Thiazide and Thiazide-like Diuretics

DRUG	ROUTE AND ADULT DOSE	REMARKS
bendroflumethiazide (Naturetin)	PO 2.5–20 mg 1–2 times/day	Intermediate acting
benzthiazide (Aquatag, Exna, Hydrex)	PO 25–200 mg daily or every other day	Intermediate acting
Pr chlorothiazide (Diuril)	PO 250–500 mg 1–2 times/day	IV form available; short acting
chlorthalidone (Hygroton)	PO 50–100 mg/day	Thiazide-like; long acting
hydrochlorothiazide (HydroDIURIL, HCTZ)	PO 12.5–100 mg 1–3 times/day	Short acting
hydroflumethiazide (Diucardin, Saluron)	PO 25–100 mg 1–2 times/day	Intermediate acting
indapamide (Lozol)	PO 2.5–5 mg/day	Thiazide-like; long acting
methylclothiazide (Aquatensin, Enduron)	PO 2.5–10 mg/day	Long acting
metolazone (Zaroxolyn, Mykrox)	PO 5–20 mg/day	Thiazide-like; intermediate acting
polythiazide (Renese)	PO 1–4 mg/day	Long acting
quinethazone (Hydromox)	PO 50–100 mg/day	Thiazide-like; intermediate acting
trichlormethiazide (Metahydrin, Naqua, Niazide, Diurese)	PO 1–4 mg 1–2 times/day	Long acting

28.6 The thiazides are the most widely prescribed class of diuretics.

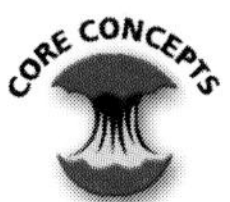

The thiazides comprise the largest, most commonly prescribed class of diuretics. These drugs act on the distal tubule to block sodium reabsorption and increase water excretion. Their primary use is for the treatment of mild to moderate hypertension. They are less effective than the loop diuretics and are not effective in patients with severe renal disease. All the thiazide diuretics have equivalent effectiveness. The thiazide and thiazide-like diuretics are listed in Table 28.2.

The frequency of adverse effects with the thiazides is much lower than that of the loop diuretics. Side effects from thiazides are generally minor and rarely cause discontinuation of therapy. As happens with other diuretics, dehydration is possible because of fluid loss, and patients may experience dizziness due to hypotension when moving from a supine to an upright position. Electrolyte levels are usually monitored periodically to prevent hypokalemia. To avoid side effects from the drug, patients taking thiazides should be taught to drink plenty of water and beverages containing electrolytes, and to eat a balanced diet.

28.7 Although less effective than the loop diuretics, potassium-sparing diuretics may help prevent hypokalemia.

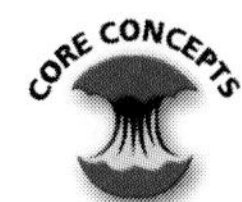

One of the most serious potential adverse effects of the thiazide and loop diuretics is potassium loss. The therapeutic advantage of the potassium-sparing diuretics is that they are able to produce diuresis without adversely affecting blood potassium levels. These diuretics are shown in Table 28.3.

Normally, sodium and potassium are exchanged in the distal tubule; Na^+ is reabsorbed back into the body and K^+ is secreted into the tubule. Potassium-sparing diuretics block this exchange, causing sodium to stay in the tubule and ultimately leave through the urine. When Na^+ is blocked, the body retains more K^+. Because most of the sodium has already been removed by the time the filtrate reaches the distal tubule, potassium-sparing diuretics produce only a mild diuresis. Their primary use is in combination with thiazide or loop diuretics to minimize potassium loss.

Unlike the loop and thiazide diuretics, patients taking potassium-sparing diuretics should not take potassium supplements or be advised to add potassium-rich foods to their diet. Intake of excess potassium when taking these medications may lead to **hyperkalemia.**

hyper = *high or above normal*
kal = *potassium*
emia = *blood condition*

TABLE 28.3 Potassium-sparing Diuretics

DRUG	ROUTE AND ADULT DOSE	REMARKS
amiloride hydrochloride (Midamor)	PO 5 mg/day (max: 20 mg/day)	Monitor serum potassium level; use with caution in diabetics
Pr spironolactone (Aldactone)	PO 25–400 mg 1–2 times/day	Often used in conjunction with other diuretics to increase the diuretic effect; monitor serum potassium level
triamterene (Dyrenium)	PO 100 mg bid (max: 300 mg/day)	Monitor serum potassium levels; often causes elevated BUN

DRUG PROFILE: Potassium-Sparing Diuretic: Pr *Spironolactone (Aldactone)*

Actions and Uses:

Spironolactone acts by blocking sodium reabsorption in the distal tubule. It accomplishes this by inhibiting **aldosterone.** Aldosterone is the hormone secreted by the adrenal cortex that is responsible for increasing the renal reabsorption of sodium in exchange for potassium, thus causing water retention. When blocked by spironolactone, sodium and water excretion is increased, and the body retains more potassium. In addition, blocking aldosterone slows the progression of heart failure (Chapter 16).

Adverse Effects and Interactions:

Spironolactone does such an efficient job of retaining potassium that hyperkalemia may develop. The probability of hyperkalemia is increased if the patient takes potassium supplements or is also taking ACE inhibitors, as described in Chapter 15. Signs and symptoms of hyperkalemia include muscle weakness, ventricular tachycardia, or fibrillation. When potassium levels are monitored carefully and maintained within normal values, side effects from spironolactone are uncommon.

Spironolactone interacts with several drugs. For example, when combined with ammonium chloride, acidosis may occur. Aspirin and other salicylates may decrease the diuretic effect of the medication. Use of spironolactone and digoxin may decrease the effects of digoxin. When taken with potassium supplements, ACE inhibitors, and angiotensin-receptor blockers, hyperkalemia may result.

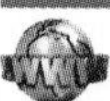
See the Companion Website for a Nursing Process Focus specific to this drug.

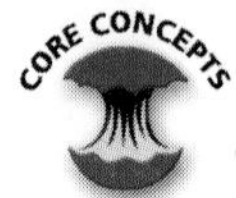

28.8 Several less commonly prescribed diuretics have specific indications.

intra = *within*
ocular = *eye*

A few diuretics cannot be classified as loop, thiazide, or potassium-sparing agents. These diuretics have very limited and specific indications. Three of these drugs inhibit **carbonic anhydrase,** an enzyme that affects acid-base balance by its ability to form carbonic acid from water and carbon dioxide. For example, acetazolamide (Diamox) is a carbonic anhydrase inhibitor used to decrease intraocular fluid pressure in patients with open-angle glaucoma (Chapter 33). Unrelated to its diuretic effect, acetazolamide also has applications as an anticonvulsant and in treating motion sickness.

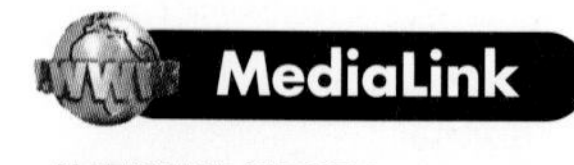

NATIONAL KIDNEY FOUNDATION

The osmotic diuretics also have very specific applications. For example, mannitol is used to maintain urine flow in patients with acute renal failure or during prolonged surgery. Mannitol can also be used to lower intraocular pressure in certain types of glaucoma. It is a very potent diuretic that is only given by the IV route. Table 28.4 lists some of the miscellaneous diuretics.

TABLE 28.4 Miscellaneous Diuretics

DRUG	ROUTE AND ADULT DOSE	REMARKS
acetazolamide (Diamox)	PO 250–375 mg/day in am	Carbonic anhydrase inhibitor; IV form available
dichlorphenamide (Daramide, Oratrol)	PO 25–50 mg 1–3 times/day	Carbonic anhydrase inhibitor
mannitol	IV 100 g infused over 2–6h	Osmotic type
methazolamide (Neptazane)	PO 50–100 mg bid or tid	Carbonic anhydrase inhibitor
urea (Ureaphil)	IV 1.0–1.5 g/kg over 1–2.5 hours	Osmotic type

28.9 Intravenous fluid therapy with crystalloids and colloids is used to replace lost fluids.

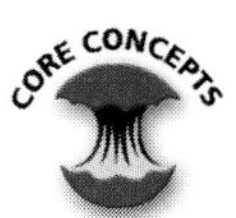

To maintain proper fluid balance in the body, the amount of fluids gained through eating and drinking must equal that lost through the urine, feces, sweating, respirations, and other excretory processes. Failure to balance intake with output can result in fluid volume disorders that are indications for pharmacotherapy. Hemorrhage, severe burns, diarrhea, vomiting, or inadequate fluid intake can lead to dehydration and death if the fluid imbalance is not corrected.

The immediate goal in treating fluid deficiencies is to replace the missing fluid. In mild cases, this may be accomplished by drinking extra water or beverages containing electrolytes. Thirst is a natural mechanism that triggers us to replace lost fluids when working outdoors in hot weather or following exercise. In acute situations, IV fluid therapy can immediately replace lost fluids. Regardless of how fluids are administered, careful attention must be paid to restoring normal levels of electrolytes, as well as fluid volume.

Intravenous replacement fluids are of two types: colloids and crystalloids. **Colloids** are proteins or other large molecules that remain suspended in the blood for a long time because they are too large to cross membranes. While circulating, they draw water molecules from the cells and tissues into the blood vessels by their ability to increase **osmotic pressure.** These agents are sometimes called *plasma* or *volume expanders.*

Crystalloids are IV solutions that contain electrolytes in concentrations resembling those of plasma. Unlike colloids, crystalloid solutions leave the blood and enter cells. They are used to replace fluids that have been lost and to promote urine output. Examples of colloids and crystalloids are listed in Table 28.5.

TABLE 28.5 Fluid Replacement Agents

AGENT	EXAMPLES
Blood products	■ Whole blood ■ Plasma protein fraction ■ Fresh frozen plasma ■ Packed red blood cells
Colloids	■ Plasma protein fraction (Plasmanate, PlasmaPlex, Plasmatein, PPF, Protenate) ■ Albumin (Albuminar, Albutein, Buminate, Plasbumin) ■ Dextran 40 (Gentran 40, Hyskon, Rheomacrodex) or dextran 70 (Macrodex) ■ Hetastarch (Hespan)
Cystalloids	■ Normal saline (0.9% sodium chloride) ■ Lactated Ringer's ■ Plasmalyte ■ Hypertonic saline (3% sodium chloride) ■ 5% dextrose in water (D_5W)

NURSING PROCESS FOCUS

Patients Receiving Fluid Replacement Therapy

ASSESSMENT

Prior to administration:
- Obtain complete health history including allergies, drug history, and possible drug interactions
- Assess vital signs, level of consciousness, skin/mucous membrane condition, and heart/lung sounds for signs of fluid volume deficit
- Obtain the following laboratory studies: CBC, serum electrolytes, serum osmolarity, and renal function (BUN and serum creatinine)

POTENTIAL NURSING DIAGNOSES

- Deficient Fluid Volume
- Risk for Decreased Cardiac Output
- Risk for Injury, related to side effects of drug therapy

PLANNING: Patient Goals and Expected Outcomes

The patient will:
- Exhibit signs of normal fluid volume such as stable blood pressure and adequate urinary output of at least 30 ml/hr
- Demonstrate an understanding of the drug's action by accurately describing drug side effects and precautions
- Immediately report effects such as itching, shortness of breath, flushing, cough, and heart palpitations

IMPLEMENTATION

Interventions and (Rationales)	Patient Education/Discharge Planning
■ Administer all fluids as ordered by physician (to ensure safety of patient).	■ Inform patient and family about the reason for and expected outcome of fluid replacement therapy.
■ Monitor intake and urine output. Report urine output if less than 30 ml/hr. (Output less than 30 ml/hr indicates fluid volume deficit.)	■ Inform the patient and family about the importance of monitoring intake and output and to report any fluids ingested. ■ Instruct patient concerning rationale for possible Foley catheter insertion.
■ Measure urine specific gravity: normal 1.010–1.035. (Specific gravity of less than 1.025 may indicate fluid volume deficit.)	■ Inform patient as to the reason for testing.
■ Monitor for hypersensitivity reactions such as urticaria, pruritus, dyspnea, flushing, and anaphylaxis.	■ Instruct patient to report itching, shortness of breath, or flushing as symptoms occur.
■ Monitor VS including peripheral pulses and capillary refill, as well as breath and heart sounds, for signs of circulatory overload such as dyspnea, cyanosis, cough, crackles, wheezes, and neck vein distention. (Effects of drugs or rapid infusion of fluids may cause fluid overload.)	Instruct patient: ■ About reason that vital signs and other assessments are monitored frequently. ■ To report shortness of breath, cough, or heart palpitation as soon as such symptoms occur.
■ Monitor lab values: electrolytes, serum osmolarity, and hematocrit. (Values may fall with rehydration. Report all abnormal values.)	■ Instruct patient of the need for frequent laboratory studies.
■ If central venous pressure monitoring devices are used, ensure that equipment is checked and patient assessments (intake and output, level of consciousness, vital signs, breath sounds) are done according to institutional policy (usually every 15–60 mins) and that CVP is within normal range (between 2–8 cm of water).	Instruct patient about: ■ Reason for using monitoring device ■ Reason that vital signs and other assessments are monitored frequently

continued...

NURSING PROCESS FOCUS

Interventions and (Rationales)	Patient Education/Discharge Planning
For colloid solutions (plasma or volume expanders): ■ Take vital signs before and during infusion (usually every 15–60 mins) to ensure patient safety.	Instruct patient: ■ About reason that vital signs and other assessments are monitored frequently.
■ Monitor for signs/symptoms of CHF or pulmonary edema. Report any of the following signs/symptoms: dyspnea, cyanosis, cough, crackles, wheezes.	■ To report shortness of breath, cough, or heart palpitation as soon as such symptoms occur.
For blood/blood products: ■ Obtain baseline vital signs. ■ Monitor for transfusion reaction. Stay with patient for first 15 minutes. If a transfusion reaction occurs, stop infusion, start NS slowly, follow institutional policy concerning the blood bag/tubing, notify the physician/charge nurse, and continue to monitor patient. ■ Ensure that vital signs are monitored and recorded according to institutional policy.	Instruct patient: ■ About reason for transfusion ■ About reason that vital signs are monitored frequently ■ To immediately report any of the following: warm feeling, chills, itching, feeling of weakness, difficulty breathing

EVALUATION OF OUTCOME CRITERIA

Evaluate the effectiveness of drug therapy by confirming that patient goals and expected outcomes have been met (see "Planning").

See Table 28.5 for a list of drugs to which these nursing actions apply.

Concept Review 28.3

- How does a colloid IV fluid differ from a crystalloid?

28.10 Acidic and basic drugs can be administered to maintain normal body pH.

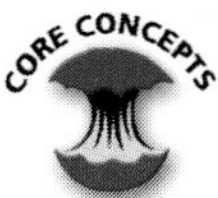

Unless quickly corrected, acidosis and alkalosis can have serious or fatal consequences. Acidic and basic agents may be given to correct pH imbalances in body fluids.

The degree of acidity or alkalinity of a solution is measured by its pH. A **pH** of 7.0 is defined as neutral, above 7.0 as basic or alkaline, and below 7.0 as acidic. To maintain homeostasis, the pH of plasma and most body fluids must be kept within the very narrow range of 7.35 to 7.45. Nearly all proteins and enzymes in the body function within this range of pH values. At pH values above 7.45, **alkalosis** develops, and symptoms of CNS stimulation occur that include nervousness and convulsions. **Acidosis** occurs below of pH of 7.35, and symptoms of CNS depression may result in coma. In either alkalosis or acidosis, death may result if large changes in pH are not corrected immediately. Acidosis and alkalosis are not diseases; they are symptoms of an underlying disorder. Primary treatment of acid-base disorders is always targeted to correcting the underlying cause. Drugs are administered to support the patient's vital functions while the disease is being treated. Common causes of alkalosis and acidosis are shown in Table 28.6.

alkal = *basic*
osis = *condition*

Alkalosis may be reversed by the IM or IV administration of acidic agents such as ammonium chloride. When this drug is metabolized in the liver, acid (H^+) is formed and the pH of body fluids decreases. Ammonium chloride will also acidify the urine, which is beneficial in treating many urinary tract infections and in promoting the excretion of alkaline drugs such as amphetamines. In less severe cases, the alkalosis may be corrected by administering sodium chloride combined with potassium chloride. This combination increases the renal excretion of bicarbonate ion (a base), which indirectly increases the acidity of the blood. The correction of acid-base imbalances is illustrated in Figure 28.4 ■.

TABLE 28.6 Causes of Alkalosis and Acidosis

ACIDOSIS	ALKALOSIS
RESPIRATORY ORIGINS OF ACIDOSIS	***RESPIRATORY ORIGIN OF ALKALOSIS***
■ hypoventilation or shallow breathing	■ hyperventilation due to asthma, anxiety, or high altitude
■ airway constriction	
■ damage to respiratory center in medulla	
METABOLIC ORIGINS OF ACIDOSIS	***METABOLIC ORIGINS OF ALKALOSIS***
■ severe diarrhea	■ constipation for prolonged periods
■ kidney failure	■ ingestion of excess sodium bicarbonate
■ diabetes mellitus	■ diuretics that cause potassium depletion
■ excess alcohol ingestion	■ severe vomiting
■ starvation	

FIGURE 28.4

Acid-base imbalances

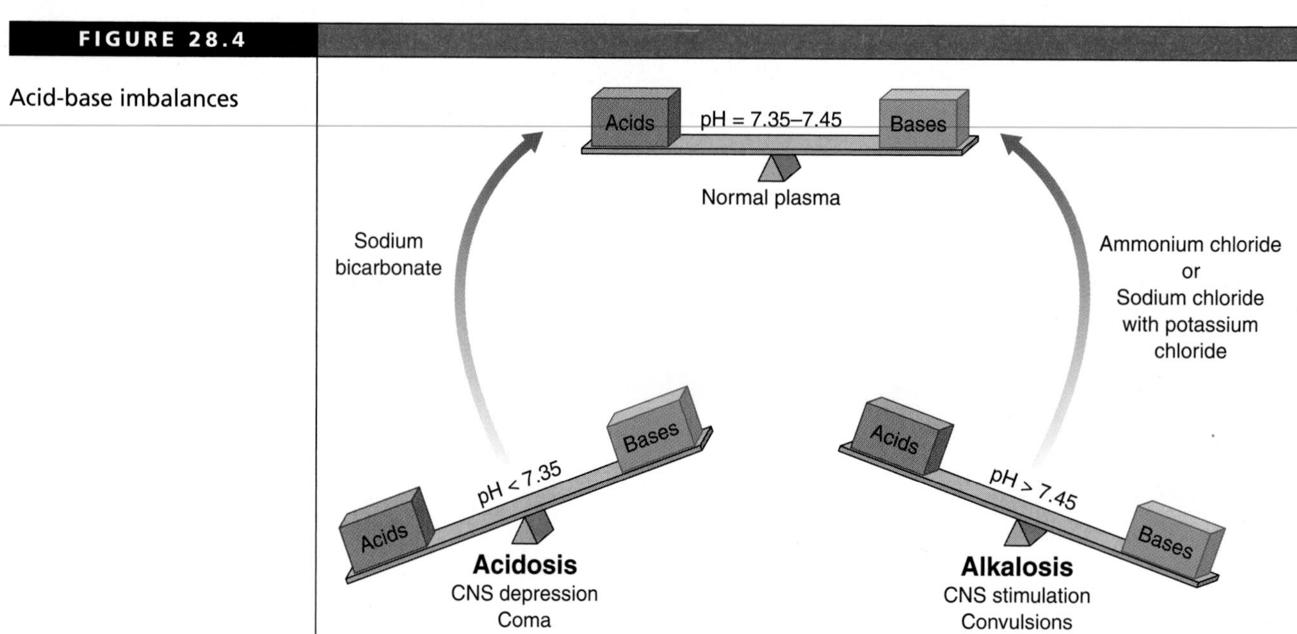

In patients with acidosis, the goal is to quickly reverse the effects of excess acids in the blood. The treatment of choice for acute acidosis is to administer infusions of sodium bicarbonate. Bicarbonate ion acts as a base to quickly neutralize acids in the blood and other body fluids. The patient must be carefully monitored during infusions because this drug can "over-correct" the acidosis, causing blood pH to turn alkaline.

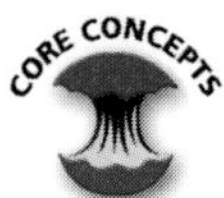

28.11 Electrolytes are charged substances that play important roles in body chemistry.

electro = *conducts electricity*
lyte = *solution*

In Chapter 27, the role of minerals in human physiology was discussed. In certain body fluids, some of these minerals become ions and possess a charge. Small, inorganic molecules possessing a positive or negative charge are called **electrolytes.** Positively charged electrolytes are called **cations;** those with a negative charge are called **anions.** They are essential to many body functions, including nerve conduction, muscle contraction, and bone growth and remodeling. Too little or too much of an electrolyte may result in serious disease and must be quickly corrected.

Levels of electrolytes in body fluids are maintained within very narrow ranges, primarily by the kidney and GI tract. As electrolytes are lost via normal excretory functions, they must be replaced by adequate intake; otherwise, electrolyte imbalances can result. Although imbalances can

DRUG PROFILE: Alkaline Agent/Electrolyte: Pr *Sodium Bicarbonate*

Actions and Uses:

Acidosis is a more common event than alkalosis, occurring during shock, cardiac arrest, or diabetes mellitus. Sodium bicarbonate is the drug of choice for correcting acidosis: the bicarbonate ion (HCO_3^-) directly raises the pH of body fluids. Sodium bicarbonate may be given orally, if acidosis is mild, or IV, in cases or acute disease. Although sodium bicarbonate neutralizes gastric acid, it is rarely used to treat peptic ulcers because of its tendency to cause gas and gastric distention. After absorption, it makes the urine more basic, which aids in the renal excretion of acidic drugs such as the barbiturates and salicylates.

Adverse Effects and Interactions:

Most of the side effects of sodium bicarbonate therapy are the result of metabolic alkalosis caused by too much bicarbonate ion. Symptoms may include confusion, irritability, slow respiration rate, and vomiting. Simply discontinuing the sodium bicarbonate infusion often reverses these symptoms; however, potassium chloride or ammonium chloride may be administered to reverse the alkalosis.

Sodium bicarbonate interacts with several drugs. For example, it may decrease absorption of ketoconazole, and may decrease elimination of dextroamphetamine; ephedrine, pseudoephedrine, and quinidine. Sodium bicarbonate may increase the elimination of lithium, salicylates, and tetracyclines.

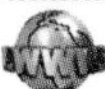 *See the Companion Website for a Nursing Process Focus specific to this drug.*

TABLE 28.7 Electrolyte Imbalances

	ION	EXCESS (ABNORMAL SERUM VALUE [mEq/L])	DEFICIENCY (ABNORMAL SERUM VALUE [mEq/L])
CATIONS			
calcium	Ca^{++}	hypercalcemia (>11)	hypocalcemia (<4)
magnesium	Mg^{++}	hypermagnesemia (>4)	hypomagnesemia (<0.8)
potassium	K^+	hyperkalemia (>5)	hypokalemia (<3.5)
sodium	Na^+	hypernatremia (>145)	hyponatremia (<135)
ANIONS			
bicarbonate	HCO_3^-	—	—
chloride	Cl^-	hyperchloremia (>112)	hypochloremia (<95)
phosphate	PO_4^- or HPO_4^{--}	hyperphosphatemia (>6)	hypophosphatemia (<1)
sulfate	SO_4^-	—	—

occur in any ion, sodium, potassium, and calcium are of greatest importance. Calcium homeostasis is presented in Chapter 31 because it is often associated with the pharmacotherapy of bone disorders. Sodium and potassium are discussed in the following paragraphs. The major electrolytes and their imbalances are shown in Table 28.7.

Because sodium is the major electrolyte in extracellular fluid, imbalances of this ion can have serious consequences. Sodium excess, or hypernatremia, is most commonly caused by kidney disease; sodium accumulates in the blood due to decreased excretion. For minor hypernatremia, a low-salt diet may be effective in returning serum sodium to normal levels. In patients with acute hypernatremia, however, IV fluids such as 5% D_5W or diuretics may be administered to quickly remove sodium from the body.

Sodium deficiency, or **hyponatremia,** may occur when sodium is lost because of disorders of the skin, GI tract, or kidneys, and in those disorders associated with excessive sweating or prolonged fever. Hyponatremia is usually treated with solutions of sodium chloride. Various concentrations of sodium chloride are available, depending on the severity of the deficiency. In most cases, concentrations of 0.45% or 0.9% are used to reverse hyponatremia.

hyper = *high or above normal*
natri = *sodium*
emia = *blood condition*

Potassium is the most abundant intracellular cation, and excess or deficiency states can be serious or fatal. Hyperkalemia may be caused by high consumption of potassium-rich foods or dietary

DRUG PROFILE: Electrolyte: 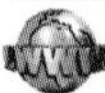 *Potassium Chloride*

Actions and Uses:

Potassium is one of the most important electrolytes in body fluids, and levels must be maintained within a narrow range of values between 3.5 and 5.5 mEq/L. Too much or too little potassium may lead to serious consequences and must be immediately corrected. Neurons and muscle fibers are most sensitive to potassium loss. Muscle weakness, dysrhythmias, and cardiac arrest are possible consequences.

Therapy with loop or thiazide diuretics is the most common cause of potassium loss. Patients taking thiazide or loop diuretics are usually instructed to take oral potassium supplements to prevent hypokalemia.

Potassium chloride is the drug of choice for treating or preventing hypokalemia. It is also used to treat mild forms of alkalosis. Dosage forms include oral and IV preparations. Oral forms include tablets, powders, and liquids, usually heavily flavored because of the unpleasant taste of the drug.

Adverse Effects and Interactions:

Nausea and vomiting are common because potassium chloride irritates the GI mucosa. The drug may be taken with meals or antacids to lessen the gastric distress.

Potassium supplements interact with potassium-sparing diuretics and ACE inhibitors to increase the risk of hyperkalemia.

See the Companion Website for a Nursing Process Focus specific to this drug.

supplements, particularly when patients are taking potassium-sparing diuretics such as spironolactone. In mild cases, potassium levels may be returned to normal by restricting major dietary sources of potassium such as bananas, dried fruits, peanut butter, broccoli, and green leafy vegetables. If the patient is taking a potassium-sparing diuretic, the dose is lowered or an alternate drug is considered. In severe hyperkalemia, serum potassium levels may be lowered by administering sodium polystyrene sulfate (Kayexalate), a resin that removes potassium ions by exchanging them for sodium ions in the large intestine. When the drug is excreted in the feces, potassium ion is eliminated. Sodium polystyrene sulfate is available in oral and enema formulations. An alternative method of treating hyperkalemia is to administer glucose and insulin, which causes potassium to leave the extracellular fluid and enter cells.

Hypokalemia is a relatively common adverse effect resulting from high doses of loop diuretics such as furosemide. Strenuous muscular activity and severe vomiting or diarrhea can also result in significant potassium loss. Mild hypokalemia is treated by increasing the dietary intake of potassium-rich foods. More severe deficiencies require oral or parenteral potassium supplements. Potassium chloride (KCl) is available in IV and a wide variety of oral formulations to increase blood potassium levels.

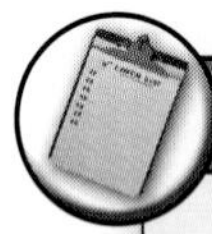

PATIENTS NEED TO KNOW

Patients treated for urinary, acid-base, and fluid disorders need to know the following:

Regarding Diuretics

1. When taking diuretics, drink plenty of water if dry mouth or thirst develops, unless otherwise directed by a healthcare provider.
2. Take diuretics at least 2 hours before bedtime to avoid nighttime diuresis.
3. If diabetes is present, monitor blood sugar levels very closely when taking loop diuretics because these drugs may elevate blood glucose levels.
4. Do not take thiazide diuretics during pregnancy or when breast-feeding.
5. When taking loop or thiazide diuretics, increase intake of potassium-rich foods such as dark, leafy vegetables, nuts, citrus fruits, bananas, and potatoes. If taking a potassium-sparing diuretic, avoid these foods unless otherwise instructed by a healthcare provider.
6. Avoid caffeinated beverages when taking diuretics. The diuretic effect of the caffeine combined with the effects of these medications may cause dehydration.

Regarding Potassium Supplements

7. Because potassium chloride tablets are irritating to the GI mucosa, they should be taken with food. Do not crush or suck the tablets. If nausea or heartburn occurs, take antacids along with the KCl. ■

CHAPTER REVIEW

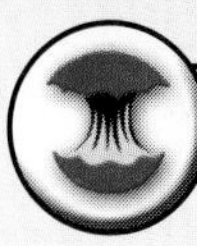

CORE CONCEPTS SUMMARY

28.1 The kidneys regulate fluid volume, electrolytes, acids, and bases.

The kidneys are essential to the overall health of the patient, controlling fluid volume, electrolyte composition, and acid-base balance. The functional unit of the kidney is the nephron.

28.2 The composition of filtrate changes dramatically as a result of the processes of reabsorption and secretion.

Filtrate entering the proximal tubule resembles plasma without proteins. Through the processes of reabsorption and secretion, the filtrate composition changes to produce urine.

28.3 Renal failure significantly impacts pharmacotherapy.

Because the kidneys excrete most drugs, a large number of medications require a significant dosage reduction in patients with moderate to severe renal failure. Renal failure is classified as acute or chronic. Pharmacotherapy of renal failure attempts to cure the cause of the dysfunction. Diuretics may be used to maintain urine output. Epoetin alfa is a form of erythropoietin used to treat anemias in which there is a deficiency in red blood cell production.

28.4 Most diuretics act by blocking sodium reabsorption in the nephron.

Diuretics are drugs that increase urine output, usually by blocking sodium reabsorption. Indications for diuretics include hypertension, heart failure, kidney failure, and liver disease.

28.5 The most effective diuretics are those that affect the loop of Henle.

The high-ceiling or loop diuretics such as furosemide act by blocking sodium reabsorption in the loop of Henle. They are the most effective diuretics, but are more likely to cause dehydration and electrolyte loss.

28.6 The thiazides are the most widely prescribed class of diuretics.

The thiazide diuretics block sodium reabsorption in the distal tubule. Although less effective than the loop diuretics, the thiazides are more frequently prescribed because of their lower incidence of serious side effects.

28.7 Although less effective than the loop diuretics, potassium-sparing diuretics may help prevent hypokalemia.

Potassium-sparing diuretics act on the distal tubule and are more effective than the loop diuretics. Their primary advantage is that they do not cause potassium loss.

28.8 Several less commonly prescribed diuretics have specific indications.

Carbonic anhydrase inhibitors and osmotic diuretics are not commonly prescribed. They have specific applications, such as decreasing intraocular pressure and maintaining urine flow during renal failure.

28.9 Intravenous fluid therapy with crystalloids and colloids is used to replace lost fluids.

Colloids are solutions such as Dextran and albumin that are used to expand plasma volume and maintain blood pressure. Crystalloids are fluids such as normal saline or lactated Ringer's that replace fluids and electrolytes that have been lost from cells and tissues.

28.10 Acidic and basic drugs can be administered to maintain normal body pH.

Ammonium chloride can be administered to quickly reverse alkalosis. Sodium chloride with potassium chloride can reverse alkalosis indirectly. Sodium bicarbonate is used to reverse acidosis.

28.11 Electrolytes are charged substances that play important roles in body chemistry.

Electrolyte imbalances can cause serious problems. Hypokalemia is a serious potential adverse effect of drug therapy with certain diuretics. Oral or IV potassium chloride can reverse symptoms of hypokalemia. Although less common, hyperkalemia may be just as serious and may be reversed by administration of glucose or insulin.

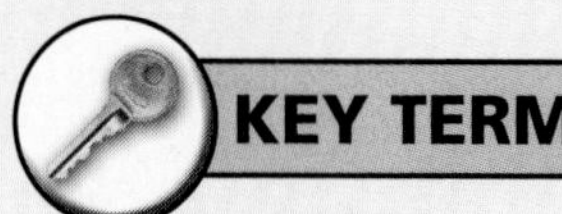

KEY TERMS

acidosis (ah-sid-OH-sis): condition of having too much acid; plasma pH below 7.35 / *page 535*

aldosterone (al-DOH-stair-own): hormone secreted by the adrenal cortex that increases sodium reabsorption in the distal tubule of the kidney / *page 532*

alkalosis (al-kah-LOH-sis): condition of having too much base; plasma pH above 7.45 / *page 535*

anions (an-EYE-ons): negatively charged ions / *page 536*

carbonic anhydrase (kar-BON-ik an-HY-drase): enzyme that forms carbonic acid by combining carbon dioxide and water / *page 532*

cations (KAT-eye-ons): positively charged ions / *page 536*

colloids (KAHL-oyds): type of IV solution consisting of large organic molecules that are unable to cross membranes / *page 533*

crystalloids (KRIS-tall-oyds): type of IV solution resembling blood plasma minus proteins that is capable of crossing membranes / *page 533*

diuretic (dye-your-ET-ik): drug that increases urine output / *page 528*

electrolytes (ee-LEK-troh-lites): small, charged ions / *page 536*

erythropoietin (ee-rith-ro-po-EE-tin): hormone secreted by the kidney that stimulates red blood cell production / *page 528*

filtrate (FIL-trate): fluid in the nephron that is filtered at Bowman's capsule / *page 526*

hyperkalemia (HY-purr-kay-LEE-mee-ah): high potassium levels in the blood / *page 531*

hypokalemia (hy-poh-kay-LEE-mee-uh): low potassium levels in the blood / *page 530*

hyponatremia (hy-po-nay-TREE-mee-uh): low levels of sodium in the blood / *page 537*

osmotic pressure (oz-MOT-ik): force exerted when there is an imbalance of solutes on each side of a semipermeable membrane / *page 533*

nephron (NEF-ron): functional unit of the kidney / *page 526*

pH: a measure of the acidity or alkalinity of a solution / *page 535*

reabsorption: movement of substances from the kidney tubule back into the blood / *page 527*

secretion: movement of substances from the blood into the kidney tubule after filtration has occurred / *page 527*

REVIEW QUESTIONS

The following questions are written in NCLEX-PN® style. Answer these questions to assess your knowledge of the chapter material, and go back and review any material that is not clear to you.

1. Which of the following is not a function of the kidneys?

1. Acid-base balance
2. Secretion of renin
3. Production of white blood cells
4. Production of calcitriol

2. When assessing for dehydration, the nurse will look for:

1. Headache and increased urinary output
2. Weight gain and edema
3. Hypertension and decreased urinary output
4. Hypotension, headache, and dry mucous membranes

3. A newly diagnosed hypertensive patient will most likely be started on which of the following medications?

1. Ethacrynic acid (Edecrin)
2. Chlorothiazide (Diuril)
3. Spironolactone (Aldactone)
4. Mannitol

4. The patient recently started on diuretic therapy should be taught to:

1. Take medication at night
2. Rise slowly from a sitting position
3. Increase sodium intake
4. Decrease fluid intake

5. When too much ammonium chloride is administered, the blood becomes:

1. Alkalotic
2. Acidotic
3. Neutralized
4. Normalized

6. The patient is exhibiting signs and symptoms of metabolic acidosis. Which of the following is not a cause of metabolic acidosis?

1. Severe diarrhea
2. Hyperventilation
3. Starvation
4. Diabetes mellitus

7. If the patient is experiencing hypernatremia, which of the following is appropriate treatment?

1. Diuretics
2. Potassium
3. IV fluids
4. Increasing fluid intake

8. The patient is receiving IV normal saline because of hyponatremia. The hyponatremia may have been caused by:

1. Constipation
2. Severe nausea and vomiting
3. Dehydration
4. Hemorrhage

9. If taking diuretics, the patient should be instructed to decrease his intake of:

1. Dark green, leafy vegetables
2. Nuts
3. Fruits
4. Caffeine

10. The patient taking torsemide (Demadex) must closely monitor his ___________ levels.

1. Glucose
2. Magnesium
3. Calcium
4. Selenium

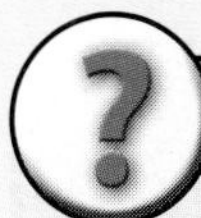

CASE STUDY QUESTIONS

For questions 1–5, please refer to the following case study, and choose the correct answer from choices 1–4.

Mr. Grant has been placed on hydrochlorothiazide (HCTZ) for high blood pressure and potassium chloride as a dietary supplement. His wife tells him to eat lots of bananas because she read that this was necessary when taking diuretics. After a few weeks, Mr. Grant becomes weak and feels as if his heart is skipping beats. His blood pressure remains high, despite the diuretic.

1. Which of the following should have been explained to Mr. Grant regarding his medication?

1. Never eat bananas when taking HCTZ.
2. Eat lots of bananas when taking HCTZ.
3. Limit potassium-rich foods when taking potassium supplements.
4. Never eat bananas and take HCTZ at the same meal.

2. Given the previous information, it is quite possible that Mr. Grant's cardiac symptoms and weakness were caused by:

1. Hyperkalemia
2. Hypokalemia
3. Hypernatremia
4. Hyponatremia

3. The physician examines Mr. Grant and decides to administer a dose of sodium polystyrene sulfonate (Kayexalate). The rationale for administering this drug is to:

1. Increase fluid volume
2. Decrease fluid volume
3. Increase serum potassium levels
4. Decrease serum potassium levels

4. After Mr. Grant's condition stabilized, the physician decided to select a more effective diuretic to treat the hypertension. Which class is more effective than the thiazides and would most likely be selected for Mr. Grant?

1. Potassium-sparing
2. Loop/high-ceiling
3. Osmotic
4. Carbonic anhydrase inhibitors

5. Crystalloids and colloids are administered to:

1. Lower serum sodium levels
2. Lower serum potassium levels
3. Make body fluids more alkaline
4. Increase the volume of body fluids

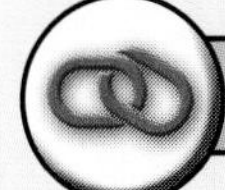

FURTHER STUDY

- Chapter 31 contains information on calcium homeostasis and on calcitriol, the active form of vitamin D, that helps maintain bone homeostasis.
- ACE inhibitors for treating hypertension are discussed in Chapter 15.
- The use of diuretics in treating hypertension and heart failure is covered in Chapters 15 and 16, respectively.
- A drug profile for furosemide is contained in Chapter 16.

- The use of acetazolamide is discussed in Chapter 33 as a drug for decreasing intraocular fluid pressure in patients with open-angle glaucoma.
- Chapter 27 includes information on the role of minerals, some of which are electrolytes, in human physiology.
- The use of spironolactone in the pharmacotherapy of heart failure is presented in Chapter 16.
- The use of diuretics in the pharmacotherapy of hypertension is discussed in Chapter 15.

EXPLORE MEDIALINK www.prenhall.com/holland

Additional resources for this chapter can be found on the CD-ROM accompanying this textbook, and on the Companion Website. Click on Chapter 28 to select activities for this chapter.

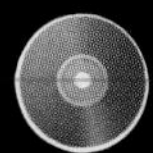

- Audio Glossary
- Concept Review
- NCLEX-PN® Review
- Nursing in Action
- Dosage Calculator

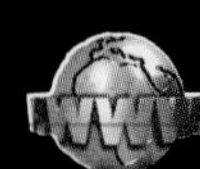

- The Nephrology Channel
- National Kidney Foundation

UNIT

1 2 3 4 5 6 7

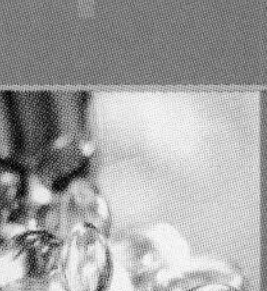

6 THE ENDOCRINE AND REPRODUCTIVE SYSTEMS

UNIT CONTENTS

CHAPTER

29 Drugs for Endocrine Disorders

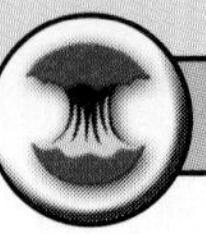

CORE CONCEPTS

29.1 The endocrine system maintains homeostasis by using hormones as chemical messengers.

29.2 Hormones are used as replacement therapy, as antineoplastics, and for their natural therapeutic effects.

29.3 The hypothalamus and the pituitary gland secrete hormones that control other endocrine organs.

29.4 Insulin and glucagon are secreted by the pancreas.

29.5 Type 1 diabetes is treated by dietary restrictions and insulin injections.

29.6 Type 2 diabetes is controlled through lifestyle changes and oral hypoglycemic agents.

29.7 The thyroid gland controls the basal metabolic rate and affects every cell in the body.

29.8 Thyroid disorders may be treated by administering thyroid hormone or by decreasing the activity of the thyroid gland.

29.9 Glucocorticoids are released during periods of stress and influence carbohydrate, lipid, and protein metabolism in most cells.

29.10 Glucocorticoids are prescribed for adrenocortical insufficiency and a wide variety of other conditions.

29.11 Of the many pituitary and hypothalamic hormones, only a few have clinical applications as drugs.

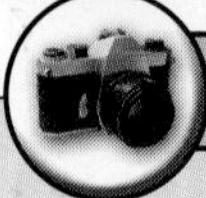

DRUG SNAPSHOT

The following drugs will be discussed in this chapter:

DRUG CLASSES	DRUG PROFILES
Insulins	Pr regular insulin (Humulin R, Novolin R, Pork Regular Iletin II, Regular Purified Pork Insulin)
Oral hypoglycemics	Pr glipizide (Glucotrol, Glucotrol XL)
THYROID DRUGS	
Thyroid agents	Pr levothyroxine (Synthroid)
Antithyroid agents	Pr propylthioracil (PTU)
ADRENAL DRUGS	
Glucocorticoids	Pr hydrocortisone (Aeroseb-HC, Alphaderm, others)

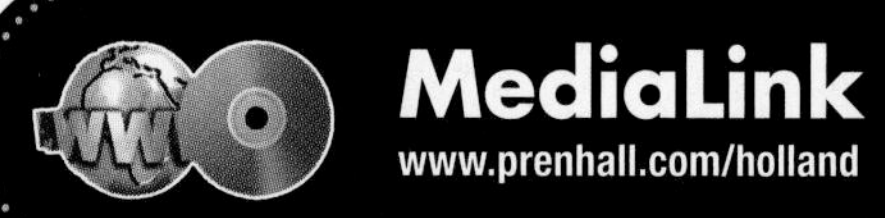

Interactive resources for this chapter can be found on the Companion Website. Click on Chapter 29 and "Begin" to select the activities for this chapter. For chapter-related animations, NCLEX-PN®-style questions, and an audio glossary, access the accompanying CD-ROM in this book.

OBJECTIVES

After reading this chapter, the student should be able to:

1. Describe the general structure and functions of the endocrine system.
2. Compare and contrast the functions of the pancreatic hormones.
3. Compare and contrast the causes, signs, symptoms, and treatment of type 1 and type 2 diabetes mellitus.
4. Identify the five types of insulin.
5. Describe the signs and symptoms of insulin overdose and underdose.
6. Explain the primary functions of the thyroid gland.
7. Identify the signs and symptoms of hypothyroidism and hyperthyroidism.
8. Explain the primary functions of the adrenal cortex.
9. Describe the signs and symptoms of Addison's disease and Cushing's syndrome.
10. For each of the following drugs or drug classes identify representative drugs, explain the mechanisms of drug action, primary actions, and important adverse effects:
    - **a.** insulin
    - **b.** oral hypoglycemics
    - **c.** thyroid hormone
    - **d.** antithyroid agents
    - **e.** glucocorticoids
    - **f.** growth hormone
    - **g.** antidiuretic hormone
11. Categorize drugs used in the treatment of endocrine disorders based on their classifications and mechanisms of action.

Like the nervous system, the endocrine system is a major controller of homeostasis. Although a nerve may exert instantaneous control over a single muscle or gland, a hormone from the endocrine system may affect all body cells and take as long as several days to produce a measurable response. Small amounts of hormones may produce very serious effects on the body. Conversely, deficiencies of small quantities may produce equally serious physiological changes. This chapter examines common endocrine disorders and their pharmacotherapy. The reproductive hormones are covered in Chapter 30.

endo = *within*
crine = *to secrete*

29.1 The endocrine system maintains homeostasis by using hormones as chemical messengers.

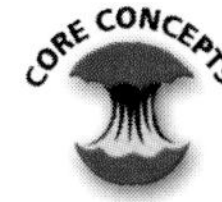

The endocrine system consists of various glands that secrete chemical messengers called **hormones.** Hormones are released in response to a change in the body's internal environment. For example, when the level of glucose in the blood rises, the pancreas secretes insulin. When blood levels of calcium fall, parathyroid hormone (PTH) is released from the parathyroid gland. The various endocrine glands are illustrated in Figure 29.1 ■.

After they are secreted, hormones enter the blood and are transported throughout the body. Some hormones, such as insulin and thyroid hormone, have receptors on nearly every cell in the body and thus produce widespread physiological changes. Others, such as parathyroid hormone and oxytocin, have receptors on only a few specific types of cells.

In the endocrine system, it is common for one hormone to control the secretion of another hormone. In addition, it is common for the last hormone or action in the pathway to provide feedback to turn off the action of the first hormone. For example, as serum calcium level falls, PTH is released. PTH causes an increase in serum calcium level, which provides feedback to the parathyroid glands to shut off PTH secretion. This is a common feature of endocrine homeostasis known as *negative feedback*.

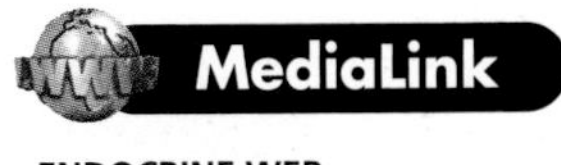

ENDOCRINE WEB

FIGURE 29.1

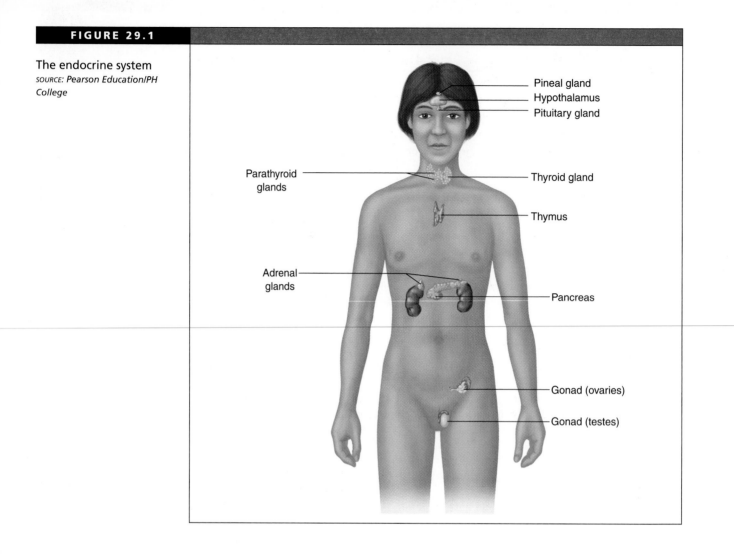

The endocrine system
SOURCE: Pearson Education/PH College

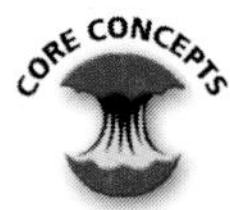

29.2 Hormones are used as replacement therapy, as antineoplastics, and for their natural therapeutic effects.

The goals of hormone pharmacotherapy vary widely. In many cases, the hormone is administered simply as replacement therapy for clients who are unable to secrete sufficient quantities of their own endogenous hormones. Examples of replacement therapy include the administration of thyroid hormone after the thyroid gland has been surgically removed or supplying insulin to a patient whose pancreas is not functioning. Replacement therapy usually supplies the same low-level amounts of the hormone that would normally be present in the body. A summary of selected endocrine disorders and their drug therapy is shown in Table 29.1.

Some hormones are used in cancer chemotherapy. Examples include testosterone for breast cancer and estrogen for testicular cancer. The antineoplastic mechanism of action of these hormones is not known. When used as antineoplastics, the doses of the hormones far exceed those levels normally present in the body (Chapter 24).

Another goal of hormone therapy may be to produce an exaggerated response that is part of the normal action of the drug to achieve some therapeutic advantage. Supplying hydrocortisone to suppress inflammation is an example of taking advantage of the normal action of the glucocorticoids, but at higher amounts than would normally be present in the body. Supplying small amounts of estrogen or progesterone at specific times during the menstrual cycle can prevent ovulation and pregnancy. In this example, the patient is supplied natural hormones; however, they are given at a time when levels in the body are normally low.

TABLE 29.1 Endocrine Disorders and Their Drug Treatment

GLAND	HORMONE(S)	DISORDER	DRUGS
adrenal cortex	glucocorticoids	hypersecretion: Cushing's syndrome	none
		hyposecretion	glucocorticoids
thyroid	thyroid hormone (T_3 and T_4)	hypersecretion: Graves' disease	propylthiouracil (PTU)
		hyposecretion: myxedema (adults) and cretinism (children)	thyroid hormone (Synthroid)
pituitary	growth hormone	hyposecretion: dwarfism	somatrem (Protropin) and somatropin (Humatrope and others)
	antidiuretic hormone	hyposecretion: diabetes insipidus	vasopressin (Pitressin), desmopressin (DDAVP, Stimate), and lypressin (Diapid)
pancreas (Islets of Langerhans)	insulin	hyposecretion: diabetes mellitus	insulin

29.3 The hypothalamus and the pituitary gland secrete hormones that control other endocrine organs.

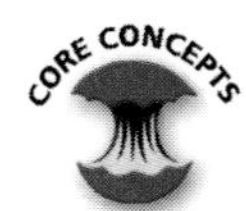

Two endocrine structures in the brain deserve special recognition because they control many other endocrine glands. The **hypothalamus** secretes chemicals called **releasing factors** or *releasing hormones* that travel via blood vessels a short distance to an area immediately below, called the anterior **pituitary gland.** These releasing factors tell the pituitary which hormone to release. After the pituitary releases the appropriate hormone, it travels to its target organ to cause its effect. For example, the hypothalamus secretes thyrotropin-releasing hormone that travels to the pituitary gland with the message to secrete thyroid-stimulating hormone (TSH). TSH then travels to its target organ—the thyroid gland—to stimulate the release of thyroid hormone. Hormones associated with the pituitary gland are shown in Figure 29.2 ■.

29.4 Insulin and glucagon are secreted by the pancreas.

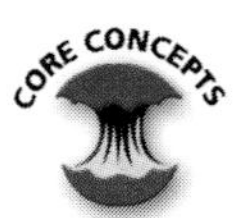

Located behind the stomach and between the duodenum and spleen, the pancreas is a gland that is essential to both the digestive and endocrine systems. It is responsible for the secretion of several enzymes into the pancreatic duct that then flow into the duodenum to assist in the chemical digestion of nutrients. This is its *exocrine* function. Certain cells in the pancreas, called **islets of Langerhans,** control its *endocrine* function: the secretion of glucagon and insulin. As with other endocrine organs, the pancreas secretes these hormones directly into blood capillaries, where they are available for transport to body tissues.

exo = *out/away from*
crine = *to secrete*

Insulin secretion is regulated by a number of chemical, hormonal, and nervous factors. One of the most important regulators is the level of glucose in the blood. After a meal, when glucose levels are high (**hyperglycemia**), the pancreas is stimulated to secrete insulin. The islet cells stop secreting insulin when blood glucose is low (**hypoglycemia**) or when high levels of insulin send the pancreas as a message to stop secreting the hormone.

hyper = *elevated*
hypo = *lowered*
glyc = *sugar*
emia = *blood*

Insulin affects carbohydrate, fat, and protein metabolism in most cells of the body. One of its most important actions is to assist in glucose transport. Without insulin, glucose cannot enter cells. A cell may be literally swimming in glucose, but it cannot enter and be used for fuel by the cell without insulin. The brain is an important exception, not requiring insulin for glucose transport. Insulin is said to have a hypoglycemic effect because its presence causes glucose to leave the blood and enter cells.

Islet cells in the pancreas also produce glucagon. Glucagon is best thought of as a blocker of insulin because its actions are opposite to those of insulin. When levels of glucose are low, glucagon is secreted. Its primary function is to maintain adequate levels of glucose in the blood

FIGURE 29.2

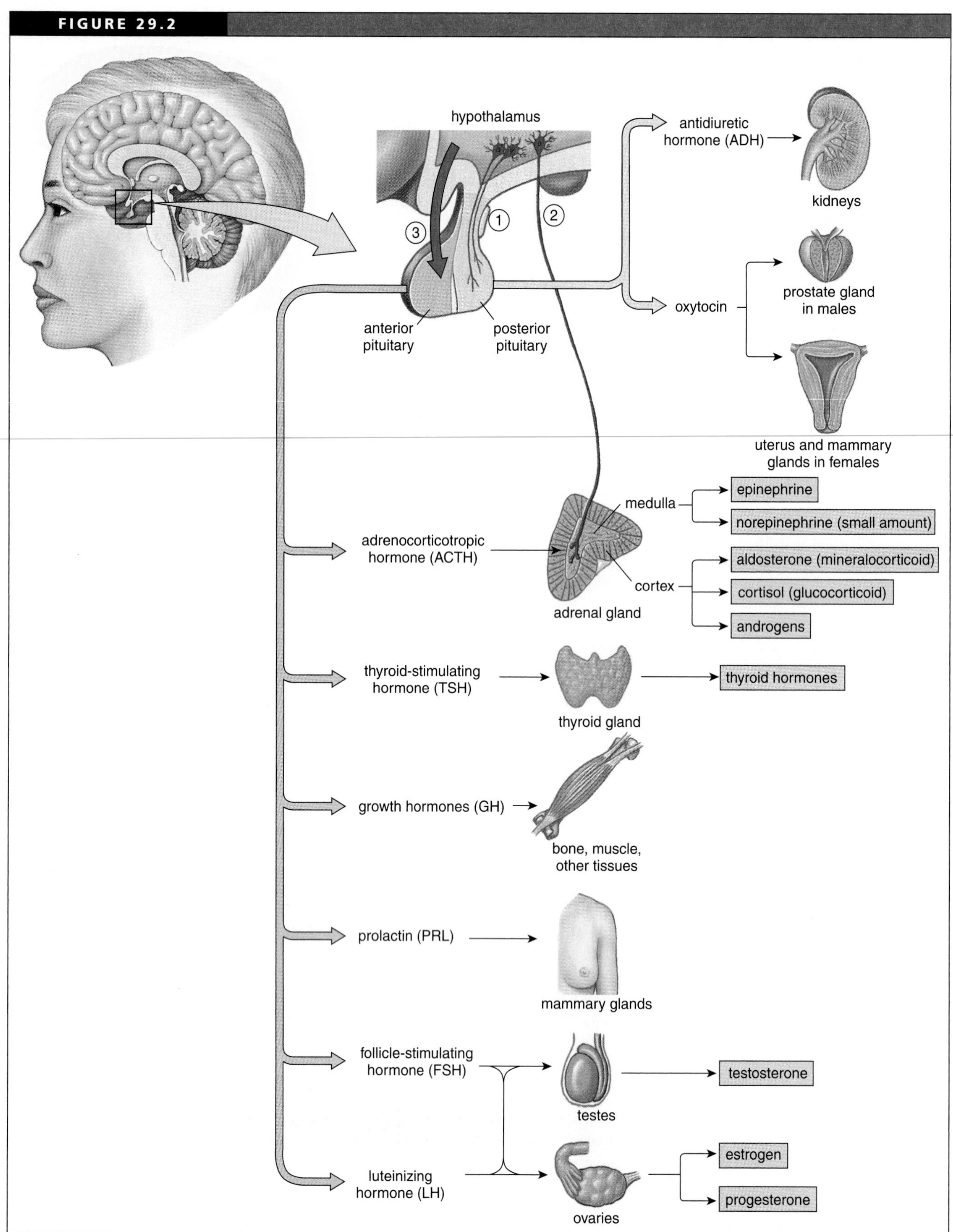

Hormones associated with the pituitary gland *Adapted by permission of Pearson Education, Inc., Upper Saddle River, NJ*

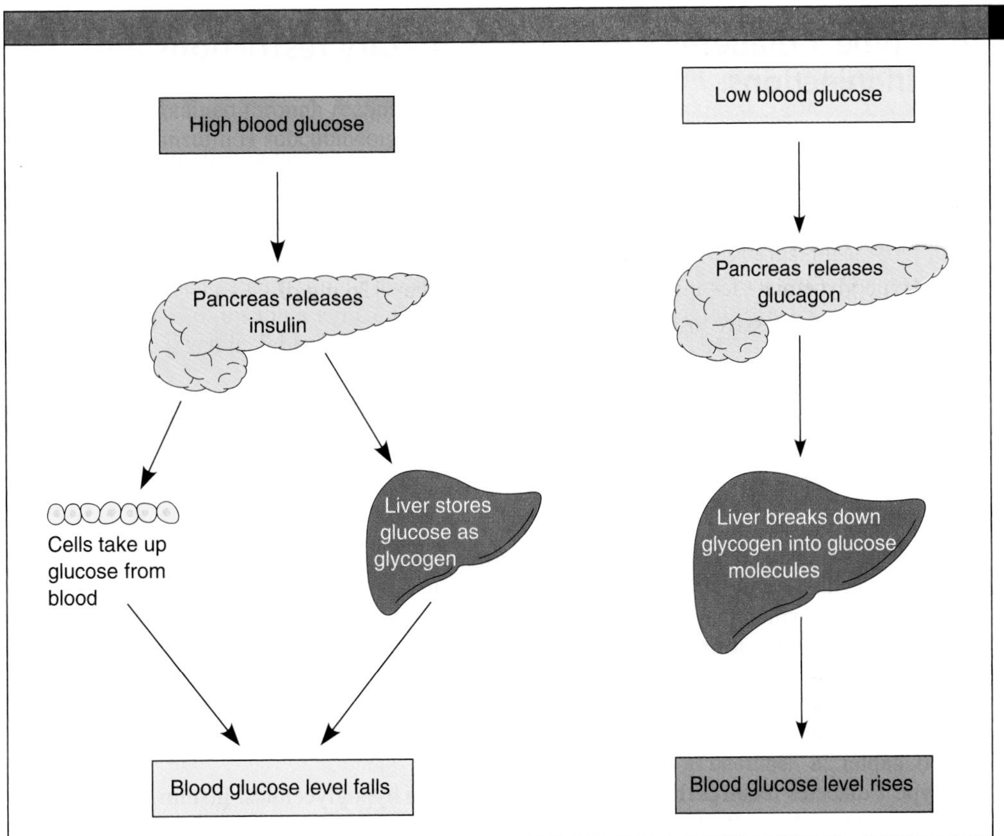

FIGURE 29.3

Insulin, glucagon, and blood glucose
SOURCE: Pearson Education/PH College

Fast Facts Diabetes Mellitus

- Of the 16 million Americans who have diabetes, 5 million probably do not know that they have the disease.
- Each day, 2200 people are diagnosed with diabetes.
- Diabetes causes more than 198,000 deaths each year; it is the sixth leading cause of death.
- Diabetes is the leading cause of blindness in adults; each year 12,000–24,000 people lose their sight because of diabetes.
- Diabetes is responsible for 50% of nontraumatic lower limb amputations; 56,000 amputations are performed each year in diabetics.
- Costs for diabetes treatment exceed $100 billion annually—one in every seven healthcare dollars.
- Diabetes is the leading cause of end-stage renal disease, accounting for about 40% of new cases.

between meals. It has a hyperglycemic effect: its presence moves glucose from cells, primarily in the liver, to the blood. Figure 29.3 ■ illustrates the relationships between blood glucose, insulin, and glucagon.

TYPE 1 DIABETES MELLITUS

dia = *through*
betes = *to go*

Type 1 diabetes mellitus is one of the most common diseases of childhood. Sometimes called *juvenile-onset diabetes* because it is often diagnosed between the ages of 11 to 13, the disease results from a lack of insulin secretion by the pancreas. There is a genetic component to type 1 diabetes, and children and siblings of people with the disease have a higher risk of acquiring the disorder.

TABLE 29.3 Oral Hypoglycemics

DRUG	ROUTE AND ADULT DOSE	REMARKS
ALPHA-GLUCOSIDASE INHIBITORS		
acarbose (Precose)	PO 25–100 mg tid (max: 300 mg/d)	Avoid use in patients with chronic intestinal diseases associated with marked disorders of digestion or absorption.
miglitol (Glyset)	PO 25–100 mg tid (max: 300 mg/d)	Use cautiously in patients with renal impairment.
BIGUANIDES		
metformin HCl (Glucophage)	PO 500 mg 1–3 times/day (max: 3 g/d)	Extended-release form available. Lactic acidosis may be a complication.
MEGLITINIDES		
nateglinide (Starlix)	PO 60–120 mg tid	Similar to second-generation sulfonylureas. Use cautiously in patients with hepatic or renal impairment.
repaglinide (Prandin)	PO 0.5–4.0 mg bid–qid	Glitazone type. Use cautiously in patients with hepatic or renal impairment.
SULFONYLUREAS, FIRST GENERATION		
acetohexamide (Dimelor, Dymelor)	PO 250 mg/day (max: 1500 mg/d)	Potential for hypersensitivity reaction.
chlorpropamide (Diabinese, Novopropamide)	PO 100–250 mg/day (max: 750 mg/d)	Known sensitivity to sulfonylureas and to sulfonamides.
tolazamide (Tolamide, Tolinase)	PO 100–500 mg 1–2 times/day (max: 1 g/d)	Known sensitivity to sulfonylureas and to sulfonamides.
tolbutamide (Orinase)	PO 250–1500 mg 1–2 times/day (max: 3 g/d)	Known sensitivity to sulfonylureas and to sulfonamides.
SULFONYLUREAS, SECOND GENERATION		
Glimepiride (Amaryl)	PO 1–4 mg/day (max: 8 mg/d)	Not recommended during pregnancy.
Pr glipizide (Glucotrol)	PO 2.5–20 mg 1–2 times/day (max: 40 mg/d)	Glucotrol XL is an extended-release form. Serious reactions may occur with overdose.
glyburide (DiaBeta, Micronase, Glynase)	PO 1.25–10 mg 1–2 times/day (max: 20 mg/d)	Glyburide combined with metformin in Glucovance. Serious reactions may occur with overdose.
THIAZOLIDINEDIONES		
pioglitazone (Actos)	PO 15–30 mg/day (max: 45 mg/d)	Glitazone type. Give without regard to meals.
rosiglitazone (Avandia)	PO 2–4 mg 1–2 times/day (max: 8 mg/d)	Glitazone type. Give without regard to meals.
COMBINATION DRUGS		
glipizide/metformin (Metaglip)	PO 2.5/250 mg/day (max: 10 mg glipizide and 2000 mg metformin/day)	Lactic acidosis is a complication in many cases if this medication is not taken properly.
glyburide/metformin (Glucovance)	PO 1.25 mg/250 mg 1–2 times/day (max: 20 mg glyburide and 2000 mg metformin/day)	Lactic acidosis is a complication in many cases if this medication is not taken properly.
rosiglitazone/metformin (Avandamet)	PO Variable dose (max: 8 mg rosiglitazone and 1000 mg metformin/day)	Lactic acidosis is a complication.

DRUG PROFILE: Oral Hypoglycemic: Pr *Glipizide (Glucotrol)*

Actions and Uses:

Glipizide belongs to the sulfonylurea group of hypoglycemics. It is a second-generation sulfonylurea that offers the advantages of higher potency, once-a-day dosing, fewer side effects, and fewer drug-drug interactions than the first-generation medications in this class. Glipizide stimulates the pancreas to secrete more insulin and also increases the sensitivity of insulin receptors in target tissues. Some degree of pancreatic function is required for glipizide to lower blood glucose. Maximum effects are achieved if the drug is taken 30 minutes prior to the primary meal of the day.

Adverse Effects and Interactions:

Hypoglycemia is less frequent with glipizide than with first-generation sulfonylureas. Patients should stay out of the sun because rashes and photosensitivity are possible. Some patients experience mild, GI-related effects such as nausea, vomiting, or loss of appetite. Glipizide and other sulfonylureas have the potential to interact with a number of drugs; thus, the patient should always consult with a healthcare practitioner before adding a new medication or herbal supplement. Ingestion of alcohol will result in distressing symptoms that include headache, flushing, nausea, and abdominal cramping.

Mechanism in Action: 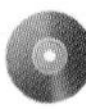

Glipizide, an oral hypoglycemic agent, lowers glucose blood levels by stimulating insulin release from pancreatic cells. This drug is used for the treatment of type 2 diabetes mellitus. Because it is a sulfonylurea drug, sensitivity reactions are possible.

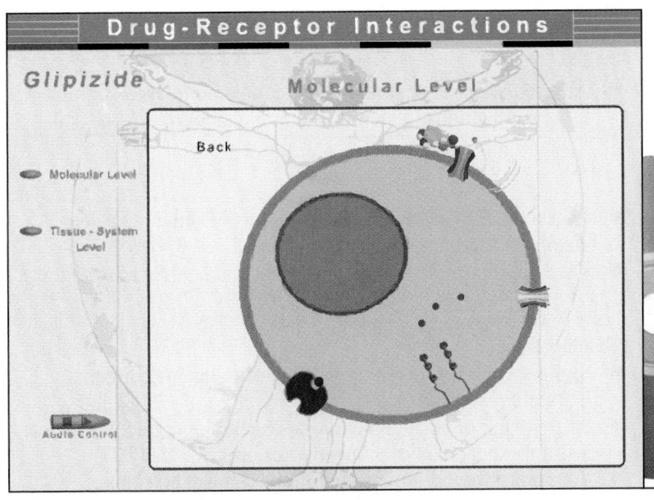

Use the student CD-ROM to see Mechanism in Action for Glipizide.

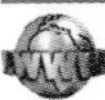 *See the Companion Website for a Nursing Process Focus specific to this drug.*

NURSING PROCESS FOCUS

Patients Receiving Oral Hypoglycemic Therapy

ASSESSMENT

Prior to administration:

- Obtain complete health history including allergies, drug history, and possible drug interactions
- Assess for pain location and level
- Assess knowledge of drug
- Assess ability to conduct blood glucose testing

POTENTIAL NURSING DIAGNOSES

- Risk for Injury (hypoglycemia), related to adverse effects of drug therapy
- Pain (abdominal), related to adverse effects of drug
- Deficient Knowledge, related to drug therapy
- Deficient Knowledge, related to blood glucose testing

PLANNING: Patient Goals and Expected Outcomes

The patient will:

- Describe signs and symptoms that should be reported immediately, including nausea, diarrhea, jaundice, rash, headache, anorexia, abdominal pain, tachycardia, seizures, and confusion
- Demonstrate an ability to accurately self-monitor blood glucose; maintain blood glucose within a normal range

continued...

NURSING PROCESS FOCUS

IMPLEMENTATION

Interventions and (Rationales)	Patient Education/Discharge Planning
■ Monitor blood glucose at least daily and monitor urinary ketones if blood glucose is over 300. (Ketones will spill into the urine at high blood glucose levels and provide an early sign of diabetic ketoacidosis.)	■ Teach patient how to monitor blood glucose and test urine for ketones, especially when ill.
■ Monitor for signs of lactic acidosis if patient is receiving a biguanide. (Mitochondrial oxidation of lactic acid is inhibited and lactic acidosis may result.)	■ Instruct patient to report signs of lactic acidosis such as hyperventilation, muscle pain, fatigue, and increased sleeping.
■ Review lab tests for any abnormalities in liver function. (These drugs are metabolized in the liver and may cause elevations in AST and LDH. Metformin decreases absorption of vitamin B_{12} and folic acid, which may result in deficiencies of these substances.)	■ Instruct patient to report the first sign of yellow skin, pale stools, or dark urine.
■ Obtain accurate history of alcohol use, especially if patient is receiving a sulfonylurea or biguanide. (These drugs may cause an Antabuse-like reaction.)	■ Advise patient to abstain from alcohol and to avoid liquid OTC medications, which may contain alcohol.
■ Monitor for signs and symptoms of illness or infection. (Illness may increase blood glucose levels.)	■ Instruct patient to report the first signs of fatigue, muscle weakness, and nausea. ■ Discuss importance of adequate rest and healthy routines.
■ Monitor blood glucose frequently, especially at the beginning of therapy and in elderly patients. ■ Monitor patients carefully who also take a beta blocker, because early signs of hypoglycemia may not be apparent.	Teach patient: ■ Signs and symptoms of hypoglycemia, such as hunger, irritability, sweating ■ At first sign of hypoglycemia, to check blood glucose and eat a simple sugar; if symptoms do not improve, call 911 ■ To monitor blood glucose before breakfast and supper ■ Not to skip meals and to follow a diet specified by the healthcare provider
■ Monitor weight, weighing at the same time of day each time. (Changes in weight will impact the amount of drug needed to control blood glucose.)	■ Instruct patient to weigh each week, at the same time of day, and report any significant loss or gain.
■ Monitor vital signs. (Increased pulse and blood pressure are early signs of hypoglycemia.)	■ Teach patient how to take accurate blood pressure, temperature, and pulse.
■ Monitor skin for rashes and itching. (These are signs of an allergic reaction to the drug.)	■ Advise patient of the importance of immediately reporting skin rashes and itching that is unaccounted for by dry skin.
■ Monitor activity level. (Dose may require adjustment with change in physical activity.)	■ Advise patient to increase activity level which will help lower blood glucose. ■ Advise patient to closely monitor blood glucose when involved in vigorous physical activity.

EVALUATION OF OUTCOME CRITERIA

Evaluate the effectiveness of drug therapy by confirming that patient goals and expected outcomes have been met (see "Planning").

See Table 29.3 for a list of drugs to which these nursing actions apply.

THYROID DISORDERS

29.7 The thyroid gland controls the basal metabolic rate and affects every cell in the body.

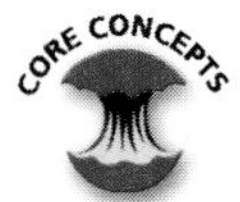

The thyroid gland lies in the neck, just below the larynx and in front of the trachea. **Follicular cells** in the gland secrete thyroid hormone, which is actually a combination of two different hormones: thyroxine (tetraiodothyronine or T_4) and triiodothyronine (T_3). Iodine is essential for the synthesis of these hormones and is provided through the dietary intake of common iodized salt. **Parafollicular cells** in the thyroid gland secrete calcitonin, a hormone that is involved with calcium homeostasis (Chapter 31).

Thyroid function is regulated through multiple levels of hormonal control. Thyroid-releasing hormone (TRH) from the hypothalamus stimulates the pituitary gland to secrete thyroid-stimulating hormone (TSH). TSH then stimulates the thyroid gland to release thyroid hormone. After thyroid hormone has reached a certain level in the blood, it operates in a negative feedback loop to shut off secretion of TRH and TSH. The negative feedback mechanism for the thyroid gland is shown in Figure 29.4 ■.

Thyroid hormone affects nearly every cell in the body by regulating *basal metabolic rate,* the baseline speed by which cells perform their functions. By increasing cellular metabolism, thyroid hormone increases body temperature. Thyroid hormone is critical to the growth of the nervous system. Deficiency during infancy may result in a combination of dwarfism and severe mental retardation known as **cretinism.**

29.8 Thyroid disorders may be treated by administering thyroid hormone or by decreasing the activity of the thyroid gland.

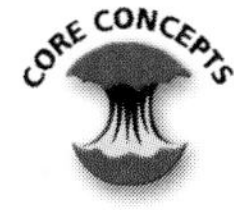

Thyroid disorders are quite common and drug therapy is often indicated. The correct dose of thyroid or antithyroid drug is highly individualized and may require periodic adjustment.

Hypothyroidism is a common disease caused by insufficient secretion of either TSH or thyroid hormone. Symptoms of hypothyroidism in adults, also known as **myxedema,** include slowed body metabolism, slurred speech, bradycardia, weight gain, low body temperature, and

Fast Facts Thyroid Disorders

- Hypothyroidism is 10 times more common in women than men; hyperthyroidism is 5–10 times more common in women.
- The two most common thyroid disorders, Graves' disease and Hashimoto's thyroiditis, are autoimmune diseases and may run in families.
- One of every 4,000 babies is born without a working thyroid gland.
- About 15,000 new cases of thyroid cancer are diagnosed each year.
- One of every five women older than age 75 has Hashimoto's thyroiditis.
- Postpartum thyroiditis occurs in 5–9% of women after giving birth and may recur in future pregnancies.
- Both hyperthyroidism and hypothyroidism can affect a woman's ability to become pregnant; both also can cause miscarriages.

DRUG PROFILE: Thyroid Agent: Pr *Levothyroxine (Synthroid)*

Actions and Uses:

Levothyroxine is a synthetic form of thyroxine (T_4) used for replacement therapy in patients with low thyroid function. Actions are those of thyroid hormone and include loss of weight, improved tolerance to environmental temperature, increased activity, and increased pulse rate. Blood levels of thyroid hormone are monitored carefully until the patient's symptoms stabilize. To achieve the proper level of thyroid function, doses may require periodic adjustments for several months or longer.

Adverse Effects and Interactions:

The difference between a therapeutic dose of levothyroxine and one that produces adverse effects is quite narrow. Adverse effects of levothyroxine resemble symptoms of hyperthyroidism and include tachycardia, anxiety, insomnia, weight loss, and heat intolerance. Menstrual irregularities may occur in women. Long-term use of levothyroxine has been associated with osteoporosis in women.

Levothyroxine interacts with many other drugs; for example, cholestyramine and colestipol decrease the absorption of levothyroxine. Using it with epinephrine and norepinephrine increases the risk of cardiac insufficiency. Oral anticoagulants may increase hypoprothrombinemia.

Herbal supplements such as lemon balm should be used cautiously. Lemon balm may interfere with thyroid hormone function.

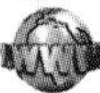
See the Companion Website for a Nursing Process Focus specific to this drug.

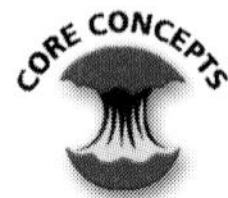

29.9 Glucocorticoids are released during periods of stress and influence carbohydrate, lipid, and protein metabolism in most cells.

The adrenal glands lie on top of each kidney. Structurally the adrenal glands are made up of two general regions—the cortex and the medulla. The outer cortex releases three important classes of hormones, called *mineralocorticoids*, *glucocorticoids*, and *androgens*. Collectively, these hormones are referred to as *corticosteroids* or *adrenocortical hormones*.

The **mineralocorticoid** aldosterone is responsible for increasing the renal absorption of sodium in exchange for potassium. Discussion of aldosterone is more relevant to the subject of diuretics because drugs or conditions may disrupt aldosterone release and alter the levels of fluids and electrolytes and important minerals in the bloodstream (see Chapter 28). Aldosterone

NURSING PROCESS FOCUS

Patients Receiving Thyroid Hormone Replacement

ASSESSMENT

Prior to administration:

- Obtain complete health history including allergies, drug history, and possible drug interactions
- Obtain complete physical examination
- Assess for the presence/history of symptoms of hypothyroidism
- Obtain EKG and laboratory studies including T_4, T_3, and serum TSH levels

POTENTIAL NURSING DIAGNOSES

- Activity Intolerance, related to disease process
- Fatigue, related to impaired metabolic status
- Deficient Knowledge, related to drug therapy
- Infective Health Maintenance, related to side effects of drug

continued...

NURSING PROCESS FOCUS

PLANNING: Patient Goals and Expected Outcomes

The patient will:

- Exhibit normal thyroid hormone levels
- Report a decrease in hypothyroid symptoms
- Experience no significant adverse effects from drug therapy
- Demonstrate an understanding of hypothyroidism and the need for life-long therapy

IMPLEMENTATION

Interventions and (Rationales)	Patient Education/Discharge Planning
■ Monitor vital signs. (Changes in metabolic rate will be manifested as changes in blood pressure, pulse, and body temperature.)	■ Instruct patient to report dizziness, palpitations, and intolerance to temperature changes.
■ Monitor for decreasing symptoms related to hypothyroidism such as fatigue, constipation, cold intolerance, lethargy, depression, and menstrual irregularities. (Decreasing symptoms will determine that drug is achieving therapeutic effect.)	■ Instruct patient about the signs of hyperthyroidism and to report symptoms.
■ Monitor for symptoms related to hyperthyroidism such as nervousness, insomnia, tachycardia, dysrhythmias, heat intolerance, chest pain, and diarrhea. (Symptoms of hyperthyroidism indicate the drug is at a toxic level.)	■ Instruct patient about the signs of hyperthyroidism and to report symptoms.
■ Monitor T_3, T_4, and TSH levels. (This helps to determine the effectiveness of pharmacotherapy.)	■ Instruct patient about the importance of ongoing monitoring of thyroid hormone levels and to keep all laboratory appointments.
■ Monitor blood glucose levels, especially in individuals with diabetes mellitus. (Thyroid hormones increase metabolic rate and may alter glucose utilization.)	■ Instruct the diabetic patient to monitor blood glucose levels and adjust insulin doses as directed by the healthcare provider.
■ Provide supportive nursing care to cope with symptoms of hypothyroidism such as constipation, cold intolerance, and fatigue until drug has achieved therapeutic effect.	Instruct patient to: ■ Increase fluid and fiber intake, as well as activity, to reduce constipation ■ Wear additional clothing and maintain a comfortable room environment for cold intolerance ■ Plan activities and include rest periods to avoid fatigue
■ Monitor weight at least weekly. (Weight loss is expected due to increased metabolic rate. Weight changes help to determine the effectiveness of drug therapy.)	■ Instruct patient to weigh weekly and to report significant changes.
■ Monitor patient for signs of decreased compliance with therapeutic regimen.	■ Instruct patient of the importance of life-long therapy, about the disease, and the importance of follow-up care.

EVALUATION OF OUTCOME CRITERIA

Evaluate the effectiveness of drug therapy by confirming that patient goals and expected outcomes have been met (see "Planning").

See Table 29.4 for a list of drugs to which these nursing actions apply.

DRUG PROFILE: Antithyroid Agent: 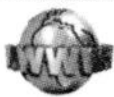 *Propylthiouracil (Propacil)*

Actions and Uses:

Propylthiouracil is administered to clients with hyperthyroidism, sometimes prior to surgery. It acts by interfering with the synthesis of T_3 and T_4. Because it does not affect thyroid hormone that has already been secreted, its action may be delayed from several days to as long as 6 to 12 weeks. Effects include a return to normal thyroid function: weight gain, reduction in anxiety, less insomnia, and slower pulse rate.

Adverse Effects and Interactions:

Overtreatment with propylthiouracil produces symptoms of hypothyroidism. In addition, a small percentage of clients display blood changes such as decreased platelet and white blood cell counts. Periodic laboratory blood counts and thyroid hormone values are necessary to establish the proper dosage.

Antithyroid medications interact with many other drugs. For example, propylthiouracil can reverse the effectiveness of drugs such as aminophylline, anticoagulants, and cardiac glycosides.

See the Companion Website for a Nursing Process Focus specific to this drug.

release is also affected by **adrenocorticotropic hormone (ACTH),** although the main action of this hormone is the direct release of the important glucocorticoid hormone cortisol.

gluco = *sweet/sugar*
corti = *cortex*
oid = *resemble*

Cortisol is one of about 30 **glucocorticoids** secreted from the outer portion, or cortex, of the adrenal gland. Glucocorticoids affect the metabolism of nearly every cell in the body. During long-term stress, these hormones mobilize the formation of glucose and increase the breakdown and use of proteins and lipids. They have a potent anti-inflammatory effect that was discussed in Chapters 21 and 25. They also serve to promote homeostasis of the cardiovascular, nervous, and musculoskeletal systems.

Control of glucocorticoid levels begins with corticotropin-releasing factor (CRF), secreted by the hypothalamus. CRF travels to the pituitary, where it causes the release of adrenocorticotropic hormone (ACTH). ACTH travels through the blood and reaches the adrenal cortex, causing it to release cortisol and other corticosteroids. When the level of cortisol in the blood rises, it provides negative feedback to the hypothalamus and pituitary to shut off further release of glucocorticoids from the adrenal gland. This negative feedback mechanism is shown in Figure 29.5 ■.

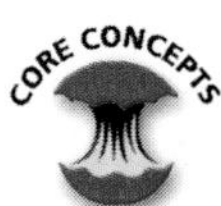

29.10 Glucocorticoids are prescribed for adrenocortical insufficiency and a wide variety of other conditions.

Lack of adequate corticosteroid production, known as *adrenocortical insufficiency*, may be caused by hyposecretion by the adrenal cortex or by inadequate secretion of ACTH from the pituitary. Symptoms include hypoglycemia, fatigue, hypotension, and GI disturbances such as anorexia, vomiting, and diarrhea. Primary adrenocortical insufficiency, known as **Addison's disease,** is quite rare and includes a deficiency of both glucocorticoids and mineralocorticoids.

Secondary adrenocortical insufficiency is relatively common and may result from long-term therapy with glucocorticoids. When glucocorticoids are taken as medications for long periods, the pituitary receives a message through the negative feedback mechanism to stop secreting ACTH. Without stimulation from ACTH, the adrenal cortex shrinks in size and stops secreting endogenous glucocorticoids, a condition known as adrenal **atrophy.** If a patient abruptly discontinues the glucocorticoid medication, the shrunken adrenal glands will not be able to secrete enough glucocorticoids, and symptoms of adrenocortical insufficiency will appear.

a = *without*
trophy = *nourishment*

The goal of replacement therapy is to achieve the same physiological level of glucocorticoids in the blood that would be present if the adrenal glands were functioning properly. Patients requiring replacement therapy may need to take glucocorticoids their entire lives.

Many glucocorticoid preparations are available via the topical, oral, IM, IV, and other routes to treat a variety of disorders. The role of corticosteroids in the treatment of inflammation and allergic rhinitis was presented in Chapters 21 and 25, respectively. Following is a list of the various disorders that may be treated with corticosteroids:

FIGURE 29.5

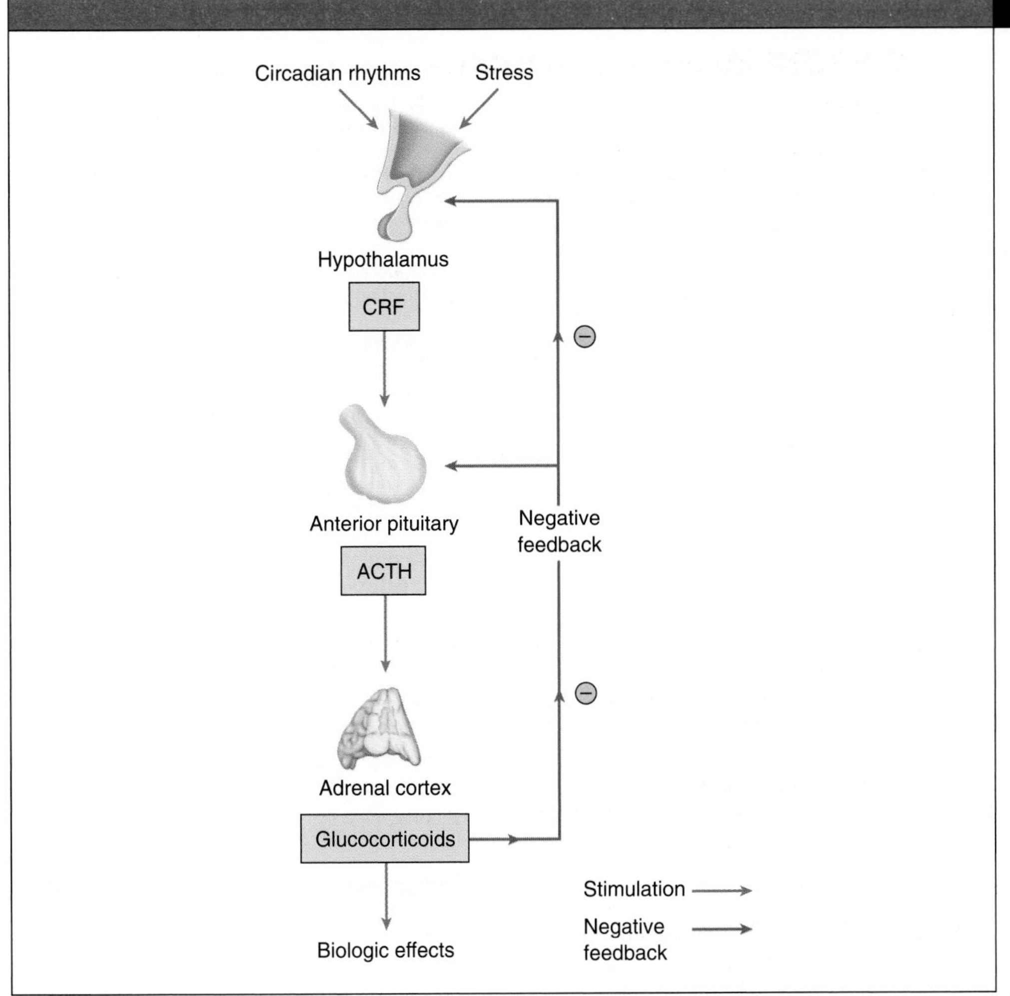

Feedback control of the adrenal cortex

- Allergies
- Asthma
- Seasonal rhinitis
- Skin disorders such as contact dermatitis and rashes
- Neoplastic disease such as Hodgkin's disease, leukemias, and lymphomas
- Shock
- Rheumatic disorders such as rheumatoid arthritis, ankylosing spondylitis, and bursitis
- Post-transplant surgery to suppress the immune system
- Chronic inflammatory bowel disease such as ulcerative colitis and Crohn's disease
- Adrenal insufficiency
- Hepatic, neurological, and renal disorders characterized by edema

Significant adverse effects can occur during long-term therapy with corticosteroids. An array of signs and symptoms known as **Cushing's syndrome** includes adrenal atrophy, osteoporosis, increased risk of infections, delayed wound healing, peptic ulcers, and a redistribution of fat around the shoulders and neck. Mood and personality changes may occur, with the patient becoming psychologically dependent on the therapeutic effects of the drug. Some of the glucocorticoids, such as hydrocortisone, also have mineralocorticoid activity and thus can cause retention of sodium and water. Alternate-day dosing, whereby the drug is administered every other day, is sometimes used to limit adrenal atrophy. Patients taking inhaled or topical corticosteroids, or who receive the drugs for 2 weeks or less, exhibit few adverse effects. Some of the glucocorticoids used in replacement therapy are shown in Table 29.5.

TABLE 29.5 Selected Glucocorticoids

DRUG	ROUTE AND ADULT DOSE	REMARKS
betamethasone (Celestone, others)	PO 0.6–7.2 mg/day	Long-acting; IV, topical, and IM forms available; has little mineralocorticoid activity
cortisone acetate (Cortistan, Cortone)	PO 20–300 mg/day	Short-acting; IM form available; also has mineralocorticoid activity
dexamethasone (Decadron, Dexasone, Hexadrol, Maxidex)	PO 0.25–4 mg bid–qid	Long-acting; IV, ophthalmic, topical, intranasal, inhalation, and IM forms available; has little mineralocorticoid activity
fludrocortisone (Florinef)	PO 0.1–0.2 mg/day	Long-acting; also has strong mineralocorticoid activity
Pr hydrocortisone (Cortef, Hydrocortone,Solu-cortef, others)	PO 2–80 mg tid–qid	Short-acting; IV, topical, and IM forms available; also has mineralocorticoid activity
methylprednisolone (Solu-medrol, Medrol)	PO 2–60 mg 1–4 times/day	Intermediate-acting; IV and IM forms available; has little mineralocorticoid activity
prednisolone (Delta-Cortef)	PO 5–60 mg 1–4 times/day	Intermediate-acting; IV and IM forms available; has little mineralocorticoid activity
prednisone (Deltasone, Meticorten, Orasone, Panasol)	PO 5–60 mg 1–4 times/day	Intermediate-acting; has little mineralocorticoid activity
triamcinolone (Aristocort, Atolone, Kenacort, Kenalog-E)	PO 4–48 mg 1–4 times/day	Intermediate-acting; IV, intra-articular, subcutaneous, topical, inhalation, and IM forms available; has little mineralocorticoid activity

DRUG PROFILE: Systemic Glucocorticoid: Pr *Hydrocortisone (Cortef, Hydrocortone, Solu-cortef, others)*

Actions and Uses:

Structurally identical to the natural hormone cortisol, hydrocortisone is a synthetic corticosteroid that is the drug of choice for treating adrenocortical insufficiency. When used for replacement therapy, it is given at physiological doses. Once proper dosing is achieved, its therapeutic effects should mimic those of natural corticosteroids. Hydrocortisone is also available for the treatment of inflammation, allergic disorders, and many other conditions. Intra-articular injections may be given to decrease severe inflammation in affected joints.

Adverse Effects and Interactions:

When used at physiological doses for replacement therapy, adverse effects of hydrocortisone should not be evident. The patient and the healthcare professional must be vigilant, however, in observing for signs of Cushing's syndrome, which can develop with high doses. If taken for longer than 2 weeks, hydrocortisone should be discontinued gradually.

Hydrocortisone interacts with many drugs. For example, barbiturates, phenytoin, and rifampin may increase liver metabolism, thus decreasing hydrocortisone levels. Estrogens increase the effects of hydrocortisone. NSAIDs increase the risk of ulcers. Cholestyramine and colestipol decrease hydrocortisone absorption. Diuretics and amphotericin B increase hypokalemia. Anticholinesterase agents may produce severe weakness. Hydrocortisone may cause a decrease in immune response to vaccines and toxoids.

Herbal supplements, such as aloe and buckthorn (a laxative), may cause potassium deficiency.

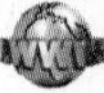
See the Companion Website for a Nursing Process Focus specific to this drug.

Concept Review 29.3

- Why does administration of glucocorticoids for extended periods result in adrenal atrophy?

NURSING PROCESS FOCUS

Patients Receiving Systemic Glucocorticoid Therapy

ASSESSMENT

Prior to administration:
- Obtain complete health history including allergies, drug history, and possible drug interactions
- Obtain complete physical examination, focusing on presenting symptoms
- Determine the reason the medication is being administered
- Obtain laboratory studies (long-term therapy) including serum sodium and potassium levels, hematocrit and hemoglobin levels, blood glucose level, and BUN

POTENTIAL NURSING DIAGNOSES

- Risk for Infection, related to immunosuppression
- Risk for Injury, related to side effects of drug therapy
- Deficient Knowledge, related to drug therapy

PLANNING: Patient Goals and Expected Outcomes

The patient will:
- Exhibit a decrease in the symptoms for which the drug is being given
- Exhibit no symptoms of infection
- Demonstrate an understanding of the drug's action, drug administration, and side effects

IMPLEMENTATION

Interventions and (Rationales)	Patient Education/Discharge Planning
■ Monitor vital signs. (Blood pressure may increase because of increased blood volume and potential vasoconstriction effect.)	■ Instruct patient to report dizziness, palpitations, or headaches.
■ Monitor for infection. Protect patient from potential infections. (Glucocorticoids increase susceptibility to infections by suppressing the immune response.)	Instruct patient to: ■ Avoid people with infection ■ Report fever, cough, sore throat, joint pain, increased weakness, and malaise ■ Consult with the healthcare provider before taking any immunizations
■ Monitor patient's compliance with drug regimen. (Sudden discontinuation of these agents can precipitate an adrenal crisis.)	Instruct patient: ■ To never suddenly stop taking the medication ■ In proper use of self-administering tapering dose pack ■ To take oral medications with food
■ Monitor for symptoms of Cushing's syndrome such as moon face, "buffalo hump" contour of shoulders, weight gain, muscle wasting, and increased deposits of fat in the trunk. (Symptoms may indicate excessive use of glucocorticoids.)	Instruct patient: ■ To weigh self daily ■ That initial weight gain is expected; provide the patient with weight gain parameters that warrant reporting ■ That there are multiple side effects to therapy and that changes in health status should be reported
■ Monitor blood glucose levels. (Glucocorticoids cause an increase in gluconeogenesis and reduce glucose utilization.)	Instruct patient to: ■ Report symptoms of hyperglycemia such as excessive thirst, copious urination, and insatiable appetite ■ Adjust insulin dose based on blood glucose level as directed by the healthcare provider

continued...

(continued from page 565)

NURSING PROCESS FOCUS

Interventions and (Rationales)	Patient Education/Discharge Planning
■ Monitor skin and mucous membranes for lacerations, abrasions, or break in integrity. (Glucocorticoids impair wound healing.)	Instruct patient to: ■ Examine skin daily for cuts and scrapes and to cover any injuries with sterile bandage ■ Watch for symptoms of skin infection such as redness, swelling, and drainage ■ Notify the healthcare provider of any nonhealing wound or symptoms of infection
■ Monitor gastrointestinal status for peptic ulcer development. (Glucocorticoids decrease gastric mucous production and predispose patient to peptic ulcers.)	■ Instruct patient to report GI side effects such as heartburn, abdominal pain, or tarry stools.
■ Monitor serum electrolytes. (Glucocorticoids cause hypernatremia and hypokalemia.)	Instruct patient to: ■ Consume a diet high in protein, calcium, and potassium but low in fat and concentrated simple carbohydrates ■ Keep all laboratory appointments
■ Monitor changes in musculoskeletal system. (Glucocorticoids decrease bone density and strength and cause muscle atrophy and weakness.)	Instruct patient: ■ To participate in exercise or physical activity, to help maintain bone and muscle strength ■ The drug may cause weakness in bones and muscles; avoid strenuous activity that may cause injury
■ Monitor emotional stability. (Glucocorticoids may produce mood and behavior changes such as depression or feeling of invulnerability.)	■ Instruct patient that mood changes may be expected and to report mental status changes to the healthcare provider.

EVALUATION OF OUTCOME CRITERIA

Evaluate the effectiveness of drug therapy by confirming that patient goals and expected outcomes have been met (see "Planning").

See Table 29.5 for a list of drugs to which these nursing actions apply.

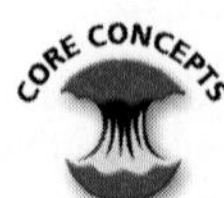

29.11 Of the many pituitary and hypothalamic hormones, only a few have clinical applications as drugs.

Of the 15 different hormones secreted by the pituitary and hypothalamus, only a few are used for drug therapy. This is because some of these hormones can only be obtained from natural sources rather than from the pituitary or hypothalamus, and it is usually easier to give drugs affecting the target organs. Two pituitary hormones, prolactin and oxytocin, affect the reproductive system and will be discussed in Chapter 30. Of those remaining, growth hormone and antidiuretic hormone have some clinical use.

Growth hormone, known as **somatotropin,** stimulates the growth of nearly every cell in the body. Deficiency of this hormone in children results in **dwarfism.** Unlike a deficiency of thyroid hormone, however, growth hormone deficiency usually does not cause mental impairment. Two preparations of human growth hormone, somatrem (Protropin) and somatropin (Humatrope and others), are available as replacement therapy in children. If therapy is begun early in life, as much as 6 inches of growth may be achieved.

As its name implies, antidiuretic hormone (ADH) conserves water in the body. ADH is secreted from the posterior pituitary gland and acts on the collecting ducts in the kidney to increase water reabsorption. A deficiency of ADH, known as **diabetes insipidus,** causes the client to lose large volumes of water. ADH is also called **vasopressin** because it has the capability to raise blood pressure when secreted in large amounts. Three preparations of ADH are available for the treatment of diabetes insipidus: vasopressin (Pitressin), desmopressin (DDAVP, Stimate), and lypressin (Diapid). Desmopressin is occasionally used by the intranasal route to treat enuresis (bedwetting).

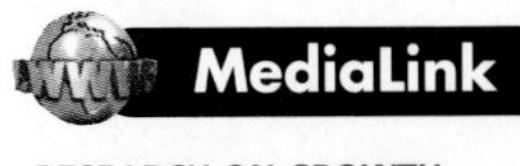

RESEARCH ON GROWTH DISORDERS

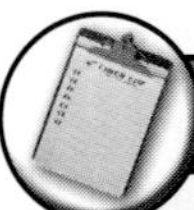

PATIENTS NEED TO KNOW

Patients treated for endocrine disorders need to know the following:

Regarding Corticosteroids

1. When taking oral corticosteroids for more than 2 weeks, do not miss doses or discontinue the drug without consulting a healthcare provider.
2. See a physician if any infections, cuts, or injuries appear to be healing abnormally slowly while on corticosteroids.
3. If taking hydrocortisone for replacement therapy, take the medication between 6:00 A.M. and 9:00 A.M. because this is the time when natural corticosteroids are released.

Regarding Diabetic Medications

4. When taking insulin or oral hypoglycemics, report any signs of hypoglycemia such as weakness, sweating, dizziness, tremor, anxiety, or tachycardia to a healthcare provider immediately. Mild symptoms may be treated with small amounts of sugar in the form of candy or fruit juice.
5. Always take insulin and oral hypoglycemics at the same time each day.
6. When self-monitoring blood glucose, recall that normal values are 80 to 120 mg/dl before meals and 100 to 140 mg/dl before bedtime.
7. Store unopened vials of insulin in the refrigerator. Do not use after the expiration date.
8. If taking insulin or oral hypoglycemics, read the directions to all medications very carefully because many drug-drug interactions are possible. Medications such as corticosteroids, thiazide diuretics, and sympathomimetics can raise blood glucose levels and inhibit the effects of insulin.
9. If diabetes in present, check with a healthcare provider before beginning a vigorous exercise program. Often, insulin doses should be reduced or extra food should be ingested just prior to intense exercise.
10. If self-injecting insulin is used, follow all instructions provided by the healthcare practitioner carefully to avoid injury or infection.

Regarding Thyroid Medications

11. As pulse rate is a good indicator of the effectiveness of thyroid medications, take it regularly. If the pulse rate consistently exceeds 100 or any other significant change is noted, contact the healthcare provider.
12. As finding the correct dosage of thyroid hormone often takes several months, do not change the prescribed dose without being advised to do so by a healthcare practitioner. ■

CHAPTER REVIEW

CORE CONCEPTS SUMMARY

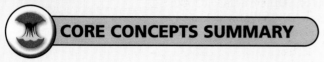

29.1 The endocrine system maintains homeostasis by using hormones as chemical messengers.

Hormones are secreted by endocrine glands in response to changes in the internal environment. The hormones act on their target cells to return the body to homeostasis. Negative feedback prevents the body from overresponding to internal changes.

29.2 Hormones are used as replacement therapy, as antineoplastics, and for their natural therapeutic effects.

Hormones are often given as replacement therapy to clients who are not able to secrete sufficient quantities of endogenous hormones. In high doses, several hormones may be used as antineoplastics. Hormones may also be used therapeutically to take advantage of their natural physiological effects.

29.3 The hypothalamus and the pituitary gland secrete hormones that control other endocrine organs.

The hypothalamus secretes releasing hormones that signal the anterior pituitary gland to release its hormones. Pituitary hormones travel throughout the body to affect many other organs.

29.4 Insulin and glucagon are secreted by the pancreas.

The pancreas secretes insulin after a meal, when blood glucose levels are high. Insulin permits glucose to leave the blood and enter cells. Glucagon has effects opposite to those of insulin, causing glucose to leave tissues and enter the blood.

29.5 Type 1 diabetes is treated by dietary restrictions and insulin injections.

Type 1 diabetes is diagnosed in late childhood and is caused by a lack of insulin secretion by the pancreas. Parenteral insulin is provided and must be carefully timed to coincide with meals. Taking too much insulin or skipping meals may result in acute hypoglycemia. Untreated diabetes leads to serious long-term consequences.

29.6 Type 2 diabetes is controlled through lifestyle changes and oral hypoglycemic agents.

Type 2 diabetes is more common than type 1, occurs in older patients, and is primarily due to a lack of sensitivity of insulin receptors. Drug therapy starts with oral hypoglycemics and may proceed to insulin injections if the disease is not controlled appropriately.

29.7 The thyroid gland controls the basal metabolic rate and affects every cell in the body.

The thyroid gland secretes thyroid hormone, which is essential for the growth and metabolism of all cells. Thyroid hormone is a combination of two different hormones, thyroxine and triiodothyronine, both of which require iodine for their synthesis.

29.8 Thyroid disorders may be treated by administering thyroid hormone or by decreasing the activity of the thyroid gland.

Hypothyroidism produces symptoms such as slowed body metabolism, slurred speech, bradycardia, weight gain, low body temperature, and intolerance to cold environments. Administration of thyroid hormone reverses these symptoms. Hyperthyroid clients exhibit the opposite symptoms. Hyperthyroidism may be treated with drugs that kill or inactivate thyroid cells.

29.9 Glucocorticoids are released during periods of stress and influence carbohydrate, lipid, and protein metabolism in most cells.

The adrenal cortex secretes glucocorticoids in response to stimulation by ACTH from the pituitary. Glucocorticoids affect the metabolism of nearly every cell in the body and have a potent anti-inflammatory effect.

29.10 Glucocorticoids are prescribed for adrenocortical insufficiency and a wide variety of other conditions.

Glucocorticoids are given to clients whose adrenal glands are unable to produce adequate amounts of these hormones, and for a wide variety of other conditions. When used at high doses, oral therapy is often limited to 2 weeks because of the potential for producing Cushing's syndrome and adrenal atrophy.

29.11 Of the many pituitary and hypothalamic hormones, only a few have clinical applications as drugs.

Growth hormone, or somatotropin, is used to increase the height in children with growth hormone deficiencies. ADH, or vasopressin, increases water reabsorption in the kidney and is used to treat diabetes insipidus.

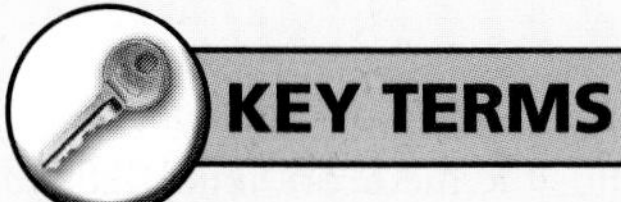

KEY TERMS

Addison's disease (ADD-iss-uns): hyposecretion of glucocorticoids and aldosterone by the adrenal cortex / ***page 562***

adrenocorticotropic hormone (ACTH) (uh-dreen-oh-kor-tik-o-TRO-pik): hormone secreted by the pituitary that stimulates the release of glucocorticoids by the adrenal cortex / ***page 562***

atrophy (AT-troh-fee): shrinkage or wasting away of a tissue / ***page 562***

cretinism (KREE-ten-izm): dwarfism and mental retardation caused by lack of thyroid hormone during infancy / ***page 557***

Cushing's syndrome (KUSH-ings): condition caused by excessive corticosteroid secretion by the adrenal glands or by overdosage with corticosteroid medication / ***page 563***

diabetes insipidus (die-uh-BEE-tees in-SIP-uh-dus): excessive urination due to lack of secretion of antidiuretic hormone / ***page 567***

diabetes mellitus, type 1 (die-uh-BEE-tees MEL-uh-tiss): disease characterized by lack of secretion of insulin by the pancreas that usually begins in the early teens / ***page 549***

diabetes mellitus, type 2: disease characterized by insufficient secretion of insulin by the pancreas or by lack of sensitivity of insulin receptors that usually begins in middle age / ***page 553***

dwarfism: below normal height caused by a deficiency in thyroid hormone or growth hormone / ***page 566***

follicular cells (fo-LIK-yu-lur): cells in the thyroid gland that secrete thyroid hormone / ***page 557***

glucocorticoid (glu-ko-KORT-ik-oyd): type of hormone secreted by the outer portion of the adrenal gland that includes cortisol / ***page 562***

Graves' disease: syndrome caused by hypersecretion of thyroid hormone / ***page 559***

hormones: chemicals secreted by endocrine glands that act as chemical messengers to affect homeostasis / ***page 545***

hyperglycemia (hi-pur-gli-SEEM-ee-uh): abnormally high level of glucose in the blood / ***page 547***

hypoglycemia (hi-po-gli-SEEM-ee-uh): abnormally low level of glucose in the blood / ***page 547***

hypothalamus (hi-po-THAL-ih-mus): region of the brain that affects emotions and drives, and that secretes releasing factors that affect the pituitary gland / ***page 547***

islets of Langerhans (EYE-lits of LANG-gur-hans): clusters of cells in the pancreas responsible for the secretion of insulin and glucagon; also called the *pancreatic islets* / ***page 547***

ketoacids (KEY-to-ass-ids): waste products of fat metabolism that lower the pH of the blood / ***page 550***

mineralocorticoid (min-ur-al-oh-KORT-ik-oyd): hormone involved in the regulation of fluid and electrolytes by its effects in the kidney / ***page 560***

myxedema (mix-uh-DEEM-uh): condition caused by insufficient secretion of thyroid hormone / ***page 557***

parafollicular cells (par-uh-fo-LIK-u-lur): cells in the thyroid gland that secrete calcitonin / ***page 557***

pituitary gland (pit-TOO-it-air-ee): endocrine gland in the brain responsible for controlling many other endocrine glands / ***page 547***

releasing factors: hormones secreted by the hypothalamus that affect secretions in the pituitary gland / ***page 547***

somatotropin (so-mat-oh-TROH-pin): another name for growth hormone / ***page 566***

vasopressin (vaz-oh-PRESS-in): another name for antidiuretic hormone / ***page 567***

REVIEW QUESTIONS

The following questions are written in NCLEX-PN® style. Answer these questions to assess your knowledge of the chapter material, and go back and review any material that is not clear to you.

1. The patient is exhibiting hypoglycemia, fatigue, hypotension, anorexia, vomiting, and diarrhea. The nurse suspects:

1. Cushing's syndrome
2. Graves' disease
3. Adrenal insufficiency
4. Diabetes mellitus

2. Which of the following is not a symptom of diabetes?

1. Polyphagia
2. Polyuria
3. Polydipsia
4. Weight gain

3. The mechanism of action of oral hypoglycemic agents is to:

1. Release insulin into the bloodstream
2. Stimulate insulin release from the pancreas
3. Increase insulin production in the pancreas
4. Decrease amount of insulin produced by the pancreas

4. The patient has a history of hypothyroidism and has been on levothyroxine (Synthroid) 250 mcg/day. The nurse recognizes the medication is being effective when:

1. The patient sleeps more hours per day
2. The patient's weight increases
3. The patient's pulse rate increases
4. The patient states she feels tired

5. The patient has been on methylprednisolone (Medrol) for an exacerbation of asthma. Which of the following instructions to the patient is of the highest priority?

1. "This medication may cause weight gain."
2. "Do not stop taking this medication abruptly."
3. "This medication can cause sleeplessness."
4. "This medication may cause restlessness."

6. The patient should be instructed to take oral glucocorticoids when?

1. In the early morning hours
2. With lunch
3. With dinner
4. At bedtime

7. The diabetic patient has decided to start an exercise program. What effect does exercise have on the body?

1. It increases the need for insulin.
2. It decreases the need for insulin.
3. Insulin is not affected.
4. Oral hypoglycemics may be required.

8. The patient has been started on desmopressin (DDAVP). The nurse understands the medication is effective when?

1. The patient's urinary output increases.
2. The patient's blood pressure is within normal limits.
3. The patient's blood sugar level is between 80 and 120 mg/dl.
4. The patient's urinary output decreases.

9. Glipizide (Glucotrol) should be administered:

1. Subcutaneously only
2. After meals
3. At bedtime
4. Just before breakfast

10. Insulin glargine (Lantus) should be administered:

1. Before meals
2. After meals
3. At bedtime
4. Before and after meals

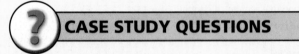

CASE STUDY QUESTIONS

For questions 1–5, please refer to the following case study, and choose the correct answer from choices 1–4.

Mr. Xonder is a 35-year-old firefighter who smokes and is somewhat overweight. Over the last 5 years, he has begun to develop slightly elevated blood pressure as determined by annual physical exams. He feels like he should lose weight and is concerned about his energy level. He has always felt fit despite the fact that he smokes, but recently, he has begun to feel sluggish and is wondering whether his physical condition is changing. He thinks to himself, "Maybe I'm just getting older." At his last visit to the doctor, lab results revealed fasting blood glucose levels above 126 mg/dl. His blood pressure was 150/90 mm Hg. Mr. Xonder has not been taking medications for any reported disorder.

1. The most likely reason for the slightly elevated blood pressure in this instance is:

1. Hypertension, a common condition associated with smokers
2. Vascular damage brought on by hypertension, a common problem with the onset of diabetes
3. High stress levels associated with the profession of firefighters
4. Hypertension, caused by the patient being overweight

2. Common signs of hyperglycemia are:

1. Pallor, weakness, and blurred vision
2. Dilated pupils and irregular pulse
3. Frequent urination, increased thirst, and flushed face
4. Loss of appetite and water retention

3. Noninsulin-dependent diabetes mellitus (NIDDM) or type 2 diabetes is a condition treated by a group of oral hypoglycemic agents that stimulate the pancreas to produce or release insulin. These agents are called:

1. Sulfonylureas
2. Biguanides
3. Alpha-glucosidase inhibitors
4. Thiazolidinediones

4. As a healthcare provider, which of the following words of advice would you give to Mr. Xonder when considering the adverse effects of oral hypoglycemic agents?

1. "Be sure to take your medication after the last meal of the day."
2. "Ingestion of alcohol will not hurt you, so go ahead . . . a few beers won't matter."
3. "You probably should avoid direct sunlight. Rashes and photosensitivity are possible."
4. "You are relatively safe if you start taking antihypertensive medication at the same time . . . don't worry."

5. Type 2 diabetes can be controlled by:

1. Lifestyle changes
2. Both hypoglycemic agents and insulin
3. a and b
4. a and hypoglycemic agents only

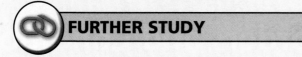

FURTHER STUDY

- High levels of ketoacids seen in diabetics change the pH of the blood, producing acidosis, as discussed in Chapter 28.
- Chapter 30 discusses reproductive hormones.
- Hormones used as antineoplastics are detailed in Chapter 24.
- Aldosterone release affects the balance of fluids, electrolytes, and minerals in the bloodstream, as discussed in Chapter 28.
- The anti-inflammatory effects of glucocorticoids are discussed in more depth in Chapters 21 and 25.
- Prolactin and oxytocin are presented in Chapter 30.
- Drugs that block the renin-angiotensin pathway also inhibit aldosterone secretion and are used to treat hypertension (Chapter 15) and heart failure (Chapter 16).

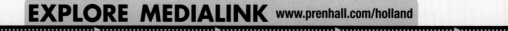

EXPLORE MEDIALINK www.prenhall.com/holland

Additional resources for this chapter can be found on the CD-ROM accompanying this textbook, and on the Companion Website. Click on Chapter 29 to select activities for this chapter.

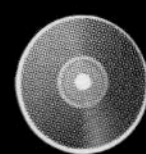

Mechanism in Action: Glipizide
Audio Glossary
Concept Review
NCLEX-PN® Review
Nursing in Action
Dosage Calculator

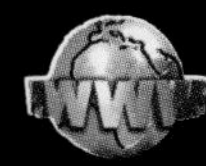

Endocrine Web
American Diabetes Association and Healthy Living
Research on Growth Disorders

CHAPTER

30 Drugs for Disorders and Conditions of the Reproductive System

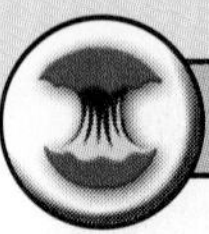

CORE CONCEPTS

30.1 Testosterone, estrogen, and progesterone are the primary hormones contributing to the growth, health, and maintenance of the reproductive system.

30.2 Low doses of estrogens and progestins are used for contraception.

30.3 Estrogens have been used for replacement therapy and in the treatment of prostate cancer.

30.4 Progestins are prescribed for dysfunctional uterine bleeding.

30.5 Oxytocin and tocolytics are drugs used to influence uterine contractions.

30.6 Androgens are used to treat hypogonadism or delayed puberty in men and breast cancer in women.

30.7 Erectile dysfunction is a common disorder that may be successfully treated with drug therapy.

30.8 In its early stages, benign prostatic hypertrophy may be treated successfully with drug therapy.

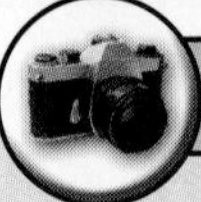

DRUG SNAPSHOT

The following drugs will be discussed in this chapter:

DRUG CLASSES	DRUG PROFILES
ORAL CONTRACEPTIVES	
Estrogen-progestin combinations	
Monophasic	Pr ethinyl estradiol with norethindrone (Ortho-Novum 1/35)
Biphasic	
Triphasic	
Progestin-only agents	
HORMONE REPLACEMENT THERAPY	
Estrogens and estrogen-progestin combinations	Pr conjugated estrogens (Premarin) and conjugated estrogens with medroxyprogesterone (Prempro)
DRUGS FOR DYSFUNCTIONAL UTERINE BLEEDING	
Progestins	Pr medroxyprogesterone (Prempro)
UTERINE STIMULANTS AND RELAXANTS	
	Pr oxytocin (Pitocin, Syntocinon)
DRUGS FOR MALE HYPOGONADISM	
Androgens	Pr testosterone base (Andro)
DRUGS FOR ERECTILE DYSFUNCTION	
	Pr sildenafil (Viagra)
DRUGS FOR BENIGN PROSTATIC HYPERTROPHY	
	Pr finasteride (Proscar)

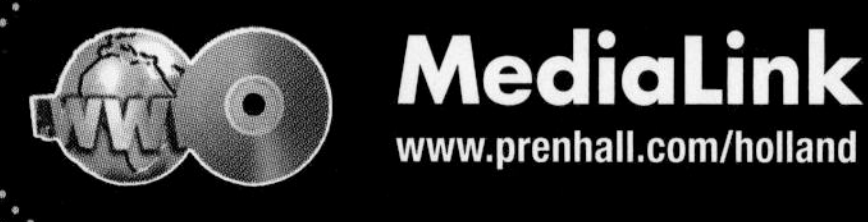

MediaLink
www.prenhall.com/holland

Interactive resources for this chapter can be found on the Companion Website. Click on Chapter 30 and "Begin" to select the activities for this chapter. For chapter-related animations, NCLEX-PN® style questions, and an audio glossary, access the accompanying CD-ROM in this book.

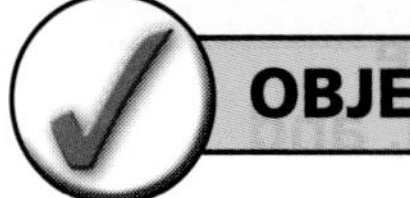

OBJECTIVES

After reading this chapter, the student should be able to:

1. Identify and describe the primary functions of the steroid sex hormones.
2. Explain the mechanisms by which estrogen and progestins prevent conception.
3. Describe the role of drug therapy in the treatment of menopausal and postmenopausal symptoms.
4. Identify the role of the steroid sex hormones in the chemotherapy of cancer.
5. Describe the uses of progestins in the therapy of dysfunctional uterine bleeding.
6. Compare and contrast oxytocin and tocolytics in antepartum and postpartum treatment.
7. Explain the role of androgens in the treatment of hypogonadism.
8. Describe the role of drug therapy in the treatment of erectile dysfunction and benign prostatic hypertrophy (BPH).
9. For each of the following drugs or drug classes, identify representative drugs, and explain the mechanisms of drug action, primary actions, and important adverse effects:
   - **a.** oral contraceptive preparations
   - **b.** estrogens
   - **c.** progestins
   - **d.** oxytocin
   - **e.** tocolytics
   - **f.** androgens
   - **g.** drugs for erectile dysfunction
   - **h.** drugs for BPH
10. Categorize drugs used in the treatment of reproductive disorders and conditions based on their classifications and mechanisms of action.

The male and female reproductive systems are regulated by a small number of hormones that are responsible for the growth and maintenance of the reproductive organs. These hormones can be supplemented with natural or synthetic hormones to achieve a variety of therapeutic goals, ranging from replacement therapy to prevention of pregnancy to milk production. This chapter examines drugs used to treat disorders and conditions of the reproductive system.

Fast Facts Reproductive Conditions and Disorders

- Erectile dysfunction affects 10 to 15 million Americans—about 1 in 4 men older than age 65.
- BPH affects 50% of men older than age 60, and 90% of men older than age 80.
- There is a wide range of ages when women reach menopause: 8 of 100 women will stop menstruating before age 40, and 5 of 100 will continue beyond age 60.
- About half the cases of dysfunctional uterine bleeding are diagnosed in women older than 45; however, 20% of cases occur in those younger than 20.
- Compared to just 10 years ago, oral contraceptives now contain 2 to 4 times less estrogen.
- The primary reason why a woman may become pregnant while on oral contraceptives is skipping a dose.
- A nonsmoking woman aged 25 to 29 has a 2 in 100,000 chance of dying from complications due to oral contraceptives. By comparison, the risk of a woman in this age group dying in an automobile accident is 74 in 100,000.
- Oral contraceptives have more benefits than simply contraception. It is estimated that each year they prevent the following:

  51,000 cases of pelvic inflammatory disease
  9,900 hospitalizations for ectopic pregnancy
  27,000 cases of iron-deficiency anemia
  20,000 hospitalizations for certain types of nonmalignant breast disease

---

Over the past 20 years, healthcare providers have commonly prescribed hormone replacement therapy (HRT) to treat unpleasant symptoms of menopause and related osteoporotic bone fractures. However, studies have raised questions regarding the safety of HRT for these conditions. Data suggests that patients may have an increased risk of coronary artery disease, stroke, and venous thromboembolism. Women are now encouraged to discuss alternatives with their healthcare provider, as discussed in Chapter 31. Undoubtedly, research will continue to provide valuable information on the long-term effects of HRT. Until then, the choice of HRT to treat menopausal symptoms will remain a highly individualized one, between the patient and her healthcare provider.

In addition to their use as oral contraceptives, estrogens are used to reduce unpleasant symptoms associated with menopause and to treat certain cancers. Higher doses are used for these conditions; thus, more side effects are observed.

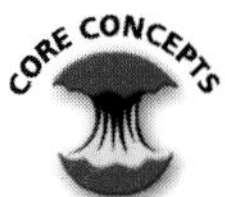

30.3 Estrogens have been used for replacement therapy and in the treatment of prostate cancer.

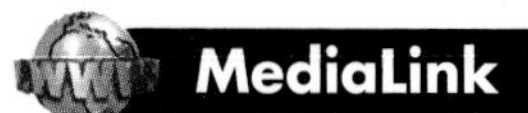

PSYCHOLOGICAL AND PHARMACOLOGICAL ASPECTS OF MENOPAUSE

When estrogen secretion becomes deficient, irregular or painful menstrual cycles may result, thus providing an indication for replacement drug therapy. In addition, surgical removal of the ovaries usually requires estrogen supplementation because the adrenal glands cannot supply sufficient quantities of estrogen. Some of the estrogen and estrogen-progesterone combinations used for replacement therapy are shown in Table 30.3.

High doses of estrogens have also been used to treat prostate and breast cancer. Prostate cancer is usually dependent on androgens for growth, and administration of estrogens will suppress androgen secretion. As an antineoplastic hormone, estrogen is rarely used alone: it is one of many agents used in combination for the chemotherapy of cancer, as discussed in Chapter 24.

TABLE 30.3 Selected Estrogens and Progestins Used for Hormone Replacement Therapy

DRUG	ROUTE AND ADULT DOSE	REMARKS
ESTROGENS		
estradiol (Estraderm, Estrace)	PO 1–2 mg/day	Available as vaginal cream and as a transdermal patch; also for breast and prostate cancer and to relieve postpartum breast engorgement
estradiol cypionate (depGynogen, Depogen)	IM 1–5 mg q3–4 weeks	Menopausal and postmenopausal symptoms
estradiol valerate (Delestrogen, Duragen-10, Valergen)	IM 10–20 mg q4 weeks	Also for breast cancer and to relieve postpartum breast engorgement
Pr estrogen, conjugated (Premarin)	PO 0.3–1.25 mg/day × 21 days each month	Also for postcoital contraception and breast cancer
estropipate (Ogen)	PO 0.75–6 mg/day × 21 days each month	Also for female hypogonadism and palliative treatment of prostate cancer; available as a vaginal cream
ethinyl estradiol (Estinyl, Feminone)	PO 0.02–0.05 mg/day × 21 days each month	Also for breast and prostate cancer and as a postcoital contraceptive
PROGESTINS		
Pr medroxyprogesterone (Provera, Cycrin)	PO 5–10 mg/day on days 1–12 of menstrual cycle	Also for endometrial and renal carcinoma; IM form available
norethindrone (Micronor, Nor-Q.D.)	PO 0.35 mg/day beginning on day 1 of menstrual cycle	Also for endometriosis
norethindrone acetate	PO 5 mg/day × 2 weeks; increase by 2.5 mg/day q2 weeks (max: 15 mg/day)	Also for endometriosis
progesterone micronized (Prometrium)	PO 400 mg at bedtime × 10 days	IM and rectal forms available; intrauterine insert available for contraception

DRUG PROFILE: Hormone Replacement Therapy, Estrogen, and Estrogen–Progestin Combination: Pr *Conjugated Estrogens (Premarin) and Conjugated Estrogens with Medroxyprogesterone (Prempro)*

Actions and Uses:

Premarin contains a mixture of different estrogens. It exerts several positive metabolic effects, including an increase in bone mass and a reduction in LDL cholesterol. It may also increase the risk of coronary artery disease and colon cancer. When used as postmenopausal replacement therapy, it is typically combined with a progestin, as in Prempro.

Adverse Effects and Interactions:

Adverse effects from Prempro or Premarin include nausea, fluid retention, breast tenderness, and weight gain. As with oral contraceptives, estrogens are contraindicated in women with a histroy of thromboembolic disease.

Estrogens, when used alone, have been associated with a higher risk of uterine cancer. Adding a progestin exerts a protective effect by lowering the risk of uterine cancer. Unfortunately, recent studies have suggested that while the progestin protects against uterine cancer, it may increase the risk of breast cancer following long-term use. The risks of adverse effects increase in women older than age 35. Conjugated estrogens are a category X drug and should not be taken during a known or suspected pregnancy.

Drug interactions include decreased effect of tamoxifen, enhanced corticosteroid effects, and decreased effects of anticoagulants, especially warfarin. The effects of estrogen may be decreased if taken with barbiturates or rifampin, and there is a possible increased effect of tricyclic antidepressants if taken with estrogens.

Use cautiously with herbal supplements. Red clover and black cohosh may interfere with estrogen therapy. Effects of estrogen may be enhanced if combined with ginseng.

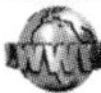

See the Companion Website for a Nursing Process Focus specific to this drug.

UTERINE ABNORMALITIES

Dysfunctional uterine bleeding is a condition in which hemorrhage occurs on a noncyclic basis or in abnormal amounts. It is the health problem most frequently reported by women and a common reason for **hysterectomy** or surgical removal of the uterus. Types of dysfunctional uterine bleeding include the following conditions:

- **Amenorrhea**—absence of menstruation
- **Oligomenorrhea**—infrequent menstruation
- **Menorrhea**—prolonged or excessive menstruation

hyster = *womb / uterus*
ectomy = *excision*

a = *lack of*
oligo = *scanty*
meno = *month*
rhea = *flow*

NURSING PROCESS FOCUS

Patients Receiving Hormone Replacement Therapy

ASSESSMENT	POTENTIAL NURSING DIAGNOSES
Prior to administration: ■ Obtain complete health history including personal or familial history of breast cancer, gallbladder disease, diabetes mellitus, and liver or kidney disease ■ Obtain drug history to determine possible drug interactions and allergies ■ Assess cardiovascular status including hypertension, history of MI, CVA, and thromboembolic disease ■ Determine if patient is pregnant or lactating	■ Excess Fluid Volume, related to edema secondary to side effect of drug ■ Ineffective Tissue Perfusion, related to development of thrombophlebitis, pulmonary, or cerebral embolism

continued...

corpus cavernosum (KORP-us kav-ver-NOH-sum): tissue in the penis that fills with blood during an erection / ***page 588***

dysfunctional uterine bleeding: hemorrhage that occurs at abnormal times or in abnormal quantity during the menstrual cycle / ***page 581***

endometrium (en-doh-MEE-tree-um): Inner lining of the uterus / ***page 574***

estrogen (ES-troh-jen): class of steroid sex hormones produced by the ovary / ***page 574***

follicles-timulating hormone (FSH): hormone secreted by the pituitary gland that regulates sperm or egg production / ***page 574***

hypogonadism (hy-poh-GO-nad-izm): below normal secretion of the steroid sex hormones / ***page 585***

hysterectomy (hiss-ter-EK-toh-mee): surgical removal of the uterus / ***page 581***

impotence (IM-poh-tense): inability to obtain or sustain an erection; also called erectile dysfunction / ***page 587***

leutinizing hormones (LH) (LEW-ten-iz-ing): hormone secreted by the pituitary gland that triggers ovulation in the female and stimulates sperm production in the male / ***page 574***

libido (lih-BEE-do): interest in sexual activity / ***page 587***

menopause (MEN-oh-paws): time when females stop secreting estrogen and menstrual cycles cease / ***page 578***

menorrhea (men-oh-REE-uh): prolonged or excessive menstruation / ***page 581***

oligomenorrhea (ol-ego-men-oh-REE-uh): infrequent menstruation / ***page 581***

ovulation (ov-you-LAY-shun): release of an egg by the ovary / ***page 574***

oxytocin (ox-ee-TOH-sin): hormone secreted by the pituitary gland that stimulates uterine contractions and milk ejection / ***page 584***

postpartum (post-PART-um): occurring after childbirth / ***page 585***

progesterone (pro-JESS-ter-own): hormone responsible for building up the uterine lining in the second half of the menstrual cycle and during pregnancy / ***page 574***

prolactin (pro-LAK-tin): hormone secreted by the pituitary gland that stimulates milk production in the mammary glands / ***page 584***

tocolytic (toh-koh-LIT-ik): drug used to inhibit uterine contractions / ***page 585***

virulization (veer-you-lih-ZAY-shun): appearance of masculine secondary sex characteristics / ***page 587***

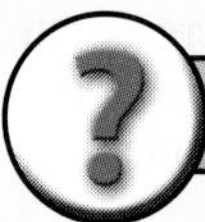

REVIEW QUESTIONS

The following questions are written in NCLEX-PN® style. Answer these questions to assess your knowledge of the chapter material, and go back and review any material that is not clear to you.

1. With which type of birth control does estrogen level remain constant throughout the cycle, although progestin level increases toward the end of the menstrual cycle?

1. Monophasic
2. Biphasic
3. Triphasic
4. Quadphasic

2. High doses of estrogen:

1. Increase androgen levels
2. Decrease androgen levels
3. Increase progestin levels
4. Decrease progestin levels

3. Which of the following patients should not be placed on medroxyprogesterone (Provera)?

1. A 37-year-old woman with dysfunctional uterine bleeding
2. A 65-year-old woman diagnosed with metastatic uterine cancer
3. A 40-year-old woman with a history of deep vein thrombosis
4. A 55-year-old woman with renal cancer

4. The patient states she had sexual intercourse yesterday and is concerned she may be pregnant. She is requesting emergency prevention. Which of the following drugs may be ordered?

1. Oxytocin (Pitocin)
2. Dinoprostone (Prepidil)
3. Medroxyprogesterone (Prempro)
4. Magnesium sulfate

5. Complications of oxytocin (Pitocin) include all of the following except:

1. Uterine rupture
2. Seizures
3. Fetal dysrhythmias
4. Termination of labor

6. Complications of testosterone therapy may include:

1. Renal failure
2. Hepatic failure
3. Decreased cholesterol levels
4. Maturation of male sex organs

7. Your patient states she has forgotten to take her birth control pills for the last 2 days. You should instruct her to:

1. Take her missed pills immediately
2. Get back on schedule as soon as possible
3. Use additional birth control until a regular schedule is established

4. Get a home pregnancy kit

8. At her yearly exam, your 37-year-old patient states she has discovered a lump in her left breast. She has been taking monophasic oral contraceptives for 5 years. You suspect the physician will:

1. Change patient to a triphasic oral contraceptive
2. Order a mammogram
3. Closely observe the patient
4. Take her off oral contraceptives

9. Your patient states she is experiencing menopausal symptoms and asks for your advice regarding hormone replacement therapy (HRT). Your best response is:

1. "HRT is dangerous and should never be prescribed."
2. "HRT is perfectly safe with no risks."
3. "You are not a candidate for HRT."
4. "You need to discuss risks versus benefits of HRT with your physician."

10. Your patient with BPH is complaining of feeling like he "cannot empty his bladder." You suspect the physician will order what?

1. Propecia
2. Sildenafil (Viagra)
3. Estrogen
4. Finasteride (Proscar)

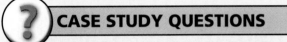

CASE STUDY QUESTIONS

For questions 1–5, please refer to the following case study, and choose the correct answer from choices 1–4.

Ms. Marge, a 29-year-old female enters the clinic with complaints of lower abdominal pain and irregular menstrual bleeding. She reports unusually painful urination and the urge to urinate more frequently. She has abnormal vaginal discharge with a pungent odor. Over the last 2 months, she has been fairly sexually active (one time per week). Vital signs reveal an elevated temperature. Blood pressure and other vital signs are normal. Ms. Marge's last physical exam was 1 year ago.

1. Which of the following disorders is most likely?

1. Toxic shock syndrome
2. Vaginosis
3. Pelvic inflammatory disease
4. Gonorrhea

2. Based on the information obtained from Ms. Marge and the vital signs assessment in this instance, dysfunctional uterine bleeding would probably be related to:

1. Thyroid disorder
2. Pelvic neoplasms
3. Pregnancy
4. Infection

3. The best course of treatment for Ms. Marge would include:

1. Progestins
2. Antibiotics and examination for reproductive scarring
3. Nonsteroidal anti-inflammatory drugs
4. High doses of conjugated estrogens

4. Prevention methods for the described disorder would include all of the following methods EXCEPT:

1. Use of condoms
2. Getting regular gynecological exams
3. Regular use of oral contraceptives
4. Prior screening of the sexual partner

5. Without effective therapy, if pregnancy were to occur later in this patient, one of the more serious complications would be:

1. Ectopic pregnancy
2. Nonmalignant breast disease
3. Iron-deficiency anemia
4. Dependence on pain medication

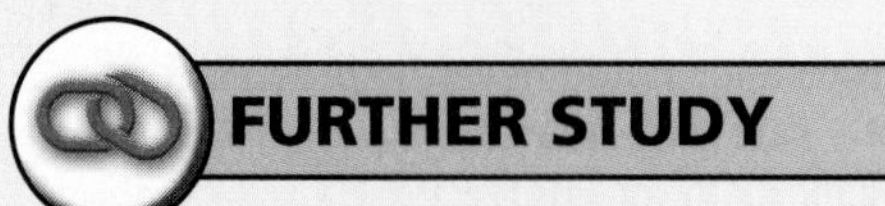

- Maintenance of bone density and alternatives to estrogen-replacement therapy are discussed in Chapter 31.
- Chapter 24 presents information on the use of reproductive hormones as antineoplastic agents.
- Chapter 15 discusses alpha blockers for use in treating hypertension.
- Nitrates used for the treatment of angina pectoris are covered in Chapter 18.

EXPLORE MEDIALINK www.prenhall.com/holland

Additional resources for this chapter can be found on the CD-ROM accompanying this textbook, and on the Companion Website. Click on Chapter 30 to select activities for this chapter.

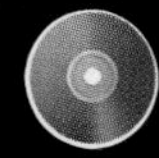

Mechanism in Action Animations:
- Ortho-Novum
- Sildenafil

Audio Glossary
Concept Review
NCLEX-PN® Review
Nursing in Action
Dosage Calculator

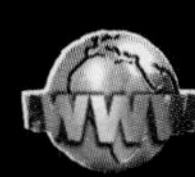

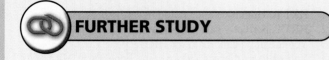

The History of Contraception
Psychological and Pharmacological Aspects of Menopause
Erectile Dysfunction Resources

UNIT

1 2 3 4 5 6 7

7 THE MUSCULOSKELETAL SYSTEM, INTEGUMENTARY SYSTEM, AND EYES AND EARS

UNIT CONTENTS

CHAPTER

31 Drugs for Muscle, Bone, and Joint Disorders

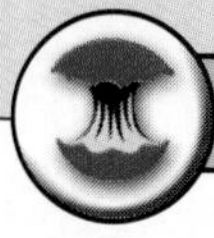

CORE CONCEPTS

31.1 Muscle spasms are caused by injury, overmedication, hypocalcemia, and debilitating disorders.

31.2 Muscle spasms can be treated with nonpharmacological and pharmacological therapies.

31.3 Many muscle relaxants treat muscle spasms by inhibiting upper motor neuron activity, causing sedation, or altering simple reflexes.

31.4 Effective treatment for spasticity includes both physical therapy and medications.

31.5 Some drugs for spasticity provide relief by acting directly on muscle tissue, interfering with the release of calcium ions.

31.6 Adequate levels of calcium, vitamin D, parathyroid hormone, and calcitonin are necessary for normal body processes.

31.7 Hypocalcemia is a serious condition that requires immediate therapy.

31.8 Treatment for osteomalacia consists of calcium and vitamin D supplements.

31.9 Treatment for osteoporosis includes calcitonin estrogen-receptor modulator drugs, and bisphosphonates.

31.10 Treatment for Paget's disease includes bisphosphonates and calcitonin.

31.11 Analgesics and anti-inflammatory drugs are important components of pharmacotherapy for osteoarthritis.

31.12 Glucocorticoids, immunosuppressants, and disease-modifying drugs are additional therapies used to treat rheumatoid arthritis.

31.13 Drug therapy for gout requires agents that inhibit uric acid buildup.

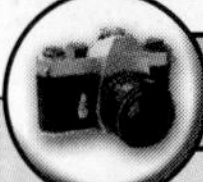

DRUG SNAPSHOT

The following drugs will be discussed in this chapter:

DRUG CLASSES	DRUG PROFILES
CENTRALLY ACTING MUSCLE RELAXANTS	
	Pr cyclobenzaprine (Cycoflex, Flexeril)
DIRECT-ACTING ANTISPASMOTICS	
	Pr dantrolene sodium (Dantrium)
CALCIUM SUPPLEMENTS AND VITAMIN D THERAPY	
	Pr calcium gluconate (Kalcinate)
	Pr calcitriol (Calcijex, Rocaltrol)
BONE RESORPTION INHIBITORS	
Hormonal agents	Pr raloxifene (Evista)
Bisphosphonates	Pr etidronate disodium (Didronel)
DISEASE-MODIFYING DRUGS OF IMPORTANCE FOR RHEUMATOID ARTHRITIS	
	Pr hydroxychloroquine sulfate (Plaquenil Sulfate)
URIC ACID INHIBITORS FOR GOUT	
	Pr colchicine

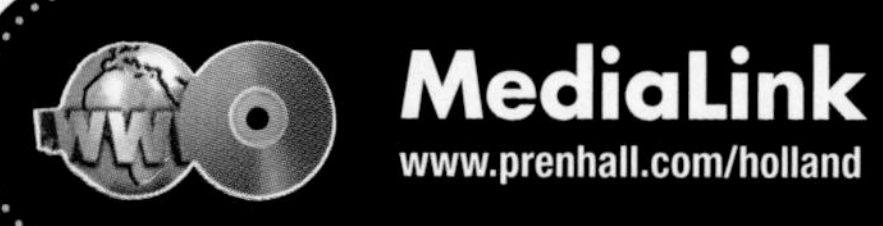

Interactive resources for this chapter can be found on the Companion Website. Click on Chapter 31 and "Begin" to select the activities for this chapter. For chapter-related animations, NCLEX-PN®-style questions, and an audio glossary, access the accompanying CD-ROM in this book.

OBJECTIVES

After reading this chapter, the student should be able to:

1. Identify the different body systems contributing to body movement.
2. Discuss nonpharmacological therapies used to treat muscle spasms, spasticity, and bone and joint disorders.
3. Explain the goals of pharmacotherapy with skeletal muscle relaxants.
4. Describe the pharmacological management of muscle spasms, disorders caused by calcium and vitamin D deficiency, and disorders related to bones and joints.
5. Compare and contrast the roles of the following drug categories in treating muscle spasms and spasticity: centrally acting skeletal muscle relaxants and direct-acting antispasmotics.
6. Identify important symptoms or disorders associated with an imbalance of calcium, vitamin D, parathyroid hormone, and calcitonin.
7. Discuss drug treatments for hypocalcemia, osteomalacia, and rickets.
8. Identify important disorders characterized by weak, fragile bones and abnormal joints.
9. For each of the drug classes, know representative drugs, and explain their mechanisms of action, primary actions, and important adverse effects.

Disorders associated with movement are some of the most difficult conditions to treat because their underlying causes can be related to at least four important systems in the body: the nervous, endocrine, muscle, and skeletal systems. Proper body movement depends on intact neural pathways and properly functioning muscles. For muscles to function properly, the body needs appropriate levels of minerals such as sodium, potassium, and calcium. The skeletal system and joints are at the core of body movement and must be free from any defect that could affect stability of the other systems. Disorders associated with bones and joints may affect a patient's ability to fulfill daily activities and lead to immobility.

This chapter focuses on the pharmacotherapy of muscle disorders associated with muscle spasms and spasticity, and skeletal disorders such as osteomalacia, osteporosis, arthritis, and gout. Many of the drugs used to treat muscle spasms are distinct from those used for spasticity. Drugs used to treat important bone and joint disorders are mentioned because of the major mobility problems that would occur without medical intervention. The importance of calcium balance and the action of vitamin D are stressed because both relate to the proper functioning of muscles and bones.

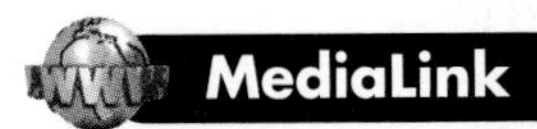

THE NATIONAL INSTITUTE OF ARTHRITIS AND MUSCULOSKELETAL AND SKIN DISEASES

MUSCLE SPASMS

Muscle spasms are involuntary contractions of a muscle or group of muscles. The muscles tighten, develop a fixed pattern of resistance, and lose functioning ability.

Fast Facts Muscle Spasms

- More than 12 million people worldwide have muscle spasms.
- Muscle spasms severe enough for drug therapy are often found in patients who have had other debilitating disorders such as stroke, injury, neurodegenerative diseases, and cerebral palsy.
- Cerebral palsy is usually associated with events that occur before or during birth, but it may be caused by head trauma or infection during the first few months or years of life.
- Dystonia affects about 250,000 people in the United States; it is the third most common movement disorder after essential tremor and Parkinson's disease.
- Researchers have recognized multiple forms of inheritable dystonia and identified at least 10 genes or chromosomal locations responsible for the various manifestations.

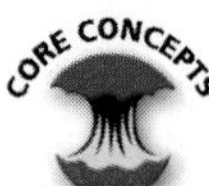

31.1 Muscle spasms are caused by injury, overmedication, hypocalcemia, and debilitating disorders.

Muscle spasms are a common condition usually associated with overuse and local injury to the skeletal muscle. Other causes of muscle spasms include overmedication with antipsychotic drugs (Chapter 10), epilepsy, hypocalcemia, pain, and debilitating neurologic disorders. Patients with muscle spasms may experience inflammation, edema, and pain at the affected muscle; loss of coordination; and reduced mobility. When a muscle goes into spasm, it freezes in a contracted state. A single, prolonged contraction is a *tonic spasm,* whereas multiple, rapidly repeated contractions are *clonic spasms.* Treatment of muscle spasms includes use of both nonpharmacological and pharmacological therapies.

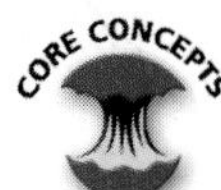

31.2 Muscle spasms can be treated with nonpharmacological and pharmacological therapies.

Patients with muscle spasms require a careful history and physical exam to determine the etiology. After a determination has been made, nonpharmacological therapies are normally used in conjunction with medications. Nonpharmacological measures may be immobilization of the affected muscle, application of heat or cold, hydrotherapy, ultrasound, supervised exercises, massage, and/or manipulation.

Pharmacotherapy for muscle spasms may include combinations of analgesics, anti-inflammatory agents, and centrally acting skeletal muscle relaxants. Most skeletal muscle relaxants relieve symptoms of muscular stiffness and rigidity that result from muscular injury. These agents also help improve mobility. Therapeutic goals are to minimize pain and discomfort, increase range of motion, and improve the patient's ability to function independently.

Concept Review 31.1

- Give several reasons why muscle spasms develop. What is the main goal of therapy for muscle spasms?

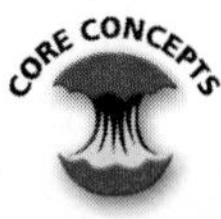

31.3 Many muscle relaxants treat muscle spasms by inhibiting upper motor neuron activity, causing sedation, or altering simple reflexes.

Antispasmodic drugs relieve symptoms of muscular stiffness and rigidity. They improve mobility in cases where patients have restricted movements.

Many antispasmodic drugs treat muscle spasms at the level of the CNS. The exact mechanisms of action are not fully known, but it is believed that these agents affect the brain and/or spinal cord by inhibiting upper motor neuron activity, causing sedation, or altering simple reflexes.

Skeletal muscle relaxants are used to treat local spasms resulting from muscular injury and may be prescribed alone or in combination with other medications to reduce pain and increase range of motion. Commonly used centrally acting medications are baclofen (Lioresal), cyclobenzaprine (Cycoflex, Flexeril), tizanidine (Zanaflex), and benzodiazepines such as diazepam (Valium), clonazepam (Klonopin), and lorazepam (Ativan) (see Table 31.1). All of the centrally acting agents can cause sedation.

Baclofen (Lioresal) is structurally similar to the inhibitory neurotransmitter gamma amino butyric acid (GABA) and produces its effect by a mechanism that is not fully known. It inhibits neuronal activity within the brain and, possibly, the spinal cord, although there is some uncertainty about whether the spinal effects of baclofen are associated with GABA. Baclofen may be used to reduce muscle spasms in patients with multiple sclerosis, cerebral palsy, or spinal cord injury. Common side effects of baclofen are drowsiness, dizziness, weakness, and fatigue. Baclofen is often a drug of first choice because of its wide safety margin.

TABLE 31.1 Centrally Acting Antispasmodic Drugs

DRUG	ROUTE AND ADULT DOSE	REMARKS
baclofen (Lioresal)	PO 5 mg tid (max: 80 mg/day)	May be administered orally or by an implantable pump, which infuses medication directly into the subarachnoid space
carisoprodol (Soma)	PO 350 mg tid	CNS depressant; does not inhibit motor activity like other conventional muscle relaxers; muscle relaxation seems to be related to sedation
chlorphenesin (Maolate)	PO 800 mg tid until effective; reduce to 400 mg qid or less	Often used in conjunction with physical therapy in cases of musculoskeletal injury and pain
chlorzoxane (Paraflex, Parafon Forte)	PO 250–500 mg tid–qid (max: 3 g/day)	Depresses nerve transmission in the brain and spinal cord, possibly by sedation; not effective for cerebral palsy
clonazepam (Klonopin)	PO 0.5 mg tid (max: 20 mg/day)	Benzodiazepine usually taken in combination with other drugs; used for the relief of skeletal muscle spasms; primarily for seizure disorders
Pr cyclobenzaprine hydrochloride (Cycoflex, Flexeril)	PO 10–20 mg bid–qid (max: 60 mg/day)	Short-term relief of muscle spasms associated with acute musculoskeletal conditions; not for cerebral palsy or central nervous system diseases
diazepam (Valium)	PO 4–10 mg bid–qid; IM/IV 2–10 mg, repeat if needed in 3–4 hours; IV pump; administer emulsion at 5 mg/min	Benzodiazepine used for the relief of skeletal muscle spasms associated with cerebral palsy, partial paralysis
lorazepam (Ativan)	PO 1–2 mg bid–tid (max: 10 mg/day)	Benzodiazepine used for extreme muscle tension
metaxalone (Skelaxin)	PO 800 mg tid–qid for max of 10 days	For acute musculoskeletal conditions; causes its effect through sedation
methocarbamol (Robaxin)	PO 1.5 grams qid for 2–3 days, then reduce to 1 g qid	Adjunct to physical therapy for acute musculoskeletal disorders and tetanus
orphenadrine citrate (Banflex, Flexon, Myolin, Norflex)	PO 100 mg bid	IM/IV forms available
tizanidine (Zanaflex)	PO 4–8 mg tid–qid (max: 36 mg/day)	To relax muscle tone associated with spasticity

Tizanidine (Zanaflex) is a centrally acting alpha$_2$-adrenergic agonist that inhibits motor neurons, mainly at the spinal cord level. Patients receiving high doses report drowsiness; thus, it also affects some neural activity in the brain. Though uncommon, one adverse effect of tizanidine is hallucinations. The drug's most frequent side effects are dry mouth, fatigue, dizziness, and sleepiness. Tizanidine is as effective as baclofen and is considered by some to be a drug of first choice.

As discussed in Chapter 11, benzodiazepines inhibit both sensory and motor neuron activity by enhancing the effects of GABA. Common adverse side effects include drowsiness and ataxia (loss of coordination). Benzodiazepines are usually prescribed for muscle relaxation when baclofen and tizanidine fail to produce adequate relief.

31.4 Effective treatment for spasticity includes both physical therapy and medications.

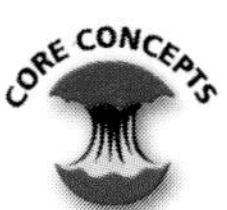

Spasticity is a condition in which certain muscle groups remain in a continuous state of contraction, usually as a result of damage to the CNS. The contracted muscles become stiff with increased muscle tone. Other signs and symptoms may include mild to severe pain, exaggerated deep tendon reflexes, muscle spasms, scissoring (involuntary crossing of the legs), and fixed joints.

DRUG PROFILE: Skeletal Muscle Relaxant, Central Acting: Pr *Cyclobenzaprine (Cycloflex, Flexeril)*

Actions and Uses:

Cyclobenzaprine relieves muscle spasms of local origin without interfering with general muscle function. This drug acts by depressing motor activity, primarily in the brain stem, with limited effects also occurring in the spinal cord. It increases circulating levels of norepinephrine, blocking presynaptic uptake. Its mechanism of action is similar to tricyclic antidepressants (Chapter 9). It causes muscle relaxation in acute muscle spasticity, but it is not effective in cases of cerebral palsy or diseases of the brain and spinal cord. This medication is meant to provide therapy for only 2 to 3 weeks.

Adverse Effects and Interactions:

Adverse reactions to cyclobenzaprine include drowsiness, blurred vision, dizziness, dry mouth, rash, and tachycardia. It should be used with caution in patients with MI, dysrhythmias, or severe cardiovascular disease. One reaction, although rare, is swelling of the tongue.

Alcohol, phenothiazines, and other CNS depressants may cause additive sedation. Cyclobenzaprine should not be used within 2 weeks of an MAO inhibitor because hyperpyretic crisis and convulsions may occur.

Mechanism in Action:

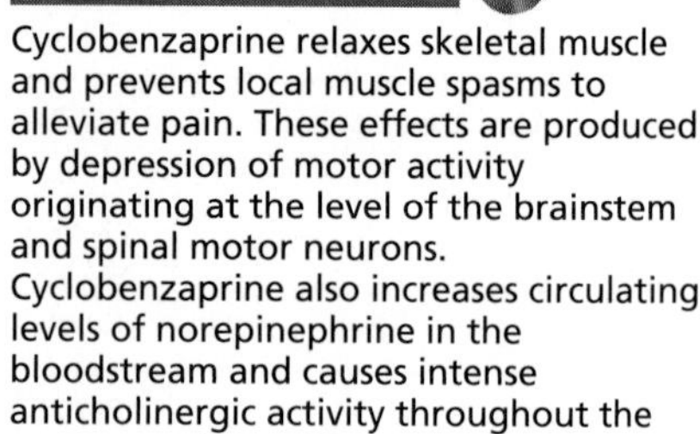

Cyclobenzaprine relaxes skeletal muscle and prevents local muscle spasms to alleviate pain. These effects are produced by depression of motor activity originating at the level of the brainstem and spinal motor neurons. Cyclobenzaprine also increases circulating levels of norepinephrine in the bloodstream and causes intense anticholinergic activity throughout the nervous system.

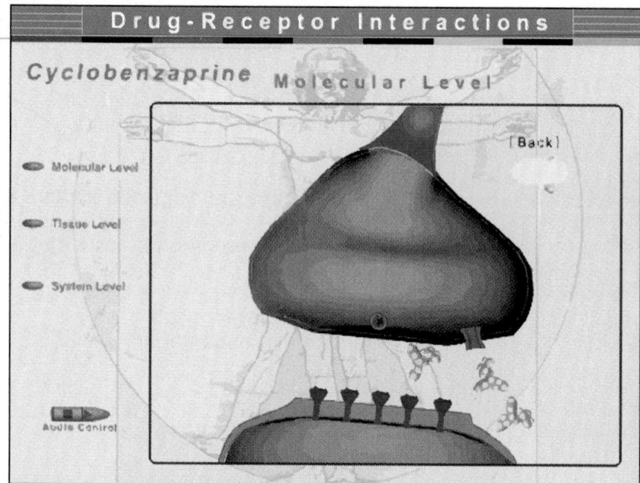

Use the student CD-ROM to see Mechanism in Action for Cyclobenzaprine.

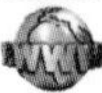

See the Companion Website for a Nursing Process Focus specific to this drug.

NURSING PROCESS FOCUS

Patients Receiving Drugs for Muscle Spasms or Spasticity

ASSESSMENT

Prior to administration:

- Obtain complete health history including allergies, drug history, and possible drug interactions
- Obtain complete physical examination
- Establish baseline level of consciousness and vital signs

POTENTIAL NURSING DIAGNOSES

- Pain (acute/chronic), related to muscle spasms
- Impaired Physical Mobility, related to acute/chronic pain
- Risk for Injury, related to drug side effects
- Deficient Knowledge, related to drug therapy

PLANNING: Patient Goals and Expected Outcomes

The patient will:

- Report a decrease in pain, increase in range of motion, and reduction of muscle spasm
- Exhibit no adverse effects from the therapeutic regimen
- Demonstrate an understanding of the therapeutic regimen

continued...

NURSING PROCESS FOCUS

IMPLEMENTATION

Interventions and (Rationales)	Patient Education/Discharge Planning
■ Monitor LOC and vital signs. (Some skeletal muscle relaxants alter the patient's LOC. Others within this class may alter blood pressure and heart rate.)	Instruct patient to: ■ Avoid driving and other activities requiring mental alertness until effects of the medication are known ■ Report any significant change in sensorium, such as slurred speech, confusion, hallucinations, or extreme lethargy ■ Report palpitations, chest pain, dyspnea, unusual fatigue, weakness, and visual disturbances ■ Avoid using other CNS depressants such as alcohol that will intensify sedation
■ Monitor pain. ■ Determine location, duration, and precipitating factors of the patient's pain. (Drugs should diminish patient's pain.)	Instruct patient: ■ To report the development of new sites of muscle pain ■ In relaxation techniques, deep breathing, and meditation methods to facilitate relaxation and reduce pain
■ Monitor for withdrawal reactions. (Abrupt withdrawal of baclofen may cause visual hallucinations, paranoid ideation, and seizures.)	■ Advise patient to not abruptly discontinue treatment.
■ Monitor muscle tone, range of motion, and degree of muscle spasm. (This will determine effectiveness of drug therapy.)	■ Instruct patient to perform gentle range of motion, only to the point of mild physical discomfort, throughout the day.
■ Provide additional pain relief measures such as positional support, gentle massage, and moist heat or ice packs. (Drugs alone may not be sufficient in providing pain relief.)	■ Instruct patient in complimentary pain interventions such as positioning, gentle massage, and the application of heat or cold to the painful area.
■ Monitor for side effects such as drowsiness, dry mouth, dizziness, nausea, vomiting, faintness, headache, nervousness, diplopia, and urinary retention (cyclobenzaprine).	Instruct the patient to: ■ Report side effects ■ Take medication with food to decrease GI upset ■ Report signs of urinary retention such as a feeling of urinary bladder fullness, distended abdomen, and discomfort
■ Monitor for side effects such as muscle weakness, dry mouth, dizziness, nausea, diarrhea, tachycardia, erratic blood pressure, photosensitivity, and urinary retention. (These adverse effects occur with certain drugs in this class.)	Instruct patient: ■ That frequent mouth rinses, sips of water, and sugarless candy or gum may help with dry mouth ■ That medication may cause a decrease in muscle strength and dosage may need to be reduced ■ To use sunscreen and protective clothing when outdoors

EVALUATION OF OUTCOME CRITERIA

Evaluate the effectiveness of drug therapy by confirming that patient goals and expected outcomes have been met (see "Planning").

See Tables 31.1 and 31.2 for lists of drugs to which these nursing actions apply.

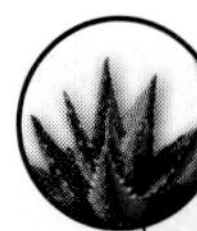

NATURAL ALTERNATIVES

Cayenne for Muscular Tension

Cayenne (*Capsicum annum*), also known as chili pepper, paprika, or red pepper, has been used as a remedy for muscle tension. Applied in a cream base, it is commonly used to relieve muscle spasms in the shoulder and areas of the arm. Capsaicin, the active ingredient in cayenne, diminishes the chemical messengers that travel through the sensory nerves, therefore decreasing the sensation of pain. Its effect accumulates over time so creams containing capsaicin need to be applied regularly to be effective. Although no known medical condition exists that would prevent the use of cayenne, it should never be applied over broken skin. External use of full-strength cayenne should be limited to no more than 2 days, because it may cause skin inflammation, blisters, and ulcers. It also needs to be kept away from eyes and mucous membranes to avoid burns. Hands must be washed thoroughly after usage. Commercial, OTC creams containing capsaicin are available. ■

dys = *abnormal*
tonia = *tension*

Spasticity usually results from damage to the motor area of the cerebral cortex, which controls muscle movement. Etiologies most commonly associated with this condition include neurologic disorders such as cerebral palsy, severe head injury, spinal cord injury or lesions, and stroke. **Dystonia,** a chronic neurologic disorder, is characterized by involuntary muscle contraction that forces body parts into abnormal, occasionally painful, movements or postures. It affects the muscle tone of the arms, legs, trunk, neck, eyelids, face, or vocal cords. Spasticity, whether short- or long-term, can be distressing and usually greatly impacts an individual's quality of life. In addition to causing pain, it also impairs physical mobility, thereby influencing the person's ability to perform activities of daily living (ADLs) and diminishing his or her sense of independence.

Effective treatment for spasticity includes both physical therapy and medications. Medications alone are not adequate to reduce the complications of spasticity, but regular and consistent physical therapy exercises have been shown to be effective in decreasing the severity of symptoms. Types of treatment include muscle stretching to help prevent contractures, muscle-group strengthening exercises, and repetitive-motion exercises for improvement of accuracy. In extreme cases, surgery for tendon release or to sever the nerve-muscle pathway has been used.

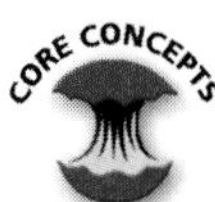

31.5 Some drugs for spasticity provide relief by acting directly on muscle tissue, interfering with the release of calcium ions.

Drugs effective in the treatment of spasticity include two centrally acting drugs, baclofen (Lioresal) and diazepam (Valium), and a direct-acting drug, dantrolene (Dantrium). The direct-acting drugs produce an antispasmodic effect at the level of the neuromuscular junction, as shown in Figure 31.1 ■.

Dantrolene relieves spasticity by interfering with the release of calcium ions in skeletal muscle. Other direct-acting drugs include botulinum toxin type A (Botox, Dysport) and botulinum toxin type B (Myobloc), used to offer significant relief of symptoms to people with dystonia, and quinine sulfate (Quinamm, Quiphile), which is used to treat leg cramps. Direct-acting drugs are summarized in Table 31.2.

Botulinum toxin is an unusual drug because, in high doses, it acts as a poison. *Clostridium botulinum* is the bacteria responsible for food poisoning or botulism. At lower doses, however, this drug is safe and effective as a muscle relaxant for patients with dystonia. It produces its effect by blocking the release of acetylcholine from cholinergic nerve terminals (Chapter 7).

Botulinum can cause extreme weakness, so its use may require the addition of other therapies to improve muscle strength. To prevent major problems with mobility or posture, botulinum toxin is often applied to small muscle groups. Sometimes this drug is administered together with centrally acting oral medications to further increase the functional use of a range of muscle groups.

Drawbacks to botulinum therapy are its delayed and limited effects. The treatment it mostly effective within 6 weeks of administration, and its effects last for only 3 to 6 months. Another drawback is the pain of injecting botulinum directly into the muscle. Local anesthetics are usually given to block this pain.

FIGURE 31.1

(a) Drugs affecting the neuromuscular junction may block the release of acetylcholine at the synaptic terminal or the action of acetylcholine at its receptor (located on the surface of muscle fibers). (b) Drugs also block the release of calcium ions from muscle tissue, preventing the muscle fibers from contracting.

HYPOCALCEMIA

Hypocalcemia, or lowered levels of calcium in the blood, is associated with a range of conditions including poor nutrition, muscle spasms, convulsions, and endocrine and bone disorders.

31.6 Adequate levels of calcium, vitamin D, parathyroid hormone, and calcitonin are necessary for normal body processes.

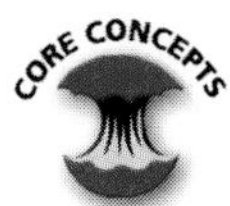

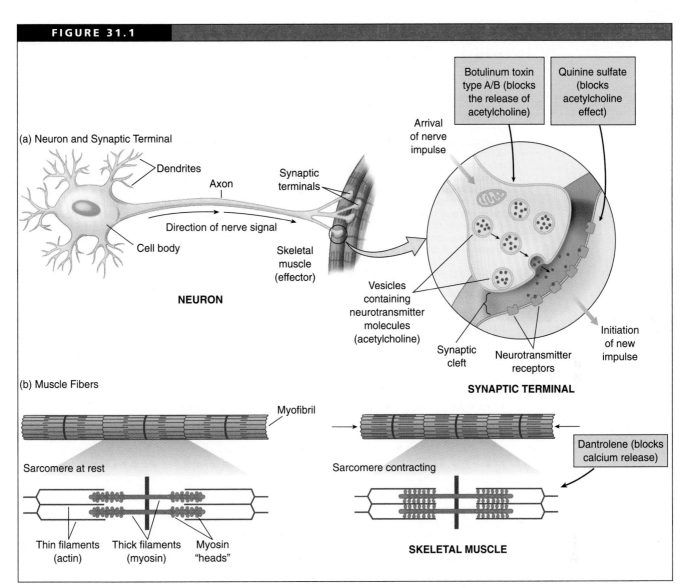

One of the most important minerals in the body responsible for muscle contraction and formation of bone is calcium. Levels of calcium in the blood are controlled by two endocrine glands: the

DRUG PROFILE: Skeletal Muscle Relaxant; Peripheral-acting: Pr *Dantrolene Sodium (Dantrium)*

Actions and Uses:

Dantrolene is often used for spasticity, especially for spasms of the head and neck. It directly relaxes muscle spasms by interfering with the release of calcium ions from storage areas inside skeletal muscle cells. It does not affect cardiac or smooth muscle. Dantrolene is especially useful for muscle spasms when they occur after spinal cord injury or stroke and in cases of cerebral palsy, multiple sclerosis, and occasionally for the treatment of muscle pain after heavy exercise. It is also used for the treatment of malignant hyperthermia.

Adverse Effects and Interactions:

Adverse effects include muscle weakness, drowsiness, dry mouth, dizziness, nausea, diarrhea, tachycardia, erratic blood pressure, photosensitivity, and urinary retention.

Dantrolene interacts with many other drugs. For example, it should not be taken with OTC cough preparations and antihistamines, alcohol, or other CNS depressants. Verapamil and other calcium channel blockers taken with dantrolene increase the risk of ventricular fibrillation and cardiovascular collapse. Patients with impaired cardiac or pulmonary function or hepatic disease should not take this drug.

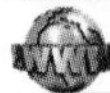

See the Companion Website for a Nursing Process Focus specific to this drug.

TABLE 31.2 Direct-Acting Antispasmodic Drugs

DRUG	ROUTE AND ADULT DOSE	REMARKS
botulinum toxin type A (Botox, Dysport)	25 units injected directly into target muscle (max: 30-day dose should not exceed 200 units)	May be used in cases of cerebral palsy, multiple sclerosis, and traumatic brain or spinal cord injury; may also be used for strabismus (crossed eyes); sometimes used for excessive sweating and wrinkles
botulinum toxin type B (Myobloc)	2500–5000 units/dose injected directly into target muscle; doses should be divided among muscle groups	May be used in cases of cervical dystonia
Pr dantrolene sodium (Dantrium)	PO 25 mg daily; increase to 25 mg bid–qid; may increase every 4–7 days up to 100 mg bid–tid	Hydantoin-like medication; also for the treatment of malignant hyperthermia; IV form available
quinine sulfate (Quinamm, Quiphile)	PO 260–300 mg at bedtime	Antimalarial drug; for nocturnal leg cramps or congenital tonic spasms

parathyroid glands, which secrete parathyroid hormone (PTH), and the thyroid gland, which secretes calcitonin, as shown in Figure 31.2 ■.

PTH stimulates bone cells called *osteoclasts.* These cells accelerate the process of **bone resorption,** the demineralization process that breaks down bone into its mineral components. Once bone is broken down or resorbed, calcium becomes available to be transported and used elsewhere in the body. The opposite of this process is **bone deposition,** or bone building. This process, which removes calcium from the blood, is stimulated by the hormone calcitonin.

PTH and calcitonin control calcium homeostasis in the body by influencing three major targets: the bones, kidneys, and gastrointestinal (GI) tract. The GI tract is mainly influenced by PTH. Vitamin D and calcium metabolism are interrelated: calcium disorders are often associated with vitamin D disorders.

Vitamin D is unique among vitamins in that the body is able to synthesize it from precursor molecules. In the skin, the inactive form of vitamin D, called **cholecalciferol,** is synthesized from cholesterol. Exposure of the skin to sunlight or ultraviolet light increases the level of cholecalciferol in the bloodstream. Cholecalciferol can also be obtained from dietary products such as milk or other foods fortified with vitamin D. Figure 31.3 ■ illustrates the metabolism of vitamin D.

Once cholecalciferol is absorbed or formed in the body, it is converted to an intermediate vitamin form called **calcifediol.** Enzymes in the kidneys metabolize calcifediol to **calcitriol,** the

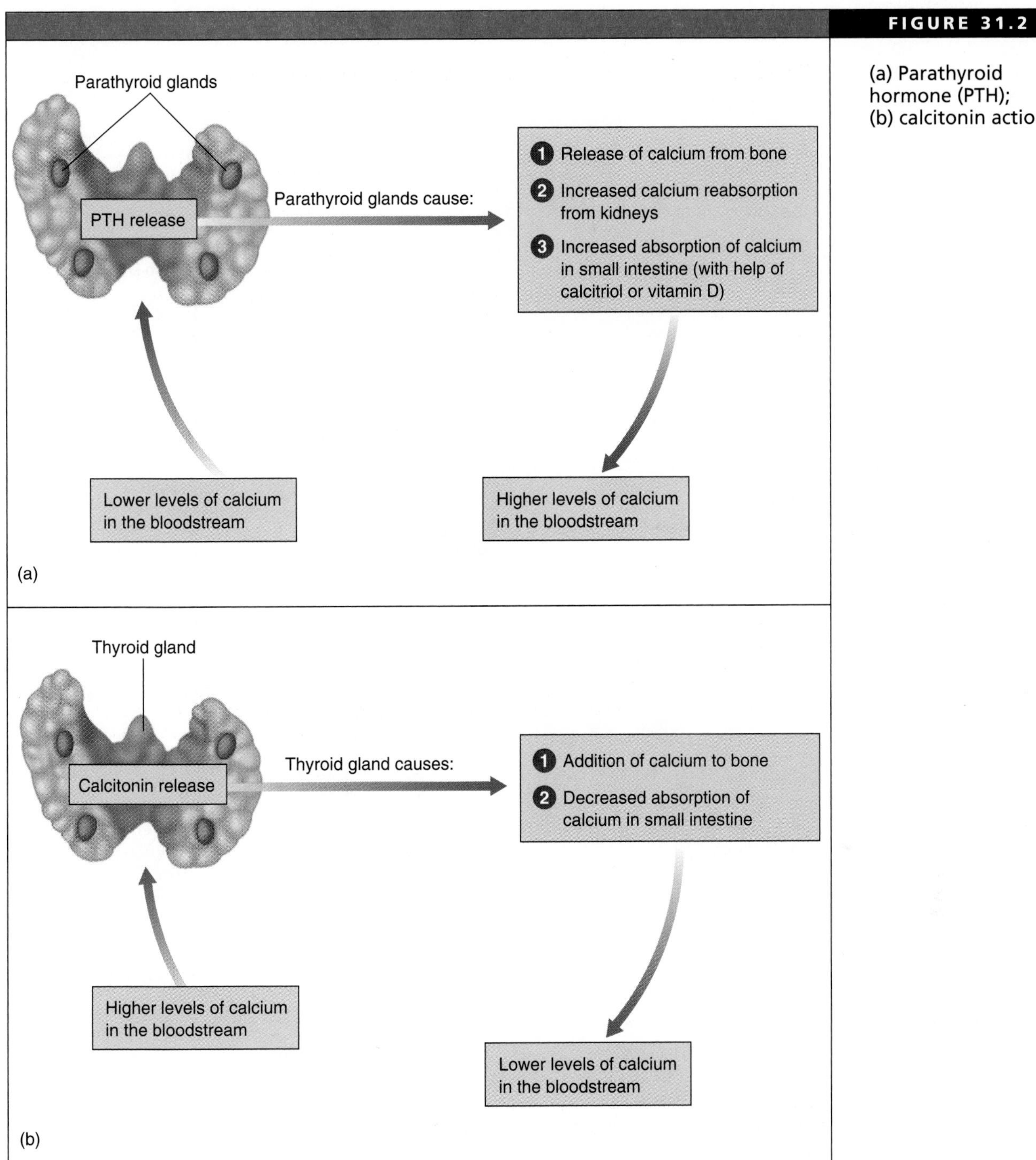

FIGURE 31.2

(a) Parathyroid hormone (PTH); (b) calcitonin action

active form of vitamin D. PTH stimulates the formation of calcitriol in the kidneys. Patients with extensive kidney disease are unable to adequately synthesize calcitriol.

The primary function of calcitriol is to increase calcium absorption from the GI tract. Dietary calcium is absorbed better in the presence of active vitamin D and PTH to produce higher levels of calcium in the bloodstream.

The importance of proper calcium balance in the body cannot be overstated. Calcium ions influence the excitability of all neurons. When calcium concentrations are too high (*hypercalcemia*), sodium permeability decreases across cell membranes. This is a dangerous state because nerve conduction depends on the proper influx of sodium into cells. When calcium levels in the bloodstream are too low (*hypocalcemia*), cell membranes become hyperexcitable. If hypocalcemia becomes severe, convulsions or muscle spasms may result. Calcium is also important for the normal functioning of other body processes such as blood coagulation, neurotransmitter release from nerve terminals, and muscle contraction.

FIGURE 31.3

Pathway for vitamin D activation and action

Sources of Vitamin D

Diet

Cholecalciferol
(inactive vitamin D)

Calcifediol
(intermediate form)

Calcitriol
(active vitamin D)

Increased absorption
of calcium in
the small intestine

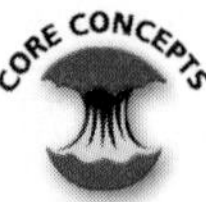

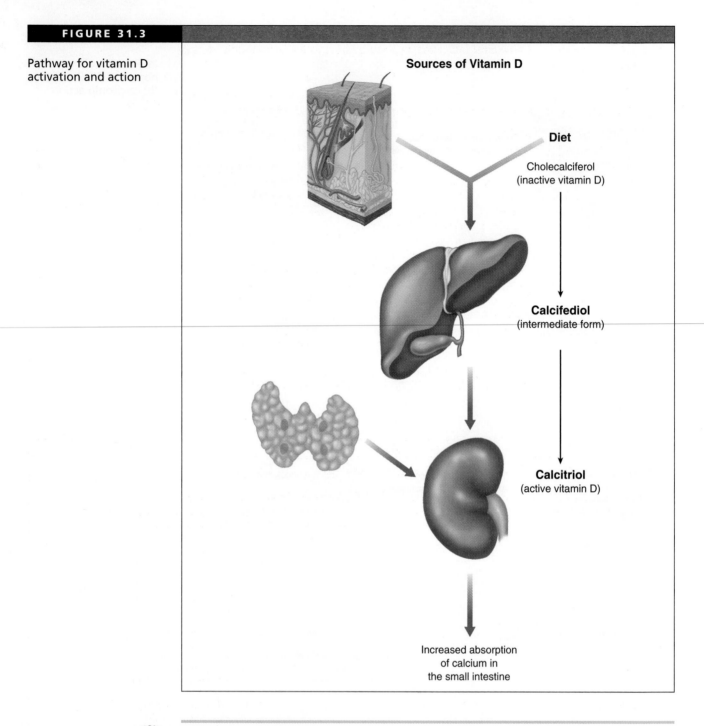

31.7 Hypocalcemia is a serious condition that requires immediate therapy.

Therapies for calcium disorders include calcium supplements, vitamin D supplements, bisphosphonates, and several miscellaneous agents. Conditions of calcium and vitamin D metabolism include hypocalcemia, osteomalacia, osteoporosis, and Paget's disease.

Hypocalcemia is not a disease, but a sign of underlying pathology; therefore, diagnosis of the cause of hypocalcemia is essential. One common cause is hyposecretion of PTH, which occurs when the thyroid and parathyroid glands are surgically removed. Digestive-related malabsorption disorders and vitamin D deficiencies also result in hypocalcemia. In cases of hypocalcemia, medical personnel assess for the adequate intake of calcium-containing foods.

Symptoms of hypocalcemia are nerve and muscle excitability. Muscle twitching, tremor, or cramping may be evident. Numbness and tingling of the extremities may occur, and convulsions are possible. A patient may be confused or behave abnormally. Severe hypocalcemia requires IV administration of calcium salts, whereas less severe hypocalcemia can often be reversed with oral supplements.

31.8 Treatment for osteomalacia consists of calcium and vitamin D supplements.

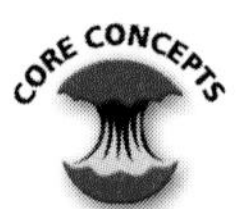

Osteomalacia, referred to as *rickets* in children, is a disorder characterized by softening of bones without alteration of basic bone structure. The cause of osteomalacia and rickets is a lack of vitamin D and calcium in the diet, usually as a result of kidney failure or malabsorption of calcium from the GI tract. Signs and symptoms include hypocalcemia, muscle weakness, muscle spasms, and diffuse bone pain, especially in the hip area. Patients may also experience pain in the arms, legs, and spinal column. Classic signs of rickets in children include bowlegs and a pigeon breast. Children may also develop a slight fever and become restless at night.

hyper = *elevated*
hypo = *lowered*
calc = *calcium*
emia = *blood level*

Tests performed to verify osteomalacia include bone biopsy; bone radiographs; computerized tomography (CT) scan of the vertebral column; and determination of serum calcium, phosphate, and vitamin D levels. Many of these tests are routine for bone disorders and are performed as needed to determine the extent of bone health.

In extreme cases, surgical correction of disfigured limbs may be required. Drug therapy for children and adults consists of calcium and vitamin D supplements. A summary of drugs used for these conditions is provided in Table 31.3.

The two major forms of calcium are complexed and elemental. Most calcium supplements are in the form of complexed calcium. These products are often compared on the basis of their

TABLE 31.3 Calcium Supplements and Vitamin D Therapy

DRUG	ROUTE AND ADULT DOSE	REMARKS
CALCIUM SUPPLEMENTS (ALL DOSES ARE IN TERMS OF ELEMENTAL CALCIUM.)		
calcium acetate (Phos-Ex, PhosLo)	PO 1–2 g bid–tid	1 gram calcium acetate equals 250 mg (12.6 mEq) elemental calcium
calcium carbonate (BioCal, Calcite-500, others)	PO 1–2 g bid–tid	1 gram calcium carbonate equals 400 mg (20 mEq) elemental calcium
calcium chloride	IV 0.5–1 g daily q3d	1 gram calcium chloride equals 272 mg (13.6 mEq) elemental calcium; may be irritating to body tissues
calcium citrate (Citracal)	PO 1–2 g bid–tid	1 gram calcium citrate equals 210 mg (12 mEq) elemental calcium
calcium gluceptate	IV 1.1–4.4 g daily IM 0.5–1.1 g daily	1 gram calcium gluceptate equals 82 mg (4.1 mEq) elemental calcium
Pr calcium gluconate (Kalcinate)	PO 1–2 g bid–qid	1 gram calcium gluconate equals 90 mg (4.5 mEq) elemental calcium
calcium lactate	PO 325 mg–1.3 g tid with meals	1 gram calcium lactate equals 130 mg (6.5 mEq) elemental calcium
calcium phosphate tribasic (Posture)	PO 1–2 g bid–tid	1 gram calcium phosphate equals 390 mg (19.3 mEq) elemental calcium
VITAMIN D SUPPLEMENTS		
calcifediol (Calderol)	PO 50–100 mcg daily or every other day	For metabolic bone disease and hypocalcemia associated with chronic kidney failure
Pr calcitriol (Calcijex, Rocaltrol)	PO 0.25 mcg daily	For hypocalcemia in chronic renal failure and with hypoparathyroidism
ergocalciferol (Deltalin, Calciferol)	PO/IM 25–125 mcg daily for 6–12 weeks	For osteomalacia; also used for vitamin D-dependent rickets and hypoparathyroidism

DRUG PROFILE: Electrolyte; Calcium Supplement: 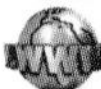 *Calcium Gluconate (Kalcinate)*

Actions and Uses:

Calcium gluconate and other calcium compounds are used to correct hypocalcemia, and for osteoporosis and Paget's disease. The objective of calcium therapy is to return serum levels of calcium to normal. People at high risk for developing these conditions include postmenopausal women, those with little physical activity over a prolonged period, and patients taking certain medications such as corticosteroids, immunosuppressive drugs, and some antiseizure medications. Calcium gluconate is available in tablets or as a 10% solution for IV injection. Calcium gluconate is pregnancy category B.

Adverse Effects and Interactions:

The most common adverse effect of calcium gluconate is hypercalcemia, brought on by taking too much of this supplement. Symptoms include drowsiness, lethargy, weakness, headache, anorexia, nausea and vomiting, increased urination, and thirst. IV administration of calcium may cause hypotension, bradycardia, dysrhythmia, and cardiac arrest.

Using this drug with cardiac glycosides increases the risk of dysrhythmias. Magnesium may compete for GI absorption. Calcium decreases the absorption of tetracyclines.

See the Companion Website for a Nursing Process Focus specific to this drug.

DRUG PROFILE: Vitamin D: *Calcitriol (Calcijex, Rocaltrol)*

Actions and Uses:

Calcitriol is the active form of vitamin D, available in both oral and IV formulations. It promotes the intestinal absorption of calcium and elevates serum levels of calcium. This medication is used in cases when patients have impaired kidney function or have hypoparathyroidism. Calcitriol reduces bone resorption and is useful in treating rickets. The effectiveness of calcitriol depends on the patient receiving an adequate amount of calcium; therefore, it is usually prescribed in combination with calcium supplements.

Adverse Effects and Interactions:

Common side effects include hypercalcemia, headache, weakness, dry mouth, thirst, increased urination, and muscle or bone pain. Thiazide diuretics may increase the effects of vitamin D, causing hypercalcemia. Too much vitamin D may cause dysrhythmias in patients who are receiving cardiac glycosides. Magnesium supplements should not be given together with calcitriol because of the increased risk of hypermagnesemia.

Mechanism in Action: 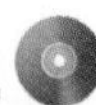

Calcitriol is an active form of vitamin D, responsible for increasing calcium absorption. Calcium is important for the proper functioning of the muscular, skeletal, and nervous systems. All three systems, as well as organs of the endocrine and renal system, play a critical role in maintaining a proper balance of calcium in the bloodstream.

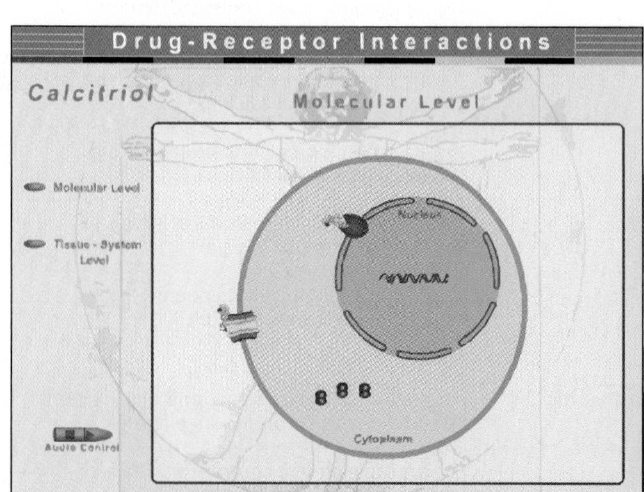

Use the student CD-ROM to see Mechanism in Action for Calcitriol.

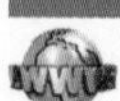 *See the Companion Website for a Nursing Process Focus specific to this drug.*

ability to release elemental calcium into the bloodstream. The greater the ability of complexed calcium to release elemental calcium, the more potent is the supplement. Elemental calcium may be obtained from dietary sources such as dark green vegetables, canned salmon, and fortified products including tofu, orange juice, and milk.

Inactive, intermediate, and active forms of vitamin D are also available as medications. The amount of vitamin D a patient needs will often vary depending on how much he or she is exposed to sunlight. After age 70, the average recommended intake of vitamin D increases from 400 to 600 units/day. Because vitamin D is needed to absorb calcium from the GI tract, many supplements combine vitamin D and calcium into a single tablet.

Concept Review 31.2

- Identify the major drug therapies used for osteomalacia, rickets, and hypocalcemia.

WEAK AND FRAGILE BONES

Two important disorders characterized by weak and fragile bones are osteoporosis and Paget's disease. Although these disorders are not the same, they share many of the same symptoms.

31.9 Treatment for osteoporosis includes calcitonin, estrogen-receptor modulator drugs, and bisphosphonates.

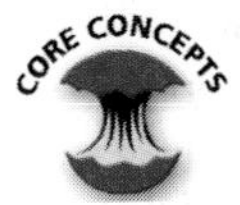

Osteoporosis, the most common metabolic bone disease, is responsible for as many as 1.5 million fractures annually. This disorder is usually asymptomatic until the bones become brittle enough to fracture or a vertebra collapses. In some cases, a lack of dietary calcium and vitamin D contribute to bone deterioration. In other cases, osteoporosis is due to disrupted bone homeostasis. Simply stated, bone resorption outpaces bone deposition and patients develop weak bones. Following are risk factors for osteoporosis:

- Postmenopause
- High alcohol or caffeine consumption
- Anorexia nervosa
- Tobacco use
- Physical inactivity
- Testosterone deficiency, particularly in elderly men
- Lack of adequate vitamin D or calcium in the diet
- Drugs such as corticosteroids, some anticonvulsants, and immunosuppressants that lower calcium levels in the bloodstream

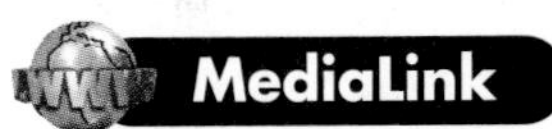

OSTEOPOROSIS AND RELATED BONE DISEASES NATIONAL RESOURCE CENTER

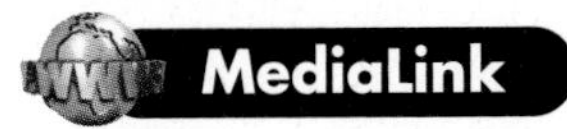

NATIONAL OSTEOPOROSIS FOUNDATION

The most common risk factor associated with the development of osteoporosis is the onset of menopause. When women reach menopause, estrogen secretion declines and bones become weak and fragile. One theory to explain this occurrence is that normal levels of estrogen may limit the life span of osteoclasts, the bone cells that resorb bone. When estrogen levels become low, osteoclast activity is no longer controlled, and bone demineralization accelerates, resulting in loss of bone density. In women with osteoporosis, fractures often occur in the hips, wrists, forearms, or spine. The metabolism of calcium in osteoporosis is illustrated in Figure 31.4 ■.

Many drug therapies are available for osteoporosis. These include calcium and vitamin D therapy, estrogen replacement therapy, estrogen-receptor modulators, statins, slow-release sodium fluoride, bisphosphonates, and calcitonin. Many of these drug classes are also used for other bone disorders or conditions unrelated to the skeletal system. Selected drugs for osteoporosis are listed in Table 31.4.

FIGURE 31.4

Calcium metabolism in osteoporosis: (a) normal calcium intake; (b) low calcium intake

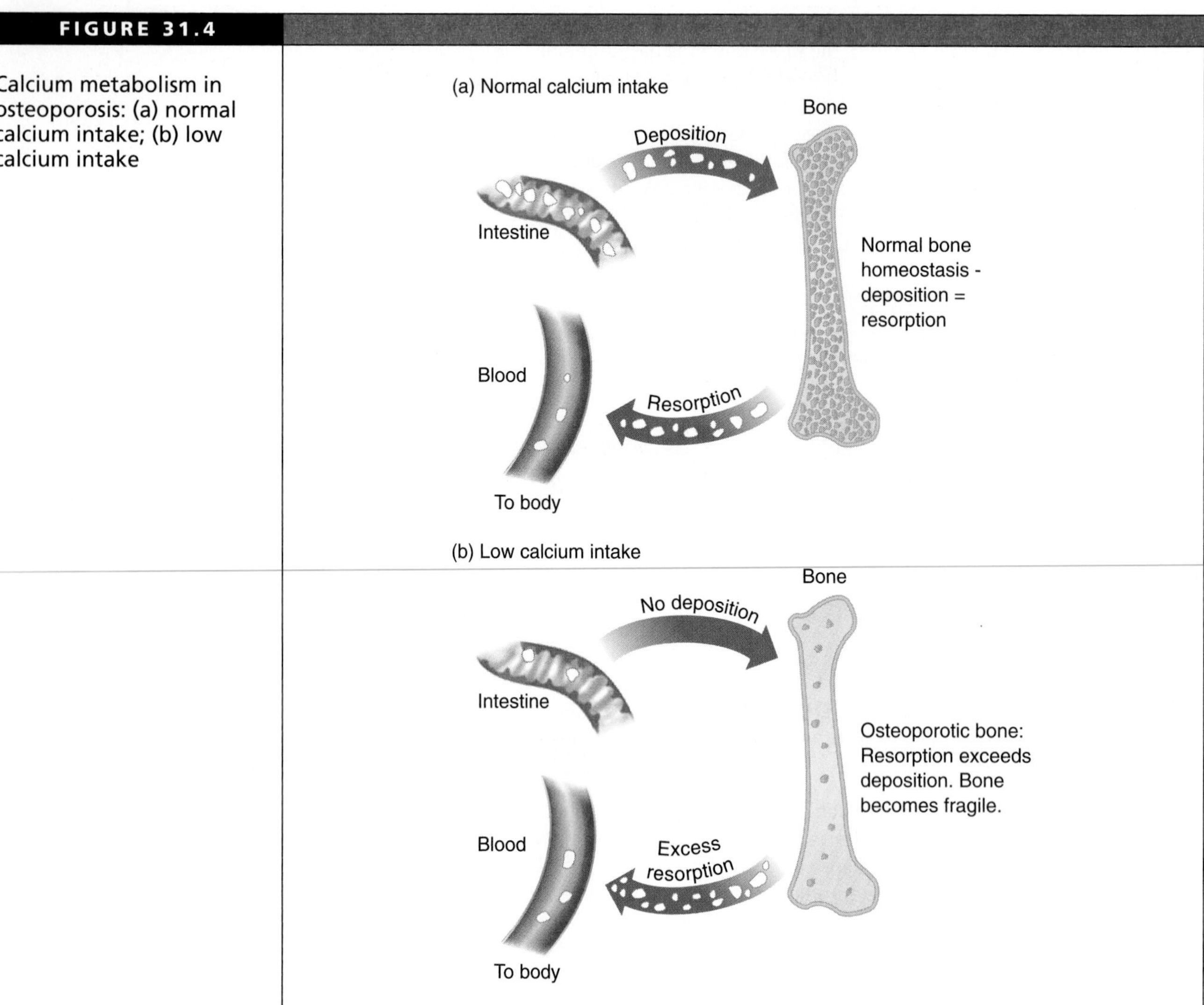

Hormonal Agents

Until recently, hormone replacement therapy (HRT) with estrogen was one of the most common treatments for osteoporosis in postmenopausal women. Because of increased risks of uterine cancer, thromboembolic disease, breast cancer, and other chronic disorders, the use of HRT in treating osteoporosis is no longer recommended. Additional information on HRT and the effects of estrogen may be found in Chapter 30.

Calcitonin

Calcitonin, a natural product obtained from salmon, is approved for the treatment of osteoporosis in women who are more than 5 years postmenopause. It is available by nasal spray or subcutaneous injection. Calcitonin increases bone density and reduces the risk of vertebral fractures. Side effects are generally minor; the nasal formulation may irritate the nasal mucosa, and allergies are possible. Parenteral forms may produce nausea and vomiting. In addition to treating osteoporosis, calcitonin is indicated for Paget's disease and hypercalcemia.

Selective Estrogen-Receptor Modulators

Selective estrogen-receptor modulators (SERMs) bind to estrogen receptors and comprise a relatively new class of drugs used in the prevention and treatment of osteoporosis. SERMs may

TABLE 31-4 Bone Resorption Inhibitor Drugs

DRUG	ROUTE AND ADULT DOSE	REMARKS
HORMONAL AGENTS		
calcitonin–human (Cibacalcin); calcitonin–salmon (Calciman; Miacalcin)	Paget's disease: subcutaneous; human, 0.5 mg daily; subcutaneous/IM salmon, 100 units daily. Hypercalcemia: subcutaneous/IM salmon, 4 units/kg bid	Used commonly for hypercalcemia and Paget's disease
Pr raloxifene hydrochloride (Evista)	PO 60 mg daily	Selective estrogen-receptor modulator; mimics the effects of estrogen on bone
BISPHOSPHONATES		
alendronate sodium (Fosamax)	Osteoporosis treatment: PO 10 mg daily Osteoporosis prevention: PO 5 mg daily Paget's disease: PO 40 mg daily for 6 months	For osteoporosis and Paget's disease
Pr etidronate disodium (Didronel)	PO 5–10 mg/kg daily for 6 months or 11–20 mg/kg daily for 3 months	For Paget's disease
pamidronate disodium (Aredia)	IV 15–90 mg in 1000 ml NS or D_5W over 4–24 hours	For Paget's disease and moderate hypercalcemia of malignancy
risedronate sodium (Actonel)	PO 30 mg daily at least 30 minutes before the first drink or meal of the day for 2 months	For Paget's disease
tiludronate disodium (Skelid)	PO 400 mg daily taken with 6–8 ounces of water 2 hours before or after food for 3 months	For Paget's disease

be estrogen agonists or antagonists, depending on the specific drug and the tissue involved. For example, raloxifene (Evista) blocks estrogen receptors in the uterus and breast; thus, it has no estrogen-like proliferative effects on these tissues that might promote cancer. Raloxifene decreases bone resorption, thus increasing bone density and making fractures less likely. Like estrogen, it has a cholesterol-lowering effect.

Bisphosphonates

The most common drug class used to treat osteoporosis is the **bisphosphonates.** These drugs are structural analogs of pyrophosphate, a natural inhibitor of bone resorption. Bisphosphonates inhibit bone resorption by suppressing osteoclast activity, thereby increasing bone density and reducing the incidence of fractures. Examples include etidronate (Didronel), alendronate (Fosamax), tiludronate (Skelid), and pamidronate (Aredia), which is available as an injectable drug. Adverse effects include GI problems such as nausea, vomiting, abdominal pain, and esophageal irritation. Because these drugs are poorly absorbed, they should be taken on an empty stomach, as tolerated by the patient. Recent studies suggest that once-weekly dosing may give the same bone-density benefits as daily dosing because of these drugs' extended duration of action.

Concept Review 31.3

- What are the major drug therapies used for the treatment of osteoporosis?

DRUG PROFILE: Estrogen-Receptor Modulator: Pr *Raloxifene (Evista)*

Actions and Uses:

Raloxifene is a selective estrogen-receptor modulator (SERM). It decreases bone resorption and increases bone mass and density by acting through the estrogen receptor. Raloxifene is primarily used for the prevention of osteoporosis in postmenopausal women. This drug also reduces serum total cholesterol and LDL (low-density lipoprotein) without lowering HDL (high-density lipoprotein) or triglycerides.

Adverse Effects and Interactions:

Common side effects are hot flashes, migraine headache, flulike symptoms, endometrial disorder, breast pain, and vaginal bleeding. Patients should not take cholesterol-lowering drugs or estrogen replacement therapy concurrently with this medication.

Use with estrogen is not recommended. Absorption is reduced by cholestyramine.

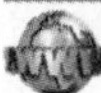
See the Companion Website for a Nursing Process Focus specific to this drug.

DRUG PROFILE: Bisphosphonate: Pr *Etidronate (Didronel)*

Actions and Uses:

Bisphosphonates are a common treatment for postmenopausal osteoporosis. Etidronate is available in oral and IV forms and has the capability of strengthening bones with continued use by slowing bone resorption. Effects begin 1 to 3 months after therapy starts and may continue for months after therapy is stopped. This drug lowers serum alkaline phosphatase, the enzyme associated with bone turnover, without causing major adverse effects. Etidronate is also used for Paget's disease and to treat hypercalcemia due to malignancy.

Adverse Effects and Interactions:

Common side effects of etidronate are diarrhea, nausea, vomiting, esophageal irritation, and a metallic or altered taste perception. Pathologic fractures may occur if the drug is taken longer than 3 months. Calcium supplements may decrease absorption of etidronate; therefore, use of these drugs together should be avoided. Food-drug interactions are common. Milk and other dairy products and medications, such as calcium, iron, antacids, and other mineral supplements, must be reviewed before beginning bisphosphonate therapy because they have the potential to decrease the effectiveness of bisphosphonates.

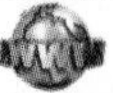
See the Companion Website for a Nursing Process Focus specific to this drug.

PAGET'S DISEASE

Paget's disease, or osteitis deformans, is a chronic, progressive condition characterized by enlarged and abnormal bones. With this disorder, the processes of bone resorption and bone formation occur at a high rate. Excessive bone turnover causes the new bone to be weak and brittle, which may result in deformity and fractures. The patient may be asymptomatic or have only vague, nonspecific complaints for many years. Symptoms include pain of the hips and femurs, joint inflammation, headaches, facial pain, and hearing loss if bones around the ear cavity are affected. Nerves along the spinal column may be pinched in the compressed vertebrae.

Paget's disease is sometimes confused with osteoporosis because some of the symptoms are similar. In fact, medical treatments for osteoporosis are similar to those for Paget's disease. The cause of Paget's disease, however, is quite different. Blood levels of the enzyme alkaline phosphatase are elevated because of the extensive bone turnover. Detection of this enzyme in the blood often provides early confirmation of the disease. Calcium blood levels are also increased. The symptoms of Paget's disease can be treated successfully when diagnosis is made early in the disease. If the diagnosis is made late in the disease's progression, permanent skeletal abnormalities may develop, and other disorders may appear, including arthritis, kidney stones, and heart disease.

31.10 Treatment for Paget's disease includes bisphosphonates and calcitonin.

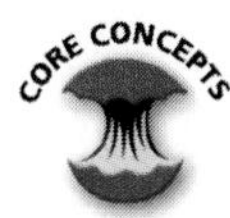

Bisphosphonates are drugs of choice for the pharmacotherapy of Paget's disease. Therapy is usually cyclic: bisphosphonates are administered until serum alkaline phosphatase levels return to normal; then a drug-free period of several months follows. When serum alkaline phosphatase levels become elevated, therapy is begun again. The pharmacological goals are to slow the rate of bone reabsorption and encourage the deposition of strong bone. Calcitonin nasal spray is used as an option for patients who cannot tolerate bisphosphonates. Surgery may be indicated in cases of severe bone deformity, degenerative arthritis, or fracture. Patients with Paget's disease should receive adequate, daily dietary intake of calcium and vitamin D. Sufficient exposure to sunlight is also important.

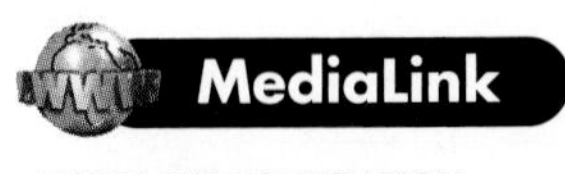

THE PAGET FOUNDATION

Concept Review 31.4

- Identify two important disorders characterized by weak and fragile bones.

ARTHRITIC DISORDERS AND GOUT

Arthritis is a general term meaning inflammation of a joint. There are several types of arthritis, each having somewhat different characteristics based on the etiology. **Osteoarthritis (OA)** is a degenerative, age-onset disease, in which the cartilage at articular joint surfaces wears away. **Rheumatoid arthritis (RA)** is a systemic autoimmune disorder that causes disfigurement and inflammation of multiple joints and usually occurs at an earlier age than osteoarthritis. **Gout,** a form of acute arthritis, is a metabolic disorder caused by the accumulation of uric acid in the bloodstream or joint cavities that causes joint pain. Because joint pain is common to all three disorders, analgesics and anti-inflammatory drugs are important components of pharmacotherapy. A few additional drugs are specific to the particular joint pathology.

osteo = *bone*
rheuma = *watery discharge*
toid = *associated*
arthr = *joint*
itis = *associated disease, often linked with inflammation*

31.11 Analgesics and anti-inflammatory drugs are important components of pharmacotherapy for osteoarthritis.

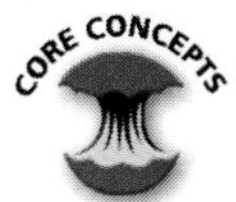

Osteoarthritis is the most common type of arthritis and produces symptoms of localized pain and stiffness, joint and bone enlargement, and limitations in movement. It is not accompanied by the degree of inflammation associated with other forms of arthritis. The cause of osteoarthritis is thought to be excessive wear and tear of weight-bearing joints; the knee, spine, and hip are particularly affected. Many consider this disorder to be a normal part of the aging process.

The goals of pharmacotherapy for osteoarthritis include reduction of pain and inflammation. The COX-2 inhibitors (see Chapter 21) were once the preferred therapy for osteoarthritis, but in 2004 their safety and effectiveness came under review by the FDA, and several of the class were removed from the market.

Topical medications (capsaicin cream and balms), NSAIDs (including aspirin), acetaminophen, and tramadol (Ultram) are valuable for treatment of pain associated with osteoarthritis. In acute cases, intra-articular glucocorticoids may be used on a temporary basis.

A new type of drug therapy for patients with moderate osteoarthritis who do not respond adequately to analgesics is now available. Sodium hyaluronate (Hyalgan) is a preparation of a chemical normally found in high amounts within synovial fluid. Administered by injection directly into the knee joint, this drug replaces or supplements the body's natural hyaluronic acid that deteriorated due to the condition of osteoarthritis. Treatment consists of 3 to 5 injections at the rate of 1 per week. By coating the articulating cartilage surface, Hyalgan helps to provide a barrier, thus preventing friction and further injury to the joint. Patients should be told that side effects can include pain and/or swelling at the injection site and that they must avoid strenuous activities for approximately 48 hours after an injection.

Rheumatoid arthritis (RA) is the second most common form of arthritis and has an autoimmune etiology. In RA, **autoantibodies,** called *rheumatoid factors,* activate complement and

auto = *self-directed*
anti = *against*
bodies = *things*

draw leukocytes into an area where they attack normal cells. This results in ongoing injury and formation of inflammatory fluid within the joints. Joint capsules, tendons, ligaments, and skeletal muscles may also be affected. Unlike OA, which causes local pain in affected joints, patients with RA may develop systemic manifestations that include infections, pulmonary disease, pericarditis, abnormal numbers of blood cells, and symptoms of metabolic dysfunction such as fatigue, anorexia, and weakness.

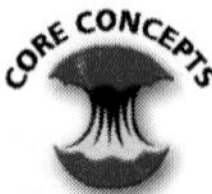

31.12 Glucocorticoids, immunosuppressants, and disease-modifying drugs are additional therapies used to treat rheumatoid arthritis.

Pharmacotherapy for RA includes the same classes of analgesics and anti-inflammatory drugs used to treat osteoarthritis. Additional drugs are sometimes prescribed to control the severe inflammation and the immune aspects of the disease.

Additional therapies, usually prescribed as a second course of treatment after analgesics and anti-inflammatories, include the following:

- Glucocorticoids
- Disease-modifying drugs: hydroxychloroquine (Plaquenil), gold salts, sulfasalazine (Azulfidine), D-penicillamine (Cuprimine)
- Immunosuppressants: methotrexate (Rheumatrex), leflunomide (Arava), azathioprine (Imuran), cyclosporine (Neoral), cyclophosphamide (Cytoxan)
- Tumor necrosis factor blockers: etanercept (Enbrel), infliximab (Remicade)

These additional therapies may require several months of treatment before maximum therapeutic effects are achieved. Because many of these drugs can be toxic, patients should be closely monitored. Adverse effects vary depending on the type of drug. These agents are shown in Table 31.5.

Nonpharmacological therapies for the pain of arthritis are common. The use of nonimpact and passive range-of-motion (ROM) exercises to maintain flexibility along with rest is encour-

TABLE 31.5 Disease-Modifying Drugs for Rheumatoid Arthritis

DRUG	ROUTE AND ADULT DOSE	REMARKS
auranofin (Ridaura)	PO 3–6 mg daily; may increase up to 3 mg tid after 6 months	Gold salt
aurothioglucose (Gold thioglucose, Solganal)	IM 10 mg wk 1, 25 mg wk 2; then 50 mg/wk to a cumulative dose of 1 g	Gold salt
azathioprine (Imuran)	PO 0.5–1.0 mg/kg/day (max: 2.5 mg/kg/day)	Immunosuppressant and anti-inflammatory; may cause bone marrow depression
gold sodium thiomalate (Myochrysine)	IM 10 mg wk 1, 25 mg wk 2; then 25–50 mg/wk to a cumulative dose of 1 g	Gold salt; expected side effects with administration: flushing, dizziness, fainting
Pr hydroxychloroquine sulfate (Plaquenil Sulfate)	PO 400–600 mg daily	Also for acute malaria and malaria suppression
leflunomide (Arava)	PO loading dose 100 mg/day for 3 days; maintenance dose 10–20 mg daily	Immunomodulator with anti-inflammatory effects, may cause Stevens-Johnson syndrome
methotrexate (Mexate, Folex)	PO 2.5–5 mg q12h for 3 doses each week	Folic acid blocker; antineoplastic and immunosuppressant; may cause liver toxicity, sudden death, and pulmonary fibrosis
penicillamine (Cuprimine, Depen)	PO 125–250 mg daily (max: 1–1.5 g/day)	Also used to promote increased excretion of excess copper; used to limit urinary excretion of cystine
sulfasalazine (Azulfidine)	PO 250–500 mg daily (max: 8 g/day)	Also for ulcerative colitis

DRUG PROFILE: Rheumatoid, Antimalarial: Pr *Hydroxychloroquine Sulfate (Plaquenil)*

Actions and Uses:

Hydroxychloroquine is prescribed for rheumatoid arthritis and lupus erythematosus in patients who have not responded well to other anti-inflammatory drugs. This agent relieves the severe inflammation characteristic of these disorders. For full effectiveness, hydroxychloroquine is most often prescribed with salicylates and glucocorticoids. This drug is also used for prophylaxis and treatment of malaria.

Adverse Effects and Interactions:

Adverse symptoms include blurred vision, GI disturbances, loss of hair, headache, and mood and mental changes. Hydroxychloroquine has possible ocular effects that include blurred vision, photophobia, diminished ability to read, and blacked out areas in the visual field.

Antacids with aluminum and magnesium may prevent absorption. This drug interferes with the patient's response to the rabies vaccine. Hydroxychloroquine may increase the risk of liver toxicity when administered with drugs that are toxic to the liver. Alcohol use should be eliminated during therapy. It also may lead to increased digoxin levels.

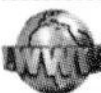

See the Companion Website for a Nursing Process Focus specific to this drug.

Fast Facts Arthritis

- Between 20 and 40 million patients in the United States are affected by osteoarthritis.
- After age 40, more than 90% of the population has symptoms of osteoarthritis in major weight-bearing joints. After 70 years of age, almost all patients have symptoms of osteoarthritis.
- Of the world's population, 1% has rheumatoid arthritis, which most often affects patients between 30 and 50 years of age. Women are 3 to 5 times more likely to develop rheumatoid arthritis than men.
- Between 1% and 3% of the U.S. population is affected by gout. Most of the patients are men between the ages of 30 and 60. Most women are affected after menopause.

aged. Splinting may help keep joints positioned correctly and relieve pain. Other therapies commonly used to relieve pain and discomfort include thermal therapies, meditation, visualization, distraction techniques, and massage therapy. Knowledge of proper body mechanics and posturing, provided by physical and occupational therapists, offer some benefit. Surgical techniques such as joint replacement and reconstructive surgery may be necessary when other methods are ineffective.

Concept Review 31.5

- Identify the major types of arthritis. What are the general differences between these disorders?

31.13 Drug therapy for gout requires agents that inhibit uric acid buildup.

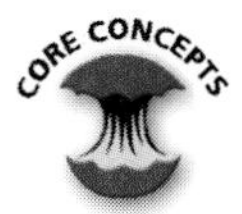

Gout is due to an accumulation of uric acid crystals that occurs when excretion of uric acid by the kidneys is reduced. Uric acid is the final breakdown product of DNA and RNA metabolism. One metabolic step that is important to the pharmacotherapy of this disease is the conversion of hypoxanthine to uric acid by the enzyme xanthine oxidase. An elevated blood level of uric acid is called *hyperuricemia.*

hyper = *elevated*
uric = *uric acid*
emia = *blood level*

Gout may be classified as primary or secondary. *Primary gout,* caused by genetic errors in uric acid metabolism, is most commonly observed in Pacific Islanders. *Secondary gout* is caused

TABLE 31.6 Uric Acid-Inhibiting Drugs for Gout and Gouty Arthritis

DRUG	ROUTE AND ADULT DOSE	REMARKS
allopurinol (Lopurin, Zyloprim)	PO (primary); 100 mg daily; may increase by 100 mg/wk (max: 800 mg/day) PO (secondary); 200–800 mg daily for 2–3 days or longer	For primary hyperuricemia, secondary hyperuricemia, and prevention of gout flare-up
Pr colchicine	PO 0.5–1.2 mg followed by 0.5–0.6 mg q1–2 h until pain relief (max: 4 mg/attack)	For acute gouty attack; may cause gastric upset at higher doses; IV form available
probenecid (Benemid, Probalan)	PO 250 mg bid for 1 wk; then 500 mg bid (max: 3 g/day)	For gout; also used as an adjunct for penicillin or cephalosporin therapy
sulfinapyrazone (Anturane)	PO 100–200 mg bid for 1 wk; then increase to 200–400 mg bid	For gout; also used for inhibition of platelet aggregation

by diseases or drugs that increase the metabolic turnover of nucleic acids or that interfere with uric acid excretion. Examples of drugs that may cause gout include thiazide diuretics, aspirin, cyclosporine, and alcohol (when ingested on a chronic basis). Conditions that can cause secondary gout include diabetic ketoacidosis, kidney failure, and diseases associated with a rapid cell turnover such as leukemia, hemolytic anemia, and polycythemia.

Acute gouty arthritis occurs when needle-shaped uric acid crystals accumulate in joints, resulting in red, swollen, and inflamed tissue. Attacks have a sudden onset, often occur at night, and may be triggered by diet, injury, or other stresses. Gouty arthritis most often occurs in the big toes, heels, ankles, wrists, fingers, knees, and elbows. About 90% of patients with gout are men.

Uric acid-inhibiting drugs block the accumulation of uric acid within the blood or uric acid crystals within the joints. The goals of gout pharmacotherapy are twofold: termination of acute attacks and prevention of future attacks. NSAIDs are the drugs of choice for treating the pain and inflammation of acute attacks. Indomethacin (Indocin) is an NSAID that has been widely used for acute gout.

The uric acid inhibitors (Table 31.6) such as colchicine, probenecid (Benemid), sulfinpyrazone (Anturane), and allopurinol (Lopurin) are also used for acute gout. Uric acid inhibitors block the accumulation of uric acid within the blood or uric acid crystals within the joints. When uric acid accumulation is blocked, symptoms associated with gout diminish. About 80% of the patients using uric acid inhibitors experience GI complaints such as abdominal cramping, nausea, vomiting, and/or diarrhea. Glucocorticoids are useful for the short-term therapy of acute gout, particularly when the symptoms are in a single joint and the medication is delivered intra-articularly.

DRUG PROFILE: Antigout Agent: Pr *Colchicine*

Actions and Uses:

Colchicine inhibits inflammation and reduces pain associated with gouty arthritis. It may be taken prophylactically for acute gout or in combination with other uric acid-inhibiting agents. Colchicine works by inhibiting the synthesis of subcellular microtubules, decreasing the movement of white blood cells into the inflammed area. It disrupts the accumulation of uric acid deposits and inhibits formation of a glycoprotein that is produced when white blood cells phagocytize the uric acid crystals.

Adverse Effects and Interactions:

Side effects such as nausea, vomiting, diarrhea, and GI upset are more likely to occur at the beginning of therapy. These side effects are related to disruption of microtubules responsible for cell proliferation. Colchicine may also directly interfere with the absorption of vitamin B_{12}.

Colchicine interacts with many drugs. For example, NSAIDs may increase GI symptoms and cyclosporine may increase bone marrow suppression. Erythromycin may increase colchicine levels. Phenylbutazone may increase the risk for blood disorders. Loop diuretics may decrease colchicine effects. Alcohol or products that contain alcohol may cause skin rashes and increased liver damage.

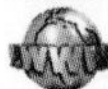
See the Companion Website for a Nursing Process Focus specific to this drug.

Prophylaxis of gout includes dietary management, avoidance of drugs that worsen gout, and treatment with antigout medications. Patients should avoid high-purine foods such as meat, legumes, alcoholic beverages, mushrooms, and oatmeal, because nucleic acids will be formed when they are metabolized. Prophylactic therapy with drugs that lower serum uric acid is used for patients who suffer frequent and acute gout attacks. Probenecid and sulfinpyrazone are *uricosuric* drugs that increase the excretion of uric acid by blocking its reabsorption in the kidney. Allopurinol blocks xanthine oxidase, thus inhibiting the formation of uric acid. Prophylactic therapy is used for patients who suffer frequent and acute gout attacks.

Concept Review 31.6

- Identify the major drug therapies for rheumatoid arthritis.

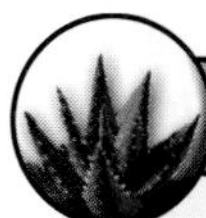

NATURAL ALTERNATIVES

Glucosamine and Chondroitin for Osteoarthritis

Glucosamine sulfate is a natural substance that is an important building block of cartilage. With aging, glucosamine is lost with the natural thinning of cartilage. As cartilage wears down, joints lose their normal cushioning ability, resulting in the pain and inflammation of osteoarthritis. Glucosamine sulfate is available as an OTC dietary supplement. Some studies have shown it to be more effective than a placebo in reducing mild arthritis and joint pain. It is claimed to promote cartilage repair in the joints. Although reliable long-term studies are not available, glucosamine is marketed as a safe and inexpensive alternative to prescription anti-inflammatory drugs.

Chondroitin sulfate is another dietary supplement claimed to promote cartilage repair. It is a natural substance that forms part of the matrix between cartilage cells. Chondroitin is usually combined with glucosamine in specific arthritis formulas. ■

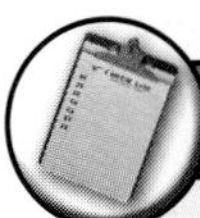

PATIENTS NEED TO KNOW

Patients taking antispasmodic drugs or drugs for bone or joint disorders need to know the following:

In General

1. When receiving treatment for problems with mobility, it often takes several weeks for effectiveness to begin. Follow the advice of a healthcare provider in order to achieve full therapeutic effect.

Regarding Antispasmodics

2. Most antispasmodic drugs produce side effects such as drowsiness and dizziness. Therefore, avoid CNS depressants and alcohol.

Regarding Bone-related Medications

3. When taking calcium or vitamin D supplements, be aware of the signs and symptoms of hypercalcemia. Check with the healthcare provider or pharmacist before taking supplements of any kind. In some cases, only proper diet and sunshine are needed for successful therapy.
4. Zinc-rich food products (nuts, seeds, tofu, and legumes) may interfere with calcium absorption. Calcium may react with some foods or interfere with the absorption of iron and bisphosphonates.
5. Be familiar with the risks and long-term effects of vitamin D therapy, corticosteroids, estrogen replacement therapy, and estrogen receptor modulators. Report any unfavorable symptoms such as bone pain, restricted mobility, inflammation, or fracture to a healthcare provider. Report any muscle pain, as muscles that have not been moved for a while may feel stiff and tender.
6. Know how to use a nasal pump if taking calcitonin by this method. Be aware that some vitamins may interfere with the pharmacological effects of calcitonin.
7. Some medications cause GI discomfort. Drugs like this can be taken after meals or with milk to minimize discomfort.

Regarding Antigout Medications

8. When taking some antigout medications, drink plenty of fluids to avoid kidney stones. To ensure proper fluid balance, monitor intake and output of fluids.
9. When taking probenecid, avoid taking aspirin for pain because it interferes with the drug's action. Take acetaminophen instead.
10. Be careful when taking sulfa drugs because they may produce unfavorable reactions. ■

CHAPTER REVIEW

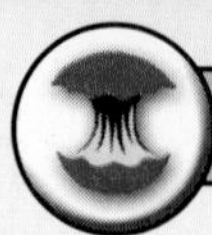

CORE CONCEPTS SUMMARY

31.1 Muscle spasms are caused by injury, overmedication, hypocalcemia, and debilitating disorders.

Muscle spasms, or involuntary contractions of a muscle or group of muscles, occur for many reasons, including overmedication with antipsychotic drugs, epilepsy, hypocalcemia, pain, and incapacitating neurologic disorders. Two types of muscle spasms are tonic and clonic.

31.2 Muscle spasms can be treated with nonpharmacological and pharmacological therapies.

After a thorough medical exam, nonpharmacological therapies such as immobilization, heat or cold, hydrotherapy, ultrasound, supervised exercises, massage, and manipulation may be used along with medications. Medications include analgesics, anti-inflammatory agents, and centrally acting skeletal muscle relaxants.

31.3 Many muscle relaxants treat muscle spasms by inhibiting upper motor neuron activity, causing sedation, or altering simple reflexes.

Skeletal muscle relaxants treat local spasms resulting from muscular injury and may be prescribed alone or in combination with medications that reduce pain and increase range of motion. These include centrally acting agents (affecting the brain and/or spinal cord) that have the potential to cause sedation and alter reflex activity.

31.4 Effective treatment for spasticity includes both physical therapy and medications.

Spasticity is a condition in which certain muscle groups remain in a state of contraction. Symptoms associated with spasticity include pain, exaggerated deep tendon reflexes, muscle spasms, scissoring, and fixed joints. Medications alone are not adequate in reducing the complications of spasticity.

31.5 Some drugs for spasticity provide relief by acting directly on muscle tissue, interfering with the release of calcium ions.

Direct-acting drugs produce an antispasmodic effect at the level of the neuromuscular junction. Drugs either affect calcium release directly from the muscle or they interfere with the release of the skeletal muscle neurotransmitter, acetylcholine.

31.6 Adequate levels of calcium, vitamin D, parathyroid hormone, and calcitonin are necessary for normal body processes.

One of the most important minerals in the body responsible for muscle contraction and bone formation is calcium. Calcium homeostasis is controlled by two important hormones, PTH and calcitonin. These hormones influence major body targets: the bones, kidneys, and GI tract. They direct the processes of bone resorption and bone deposition. Active vitamin D increases calcium absorption from the GI tract and helps to keep proper calcium balance in the body.

31.7 Hypocalcemia is a serious condition that requires immediate therapy.

Hypocalcemia, or lowered calcium levels in the bloodstream, is a sign of an underlying disorder; therefore, identifying its cause is essential. Signs of hypocalcemia are nerve and muscle excitability, muscle twitching, tremor, or cramping. These conditions are often reversed with calcium supplements. Calcium supplements consist of complexed and elemental calcium. Elemental calcium may be obtained from dietary sources.

31.8 Treatment for osteomalacia consists of calcium and vitamin D supplements.

Osteomalacia, called rickets in children, is a disorder characterized by softening of bones without alteration of basic bone structure. Drug therapy for children and adults consists of calcium supplements and vitamin D.

31.9 Treatment for osteoporosis includes calcitonin, estrogen-receptor modulator drugs, and bisphosphonates.

Osteoporosis, or weak bones caused by disrupted bone homeostasis, is the most common metabolic bone disease. The onset of menopause is the most frequent risk factor. Many drug therapies are available for this disorder including calcium and vitamin D therapy, estrogen replacement therapy, estrogen receptor modulators, statins, slow-release sodium fluoride, bisphosphonates, and calcitonin.

31.10 Treatment for Paget's disease includes bisphosphonates and calcitonin.

Paget's disease is a chronic progressive condition characterized by enlarged and abnormal bones. Although the cause of Paget's disease is different from that of osteoporosis, medical treatments are similar. Bisphosphonates are drugs of choice for the pharmacotherapy of Paget's disease.

31.11 Analgesics and anti-inflammatory drugs are important components of pharmacotherapy for osteoarthritis.

Arthritis is a general term meaning inflammation of the joints. The goals of pharmacotherapy for osteoarthritis include reduction of pain and inflammation.

31.12 Glucocorticoids, immunosuppressants, and disease-modifying drugs are additional therapies used to treat rheumatoid arthritis.

Rheumatoid arthritis (RA) is the second most common form of arthritis and has an autoimmune etiology. Pharmacotherapy for RA includes these same classes of analgesics and anti-inflammatory drugs plus additional therapies of glucocorticoids, disease-modifying drugs, immunosuppressants, and tumor necrosis factor blockers.

31.13 Drug therapy for gout requires agents that inhibit uric acid buildup.

Gout is caused by an accumulation of uric acid in the bloodstream. Gout may be classified as primary or secondary gout. Acute gouty arthritis occurs when needle-shaped uric acid crystals accumulate in the joints. The goals of gout pharmacotherapy include termination of acute attacks and prevention of future attacks with the use of uric acid inhibitors.

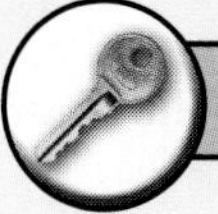

KEY TERMS

acute gouty arthritis (ah-CUTE GOW-ty are-THRYE-tis): condition where uric acid crystals quickly accumulate in the joints of the big toes, heels, ankles, wrists, fingers, knees, or elbows, resulting in red, swollen, or inflamed tissue / *page 616*

autoantibodies (AW-tow-ANN-tee-BAH-dees): proteins called rheumatoid factors released by B lymphocytes; these tear down the body's own tissue / *page 613*

bisphosphonates (bis-FOSS-foh-nayts): family of drugs that block bone resorption by inhibiting osteoclast activity / *page 611*

bone deposition: the opposition of bone resorption; the process of depositing mineral components into bone / *page 604*

bone resorption (ree-SORP-shun): process of bone demineralization or the breaking down of bone into mineral components / *page 604*

calcifediol (kal-SIF-eh-DYE-ol): intermediate form of vitamin D / *page 604*

calcitonin therapy (kal-sih-TOH-nin): treatment typically administered to women who cannot take estrogen or bisphosphonate therapy or for clients with Paget's disease / *page 610*

calcitriol (kal-si-TRY-ol): substance that is transformed in the kidneys during the second step of the conversion of vitamin D to its active form / *page 604*

cholecalciferol (KOH-lee-kal-SIF-er-ol): inactive form of vitamin D / *page 604*

dystonia (diss-TONE-ee-ah): muscle spasm characterized by abnormal, occasionally painful, movements or postures / *page 602*

gout (GOWT): metabolic disorder characterized by the accumulation of uric acid in the bloodstream or joint cavities / *page 613*

osteoarthritis (OA) (OSS-tee-oh-are-THRYE-tis): disorder characterized by degeneration of joints such as the fingers, spine, hips, and knees / *page 613*

osteomalacia (OSS-tee-oh-muh-LAY-shee-uh): rickets in children; disease characterized by softening of the bones without alteration of basic bone structure / *page 607*

osteoporosis (OSS-tee-oh-poh-ROH-sis): condition where bones become brittle and susceptible to fracture / *page 609*

Paget's disease: (PAH-jets): disorder characterized by weak, enlarged, and abnormal bones / *page 612*

rheumatoid arthritis (RA) (ROO-mah-toyd are-THRYE-tis): systemic autoimmune disorder characterized by inflammation of multiple joints / *page 613*

selective estrogen-receptor modulators (SERMs): drugs that directly produce an action similar to estrogen in body tissues; used for the treatment of osteoporosis in postmenopausal women / *page 610*

spasticity (spas-TISS-ih-tee): condition in which certain muscle groups remain in a continuous contracted state / *page 599*

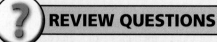

REVIEW QUESTIONS

The following questions are written in NCLEX-PN® style. Answer these questions to assess your knowledge of the chapter material, and go back and review any material that is not clear to you.

1. This medication lowers serum alkaline phosphatase.

1. Sulfasalzine (Azulfidine)
2. Etidoronate (Didronel)
3. Colchicine
4. Baclofen (Lioresal)

2. The patient on raloxifene (Evista) has had warfarin (Coumadin) ordered. The nurse understands the patient may experience:

1. Decreased effectiveness of raloxifene
2. Increased effectiveness of raloxifene
3. Increased clotting times
4. Decreased clotting times

3. The patient taking calcitriol should be assessed for:

1. Dysrhythmias
2. Hypocalcemia
3. Fluid overload
4. Flu-like symptoms

4. Which of the following statements demonstrates the patient with gout needs additional instructions?

1. "I will take my allopurinol as prescribed by my physician."
2. "I will stop having alcoholic beverages."
3. "I will avoid high purine foods."
4. "I will continue my aspirin therapy."

5. Because esophageal irritation can occur, this medication should not be used if the patient cannot remain in an upright position for 30 minutes after taking it.

1. HRT
2. Calcitonin
3. Alendronate (Fosamax)
4. Raloxifene (Evista)

6. This medication, when used intranasally, may cause irritation of the nasal mucosa.

1. Calcitonin
2. Vitamin D
3. Calcium
4. Raloxifene (Evista)

7. Your patient has had a total thyroidectomy. The nurse will assess for all of the following except:

1. Cramping
2. Confusion
3. Tingling of extremities
4. Bone pain

8. Adequate calcium levels in the body are maintained by:

1. Calcitriol
2. Parathyroid
3. Thyroid
4. Vitamin D

9. Calcitonin is not indicated for which of the following?

1. Paget's disease
2. Hypercalcemia
3. Hypocalcemia
4. Osteoporosis

10. The patient taking calcium channel blockers should not take:

1. Dantrolene sodium (Dantrium)
2. Calcifediol (Calderol)
3. Ergocalciferol (Deltalin)
4. Calcium gluconate (Kalcinate)

CASE STUDY QUESTIONS

For questions 1–5, please refer to the following case study, and choose the correct answer from choices 1–4.

Mr. Wung, a 75-year-old man, has persistent pain in his right hip and comes in for treatment. He explains that he has been taking enteric-coated aspirin for several weeks. He has also been experiencing muscle twitches (multiple, rapidly repeating contractions) in his right hamstring. The muscle twitches have not been severe, but he is concerned that his condition will worsen if he doesn't receive therapy. Lab values show slight hypocalcemia. The patient explains that he hasn't had any trouble with his diet. No abnormalities in bone structure or inflammatory symptoms are observed on examination.

1. Mr. Wung most likely has which of the following disorders?

1. Paget's disease
2. Gouty arthritis
3. Osteoarthritis
4. Rheumatoid arthritis

2. Which of the following medications will most likely be effective in treating Mr. Wung's disorder?

1. Calcitriol (Calcijex, Rocaltrol)
2. Azathioprine (Imuran)
3. Allopurinol (Lopurin, Zyloprim)
4. Raloxifene (Evista)

3. Symptoms of Mr. Wung's disorder are more correctly classified as:

1. Tonic spasms
2. Clonic spasms
3. Spasticity
4. Dystonia

4. Treatment with direct-acting antispamotics in this case would:

1. Improve Mr. Wung's condition.
2. Make Mr. Wung's condition worse.
3. Cause Mr. Wung to be sedated.
4. Both 2 and 3 are correct answers to this question.

5. In this case, the relief experienced by Mr. Wung from the enteric-coated aspirin is probably explained by its:

1. Anti-inflammatory properties.
2. Analgesic properties.
3. Protective coating in the stomach.
4. None of the above choices is correct; aspirin in this case is acting as a placebo.

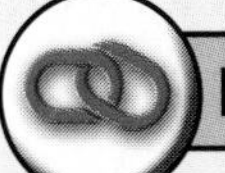

FURTHER STUDY

- Other causes of muscle spasms can include overmedication with antipsychotic drugs, which are discussed in Chapter 10.
- As discussed in Chapter 11, benzodiazepines inhibit both sensory and motor neuron activity by enhancing the effects of GABA.
- Acetylcholine is discussed in detail in Chapter 7.
- Additional information on HRT and the effects of estrogen may be found in Chapter 30.
- Drugs for relieving pain are discussed in Chapter 12.
- Antiinflammatory agents are presented in Chapter 21.

EXPLORE MEDIALINK www.prenhall.com/holland

Additional resources for this chapter can be found on the CD-ROM accompanying this textbook, and on the Companion Website. Click on Chapter 31 to select activities for this chapter.

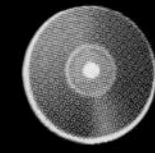

Mechanism in Action Animations:
- Cyclobenzaprine
- Calcitriol

Audio Glossary
Concept Review
NCLEX-PN® Review
Nursing in Action
Dosage Calculator

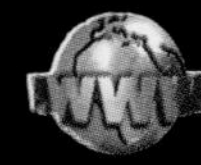

The National Institute of Arthritis and Musculoskeletal and Skin Diseases
Osteoporosis and Related Bone Diseases National Resource Center
National Osteoporosis Foundation
The Paget Foundation

CHAPTER

32 Drugs for Skin Disorders

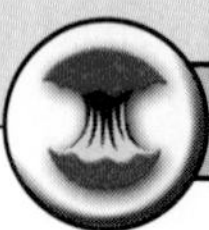

CORE CONCEPTS

32.1 Three layers of skin provide protection to the body.

32.2 The major causes of skin disorders are injury, aging, inherited factors, and other medical conditions.

32.3 Scabicides and pediculicides treat parasitic mite and lice infestation.

32.4 The goal of drug therapy for sunburn is to eliminate discomfort until healing occurs.

32.5 Problems of acne and rosacea are treated by a combination of OTC and prescription drugs.

32.6 Topical glucocorticoids are used mainly to treat dermatitis and related symptoms.

32.7 Several topical and systemic medications are used to treat psoriatic symptoms.

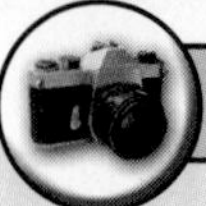

DRUG SNAPSHOT

The following drugs will be discussed in this chapter:

DRUG CLASSES	DRUG PROFILES
ANTIPARASITES	Pr lindane (Kwell)
DRUGS FOR SUNBURN AND MINOR IRRITATIONS	
Local anesthetics	Pr benzocaine (Solarcaine, others)
DRUGS FOR ACNE AND ROSACEA	
OTC agent	Benzoyl peroxide
Retinoids	Pr isotretinoin/13-cis-retinoic acid (Accutane)
Hormones	ethinyl estradiol
Antibiotics	
DRUGS FOR DERMATITIS AND ECZEMA	
Topical glucocorticoids	
DRUGS FOR PSORIASIS	
Topical glucocorticoids	
Topical immunomodulators	
Retinoids	
Systemic agents	

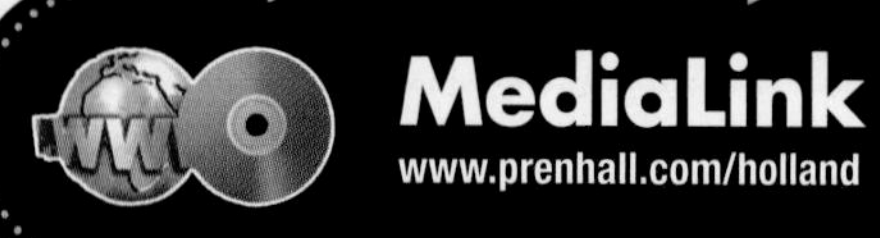

Interactive resources for this chapter can be found on the Companion Website. Click on Chapter 32 and "Begin" to select the activites for this chapter. For chapter-related animations, NCLEX-PN®-style questions, and an audio glossary, access the accompanying CD-ROM in this book.

OBJECTIVES

After reading this chapter, the student should be able to:

1. Identify important skin layers and explain how superficial skin cells must be replaced after they become damaged or lost.
2. Describe major symptoms associated with stress and injury to the skin versus those associated with a patient's changing age or health.
3. Identify important drug therapies for the following disorders, distinguishing between topical and systemic medications:
   - **a.** scabies (mites) and *Pediculus* (lice) infestation
   - **b.** sunburn, minor irritations, and insect bites
   - **c.** acne and acne-related disorders (blackheads, whiteheads, rosacea)
   - **d.** dermatitis (eczema, contact dermatitis, seborrheic dermatitis, stasis dermatitis)
   - **e.** psoriasis
4. Identify the major actions of the following types of drugs as they pertain to treatment of skin disorders: scabicides, pediculicides, topical anesthetics, antibiotics, retinoids, keratolytic agents, glucocorticoids, emollients, and psoralens.
5. Describe popular treatments used in conjunction with available drug therapies for skin disorders.

The integumentary system consists of the skin, hair, nails, sweat glands, and oil glands. The largest of all organs is the skin. Because of its large surface area, it normally provides an effective barrier between extreme conditions in the outside environment and the body's internal organs. At times, however, external conditions become too extreme or conditions within the body change, resulting in unhealthy skin. When this happens, either the body's natural defense system must try to correct the problem or therapy may be provided to improve the skin's condition. The relationship between the integumentary system and other body systems is depicted in Figure 32.1 ■.

The purpose of this chapter is to examine the broad scope of skin disorders and the medications used for skin therapy. Particular attention is given to drugs that are of direct benefit to lice and mite infestation, sunburn, acne, inflammation, and dry, scaly skin. Pharmacotherapy of these conditions provides the basis for a more complete understanding of the many drugs applied to the skin's surface.

32.1 Three layers of skin provide protection to the body.

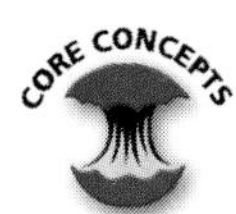

The skin has three major layers: the epidermis, dermis, and a subcutaneous layer called the hypodermis. Each layer is distinct in form and function and provides the basis for how drugs are injected or applied to the surface of the skin (Chapter 3). The most superficial skin layer is the epidermis. Depending on its thickness, the epidermis has either four or five sublayers. The strongest and outermost sublayer is the stratum corneum, or horny layer. It is called this because of the abundance of the protein keratin, also found in the hair, hooves, and horns of many vertebrate mammals. Not every part of the skin has a large amount of keratin—only those areas that are subject to mechanical stress, for example, the soles of the feet and the palms of the hands.

The deepest sublayer of the epidermis is the stratum germanitivum. It supplies the epidermis with new cells after older, superficial cells have been damaged or lost by normal wear. Cells must migrate over their lifetime to the outermost layers of the skin, where they eventually fall off. As these cells are pushed to the surface, they are flattened and covered with a water-insolube material, forming a protective seal. The average time it takes for a cell to move from the germanitivum layer to the outer body surface is about 3 weeks. Specialized cells within the deeper layers of the epidermis celled *melanocytes* secrete the dark pigment melanin, which offers a degree of protection from the sun's ultraviolet rays.

The next major layer of skin, the dermis, is made up of dense, irregular connective tissue, named this way because of its irregular arrangement of thick protein fibers. The dermis provides a foundation for the epidermis and appendages such as hair and nails. Most receptor nerve endings, sweat glands, oil glands, and blood vessels are found within the dermis.

FIGURE 32.1

The integumentary system

Endocrine system
Hormones influence glandular activity, calcium homeostasis, and skin health.

Nervous system
Emotions affect skin coloration. The skin is a sensory organ.

Muscular system
The skin and muscles are important for proper body movement and expression.

Cardiovascular system
The blood carries oxygen and carbon dioxide, factors that influence skin health and coloration.

Lymphatic system
Helps fight diseases and infections of the skin.

Respiratory system
The lungs provide oxygen to all cells in the body.

Digestive system
Proper nutrition is important for healthy skin.

Skeletal system
The bones are a storage site for calcium, an important mineral connected with vitamin D function.

Urinary system
The accumulation of toxic substances in the bloodstream will affect the skin adversely.

For all systems
The skin forms a protective barrier against hazardous conditions.

Reproductive system
The skin covers external genitalia. Sex hormones influence skin health.

The integumentary system (skin) and how the other body systems affect it

The deepest of the skin layers is the subcutaneous layer, or hypodermis. This layer is composed mainly of adipose tissue or fat that cushions, insulates, and provides a source of energy for the body. The hypodermis is involved with the maintenance of body homeostasis, temperature regulation, and metabolism.

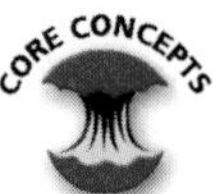

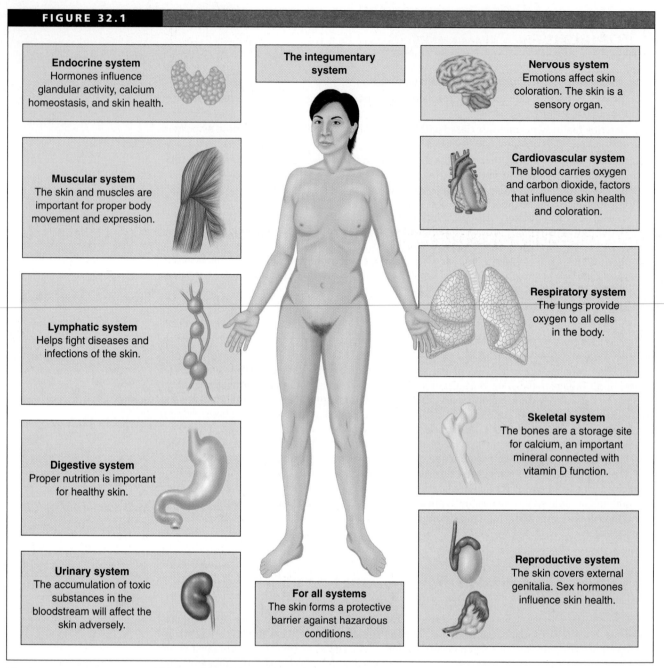

32.2 The major causes of skin disorders are injury, aging, inherited factors, and other medical conditions.

prur = *itching*
itus = *condition*

Skin that is dry, cracked, scaly, or worn represents a disturbance in the outermost skin layer. **Pruritus,** or itching, is a symptom often associated with dry, scaly skin, or it may be a symptom of infestation with mites and lice. The thick, horny layer is designed to protect the skin and keep it from drying out.

Some forceful or noxious stresses may damage deeper layers of the epidermis. When this happens, the role of the germanitivum layer is to replace any skin that might be lost or damaged due to special stresses.

Burns are a unique type of stress that may affect all layers of the skin. They are classified according to the degree of skin damage. First-degree burns affect only the outer layers of the epidermis, are characterized by redness, and are analogous to sunburn. Second-degree burns affect most of the epidermis and part of the dermis, resulting in inflammation and blisters. Third-degree burns are full-thickness burns; all layers of the skin are damaged. With full-thickness burns, the skin cannot regenerate, and skin grafting is required.

Inflammation, a characteristic of burns and other traumatic disorders, occurs when damage to the skin is extensive. Signs accompanying inflammation include **erythema** or redness, irritation, and pain. Symptoms including bleeding, bruises, and infections may accompany trauma to deeper tissues. Common symptoms of stress or skin injury are shown in Table 32.1.

eryth = *red*
ema = *appears*

Not all skin disorders are associated with a stressful environment. Many common skin disorders are related to inherited factors or the normal aging process. Sometimes the skin may appear unhealthy because of another medical condition, or, in some cases, the reason for skin irritation may be unclear and indirect. Common symptoms associated with a range of conditions are shown in Table 32.2.

As shown in Table 32.3, the reasons for skin conditions are many. They can be grouped based on whether they are infectious disorders, inflammatory disorders, or cancer-related disorders.

Although there are many skin disorders, a limited number are less debilitating and require only intermittent drug therapy. A few irritating disorders are of particular importance to patients who require healthcare on a walk-in basis. Examples include lice infestation, sunburn with minor irritation, and acne. Eczema, dermatitis, and psoriasis are more serious disorders requiring therapy for a longer time. Figure 32.2 ■ shows examples of regions in the body where irritating symptoms are most likely to occur.

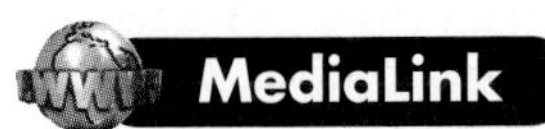

NATIONAL INSTITUTE OF ALLERGIES AND INFECTIOUS DISEASES

TABLE 32.1 Symptoms Associated with Stress or Injury to the Skin

SYMPTOM	DESCRIPTION
blisters and calluses	Improperly fitting shoes or clothing may cause mechanical stress and abrasion leading to these symptoms.
bruises, scrapes, and small-impact injuries	Increased physical activity sometimes wears away at the skin and results in minor skin damage.
crusty and cracked areas	These may be caused by lack of moisture, extremely dry conditions, or hot temperatures; areas affected by lack of moisture include the lips, corners of the mouth, nose, between the fingers and toes, and joint areas.
cuts, abrasions, and larger wounds	These signs may accompany more dramatic stress, such as sudden trauma or serious accidental injury.
infections and infestations	There are many types of bacterial, fungal, parasitic, and viral infections that occur throughout the body; ticks, lice, and mites are common problems associated with hairy skin.
inflammation and redness	Tissue damage almost always results in inflammation; other signs may also accompany inflammation as with some allergies, drugs, insect bites, stings, and plant toxins.
irritated areas	Burning and itching are common symptoms of irritated skin; many chemical agents (for example, household or industrial detergents, greases, and volatile organic agents) may cause skin irritation.
rash	Exposure to wet conditions for long periods may cause rash; examples are an infant's wet diaper or someone staying in a wet bathing suit for too long.
sores and lesions	Lack of attention to an area of the body for a long time may cause unhealthy skin, as occurs in elderly, bedridden patients or those who are wheelchair-bound.
sunburn	The sun's hazardous rays may damage the skin; also, prolonged sun exposure may cause some types of skin cancer.

TABLE 32.2 Signs and Symptoms Associated with a Patient's Changing Health, Age, or Weakened Immune System

SYMPTOM	DESCRIPTION
delicate skin, wrinkles, and hair loss	Many degenerative changes occur in the skin; some are found in elderly patients; others are genetically related (fragile epidermis, wrinkles, reduced activity of oil and sweat glands, male pattern baldness, poor blood circulation); hair loss may also be linked to some medical procedures; for example, radiation and chemotherapy.
discoloration of the skin	Discoloration is often a useful sign of another medical disorder (for example, anemia, cyanosis, fever, jaundice, and Addison's disease); some medications have photosensitive properties, making a patient's skin sensitive to the sun and causing erythema.
scales, patches, and itchy areas	Some symptoms may be related to a combination of genetics, stress, and immunity other symptoms may be related to a fast turnover of skin cells; some symptoms develop for unknown reasons.
seborrhea/oily skin and bumps	This condition is usually associated with a younger age group; examples include cradle cap in infants and an oily face, chest, arms, and back in teenagers and young adults; pustules, cysts, papules, and nodules represent lesions connected with oily skin.
tumors	Tumors may be genetic or may occur because of exposure to harmful agents or conditions.
warts, skin marks, and moles	Some skin marks are congenital; others are acquired or may be linked to environmental factors.

TABLE 32.3 Classification of Skin Disorders

DISORDER	EXAMPLE
infectious disorders	Bacterial infections such as boils, impetigo, infected hair follicles; fungal infections such as ringworm, athlete's foot, jock itch, nail infection; parasitic infections such as mosquito bites, ticks, mites, lice; viral infections such as cold sores, fever blisters (herpes simplex), chickenpox, warts, shingles (herpes zoster), measles (rubeola), and German measles (rubella). (See Chapter 22 for information on anti-infectives.)
inflammatory disorders	Injury and exposure to the sun such as sunburn and other environmental stresses; disorders marked by a combination of overactive glands, increased hormone production, or infection such as acne, blackheads, whiteheads, rosacea; disorders marked by itching, cracking, and discomfort such as eczema (atopic dermatitis), other forms of dermatitis (contact dermatitis, seborrheic dermatitis, stasis dermatitis), and psoriasis.
skin cancers	There are several types of malignant skin cancers: squamous cell carcinoma, basal cell carcinoma, and malignant melanoma. Malignant melanoma is the most dangerous. Other types of cancer (benign type) include keratosis and keratoacanthoma.

Fast Facts Skin Disorders

- An estimated 3 million people with new cases of lice infestation are treated each year in the United States.
- Nearly 17 million people in the United States have acne, making it the most common skin disease.
- More than 15 million people in the United States have symptoms of dermatitis.
- Ten percent of infants and young children experience symptoms of dermatitis. Roughly 60% of these infants continue to have symptoms into adulthood.
- Psoriasis affects 1–2% of the U.S. population. This disorder occurs in all age groups—adults mainly—affecting about the same number of men as women.

Concept Review 32.1

- Identify the three skin layers protecting the body. Give examples of layers specifically affected by minor or major external stresses. What skin disorders are not related to the external environment? How would you categorize most skin disorders?

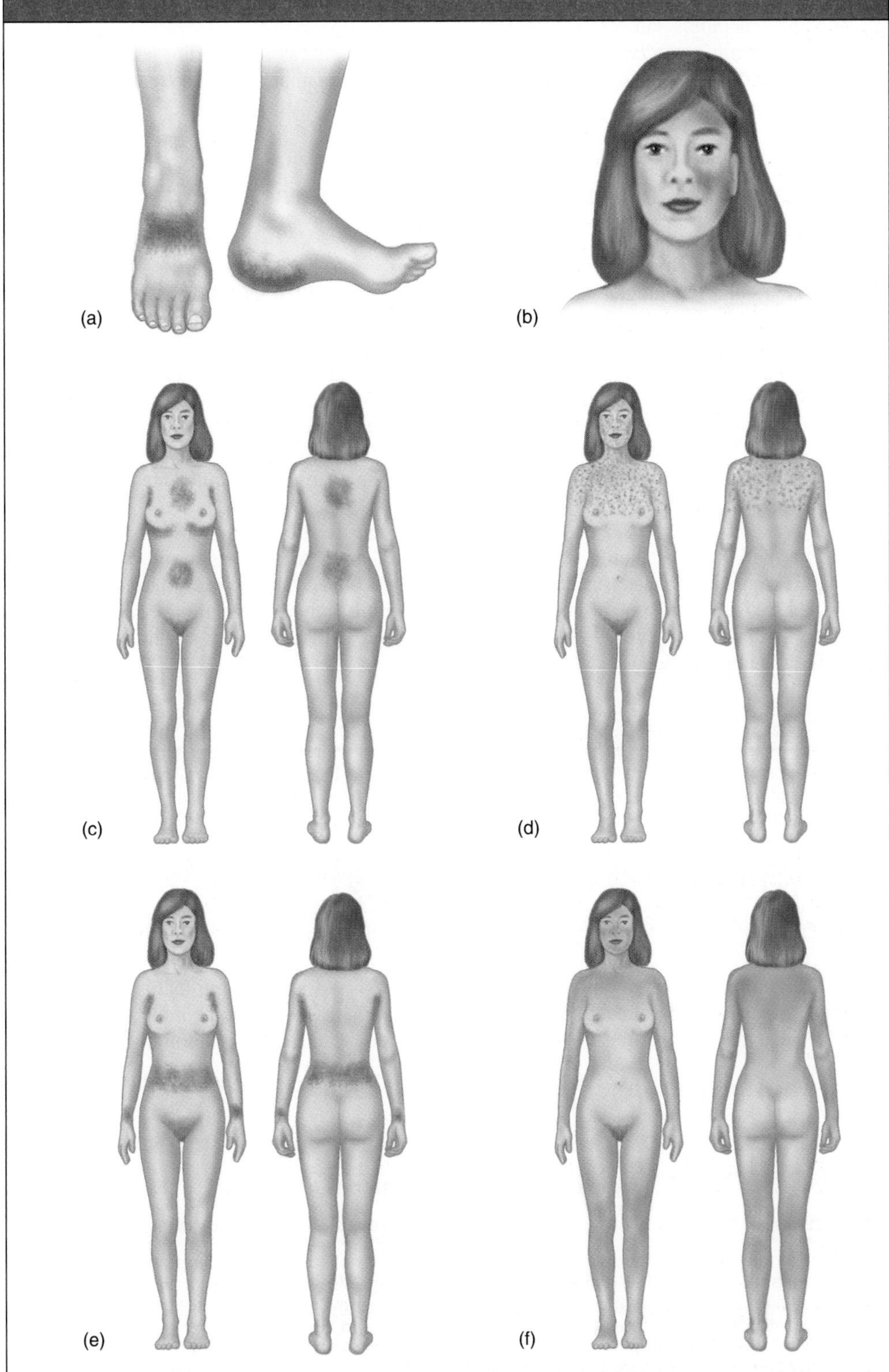

FIGURE 32.2

Anatomical distribution of common skin disorders: (a) contact dermatitis due to footwear or (b) cosmetics; (c) seborrheic dermatitis; (d) acne; (e) scabies; (f) sunburn

SKIN PARASITES

Common skin parasites include mites and lice. Mites cause a skin disorder called **scabies,** based on their scientific name, *Sarcoptes scabiei.* Scabies in an eruption of the skin caused by the female mite burrowing into the skin and laying eggs. This causes intense itching most commonly between the fingers, extremities, and around the trunk and pubic area. Scabies is readily spread among family members and sexual partners.

Lice, scientific name *Pediculus,* are another type of skin parasite readily passed on by infected clothing or close personal contact. Lice often infest the pubic area or the scalp and lay eggs that attach to body hairs.

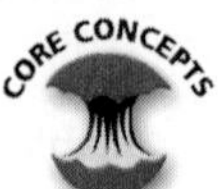

32.3 Scabicides and pediculicides treat parasitic mite and lice infestation.

Scabicides are pharmacological agents that kill mites; **pediculicides** kill lice. Either treatment may be effective for both types of parasites. The choice of drug often depends on where the infestation has occurred.

Three important drugs kill lice and mites. These are lindane (Kwell, Scabene), sometimes referred to by its chemical name, gamma benzene hexachloride; crotamiton (Eurax); and permethrin (Nix). Unlike lindane or crotamiton, permethrin is an insecticide and should be rinsed from the body within 10 minutes after being applied. Permethrin is most often applied to the pubic or scalp area. Patients should be cautioned against applying any lice or mite medication to the mouth, open skin lesions, or eyes.

Lice lay eggs called *nits.* Fine-toothed nit combs are useful in removing nits after the lice have been killed. Patients should comb the infested area after the hair has been dried. To ensure that drug therapy using lindane, crotamiton, or permethrin is effective, patients should inspect hair shafts daily for at least 1 week after treatment. Because nits may be present in bedding and other upholstery material, all material coming in close contact with the patient should be washed or treated with the medication.

Concept Review 32.2

- Name examples of medications used to treat mite and lice infestations. What precautions should be taken when using these medications?

SUNBURN AND MINOR IRRITATION

Sunburn, a common problem among the general public, is associated with factors such as light skin complexion and lack of proper sun protection. Nonpharmacological approaches to sun protection include the appropriate use of sunscreens, sunglasses, and sufficient clothing. Limiting the

DRUG PROFILE: Antiparasitic, Scabicide: Pr *Lindane (Kwell)*

Actions and Uses:

Lindane for mites is marketed as a cream or lotion. Lindane for head lice is available as a shampoo. Lindane cream or lotion takes longer to produce its effect; therefore, it is usually left on the body for about 8 to 12 hours before rinsing. Lindane shampoo is usually applied and left on for at least 5 minutes before rinsing. Patient should be aware that penetration of the skin with mites causes itching, which lasts for up to 2 or 3 weeks even after the parasites have been killed. Thus, a persistent itch is not unusual. Lindane kills mites and lice by overstimulating their nervous system.

Adverse Effects and Interactions:

If lindane is accidentally ingested in high enough doses, symptoms may include restlessness, dizziness, tremors, or convulsions. If inhaled, lindane may cause headaches, nausea, vomiting, or irritation of the ears, nose, or throat. A substantial number of lice and mite strains have become resistant to lindane; therefore, one should check carefully over the course of several weeks to make sure the medication is working.

No clinically significant interactions have been established.

NURSING PROCESS FOCUS

Patients Receiving Lindane (Kwell)

ASSESSMENT

Prior to administration:

- Obtain complete health history including allergies, drug history, and possible drug interactions
- Assess vital signs
- Assess skin for presence of lice and/or mite infestation, skin lesions, raw or inflamed skin, and open cuts
- Obtain history of seizure disorders
- Obtain patient's age
- Assess pregnancy and lactation status
- Obtain social history of close contacts, including household members and sexual partners

POTENTIAL NURSING DIAGNOSES

- Deficient Knowledge, related to no previous contact with lice or mites or treatment
- Treatment Regimen Noncompliance, related to knowledge deficit, embarrassment
- Risk for Impaired Skin Integrity, related to lesions and itching

PLANNING: Patient Goals and Expected Outcomes

- Patient and significant others will be free of lice or mites and experience no reinfestation.
- Patient will express an understanding of how lice and mites are spread, proper administration of lindane, necessary household hygiene, and the need to notify household members, sexual partners, and other close contacts such as classmates of infestation.
- Skin will be intact and free of secondary infection and/or irritation.

IMPLEMENTATION

Interventions and (Rationales)	Patient Education/Discharge Planning
■ Monitor for presence of lice or mites. (This determines the effectiveness of drug therapy.)	Instruct patient and caregiver to: ■ Examine for nits on hair shafts; lice on skin or clothes, inner thigh areas, seams of clothes that come in contact with axilla, neckline, or beltline ■ Examine for mites between the fingers, on the extremities, in the axillary and gluteal folds, around the trunk, and in the pubic area
■ Apply lindane properly. (Proper application is critical to elimination of infestation.)	Instruct patient and caregiver: ■ To wear gloves during application, especially if applying lindane to more than one person, or if pregnant ■ That all skin lotions, creams, and oil-based hair products should be removed completely by scrubbing the whole body well with soap and water, and drying the skin prior to application ■ To apply lindane to clean and dry affected body area as directed, using no more than 2 oz per application ■ That eyelashes can be treated with the application of petroleum jelly twice a day for 8 days followed by combing to remove nits ■ To use fine-tooth comb to comb affected hair following lindane application to the hair and scalp; to treat all household members and sexual contacts simultaneously ■ To recheck affected hair or skin daily for 1 week after treatment
■ Inform patient and caregivers about proper care of clothing and equipment. (Contaminated articles can cause reinfestation.)	Instruct patient and caregiver to: ■ Wash all bedding and clothing in hot water, and to dry-clean all nonwashable items which came in close contact with patient ■ Clean combs and brushes with lindane shampoo and rinse thoroughly

EVALUATION OF OUTCOME CRITERIA

Evaluate the effectiveness of drug therapy by confirming that patient goals and expected outcomes have been met (see "Planning").

DRUG PROFILE: Local Anesthetic: 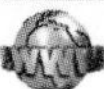 *Benzocaine (Solarcaine and Others)*

Actions and Uses:

Benzocaine provides temporary relief for pain and discomfort in cases of sunburn, pruritis, minor wounds, and insect bites. Its pharmacological action is caused by local anesthesia of skin receptor nerve endings. Preparations are also available to treat the skin and other areas such as the ear, mouth, throat, rectal, and genital areas.

Adverse Effects and Interactions:

Benzocaine should not be used for treatment of patients with open lesions, traumatized mucosal areas, or a history of drug sensitivity. Benzocaine may interfere with the activity of some antibacterial sulfonamides. Patients should use preparations only in areas of the body for which the medication is intended.

See the Companion Website for a Nursing Process Focus specific to this drug.

amount of time spent directly in the sun is essential to avoiding sunburn. Many dangers result from sun exposure, including eye injury and skin cancer. Some of these disorders may not appear until years after the exposure.

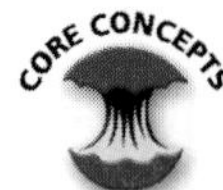

32.4 The goal of drug therapy for sunburn is to eliminate discomfort until healing occurs.

Drugs for sunburn and minor irritation include mild lotions and topical anesthetic medications. These are meant to provide temporary relief of painful symptoms.

Pharmacological treatments for sunburn may not be necessary. Remaining calm until the minor irritation passes is one common approach to mild sunburn. In cases where pharmacological intervention is necessary, topical anesthetics such as benzocaine (Solarcaine, others), dibucaine (Nupercainal), and tetracaine (Pontocaine) may be applied. Some of these medications may also provide minor relief from insect bites and pruritis. In cases of more lengthy sun exposure, more potent pain medications may be administered (Chapters 12 and 21), or tetanus toxoid might be administered to prevent infection (Chapter 22).

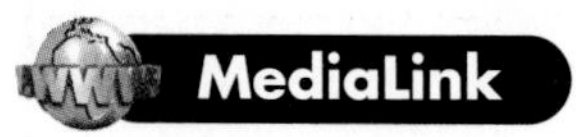

THE AMERICAN ACADEMY OF DERMATOLOGY

Concept Review 32.3

- What is the major purpose of drugs used to treat sunburn, insect bites, and related injuries? What major class of drugs would be used for this purpose?

ACNE AND ACNE-RELATED DISORDERS

sebor = *oil*
rhea = *flow*

Acne is a common condition found most often in adolescents and young adults. The disorder usually begins 1 or 2 years before puberty and is caused by overproductive oil glands or **seborrhea.** Acne is also caused by abnormal **keratinization** or development of the horny layer of the epithelial tissue. This activity results in blocked oil glands. Administration of androgens or testosterone-like hormones may cause extensive acne by increasing keratinization and the production of sebum (oil). Following this, the bacterium *Propionibacterium acnes* grows within gland openings and modifies the sebum into an acidic and irritating substance. As a result, small inflamed bumps appear on the surface of the skin.

Blackheads, or **open comedones,** are a type of acne in which sebum has plugged the oil gland, causing it to become black because of the presence of melanin granules. Whiteheads, or **closed comedones,** are a type of acne that develop just beneath the surface of the skin and appear white rather than black. In more severe cases of acne, deeper bumps called *nodules* may appear and become very painful because of the intense inflammation and pus found within pore pockets.

Another related skin disorder characterized by inflammation without pus is **rosacea.** Unlike pimples or **pustules,** the technical name given to pus-filled bumps, rosacea is characterized by small **papules** or inflammatory bumps without pus that swell, thicken, and become very painful. Associated with rosacea is swelling that occurs just beneath the surface of the skin. The face of a client with rosacea may take on a flushed appearance, particularly around the nose and cheek area. Rosacea is exacerbated by many factors including sunlight, stress, increased temperature, and agents that dilate facial blood vessels including alcohol, spicy foods, and warm beverages.

32.5 Problems of acne and rosacea are treated by a combination of OTC and prescription drugs.

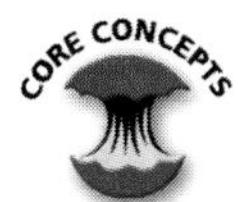

Most acne drugs slow down the turnover of skin cells, especially those surrounding pore openings. Some inhibit bacterial growth because they are combined with antibiotics such as doxycycline and tetracycline (Chapter 22). Some drugs must be used carefully because of their ability to dramatically reduce oil gland activity and skin cell turnover.

Important medications for acne-related disorders are summarized in Table 32.4. Benzoyl peroxide (Benzaclin, Benzamycin, and others) is the main OTC medication used to treat acne-related disorders. This medication may be dispensed as a lotion, cream, or gel and is available in various concentrations. Benzoyl peroxide decreases symptoms of acne by inhibiting bacterial growth and suppressing the turnover of skin cells at the pore's opening. Sometimes benzoyl peroxide is combined with antibiotics to directly fight bacterial infections.

TABLE 32.4 Drugs for Acne and Acne-related Disorders

DRUG	REMARKS
ACNE-RELATED DRUGS	
OTC MEDICATION—TOPICAL PREPARATION	
benzoyl peroxide (Benzaclin, Benzamycin, others)	Often combined with erythromycin or clindamycin to fight bacterial infection; refer to Chapter 22.
PRESCRIPTION MEDICATION—TOPICAL PREPARATIONS	
adapalene (Differin)	Retinoid-like compound used to treat acne formation.
azelaic acid (Alzelex)	For mild to moderate inflammatory acne.
sulfacetamide sodium (AK-Sulf, Cetamide)	For sensitive skin; sometimes combined with sulfur to promote peeling, as in rosacea; also used for conjunctivitis.
tretinoin (Retin-A, others)	Used to prevent clogging of pore follicles; also used for the treatment of acute promyelocytic leukemia and wrinkles.
PRESCRIPTION MEDICATION—ORAL PREPARATIONS	
doxycycline (Doryx, Vibramycin)	Antibiotic; refer to Chapter 22.
ethinyl estradiol (Estinyl)	Oral contraceptives are sometimes used for acne treatment; combination drugs may be helpful, for example, ethinyl estradiol plus norgestimate (Ortho Tri-Cyclen -28).
Pr isotretinoin/13-cis-retinoic acid (Accutane)	For acne with cysts or acne formed in small, rounded masses; category X drug.
tetracycline hydrochloride (Achromycin, Panmycin, Sumycin)	Antibiotic; refer to Chapter 22.

Retinoids are vitamin A-like compounds. Vitamin A provides improved resistance to bacterial infection by reducing oil production and the occurrence of clogged pores. Retinoids are not recommended during pregnancy because of possible harmful effects to the fetus. A common reaction to retinoids is sensitivity to sunlight.

Prescription medications for acne include adapalene (Differin), a retinoid-like compound, and related compounds such as azelaic acid (Alzelex), sulfacetamide (Klaren), and tretinoin (Retin-A). Tretinoin is sometimes used for wrinkle removal. When acne is particularly severe, resorcinol, salicylic acid, or sulfur may be used as additional treatments to promote shedding of old skin. These are called **keratolytic agents.**

kerato = *horny layer*
lytic = *loosening*

Some drugs may be taken in combination with or in lieu of other acne medications, including doxycycline (Vibramycin and others), tetracycline (Achromycin), and ethinyl estradiol (Estinyl, Feminone). Doxycycline and tetracycline are antibiotics. Ethinyl estradiol is an estrogen commonly found in birth control medications.

Concept Review 32.4

- What is the major purpose of drugs used to treat acne and related skin conditions? Give examples of both topical and systemic medications. Which medications are OTC, and which are prescription medications?

DERMATITIS AND ECZEMA

atopic = *out of place*

Eczema also called *atopic dermatitis,* is skin disorder with symptoms resembling an allergic reaction, including inflammation, itching, and rash. Long-term itching and scaling may cause the skin to appear thickened and leathery. Exposure to environmental irritants may make these symptoms worse. Other conditions, including stress, too little or too much moisture, and extreme tem-

DRUG PROFILE: Antiacne Agent; Retinoid: Pr *Isotretinoin/13-Cis-Retinoic Acid (Accutane)*

Actions and Uses:

The principal action of isotretinoin is regulation of skin growth and turnover. As cells from the germanitivum grow toward the skin's surface, skin cells are lost from the pore openings, and their replacement is slowed down. Isotretinoin also decreases oil production by reducing the size and number of oil glands. This drug is most often used in cases of cystic acne or severe keratinization disorders.

Adverse Effects and Interactions:

Isotretinoin is a highly toxic metabolite of **retinol** or vitamin A. Therefore it must be used carefully. Common effects are conjunctivitis (visual disturbance), dry mouth, inflammation of the lip, dry nose, increased serum concentrations of triglycerides (by 50 to 70%), bone and joint pain, and photosensitivity. Liver function, serum glucose, and serum triglyceride tests should be performed when taking isotretinoin. Vitamin A supplements should be avoided. Patients should not take this drug while pregnant.

Isotretinoin interacts with vitamin A supplements, which increase toxicity. In addition, tetracycline or minocycline use may increase risk of pseudotumor cerebri. Using it together with hypoglycemic agents may lead to loss of glycemic control as well as increased risk of cardiovascular disease because of elevated triglyceride levels. Blood levels of carbamazepine will be decreased if the two drugs are used together, which may lead to increased seizure activity.

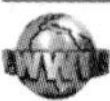
See the Companion Website for a Nursing Process Focus specific to this drug.

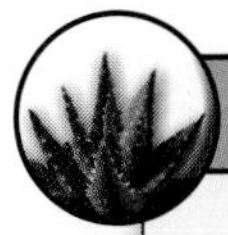

NATURAL ALTERNATIVES

Burdock Root for Acne and Eczema

Burdock root, *Arcticum lappa,* comes from a thick, flowering plant sometimes found on the roadsides of Britain and North America. It contains several active substances such as bitter glycosides and flavenoids, and it has a range of properties in the body: anti-infective, diuretic, mild laxative, and skin detoxifier. It is sometimes described as an attacker of skin disorders from within because it fights bacterial infections, reduces inflammation, and treats some stages of eczema, particularly the dry and scaling phases. Some claim that it is also effective against boils and sores.

In many cases, burdock root is combined with other natural products for a better range of effectiveness. Such products include sarsaparilla (*Smilax officinalis*), yellow dock (*Rumex crispus*), licorice root (*Glycyrrhiza glabra*), echinacea (*Echinacea purpurea*), and dandelion (*Taraxacum officinale*). ■

perature fluctuations, may worsen symptoms. Blisters and other lesions may also develop. In infants and small children, lesions usually begin on the face and progress to other parts of the body. The skin may become raw and infected from scratching.

Contact dermatitis is a delayed type of allergic reaction resulting from exposure to specific allergens, for example, perfume, cosmetics, detergents, latex, or jewelry. Accompanying the allergic reaction may be various degrees of cracking, bleeding, or small blisters.

Seborrheic dermatitis is a disorder caused by overactive oil glands. This condition is sometimes seen in newborns and in teenagers after puberty. Oily and scaly patches of skin appear in areas of the face, scalp, chest, back, or pubic area. Bacterial infection or dandruff may accompany these symptoms.

Stasis dermatitis is seen more commonly in older women. It is found primarily in the lower extremities. Redness and scaling may be observed in areas where venous circulation is impaired or where deep venous blood clots have formed.

32.6 Topical glucocorticoids are used mainly to treat dermatitis and related symptoms.

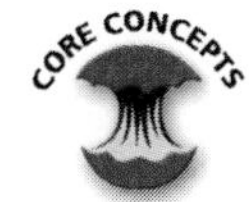

Topical glucocorticoids or corticosteroids are used in cases of **dermatitis** and eczema to treat symptoms of inflammation, burning, and pruritis. In conjunction with other medical therapies, topical corticosteroids are also used for the treatment of psoriasis.

dermat = *skin*
itis = *inflammation*

Topical glucocorticoids are the most effective treatment for dermatitis. As shown in Table 32.5, there are many varieties of glucocorticoids supplied at different levels of potency. Creams, lotions, solutions, gels, and pads are specially formulated to cross skin membranes. These medications are especially intended for the relief of local inflammation and itching. In cases of long-term use, however, adverse affects such as irritation, redness, and thinning of the skin membranes may occur. If absorption occurs, topical glucocorticoids may produce undesirable systemic effects including adrenal insufficiency, mood changes, serum imbalances, and bone defects as discussed in Chapter 21.

PSORIASIS

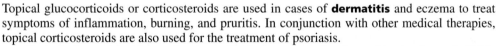

Psoriasis is a chronic disorder characterized by red patches of skin covered with flaky, silver-colored scales. The silver-colored scales are called *plaques.* The reason for the appearance of plaques is an extremely fast skin turnover rate. The skin reacts as if it has been injured but skin cells reach the surface much more quickly than usual, in about 4 days, which is 6 to 7 times faster than usual. The reason for this kind of reaction is not known, although scientists believe that it may be a genetic immune reaction. Plaques are ultimately shed from the skin's surface, while the underlying skin becomes inflamed and irritated.

TABLE 32.5 Topical Glucocorticoids Used to Treat Dermatitis and Related Symptoms

GENERIC NAME	TRADE NAMES
HIGHEST LEVEL OF POTENCY	
betamethasone	Benisone, Diprosone, Valisone
clobetasol	
diflorasone	Florone, Maxiflor, Psorcon
MIDDLE LEVEL OF POTENCY	
amcinonide	Cyclocort
desoximetasone	Topicort, Topicort LP
fluocinonide	Lidex, Lidex-E
halcinonide	Halog
mometasone	Elocon
triamcinolone	Aristocort, Kenalog, others
LOWER LEVEL OF POTENCY	
clocortilone	Cloderm
fluocinolone	Symalar
flurandrenolide	Cordran
fluticasone	Flonase
hydrocortisone	Hytone, Locoid, Westcort
LOWEST LEVEL OF POTENCY	
aclometasone	Aclovate
desonide	DesOwen, Tridesilon
dexamethasone	Decaderm, Decadron

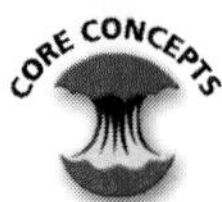

32.7 Several topical and systemic medications are used to treat psoriatic symptoms.

emolli = *to soften*
ent = *causing*

Because psoriatic symptoms may be extreme, numerous drugs are employed to soothe the patient's symptoms including **emollients,** topical glucocorticoids, and immunosuppressant medications.

Drugs used for the treatment of psoriasis include topical and systemic medications. Examples are provided in Table 32.6. One of the main treatments for psoriasis is topical glucocorticoids, which reduce the inflammation associated with fast skin turnover. Other agents applied topically are retinoid-like compounds such as calcipotriene (Dovonex) and tarzarotene (Tazorac). These drugs provide the same benefits as topical glucocorticoids, but they are much less toxic. Calcipotriene produces elevated levels of calcium in the bloodsteam, so this medication is not used on an extended basis.

Systemic medications for psoriasis include acitreten (Soriatane) and etretinate (Tegison). These drugs are taken orally to inhibit skin cell growth. Methotrexate (Amethopterin and others) produces similar effects in the body (Chapter 24). Other medications used for different disorders, but which provide relief of severe psoriatic symptoms, are hydroxyurea (Hydrea) and cyclosporine (Sandimmune, Neoral). Hydroxyurea is a sickle cell anemia medication. Cyclosporine is an immunosuppressive agent, discussed in Chapter 21.

Skin therapy techniques may be used with or without other psoriasis medications. These include various forms of tar treatment (coal tar) and a material called *anthralin.* Both substances are applied to the skin's surface. Tar and anthralin inhibit DNA synthesis and arrest abnormal cell growth.

UVB (ultraviolet B) and UVA (ultraviolet A) phototherapy are techniques used in cases of severe psoriasis. UVB therapy is less hazardous than UVA therapy. UVB light has a wavelength similar to sunlight; it reduces widespread lesions that normally resist topical treatments. With close supervision, this type of phototherapy can be administered at home. Keratolytic pastes are

TABLE 32.6 Drugs for Psoriasis and Related Disorders

DRUG	ROUTE AND ADULT DOSE	REMARKS
TOPICAL MEDICATIONS		
calcipotriene (Dovonex)	Topically to lesions once or twice daily	Synthetic form of vitamin D_3; may raise the level of calcium in the body to unhealthy levels
tazarotene (Tazorac)	Acne: Apply thin film to clean dry area daily; plaque psoriasis: apply thin film daily in the evening	Topical retinoid; less toxic than corticosteroids
SYSTEMIC MEDICATIONS		
acitretin (Soriatane)	PO 10–50 mg/day with the main meal	Retinoid; category X drug
cyclosporine (Sandimmune, Neoral)	PO 1.25 mg/kg bid (max: 4 mg/kg/day)	Immunosuppressant drug
etretinate (Tegison)	PO 0.75–1 mg/kg daily (max: 1.5 mg/kg/day)	Second-generation retinoid; category X drug
hydroxyurea (Hydrea)	PO 80 mg/kg q3 days or 20–30 mg/kg daily	Unlabeled use for psoriasis; also used for sickle cell anemia
methotrexate (Amethopterin, Folex, Rheumatrx)	PO 2.5–5 mg bid × 3 doses each week (max: 25–30 mg/week)	Also for rheumatoid arthritis and neoplasia

often applied between treatments. The second type of phototherapy is often referred to as PUVA therapy because **psoralens** are often administered in conjuntion with phototherapy. Psoralens are oral or topical agents that, when exposed to UV light, produce a photosensitive reaction. This reaction seems to provide benefit to the patient by reducing the number of lesions, but unpleasant side effects such as headache, nausea, and skin sensitivity still occur, limiting the effectiveness of this therapy. Immunosuppressant drugs such as cyclosporine are not used in conjunction with PUVA therapy because they increase the risk of skin cancer.

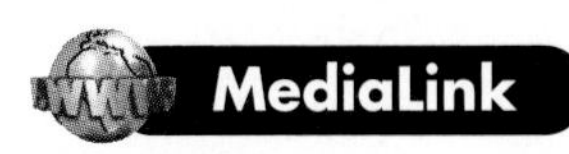

THE NATIONAL PSORIASIS FOUNDATION

Concept Review 32.5

- In most cases, which drug category is used to treat symptoms of dermatitis and psoriasis? What other drug therapies and techniques are used to provide a measure of relief for these symptoms?

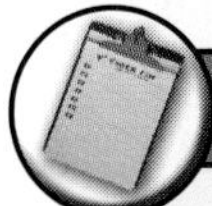

PATIENTS NEED TO KNOW

Patients taking medications for skin disorders need to know the following:

1. Inform family members, sexual partners, school personnel, and any other persons with whom close contact has occurred about skin infestations. Treat clothes, bed linens, and personal items properly to avoid reinfestation.
2. Be informed and understand the proper way to apply medication or to remove nits if necessary. Scabicides and pediculicides should not be applied to the face, mouth, open skin lesions, or the eyes.
3. For acne and related disorders, apply medication only to areas where it is supposed to be applied. Follow instructions in package inserts, and do not deviate from the precautions communicated by medical staff.
4. Do not share skin medications with family or friends. Be familiar with medication side effects, especially those of retinoids, retinoid-like products, or medications used to treat severe skin disorders.
5. Use medications only during the time for which they are intended. With extended use, some medications (for example, corticosteroids) may cause adverse side effects. Take a medication suitable for the disorder: avoid those that are too potent or not potent enough.
6. Give medications a chance to work. Some systemic medications must be taken exactly as prescribed without skipping or stopping early.
7. Avoid contact with agents that are known to cause allergy or dermatitis. Try to avoid scratching, if possible. For severe skin disorders, see a dermatologist. ■

CHAPTER REVIEW

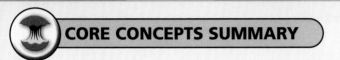

CORE CONCEPTS SUMMARY

32.1 Three layers of skin provide protection to the body.

Three layers of skin protect the body: the epidermis, dermis, and hypodermis. The most superficial layer is the epidermis, where skin cells are replenished every 3 weeks. New cells arise from the bottom layer, called the germanitivum, and are pushed to the outermost layer.

32.2 The major causes of skin disorders are injury, aging, inherited factors, and other medical conditions.

Many symptoms are associated with skin stress and injury. Others are associated with a patient's changing age or health. Skin disorders fit into three main categories: infectious, inflammatory, and cancerous disorders.

32.3 Scabicides and pediculicides treat parasitic mite and lice infestation.

Mites affect the skin and hair, whereas lice remain localized in hairy regions of the body. Both conditions are treatable with medications. Scabicides kill mites; pediculicides kill lice.

32.4 The goal of drug therapy for sunburn is to eliminate discomfort until healing occurs.

Local anesthetics are the primary medication used to treat mild sunburn and irritation. Often drugs are used for temporary relief of minor discomfort; in some cases, drugs may not be needed at all.

32.5 Problems of acne and rosacea are treated by a combination of OTC and prescription drugs.

Blackheads, whiteheads, and rosacea are disorders in which pores become blocked, inflamed, or infected because of accelerated skin processes. Topical drugs for acne are those that inhibit bacterial growth (antibiotics) or promote shedding of old skin (keratolytic agents). Vitamin A-like compounds (retinoids) provide an improved resistance to bacterial infections by reducing oil production and the occurrence of clogged pores.

32.6 Topical glucocorticoids are used mainly to treat dermatitis and related symptoms.

Dermatitis is treated by agents that reduce symptoms of inflammation, itchiness, flaking, cracking, bleeding, and lesions. Topical corticosteroids are the primary drug treatment for dermatitis. Potency depends on the type of drug formulation and whether it is packaged as a cream, lotion, solution, gel, or pad.

32.7 Several topical and systemic medications are used to treat psoriatic symptoms.

Psoriasis is a chronic disorder characterized by extreme discomfort and flaky areas called plaques. The treatments for psoriasis include topical glucocorticoids, retinoid-like compounds, drugs that arrest skin cell growth, and immunosuppressants. Skin therapy techniques are also used; including keratolytic agents, coal tar, anthralin, psoralens, and phototherapy.

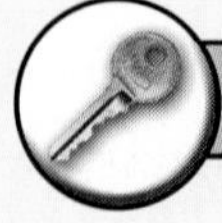

KEY TERMS

closed comedones (KOME-eh-dones): commonly called whiteheads, this type of acne develops just beneath the surface of the skin / ***page 630***

dermatitis (dur-mah-TIE-tiss): inflammatory condition of the skin characterized by itching and scaling / ***page 633***

eczema (ECK-zih-mah): also called *atopic* dermatitis, a skin disorder with unexplained symptoms of inflammation, itching, and scaling / ***page 632***

emollients (ee-MOLE-ee-ents): agents used to soothe and soften the skin / ***page 634***

erythema (ear-ih-THEE-mah): redness associated with skin irritation / ***page 625***

keratinization (keh-RAT-en-eye-zay-shun): development of the stratum corneum or horny layer of epithelial tissue / ***page 630***

keratolytic agents (keh-RAT-oh-lih-tik): drugs used to promote shedding of old skin / ***page 632***

open comedones: type of acne where sebum has plugged the oil gland; commonly called blackheads / ***page 630***

papules (PAP-yools): inflammatory bumps without pus that swell, thicken, and become painful / ***page 631***

pediculicides (puh-DIK-you-lih-sides): medications that kill lice / *page 628*

pruritus (proo-RYE-tus): itching symptom associated with dry, scaly skin / *page 624*

psoralen (SOR-uh-len): drug used along with phototherapy for the treatment of psoriasis and other severe skin disorders / *page 635*

pustules (PUSS-chools): inflammatory bumps with pus / *page 631*

retinoids (RETT-ih-noydz): Vitamin A-like compounds used in the treatment of severe acne and psoriasis / *page 632*

retinol (RETT-in-nall): chemical name for vitamin A / *page 632*

rosacea (roh-ZAY-shee-uh): skin disorder characterized by clusters of papules / *page 631*

scabicides (SKAY-bih-sides): drugs that kill scabies and mites / *page 628*

scabies (SKAY-beez): skin disorder caused by the female mite burrowing into the skin and laying eggs / *page 627*

seborrhea (seb-oh-REE-ah): condition characterized by overactivity of oil glands / *page 630*

REVIEW QUESTIONS

The following questions are written in NCLEX-PN® style. Answer these questions to assess your knowledge of the chapter material, and go back and review any material that is not clear to you.

1. This skin disorder may be caused by lack of moisture and extremely dry conditions.

1. Sunburn
2. Crusty and cracked areas
3. Blisters and calluses
4. Sores and lesions

2. With this type of burn, there is inflammation and blisters.

1. Full thickness
2. First degree
3. Second degree
4. Third degree

3. This medication must be rinsed from the body within 10 minutes after being applied.

1. Lindane (Kwell)
2. Crotamiton (Eurax)
3. Hexachloride
4. Permethrin (Nix)

4. The patient is complaining of discomfort related to minor sunburn. Which of the following would be recommended?

1. Benzocaine (Solarcaine)
2. Hexachloride
3. Benzoyl peroxide
4. Doxycycline

5. Patients that are or may become pregnant should not take this medication.

1. Ethinyl estradiol
2. Tretinoin (Retin-A)
3. Benzoyl peroxide
4. Isotretinoin/13-cis-retinoic acid (Accutane)

6. The patient is using topical glucocorticoids. The nurse will assess for all the following systemic effects of the medication except:

1. Mood changes
2. Osteoporosis
3. Liver toxicity
4. Adrenal insufficiency

7. Which of the following drugs would be used to treat severe psoriasis?

1. Calcipotriene (Dovonex)
2. Tarzarotene (Tazorac)
3. Acitreten (Soriatane)
4. Cyclosporine (Sandimmune)

8. This group of medications promotes shedding of old skin.

1. Pediculicides
2. Keratolytic agents
3. Retinoids
4. Glucocorticoids

9. Patients with this skin disorder exhibit bumps without pus that are swollen, thick, and painful.

1. Pustules
2. Erythema
3. Rosacea
4. Papules

10. Within which of the following areas would you expect to identify a more unique organization of keratin?

1. Legs
2. Hair
3. Feet
4. Palms of hands

CASE STUDY QUESTIONS

For questions 1–5, please refer to the following case study, and choose the correct answer from choices 1–4.

Burt is a 16-year-old white male with a family history of various allergy disorders. He is complaining of itching (pruritus), dryness, and general irritation around the face, neck, and forearm. On examination, the nurse pays close attention to the scalp, forehead, behind the ears, and eyes. Nothing unusual is observed–only a slight case of acne in the face, no excessive oil, no erythema, no lesions, no burrows, nor nits. Although areas around the neck and forearm are inflamed, these do not appear to be infected.

1. The condition described is probably:

1. Seborrheic dermatitis
2. Condition of scabies
3. Sunburn
4. Atopic dermatitis

2. Effective treatment of the neck and arms would include:

1. Cleansing of the skin with antibacterial soap
2. Application of topical benzocaine (Solarcaine)
3. Short-term application of topical glucocorticoids
4. Chloramphenicol (Chloromycetin) cream

3. Undesirable systemic effects from the medication used to treat Burt's condition would include:

1. Cardiac arrest
2. Adrenal insufficiency
3. Irritation to the eyes and mucous membranes
4. Adverse CNS effects including restlessness, dizziness, and tremors

4. In a plan to care for the appearance of acne, which of the following interventions would not be helpful?

1. Establish rapport with the patient
2. Tell the patient to avoid products that will irritate the skin such as cologne, perfumes, and other alcohol-based products
3. Encourage use of non-oily face creams
4. Tell the patient to avoid foods that make the acne worse

5. A more practical medication for Burt's minor acne problem might be:

1. Benzoyl peroxide
2. Sulfacetamide
3. Isotretinoin
4. A patch test should be done before any acne medication is used

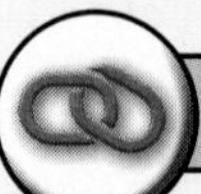

FURTHER STUDY

- A discussion of topical drug administration is detailed in Chapter 3.
- Chapters 11 and 21 cover pain medications that may be of use in severe sunburn.
- Tetanus toxoid, which is discussed in Chapter 22, may be needed to prevent infection in severe sunburn.
- Detailed information on the systemic effects that topical glucocorticoids can cause are discussed in Chapter 21.
- Systemic medications that are used for psoriasis, such as methotrexate and cyclosporine, are also presented in Chapters 24 and 21, respectively.
- Anti-infective agents, used for skin infections, are covered in Chapter 22.
- Local anesthetics such as benzocaine are presented in Chapter 13.

EXPLORE MEDIALINK www.prenhall.com/holland

Additional resources for this chapter can be found on the CD-ROM accompanying this textbook, and on the Companion Website. Click on Chapter 32 to select activities for this chapter.

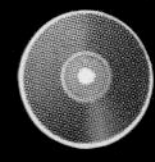

Audio Glossary
Concept Review
NCLEX-PN® Review
Nursing in Action
Dosage Calculator

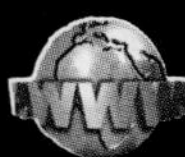

National Institute of Allergies and Infectious Diseases
The American Academy of Dermatology
The National Psoriasis Foundation

CHAPTER

33 Drugs for Eye and Ear Disorders

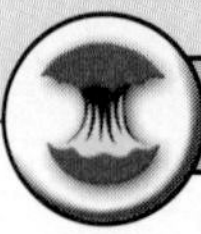

CORE CONCEPTS

33.1 Knowledge of basic eye anatomy is required for an understanding of eye disorders and drug therapy.

33.2 Glaucoma is one of the leading causes of blindness.

33.3 Glaucoma therapy centers on adjusting the circulation of aqueous humor.

33.4 Some antiglaucoma medications increase the outflow of aqueous humor.

33.5 Other antiglaucoma medications decrease the formation of aqueous humor.

33.6 Drugs provide relief for minor eye conditions and are used for eye exams.

33.7 Otic preparations treat infections, inflammation, and earwax buildup.

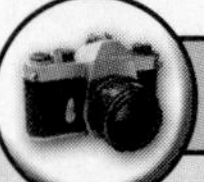

DRUG SNAPSHOT

The following drugs will be discussed in this chapter:

DRUG CLASSES	DRUG PROFILES
DRUGS FOR GLAUCOMA THAT INCREASE THE OUTFLOW OF AQUEOUS HUMOR	
Direct-acting miotics (Cholinergic agents)	
Indirect-acting miotics (Cholinesterase inhibitors)	
Sympathomimetics	
Prostaglandins and Prostamides	Pr latanoprost (Xalatan)
DRUGS FOR GLAUCOMA THAT DECREASE THE FORMATION OF AQUEOUS HUMOR	
Beta-adrenergic blockers	Pr timolol (Timoptic, Timoptic XE)
$Alpha_2$-adrenergic agents	
Carbonic anhydrase inhibitors	
Osmotic diuretics	
DRUGS FOR EYE EXAMINATIONS AND MINOR EYE CONDITIONS	
Mydriatics—sympathomimetics	
Cycloplegics—anticholinergics	
Lubricants	
DRUGS FOR EAR CONDITIONS	
Antibiotics	
Earwax (cerumen) softeners	

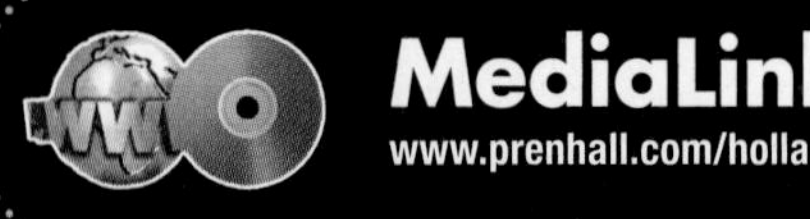

MediaLink
www.prenhall.com/holland

Interactive resources for this chapter can be found on the Companion Website. Click on Chapter 33 and "Begin" to select the activities for this chapter. For chapter-related animations, NCLEX-PN®-style questions, and an audio glossary, access the accompanying CD-ROM in this book.

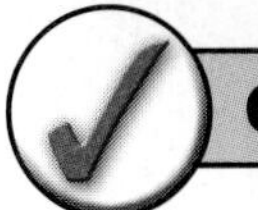

OBJECTIVES

After reading this chapter, the student should be able to:

1. Describe important eye anatomy relevant to glaucoma development.
2. Identify the major risk factors associated with glaucoma.
3. Explain how intraocular pressure is related to nerve damage in the eye.
4. Compare and contrast the two principal types of glaucoma and explain their reasons for development.
5. Explain two major mechanisms by which drugs reduce intraocular pressure.
6. Identify examples of important drugs for treating glaucoma and explain their basic actions and adverse effects.
7. Identify examples of drugs that dilate or constrict pupils, relax ciliary muscles, constrict ocular blood vessels, or moisten eye membranes.
8. Identify examples of drugs for treating ear infections, earaches, or a buildup of earwax.

The eye is one of the most precious sensory organs. A simple scratch can cause the patient almost unbearable discomfort. Other eye disorders may be more bearable, but are extremely dangerous—including glaucoma, one of the leading causes of blindness. The first part of this chapter covers various drugs used for the treatment of glaucoma. Drugs used routinely by ophthalmic practitioners are also discussed. The remaining part of the chapter covers examples of drugs used for treatment of ear disorders, including infections, inflammation, and the buildup of earwax (cerumen).

33.1 Knowledge of basic eye anatomy is required for an understanding of eye disorders and drug therapy.

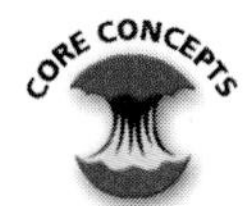

To understand eye disorders and drug action, one must be familiar with basic eye anatomy. As shown in Figure 33.1 ■, a watery fluid called *aqueous humor* is found in the anterior cavity of the eye. The anterior cavity has two major subcavities: the anterior chamber and the posterior chamber. In the posterior chamber (Figure 33.2 ■), aqueous humor originates from an important muscle structure called the *ciliary body*. From there, aqueous humor flows through the pupil and into the anterior chamber. Within the anterior chamber and around the periphery is a network of spongy connective tissue called *trabecular meshwork*. Connected with trabecular meshwork is an opening called the canal of Schlemm, the location where aqueous humor drains from the anterior cavity.

trabecular = *strut-like*

GLAUCOMA

Glaucoma is one of the most dreaded eye disorders. In some cases, glaucoma is genetic; in other cases, glaucoma may be caused by nongenetic factors including eye injury and disease. Some medications may contribute to the development of glaucoma, including long-term use of topical glucocorticoids, some antihypertensives, antihistamines, and antidepressants. The major risk factors associated with glaucoma include high blood pressure, migraine headaches, refractive disorders such as nearsightedness or farsightedness, and older age.

33.2 Glaucoma is one of the leading causes of blindness.

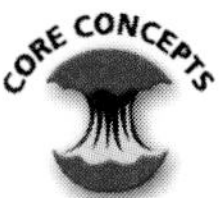

Tests such as tonometry may confirm the presence of glaucoma. **Tonometry** is an ophthalmic technique for measuring increased pressure inside the eye. Other routine refractory and visual field tests may uncover glaucoma signs. One problem with testing is that patients with glaucoma typically do not experience symptoms and therefore do not seek medical attention. In some cases, glaucoma occurs so gradually that patients do not notice a problem until later in the disease process.

tono = *pressure*
metry = *measurement*

FIGURE 33.1

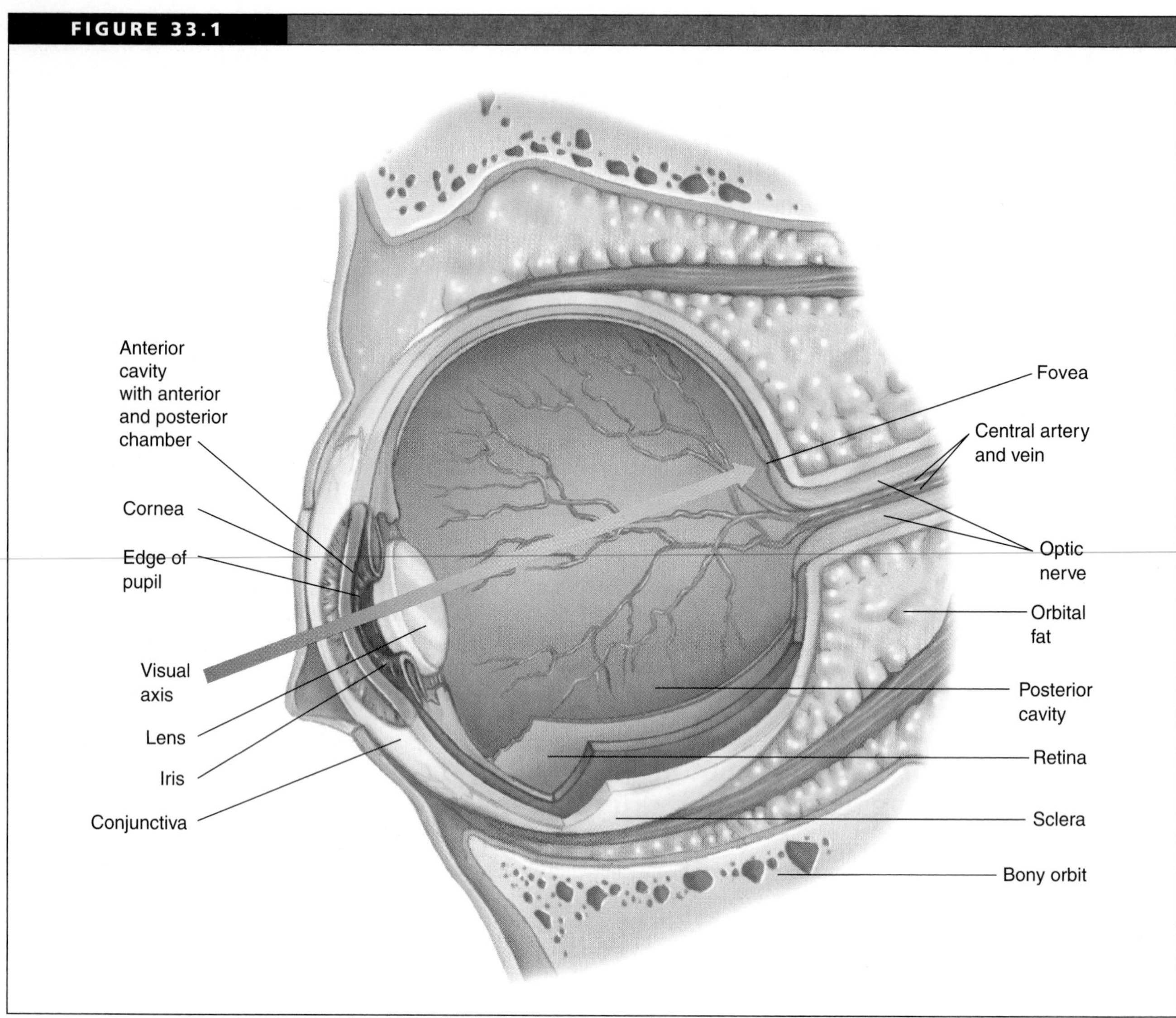

Internal structures of the eye *SOURCE: Pearson Education/PH College*

Fast Facts Glaucoma

- Worldwide, more than 5 million people have lost their vision as a result of glaucoma. More than 50,000 are in the United States.
- Patients of African heritage are affected more by glaucoma than any other ethnic group.
- Glaucoma is most common in patients older than 60 years of age.
- Acute glaucoma is often caused by head trauma, cataracts, tumors, or hemorrhage.
- Chronic simple glaucoma accounts for 90% of all glaucoma cases.

intra = *inside*
ocular = *eye*

Glaucoma is characterized by increased pressure inside the eyeball, termed *intraocular pressure* (IOP). The reason why IOP develops is because the flow of aqueous humor becomes blocked. Over time, pressure around the optic nerve can build, leading to blindness. In some cases, eye injury may be sudden, but in most cases it is gradual.

As shown in Figure 33.2 ■, the two principal types of glaucoma are **closed-angle glaucoma** and **open-angle glaucoma.** Both disorders result from the same problem: pressure inside the anterior cavity puts pressure on the posterior cavity, leading to progressive damage of the optic nerve. The difference between these two disorders includes how quickly the IOP develops.

FIGURE 33.2

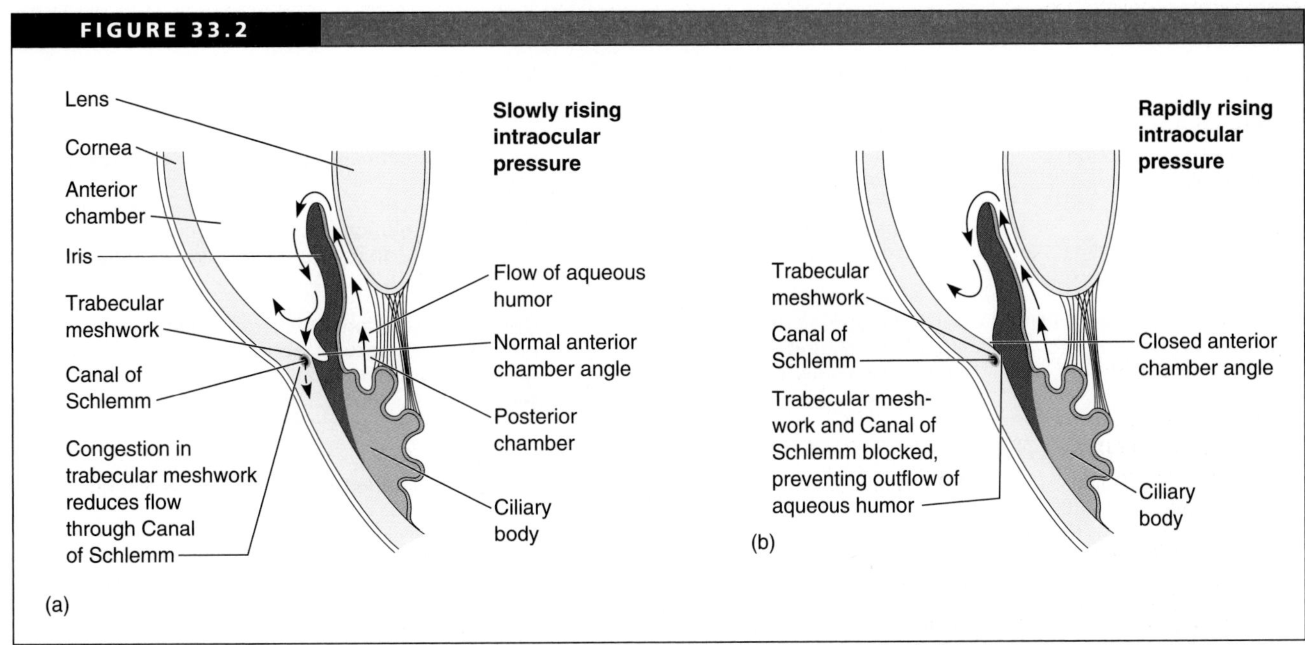

Forms of primary adult glaucoma: (a) in chronic open-angle glaucoma, the anterior chamber angle remains open, but drainage of aqueous humor through the canal of Schlemm is impaired; (b) in acute angle-closure glaucoma, the angle of the iris and anterior chamber narrows, obstructing the outflow of aqueous humor *SOURCE: Pearson Education/PH College*

Open-angle, or *chronic simple glaucoma,* is the most common type of glaucoma. With this disorder, intraocular pressure develops more slowly. It is called "open-angle" because the iris does not cover trabecular meshwork (Figure 33.2a ■).

Closed-angle glaucoma, sometimes referred to as *acute glaucoma,* is usually caused by stress, impact injury, or medications. Pressure inside the anterior chamber increases suddenly because the iris is pushed over the area where the aqueous fluid normally drains. Symptoms include intense headaches, difficulty concentrating, bloodshot eyes, and blurred vision (Figure 33.2b ■).

33.3 Glaucoma therapy centers on adjusting the circulation of aqueous humor.

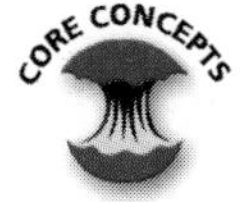

There are several approaches to glaucoma therapy. In cases of acute gluacoma, conventional or laser surgery might be performed to return the iris back to its original position. Most therapies focus on reducing the amount of aqueous humor formed or unblocking its drainage. Specifically, drug therapy for glaucoma works by either increasing the outflow of aqueous humor at the canal of Schlemm or by decreasing the formation of aqueous humor at the ciliary body.

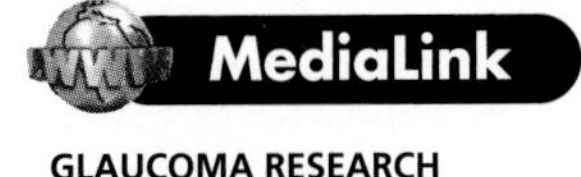

GLAUCOMA RESEARCH FOUNDATION

Concept Review 33.1

- Which components of the eye are specifically affected by glaucoma? Why is glaucoma such a dreaded eye disease? Drug therapy for glaucoma centers around which major approach?

33.4 Some antiglaucoma medications increase the outflow of aqueous humor.

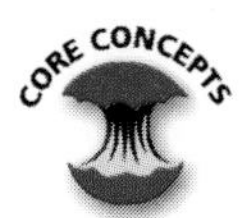

Drugs increasing the outflow of aqueous humor include miotics, sympathomimetics, prostaglandins, and prostamides. **Miotics** are drugs that cause the pupils to constrict. Sympathomimetics are drugs that mimic activation of the sympathetic nervous system (Chapter 7).

TABLE 33.1 Antiglaucoma Drugs That Increase the Outflow of Aqueous Humor

DRUG	ROUTE AND ADULT DOSE	REMARKS
MIOTICS, DIRECT-ACTING CHOLINERGIC AGENTS		
acetylcholine chloride (Miochol)	0.5–2 ml 1% intraocular solution instilled into eye	Intraocular treatment before surgery; cholinergic agent
carbachol (Isopto Carbachol, Miostat)	1–2 drops 0.75–3% solution in lower conjunctival sac q4h–tid	Ophthalmic solution; cholinergic agent; less useful in glaucoma than other drugs; causes stinging of the eyes
pilocarpine hydrochloride (Adsorbocarpine, Isopto Carptine, others)	acute glaucoma: 1 drop 1–2% solution every 5–10 minutes for 3–6 doses; chronic glaucoma: 1 drop 0.5–4% solution every 4–12 hours	Ophthalmic solution; cholinergic agent; may be prescribed as an ocular therapeutic system, a slow-release delivery method (Ocusert); Ocusert effects can last up to 7 days
MIOTICS, CHOLINESTERASE INHIBITORS		
demecarium bromide (Humorsol)	1–2 drops 0.125–0.25% solution 2 × per week	Ophthalmic solution; longer-acting medication (2–3 days)
echothiophate iodide (Phosphaline iodide)	1 drop 0.03–0.25% solution once or twice daily	Ophthalmic solution; must be prepared immediately before use because of instability
physostigmine salicylate (Eserine sulfate)	1 drop 0.25–0.5% solution 1–4 times/day	Ophthalmic solution; also constricts ciliary muscle, decreasing intraocular pressure
SYMPATHOMIMETICS		
dipivefrin HCl (Propine)	1 drop 0.1% solution bid	Ophthalmic solution; converted to epinephrine in the eye
epinephrine borate (Ipinal, Eppy/N)	1–2 drops 0.25–2% solution once or twice daily	Ophthalmic solution; causes mydriasis
PROSTAGLANDINS AND PROSTAMIDES		
bimatoprost (Lumigan)	1 drop 0.03% solution daily in the evening	Ophthalmic solution; prostamide; approved by the FDA, March 2001
Pr latanoprost (Xalatan)	1 drop (1.5 mg) solution daily in the evening	Ophthalmic solution; prostaglandin
travoprost (Travatan)	1 drop 0.004% solution daily in the evening	Ophthalmic solution; prostamide; maximum effect after about 12 h
unoprostone isopropyl (Rescula)	1 drop 0.15% solution bid	Ophthalmic solution; prostaglandin

Prostaglandins and prostamides are chemical agents that change vascular permeability in selected body tissues. Drugs that increase the outflow of aqueous humor are summarized in Table 33.1.

miosis = *shortening*

Miotic drugs produce an effect like acetylcholine; sympathomimetic drugs produce an effect like norepinephrine. Acetylcholine normally causes constriction of pupils or **miosis.** Norepinephrine causes dilation of pupils or **mydriasis.** (Review Chapter 7.) Although no antiglaucoma agents are intended to directly alter pupil diameter, they often produce this effect because of their physiological properties. Prostaglandins do not affect pupil diameter at all, but rather directly dilate trabecular meshwork within the anterior chamber. One of the drawbacks of prostaglandins is that they change pigmentation of the eyes. A related class of drugs called *prostamides* also directly affects trabecular meshwork but with less dramatic effects on iris pigmentation. Although their long-term effectiveness remains to be established, prostamides represent a promising class of drug for the treatment of open-angle glaucoma.

Direct-acting Miotics (Cholinergic Agents)

Acetylcholine chloride (Miochol), carbachol (Isopto Carbachol, Miostat), and pilocarpine (Adsorbocarpine, Isopto Carptine, and others) are cholinergic agents. These agents directly activate the cholinergic receptor, producing various responses in the eye including dilation of trabecular meshwork so that the canal of Schlemm can absorb more aqueous humor. When more aqueous

DRUG PROFILE: Prostaglandin: Pr *Latanoprost (Xalatan)*

Actions and Uses:

Latanoprost is a prostaglandin analog believed to reduce intraocular pressure (IOP) by increasing the outflow of aqueous humor. The recommended dose is one drop in the affected eye(s) in the evening. It is metabolized to its active form in the cornea, reaching its peak effect in about 12 hours. It is used to treat open-angle glaucoma and elevated IOP.

Adverse Effects and Interactions:

Adverse effects include ocular symptoms such as conjunctival edema, tearing, dryness, burning, pain, irritation, itching, sensation of foreign body in eye, photophobia, and visual disturbances. The eyelashes on the treated eye only may grow, thicken, and darken. Changes may occur in pigmentation of the iris of the treated eye and in the periocular skin. The most common systemic side effect is a flulike upper respiratory infection. Rash, asthenia, or headache may occur.

Latanoprost interacts with thimerosal: If mixed with eye drops containing thimerosal, precipitation may occur.

See the Companion Website for a Nursing Process Focus specific to this drug.

humor is absorbed, IOP is reduced. Side effects, however, include temporary **cycloplegia,** or blurred vision, and accommodation defects.

cyclop = *round eye*
plegia = *paralysis*

Indirect-acting Miotics (Cholinesterase Inhibitors)

Demecarium bromide (Humorsol), echothiophate iodide (Phosphaline iodide), and physostigmine salicylate (Eserine sulfate) are indirect-acting cholinergic agents. They produce about the same effects as direct-acting drugs, except that they block cholinesterase, the enzyme responsible for breaking down the natural neurotransmitter acetylcholine.

Sympathomimetics

Dipivefrin (Propine) and epinephrine borate (Ipinal and others) are sympathomimetic drugs. Dipiverdin is converted to epinephrine; epinephrine produces mydriasis, increased outflow of aqueous humor, and the subsequent fall of IOP. As discussed in Chapter 19, when epinephrine is released into the general circulation, it increases blood pressure and heart rate.

Prostaglandins and Prostamides

Bimatoprost (Lumigan), latanoprost (Xalatan), travaprost (Travatan), and unoprostone isopropyl (Rescula) also increase aqueous humor outflow by reducing congestion in trabecular meshwork. Their main side effect is heightened pigmentation, usually brown color of the iris in patients with lighter colored eyes. These medications cause cycloplegia, local irritation, and stinging of the eyes. Because of these effects, prostaglandins are normally administered just before the patient goes to bed. Although prostaglandins can be irritating to the eyes, they usually do not prevent the patient from falling asleep.

33.5 Other antiglaucoma medications decrease the formation of aqueous humor.

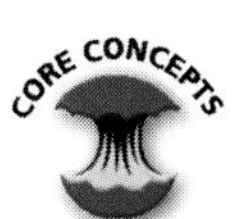

Beta-adrenergic blockers, $alpha_2$-adrenergic agents, carbonic-anhydride inhibitors, and osmotic diuretics are drug classes that decrease the formation of aqueous humor. These are summarized in Table 33.2. Beta blockers do not alter pupil diameter or produce cycloplegic effects. Similarly, $alpha_2$ agents produce fewer ocular symptoms. For patients who cannot use beta-blocking agents, carbonic-anhydrase inhibitors and osmotic diuretics are other alternatives.

Beta-blocking agents are used more often than the other antiglaucoma medications. These include betaxolol (Betaoptic), carteolol (Ocupress), levobunolol (Betagan), metipranolol (OptiPranolol),

TABLE 33.2 Antiglaucoma Drugs That Decrease the Formation of Aqueous Humor

DRUG	ROUTE AND ADULT DOSE	REMARKS
BETA-ADRENERGIC BLOCKERS		
betaxolol (Betaoptic)	1 drop 0.5% solution bid	Ophthalmic solution; available as ophthalmic suspension; beta$_1$ blocker; reduces blood pressure, heart rate
carteolol (Ocupress)	1 drop 1% solution bid	Ophthalmic solution; nonspecific beta blocker; causes bronchoconstriction
levobunolol (Betagan)	1–2 drops 0.25–0.5% solution one or twice daily	Ophthalmic solution; nonspecific beta blocker
metipranolol (OptiPranolol)	1 drop 0.3% solution bid	Ophthalmic solution; nonspecific beta blocker
Pr timolol (Timoptic, Timoptic XE)	drops: 1–2 drops of 0.25–0.5% solution once or twice daily; gel (salve): apply daily	Ophthalmic solution; nonspecific beta blocker
ALPHA$_2$-ADRENERGIC AGENTS		
apraclonidine (Iopidine)	1 drop 0.5% solution bid	Ophthalmic solution
brimonidine tartrate (Alphagan)	1 drop 0.2% solution tid	Ophthalmic solution
CARBONIC ANHYDRASE INHIBITORS		
acetazolamide (Diamox)	PO 250 mg 1–4 times/day	Oral diuretic; sulfonamide; also for seizures, high altitude sickness, and renal impairment
brinzolamide (Azopt)	1 drop 1% solution tid	Ophthalmic solution; sulfonamide
dichlorphenamide (Duranide, Oratrol)	PO 100–200 mg followed by 100 mg bid	Oral sulfonamide
dorzolamide hydrochloride (Trusopt)	1 drop 2% solution tid	Ophthalmic solution; sulfonamide
methazolamide (Neptazane)	PO 50–100 mg bid or tid	Oral sulfonamide; less diuretic activity than acetazolamide
OSMOTIC DIURETICS		
glycerin anhydrous (Ophthalagen)	PO 1–1.8 g/kg 1–1.5 h before ocular surgery; may repeat q5h	Often used for eye surgery in cases of injury
isosorbide (Ismotic)	PO 1–3 g/kg bid–qid	Used before and after eye surgery
mannitol (Osmitrol)	IV 1.5–2 mg/kg as a 15–25% solution over 30–60 minutes	Raises osmotic pressure causing diuresis; IV medication
urea (Ureaphil)	IV 1–1.5 g/kg of 30% solution infused slowly over 1–2.5 h at a rate not to exceed 4 ml/min (max: 120 g/24 h)	For cases of prolonged surgery to reduce intracranial and intraocular pressure associated with head injury

and timolol (Timoptic, Timoptic XE). The exact mechanism by which these drugs produce their effects is not fully understood. However, they all reduce IOP effectively without the ocular side effects of miotic and sympathomimetic drugs. Systemic beta-blocker effects can be problematic; however, the doses of beta-blockers used for glaucoma treatment are generally not high enough to enter the general circulation. Systemic side effects, if they occur, include bronchoconstriction, bradycardia, and hypotension.

Alpha$_2$-adrenergic agents are less frequently prescribed than the other antiglaucoma medications. These medications include apraclonidine (Iopidine) and brimonidine (Alphagan). They produce minimal cardiovascular and pulmonary side effects. The most significant side effects are headache, drowsiness, dry mucosal membranes, blurred vision, and irritated eyelids.

Carbonic-anhydrase inhibitors may be administered topically or systemically to reduce IOP. Usually these medications are used as a second choice if beta blockers are not effective. Examples include acetazolamide (Diamox), brinzolamide (Azopt), dichlorphenamide (Duranide, Oratrol), dorzolamide (Trusopt), and methazolamide (Neptazane). These medications are more effective in cases of open-angle glaucoma. Patients must be cautioned when taking these medications because they are *sulfonamides*—agents that may cause an allergic reaction. All of these drugs are diuretics, which means they can reduce IOP rather quickly and dramatically, altering serum electrolytes with continuous treatment.

Osmotic diuretics are most often used in cases of eye surgery or acute closed-angle glaucoma. Examples include glycerin anhydrous (Ophthalagen), isosorbide (Ismotic), mannitol (Osmitrol), and urea (Ureaphil and others). Because they have an ability to reduce plasma volume very quickly (Chapter 28), they may produce unpleasant side effects including headache, tremors, dizziness, dry mouth, fluid and electrolyte imbalance, and *thrombophlebitis* or venous clot formation near the site of IV administration.

thrombo = *clot*
phleb = *vein*
itis = *inflammation*

Concept Review 33.2

- Describe two major approaches for controlling intraocular pressure in glaucoma clients. What major drug classes are used in each case?

EYE EXAMINATIONS AND MINOR EYE CONDITIONS

Drugs for minor irritation and injury come from a broad range of classes including antimicrobials, local anesthetics, glucocorticoids, and NSAIDs.

33.6 Drugs provide relief for minor eye conditions and are used for eye exams.

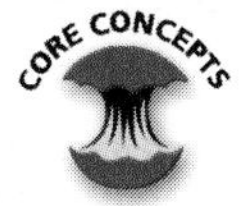

A range of drug preparations may be used including drops, salves, optical inserts, and injectable formulations. Some agents only provide moisture to the eye's surface. Others penetrate and affect a specific area of the eye.

DRUG PROFILE: Beta-adrenergic Blocker: Pr *Timolol (Timoptic, Timoptic XE)*

Actions and Uses:

Timolol is a nonselective beta-adrenergic blocker available as a 0.25% or 0.5% ophthalmic solution. Timolol reduces elevated intraocular pressure (IOP) in chronic open-angle glaucoma by reducing the formation of aqueous humor. The usual dose is one drop in the affected eye(s) twice a day. Timoptic XE allows for once-a-day dosing. Treatment may require 2 to 4 weeks for maximum therapeutic effect. It is also available in tablets, which are prescribed to treat mild hypertension.

Adverse Effects and Interactions:

The most common side effects are local burning and stinging on instillation. In most patients there is no significant systemic absorption to cause adverse effects as long as timolol is applied correctly. If significant systemic absorption occurs, however, drug interactions could occur. Anticholinergics, nitrates, reserpine, methyldopa, and/or verapamil use could lead to increased hypotension and bradycardia. Indomethacin and thyroid hormone use could lead to decreased antihypertensive effects of timolol. Epinephrine use could lead to hypertension followed by severe bradycardia. Theophylline use could lead to decreased bronchodilation.

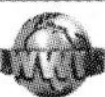
See the Companion Website for a Nursing Process Focus specific to this drug.

NURSING PROCESS FOCUS

Patients Receiving Ophthalmic Solutions for Glaucoma

ASSESSMENT

Prior to drug administration:

- Obtain complete health history including allergies, drug history, and possible drug interactions
- Obtain complete physical examination focusing on visual acuity and visual field assessments
- Assess for the presence/history of ocular pain

POTENTIAL NURSING DIAGNOSES

- Risk for Injury, related to visual acuity deficits
- Self-Care Deficit, related to impaired vision
- Pain, related to disease process

PLANNING: Patient Goals and Expected Outcomes

The patient will:

- Exhibit no progression of visual impairment
- Demonstrate an understanding of the disease process
- Safely function within own environment without injury
- Report absence of pain

IMPLEMENTATION

Interventions and (Rationales)	Patient Education/Discharge Planning
■ Monitor visual acuity, blurred vision, papillary reactions, extraocular movements, and ocular pain.	■ Instruct patient to report changes in vision and headache.
■ Monitor the patient for specific contraindications for prescribed drug. (There are many physiologic conditions in which ophthalmic solutions may be contraindicated.)	■ Instruct patient to inform healthcare provider of all health-related problems and prescribed medications.
■ Remove contact lenses before administration of ophthalmic solutions.	■ Instruct patient to remove contact lenses prior to administering eye drops and wait 15 minutes before reinsertion.
■ Administer ophthalmic solutions using proper technique.	Instruct patient in the proper administration of eye drops: ■ Wash hands prior to eye drop administration ■ Avoid touching the tip of the container to the eye, which may contaminate the solution ■ Administer the eye drop in the conjunctival sac ■ Apply pressure over the lacrimal sac for 1 minute ■ Wait 5 minutes before administering other ophthalmic solutions ■ Schedule glaucoma medications around daily routines such as waking, mealtimes, and bedtime to lessen the chance of missed doses
■ Monitor for ocular reaction to the drug such as conjunctivitis and lid reactions.	■ Instruct patient to report itching, drainage, ocular pain, or other ocular abnormalities.
■ Assess intraocular pressure readings. (These are used to determine effectiveness of drug therapy.)	■ Instruct patient that intraocular pressure readings will be done prior to beginning treatment and periodically during treatment.
■ Monitor color of iris and periorbital tissue of treated eye.	Instruct patient that: ■ More brown color may appear in the iris and in the periorbital tissue of the treated eye only ■ Any pigmentation changes develop over months to years

continued...

NURSING PROCESS FOCUS

Interventions and (Rationales)	Patient Education/Discharge Planning
■ Monitor for systemic absorption of ophthalmic preparations. (Ophthalmic drugs for glaucoma can cause serious cardiovascular and respiratory complications if the drug is systemically absorbed.)	■ Instruct patient to immediately report palpitations, chest pain, shortness of breath, and irregularities in pulse.
■ Monitor and adjust environmental lighting to aid in patient's comfort. (People who have glaucoma are sensitive to excessive light, especially extreme sunlight.)	Instruct patient to: ■ Adjust environmental lighting as needed to enhance vision or reduce ocular pain ■ Wear darkened glasses as needed
■ Encourage compliance with treatment regimen.	Instruct patient: ■ To adhere to medication schedule for eye drop administration ■ About the importance of regular follow-up care with ophthalmologist

EVALUATION OF OUTCOME CRITERIA

Evaluate the effectiveness of drug therapy by confirming that patient goals and expected outcomes have been met (see "Planning").

See Tables 33.1 and 33.2 for lists of drugs to which these nursing actions apply.

Some drugs are specifically designed for ophthalmic examinations. These include **cycloplegic drugs** to relax ciliary muscles and **mydriatic drugs** to dilate the pupils. One has to be especially careful with anticholinergic mydriatics because these drugs can increase IOP and worsen the condition of patients with glaucoma. In addition, anti-cholinergic agents have the potential for producing unfavorable central side effects such as confusion, unsteadiness, or drowsiness in adults. Children generally become restless and spastic. Examples of cycloplegic, mydriatic, and lubricant drugs are listed in Table 33.3.

Concept Review 33.3

- List examples of commonly used drugs for minor eye irritation and injury. What are the major actions of cycloplegic and mydriatic drugs?

EAR CONDITIONS

The ear has two major sensory functions: hearing and maintenance of equilibrium and balance. Three important structural areas—the outer ear, middle ear, and inner ear—carry out these functions (Figure 33.3).

Otitis, inflammation of the ear, most often occurs in the outer and middle ear compartments. **External otitis,** commonly called *swimmer's ear,* is inflammation of the outer ear; **otitis media** is inflammation of the middle ear. Outer ear infections most often occur with water exposure. Middle ear infections most often occur with upper respiratory infections, allergies, or auditory tube irritation. Of all ear infections, the most difficult ones to treat are inner ear infections. **Mastoiditis,** or inflammation of the mastoid sinus, can be a serious problem because if left untreated, it can result in hearing loss.

ot = *ear*
itis = *inflammation*

TABLE 33.3 Drugs for Eye Examinations and Moistening Eye Membranes

DRUG	ROUTE AND ADULT DOSE	REMARKS
MYDRIATICS: SYMPATHOMIMETICS		
hydroxyamphetamine (Paredrine)	1 drop 1% solution before eye exam	Used to dilate pupils in closed-angle glaucoma
phenylephrine hydrochloride (Mydfrin, Neo-Synephrine)	1 drop 2.5% or 10% solution before eye exam	Decongestant and vasoconstriction properties; smaller doses provide temporary relief of eye redness; also for pupil dilation in closed-angle glaucoma
CYCLOPLEGICS: ANTICHOLINERGICS		
atropine sulfate (Isopto Atropine, others)	1 drop 0.5% solution daily	Also provided as ointment; should not be administered to patients with glaucoma; effects may be prolonged
cyclopentolate (Cyclogyl, Pentalair)	1 drop 0.5–2% solution 40–50 minutes before procedure	Not for glaucoma patients; causes burning and irritation; possible central side effects with higher doses
homatropine (Isopto Homatropine, others)	1–2 drops 2% or 5% solution before eye exam	Not for glaucoma patients; effects may be prolonged after treatment
scopolamine hydrobromide (Isopto Hyoscine)	1–2 drops 0.25% solution 1 hour before eye exam	Not for glaucoma patients; effects may be prolonged after treatment; possible central side effects with higher doses
tropicamide (Mydriacyl, Tropicacyl)	1–2 drops 0.5–1% solution before eye exam	Not for glaucoma patients; central side effects with higher doses
LUBRICANTS CAUSING OCULAR VASOCONSTRICTION		
naphazoline hydrochloride (Albalon, Allerest, ClearEyes, others)	1–3 drops 0.1% solution every 3–4 hours prn	OTC and prescription medications available
oxymetazoline hydrochloride (OcuClear, Visine LR)	1–2 drops 0.025% solution qid	OTC and prescription medications available
tetrahydrozoline hydrochloride (Collyrium, Murine Plus, Visine, others)	1–2 drops 0.05% solution bid–tid	Primarily OTC medication
GENERAL PURPOSE LUBRICANTS		
lanolin alcohol (Lacri-lube)	Apply a thin film to the inside of the eyelid	Mixed with mineral oil and petroleum jelly as a salve
methylcellulose (Methulose, Visculose, others)	1–2 drops prn	Artificial tear solution
polyvinyl alcohol (Liquifilm. others)	1–2 drops prn	Artificial tear solution

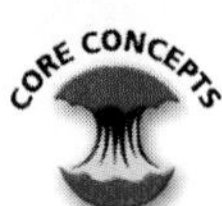

33.7 Otic preparations treat infections, inflammation, and earwax buildup.

Combination drugs effectively treat many different types of ear conditions including infections, earaches, edema, and earwax.

The basic treatment for ear infection is essentially the same as in all places of the body: antibiotics. Topical antibiotics in the form of ear drops may be administered for external ear infections. Systemic antibiotics (Chapter 13) may be needed in cases in which outer ear infections are extensive or in cases of middle or inner ear infections. Medications for pain, edema, and itching may also be necessary. Glucocorticoids are often combined with antibiotics or with other drugs when inflammation is present. Examples of these drugs are listed in Table 33.4.

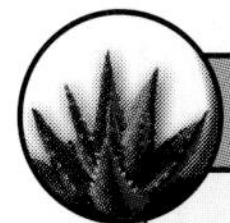

NATURAL ALTERNATIVES

Aloe Vera for Improving Eye and Ear Health

For centuries, *Aloe vera* has been hailed as the "medicine plant" because of its ability to treat burns, cuts, scrapes, rashes, and abrasions. It has a reputation for treating inflammation and acid indigestion, and even lowering blood cholesterol. *Aloe* may be able to treat eye irritation and conjunctivitis in addition to many other disorders.

One does not have to put *Aloe* directly into the eyes to obtain its therapeutic effect. The benefit comes from treating areas around the eyes, including the bridge of the nose and the outside of the eyelids and cheeks. The skin around the ears may also be treated. The antiseptic properties of *Aloe* probably come from the many agents found within its sap and leaves. Other agents have a reputation for killing microorganisms, including salicylic acid, urea nitrogen, cinnamonic acid, phenols, sulphur, and lupeol. Other groups of agents that qualify as substances with healing properties include plant sterols, immune modulating peptides, anti-inflammatory fatty acids, and viscous-like polysaccharides. ■

FIGURE 33.3

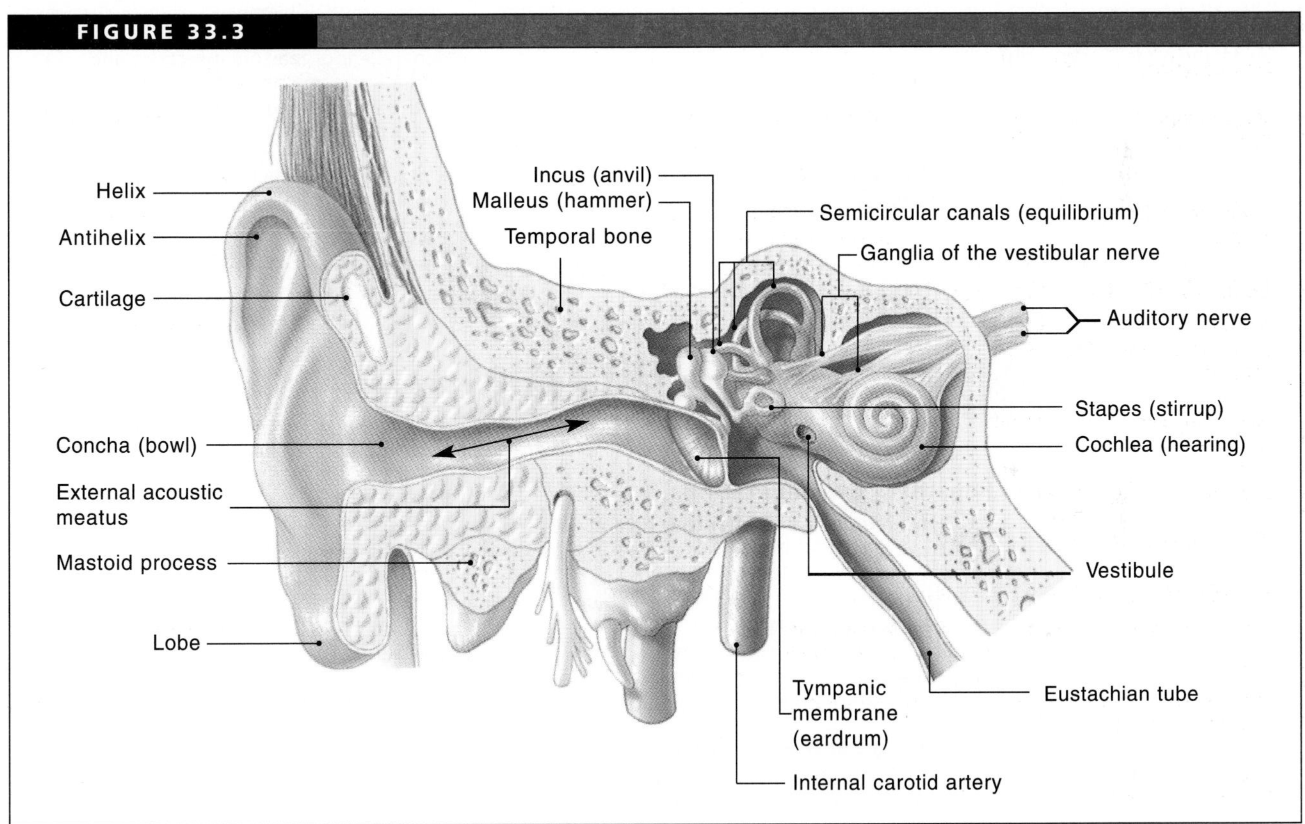

Structures of the external ear, middle ear, and inner ear *SOURCE: Pearson Education/PH College*

Mineral oil, earwax softeners, and commercial products are also used for proper ear health. When earwax accumulates, it narrows the ear canal, and may interfere with hearing. This is especially true for older patients who are not able to properly groom themselves. Healthcare providers working with elderly patients are trained to take appropriate measures when removing impacted earwax.

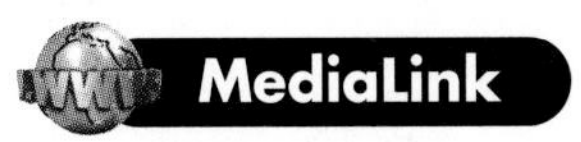

U.S. NATIONAL LIBRARY OF MEDICINE

Concept Review 33.4

- Identify areas of the ear where microbial infections are most likely. What kind of otic preparations treat infections, inflammation, and earwax buildup?

TABLE 33.4 Otic Preparations

DRUG	ROUTE AND ADULT DOSE	REMARKS
acetic acid and hydrocortisone (Vosol HC)	3–5 drops in the affected ear q4h–qid × 24 hours, then 5 drops tid–qid	Combination of acetic acid and glucocorticoid; for general ear infections and inflammation; prescription medication
aluminum sulfate and calcium acetate (Domeboro)	2 drops 2% solution tid–qid	For general ear infections and the prevention of swimmer's ear; may be administered using an ear wick; OTC medication
benzocaine and antipyrine (Auralgan)	Fill ear canal with solution tid × 2 for 3 days	For acute otitis media and the removal of earwax; reduces earache associated with the infection; prescription medication
carbamide peroxide (Debrox)	1–5 drops 6.5% solution bid × 4 days	To soften, loosen, and remove excessive earwax; OTC medication
ciprofloxacin hydrochloride and hydrocortisone (Cipro)	3 drops of the suspension instilled into the affected ear bid × 7 days	Combination of fluoroquinolone antibiotic and glucocorticoid; for ear infections and inflammation; prescription medication
polymixin B, neomycin and hydrocortisone (Cortisporin)	4 drops in ear tid–qid	Combination of antibiotics and glucocorticoid; for general ear or mastoid infections and inflammation; some patients may develop dermatitis as a result of sensitivity to neomycin; prescription medication
triethanolamine polypeptide oleate 10% condensate (Cerumenex)	Fill ear canal with solution; wait 10–20 minutes	Drug dissolved in propylene glycerol; breaks apart earwax; small risk of sensitivity; OTC medication

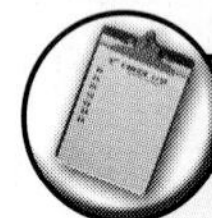

PATIENTS NEED TO KNOW

Patients taking medications for eye and ear disorders need to know the following:

Regarding Eye Medications

1. Have regular eye exams after the age of 40.
2. Do not strain or lift heavy objects if risk for glaucoma is present. Any effort that might produce eyestrain should be avoided.
3. Make sure that all allergies or sensitivities, including those to sulfa drugs, are known to the healthcare providers.
4. Do not take OTC medications that "get the red out" for longer than 24 hours. Use eye lubricants instead. Persistent irritation should be reported immediately.
5. Keep eye solutions clear and sterile, do not actually touch the eye when instilling drops.

Regarding Ear Medications

6. Take precautions to keep the ear canal dry when in or around water for an extensive time. Use appropriate earplugs or a bathing cap.
7. Apply 2% acetic acid to the ear canal after swimming. Acetic acid acts as a drying agent and restores the ear canal to its normal acidic condition.
8. Avoid using glucocorticoids for long periods. They could cause eye or ear damage.
9. Rather than placing objects like cotton swabs in the ear canal, use a bulb syringe approved for removing debris and warm water. Use any cerumen dissolving agent responsibly. ■

CHAPTER REVIEW

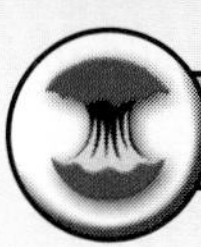

CORE CONCEPTS SUMMARY

33.1 Knowledge of basic eye anatomy is required for an understanding of eye disorders and drug therapy.

The anterior cavity of the eye is the place where aqueous humor is circulated. Aqueous humor originates from the ciliary body located in the posterior chamber and drains into the canal of Schlemm found in the anterior chamber.

33.2 Glaucoma is one of the leading causes of blindness.

Glaucoma develops because the flow of aqueous humor in the anterior eye cavity becomes disrupted, leading to increasing intraocular pressure (IOP). Two principal types of glaucoma are closed-angle glaucoma and open-angle glaucoma.

33.3 Glaucoma therapy centers on adjusting the circulation of aqueous humor.

Glaucoma therapy generally works by increasing the outflow of aqueous humor or decreasing aqueous humor formation.

33.4 Some antiglaucoma medications increase the outflow of aqueous humor.

Drugs that increase the outflow of aqueous humor include miotics, sympathomimetics, prostaglandins, and prostamides.

33.5 Other antiglaucoma medications decrease the formation of aqueous humor.

Medications that decrease the formation of aqueous humor include beta blockers, alpha$_2$-adrenergic agents, carbonic-anhydrase inhibitors, and osmotic diuretics. The beta-adrenergic blockers are the most commonly prescribed drug class.

33.6 Drugs provide relief for minor eye conditions and are used for eye exams.

Mydriatic or pupil-dilating drugs and cyclopegic or ciliary-muscle relaxing drugs are routinely used for eye examinations. Some drugs constrict local blood vessels. Others lubricate the eyes.

33.7 Otic preparations treat infections, inflammation, and earwax buildup.

Combination drugs provide relief of ear conditions associated with the outer, middle, and inner ear. Drugs include antibiotics, corticosteroids, and earwax dissolving agents.

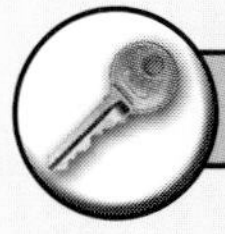

KEY TERMS

closed-angle glaucoma (glaw-KOH-mah): called acute glaucoma, this type of glaucoma is caused by the iris blocking trabecular meshwork, hindering outflow of aqueous fluid / ***page 642***

cycloplegia (sy-kloh-PLEE-jee-ah): blurred vision / ***page 645***

cycloplegic drug (sy-kloh-PLEE-jik): drugs that relax or temporarily paralyze ciliary muscles / ***page 649***

external otitis (oh-TYE-tiss): commonly called swimmer's ear, this is inflammation of the outer ear / ***page 649***

mastoiditis (mass-toy-DYE-tuss): inflammation of the mastoid sinus / ***page 649***

miosis (my-OH-sis): constriction of the pupil / ***page 644***

miotics (my-AH-tiks): drugs that cause pupilc constriction / ***page 643***

mydriasis (mih-DRY-uh-siss): dilation of the pupil / ***page 644***

mydriatic drugs (my-DRY-at-tik): drugs that cause pupil dilation / ***page 649***

open-angle glaucoma (glaw-KOH-mah): also called chronic simple glaucoma, this type of glaucoma is caused by congestion in trabecular meshwork, hindering outflow of aqueous fluid / ***page 642***

otitis media (oh-TYE-tuss MEE-dee-ah): inflammation of the middle ear / ***page 649***

tonometry (toh-NAHM-uh-tree): technique for measuring eye tension and pressure / ***page 641***

REVIEW QUESTIONS

The following questions are written in NCLEX-PN® style. Answer these questions to assess your knowledge of the chapter material, and go back and review any material that is not clear to you.

1. This classification of drugs causes the pupils to constrict.

1. Miotics
2. Mydriatics
3. Constrictors
4. Glucocorticoids

2. This medication relieves pressure in the eye by increasing the outflow of aqueous humor.

1. Timolol (Timoptic)
2. Betaxolol (Betaoptic)
3. Pilocarpine (Ocusert)
4. Ciprofloxacin (Cipro)

3. This medication relieves pressure by decreasing production of aqueous humor.

1. Timolol (Timoptic)
2. Atropine sulfate
3. Pilocarpine (Ocusert)
4. Ciprofloxacin (Cipro)

4. Patients with glaucoma should not take which of the following classifications of medications?

1. Osmotic diuretics
2. Beta-adrenergic blockers
3. Anticholinergics
4. $Alpha_2$-adrenergic blockers

5. If the patient has an ear infection with inflammation, which of the following medications may be added?

1. Glucocorticoids
2. Aluminum sulfate and calcium acetate (Domeboro)
3. Osmotic diuretics
4. Carbonic-anhydrase inhibitors

6. Prior to administering ear drops, the nurse should instruct the patient that:

1. The solution should stay in the ear for 1 hour.
2. The solution will be removed within 1 hour.
3. There may be a decrease in hearing for a few minutes.
4. The medication will take effect immediately.

7. If the patient has closed-angle glaucoma, the nurse will assess for:

1. Blindness
2. Blurred vision
3. Loss of consciousness
4. Hyperactivity

8. The goal of treatment in glaucoma patients is to:

1. Decrease aqueous humor production and increase outflow of aqueous humor
2. Increase aqueous humor production and decrease outflow of aqueous humor
3. Decrease aqueous humor production and decrease outflow of aqueous humor
4. Increase aqueous humor production and increase outflow of aqueous humor

9. The patient started on travoprost (Travatan) should be instructed that:

1. This medication is administered in the morning only.
2. Due to pupil constriction, visual acuity may be affected.
3. This medication may change the pigmentation of the eyes.
4. Due to dilation of the pupils, visual acuity may be affected.

10. If the patient is allergic to sulfonamides, he should not take:

1. Methazolamide (Neptazane)
2. Betaxolol (Betaoptic)
3. Carteolol (Ocupress)
4. Beta blockers

CASE STUDY QUESTIONS

For questions 1–5, please refer to the following case study, and choose the correct answer from choices 1–4.

Ms. Saunders is a 45-year-old black female presenting with severe pain in the right eye, headache, and blurred vision. She has a history of primary hypertension. Her blood pressure is 140/90 mm Hg. No other obvious signs are noted. In the course of the examination, she mentions that she and her family have recently relocated. It has been a particularly stressful time because she has not had much help from her family. She has not been taking her medication. At a recent hospital visit, she was prescribed the beta blocker, timolol (Timoptic).

1. The primary diagnosis of Ms. Saunders is:

1. Diabetes
2. Myopia
3. Glaucoma
4. Fibroplasia

2. The nurse examining the eye of Ms. Saunders should be cautious of the potential adverse reactions to which of the following drugs?

1. Cholinergic-blocking drugs
2. Miotic medication
3. Prostaglandins
4. Antibiotic drops

3. Which of the following could be a potential contraindication to the use of timolol (Timoptic)?

1. Hyperthyroidism
2. Liver disease
3. Organic nitrates for angina
4. Theophylline for asthma

4. In the counseling of Ms. Saunders, the nurse explains that if left untreated pharmacologically, the condition could lead to:

1. Mydriasis
2. Cycloplegia
3. Blindness
4. Vertigo

5. The severe eye pain, headache, and blurred vision most likely have something to do with:

1. Intraocular pressure
2. Hypertension
3. Lifting heavy objects
4. All of the above are possible causes

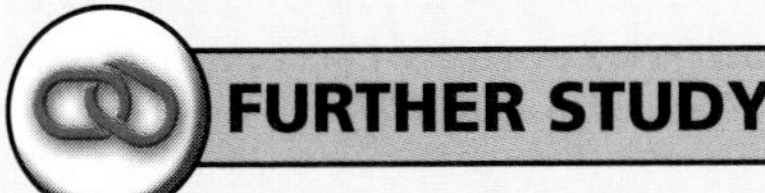

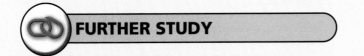

FURTHER STUDY

- Sympathomimetics, cholinergic agents, and cholinesterase inhibitors are autonomic agents that are discussed in Chapter 7.
- Chapter 19 presents details of epinephrine's effect on blood pressure and heart rate.
- Osmotic diuretics are discussed in Chapter 28.
- Chapter 13 discusses the use of systemic antibiotics that may be utilized for eye or ear infections.
- Use of the beta blocker timolol in the treatment of hypertension is presented in Chapter 15.

EXPLORE MEDIALINK www.prenhall.com/holland

Additional resources for this chapter can be found on the CD-ROM accompanying this textbook, and on the Companion Website. Click on Chapter 33 to select activities for this chapter.

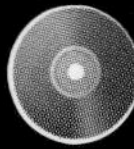

Audio Glossary
Concept Review
NCLEX-PN® Review
Nursing in Action
Dosage Calculator

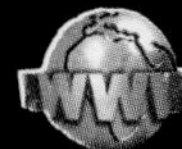

Glaucoma Research Foundation
U.S. National Library of Medicine

APPENDIX A: References

General References

Audesirk, T., Audesirk, G., & Beyers, B. E. (2005). *Biology: Life on earth* (7th ed.). Upper Saddle River, NJ: Prentice Hall.

Beers, M. H., & Berkow, R. (Eds.). (2001). *Merck manual: Diagnosis and therapy* (17th ed.). Whitehouse Station, NJ: Merck & Co., Inc.

Brunton, L. L., Lazo, J. S., & Parker, K. L. (Eds.). (2006). *The pharmacological basis of therapeutics* (11th ed.). New York: McGraw-Hill.

Krogh, D. (2005). *Biology: A guide to the natural world.* Upper Saddle River, NJ: Prentice Hall.

LeMone, P., & Burke, K. M. (2004). *Medical-surgical nursing: Critical thinking in client care* (3rd ed.). Upper Saddle River, NJ: Prentice-Hall.

Martini, F. H. (2001). *Fundamentals of human anatomy and physiology* (5th ed.). Upper Saddle River, NJ: Prentice Hall.

Medical Economics Staff. (Ed.). (2001). *Physicians' desk reference for non-prescription drugs and dietary supplements.* Montvale: Medical Economics.

Medical Economics Staff. (Ed.). (2006). *Physicians' desk reference* (60th ed.). Montvale: Medical Economics.

Mulvihill, M. L., Zelman, P., Holdaway, P., Tompary, E., & Turchany, J. (2006). *Human diseases: A systemic approach* (6th ed.). Upper Saddle River, NJ: Prentice Hall.

Rice, J. (2005). *Medical terminology with human anatomy.* Upper Saddle River, NJ: Prentice Hall.

Silverthorn, D. U. (2004). *Human physiology: An integrated approach.* Upper Saddle River, NJ: Benjamin-Cummings.

Wilson, B. A., Shannon, M. T., & Strang, C. L. (2006). *Nurse's drug guide 2006.* Upper Saddle River, NJ: Prentice Hall.

CHAPTER 1
Introduction to Pharmacology: Drug Regulation and Approval

Bond, C. A., Raehl, C. L., & Franke, T. (2001). Medication errors in United States hospitals. *Pharmacotherapy, 21*(9), 1023–1036.

Brown, S. D., & Landry, F. J. (2001). Recognizing, reporting, and reducing adverse drug reactions. *Southern Medical Journal, 94*(4), 370–373.

Carrico, J. M. (2000). Human Genome Project and pharmacogenomics: Implications for pharmacy. *Journal of American Pharmacology Association, 40*(1), 115–116.

Gaither, C. A., Kirking, D. M., Ascione, F. J., & Welage, L. S. (2001). Consumers' views on generic medications. *Journal of American Pharmacology Association, 41*(5), 729–736.

Kacew, S. (1999). Effects of over-the-counter drugs on the unborn child: What is known and how should this influence prescribing? *Pediatric Drugs, 1*(2), 75–80.

Kohn, L. T., Corrigan, J. M., & Donaldson, M. S. (Eds.). (1999). *To err is human: Building a safer system.* Washington, DC: The National Academy of Sciences, National Academy Press.

Lazarou, J., Pomeranz, B. H., & Corey, P. N. (1998). Incidence of adverse drug reactions in hospitalized patients. *Journal of American Medical Association, 279*(15), 1200–1205.

Newton, G. D., Pray, W. S., & Popovich, N. G. (2001). New OTC drugs and devices 2000: A selective review. *Journal of American Pharmacology Association, 41*(2), 273–282.

Phillips, K. A., Veenstra, D. L., Oren, E., Lee, J. K., & Sardee, W. (2001). Potential role of pharmacogenomics in reducing adverse drug reactions: A systematic review. *Journal of American Medical Association, 286,* 2270–2279.

CHAPTER 2
Drug Classes, Schedules, and Categories

Brass, E. P. (2001). Drug therapy: Changing the status of drugs from prescription to over-the counter availability. *New England Journal of Medicine, 345,* 810–816.

Drug Enforcement Agency. (2005). *Drugs of abuse* (2005 ed.). Retrieved May 27, 2005, from *http://www.usdoj.gov/dea/pubs/abuse/doa-p.pdf*

Smith, S. F., Duell, D. J., & Martin, B. C. (2004). *Clinical nursing skills* (6th ed.). Upper Saddle River, NJ: Prentice Hall.

CHAPTER 3
Methods of Drug Administration

Berman, A., Snyder, S., Kozier, B., & Erb, G. (2004). *Kozier and Erb's techniques in clinical nursing* (5th ed.). Upper Saddle River, NJ: Prentice Hall.

Institute for Safe Medical Practices. (2003). List of error-prone abbreviations, symbols, and dose designations. *ISMP MedicationSafetyAlert!, 8.*

Joint Commission on Accreditation of Healthcare Organizations. (2002). *The official "do not use" list.* Retrieved June 2, 2005, from *http://www.jcaho.org/accredited+organizations/patient+safety/dnu.htm*

Rosenthal, K. (2003). Keeping I.V. therapy safe with needleless systems. *Nursing Management, 34,* 16–20.

Smith, S. F., Duell, D. J., & Martin, B. C. (2002). *PhotoGuide of nursing skills.* Upper Saddle River, NJ: Prentice Hall.

CHAPTER 4
What Happens After a Drug Has Been Administered

Bateman, D. N. (2001). Introduction to pharmacokinetics and pharmacodynamics. *Journal of Toxicology—Clinical Toxicology, 39*(3), 207.

Buxton, I. L. (2006). Pharmacokinetics and pharmacodynamics: The dynamics of drug absorption, distribution, action and elimination. In L. L. Brunton, J. S. Lazo, and K. L. Parker. (Eds.), *The pharmacological basis of therapeutics* (11th ed.), (pp. 1–39). New York: McGraw-Hill.

Consider racial, ethnic, and cultural differences in cardiovascular drug effectiveness. (2001). *Progress in Cardiovascular Nursing, 16*(4), 152–160+.

Levy, R. H., Thummel, K. E., Trager, W. F., Hansten, P. D., & Eichelbaum, M. (Eds.). (2000). *Metabolic drug interactions.* Philadelphia: Lippinott Williams & Wilkins.

CHAPTER 5
Herbs and Dietary Supplements

Blumenthal, M. (Ed.). (2000). *Herbal medicine: Expanded Commission E monographs.* Austin, TX: American Botanical Council.

Ebadi, M. (2002). *Pharmcodynamic basis of herbal medicine.* Boca Raton, FL: CRC Press.

Eisenberg, D. M., Davis, R. B., Ettner, S. L., Appel, S., Wilkey, S., Van Rompay, M., & Kessler, R. C. (1998). Trends in alternative medicine use in the United States, 1990–1997. *Journal of American Medical Association, 280,* 1569–1575.

Fontaine, K. L. (2005). *Complementary and alternative therapies for nursing practice.* Upper Saddle River, NJ: Prentice Hall.

Foster, S., & Hobbs, C. (2002). *A field guide to western medicinal plants and herbs.* Boston and New York: Houghton Mifflin Co.

Goldman, P. (2001). Herbal medicines today and the roots of modern pharmacology. *Annals of Internal Medicine, 135*(8), 594–597.

Hardy, M. L. (2000). Herbs of special interest to women. *American Pharmacology Association, 40*(2), 234–242.

Hatcher, T., Dokken, D., & Sydnor-Greenberg, N. (2000). Exploring complementary and alternative medicine in pediatrics: Parents and professionals working together for new understanding. *Pediatric Nursing, 26*(4), 383.

Medical Economics Staff. (Ed.). (2006). *Physicians' desk reference for herbal medicines* (3rd ed.).

Montvale: Medical Economics. *The review of natural products: 2002.* Missouri: Facts and Comparisons®, Publisher.

Scott, G. N., & Elmer, G. W. (2002). Update on natural product-drug interactions. *American Journal of Health-System Pharmacy, 59*(4), 339–347.

Sierpina, V. S., Wollschlaeger, B., & Blumenthal, M. (2003). Ginkgo biloba. *American Family Physician, 68*(5), 923–926.

White, L. B., & Foster, S. (2000). *The herbal drugstore.* Emmaus, PA: Rodale.

White House Commission on Complementary and Alternative Medicine Policy. (2002, March). Final report, *http://govinfo.library.unt.edu/whccamp/*

CHAPTER 6
Substance Abuse

Haseltine, E. (2001). The unsatisfied mind: Are reward centers in your brain wired for substance abuse? *Discover, 22*(11), 88.

Jason, L. A., Davis, M. I., Ferrari, J. R., & Bishop, P. D. (2001). A review of research and implications for substance abuse recovery and community research. *Journal of Drug Education, 31*(1), 1–28.

Manoguerra, A. S. (2001). Methamphetamine abuse. *Journal of Toxicology Clinical Toxicology, 38*(2), 187.

Naegle, M. A., & D'Avanzo, C. E. (2001). *Addictions and substance abuse: Strategies for advanced practice nursing.* Upper Saddle River, NJ: Prentice Hall.

O'Brien, C. P. (2006). Drug addiction and drug abuse. In L. L. Brunton, J. S. Lazo, and K. L. Parker. (Eds.). *The pharmacological basis of therapeutics* (11th ed.), (pp. 607–627). New York: McGraw-Hill.

Sindelar, J. L., & Fiellin, D. A. (2001). Innovations in treatment for drug abuse: Solutions to a public health problem. *Annual Review of Public Health, 22,* 249.

Wasilow-Mueller, S., & Erickson, C. K. (2001). Drug abuse and dependency: Understanding gender differences in etiology and management. *Journal of American Pharmacology Association, 41*(1), 78–90.

CHAPTER 7
Drugs Affecting Functions of the Autonomic Nervous System

Westfall, T. C., & Westfall, D. P. (2006). Neurotransmission: The autonomic and somatic nervous systems. In L. L. Brunton, J. S. Lazo, and K. L. Parker. (Eds.). *The pharmacological basis of therapeutics* (11th ed.), (pp. 137–181). New York: McGraw-Hill.

CHAPTER 8
Drugs for Anxiety and Insomnia

Baldessarini, R. J. (2006). Drug therapy of depression and anxiety disorders. In L. L. Brunton, J. S. Lazo, and K. L. Parker. (Eds.). *The pharmacological basis of therapeutics* (11th ed.), (pp. 429–460). New York: McGraw-Hill.

Charney, D. S., Mihic, J., & Harris, A. (2006). Hypnotics and sedatives. In L. L. Brunton, J. S. Lazo, and K. L. Parker. (Eds.). *The pharmacological basis of therapeutics* (11th ed.), (pp. 401–438). New York: McGraw-Hill.

Fontaine, K. L., & Fletcher, J. S. (2003). *Mental health nursing* (5th ed.). Upper Saddle River, NJ: Prentice Hall.

Gorman, J. N. (2001). Generalized anxiety disorder. *Clinical Corner, 3*(3), 37–46.

Lippmann, S., Mazour, I., & Shahab, H. (2001). Insomnia: Therapeutic approach. *Southern Medical Journal, 94*(9), 866–873.

Smock, T. K. (2001). *Physiological psychology: A neuroscience approach.* Upper Saddle River, NJ: Prentice Hall.

Stahl, S. M. (1999). Antidepressants: The blue chip psychotropic for the modern treatment of anxiety disorders. *Journal of Clinical Psychiatry, 60,* 6.

Vitiello, M. V. (2000). Effective treatment of sleep disturbances in older adults. *Clinical Corner, 2*(5), 16–27.

CHAPTER 9
Drugs for Emotional and Mood Disorders

American Academy of Pediatrics. (2000). Diagnosis and evaluation of the child with attention deficit-hyperactivity disorder. *Pediatrics, 105*(5), 1158–1170.

Baldessarini, R. J., & Tarazi, F. I. (2006). Pharmacotherapy of psychosis and mania. In L. L. Brunton, J. S. Lazo, and K. L. Parker. (Eds.). *The pharmacological basis of therapeutics* (11th ed.), (pp. 461–500). New York: McGraw-Hill.

Desai, H. D., & Jann, M. W. (2000). Major depression in women: A review of the literature. *Journal of American Pharmacology Association, 40*(4), 525–537.

Emslie, G. J., & Mayes, T. L. (1999). Depression in children and adolescents: A guide to diagnosis and treatment. *CNS Drugs, 11*(3), 181–189.

Janicak, P. G., Dowd, S. M., Martis, B., Alam, D., Beedle, D., Krasuski, J., Strong, M. J., Sharma, R., Rosen, C., & Viaha, M. (2002, April 15). Repetitive transcranial magnetic stimulation versus electroconvulsive therapy for major depression: Preliminary results of a randomized trial *Biological Psychiatry, 51*(8), 659–667.

Nelson, J. C. (2000). Augmentation strategies in depression. *Journal of Clinical Psychiatry, 61,* 13–19.

Rosenburg, P. B., Mehndiratta, R. B., Mehndiratta, Y. B., Wamer, A., Rosse, R. B., & Balish, M. (2002). Repetitive transcranial magnetic stimulation treatment of comorbid posttraumatic stress disorder and major depression. *Journal of Neuropsychiatry and Clinical Neurosciences, 14*(3), 270–276.

CHAPTER 10
Drugs for Psychoses and Degenerative Diseases of the Nervous System

Bailey, K. (2003). Aripiprazole: The newest antipsychotic agent for the treatment of schizophrenia. *Pyschological Nursing and Mental Health Services, 41*(2), 14–18.

Baldessarini, R. J., & Tarazi, F. I. (2006). Pharmacotherapy of psychosis and mania. In L. L. Brunton, J. S. Lazo, and K. L. Parker. (Eds.). *The pharmacological basis of therapeutics* (11th ed.), (pp. 461–500). New York: McGraw-Hill.

Brown, C. S., Markowitz, J. S., Moore, T. R., & Parker, N. G. (1999). Atypical antipsychotics: Part II. Adverse effects, drug interactions, and costs. *Annals of Pharmacotherapy, 33,* 210–217.

Burns, M. J. (2001). The pharmacology and toxicology of atypical antipsychotic agents. *Journal of Toxicology—Clinical Toxicology, 39*(1), 1.

Canales, P. L., Olsen, J., Miller, A. L., & Crismon, M. L. (1999). Role of antipsychotic polypharmacotherapy in the treatment of schizophrenia. *CNS Drugs, 12,* 179–188.

Markowitz, J. S., Brown, C. S., & Moore, T. R. (1999). Atypical antipsychotics: Part I. Pharmacology, pharmacokinetics, and efficacy. *Annals of Pharmacotherapy, 33,* 73–85.

Owen, W., & Castle, D. J. (1999). Late-onset schizophrenia: Epidemiology, diagnosis, management, and outcomes. *Drugs and Aging, 15*(2), 81–89.

Tandon, R., Milner, K., & Jibson, M. D. (1999). Antipsychotics from theory to practice: Integrating clinical and basic data. *Journal of Clinical Psychiatry, 8,* 21–28.

Vitiello, B. (2001). Psychopharmacology for young children: Clinical needs and research opportunities. *Pediatrics, 108*(4), 983.

CHAPTER 11
Drugs for Seizures

Bourdet, S. V., Gidal, B. E., & Alldredge, B. K. (2001). Pharmacologic management of epilepsy in the elderly. *Journal of American Pharmacology Association, 41*(3), 421–436.

Landover, M. D. (1999). *Epilepsy: A report to the nation* [on-line]. Available: *http://www.efa.org/epusa/nation/nation/html*

McNamara, J. O. (2006). Pharmacotherapy of the epilepsies. In L. L. Brunton, J. S. Lazo, and K. L. Parker. (Eds.). *The pharmacological basis of therapeutics* (11th ed.), (pp. 501–526). New York: McGraw-Hill.

Schachter, S. C. (2000). The next wave of anticonvulsants: Focus on levetiracetam, oxcarbazepine, and zonisamide. *CNS Drugs, 14*(3), 229–249.

Stahl, S. M. (1999). Antidepressants: The blue chip psychotropic for the modern treatment of anxiety disorders. *Journal of Clinical Psychiatry, 60,* 6.

Tatum, W. O., Galvez, R., Benbadis, S., & Carrazana, E. (2000). New antiepileptic drugs: Into the new millennium. *Archives of Family Medicine, 9,* 1135–1141.

Winkelman, C. (1999). Pharmacology update: A review of pharmacodynamics and pharmacokinetics in seizure management. *Journal of Neuroscience Nursing, 31*(1), 50–53.

CHAPTER 12
Drugs for Pain Control

Bannwarth, B. (1999). Risk-benefit assessment of opioids in chronic noncancer pain. *Drug Safety, 21*(4), 283–296.

Barkin, R. L., & Barkin, D. (2001). Pharmacologic management of acute and chronic pain: Focus on drug interactions and patient-specific pharmacotherapeutic selection. *Southern Medical Journal, 94*(8), 756–812.

Broadbent, C. (2000). The pharmacology of acute pain—Part 3. *Nursing Times, 96*(26), 39. elt-Hansen, P., DeVries, P., & Sexena, P. R. (2000). Triptans in migraine: A comparative review of pharmacology, pharmacokinetics, and efficacy. *Drugs, 60*(6), 1259–1287.

FDA News. (2004, September 30). *FDA issues Public Health Advisory on Vioxx as its manufacturer voluntarily recalls the product.* Retrieved June 8, 2005, from *http://www.fda.gov/bbs/topics/news/2004/NEW01122.html*

Glajchen, M. (2001). Chronic pain: Treatment barriers and strategies for clinical practice. *Journal of the American Board of Family Practice, 14*(3), 178–183.

Guay, D.R.P. (2001). Adjunctive agents in the management of chronic pain. *Pharmacotherapy, 21*(9), 1070–1081.

Gunstein, H. B., & Akil, H. (2006). Opioid analgesics. In L. L. Brunton, J. S. Lazo, and K. L. Parker. (Eds.). *The pharmacological basis of therapeutics* (11th ed.), (pp. 547–590). New York: McGraw-Hill.

Khouzam, H. R. (2000). Chronic pain and its management in primary care. *Southern Medical Journal, 93*(10), 946–952.

Tepper, S. J., & Rapoport, A. M. (1999). The triptans: A summary. *CNS Drugs, 12*(5), 403–417.

CHAPTER 13
Drugs for Anesthesia

Catterall, W. A., & Mackie, K. (2006). Local anesthetics. In L. L. Brunton, J. S. Lazo, and K. L. Parker. (Eds.). *The pharmacological basis of therapeutics* (11th ed.), (pp. 369–386). New York: McGraw-Hill.

Colbert, B. J., & Mason, B. J. (2002). *Integrated cardiopulmonary pharmacology.* Upper Saddle River, NJ: Prentice Hall.

Evers, A. S., Crowder, C. M., & Balser, J. R. (2006). General anesthetics. In L. L. Brunton, J. S. Lazo, and K. L. Parker. (Eds.). *The pharmacological basis of therapeutics* (11th ed.), (pp. 341–368). New York: McGraw-Hill.

Nagelhout, J. J., Nagelhout, K., & Zaglaniczny, V. H. (2001). *Handbook of nurse anesthesia* (2nd ed.). Philadelphia: W. B. Saunders.

Omoigui, S. (2001). *Sota Omogui's anesthesia drugs handbook* (4th ed.). Hawthorne, CA: State of the Art Technologies.

Stoelting, R. K. (2006). *Pharmacology and physiology in anesthetic practice* (4th ed.). Philadelphia: Lippincott, Williams, and Wilkins.

Waugaman, W. R., Foster, S. D., & Rigor, B. M. (1999). *Principles and practice of nurse anesthesia* (3rd ed.). Upper Saddle River, NJ: Prentice Hall.

CHAPTER 14
Drugs for Coagulation Disorders

Adams, M., Josephson, D., & Holland, N. (2005). *Pharmacology for nurses: A pathophysiologic approach.* Upper Saddle River, NJ: Prentice Hall.

Ageno, W., Crotti, S., & Turpie, A. G. (2004, March). The safety of antithrombotic therapy during pregnancy. *Expert Opinion on Drug Safety, 3*(2), 113–118.

Alligood, K. A., & Iltz, J. L. (2001). Update on antithrombotic use and mechanism of action. *Progess in Cardiovascular Nursing, 16*(2), 81–85.

Bates, S. M., & Hinsberg, J. S. (2004, July 15). Clinical practice. Treatment of deep-vein thrombosis. *New England Journal of Medicine, 351*(3), 268–277.

Berge, E., & Sandercock, P. (2004). Anticoagulants versus antiplatelet agents for acute ischemic stroke. *Cochrane Review Abstracts,* July 1, 2004.

Brouwer, M. A., Clappers, N., & Verheugt, F. W. (2004, May). Adjunctive treatment in patients treated with thrombolytic therapy. *Heart, 90*(5), 581–588.

Ferguson, J. (2004, March). Low-molecular-weight heparins and glycoprotein IIb/IIIa antagonists in acute coronary syndromes. *Journal of Invasive Cardiology, 16*(3), 136–144.

HealthSquare.com (2003). *Coumadin: Prescription Drug Reference* [on-line]. *www.healthsquare.com*

Hiatt, W. R. (2001). Drug therapy: Medical treatment of peripheral arterial disease and claudication. *New England Journal of Medicine, 344,* 1608–1621.

Lie, D. (2004). Ginseng reduces warfarin efficacy. *Medscape Medical News,* July 6.

Majerus, P. W., & Tollefson, D. M. (2006). Blood coagulation and anticoagulant, thrombolytic, and antiplatelet drugs. In L. Brunton, J. Lazo, and K. Parker. (Eds.), *The pharmacological basis of therapeutics* (pp. 1467–1487). New York: McGraw-Hill.

McGlasson, D. L. (2004, Spring). Oral anticoagulants. *Clinical Laboratory Science, 17*(2), 107–112.

Medical Economics Staff. (Ed.). (2000). *PDR for herbal medicines.* Montvale, NJ: Author.

Medical Economics Staff. (Ed.). (2001). *PDR for nutritional supplements.* Montvale, NJ: Author.

Wilson, B. A., Shannon, M. T., & Stang, C. L. (2005). *Nurse's drug guide 2005.* Upper Saddle River, NJ: Prentice Hall.

CHAPTER 15
Drugs for Hypertension

Chaudhry, S. I., Krumholz, H. M., & Foody, J. M. (2004). Systolic hypertension in older persons. *Journal of American Medical Association, 292*(9), 1074–1080.

Colbert, B. J., & Mason, B. J. (2001). *Integrated cardiopulmonary pharmacology.* Upper Saddle River, NJ: Prentice Hall.

Hajjar, I. M., Grim, C. E., George, V., & Theodore, A. (2001). Impact of diet on blood pressure and age-related changes in blood pressure in the U.S. population: Analysis of NHANES III. *Archive of Internal Medicine, 161,* 589.

Hoffman, B. B. (2006). Therapy of hypertension. In L. L. Brunton, J. S. Lazo, and K. L. Parker. (Eds.). *The pharmacological basis of therapeutics* (11th ed.), (pp. 845–868). New York: McGraw-Hill.

National High Blood Pressure Education Program Working Group on High Blood Pressure in Children and Adolescents. (2004). The fourth report on the diagnosis, evaluation, and treatment of high blood pressure in children and adolescents. *Pediatrics, 114*(2 Suppl), 555–576.

National Institues of Health. (2003). NHLBI issues new high blood pressure clinical practice guidelines. *NIH NEWS.* Retrieved June 14, 2005, from *http://www.nhlbi.nih.gov*

Nurko, S. (2001). At what level of hyperkalemia or creatinine elevation should ACE inhibitor therapy be stopped or not started? *Cleveland Clinical Journal of Medicine, 68*(9), 754–760.

Poudre Valley Health System. (2003). Herbal medicines and dietary supplements: Information for people with heart disease. Retrieved June 14, 2005, from *http://www.pvhs.org*

Saunders, E. (2004). Managing hypertension in African-American patients. *Journal of Clinical Hypertension, 6*(4 Suppl 1), 19–25.

Shah, S. U., Anjum, S., & Littler, W. A. (2004). Use of diuretics in cardiovascular disease: (2) hypertension. *Postgraduate Medical Journal, 80*(943), 271–276.

Simpson, C. (2003). Autonomic nervous system agents: Adrenergics and adrenergic blocking agents. Retrieved June 14, 2005, from *http://www.cotc.tech.oh.us*

Thadhani, R., Camargo, C. A., Jr., Stampfer, M. J., Curhan, G. C., Willett, W. C., & Rimm, E. B. (2002). Prospective study of moderate alcohol consumption and risk hypertension in young women. *Archive of Internal Medicine, 162,* 569–574.

U.S. Department of Health and Human Services. (2003). *JNC-7 Express: The seventh report of the Joint National Committee on Prevention, Detection Evaluation and Treatment of High Blood Pressure* (NIH Publication No.03-5233). Bethesda, MD: Author.

CHAPTER 16

Drugs for Heart Failure

Albrant, D. H. (2001). Drug treatment protocol: Management of chronic systolic heart failure. *Journal of American Pharmacology Association, 41*(5), 672–681.

Amabile, C. M., & Spencer, A. P. (2004). Keeping your patient with heart failure safe: A review of potentially dangerous medications. *Archive of Internal Medicine, 164*(7), 709–720.

Dec, G. W. (2003). Digoxin remains useful in the management of chronic heart failure. *Medical Clinics of North America, 87*(2), 317–337.

Gomberg-Maitland, M., Baran, D. A., & Fuster, V. (2001). Treatment of congestive heart failure: Guidelines for the primary care health care provider and the heart failure specialist. *Archive of Internal Medicine, 161,* 342–352.

Jamali, A. H., Tang, A. H. W., Khot, U. N., & Fowler, M. B. (2001). The role of angiotensin receptor blockers in the management of chronic heart failure. *Archive of Internal Medicine, 161,* 667–672.

Opie, L. H., & Gersh, B. J. (Eds.). (2001). *Drugs for the heart* (5th ed.). Philadelphia: W. B. Saunders.

Paul, S. (2002). Balancing diuretic therapy in heart failure: Loop diuretics, thiazides, and antagonists. *CHF, 8*(6), 307–312.

Richardson, L. G. (2003). Psychosocial issues in patients with congestive heart failure. *Progressive Cardiovascular Nursing, 18*(1), 19–27.

Rocco, T. P. & Fang, J. C. (2006). Pharmacotherapy of congestive heart failure. In L. L. Brunton, J. S. Lazo, & K. L. Parker. (Eds.). *The pharmacological basis of therapeutics* (11th ed.), (pp. 869–898). New York: McGraw-Hill.

Sperelakis, N., Kurachi, Y., Terzic, A., & Cohen, M. (Eds.). (2001). *Heart physiology and pathophysiology* (4th ed.). San Diego: Academic Press.

Tang, W. H. & Francis, G. S. (2003). Novel pharmacological treatments for heart failure. *Expert Opinion on Investigational Drugs, 12*(11), 1791–1801.

CHAPTER 17

Drugs for Dysrhythmias

Berry, C., Rankin, A. C., & Brady, A. (2004). Bradycardia and tachycardia occurring in older people: An introduction. *British Journal of Cardiology, 11*(1), 61–64.

Dayer, M., & Hardman, S. (2002). Special problems with antiarrhythmic drugs in the elderly: Safety, tolerability, and efficacy. *American Journal of Geriatric Cardiology, 11*(6), 370–375.

Ellison, K. E., Stevenson, W. G., Sweeney, M. O., Epstein, L. M., & Maisel, W. H. (2003). Management of arrhythmias in heart failure. *Congestive Heart Failure, 9*(2), 91–99.

Haugh, K. H. (2002). Antidysrhythmic agents at the turn of the twenty-first century: A current review. *Critical Care Nursing Clinics of North America, 14*(1), 53–69.

Huikuri, H. V., Castellanos, A., & Myerburg, R. J. (2001). Medical progress: Sudden death due to cardiac arrhythmias. *New England Journal of Medicine, 345,* 1473–1482.

Kern, L. S. (2004). Postoperative atrial fibrillation: New directions in prevention and treatment. *Journal of Cardiovascular Nursing, 19*(2), 103–115.

Kudzma, E. C. (2001). Cultural competence: Cardiovascular medications. *Medscape DrugInfo* (2003) *Inderal.* Available at *www.medscape.com/druginfo/*

Podrid, P. J., & Kowey, P. R. (Eds.). (2001). *Cardiac arrhythmia: Mechanisms, diagnosis, and management* (2nd ed.). Philadelphia: Lippincott, Williams, and Wilkins.

Roden, D. M. (2006). Antiarrhythmic drugs. In L. L. Brunton, J. S. Lazo, and K. L. Parker. (Eds.). *The pharmacological basis of therapeutics* (11th ed.), (pp. 899–932). New York: McGraw-Hill.

CHAPTER 18

Drugs for Angina Pectoris, Myocardial Infarction, and Cerebrovascular Accident

Demaerschalk, B. M. (2003). Diagnosis and management of stroke (brain attack). *Seminars in Neurology, 23*(3), 241–252.

Harvey, S. (2004). The nursing assessment and management of patients with angina. *British Journal of Nursing, 13*(10), 598–601.

Jain, A., Wadehra, V., & Timmis, A. D. (2003). Management of stable angina. *Postgraduate Medical Journal, 79*(932), 332–336.

Kreisberg, R. A. (2000). Overview of coronary heart disease and selected risk factors. *Clinical Review* (Spring), 4–9.

Levine, G. N., Ali, M. N., & Schafer, A. I. (2001). Antithrombotic therapy in patients with acute coronary syndromes. *Archive of Internal Medicine, 161,* 937–948.

McGovern, R., & Rudd, A. (2003). Management of stroke. *Postgraduate Medical Journal, 79*(928), 87–92.

Michel, T. (2006). Treatment of myocardial ischemia. In L. L. Brunton, J. S. Lazo, and K. L. Parker. (Eds.). *The pharmacological basis of therapeutics* (11th ed.), (pp. 823–844). New York: McGraw-Hill.

Noronha, B., Duncan, E., & Byrne, J. A. (2003). Optimal medical management of angina. *Current Cardiology Report, 5*(4), 259–265.

Parchure, N., & Brecker, S. J. (2002). Management of acute coronary syndromes. *Current Opinions on Critical Care, 8*(3), 230–235.

Quinn, T. (2004). Managing acute myocardial infarction. *Emerging Nurse, 12*(3), 17–19.

Staniforth, A. D. (2001). Contemporary management of chronic stable angina. *Drugs & Aging, 18*(2), 109–121.

Vega, C. (2004). Angina guidelines recommend treatment and follow-up. *Medscape Medical News.* Available at: *http://www.medscape.com/viewarticle/491419*

CHAPTER 19

Drugs for Shock and Anaphylaxis

Bench, S. (2004). Clinical skills: Assessing and treating shock: a nursing perspective. *British Journal of Nursing, 13*(12), 715–721.

Crusher, R. (2004). Anaphylaxis. *Emerging Nurse, 12*(3), 24–31.

Dellinger, R. P. (2003). Cardiovascular management of septic shock. *Critical Care Medicine, 31*(3), 946–955.

Kolecki, P., & Menckhoff, C. R. (2001, December 11). Hypovolemic shock. *eMedicine Journal, 2*(12).

Liolios, A. (2004). Volume resuscitation: The crystalloid vs. colloid debate revisited paper given at the 24th International Symposium on

Intensive Care and Emergency Medicine. *Medscape Today.* Retrieved July 13, 2005, from *http://www.medscape.com/viewarticle/480288*

Menon, V., & Fincke, R. (2003, Jan–Feb). Cardiogenic shock: A summary of the randomized SHOCK trial. *Congestive Heart Failure, 9*(1), 35–39.

Moser-Wade, D. M., Bartley, M. K., & Chiari-Allwein, H. L. (2000). Shock: Do you know how to respond? *Nursing 2000, 30*(10), 34–40.

Tang, A. W. (2003). A practical guide to anaphylaxis. *American Family Physician, 68*(7), 1325–1332.

von Rosenstiel, N., von Rosenstiel, I., & Adam, D. (2001). Management of sepsis and septic shock in infants and children. *Paediatric Drugs, 3*(1), 9–27.

CHAPTER 20
Drugs for Lipid Disorders

Gylling, H., & Miettinen, T. A. (2002). Combination therapy with statins. *Current Opinion on Investigating Drugs, 3*(9), 1318–1323.

Mahley, R. W., & Bersot, T. P. (2006). Drug therapy for hypercholesterolemia and dyslipidemia. In L. L. Brunton, J. S. Lazo, and K. L. Parker. (Eds.). *The pharmacological basis of therapeutics* (11th ed.), (pp. 933–964). New York: McGraw-Hill.

Maltin, L. J. (2002, April 9). Statin drugs may fight Alzheimer's, too. *WebMD Medical News.*

McLoughlin, C. (2004). Statins. *Professional Nurse, 19*(11), 51–52.

Nichols, N. (2004). Clinical practice guidelines for the management of dyslipidemia. *Canadian Journal of Cardiovascular Nursing, 14*(2), 7–10.

Nutrition and Metabolism Advisory Committee, Heart Foundation. (2001). *Plant sterols and stanols, a position statement.*

Robinson, A. W., Sloan, H. L., & Arnold, G. (2001). Use of niacin in the prevention and management of hyperlipidemia. *Progressive Cardiovascular Nursing, 16*(1), 14–20.

U.S. Food and Drug Administration Center for Food Safety and Applied Nutrition Office of Nutritional Products, Labeling, and Dietary Supplements. (February 2001). (Updated September 10, 2001). *New dietary ingredients in dietary supplements.*

Xydakis, A. M., & Ballantyne, C. M. (2002). Combination therapy for combined dyslipidemia. *American Journal of Cardiology, 20, 90*(10B), 21K–29K.

Xydakis, A. M., & Ballantyne, C. M. (2004). Management of metabolic syndrome: Statins. *Endocrinology and Metabolism Clinics of North America, 33*(3), 509–523.

Young, K. L., Allen, J. K., & Kelly, K. M. (2001). HDL cholesterol: Striving for healthier levels. *Clinical Review, 1*(5), 50–61.

CHAPTER 21
Drugs for Inflammation, Allergies, and Immune Disorders

Braunstahl, G., & Hellings, P. W. (2003). Allergic rhinitis and asthma: The link further unraveled. *Current Opinion in Pulmonary Medicine, 9*(1), 46–51.

Capriotti, T. (2001). Monoclonal antibodies: Drugs that combine pharmacology and biotechnology. *MedSurg Nursing, 10*(2), 89.

Centers for Disease Control and Prevention. (2003). *National vaccine program office: Immunization laws.* Retrieved July 9, 2005, from *http://wwwcdc.gov/od/nvpo/law.htm*

Centers for Disease Control and Prevention. (2005). Fact sheet: Eliminating racial and ethnic health disparities. U.S. Department of Health and Human Services. Available at: *http://www.cdc.gov/omh/AboutUs/disparities.htm*

Children's Defense Fund. (2003). Child health: Immunizations. Retrieved July 13, 2005, from *http://www.childrensdefense.org/childhealth/immunizations/default.aspx*

Fitzgerald, G. A., & Patrono, C. (2001). Drug therapy: The coxibs, selective inhibitors of cyclooxygenase-2. *New England Journal of Medicine, 345,* 433–442.

Fitzgerald, K. A., O'Neill, L. A. J., & Gearing, A. J., & Callard, R. E. (Eds.). (2001). *The Cytokine FactsBook* (2nd ed.). New York: Academy Press.

Galley, H. F. (2003). *Critical care focus: Inflammation and immunity,* Vol. 10. London: BMJ Publishing Group.

Karam, U. S., & Reddy, K. R. (2003). Pegylated interferons. *Clinical Liver Disease, 7*(1), 139–148.

Krensky, A. M., Vincenti, F., & Bennett, W. M. (2006). Immunosuppressants, tolerogens, and immunostimulants. In L. L. Brunton, J. S. Lazo, and K. L. Parker. (Eds.). *The pharmacological basis of therapeutics* (11th ed.), (pp. 1405–1431). New York: McGraw-Hill.

Neuzil, K. M. (2003). Adult immunizations: A review of current recommendations. Retrieved July 12, 2005, from *http://www.medscape.com/viewprogram/2237*

Raeburn, D., & Giembycz, M. A. (Eds). (2001). *Rhinitis: Immunopathology and pharmacotherapy.* Boston: Birkhauser.

Santamaria, P. (2003). *Cytokines and autoimmune disease.* New York: Plenum Publishing Corp.

Sklar, G. E. (2002). Hemolysis as a potential complication of acetaminophen overdose in a patient with glucose-6-phosphate dehydrogenase deficiency. *Pharmacotherapy, 22*(5), 656–658.

CHAPTER 22
Drugs for Bacterial Infections

Barclay, L. (2002). *Linezolid as effective as vancomycin for MRSA.* Medscape Medical News 2002: June 14, 2002.

Bartlett, J. G. (2004). *Antimicrobial drug resistance update.* 44th Interscience Conference on Antimicrobial Agents & Chemotherapy: Antimicrobial Drug Resistance and Emerging Infectious Threats.

Chambers, H. F. (2006). General considerations of antimicrobial therapy. In L. L. Brunton, J. S. Lazo, and K. L. Parker. (Eds.). *The pharmacological basis of therapeutics* (11th ed.), (pp. 1095–1110). New York: McGraw-Hill.

Diekema, D., & Jones, R. (2001). Oxazolidinones: A review. *Drugs, 59*(1), 7–16.

Gilbert, D. N., Moellering, R. C., & Sande, M. A. (2001). *The Sanford guide to antimicrobial therapy 2001* (31st ed.). Hyde Park, VT: Antimicrobial Therapy, Inc.

Gleckman, R. A. (2004). Selected issues in antibiotic resistance. *Infections in Medicine, 21*(3), 114–122.

Kenyon, N. J., & Albertson, T. E. (2004). Current issues in treatment of respiratory infections. *Infections in Medicine, 21*(4), 167–173.

Petri, W. A. (2006). Chemotherapy of tuberculosis, *Mycobacterium avium* complex disease, and leprosy. In L. L. Brunton, J. S. Lazo, and K. L. Parker. (Eds.). *The pharmacological basis of therapeutics* (11th ed.), (pp. 1203–1224). New York: McGraw-Hill.

Petri, W. A. (2006). Penicillins, cephalosporins, and other beta-lactam antibiotics. In L. L. Brunton, J. S. Lazo, and K. L. Parker. (Eds.). *The pharmocological basis of therapeutics* (11th ed.), (pp. 1127–1154). New York: McGraw-Hill.

Petri, W. A. (2006). Sulfonamides, trimethoprim-sulfamethoxazole, quinolones, and agents for urinary tract infections. In L. L. Brunton, J. S. Lazo, and K. L. Parker. (Eds.). *The pharmacological basis of therapeutics* (11th ed.), (pp. 1111–1126). New York: McGraw-Hill.

Small, P. M., & Fujiwara, P. I. (2001). Medical progress: Management of tuberculosis in the United States. *New England Journal of Medicine, 345,* 189–200.

Tortora, G. J., Funke, B. R., & Case, C. L. (2001). *Microbiology: An introduction* (7th ed). Menlo Park, CA: Benjamin Cummings.

Wooten, J., & Sakind, A. (2003). *Superbugs: Unmasking the threat. RN, 3*(66), 37–43.

CHAPTER 23
Drugs for Fungal, Viral, and Parasitic Diseases

Bennet, J. E. (2006). Antifungal agents. In L. L. Brunton, J. S. Lazo, and K. L. Parker. (Eds.). *The pharmacological basis of therapeutics* (11th ed.), (pp. 1225–1242). New York: McGraw-Hill.

Centers for Disease Control and Prevention. (2002a). Recommendations of the International Task Force of Disease Eradication. *MMWR,* U.S. Department of Health and Human Services.

Centers for Disease Control and Prevention. (2002b). Sexually transmitted diseases treatment guidelines. *MMWR,* 51, 1–80. U.S. Department of Health and Human Services.

Dickson, R., Awasthi, S., Dimellweek, C., & Williamson, P. (2003). Antihelmintic drugs for treating worms in children: Effects on growth and cognitive performance. *Cochrane Review.* Retrieved from *http://www.medscape.com*

Dismukes, W. E., Pappas, P. G., & Sobel, J. D. (2003). *Clinical mycology.* Oxford University Press.

Jucker, E., Muller, J., Polak, A., Kappe, R., Rimek, D., Seibold, M., & Tintelnot, K. (2004). *Antifungal agents: Advances and problems (Progress in Drug Research. Special Topic).* Boston: Birkhauser.

Shapiro, T. A., & Goldberg, D. E. (2006). Chemotherapy of protozoal infections: malaria In L. L. Brunton, J. S. Lazo, and K. L. Parker. (Eds.). *The pharmacological basis of therapeutics* (11th ed.), (pp. 869–898). New York: McGraw-Hill.

Steile, R. W. (2002). Focus on infection: Prevention, detection and treatment. *http://www.medscape.com*

Turness, B. W., Beach, M. J., and Roberts, J. M. (2000). Giardiasis surveillance. *MMWR,* Centers for Disease Control and Prevention.

van Voorhis, W. C., & Weller, P. F. (2004). Protozoan infections. *ACP Medicine,* posted 11/19/2004.

CHAPTER 24
Drugs for Neoplasia

Birner, A. (2003). Safe administration of oral chemotherapy. *Clinical Journal of Oncological Nursing, 7*(2), 158–162.

Chabner, B. A., Amrein, P. C., Druker, B., Michaelson, M. D., Mitsiades, C. S., Goss, P. E., et al. (2006). Chemotherapy of neoplastic diseases. In L. L. Brunton, J. S. Lazo, and K. L. Parker. (Eds.). *The pharmacological basis of therapeutics* (11th ed.), (pp. 1315–1403). New York: McGraw-Hill.

Fortenbaugh, C., & Rummel, M. (2004). Chemotherapy safety. *Clinical Journal of Oncological Nursing, 8*(4), 424–425.

Hood, L. E. (2003). Chemotherapy in the elderly: Supportive measures for chemotherapy-induced myelotoxicity. *Clinical Journal of Oncological Nursing, 2*(7), 185–190.

Kirsner, K. M. (2003). Cancer: New therapies and new approaches to recurring problems. *American Association of Nurse Anesthetists Journal, 71*(1), 55–62.

Marek, C. (2003). Antiemetic therapy in patients receiving cancer chemotherapy. *Oncological Nursing Forum, 30*(2), 259–271.

Oh, W. K. (2002). The evolving role of estrogen therapy in prostate cancer. *Clinical Prostate Cancer, 1*(2), 81–89.

Smith, B., Waltzman, R., & Rugo, H. (2002). Living longer with cancer: Preserving quality of life. Produced 12/10/02. *http://healthology.com*

CHAPTER 25
Drugs for Pulmonary Disorders

Altman, E. E. (2004). Update on COPD. Today's strategies improve quality of life. *Advanced Nursing Practices, 12*(3), 49–54.

Celli, B. (2003). *Pharmacotherapy in chronic obstructive pulmonary disease.* New York: Marcel Dekker.

Colbert, B. J., & Mason, B. J. (2002). *Integrated cardiopulmonary pharmacology.* Upper Saddle River, NJ: Prentice Hall.

Luggen, A. S. (2004). Pharmacology tips: Medications that complicate asthma control in older people. *Geriatric Nursing, 25*(3), 184.

Rogers, D. F. (2003). Airway hypersecretion in allergic rhinitis and asthma: New pharmacotherapy. *Current Allergy Asthma Report, 3*(3), 238–248.

Rosenwasser, L. J. (2002). Treatment of allergic rhinitis. *American Journal of Medicine, 16*(113 Suppl 9A), 17S–24S.

Roy, S. R. (2003). Asthma. *Southern Medical Journal, 96*(11), 1061–1067.

Stevens, N. (2003). Inhaler devices for asthma and COPD: Choice and technique. *Professional Nurse, 18*(11), 641–645.

Undem, B. J. (2006). Pharmacotherapy of asthma. In L. L. Brunton, J. S. Lazo, and K. L. Parker. (Eds.). *The pharmacological basis of therapeutics* (11th ed.), (pp. 717–735). New York: McGraw-Hill.

Vega, C. (2005). Budesonide/formoterol may be effective for maintenance and acute relief of asthma. *American Journal of Respiratory Critical Care Medicine, 171,* 129–136.

Weir, P. (2004). Quick asthma assessment. A stepwise approach to treatment. *Advanced Nurse Practioner, 12*(1), 53–56.

Wheeler, L. (2003, Mar–Apr). The last word: Asthma management in schools. *FDA Consumer, 37*(2).

CHAPTER 26
Drugs for Gastrointestinal Disorders

Hoogerwerf, W. A., & Pasricha, P. J. (2006). Pharmacotherapy of gastric acidity, peptic ulcers and gastroesophageal reflux disease. In L. L. Brunton, J. S. Lazo, and K. L. Parker. (Eds.). *The pharmacological basis of therapeutics* (11th ed.), (pp. 967–982). New York: McGraw-Hill.

Huggins, R. M., Scates, A. C., & Latour, J. K. (2003). Intravenous proton-pump inhibitors versus H_2-antagonists for treatment of GI bleeding. *Annals of Pharmacotherapy, 37*(3), 433–437.

Meurer, L. N., & Bower, D. J. (2002). Management of *Helicobacter pylori* infection. *American Family Physician, 65,* 1327–1336, 1339.

Patel, A. S., Pohl, J. F., & Easley, D. J. (2003). What's new: Proton pump inhibitors and pediatrics. *Pediatric Review, 24*(1), 12–15.

Petersen, A. M. (2003). *Helicobacter pylori:* An invading microorganism? A review. *FEMS Immunology and Medical Microbiology, 36*(3), 117–126.

Sharma, P., & Vakil, N. (2003). *Helicobacter pylori* and reflux disease. *Alimentary Pharmacology and Therapeutics, 17*(3), 297–305.

Stanghellini, V. (2003). Management of gastroesophageal reflux disease. *Drugs Today, 39* (Suppl A), 15–20.

Vanderhoff, B. T., & Tahboub, R. M. (2002).Proton pump inhibitors: An update. *American Family Physician, 66,* 273–280.

CHAPTER 27
Vitamins, Minerals, and Nutritional Supplements

Bhagavan, N. V. (2002). *Medical biochemistry.* Burlington, MA: Harcourt/Academic Press.

Kaushansky, K., & Kipps, T. J. (2006). Hematopoietic agents: growth factors, minerals and vitamins. In L. L. Brunton, J. S. Lazo, and K. L. Parker. (Eds.). *The pharmacological basis of therapeutics* (11th ed.), (pp. 1433–1466). New York: McGraw-Hill.

Oh, R. C., & Brown, D. L. (2003). Vitamin B_{12} deficiency. *American Family Physician, 67,* 979–986, 993–994.

Padayatty, S. J., Katz, A., Wang, Y., Eck, P., Kwon, O., Lee, J. H., et al. (2003). Vitamin C as an antioxidant: Evaluation of its role in disease prevention. *Journal of American College of Nutrition, 22*(1), 18–35.

Perrotta, S., Nobili, B., Rossi, F., Di Pinto, D., Cucciolla, V., Borriello, A., et al. (2003). Riboflavin (vitamin B-2) and health. *American Journal of Clinical Nursing, 77*(6), 1352–1360.

Ragione, F. (2003). Vitamin A and infancy. Biochemical, functional, and clinical aspects. *Vitamins and Hormones, 66,* 457–591.

Rampersaud, G. C., Kauwell, G. P., & Bailey, L. B. (2003). Folate: A key to optimizing health and reducing disease risk in the elderly. *Journal of American College of Nutrition, 22*(1), 1–8.

CHAPTER 28
Drugs for Fluid, Acid-Base, and Electrolyte Disorders

Bard, R. L., Bleske, B. E., & Nicklas, J. M. (2004). Food: An unrecognized source of loop diuretic resistance. *Pharmacotherapy, 24*(5), 630–637.

Bunn, F., Alderson, P., & Hawkins, V. (2004). Colloid solutions for fluid resuscitation. *Cochrane Reviews Abstract.*

Burke, K. M., LeMone, P., & Mohn-Brown, E. L. (2003). *Medical surgical nursing care.* Upper Saddle River, NJ: Prentice Hall.

Chio, P. T. L., Gordon, Y., Quinonez, L. G., et al. (1999). Crystalloids vs. colloids in fluid resuscitation: A systemic review. *Critical Care Medicine, 27*(1), 200–203.

Costello-Boerrigter, L. C., Boerrigter, G., & Burnett, J. C. (2003). Revisiting salt and water retention: New diuretics, aquaretics, and natriuretics. *Medical Clinics of North America, 87*(2), 475–491.

Jackson, E. K. (2006). Diuretics. In L. L. Brunton, J. S. Lazo, and K. L. Parker. (Eds.). *The pharmacological basis of therapeutics* (11th ed.), (pp. 737–770). New York: McGraw-Hill.

Josephson, D. L. (2004). *Intravenous fluid therapy for nurses: Principles and practice.* (2nd ed.) Clifton Park, NY: Delmar Publishers.

Rose, B. D. (2000). *Clinical physiology of acid-base and electrolyte disorders* (5th ed.). New York: McGraw-Hill.

Sica, D. A. (2004). Diuretic-related side effects: Development and treatment. *Journal of Clinical Hypertension, 6*(9), 532–540.

Wilmore, D. (2000). Nutrition and metabolic support in the 21st century. *Journal of Parenteral and Enteral Nutrition, 4*(1), 1–4.

CHAPTER 29
Drugs for Endocrine Disorders

American Diabetes Association. (2000). Clinical practice recommendations. *Diabetes Care, 23*(Suppl. 1), S1–S16.

American Diabetes Association. (2001). Standards of care. *Diabetes Care, 24*(Suppl. 1), S33–S43.

Bell, D. S. H., & Ovalle, F. (2000). Management of type 2 diabetes. *Clinical Reviews,* Spring, 93–96.

Chehade, J. M., & Mooradian, A. D. (2000). A rational approach to drug therapy of type 2 diabetes mellitus. *Drugs, 60*(1), 95–113.

Davis, S. N. (2006). Insulin, oral hypoglycemic agents, and the pharmacology of the endocrine pancreas. In L. L. Brunton, J. S. Lazo, and K. L. Parker. (Eds.). *The pharmacological basis of therapeutics* (11th ed.), (pp. 1613–1646). New York: McGraw-Hill.

Demester, N. (2001). Diseases of the thyroid: A broad spectrum. *Clinical Reviews, 11*(7), 58–64.

Farwell, A. P., & Braverman, L. E. (2006). Thyroids and antithyroid drugs. In L. L. Brunton, J. S. Lazo, and K. L. Parker. (Eds.). *The pharmacological basis of therapeutics* (11th ed.), (pp. 1511–1540). New York: McGraw-Hill.

Harrigan, R. A., Nathan, M. S., & Beattie, P. (2001). Oral agents for the treatment of type 2 diabetes mellitus: Pharmacology, toxicity, and treatment. *Annals of Emergency Medicine, 38*(1), 68.

Margioris, A. N., & Chrousos, G. P. (Eds.). (2001). *Adrenal disorders.* New Jersey: Humana Press.

Mokdad, A. H., Bowman, B. A., Ford, E. S., Vinicor, F., Marks, J. S., & Koplan, J. P. (2001). The continuing epidemics of obesity and diabetes in the United States. *Journal of American Medical Association, 286,* 1195–1200.

Parker, K. L., & Schimmer, B. P. (2006). Pituitary hormones and their hypothalamic releasing factors. In L. L. Brunton, J. S. Lazo, and K. L. Parker. (Eds.). *The pharmacological basis of therapeutics* (11th ed.), (pp. 1489–1510). New York: McGraw-Hill.

Winqvist, O., Rorsman, F., & Kampe, O. (2000). Autoimmune adrenal insufficiency: Recognition and management. *BioDrugs, 13*(2), 107–114.

CHAPTER 30
Drugs for Disorders and Conditions of the Reproductive System

Basaria, S., & Dobs, A. S. (1999). Risk versus benefits of testosterone therapy in elderly men. *Drugs and Aging, 15*(2), 131–142.

Frackiewicz, E. J., & Shiovitz, T. M. (2001). Evaluation and management of premenstrual syndrome and premenstrual dysphoric disorder. *Journal of American Pharmacological Association, 41*(3), 437–447.

Loose, D. S., & Stancel, G. M. (2006). Estrogens. In L. L. Brunton, J. S. Lazo, and K. L. Parker. (Eds.). *The pharmacological basis of therapeutics* (11th ed.), (pp. 1541–1572). New York: McGraw-Hill.

Nelson, A. (2000). Contraceptive update Y2K: Need for contraception and new contraceptive options. *Clinic Corner, 3*(1), 48–62.

Rozenberg, S., Vasquez, J. B., Vandromme, J., & Kroll, M. (1998). Educating patients about the benefits and drawbacks of hormone replacement therapy. *Drugs and Aging, 13*(1), 33–41.

Shepherd, J. E. (2001). Effects of estrogen on cognition, mood, and degenerative brain diseases. *Journal of American Pharmacological Association, 41*(2), 221–228.

Snyder, P. J. (2006). Androgens. In L. L. Brunton, J. S. Lazo, and K. L. Parker. (Eds.). *The pharmacological basis of therapeutics* (11th ed.), (pp. 1573–1586). New York: McGraw-Hill.

CHAPTER 31
Drugs for Muscle, Bone, and Joint Disorders

Burke, A., Smyth, E. M., & Fitzgerald, G. A. (2006). Analgesic-antipyretic agents; pharmacotherapy of gout. In L. L. Brunton, J. S. Lazo, and K. L. Parker. (Eds.). *The pharmacological basis of therapeutics* (11th ed.), (pp. 671–716). New York: McGraw-Hill.

Cashman, J. N. (2000). Current pharmacotherapeutic strategies in rheumatic diseases and other pain states. *Clinical Drug Investigation, 19*(Suppl. 2), 9–20.

Clemett, D., & Goa, K. L. (2000). Celecoxib: A review of its use in osteoarthritis, rheumatoid arthritis, and acute pain. *Drugs, 59*(4), 957–980.

Friedman, P. A. (2006). Agents affecting mineral ion homeostasis and bone turnover. In L. L. Brunton, J. S. Lazo, and K. L. Parker. (Eds.). *The pharmacological basis of therapeutics* (11th ed.), (pp. 1647–1677). New York: McGraw-Hill.

Jelley, M. J., & Wortmann, R. (2000). Practical steps in the diagnosis and management of gout. *Biodrugs, 14*(2), 99–107.

Lacki, J. K. (2000). Management of the patient with severe refractory rheumatoid arthritis: Are the newer treatment options worth considering? *BioDrugs, 13*(6), 425–435.

Orwoll, E. S. (1999). Osteoporosis in men. *New Dimensions in Osteoporosis, 1*(5), 2–8, 12.

Prestwood, K. M. (2000). Prevention and treatment of osteoporosis. *Clinic Corner, 2*(6), 34–44.

Watts, N. B. (1999). Treatment of postmenopausal osteoporosis. *New Dimensions in Osteoporosis, 1*(4), 2–6.

CHAPTER 32
Drugs for Skin Disorders

Fox, L. P., Merk, H. F., & Bickers, D. R. (2006). Dermatological pharmacology. In L. L. Brunton, J. S. Lazo, and K. L. Parker. (Eds.). *The pharmacological basis of therapeutics* (11th ed.), (pp. 1679–1706). New York: McGraw-Hill.

Feldman, S. (2000). Advances in psoriasis treatment. *Dermatology Online, 6*(1), 4.

Roos, T. C., & Merk, H. F. (2000). Important drug interactions in dermatology. *Drugs, 59*(2), 181–192.

CHAPTER 33
Drugs for Eye and Ear Disorders

APhA drug treatment protocols: Management of pediatric acute otitis media. *Journal of American Pharmacology Association, 40*(5), 599–608.

Brook, I. (1999). Treatment of otitis externa in children. *Paediatric Drugs, 1*(4), 283–289.

Camras, C. B., & Tamesis, R. R. (1999). Efficacy and adverse effects of medications used in the treatment of glaucoma. *Drugs and Aging, 15*(5), 377–388.

Henderer, J. D. & Rapuano, C. J. (2006). Ocular pharmacology. In L. L. Brunton, J. S. Lazo, and K. L. Parker. (Eds.). *The pharmacological basis of therapeutics* (11th ed.), (pp. 1707–1737). New York: McGraw-Hill.

Hoyng, P. F. J., & van Beek, L. M. (2000). Pharmacological therapy for glaucoma: A review. *Drugs, 59*(3), 411–434.

Leibovitz, E., & Dagan, R. (2001a). Otitis media therapy and drug resistance: Current concepts and new directions. *Infections in Medicine, 18*(5), 263–270.

Leibovitz, E., & Dagan, R. (2001b). Otitis media therapy and drug resistance: Management principles. *Infections in Medicine, 18*(4), 212–216.

Pray, S. (2001). Swimmer's ear: An ear canal infection. *U. S. Pharmacist, 26*(8).

APPENDIX B: Answers to NCLEX-PN® and Case Study Questions

Rationales are provided for all of the NCLEX-PN® questions in the Instructor's Manual.

Chapter 1

Answers to NCLEX-PN® Questions

1. 4
2. 3
3. 4
4. 4
5. 2
6. 4
7. 2
8. 4
9. 3
10. 4

Chapter 2

Answers to NCLEX-PN® Questions

1. 1
2. 2
3. 4
4. 4
5. 4
6. 2
7. 2
8. 3
9. 2
10. 3

Chapter 3

Answers to NCLEX-PN® Questions

1. 3
2. 2
3. 1
4. 3
5. 2
6. 1
7. 4
8. 4
9. 2
10. 3
11. 4
12. 1

Chapter 4

Answers to NCLEX-PN® Questions

1. 3
2. 2
3. 4
4. 3
5. 1
6. 4
7. 2
8. 3
9. 2
10. 1

Chapter 5

Answers to NCLEX-PN® Questions

1. 2, 3
2. 2
3. 2
4. 1
5. 3
6. 3
7. 2
8. 4
9. 3
10. 4

Chapter 6

Answers to NCLEX-PN® Questions

1. 3
2. 2
3. 4
4. 1
5. 2
6. 2
7. 3
8. 1
9. 3
10. 2

Chapter 7

Answers to NCLEX-PN® Questions

1. 4
2. 2
3. 4
4. 3
5. 2
6. 2
7. 3
8. 2
9. 4
10. 3

Answers to Case Study Questions

1. 3
2. 1
3. 3
4. 4

Chapter 8

Answers to NCLEX-PN® Questions

1. 4
2. 2
3. 3
4. 3
5. 2
6. 4
7. 3
8. 2
9. 2
10. 1

Answers to Case Study Questions

1. 4
2. 1

Chapter 9

Answers to NCLEX-PN® Questions

1. 3
2. 3
3. 4
4. 1
5. 1
6. 2
7. 2
8. 3
9. 2
10. 3

Answers to Case Study Questions

1. 1
2. 4
3. 3
4. 2
5. 4

Chapter 10

Answers to NCLEX-PN® Questions

1. 2
2. 4
3. 3
4. 3
5. 2
6. 3
7. 2
8. 2
9. 4
10. 3

Answers to Case Study Questions

1. 1
2. 2
3. 2

Chapter 11

Answers to NCLEX-PN® Questions

1. 4
2. 3
3. 4
4. 1
5. 2
6. 3
7. 4
8. 4
9. 3
10. 1

Answers to Case Study Questions

1. 3
2. 3
3. 3
4. 4

Chapter 12

Answers to NCLEX-PN® Questions

1. 4
2. 1
3. 1
4. 4
5. 3
6. 2
7. 3
8. 1
9. 2
10. 2

Answers to Case Study Questions

1. 3
2. 2
3. 4
4. 1
5. 2

Chapter 13

Answers to NCLEX-PN® Questions

1. 4
2. 2
3. 1
4. 2
5. 3
6. 2
7. 1
8. 2
9. 3
10. 3

Answers to Case Study Questions

1. 2
2. 3
3. 1
4. 4
5. 4

Chapter 14

Answers to NCLEX-PN® Questions

1. 4
2. 2
3. 3
4. 2
5. 4
6. 2
7. 3
8. 1
9. 4
10. 3

Answers to Case Study Questions
1. 4
2. 3
3. 3
4. 2
5. 1

Chapter 15

Answers to NCLEX-PN® Questions
1. 4
2. 1
3. 2
4. 2
5. 4
6. 3
7. 2
8. 3
9. 4
10. 2

Answers to Case Study Questions
1. 3
2. 2
3. 2
4. 1
5. 4

Chapter 16

Answers to NCLEX-PN® Questions
1. 2
2. 4
3. 2
4. 1
5. 2
6. 3
7. 1
8. 1
9. 2
10. 3

Answers to Case Study Questions
1. 2
2. 2
3. 1
4. 3
5. 3

Chapter 17

Answers to NCLEX-PN® Questions
1. 3
2. 2
3. 4
4. 3
5. 2
6. 2
7. 1
8. 3
9. 2
10. 1

Answers to Case Study Questions
1. 4
2. 2
3. 1
4. 2
5. 3

Chapter 18

Answers to NCLEX-PN® Questions
1. 2
2. 1
3. 2
4. 2
5. 3
6. 4
7. 3
8. 2
9. 3
10. 3

Answers to Case Study Questions
1. 2
2. 2
3. 1
4. 1
5. 3

Chapter 19

Answers to NCLEX-PN® Questions
1. 2
2. 4
3. 2
4. 4
5. 1
6. 4
7. 2
8. 3
9. 2
10. 2

Answers to Case Study Questions
1. 4
2. 1
3. 4
4. 1
5. 4

Chapter 20

Answers to NCLEX-PN® Questions
1. 3
2. 3
3. 2
4. 4
5. 1
6. 3
7. 1
8. 1
9. 3
10. 1

Answers to Case Study Questions
1. 1
2. 2
3. 4
4. 1
5. 3
6. 4

Chapter 21

Answers to NCLEX-PN® Questions
1. 4
2. 3
3. 2
4. 1
5. 2
6. 4
7. 2
8. 4
9. 2
10. 3

Answers to Case Study Questions
1. 2
2. 3
3. 1
4. 3
5. 2

Chapter 22

Answers to NCLEX-PN® Questions
1. 4
2. 2
3. 3
4. 1
5. 3
6. 3
7. 4
8. 3
9. 4
10. 2

Answers to Case Study Questions
1. 4
2. 2
3. 1
4. 3
5. 1

Chapter 23

Answers to NCLEX-PN® Questions
1. 3
2. 4
3. 3
4. 1
5. 3
6. 4
7. 4
8. 2
9. 3
10. 4

Answers to Case Study Questions
1. 3
2. 2
3. 1
4. 2
5. 4

Chapter 24

Answers to NCLEX-PN® Questions
1. 3
2. 2
3. 4
4. 2
5. 1
6. 4
7. 2
8. 3
9. 3
10. 2

Answers to Case Study Questions
1. 2
2. 3
3. 2
4. 4
5. 3

Chapter 25

Answers to NCLEX-PN® Questions
1. 3
2. 1
3. 4
4. 4
5. 3
6. 2
7. 2
8. 4
9. 1
10. 4

Answers to Case Study Questions
1. 4
2. 3
3. 1
4. 1
5. 2

Chapter 26

Answers to NCLEX-PN® Questions
1. 3
2. 1
3. 1
4. 2
5. 1
6. 2
7. 2
8. 1
9. 3
10. 1

Answers to Case Study Questions

1. 1
2. 4
3. 1
4. 4
5. 2

Chapter 27

Answers to NCLEX-PN® Questions

1. 3
2. 4
3. 1
4. 2
5. 3
6. 4
7. 2
8. 4
9. 3
10. 4

Answers to Case Study Questions

1. 2
2. 3
3. 3
4. 1
5. 4

Chapter 28

Answers to NCLEX-PN® Questions

1. 3
2. 4
3. 2
4. 2
5. 2
6. 2
7. 1
8. 2
9. 4
10. 1

Answers to Case Study Questions

1. 1
2. 1
3. 4
4. 2
5. 4

Chapter 29

Answers to NCLEX-PN® Questions

1. 3
2. 4
3. 2
4. 3
5. 2
6. 1
7. 2
8. 2
9. 4
10. 3

Answers to Case Study Questions

1. 2
2. 3
3. 1
4. 3
5. 2

Chapter 30

Answers to NCLEX-PN® Questions

1. 2
2. 2
3. 3
4. 2
5. 4
6. 2
7. 3
8. 2
9. 4
10. 4

Answers to Case Study Questions

1. 3
2. 4
3. 2
4. 3
5. 1

Chapter 31

Answers to NCLEX-PN® Questions

1. 2
2. 4
3. 1
4. 4
5. 3
6. 1
7. 4
8. 2
9. 3
10. 1

Answers to Case Study Questions

1. 3
2. 1
3. 2
4. 2
5. 2

Chapter 32

Answers to NCLEX-PN® Questions

1. 2
2. 3
3. 4
4. 1
5. 4
6. 3
7. 4
8. 2
9. 4
10. 1

Answers to Case Study Questions

1. 4
2. 3
3. 2
4. 3
5. 4

Chapter 33

Answers to NCLEX-PN® Questions

1. 1
2. 3
3. 1
4. 3
5. 1
6. 3
7. 2
8. 1
9. 3
10. 1

Answers to Case Study Questions

1. 3
2. 1
3. 1
4. 3
5. 4

APPENDIX C: Top 100 Drugs Ranked by Number of Prescriptions in 2004

Rank	Brand Name (if applicable)	Generic Name
1	Hydrocodone w/APAP	Hydrocodone w/APAP
2	Lipitor	Atorvastatin
3	Lisinopril	Lisinopril
4	Atenolol	Atenolol
5	Synthroid	Levothyroxine
6	Amoxicillin	Amoxicillin
7	Hydrochlorothiazide	Hydrochlorothiazide
8	Zithromax	Azithromycin
9	Furosemide	Furosemide
10	Norvasc	Amlodipine
11	Toprol-XL	Metoprolol
12	Alprazolam	Alprazolam
13	Albuterol Aerosol	Albuterol
14	Zoloft	Sertraline
15	Zocor	Simvastatin
16	Metformin	Metformin
17	Ibuprofen	Ibuprofen
18	Triamterene/HCTZ	Triamterene/HCTZ
19	Ambien	Zolpidem
20	Cephalexin	Cephalexin
21	Nexium	Esomeprazole
22	Prevacid	Lansoprazole
23	Lexapro +	Escitalopram Oxalate
24	Prednisone	Prednisone
25	Zyrtec	Cetirizine
26	Singulair	Montelukast
27	Celebrex	Celecoxib
28	Fluoxetine	Fluoxetine
29	Fosamax	Alendronate
30	Metoprolol tartrate	Metoprolol
31	Premarin	Conjugated Estrogens
32	Levoxyl	Levothyroxine
33	Lorazepam	Lorazepam
34	Allegra	Fexofenadine
35	Plavix	Clopidogrel
36	Effexor XR	Venlafaxine
37	Potassium Chloride	Potassium Chloride
38	Protonix	Pantoprazole
39	Propoxyphene N/APAP	Propoxyphene N/APAP
40	Advair Diskus	Salmeterol/Fluticasone
41	Warfarin	Warfarin
42	Acetaminophen/Codeine	Acetaminophen/Codeine
43	Clonazepam	Clonazepam
44	Neurontin	Gabapentin
45	Flonase	Fluticasone
46	Amitriptyline	Amitriptyline
47	Ranitidine HCl	Ranitidine
48	Trazodone	Trazodone
49	Naproxen	Naproxen
50	Amox TR/Potassium/ Clavulanate	Amox TR/Potassium/Clavulanate
51	Enalapril	Enalapril

Rank	Brand Name (if applicable)	Generic Name
52	Paroxetine HCl	Paroxetine HCl
53	Pravachol	Pravastatin
54	Viagra	Sildenafil Citrate
55	Cyclobenzaprine	Cyclobenzaprine
56	Vioxx	Rofecoxib
57	Altace	Ramipril
58	Diovan	Valsartan
59	Lotrel	Amlodipine/Benazepril
60	Levaquin	Levofloxacin
61	L-thyroxine sodium	Levothyroxine Sodium
62	Bextra	Valdecoxib
63	Oxycodone/APAP	Oxycodone/APAP
64	Diazepam	Diazepam
65	Tramadol	Tramadol
66	Verapamil HCl	Verapamil
67	Diovan HCT	Valsartan / HCTZ
68	Albuterol Sulfate	Albuterol
69	Lisinopril/HCTZ	Lisinopril/HCTZ
70	Ortho-evra +	Norelgestromin / Ethinyl Estradiol (transdermal)
71	Celexa	Citalopram
72	Accupril	Quinapril
73	Carisoprodol	Carisoprodol
74	Actos	Pioglitazone
75	Promethazine	Promethazine
76	Actonel	Risedronate
77	Isosorbide Mononitrate	Isosorbide Mononitrate S.A.
78	Allopurinol	Allopurinol
79	Paxil	Paroxetine
80	Cozaar	Losartan
81	Clonidine	Clonidine
82	Cipro	Ciprofloxacin
83	Wellbutrin XL	Bupropion HCL
84	Glyburide	Glyburide
85	Avandia	Rosiglitazone Maleate
86	Penicillin VK	Penicillin VK
87	Zetia +	Ezetimibe
88	Trimox	Amoxicillin
89	Methylprednisolone	Methylprednisolone
90	Folic Acid	Folic Acid
91	Aciphex	Rabeprazole
92	Glipizide ER	Glipizide ER
93	Flomax	Tamsulosin
94	Diltiazem	Diltiazem
95	Risperdal	Risperidone
96	Omeprazole	Omeprazole
97	Yasmin 28 +	Drospirenone and Ethinyl Estradiol
98	Doxycycline Hyclate	Doxycycline
99	Tricor	Fenofibrate
100	Seroquel	Quetiapine

Source: http://www.rxlist.com/top200.htm

+ Indicates a drug added to the top 100 list from 2002–2004.

INDEX

Indexing style is as follows: **Prototype generic drugs appear in boldface and lowercase; prototype Trade drugs appear in boldface with initial cap(s).** Non-prototype generic drugs appear in plain type and lowercase; non-prototype Trade drugs appear in plain type with initial cap(s). DRUG CLASSIFICATIONS APPEAR IN SMALL CAPS. Diseases, disorders, and conditions appear in green. Figures and tables are denoted respectively by f and t following the page number.

A

B

D

G

I

J

K

O

Q

R

S

Pearson Education, Inc.

YOU SHOULD CAREFULLY READ THE TERMS AND CONDITIONS BEFORE USING THE CD-ROM PACKAGE. USING THIS CD-ROM PACKAGE INDICATES YOUR ACCEPTANCE OF THESE TERMS AND CONDITIONS.

Pearson Education, Inc. provides this program and licenses its use. You assume responsibility for the selection of the program to achieve your intended results, and for the installation, use, and results obtained from the program. This license extends only to use of the program in the United States or countries in which the program is marketed by authorized distributors.

LICENSE GRANT

You hereby accept a nonexclusive, nontransferable, permanent license to install and use the program ON A SINGLE COMPUTER at any given time. You may copy the program solely for backup or archival purposes in support of your use of the program on the single computer. You may not modify, translate, disassemble, decompile, or reverse engineer the program, in whole or in part.

TERM

The License is effective until terminated. Pearson Education, Inc. reserves the right to terminate this License automatically if any provision of the License is violated. You may terminate the License at any time. To terminate this License, you must return the program, including documentation, along with a written warranty stating that all copies in your possession have been returned or destroyed.

LIMITED WARRANTY

THE PROGRAM IS PROVIDED "AS IS" WITHOUT WARRANTY OF ANY KIND, EITHER EXPRESSED OR IMPLIED, INCLUDING, BUT NOT LIMITED TO, THE IMPLIED WARRANTIES OR MERCHANTABILITY AND FITNESS FOR A PARTICULAR PURPOSE. THE ENTIRE RISK AS TO THE QUALITYAND PERFORMANCE OF THE PROGRAM IS WITH YOU. SHOULD THE PROGRAM PROVE DEFECTIVE, YOU (AND NOT PRENTICE-HALL, INC. OR ANY AUTHORIZED DEALER) ASSUME THE ENTIRE COST OF ALL NECESSARY SERVICING, REPAIR, OR CORRECTION. NO ORAL OR WRITTEN INFORMATION OR ADVICE GIVEN BY PRENTICE-HALL, INC., ITS DEALERS, DISTRIBUTORS, OR AGENTS SHALL CREATE A WARRANTY OR INCREASE THE SCOPE OF THIS WARRANTY.

SOME STATES DO NOT ALLOW THE EXCLUSION OF IMPLIED WARRANTIES, SO THE ABOVE EXCLUSION MAY NOT APPLY TO YOU. THIS WARRANTY GIVES YOU SPECIFIC LEGAL RIGHTS AND YOU MAY ALSO HAVE OTHER LEGAL RIGHTS THAT VARY FROM STATE TO STATE.

Pearson Education, Inc. does not warrant that the functions contained in the program will meet your requirements or that the operation of the program will be uninterrupted or error-free.

However, Pearson Education, Inc. warrants the diskette(s) or CD-ROM(s) on which the program is furnished to be free from defects in material and workmanship under normal use for a period of ninety (90) days from the date of delivery to you as evidenced by a copy of your receipt.

The program should not be relied on as the sole basis to solve a problem whose incorrect solution could result in injury to person or property. If the program is employed in such a manner, it is at the user's own risk and Pearson Education, Inc. explicitly disclaims all liability for such misuse.

LIMITATION OF REMEDIES

Pearson Education, Inc.'s entire liability and your exclusive remedy shall be:

1. the replacement of any diskette(s) or CD-ROM(s) not meeting Pearson Education, Inc.'s "LIMITED WARRANTY" and that is returned to Pearson Education, or
2. if Pearson Education is unable to deliver a replacement diskette(s) or CD-ROM(s) that is free of defects in materials or workmanship, you may terminate this agreement by returning the program.

IN NO EVENT WILL PRENTICE-HALL, INC. BE LIABLE TO YOU FOR ANY DAMAGES, INCLUDING ANY LOST PROFITS, LOST SAVINGS, OR OTHER INCIDENTAL OR CONSEQUENTIAL DAMAGES ARISING OUT OF THE USE OR INABILITY TO USE SUCH PROGRAM EVEN IF PRENTICE-HALL, INC. OR AN AUTHORIZED DISTRIBUTOR HAS BEEN ADVISED OF THE POSSIBILITY OF SUCH DAMAGES, OR FOR ANY CLAIM BY ANY OTHER PARTY.

SOME STATES DO NOT ALLOW FOR THE LIMITATION OR EXCLUSION OF LIABILITY FOR INCIDENTAL OR CONSEQUENTIAL DAMAGES, SO THE ABOVE LIMITATION OR EXCLUSION MAY NOT APPLY TO YOU.

GENERAL

You may not sublicense, assign, or transfer the license of the program. Any attempt to sublicense, assign or transfer any of the rights, duties, or obligations hereunder is void.

This Agreement will be governed by the laws of the State of New York.

Should you have any questions concerning this Agreement, you may contact Pearson Education, Inc. by writing to:

Director of New Media
Higher Education Division
Pearson Education, Inc.
One Lake Street
Upper Saddle River, NJ 07458

Should you have any questions concerning technical support, you may contact:

Product Support Department: Monday–Friday 8:00 A.M.–8:00 P.M. and Sunday 5:00 P.M.-12:00 A.M. (All times listed are Eastern). 1-800-677-6337

You can also get support by filling out the web form located at http://247.prenhall.com

YOU ACKNOWLEDGE THAT YOU HAVE READ THIS AGREEMENT, UNDERSTAND IT, AND AGREE TO BE BOUND BY ITS TERMS AND CONDITIONS. YOU FURTHER AGREE THAT IT IS THE COMPLETE AND EXCLUSIVE STATEMENT OF THE AGREEMENT BETWEEN US THAT SUPERSEDES ANY PROPOSAL OR PRIOR AGREEMENT, ORAL OR WRITTEN, AND ANY OTHER COMMUNICATIONS BETWEEN US RELATING TO THE SUBJECT MATTER OF THIS AGREEMENT.

QUICK GUIDE TO SPECIAL FEATURES

BIOTERRORISM

Fast Facts

Life Span Facts

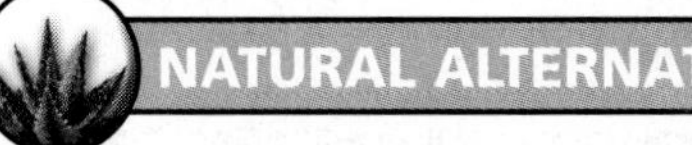

QUICK GUIDE TO SPECIAL FEATURES *(continued)*

NURSING PROCESS FOCUS

Patients Receiving . . .

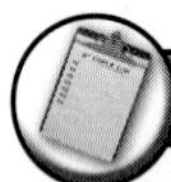

PATIENTS NEED TO KNOW